# THE
# AMERICAN
# MEDICAL
# ASSOCIATION

# HOME MEDICAL
# ENCYCLOPEDIA

The information in this encyclopedia reflects current
medical knowledge. The recommendations and
information are appropriate in most cases; however,
they are not a substitute for medical diagnosis. For
specific information concerning your personal
medical condition, the AMA suggests that you
consult a physician.

The names of organizations, products, or alternative
therapies appearing in this encyclopedia are given for
informational purposes only. Their inclusion does not
imply AMA endorsement, nor does the omission of any
organization, product, or alternative therapy indicate
AMA disapproval.

Library of Congress Cataloging in Publication Data

The American Medical Association home medical
    encyclopedia.

    Includes index.
    1. Medicine, Popular—Dictionaries. I. American
Medical Association. II. Title: Home medical
encyclopedia.
RC81.A2A522    1989    610′.3    89-10589
ISBN 0-394-58248-9 (set)
ISBN 0-394-58246-2 (v. 1)
ISBN 0-394-58247-0 (v. 2)

Manufactured in the United States of America

Computerset by M. F. Graphics Limited, England
Reproduction by Mandarin Offset Limited, Hong Kong

# THE
# AMERICAN
# MEDICAL
# ASSOCIATION

# HOME MEDICAL
# ENCYCLOPEDIA

## VOLUME TWO · I – Z

### MEDICAL EDITOR
Charles B. Clayman, MD

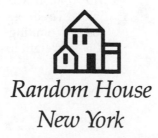

*Random House*
*New York*

Published by The Reader's Digest Association, Inc.,
with permission of Random House, Inc.

# EMERGENCY FIRST-AID TECHNIQUES

Use this quick-reference list to find illustrated first-aid boxes containing step-by-step instructions for performing emergency techniques.

| | | | |
|---|---|---|---|
| Artificial respiration | 134 | Hypothermia | 563 |
| Bleeding, treating | 179 | Poisoning | 805 |
| Burns, treating | 220 | Pressure points | 820 |
| Cardiopulmonary resuscitation | 237 | Recovery position | 855 |
| Childbirth, emergency | 266 | Shock | 902 |
| Choking (adult) | 271 | Snakebite | 921 |
| Choking (infant and child) | 272 | Suffocation | 953 |
| Electrical injury | 395 | Unconsciousness | 1022 |
| Frostbite | 469 | Wounds | 1079 |
| Heat stroke | 526 | | |

# SYMPTOM CHARTS

Use this quick-reference list to find question-and-answer flow charts that indicate the possible causes and significance of many common symptoms.

| | | | |
|---|---|---|---|
| Abdomen, swollen | 56 | Headache | 508 |
| Abdominal pain | 51 | Hoarseness or loss of voice | 542 |
| Abdominal pain, recurrent | 53 | Intercourse, painful (men) | 596 |
| Backache | 151 | Intercourse, painful (women) | 597 |
| Breathing difficulty | 211 | Menstruation, irregular | 679 |
| Chest pain | 260 | Numbness and tingling | 734 |
| Constipation | 299 | Rash with fever | 851 |
| Cough | 315 | Rash with itching | 852 |
| Diarrhea | 355 | Tiredness | 990 |
| Dizziness | 368 | Vomiting | 1063 |
| Feeling faint and fainting | 436 | Weight loss | 1074 |
| Fever | 450 | | |

# CONTENTS

HOW TO USE THE ENCYCLOPEDIA —— 10

MEDICINE TODAY —————— 15

THE A to Z OF MEDICINE ———— 49

SELF-HELP ORGANIZATIONS ——— 1090

DRUG GLOSSARY —————— 1096

INDEX ————————— 1118

**I**

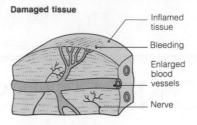

**Damaged tissue**
- Inflamed tissue
- Bleeding
- Enlarged blood vessels
- Nerve

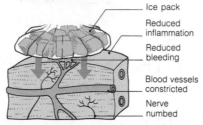

**Ice pack application**
- Ice pack
- Reduced inflammation
- Reduced bleeding
- Blood vessels constricted
- Nerve numbed

**Use of an ice pack**
Applying an ice pack to an area of damaged tissue helps relieve pain, reduce inflammation and further tissue damage, and minimize bleeding and swelling.

## Iatrogenic

Meaning literally "physician produced," the term iatrogenic can be applied to any medical condition, disease, or other adverse occurrence that results from medical treatment. The development of an iatrogenic condition does not necessarily imply a lack of care or knowledge on the part of the physician. Effective forms of treatment are seldom, if ever, entirely free of possible unwanted effects. The drowsiness produced by some groups of antiallergy drugs is one example.

## Ibuprofen

A *nonsteroidal anti-inflammatory drug* (NSAID) used as an *analgesic* (painkiller) in the treatment of headache, menstrual pain, and painful injury to soft tissues (such as muscles and ligaments). The anti-inflammatory effect of ibuprofen helps reduce joint pain and stiffness occurring in some types of arthritis, such as *rheumatoid arthritis* and *osteoarthritis*.

Ibuprofen may cause abdominal pain, diarrhea, nausea, heartburn, and, rarely, dizziness. It may also cause a *peptic ulcer*, but is less likely to do so than some other NSAIDs.

## Ice packs

Means of applying ice (in a towel or other material) to the skin to relieve pain, stem bleeding, or reduce inflammation. Cold causes the blood vessels to contract, reducing blood flow.

**WHY IT IS DONE**

Ice treatment is used to relieve pain in a variety of disorders, including severe *headache*, *hemorrhoids*, and pain in the throat after a *tonsillectomy*. Another common use is after sports injuries to minimize swelling, bruising, and further tissue damage. In sports injuries, ice is usually combined with the application of a pressure bandage and the raising of the injured part. Ice may also be used to stop bleeding from small vessels, as in a nosebleed.

**HOW IT IS DONE**

Ice is wrapped in a wet cloth (to prevent it from burning the skin) and applied to the skin's surface. Chemical packs are also available; striking or shaking the pack mixes the chemicals within, producing a liquid with a very low temperature.

## Ichthyosis

A rare, inherited condition in which the skin is dry, thickened, scaly, and darker than normal due to an abnormality in the production of *keratin* (a protein that is the main component of skin). The name ichthyosis is taken from the Greek word "ichthus" (meaning fish); the condition is commonly called fish skin disease.

Ichthyosis usually appears at or shortly after birth and generally improves during childhood. The areas most commonly affected are the thighs, arms, and backs of the hands.

There is no special treatment, although lubricants and emulsifying ointments help the dryness and bath oils moisten the skin. Washing with soap makes ichthyosis worse and should be avoided. The condition improves in a warm, humid atmosphere. Ichthyosis is at its worst in cold weather (when the sufferer should wear additional layers of protective, warm clothing).

## Icterus

Another term for *jaundice*.

## Id

One of the three parts of the personality (with the *ego* and *superego*) described by Sigmund Freud. The id is the primitive, unconscious store of energy from which come the instincts for food, love, sex, and other basic needs. The id seeks simply to gain pleasure and to avoid pain. (See also *Psychoanalytic theory*.)

## Idiocy

An outdated term for severe *mental retardation*. Idiots were defined as having an IQ of under 35.

## Idiopathic

Of unknown cause. For example, epilepsy in which no specific cause can be found is referred to as idiopathic epilepsy. The word idiopathic comes from the Greek "idio-" meaning "one's own" and "pathos" meaning disease.

## Idoxuridine

An *antiviral drug*. Idoxuridine is used to treat *herpes simplex* infections affecting the eyelids or cornea of the eye. It is occasionally given to prevent a recurrence of herpes simplex infection in people receiving *corticosteroid drug* treatment for a different eye disorder.

Idoxuridine may cause irritation of the eye and, in rare cases, photophobia (abnormal sensitivity to light), swollen eyelids, or blurred vision.

## Ileostomy

An operation in which the ileum (lower part of the small intestine) is brought through an incision in the abdominal wall and formed into an artificial outlet for the bowel to allow the discharge of feces into a bag attached to the skin. An ileostomy is usually permanent.

**WHY IT IS DONE**

Permanent ileostomy is usually performed for people with *ulcerative colitis* or *Crohn's disease* whose health, despite drug treatment, continues to deteriorate because of chronic inflammation of the colon. For these people, the only means of restoring health is to perform a *colectomy* (an operation to remove the colon and rectum) followed by an ileostomy.

Temporary ileostomy is sometimes required at the time of partial colectomy (removal of part of the colon) to allow the repair of the colon to heal before waste material passes through it. Temporary ileostomy may also be carried out as an emergency measure in a person who is very ill due to an

## PROCEDURE FOR ILEOSTOMY

Two incisions are made in the abdominal wall (usually on the right side)—a small circular cut for the stoma (most often located about 2 inches below the waist and away from the hipbone and groin crease) and a vertical cut to give access to the intestine and *mesentery*.

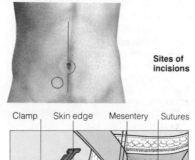

**Sites of incisions**

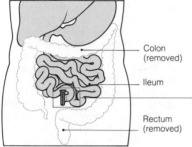

Colon (removed)

Ileum

Rectum (removed)

**1** After removal of the colon, the cut end of the ileum is clamped and part of the mesentery is cut to free a short length of ileum for the stoma.

Clamp  Skin edge  Mesentery  Sutures

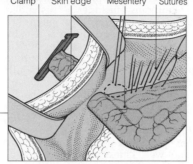

**2** The free end of the ileum is pushed out through the circular incision in the abdomen; the mesentery is then stitched to the inner abdominal wall.

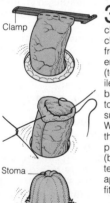

Clamp

Stoma

**3** The main vertical incision is closed, and the clamp is removed from the protruding end of the ileum (top). The end of the ileum is then turned back and attached to the abdomen with sutures (middle). When completed, this creates a small protruding stoma (bottom). A temporary ileostomy appliance is usually fitted immediately.

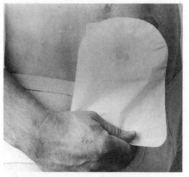

**4** After the intestine begins to function normally, an ileostomy bag is fitted around the stoma. The bag attaches closely to the skin with adhesive seals.

obstruction high in the large intestine that is preventing the normal passage of feces. The ileostomy is made above the obstruction and, by allowing waste material to discharge, enables the patient to recover sufficiently to undergo a partial colectomy to remove the obstruction. Temporary ileostomies are closed when the rejoined colon has healed.

### HOW IT IS DONE

When the whole of the colon and rectum has been removed, the cut end of the ileum is brought to the surface of the skin through an incision in the abdominal wall. In the case of a temporary ileostomy, a loop of bowel is brought to the surface and opened so that waste material can pass through. The edges of this opening are then stitched to the skin at the edge of the abdominal incision to create a stoma (an artificial opening). The stoma is usually located on the right side about 2 inches (5 cm) below the natural waist and away from the hipbone.

### POSTOPERATIVE CARE

For a few days, patients may need to be fed by *intravenous infusion*. After that, the intestine starts to function normally again; liquid waste is discharged through the stoma into a bag that is closely attached to the skin by adhesive seals.

During the convalescent period, patients with permanent ileostomies are given counseling to help them come to terms with an altered body image and the appearance of the stoma. They are also taught the practical aspects of stoma care. There is no muscle control over evacuation of body wastes through the stoma. These wastes are semiliquid and contain enzymes that can damage the skin around the stoma. For these reasons, it is usually necessary for the bag to be worn at all times. The nursing staff (ideally a stoma-care nurse clinician) teaches the patient how to empty, change, and dispose of the bag, and how to maintain a good seal between bag and body to protect the skin and prevent leaks.

Full recovery from the operation takes about six weeks, during which time patients should avoid vigorous physical activity.

### OUTLOOK

The condition of patients who are given ileostomies after removal of a chronically inflamed colon usually improves dramatically. Because their ability to be active is enhanced, many of these people say they wish they had had the operation years earlier.

Following convalescence, patients should be able to return to their usual employment, life-style, and family and social activities. After an ileostomy it is necessary to drink increased amounts of water and to ensure that the intake of salt is adequate, thus compensating for the lack of a colon (the main functions of which are the absorption of water and salt). Apart from this recommendation, it is generally possible to eat a normal diet.

Only an occasional medical checkup is needed to make sure that the stoma is in good condition, although the physician should always be informed of any change in the function or appearance of the stoma. Occasionally, the channel of the stoma becomes narrowed or prolapses (protrudes too far from the abdomen), requiring surgical correction.

Various attempts have been made to devise ileostomies that require emptying only once or twice a day at fixed times and do not require an external appliance. These devices include internal reservoirs made from loops of small intestine, magnetic closures, and carbon filter systems for gas. However, none has yet proved consistently reliable, and most patients are still offered a conventional ileostomy.

## Ileum

The final, longest, and narrowest section of the small intestine. It is joined at its upper end to the *jejunum* and at its lower end to the large intestine.

The function of the ileum is to absorb nutrients from food that has been digested in the stomach and first two sections of the small intestine. The millions of *villi* (minute fingerlike projections) that line the ileum considerably increase its surface area and thus its powers of absorption.

**LOCATION OF THE ILEUM**
The ileum (the final part of the small intestine) joins the jejunum and cecum (the first part of the large intestine).

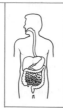

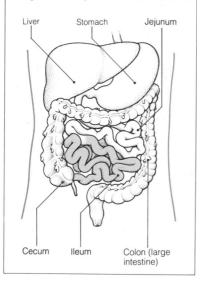

Liver    Stomach    Jejunum

Cecum    Ileum    Colon (large intestine)

**DISORDERS**
Occasionally, the ileum becomes obstructed—by pushing through a weakness in the abdominal wall (see *Hernia*) or by becoming caught up with scar tissue following abdominal surgery, for example.

Other disorders of the ileum include *Meckel's diverticulum* (a pouch in the ileum wall that may become ulcerated), *Crohn's disease,* and diseases in which absorption of nutrients is impaired, such as *celiac sprue,* tropical *sprue,* and *lymphoma.*

## Ileus, paralytic

A failure, usually temporary, of the normal contractility of the muscles of the intestine. As a result, intestinal contents can no longer pass out of the body and the bowel becomes obstructed. This condition commonly follows abdominal surgery and may also be induced by severe abdominal injury, *peritonitis* (inflammation of the membrane lining the abdomen), internal extraintestinal bleeding, acute *pancreatitis* (inflammation of the pancreas), or interference with the blood or nerve supply to the intestine.

Symptoms include a distended abdomen, vomiting, and failure to pass stools. The condition is usually successfully treated by sucking out the intestinal contents through a tube passed through the nose or mouth into the stomach or intestine and by maintaining body fluid levels by *intravenous infusion* (drip).

## Illness

Perception by a person that he or she is not well. Illness is a subjective sensation and may have physical or psychological causes; illness is not synonymous with disease or disorder.

## Illusion

A distorted sensation. An illusion is based on misinterpretation of a real stimulus (for example, a pen is seen as a dagger or the sound of a screeching brake is heard as a scream). This is not the same as a *hallucination*, in which a perception occurs with no stimulus.

Usually, illusions are brief and can be understood when explained. They may be due to tiredness or anxiety, to drugs of many sorts, or to certain forms of brain damage. *Delirium tremens* is a classic inducer of illusions.

## Imaging techniques

Techniques that produce images of structures within the body that cannot otherwise be seen. Imaging techniques are an invaluable aid in diagnosing abnormalities and disease.

**X RAYS**
In 1895 the discovery of *X rays* revolutionized medical diagnosis by making it possible for the first time to visualize bone, organs, and other internal tissue without opening up the body. The rays are electromagnetic waves of short wavelength. Some are absorbed and others pass through tissues; the shadow that is cast is projected onto a fluorescent screen or a film.

**CONTRAST MEDIA** X-ray images of bones are distinct, but soft tissues show up less clearly. To overcome this, radiologists from the 1920s onward began using substances opaque to radiation as part of certain X-ray procedures.

When such substances (known as contrast media) are introduced into internal organs, blood vessels, or ducts, they produce (on the X-ray screen or film) an outline of the cavities they fill.

A contrast medium can be introduced into the body in various ways. In *cholecystography* (carried out to examine the gallbladder and common bile duct) and in some *barium X-ray examinations* of the esophagus, the stomach, and the small bowel, the medium is swallowed in tablet or liquid form. In *bronchography* (used to diagnose various chest disorders) the contrast medium is placed into the airways (bronchi) connecting the windpipe to the lungs. In *angiography* and *venography*, it is injected into an artery or vein, respectively, to provide images of the blood vessels. In intravenous *pyelography*, contrast medium injected into a vein in the arm travels to the kidneys and urinary tract. In *ERCP* (by which the pancreatic duct and biliary system are examined), the medium is passed into the ducts by means of a catheter (tube) passed through a channel in an endoscope (a flexible viewing instrument).

**SCANNING TECHNIQUES**
Since the 1970s many X-ray imaging techniques have been superseded by newer procedures that are simpler to perform and are safer and more comfortable for the patient. *Ultrasound scanning* consists of passing high-frequency sound waves through the body with a transducer placed against the skin. The waves are reflected to varying degrees by structures of different density, and the pattern of the echoes is electronically recorded on a screen. Ultrasound scanning is the first choice for diagnostic imaging of the gallbladder, female genital tract, and fetus. It also provides remarkably clear pictures of the kidney.

**COMPUTERS** Many scanning techniques use a computer to provide images. In *CT scanning* (computerized tomography scanning), X rays are passed through the body at different angles. The computer produces cross-sectional images ("slices") of the tissues being examined. In *MRI* (magnetic resonance imaging), the patient is placed in a strong magnetic field and radio-frequency waves are passed through the body. A computer analyzes changes in the magnetic alignment of the hydrogen protons of the cells to give an image of the tissues.

CT scanning and MRI are particularly valuable in the diagnosis of brain disorders. So, too, is a more recent

## IMAGING THE BODY

Over the past decade, many new methods of imaging the body have been developed. These new imaging techniques have made it possible to visualize internal structures in a variety of different ways. Today, in addition to conventional X rays (which show primarily bones), techniques such as CT scanning, radionuclide scanning, ultrasound scanning, MRI, and PET scanning are used to provide detailed diagnostic pictures of soft tissues and organs. The examples given here show some of the different ways in which the kidneys can be imaged. Annotated diagrams and explanatory text will help you interpret the images.

### X RAYS

Radiopaque contrast media may be utilized to give distinct X-ray images of soft tissues, as in intravenous pyelography, which is used to clearly visualize the kidneys and urinary tracts.

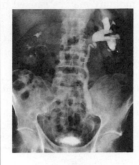
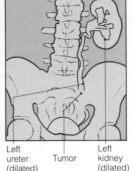

Left ureter (dilated)    Tumor    Left kidney (dilated)

**Intravenous pyelogram**
The intravenous pyelogram (far left) shows the left kidney and ureter, which are visible because they are filled with contrast medium that has been retained due to a tumor obstructing the ureter (see left).

## SCANNING TECHNIQUES

Many new techniques have been developed for imaging the body, particularly the soft tissues. Some of these techniques, such as CT scanning, rely on computers to process the raw imaging data and produce the actual image. Others, such as ultrasound scanning and radionuclide scanning, can produce images without a computer, although one may be used for image enhancement.

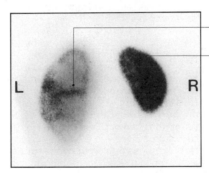

Damaged left kidney

Normal right kidney

**Radionuclide scanning**
A radioactive substance is introduced into the body, and the radiation emitted is detected by a gamma camera, which converts it into an image. In the scan of the kidneys (left), the left one has taken up little of the radioactive substance (and thus appears faint), which indicates that it is damaged.

### Ultrasound scanning

Ultrahigh frequency sound waves reflected from tissues in the body are converted into an image by special electronic equipment. The scan (below left) shows a section through a diseased kidney; the inner tissues (calyx and pelvis) are greatly dilated, and the outer cortex is abnormally thin (see diagram, below right).

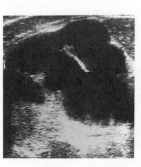
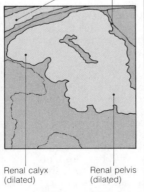

Back    Thin cortex

Renal calyx (dilated)    Renal pelvis (dilated)

### CT scanning

A CT scanner produces cross-sectional images (slices) of the body. The CT scan (right) shows a greatly dilated right kidney (see diagram, below right).

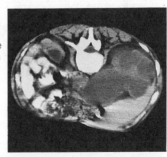
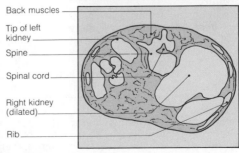

Back muscles

Tip of left kidney

Spine

Spinal cord

Right kidney (dilated)

Rib

technique called *PET* (positron emission tomography) *scanning*, in which very short-lived radioisotopes are introduced into tissues; the paths of gamma rays emitted are analyzed by a computer, giving information about brain function and structure.

In *radionuclide scanning*, a gamma camera records, and a computer transforms into images, radiation emitted from tissues into which a radioactive substance has been introduced. The computer may be used to obtain more information.

## Imipramine

A tricyclic *antidepressant drug*. Imipramine is most commonly used as a long-term treatment for *depression*, but may take up to six weeks to have a beneficial effect.

Possible adverse effects include excessive sweating, blurred vision, dry mouth, dizziness, constipation, nausea, and difficulty passing urine in older men. Overdose, particularly in a child, can be fatal.

## Immersion foot

A condition that occurs in shipwreck survivors and soldiers (in whom it is known as trench foot) resulting from the feet being wet and cold for a long time. Initially, the feet turn pale and have no detectable pulse; later, they become red, swollen, and painful, and have a strong pulse.

**TREATMENT**
If the feet are at the pale stage, they should be gradually and carefully rewarmed; overheating may lead to *gangrene* (tissue death). Conversely, if they are red and swollen, they should be gradually cooled.

If the condition is ignored and becomes severe, muscle weakness, skin ulcers, or gangrene may develop. Even with mild cases, the feet may be painful and sensitive to cold for several years afterward.

## Immobility

Reduced physical activity and movement. Immobility is particularly harmful in the elderly because it causes muscle wasting and progressive loss of function.

**CAUSES**
Total immobility is rare; it occurs in coma, which is sometimes the result of *stroke*, *brain tumor*, or major *head injury*. *Catatonia* is associated with varying degrees of immobility.

Temporary loss of mobility, lasting a few days, occurs during recovery from any serious illness, such as a myocardial infarction, or from a major surgical procedure.

Fractures in a lower limb may be treated by *traction*, which requires several weeks in bed, or by use of a *cast*, which also hinders mobility.

Loss of mobility may be caused by the symptoms of a specific medical disorder, such as *asthma* or *angina pectoris* (chest pain due to reduced blood supply to the heart muscle). Both these conditions may, in severe cases, be aggravated by exercise. *Arthritis* (inflammation of joints) limits mobility if the hips, knees, ankles, or feet are affected by pain and stiffness. Nervous system disorders that restrict mobility include *hemiplegia* (paralysis on one side of the body), *Parkinson's disease*, and *multiple sclerosis*.

A person may find it difficult to move around because of deteriorating eyesight, or may lack motivation due to *depression* or the effects of alcohol or other drugs (such as tranquilizers).

**COMPLICATIONS**
Total immobility can cause *bedsores*, *pneumonia* caused by secretions building up in the lungs, or *contractures*.

A common complication of partial immobility is *edema* (abnormal retention of fluid in body tissues), which causes swelling of the legs as a result of the calf muscles not working to pump the fluid back to the heart in the circulation. Rarely, a *thrombosis* (blood clot) forms in one of the veins in the leg because of this lack of blood flow.

Obesity is more likely to occur in people who do not exercise. Stiffness tends to develop in any joint not being used properly. Muscle wasting and *osteoporosis* are common problems caused by immobility in the elderly.

**TREATMENT**
Regular *physical therapy* and adequate nursing care are important for any person who is totally immobile. Regular turning and the use of a special mattress and bed reduce the risk of bed sores. Stretching exercises may prevent contractures.

Early mobilization after serious illness or major surgery is usually encouraged to avoid the problems of prolonged bed rest. After a lower limb fracture, walking with the aid of crutches is started as soon as possible.

Aids for the disabled (see *Disability*) can increase mobility that is impaired by leg weakness, stiffness, loss of balance, or poor coordination. If the person is unable to walk despite assistance, exercises may be done in a chair or in bed to keep the muscles and joints in reasonable working order.

## Immobilization

An orthopedic term for techniques used to prevent movement of joints or displacement of fractured bones so that the bones can unite properly. (See also *Fracture*.)

## Immune response

A defensive reaction of the body to invading microorganisms, cancer cells, transplanted tissue, and other substances or materials that are recognized as antigenic or "foreign" (that is, different from normal body components). The response consists of the production of substances called *antibodies* or *immunoglobulins*, sensitized cells called *lymphocytes*, and other substances and cells that act to destroy the antigenic material. (See also *Immune system*.)

## Immune serum globulin

A preparation of *antibodies*, also known as immune globulin and gamma globulin, used to prevent and sometimes treat infectious diseases.

Its main use is in the prevention of viral *hepatitis* (e.g., before traveling to a country where the disease is common). It is also given to prevent *measles* and *rubella* in people who are exposed to these infections and are not already immune to them from previous infection or *immunization*.

Immune serum globulin is also given to people with *immunodeficiency disorders* (impaired natural defenses).

**HOW IT WORKS**
Immune serum globulin provides immunity to a range of common infectious diseases. It works by passing on antibodies obtained from the blood of large numbers of people who have previously been exposed to these diseases and thus have developed antibodies to them.

**POSSIBLE ADVERSE EFFECTS**
Immune serum globulin may cause rash, fever, and pain and tenderness at the injection site.

## Immune system

A collection of cells and proteins that works to protect the body from potentially harmful, infectious microorganisms (microscopic life-forms), such as bacteria, viruses, and fungi. The immune system also plays a role in the control of cancer and is responsible for the phenomena of *allergy*, *hypersensitivity*, and rejection problems when organs or tissue are transplanted.

Some of the main components of the body's immune system are described in the illustrated boxes.

A newborn child is, to some extent, protected against infection by barriers (such as the skin), by substances in the mouth, in the urinary tract, or on the eye surface that destroy microorganisms, and by *antibodies* or *immunoglobulins* (protective proteins) that have been passed to the child from the mother (including those received in breast milk).

This natural, or innate, immunity cannot guard against all disease-causing organisms. As the child grows, he or she encounters organisms that overcome the innate defenses and thus cause disease. The second line of immune defense, called the adaptive immune system, then comes into play. As the name implies, this system adapts its response specifically to fight the invading organism. In addition, it retains a memory of the invader so that defenses can be rallied instantly in the future. The person is then said to have acquired immunity to the infection. If these microorganisms invade again, they are quickly recognized and dealt with (which explains why diseases such as measles and diphtheria rarely affect the same person twice).

The acquisition of immunity in response to an infection can take a few days or weeks to develop; in the interim, a child or adult can become very ill or even die. In the past, many did die. Today, our chance of surviving, recovering, or totally avoiding infectious diseases is much improved, partly as a result of better general health and nutrition (which bolsters the immune system) and partly through *immunization* against specific disease-causing microorganisms.

### INNATE IMMUNITY
The skin provides an impenetrable barrier to the vast majority of infectious agents, most of which can gain entry only via the mucous membranes (e.g., in the mouth, throat, eyes, intestines, vagina, or urinary tract). These areas are protected by the movement of mucus and other fluids (such as tears) and the presence of enzymes (such as lysozyme) that destroy bacteria.

If microorganisms are able to penetrate the outer layer of the skin or a mucous membrane, they soon encounter white blood cells called phagocytes (literally, "engulfing" cells), which attempt to destroy them, and other types of white cells, such as natural killer (cytotoxic) cells. Microorganisms may also meet naturally produced substances (such

as *interferon*) or a system of blood proteins known as the complement system, which act to destroy the invading microorganisms.

### ADAPTIVE IMMUNITY
The adaptive part of the immune system is extremely complex and only partly understood. Its function is to produce specific defenses against a range of different invading organisms or tumor cells. Broadly, however, it first must recognize part of an invading organism or tumor cell as an *antigen* (a protein that is foreign or different from any natural body protein).

A response (either humoral or cellular) is then mounted against the antigen. The humoral response consists of the production of soluble proteins, called antibodies or immunoglobulins, manufactured by cells called B-lymphocytes. Cellular responses center around the activities of the cells called T-lymphocytes.

**HUMORAL IMMUNITY** This type of immunity is particularly important in the defense against bacteria. After a complex recognition process, certain B-lymphocytes are stimulated to multiply. These cells then begin to produce vast numbers of antibodies that are able to bind to the antigens. Once this has occurred, the organisms bearing the antigens are easy prey to phagocytic ("engulfing") white cells. Binding of antibody and antigen may also activate the complement system, which increases the efficiency with which phagocytes engulf and destroy the invading organisms.

**CELLULAR IMMUNITY** This is particularly important in the defense against viruses, some types of parasites that hide within cells, and, possibly, cancer cells. The T-lymphocytes at the center of cellular immunity are of two types, called helper cells and killer cells. The helper cells play a role in the recognition of antigens. Along with various other functions, they activate the killer cells. Killer lymphocytes lock onto cells that have been invaded by viruses or other parasites that have left recognizable antigens on the cell surfaces. The killer lymphocytes then destroy these parasitized cells. They may act in a similar way against tumor cells and against the cells in transplanted tissue.

The memory of the immune system (which provides acquired immunity to certain diseases) relies on the long-term survival of lymphocytes that were activated or sensitized to antigens when these antigens were first encountered.

### IMMUNE SYSTEM DEFECTS
The immune system is an essential asset for the protection of the body from infectious agents and probably cancer. In certain circumstances, however, it may itself be a cause of disease or other undesirable consequences. In some cases, the body's own proteins are misidentified as antigens, and an immunological attack is mounted against them, causing *autoimmune disorders*. In other cases, the immune system mounts an inappropriate response to what are usually innocuous antigens, such as pollen, causing *hypersensitivity* or *allergy*.

### SUPPRESSION OF THE IMMUNE SYSTEM
In certain circumstances, such as after transplantation of tissues (see *Transplant surgery*) and in people with an autoimmune disorder, it is advantageous to suppress the immune system (especially the adaptive part of the immune system) through use of drugs. This prevents the rejection of the donor organ by lymphocytes and other cells that recognize proteins in the transplanted tissue as antigens. Immunosuppression can also occur as an inherited disorder or after infection with certain viruses, including HIV, the virus that causes *AIDS* (see *Immunodeficiency disorders*).

## Immunity
A state of protection against a disease or diseases through the activities of the *immune system*. Natural, or innate, immunity is present from birth and is the first line of defense against the vast majority of infectious agents. Acquired immunity is the second line of defense. It develops either through exposure to invading microorganisms (after they have broken through the innate immune defenses) or as a result of *immunization*.

## Immunization
The process of inducing *immunity* as a preventive measure against certain infectious diseases. The incidence of a number of diseases (*diphtheria* and *measles*, for example) has declined dramatically since the introduction of effective immunization programs; one disease (*smallpox*) has been eradicated worldwide.

Although diseases such as diphtheria, measles, *mumps*, rubella (German measles), *poliomyelitis*, and *pertussis* (whooping cough) are today rare in the US, routine immunization against them must continue. If a large proportion of the population were nonimmunized, there would be a risk

## THE INNATE IMMUNE SYSTEM

Each of us has many inborn defenses against infection, including external barriers (below), the inflammatory response (right), and phagocyte action (below right). Others include chemicals called complement (which is activated by and attacks bacteria) and *interferon* (which has antiviral effects).

All these defenses are nonspecific and quick-acting. By contrast, the adaptive immune system (next page) mounts specific attacks against particular microbes. These cells are most effective on second exposure to the organisms.

The two parts of the immune system work together; antibodies produced by the adaptive immune system assist phagocyte action.

## THE INFLAMMATORY RESPONSE

If microbes break through the body's outermost barriers, inflammation is the second line of defense. Chemicals (such as histamine) are released, prompting the effects shown below, including the attraction of phagocytes to the microbes. The symptoms of inflammation are redness, pain, swelling, and heat.

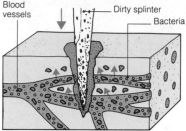

Following tissue injury (here caused by a splinter) and entry of bacteria or other microbes, blood vessels in the area widen and there is increased leakage of fluid from the blood into the tissues. This

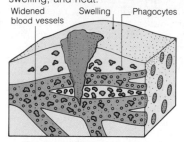

allows easier access for immune system components that fight the invaders, including phagocytes and soluble factors (such as the group of chemicals known as complement).

### Physical and chemical barriers

These barriers, summarized below, provide the first line of defense against harmful microbes (bacteria, viruses, and fungi).

### Eyes

Tears produced by the lacrimal apparatus help wash away microorganisms; tears contain an enzyme (lysozyme) that can destroy bacteria.

### Mouth

Lysozyme present in saliva destroys bacteria.

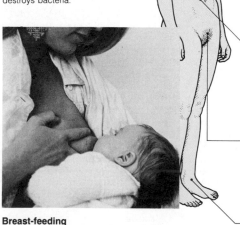

### Breast-feeding

Antibodies (proteins with a protective role) formed by the mother against certain microbes are transferred to the baby in breast milk. This action provides some extra immunity until the baby can form his or her own specific antibodies.

### Nose

Hairs in the nose help prevent entry of microorganisms on dust particles. This process is assisted by the sneeze reflex.

### Respiratory tract

Mucus secreted by cells lining the throat, windpipe, and bronchi traps microbes, which are then swept away by cilia (hairs on cells in the lining) or engulfed by phagocytes (types of white cells). The cough reflex also helps to expel microbes.

### Stomach and intestines

Stomach acid destroys the vast majority of microorganisms. The intestines contain harmless bacteria (commensals) that compete with and control the harmful organisms.

### Genitourinary system

The vagina and urethra also contain commensals and are protected by mucus. Spermine in semen may exert some antimicrobial action.

### Skin

Intact skin provides an effective barrier against most microbes. The sebaceous glands secrete chemicals that are highly toxic to many bacteria.

## ACTION OF PHAGOCYTES

These white blood cells are attracted to infection sites, where they engulf and digest microorganisms and debris.

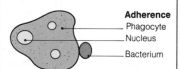

**Adherence**
- Phagocyte
- Nucleus
- Bacterium

**1** The phagocyte must first contact and recognize a microbe as foreign. This process is assisted by chemicals released during inflammation.

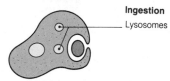

**Ingestion**
- Lysosomes

**2** The phagocyte engulfs the microbe in a pouch formed in its membrane. Fluid-filled particles called lysosomes move toward the microbe.

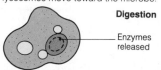

**Digestion**
- Enzymes released

**3** Enzymes within the lysosome are released into the pouch to help digest the microbe. Debris from this process is later ejected.

# THE ADAPTIVE IMMUNE SYSTEM

This system is based on cells called lymphocytes. It has two parts. Humoral immunity relies on the production, by B-lymphocytes, of antibodies, which circulate and attack specific microbes. In cellular immunity, cells called T-lymphocytes are activated and attack specific microbes or abnormal cells (such as virally infected or tumor cells).

## HUMORAL IMMUNITY

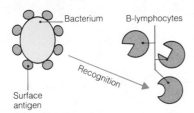

**1** A humoral response is started when an antigen (foreign protein)—here on the surface of a bacterium—activates one type of B-lymphocyte.

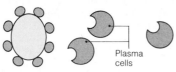

**2** The particular type of B-lymphocyte multiplies, forming cells called plasma cells, which make antibodies designed specifically to attack the bacterium.

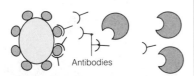

**3** After a few days, the antibodies are released and travel to and attach to the antigen. This triggers more reactions, which ultimately destroy the bacterium.

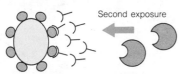

**4** Some B-lymphocytes remain in the body as memory cells; if the bacterium enters the body again, they rapidly produce antibodies to halt the infection.

## CELLULAR IMMUNITY

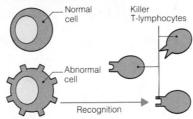

**1** An antigen, here on the surface of an abnormal cell (such as a virus-infected or tumor cell), is identified by, and activates, specific killer (cytotoxic) T-lymphocytes.

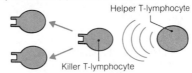

**2** With the assistance of helper T cells (another type of T-lymphocyte), the killer T-lymphocytes begin to multiply.

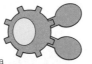

**3** The killer T-lymphocytes travel to, and attach to, the abnormal cells (a), leading to their destruction (b). The T-lymphocytes survive and may go on to kill more targets.

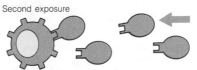

**4** Some of the killer T-lymphocytes remain as memory cells, and quickly attack abnormal cells should they reappear (e.g., after reinfection with a virus).

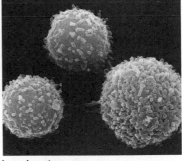

**Lymphocyte**
Lymphocytes are found in the blood and lymphoid organs (lymph nodes, spleen, and thymus). The two main types—B- and T-lymphocytes—have different functions but look identical under the microscope.

## AIDS AND CELLULAR IMMUNITY

HIV—the virus responsible for AIDS—causes illness by disrupting the cellular part of the adaptive immune system.

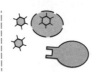

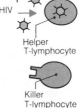

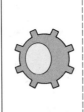

**1** HIV invades and destroys the helper T-lymphocytes, thus preventing the assistance they normally give to killer T-lymphocytes.

**2** As a result, the killer T-lymphocytes fail to multiply and attack in response to abnormal cells or invading microorganisms.

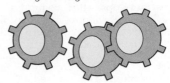

**3** Opportunistic viruses and other microbes or tumor cells may thus proliferate unchecked, causing the features of AIDS.

## EXAMPLES OF INFECTIOUS ORGANISMS COMBATTED

| Humoral immunity particularly important against: | Cell-mediated immunity particularly important against: |
| --- | --- |
| Some viruses (e.g., measles) | Many viruses (e.g., herpes simplex) |
| Many bacteria (e.g., cholera) | Some bacteria (e.g., tuberculosis) |
| Some parasites (e.g., malaria) | Some fungi (e.g., candidiasis) |

of a new epidemic because there is still a steady flow of cases of infectious diseases (many imported).

## IMMUNIZATION AND VACCINATION

Immunization may be active or passive (see diagram). The terms vaccination and active immunization are used interchangeably. The word vaccination is derived from the vaccinia virus (which is similar to the smallpox virus), which was used for vaccination against smallpox.

## WHO SHOULD BE IMMUNIZED

Some types of immunization, such as against polio and DPT (diphtheria, pertussis, and *tetanus*), are aimed at the general population, primarily young children. Others are intended for specific people, such as those exposed to dangerous infections during local outbreaks or those who are at risk of contracting unusual infections through occupational exposure (e.g., laboratory workers or veterinarians).

Immunization before foreign travel may be necessary for entry into certain countries (today, this usually applies only to immunization against *yellow fever*) and to protect the traveler against infection. The traveler should determine a few months before departure which immunizations are necessary or recommended.

The accompanying table gives details of a typical immunization schedule during childhood. (See also *Travel immunization*.)

## HOW IMMUNIZATION IS DONE

Most immunizations are given by injection, either into the muscle or into the tissues under the skin in the upper arm. If the injection contains a large volume of fluid, it may be given in the buttock. Polio vaccine is almost always given orally.

## ADVERSE REACTIONS

Usually there are no aftereffects following immunization. Some vaccines cause pain and swelling at the injection site and may produce a slight fever and a feeling of irritability and malaise. Acetaminophen should be given to young children in whom fever develops after being immunized. Some vaccines, such as the measles vaccine, may produce a mild form of the disease.

In very rare cases, severe reactions (such as seizures) occur following immunization. This has led to controversy about the advisability of some types of vaccination, notably against pertussis (whooping cough). However, for most people, the risks of vaccination are much smaller than the risk of damage through the disease.

### TYPICAL CHILDHOOD IMMUNIZATION SCHEDULE

| Age | Disease | |
|---|---|---|
| 2 months | Diphtheria, pertussis (whooping cough), tetanus* | Poliomyelitis† |
| 4 months | Diphtheria, pertussis, tetanus* | Poliomyelitis† |
| 6 months | Diphtheria, pertussis, tetanus* | |
| 15 months | Measles, mumps, rubella (German measles)* | |
| 18 months | Diphtheria, pertussis, tetanus* | Poliomyelitis† |
| 4 to 6 years | Diphtheria, pertussis, tetanus* | Poliomyelitis† |
| | * Combined injection | † Oral |

Although most modern vaccines provide a reliable method of preventing disease, they do not all provide 100 percent protection. *Cholera* and *typhoid fever* vaccinations, in particular, give only partial protection, so other precautions (principally food and water hygiene) must be observed during travel to areas where there is a risk of these diseases.

## WHO SHOULD NOT BE IMMUNIZED

Immunization should not be given to any person who suffers from an *immunodeficiency disorder* or a cancer

## TYPES OF IMMUNIZATION

There are two main types. In passive immunization, antibodies (protective proteins) are injected and provide immediate, but short-lived, protection against specific disease-causing bacteria, viruses, or toxins. Active immunization primes the body to make its own antibodies against such microorganisms and confers longer-lasting immunity.

### PASSIVE IMMUNIZATION

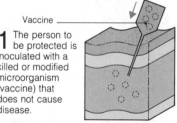

**1** Blood is taken from a person or, rarely, an animal previously exposed to a specific microorganism. The blood contains antibodies against that organism.

Antibodies

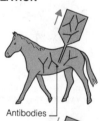

**2** An extract of the blood containing the antibodies (called immune serum or antiserum) is injected into the person to be protected.

Serum

Bloodstream

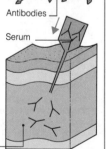

**3** The antibodies help destroy the microorganism if it is present in the blood or enters it over the following few days.

Microorganism

### ACTIVE IMMUNIZATION

Vaccine

**1** The person to be protected is inoculated with a killed or modified microorganism (vaccine) that does not cause disease.

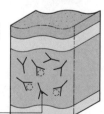

**2** The immune system is provoked to make antibodies against the modified microorganism; it also retains a "memory" of the organism.

Antibodies

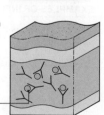

**3** If the real microorganism then enters the blood, antibodies are produced in large numbers to halt the infection.

Disease-causing microorganism

that has spread. Any person who is taking *corticosteroid drugs* or who has previously had a severe reaction to the same vaccine should not be vaccinated. Some vaccines, such as those for typhoid and yellow fever, should not be given to very young children. Vaccination should be deferred if the person has a fever or infection. A number of vaccines, particularly the rubella vaccine, should not be given during pregnancy due to the risk of affecting the fetus.

## Immunoassay

A group of laboratory techniques that includes ELISA (enzyme-linked immunosorbent assay) and radioimmunoassay. Both are used in the diagnosis of infectious diseases; variants of radioimmunoassay, such as the radioallergosorbent test (RAST) and the radioimmunosorbent test (RIST), are also used in the diagnosis of allergies and in the measurement of blood hormone concentrations.

Either technique can determine the presence or absence in a person's blood of a specific protein—such as an *antigen* (a protein on the surface of a microorganism or an allergen), a specific *antibody* (a protein formed by the body's immune system to protect against a particular type of microorganism or allergen), or other protein, such as a hormone.

The principle underlying these techniques is that, for any specific antibody, there is a specific antigen. If molecules of these two proteins come in close contact, they will bind strongly to each other. Any specific antibody will bind only to its own antigen, and vice versa.

### HOW IT IS DONE

First, the surface of a plate or the inside of a test tube is prepared with a covering of the specific protein (antigen or antibody) that will bind to the antibody or antigen whose presence in the blood is to be tested. For example, in the ELISA test for antibody to *HIV* (the virus responsible for *AIDS*), the inside of a test tube is lined with small amounts of antigen from HIV.

This surface is then exposed to plasma of the blood; if the antibody (or antigen) under test is present, it will stick strongly to the surface. The surface is then washed and a chemical added that will bind to the bound protein. This chemical is itself linked either to an enzyme called peroxidase (in the ELISA test) or to a radioactive isotope (in radioimmunoassay).

Any excess chemical is washed away, and, if the antibody or antigen was present, either peroxidase or radioactivity is left on the surface. Peroxidase can be detected by adding another chemical that changes color in its presence; radioactivity can be measured by a gamma counter.

The RIST differs from other types of radioimmunoassay in that the blood serum containing the substance being tested is first mixed with a solution containing the same substance, which has been radioactively labeled. The radioactive and the test versions compete to bind to the test plate. The result is that, after washing, the less radioactivity found on the test plate, the more test substance must have been present in the blood serum.

## Immunodeficiency disorders

Disorders in which there is a failure of the *immune system's* defenses to fight infection and tumors. Immunodeficiency may be the result of an inherited or congenital defect that interferes with the normal development of the immune system or the result of acquired disease that damages the system's function. The result, in either case, is the appearance of persistent or recurrent infection by organisms that would not ordinarily cause disease, incomplete recovery from illness with poor response to customarily effective treatment, and an undue susceptibility to certain forms of cancer.

The infections seen in people with immunodeficiency disorders sometimes are called *opportunistic infections* because the microorganisms take advantage of the person's lowered defenses. Infections of this type include pneumonia caused by *PNEUMOCYSTIS CARINII*, widespread *herpes simplex* infections, and many *fungal infections*.

### INHERITED IMMUNODEFICIENCY

The adaptive part of the immune system (which mounts specific defenses against particular microorganisms or tumor cells) has two major prongs. One of these, the humoral system, relies on the production of antibodies, or immunoglobulins, manufactured by B-*lymphocytes*. The other prong is called the cellular system and relies on the activity of T-lymphocytes. Congenital or inherited deficiencies can occur in either of these systems.

Deficiencies of the humoral system include hypogammaglobulinemia (in which the production of one or more types of immunoglobulin is interfered

with) and agammaglobulinemia (in which there is an almost complete absence of B-lymphocytes and immunoglobulins). The most common type of hypogammaglobulinemia affects about one person in 600 and may cause no more than repeated mild attacks of respiratory infection. Agammaglobulinemia is a rare, grave condition that often has a fatal outcome in infancy or childhood.

Congenital deficiencies of the T-lymphocytes may lead to problems such as persistent and widespread *candidiasis* (thrush) affecting the skin, mouth, throat, and vagina. Problems of this type are caused by the inability of the immune system to fight fungi.

A combined deficiency of both prongs of the immune system is also known. It is called severe combined immunodeficiency. Infants with this combined deficiency usually die within the first year of life.

### ACQUIRED IMMUNODEFICIENCY

Acquired deficiency of the immune system may occur in either of two ways—by damage to the immune system as a result of its suppression with drugs or by disease processes.

Deliberate suppression of the immune system with *immunosuppressant drugs* and *corticosteroid drugs* is usually carried out as part of the treatment of *autoimmune disorders* and after transplantation to minimize the risk of organ rejection.

Diseases that cause immunodeficiency include infection with *HIV* (human immunodeficiency virus), which leads to *AIDS* (acquired immunodeficiency syndrome). Severe malnutrition, especially with protein deficiency, and many types of cancer can also cause immunodeficiency.

### IMMUNODEFICIENCY IN THE ELDERLY

A degree of immunodeficiency arises simply as a consequence of age. The thymus, which plays an important part in the production of T-lymphocytes, reaches peak size in puberty and steadily shrinks thereafter. This results in a decline in the number and activity of T-lymphocytes with age; there is also a decline in the numbers of B-lymphocytes.

## Immunoglobulins

Proteins found in the blood serum and in tissue fluids, also known as *antibodies*. Immunoglobulins are produced by cells of the *immune system* called B-lymphocytes. Their function is to bind to substances in the body that are recognized as foreign antigens (often proteins on the surface of bacteria and viruses). This binding is a crucial event in the destruction of the microorganisms that bear the antigens. Immunoglobulins also play a central role in *allergies* and *hypersensitivity* reactions. In this case they bind to antigens that are not necessarily a threat to health, which may provoke an inflammatory reaction.

There are five classes of immunoglobulins; of these, immunoglobulin G (IgG) is the major immunoglobulin in human blood serum. The IgG molecule consists of two parts, one of which binds to antigen; the other binds to other cells of the immune system. These other cells are principally white cells called phagocytes, which then engulf the microorganisms bearing the antigen. The antigen-binding site of the IgG molecule is variable in its structure, the different versions of the molecule being capable of binding to an almost infinite number of antigens.

Immunoglobulins can be extracted from blood of recovering patients and used for passive *immunization* against certain infectious diseases.

## Immunologist

A specialist in the functioning of the *immune system* who may also devise ways in which the immune system can be stimulated to provide immunity (principally through the use of *vaccines*) and who investigates and treats problems related to the immune system. The latter include *allergies*, *autoimmune disorders*, and *immunodeficiency disorders* such as *AIDS*.

Immunologists also play an important part in *transplant surgery*, looking preoperatively for a good immunological match between recipient and donor organ, and suppressing the recipient's immune system after transplantation to minimize the chances of organ rejection.

## Immunology

The study of the functioning and disorders of the *immune system*.

## Immunostimulant drugs

A group of drugs that increases the efficiency of the body's *immune system* (natural defenses against infection and abnormal cells). Immunostimulant drugs include *vaccines*, which protect against specific infectious diseases (see *Immunization*). Two drugs belonging to this group are *interferon* (used to treat viral infections and certain types of cancer) and *zidovudine* (used to treat *AIDS*).

Some immunostimulant drugs enhance the ability of a vaccine to stimulate the immune system and are added to the vaccine for this reason. Aluminum phosphate, for example, increases the effectiveness of the *tetanus* vaccine.

## Immunosuppressant drugs

| COMMON DRUGS |
| --- |
| Anticancer drugs |
| *Azathioprine Chlorambucil* |
| *Cyclophosphamide Methotrexate* |
| Corticosteroid drugs |
| *Dexamethasone Prednisone* |
| Others |
| *Cyclosporine* |

A group of drugs that reduces the activity of the body's *immune system* (natural defenses against infection and abnormal cells).

Immunosuppressant drugs are prescribed after *transplant surgery* to prevent the rejection of foreign tissues. They are also given to halt the progress of *autoimmune disorders* (in which the body's immune system attacks its own tissues) when other treatments are ineffective. They are unable, however, to restore tissue that has already been damaged.

**HOW THEY WORK**

Immunosuppressant drugs work by suppressing the production and activity of *lymphocytes*, a type of white blood cell that plays an important part in fighting infection and in eliminating abnormal cells that may form a malignant tumor.

**POSSIBLE ADVERSE EFFECTS**

Apart from the individual effects of each type, these drugs increase the risk of infection and of the development of certain cancers.

## Immunotherapy

A preventive treatment of allergy to substances such as grass pollens, house-dust mites, and wasp and bee venom. Immunotherapy involves giving gradually increasing doses of the substance, or allergen, to which the person is allergic. This works by making the *immune system* less sensitive to that substance, probably by causing production of a particular "blocking" *antibody*, which reduces the symptoms of allergy when the substance is encountered in the future.

Before starting treatment, the physician and patient try to identify trigger factors for allergic symptoms. Skin or sometimes blood tests are per-

formed to confirm the specific allergens to which the person has antibodies. Immunotherapy is usually recommended only if the person seems to be selectively sensitive to several allergens (such as grass).

**HOW IT IS DONE**

A purified extract of a small amount of the allergen is injected into the skin of the arm. An injection is given once a week for about 30 weeks, after which injections can be administered every two weeks. Eventually, injections can be given every four weeks; the duration of therapy is three to four years.

**RISKS**

There is a danger of *anaphylactic shock* (a severe allergic reaction) shortly after an injection. Therefore, immunotherapy requires medical supervision and is not done at times of exposure to the substance causing the allergy.

**IMMUNOTHERAPY IN CANCER TREATMEMT**

Another use of the term immunotherapy refers to stimulation of the immune system to treat cancer. It is still largely experimental, but it may prove a useful adjunct to other therapies, such as *chemotherapy*, in the treatment of *leukemia*, *lymphoma*, and some other cancers.

One type of immunotherapy relies on the use of immunostimulants, substances that cause general stimulation of the immune system.

Another technique is to inoculate the patient with tumor cells or cellular extracts, rendered harmless by irradiation, that have been taken from another person suffering from the same disease. The patient's immune system then produces its own *antibodies*, which attack the tumor cells. Alternatively, immunoglobulins (ready-made antibodies) from another person with the same type of tumor can be given to the patient. More recently, monoclonal antibodies (see *Antibodies, monoclonal*) to be directed against tumors have been produced artificially by *genetic engineering*. *Interferon* or chemical poisons can be linked to these antibodies to increase their ability to destroy tumor cells.

One drawback to the administration of some of these anticancer treatments is that they, too, may be recognized as foreign by the person's immune system, causing either allergic reactions (serum sickness) or new antibody production, which interferes with the activity against cancer.

## Impaction, dental

Failure of a tooth to emerge fully or at all from the gum when, because of

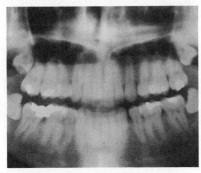

**Impacted wisdom teeth**
This X ray shows impacted wisdom teeth lying horizontally in the lower jaw. The impacted teeth are wedged against the adjacent molars and are not able to erupt normally.

mechanical impediment, it is embedded in bone or soft tissue beyond its normal eruption time.

Impaction is caused by overcrowding of the teeth in places where little room is left for the teeth that erupt last (the wisdom teeth and the upper canines). It is also caused by the tooth traveling in the wrong direction and by dense bone that impedes the tooth's progress.

**IMPACTED WISDOM TEETH**
These are common, but usually cause no trouble unless they partially penetrate the gum, leaving a flap of tissue over most of the crown. Plaque bacteria and food debris then collect between the tooth and the gum, which often becomes inflamed and painful. There may also be swollen lymph nodes in the upper neck and difficulty opening the mouth.

Rinsing the area with warm, salt water and taking *analgesics* (painkillers) can relieve some symptoms of the condition, but, if it is severe, *antibiotic drugs* are required to clear up the infection. A dentist may decide that the tooth requires extraction to prevent more trouble.

**IMPACTED UPPER CANINES**
These teeth play a much more important part than do wisdom teeth in biting and chewing. If they are impacted, they are not usually removed, but instead are trained into the correct position by means of an *orthodontic appliance*.

## Impetigo

A highly contagious skin infection, common in children, that usually occurs around the nose and mouth.

**CAUSES AND INCIDENCE**
Impetigo is caused by bacteria entering the skin through a broken area, such as a cut, cold sore, or an area affected by *eczema*. The infection is more common in warm weather. Impetigo was once extremely common, but occurs less frequently now because of improved standards of personal hygiene. Small epidemics occasionally occur in schools.

**SYMPTOMS AND SIGNS**
The skin reddens and small, fluid-filled blisters appear on the surface. The blisters tend to burst, leaving moist, weeping areas underneath; the released fluid dries to leave honey-colored crusts on the skin. The infected area may spread at the edges or another patch may develop nearby.

In severe cases there may be swelling of the *lymph nodes* in the face or neck, accompanied by a fever. Very occasionally, complications such as *septicemia* (blood poisoning) or *glomerulonephritis* (inflammation of the kidneys) develop.

**TREATMENT**
Because impetigo spreads rapidly, it is advisable to consult a physician. *Antibiotic drugs* in tablet or ointment form usually clear up the problem in about

## TYPES OF IMPLANTS

Implants may be inserted into various parts of the body. They can be used to replace a diseased structure, to improve appearance, to maintain proper functioning of an internal organ, to treat certain disorders, or to deliver drugs or hormones.

**Hormonal**
Some hormonal drugs (particularly hormonal contraceptives) can be placed in implants that are inserted under the skin to release the drug slowly over time. Alternatively, such drugs can be incorporated in some IUDs (intrauterine contraceptive devices).

**Breast**
Silicone implants can be used to restore breast shape after mastectomy (breast removal) for cancer or to increase breast size for cosmetic purposes (augmentation mammoplasty).

**Therapeutic**
Radioactive materials in sealed containers can be inserted into tissue to treat malignant tumors, for example, a cancer of the cervix.

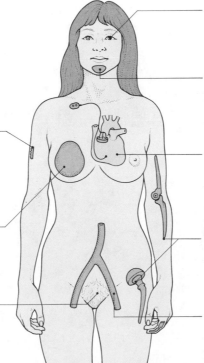

**Eye**
An implant can be used to replace the lens of the eye after cataract removal, or the entire eyeball if it requires removal because of injury or disease.

**Face**
Pieces of bone taken from another part of the body, or shaped pieces of silicone, can be implanted on the face to make a receding chin more prominent or to improve the contour at a fracture site.

**Heart**
Cardiac pacemakers (battery-powered electronic devices connected by wires to the heart muscle) can be implanted in the chest to regulate the heart beat; diseased heart valves may be replaced with artificial or natural substitutes.

**Joints**
Diseased joints can be replaced with artificial substitutes to help restore full function. The elbow, the hip, the knee, the finger joints, and the shoulder can all now be treated in this way.

**Artery**
Diseased sections of artery, such as the lower aorta and upper iliac arteries (shown here), can be replaced or bypassed with artificial tubular materials made from woven or knitted synthetic fibers.

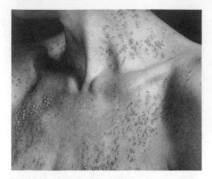

**The appearance of impetigo**
Fluid-filled blisters appear on the skin (in this case, on the neck and chest). The blisters often burst, releasing fluid that dries to leave pale-brown crusts.

five days. Any loose crusts should be gently washed off with soap and water and the area dabbed dry.

To prevent spreading, pillowcases, towels, and washcloths should not be shared and should be boiled after use. Children should not touch affected skin and should stay out of school until the infection clears.

## Implant
Any material, natural or artificial, inserted into the body (see box on the previous page).

## Implantation, egg
 Attachment of a fertilized ovum to the wall of the uterus. About six days after fertilization, the developing *embryo* comes into contact with the wall of the uterus and attaches to it. As the cells of the embryo divide, the outer cell layer grows into the lining of the uterus to obtain oxygen and nutrients from the mother's blood; later, this layer develops into the *placenta*.

The embryo usually implants in the upper part of the uterus; if it implants low down near the cervix, *placenta previa* may develop. Rarely, the embryo does not reach the uterus and implants in a fallopian tube, resulting in an *ectopic pregnancy*.

## Impotence
The inability to achieve or maintain an *erection*. Impotence is the most common male sexual disorder, affecting most men at some time in their lives.
**CAUSES**
In the majority of men, impotence is caused by psychological factors. They may be temporary (caused by stress or fatigue) or long-standing (caused by anxiety and guilt that originated in childhood). Impotence may be a symptom of *depression*.

Approximately 10 percent of impotence is caused by a physical disorder (including *diabetes mellitus* or hormonal imbalance) or by a neurological disorder (such as spinal cord damage or chronic alcohol abuse). Impotence may be caused by taking various drugs—particularly antipsychotics, antidepressants, antihypertensives, and diuretics. Impotence is also more common as men get older, possibly because of altered circulation or, less often, lowered levels of the male sex hormone *testosterone*.
**DIAGNOSIS AND TREATMENT**
If the cause is psychological, counseling or *sex therapy* (preferably with the person's partner) is successful in more than half the cases of long-term impotence. To eliminate the possibility of any physical disorder, tests may be performed. The physician may stop medication or alter the dose to aid in diagnosis; attempts are also made to treat any depression or alcohol abuse. *Penile implants* help some men whose impotence is caused by disease.

## Impression, dental
A mold taken of the teeth, gums, and sometimes the palate. A quick-setting material, such as alginate or a rubber compound, is placed in a shaped tray that is eased over the area of which a replica is to be made and left in position until the material has set. After the mold has been removed, plaster of Paris is poured into it to obtain a model of the area. This is then used as a base on which to build a *denture*, *bridge*, *inlay*, or *onlay*.

Impressions are also used in *orthodontics* to study the position of the teeth and the structure of the mouth, and to make any orthodontic appliances to correct the irregularities.

## Impulse control disorders
A group of psychiatric disorders characterized by the inability to resist an impulse or temptation to do some-

### INCIDENCE OF RELATIVELY SHORT-LIVED CONDITIONS* IN THE US

| Incidence (new cases per 100,000 people per year) | Categorization | Examples |
|---|---|---|
| More than 10,000 | Extremely common | Common cold |
| 1,000 to 10,000 | Very common | Sexually transmitted infection (all types) |
| 100 to 1,000 | Common | Basal cell carcinoma, gonorrhea, lung cancer, myocardial infarction, shingles, stroke |
| 20 to 100 | Fairly common | Breast cancer, viral hepatitis, intestinal cancer, symptomatic kidney stones |
| 5 to 20 | Uncommon | AIDS, brain tumor, acute leukemia, malignant melanoma, syphilis (primary and secondary), tuberculosis |
| 0.5 to 5 | Rare | Amebiasis, gallbladder cancer, Guillain-Barré syndrome, Hodgkin's disease, measles, motor neuron disease, pertussis |
| 0.005 to 0.5 | Very rare | Botulism, leptospirosis, lymphogranuloma venereum, malaria |
| Less than 0.005 | Extremely rare | Cholera, diphtheria, rabies |

\* conditions that are self-resolving, curable, or fatal

thing that ultimately proves harmful to oneself. The group includes pathological *gambling*, *kleptomania*, *pyromania*, and *explosive disorders*.

## Incest

Legally defined as sexual intercourse between close relatives (parent-child or brother-sister intercourse is regarded as first degree; with a grandparent, aunt, or uncle, it is regarded as second degree; with a cousin it is regarded as third degree).

Marriage between close kin is forbidden by law in certain jurisdictions and religions, but permitted in others. Incest prohibitions are widespread and are probably based on concerns over the higher risk of certain congenital problems due to inbreeding.

The actual prevalence of incest is unknown. Recent estimates state that 5 to 10 percent of girls experienced sexual contact with a brother, father, or other male relative, as did 1 to 2 percent of boys with either a male or a female relative.

The 1978 Federal Child Abuse Laws mandate reporting to child protection authorities "any sexual act" (not just intercourse) between an adult and a child inside or outside the family; this aberrant and psychologically damaging behavior is regarded as criminal.

Incest was customary in the royal families of ancient Egypt and contemporary Hawaii. It is more common in isolated mountain and rural communities, where incest-accepting families remain unaware of the law. Education and individual and family therapy are useful.

## Incidence

One of the two principal measures (the other is prevalence) of how common a disease is in a defined population. The incidence of a disease is the number of new cases that occurs during a given period (e.g., 17 cases per 100,000 people per year). Prevalence is the total number of cases of a disease in existence at any one time; it includes both new and old cases. Thus, in 100,000 people, there may be an incidence of, say, 400 cases of a specific type of cancer per year, but a prevalence of 4,000 cases, because the disease lasts an average of 10 years before being cured or causing death.

## Incision

A cut made into the tissues of the body by a scalpel (surgical knife). Most incisions are made to gain access to tissue inside the body (usually to repair or

---

### ABDOMINAL INCISIONS

Surgery is frequently performed on the abdomen. Standard incision sites provide access to the diseased portion with minimum weakening of the abdominal wall. The most commonly used of these standard incision sites are shown in the diagram below.

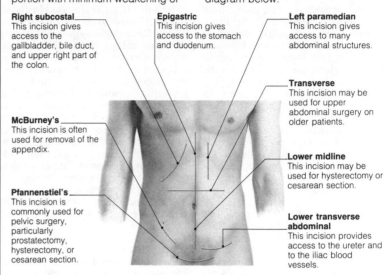

**Right subcostal**
This incision gives access to the gallbladder, bile duct, and upper right part of the colon.

**Epigastric**
This incision gives access to the stomach and duodenum.

**Left paramedian**
This incision gives access to many abdominal structures.

**McBurney's**
This incision is often used for removal of the appendix.

**Transverse**
This incision may be used for upper abdominal surgery on older patients.

**Pfannenstiel's**
This incision is commonly used for pelvic surgery, particularly prostatectomy, hysterectomy, or cesarean section.

**Lower midline**
This incision may be used for hysterectomy or cesarean section.

**Lower transverse abdominal**
This incision provides access to the ureter and to the iliac blood vessels.

---

remove a diseased organ) or to relieve pressure (e.g., from pus in an abscess). Standard incision sites for abdominal surgery are shown in the illustrated box.

## Incisor

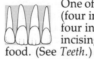 One of the eight front teeth (four in the upper jaw and four in the lower) used for incising (cutting through) food. (See *Teeth*.)

## Incompetent cervix

See *Cervical incompetence*.

## Incontinence, fecal

Inability to retain feces in the rectum.
**CAUSES**
The most common cause of fecal incontinence in the elderly and in children who have been toilet trained is *fecal impaction*. The feces lodged in the rectum irritate and inflame its lining and, as a result, fecal fluid and small pieces of feces are passed involuntarily. Temporary loss of continence may occur at any age with severe *diarrhea* when the need to evacuate the bowel becomes too great to contain.

Less common causes include injury to the anal muscles (for example, during childbirth or surgery), *paraplegia* (paralysis of the legs and lower trunk), mental handicap, and *dementia*.

**TREATMENT**
Impaction, often caused by constipation, may be prevented by a high-fiber diet. Glycerin suppositories taken daily (or laxative suppositories taken occasionally) may be used if the constipation has persisted for several days. Incontinence due to dementia or nerve injury can be avoided by regularly using enemas or suppositories to empty the rectum.

## Incontinence, urinary

Uncontrollable, involuntary urination, often due to injury or disease of the *urinary tract*. This disorder often affects the elderly because the efficiency of the sphincter muscles surrounding the *urethra* declines with age. Women are affected more often than men.

**TYPES AND SYMPTOMS**
**STRESS INCONTINENCE** This refers to the involuntary escape of a small amount of urine when a person coughs, laughs, picks up a heavy package, or moves excessively (such as during athletic activity). Stress incontinence is very common in women, particularly after childbirth when the urethral sphincter muscles are stretched.
**URGE INCONTINENCE** In this type, an urgent desire to urinate is accompanied by inability to control the bladder. Urge incontinence may occur when walking or sitting, but is fre-

quently triggered by a sudden change in position. Once urination starts, it continues until the bladder is empty.

**TOTAL INCONTINENCE** This refers to a complete lack of bladder control resulting from the total absence of sphincter activity. In rare cases, total incontinence occurs because the urine bypasses the sphincter, as in a vesicovaginal fistula (a hole between the bladder and vagina) or an ectopic ureter (in which the ureter enters the urethra rather than the bladder).

**OVERFLOW INCONTINENCE** This occurs in chronic *urine retention*, a condition in which the sufferer is unable to empty the bladder normally, often because of an obstruction such as an enlarged *prostate gland*. The bladder is always full, leading to constant dribbling of the overflow. Relief of the obstruction restores continence.

**CAUSES**

Incontinence may be caused by localized disorders of the urinary tract (including infections, bladder stones, or tumors) or by *prolapse* of the uterus or vagina. Incontinence due to lack of control by the brain commonly occurs in the young (see *Enuresis*), the elderly, and those with mental impairment. Damage to the brain or spinal cord by injury or disease also affects bladder control, as does stress, anger, and anxiety. Weak pelvic muscles, a fractured pelvis, or cancer of the prostate can cause incontinence. *Irritable bladder*, in which the bladder muscle twitches intermittently, raises the pressure in the bladder to push some urine out of the urethra; this causes an intense desire to urinate.

**DIAGNOSIS**

*Urinalysis* (examination of the urine) is performed to eliminate the possibility of infection, inflammation, diabetes, or protein loss. *Ultrasound scanning*, intravenous *pyelography* (X rays of the kidney and ureters after injection of a dye), and a voiding *cystourethrogram* (X rays taken while the patient is urinating) are used to investigate the possibility of an obstruction. *Cystometry*, which measures the pressure within the bladder, can determine if the bladder is functioning normally or if there is any abnormality of the nerves supplying the bladder. *Cystoscopy* (examination of the urethra and bladder through a rigid or flexible viewing tube) is performed to look for the presence of bladder *calculi*, tumors, or cysts.

**TREATMENT**

If weak pelvic muscles are causing stress incontinence, *pelvic floor exercises* may help to restore sphincter function. Sometimes an operation is performed to tighten the urethra. In severe cases, an inflatable artificial plastic sphincter may be placed around the urethra; when urination is required, a trigger is pressed to deflate the mechanism to allow urine to flow.

*Anticholinergic drugs* are sometimes used to relax the spastic bladder muscle if irritable bladder is the cause.

If normal bladder function cannot be restored, special incontinence underpants (with an internal pad to absorb the urine) can alleviate discomfort. Men can wear a sheath over the penis; the sheath leads into a tube connected to a portable urine bag. Some people are able to pass a catheter into the bladder four or five times a day to empty it and avoid incontinence.

If these measures are unsuccessful and the condition is severe, a *urinary diversion* operation to bypass the bladder may be necessary.

## Incoordination

Loss of the ability to produce smooth, harmonious muscular movements, leading to clumsiness and unsteady balance. Incoordination can also mean the failure of a group of organs to work together successfully. (See *Ataxia*.)

## Incubation period

The time during which any infectious disease develops, from the point when the infecting organism enters the body until the appearance of symptoms. Different infections have characteristic incubation periods—for example, 14 to 21 days for chickenpox and seven to 14 days for measles. The incubation period for cholera may be as short as several hours. (See also *Infectious disease* table.)

## Incubator

A transparent plastic container in which oxygen, temperature, and

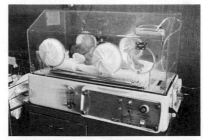

**Premature infant in an incubator**
Portholes make it possible to handle the infant without disturbing the special conditions provided by the incubator.

humidity levels are controlled to provide premature or sick infants with ideal conditions for survival. An incubator also provides some protection from airborne infection.

Incubators have portholes to allow handling of the baby and smaller holes through which monitoring cables and intravenous and respiratory tubing can pass. The air temperature within the incubator is carefully regulated.

## Indian medicine

In contrast to Chinese medicine, traditional East Indian medicine was based on empirical observation and practice rather than on philosophy. The earliest Indian literature, the Vedas, which date from about 1500 BC, contain detailed descriptions of numerous disorders and their treatments. Ayurvedism, as Vedic medicine is known, was based largely on herbal treatment, although early Vedic physicians also used simple surgical techniques and invented artificial limbs and eyes.

The Vedic era ended in about 800 BC, but the medical traditions of ayurvedism survived and were further developed (especially the surgical aspect) under the Brahmans, the caste of wise men. As a result, by about 500 AD, Indian medicine had become a scientifically based system with a wide range of surgical techniques available (such as operations for cataracts and kidney stones) along with the herbal tradition. The Brahmans, however, cloaked their medical knowledge in theology and superstition and traditional Indian medicine stagnated. Today, most Indian medicine follows Western practices.

## Indigestion

A term covering a variety of symptoms brought on by eating, including *heartburn*, *abdominal pain*, *nausea*, and *flatulence* (excessive gas in the stomach or intestine, causing belching or discomfort).

Indigestion refers to a burning discomfort in the upper abdomen, often brought on by eating too much, too quickly, or by eating very rich, spicy, or fatty foods. Nervous indigestion is a common effect of stress. Occasionally, persistent or recurrent indigestion is associated with a *peptic ulcer*, *gallstones*, or *esophagitis* (inflammation of the esophagus).

**TREATMENT**

Self-help treatment includes avoiding foods and situations that bring on symptoms and finding time to eat three or four times a day, at regular times, without rushing. Taking *antacid drugs* or drinking milk may make symptoms subside.

Anyone who takes antacid drugs regularly should see a physician so that the underlying cause of the problem can be investigated. If abdominal pain persists for more than six hours, or if there are other symptoms, such as prolonged vomiting, vomiting blood (which may appear brown), passing very dark or black feces, or feeling weak or faint, a physician should be consulted immediately.

## Indomethacin
A *nonsteroidal anti-inflammatory drug* (NSAID) used to relieve pain, stiffness, and inflammation in disorders such as *osteoarthritis*, *rheumatoid arthritis*, *gout*, *ankylosing spondylitis*, and *tendinitis*. Indomethacin is also prescribed to relieve pain caused by injury to soft tissues, such as muscles and ligaments.

Treatment with indomethacin may cause abdominal pain, nausea, heartburn, headache, dizziness, and an increased risk of *peptic ulcer*.

## Induction of labor
Use of artificial means to initiate the process of childbirth. Labor is induced if the health of the mother or baby would be endangered by allowing the pregnancy to continue. If the pregnancy is not at full term, the risks of induction are weighed against the risks of a premature delivery.

**WHY IT IS DONE**

The primary reason for inducing labor is that the pregnancy has continued past the estimated delivery date, which increases the chance of both maternal and fetal complications during childbirth. Most obstetricians induce labor if the delivery is more than two weeks overdue.

Labor is induced early if the mother is suffering from *eclampsia* or *preeclampsia*, or if she has chronic *hypertension*. Labor may also be induced if there is Rh incompatibility between the mother and baby (because of the risk of *hemolytic disease of the newborn*) or if there are indications of *intrauterine growth retardation*.

**HOW IT IS DONE**

The most common technique of inducing labor is to rupture the membrane around the baby to release some of the amniotic fluid. This is usually sufficient to start labor. If not, vaginal suppositories containing prostaglandin (a hormone that stimulates the uterus to

contract) may be inserted high in the vagina. If this is unsuccessful, an intravenous infusion of *oxytocin* (another hormone that stimulates uterine contractions) may be necessary. If the uterus fails to respond to any of these treatments, the baby may be delivered by cesarean section.

**COMPLICATIONS**

The conditions of both the mother and baby are monitored closely during an induced labor because of the danger that *hypoxia* (reduced oxygen supply) may develop in the baby. Special care facilities are needed if the baby is born prematurely.

## Industrial diseases
See *Occupational disease and injury*.

## Infant
A baby up to the age of 12 months; sometimes this description also includes the period up to 24 months.

## Infantile spasms
A rare type of recurrent seizure that affects babies. Infantile spasms are a form of *epilepsy* in which the baby suddenly stiffens, bending the trunk, limbs, and neck. There may be several hundred such spasms per day, each lasting a few seconds and sometimes preceded by a cry. In most cases the seizures are a sign of brain damage and affected babies grow up with severe mental retardation.

## Infant mortality
The number of infants who die during the first year of life per 1,000 live births. About two thirds of all infant deaths occur during the neonatal period (the first month of life). Most of those who die are very premature (born before the 30th week of pregnancy) or have severe birth defects.

Infant mortality varies greatly among different countries and among different racial and social groups. For example, in Sweden (in the early 1980s), the mortality was low, at eight deaths per 1,000 live births, whereas, in certain African countries, it was as high as 150 per 1,000. In the US, the mortality was 19 per 1,000 live births for black infants, compared with 10 per 1,000 for white infants.

In most developed countries, there has been an overall decline in infant mortality since about the turn of the century. This is largely due to improvements in nutrition and in social conditions and to medical advances, particularly in *prenatal care* and neonatal intensive care.

## Infarction
Death of an area of tissue caused by *ischemia* (lack of blood supply). Common examples include *myocardial infarction* (heart attack) and pulmonary infarction, which is lung damage caused by a *pulmonary embolism* (a blood clot that has moved into a vessel in the lung and is obstructing the flow of blood). See also *Necrosis*.

## Infection

The establishment of a colony of disease-causing microorganisms (such as bacteria, viruses, or fungi) in the body. The organisms actively reproduce and cause disease directly by damage to cells or indirectly by toxins they release. Infection normally provokes a response from the *immune system*, which accounts for many of the features of the infection.

Toxic symptoms, such as fever, weakness, and joint aches, are expressions of *infectious disease*. In such cases, the microorganisms are often spread throughout the body (this is called "systemic" infection). Infection may also be localized within a particular tissue or area, often through spread of organisms from parts of the body where they are harmless to parts where they are harmful (e.g., through leakage from the intestines into the abdomen to cause *peritonitis*).

Entry of microorganisms from soil into wounds or during the course of surgical operations and procedures is another common cause of localized infection. In the early days of surgery, infection of internal body cavities was the major (and frequently fatal) risk to the patient. Antiseptic surgical techniques have largely eliminated this problem.

**AVOIDANCE**

Localized infections (as opposed to infectious diseases) can be avoided by standard hygienic measures, such as keeping the hands clean, not picking at blemishes, washing and covering cuts and grazes, having wounds attended to by a physician, and seeking regular dental treatment.

**SYMPTOMS, DIAGNOSIS, AND TREATMENT**

Localized infection is generally followed by *inflammation*, which increases the flow of blood to the infected area, bringing white blood cells and other components of the immune system. Symptoms and signs usually include pain, redness, swelling, formation of a pus-filled abscess at the site of infection, and sometimes a rise in temperature.

Any suspected infection should be brought to the attention of a physician. Once the nature of the causative microorganism has been discovered, treatment consists of an antimicrobial drug, such as an *antibiotic*.

## Infection, congenital

Any infection present at birth that was acquired by the infant either in the uterus or during passage through the birth canal.

### INFECTIONS ACQUIRED IN THE UTERUS

Many viruses, bacteria, and other microorganisms can pass from the mother's blood through the placenta and into the circulation of the growing fetus. Particularly serious are organisms responsible for *rubella* (German measles), *syphilis*, and *toxoplasmosis*, and the *cytomegalovirus*. Any of these infections may cause *intrauterine growth retardation*. Further effects depend on the stage of pregnancy at which the infection was acquired. Thus, rubella occurring at around nine to 10 weeks (the stage at which various organs are beginning to develop) may cause *deafness*, congenital *heart disease*, and other damage. If infection occurs much later in pregnancy, it may cause no serious harm.

A woman who is infected with the HIV virus (responsible for *AIDS*) risks passing the infection on to her baby during pregnancy. AIDS usually develops within the first two years of life in infants infected with HIV.

### INFECTIONS ACQUIRED DURING BIRTH

These infections are almost always acquired from the mother's vaginal secretions or uterine fluid that has become infected with microorganisms. If the membranes rupture prematurely, the baby is at risk of infection from organisms ascending into the uterus from the birth canal.

Conditions acquired in this way include *conjunctivitis* (caused by infection with the organisms responsible for *gonorrhea*), genital *herpes*, a *chlamydial infection*, and infantile *diarrhea* (caused by salmonella or other bacteria). *Meningitis*, *hepatitis B*, *listeriosis*, and staphylococcal and streptococcal bacterial infections may also be acquired in this way. Babies who inhale infected maternal secretions may develop *pneumonia*.

### PREVENTION

The risk of a baby acquiring an infection in the uterus is minimized by all girls being immunized against rubella in childhood and by pregnant women avoiding sexually transmitted disease (or by having any such disease treated promptly).

If a woman has an active genital herpes infection close to the time of delivery, cesarean section is usually performed, because infection of the newborn baby with herpes simplex virus is particularly serious and commonly fatal.

### TREATMENT

If a baby is diagnosed as having an infection at birth, treatment against the infecting agent is started. Any stunting of growth that has occurred due to infection in the uterus cannot usually be reversed. Some types of birth defects caused by infection (e.g., heart defects) are treatable; others (such as deafness) usually are not.

## Infectious disease

Any illness that is caused by a specific microorganism.

### INCIDENCE

Infectious diseases are a large and important group of conditions and, until recently, were the major cause of illness and death throughout the world. (In many developing countries, they remain a major cause of death.) Over the last century or so, this situation has changed in the more developed countries as a result of four important advances. First, better methods are employed for controlling the spread of disease organisms—including better sanitation, water purification, housing, pest control, personal hygiene, and quarantining procedures (see *Public health*). Second, many effective antimicrobial drugs have been developed. Third, vaccines and other preparations have been developed to provide immunity to certain infectious diseases (see *Immunization*). Fourth, better general health and nutrition have bolstered immunity and improved survival.

In developed countries, such measures have brought about a dramatic decline in the incidence of some serious diseases (such as *poliomyelitis*, *smallpox*, *diphtheria*, and *tuberculosis*). In poorer countries, however, infectious diseases remain a huge problem, for reasons that include lack of resources, ignorance, low standards of public and personal hygiene, the presence of insect transmitters of disease, and, perhaps most importantly, malnutrition. Diseases such as measles have a mortality of 20 percent or more in malnourished children.

---

## HOW INFECTIOUS DISEASES ARE TRANSMITTED

In developed countries, infectious diseases are usually spread by sexual transmission, airborne transmission, blood-borne transmission, or direct skin contact. In poorer countries, insect-borne, food-borne, and waterborne infection are other important mechanisms of transmission. Certain infections can also pass from a pregnant woman's blood across the placenta into the blood of the fetus.

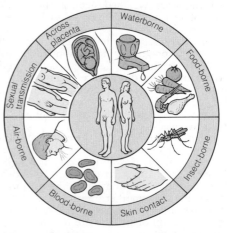

**Cholera bacteria**
The comma-shaped bacteria that cause the dangerous infectious disease cholera are spread by contamination of water.

---

### CAUSES

Disease-causing organisms fall into a number of well-defined groups. Among the most important are the *viruses*, *bacteria*, and *fungi*, along with three smaller groups, the rickettsiae, chlamydiae, and mycoplasmas. All are relatively simple organisms that can readily multiply in a host's tissues when defenses are low. Other groups include the *protozoa* (single-celled animal parasites), *worms*, and *flukes*. These more complex parasites may spend only part of their life cycle in human tissues; the rest of their lives is spent in another animal or in soil. Colonization of the body by worms and flukes (along with external parasites, such as *scabies* and *lice*) is generally referred to as an *infestation* rather than an infection.

See table, below, for examples of transmission mechanisms.

**AVOIDANCE**
Serious infectious diseases can largely be avoided by measures such as *immunization*, good hygiene with respect to food and drink and washing the

## SOME IMPORTANT INFECTIOUS DISEASES

### VIRAL INFECTIONS

| Infective agent | Transmission | Incubation period | Symptoms | Treatment |
|---|---|---|---|---|
| **AIDS virus infection** | | | | |
| Human immuno-deficiency virus (HIV) | Sexual contact; sharing hypodermic needles; mother to child; blood product infusion before March 1985 | Variable, usually several years | Fever; weight loss; fatigue; diarrhea; swollen lymph nodes; shortness of breath | Treatment of complicating infections; zidovudine can prolong life expectancy |
| **Chickenpox** | | | | |
| Varicella-zoster virus (herpes zoster virus) | Airborne droplets; direct contact | 11 to 21 days | Slight fever; malaise; characteristic rash | Relief of symptoms; acyclovir beneficial in adults |
| **Common cold** | | | | |
| Numerous rhino-viruses; corona-viruses | Airborne droplets; hand-to-hand contact | 1 to 3 days | Sneezing; chills; muscle aches; runny nose; cough | Relief of symptoms |
| **Hepatitis, viral** | | | | |
| Hepatitis virus types A and B; others | Infected food or water (type A); sexual contact; blood-borne transmission; sharing hypodermic needles (type B) | 3 to 6 weeks (type A); a few weeks to several months (type B) | Influenzalike illness; jaundice; many people are asymptomatic | Relief of symptoms; interferon may be beneficial in some cases |
| **Influenza** | | | | |
| Influenza viruses types A, B, or C | Airborne droplets | 1 to 3 days | Fever; chills; aches; headache; sore throat; cough; runny nose | Relief of symptoms; fluids |
| **Measles** | | | | |
| Measles virus (a paramyxovirus) | Airborne droplets | 7 to 14 days | Fever; coldlike symptoms; characteristic rash; conjunctivitis | Relief of symptoms |
| **Meningitis, viral** | | | | |
| Various viruses | Various methods, including via rodents | Variable | Fever; headache; drowsiness; confusion | Relief of symptoms; acyclovir in some cases |
| **Mononucleosis, infectious** | | | | |
| Epstein-Barr virus | Possibly via saliva | 1 to 6 weeks | Swollen glands; fever; sore throat; headache; malaise; lethargy | Relief of symptoms; rest; fluids |
| **Poliomyelitis** | | | | |
| 3 polioviruses | From feces to mouth via hands; airborne droplets | Minor illlness—3 to 5 days. Major illness—7 to 14 days | Minor illness—sore throat; headache; vomiting. Major illness—fever; stiff neck and back; muscle aches; paralysis | Relief of symptoms |
| **Rabies** | | | | |
| Rabies virus (a rhabdovirus) | Bite from infected animal | 10 days to 8 months | Fever; general malaise; irrationality; throat spasms; hydrophobia | No effective treatment |
| **Rubella** | | | | |
| Rubella virus | Airborne droplets; mother to child | 2 to 3 weeks | Low fever; characteristic rash | Relief of symptoms |

## CHLAMYDIAL INFECTIONS

| Infective agent | Transmission | Incubation period | Symptoms | Treatment |
| --- | --- | --- | --- | --- |
| **Nonspecific urethritis** | | | | |
| *Chlamydia trachomatis* | Sexual contact | 1 to 4 weeks | Pain on passing urine; watery, mucus discharge | Antibiotics |
| **Psittacosis** | | | | |
| *Chlamydia psittaci* | Inhalation of dust containing feces from infected birds | 1 to 3 weeks | Flulike and feverish symptoms, shortness of breath | Antibiotics |

## RICKETTSIAL INFECTIONS

| Infective agent | Transmission | Incubation period | Symptoms | Treatment |
| --- | --- | --- | --- | --- |
| **Q fever** | | | | |
| *Coxiella burnetti* | Inhalation of infected dust | 7 to 14 days | Sudden onset of fever and sweating; cough; chest pains; headache | Antibiotics |
| **Rocky Mountain spotted fever** | | | | |
| *Rickettsia rickettsii* | Bite from infected tick | 2 to 7 days | Severe headache; high fever; muscle aches; weakness; rash | Antibiotics |

## BACTERIAL INFECTIONS

| Infective agent | Transmission | Incubation period | Symptoms | Treatment |
| --- | --- | --- | --- | --- |
| **Gonorrhea** | | | | |
| *Neisseria gonorrhoeae* | Sexual contact; mother to baby | 2 to 6 days | Pain on passing urine; discharge; pain in abdomen | Penicillin; ampicillin; other antibiotics for resistant forms |
| **Meningitis, bacterial** | | | | |
| *Neisseria meningitidis* (meningococcus); *Streptococcus pneumoniae*; others | Mother to baby via vagina; infection reaching bloodstream from another organ | Less than 3 weeks, could be less than 24 hours | High fever; stiff neck; nausea; confusion | Antibiotic treatment |
| **Pertussis** (whooping cough) | | | | |
| *Bordetella pertussis* | Airborne droplets | 1 to 2 weeks | Runny nose and moderate fever; slight cough leading to characteristic cough spasms | Erythromycin in early stage; small children may require hospitalization |
| **Pneumonia** | | | | |
| *Streptococcus pneumoniae*; *Legionella pneumophila*; others | Airborne droplets | 1 to 3 weeks | Cough; fever; chest pain; shortness of breath | Antibiotics |
| **Tuberculosis** | | | | |
| *Mycobacterium tuberculosis* | Airborne transmission; cow's milk | Several weeks to several years | Malaise; weight loss; cough; shortness of breath; chest pain | Various antibiotics; possibly surgery |
| **Typhoid fever** | | | | |
| *Salmonella typhosa* | Food or water contaminated with infected feces | 1 to 2 weeks, sometimes longer | Headache; lethargy, intestinal upsets; very high, prolonged fever | Several effective drugs, but fever takes a long time to control |

## FUNGAL INFECTIONS

| Infective agent | Transmission | Incubation period | Symptoms | Treatment |
|---|---|---|---|---|
| **Histoplasmosis** | | | | |
| *Histoplasma capsulatum* | Inhalation of fungus from soil; bird or bat droppings, mostly in Ohio river valley region | 2 to 3 weeks | Headache; chills; fever; cough; possible chest pain | Antifungal drugs |
| **Meningitis, fungal** | | | | |
| *Cryptococcus neoformans* | Inhalation of fungus from pigeon droppings | Unknown | Headache; stiff neck; photophobia | Antifungal drugs |

## PROTOZOAL INFECTIONS

| Infective agent | Transmission | Incubation period | Symptoms | Treatment |
|---|---|---|---|---|
| **Amebiasis** | | | | |
| *Entamoeba histolytica* | Food or water contaminated by feces | A few weeks to many years | Severe diarrhea | Antiprotozoal drugs (e.g., metronidazole) |
| **Giardiasis** | | | | |
| *Giardia lamblia* | Food or water contaminated by feces; sexual contact | 3 to 40 days | Diarrhea; abdominal discomfort; bloating | Antiprotozoal drugs (e.g., metronidazole) |
| **Malaria** | | | | |
| *Plasmodium falciparum*; *Plasmodium vivax*; others | Bite from infected mosquito | 10 to 40 days | Chills; high fever; sweating; headache; fatigue | Various drugs (e.g., chloroquine) |

hands after using the toilet, avoiding contact with animal feces and secretions, and prudence in choice of sexual partners (or precautions, such as the use of condoms). For travel outside of the US, Canada, Northern Europe, Australia, and New Zealand, extra immunizations, and, in some cases, antimalarial tablets and protective measures against insects, may be recommended by your travel agent and confirmed by your physician.

### SYMPTOMS AND DIAGNOSIS

The symptoms of an infectious disease are caused in part by microorganisms damaging cells and tissues, releasing toxins, and drawing on their host's reserves of nutrients; symptoms are also caused by the efforts of the body's defenses (including the *immune system*) to destroy the microorganisms. The outcome depends on whether the microorganisms or the defenses (sometimes aided by drug therapy) gain the upper hand. The strength of a person's immune system, which reflects his or her general health, strongly influences this outcome.

Fever is a feature in many infectious diseases; symptoms generally are related to the system or organ attacked—for example, cough, diarrhea, or skin rash.

Apart from diseases in which the symptoms and signs are usually easily recognizable (such as *chickenpox*), diagnosis relies on identifying the causative microorganism; testing may be by direct microscope examination of a specimen of infected tissue or body fluid, by *culture* techniques, or by detecting antibodies (proteins manufactured by the body to defend against a particular organism) in blood serum (see *Immunoassay*).

A particular problem with infectious diseases is that there is always a time gap (the incubation period) between entry of the microorganisms into the body and the first appearance of symptoms. The incubation period may last from a few hours to several years; during this time, the infected person is likely to pass the microorganism to other people. Moreover, symptoms may never develop in some infected people, but they nonetheless continue to carry the disease organisms and unwittingly transmit them to others.

As a result, an epidemic can be well established before it is recognized and control measures introduced. This can be particularly devastating when the disease is a new one and has a long incubation period and a high mortality (*AIDS* is a classic example).

### TREATMENT

The mainstay of treatment is the use of *antibiotic* and other antimicrobial drugs. Drug treatment must be carefully selected through culture and identification of organisms because certain microorganisms are susceptible only to certain antibiotics. For many viruses, no effective antiviral drug is available and treatment relies on supportive measures, such as reducing temperature, maintaining food and fluid intake, and so on.

### OUTLOOK

Although great strides have been made in the fight against infectious diseases, many problems remain, even in developed countries. The spread of certain diseases (such as sexually transmitted infections) is difficult to control except by modifying human behavior. For many infections, no effective vaccine has been developed. The majority of viral illnesses cannot be effectively combated with drugs, and some bacteria have developed *resistance* to the drugs available. When a new infectious disease appears, it may be years before an effective vaccine or drug treatment can be devised. In the meantime, large numbers of people may die (AIDS again provides the most recent example).

## Infectious mononucleosis

See *Mononucleosis, infectious.*

## Inferiority complex

A neurotic state of mind that develops because of repeated hurts or failures in the past. Inferiority complex arises from a conflict between the positive wish to be recognized as someone worthwhile and the haunting fear of frustration and failure. Attempts to compensate for the sense of worthlessness may take the form of aggression and violence, or of overzealous involvement in activities. (See also *Superiority complex.*)

## Infertility

The inability of a couple to conceive. Conception depends on the production of healthy sperm by the man, healthy eggs by the woman, and sexual intercourse so that the sperm reach the woman's fallopian tubes. There must not be a mechanical obstruction to prevent the sperm from reaching the egg, and the sperm must be able to fertilize the egg when they meet (see *Fertilization*). Next, the fertilized egg must be able to become implanted in the uterus (see *Implantation, egg*). Finally, the developing embryo must be healthy and its hormonal environment must be adequate for further development so that the pregnancy can continue to full term. Infertility may result from a disturbance of one or more of these factors.

### INCIDENCE

Infertility is a common problem. As many as one in six couples requires help from a specialist. Infertility increases with age; the older a couple is when trying to conceive, the more difficult it may be.

### INFERTILITY FACTORS

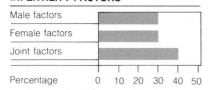

| | Percentage | | | | | |
|---|---|---|---|---|---|---|
| Male factors | | | | | | |
| Female factors | | | | | | |
| Joint factors | | | | | | |
| Percentage | 0 | 10 | 20 | 30 | 40 | 50 |

**Factors responsible for infertility**
In rough terms, about 30 percent of infertility cases are due to factors that affect the man; another 30 percent are due to factors that affect the woman. In the remaining 40 percent of cases, infertility is due to factors that affect both partners.

### CAUSES

**MALE INFERTILITY** The major cause of male infertility is failure to produce enough healthy sperm. *Azoospermia* (in which there is no sperm) and *oligospermia* (in which few sperm are produced) both cause infertility.

In some cases the sperm are malformed or their life span after ejaculation is too short for them to travel far enough to reach the egg. Defects in the sperm may be due to a blockage of the spermatic tubes or damage to the spermatic ducts, usually due to a sexually transmitted disease, such as *gonorrhea*. A *varicocele* (varicose veins in the scrotum) may also be a factor. Abnormal development of the testes due to an endocrine disorder (see *Hypogonadism*) or damage to the testes by *orchitis* (inflammation of the testes) may also cause defective sperm. Toxins such as alcohol, cigarettes, or various drugs can lower the sperm count.

Infertility in men may also be caused by a failure to deliver the sperm into the vagina, as occurs in *impotence* or in disorders affecting ejaculation, such as inhibited ejaculation or retrograde ejaculation (see *Ejaculation, disorders of*).

In rare cases, there may be a chromosomal abnormality (such as *Klinefelter's syndrome*) or a genetic disease (such as *cystic fibrosis*) that causes infertility in men.

**FEMALE INFERTILITY** Anovulation (failure to ovulate) is the most common cause of female infertility. Failure to ovulate often occurs for no obvious reason. It can be caused by a hormonal imbalance, stress, or a disorder of the *ovary*, such as a tumor or cyst.

Blocked *fallopian tubes*, which frequently occur after *pelvic inflammatory disease*, may prevent the sperm from reaching the egg. The woman may have one tube or no tubes because of a congenital defect or because they were removed during surgery for *ectopic pregnancy*. Disorders of the uterus (such as *fibroids*) often cause infertility, as can *endometriosis*.

Infertility also occurs if the woman's cervical mucus provides a hostile environment to her partner's sperm by producing antibodies that kill or immobilize them.

Rarely, a chromosomal abnormality or allergy to her partner's sperm may cause a woman's infertility.

### DIAGNOSIS

If pregnancy has not resulted after a year of unprotected intercourse (about 90 percent of women trying to get pregnant do so within a year), the couple may seek professional help.

A physical examination of both the man and the woman will be performed to determine the general state of their health, and to eliminate untreated physical disorders that may be causing the infertility. The couple is also interviewed, separately and together, regarding their sexual habits to determine if intercourse is taking place correctly for conception. If the cause of infertility remains undiagnosed after these examinations, special tests may be performed (see illustrated box).

### TREATMENT

When no specific cause can be found, improving the general state of health may help. The physician may suggest changes in diet, such as reducing alcohol intake, and may suggest relaxing and eliminating stress.

Treatment of male infertility is limited. When azoospermia exists, the couple must accept their childless state or consider adoption or *artificial insemination* by donor. If the sperm count is low, artificial insemination by the husband may be tried, although its success rate varies. In some cases of male infertility due to an endocrine imbalance, drugs such as *clomiphene* or *gonadotropin hormone* therapy may prove useful.

For female infertility, failure to ovulate requires ovarian stimulation with a drug such as clomiphene with or without a gonadotropin hormone. Microsurgery can sometimes repair damage to the fallopian tubes if it is not too severe. If surgery on the fallopian tubes is unsuccessful, *in vitro fertilization* is the only way that pregnancy will be possible. Uterine abnormalities or disorders, such as fibroids, may require treatment. If the cervical mucus has proved hostile, artificial insemination of the husband's semen directly into the cervix can prevent the sperm from coming into contact with the mucus.

### OUTLOOK

Only about half the couples professionally treated for infertility achieve a pregnancy, but the chances vary according to cause.

## Infestation

The presence of animal parasites (such as mites, ticks, or lice) in the skin or hair or of worms (such as tapeworms) inside the body.

## Infiltrate

Accumulation of substances or cells within a tissue that are either not normally found in it or are usually present only in smaller amounts. Infiltrate

# INVESTIGATING INFERTILITY

If no cause for infertility is found after a general checkup and/or a personal interview regarding sexual behavior, more specialized tests may be performed. Both partners may require testing because infertility can be attributed to one person, to both of them, or to mutual incompatibility.

## CAUSES OF INFERTILITY

Conception is a complicated process; the organs involved can be affected in numerous ways, resulting in infertility. Some of the principal underlying causes of infertility—in men and women—are illustrated at right.

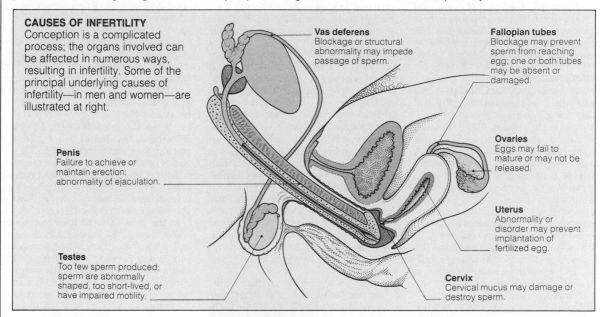

**Vas deferens**
Blockage or structural abnormality may impede passage of sperm.

**Fallopian tubes**
Blockage may prevent sperm from reaching egg; one or both tubes may be absent or damaged.

**Penis**
Failure to achieve or maintain erection; abnormality of ejaculation.

**Ovaries**
Eggs may fail to mature or may not be released.

**Uterus**
Abnormality or disorder may prevent implantation of fertilized egg.

**Testes**
Too few sperm produced; sperm are abnormally shaped, too short-lived, or have impaired motility.

**Cervix**
Cervical mucus may damage or destroy sperm.

## FEMALE INFERTILITY

Investigations to discover the cause of a woman's infertility may include taking a menstrual history, a study of body temperature during the menstrual cycle (below) and/or blood and urine tests to discover whether ovulation is normal, hysterosalpingography (right), or laparoscopy (below right).

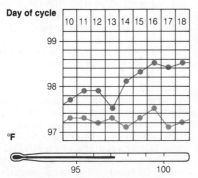

**Day of cycle**

**Body temperature and ovulation**
Charting a woman's body temperature during her menstrual cycle can indicate abnormalities of ovulation. The chart above shows typical temperature fluctuations during a normal cycle (black line) and those associated with failure to ovulate (red line).

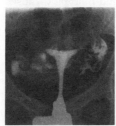

**Hysterosalpingography**
This X-ray technique is used to visualize the uterus and/or fallopian tubes. The image (left) shows a blockage of the left fallopian tube.

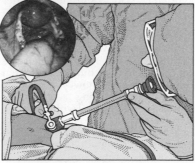

**Laparoscopy**
In this technique, a laparoscope (a type of viewing tube) is inserted through the abdominal wall to examine the woman's reproductive organs and determine whether an abnormality, such as a cyst or tumor, is present. The laparoscope view (above) shows a tumor in the left ovary.

## MALE INFERTILITY

The first test for investigating male infertility is a semen analysis (below). If it reveals a low sperm count, more tests may be needed to investigate the underlying cause.

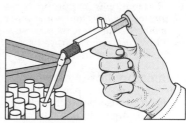

**Semen analysis**
Semen produced by masturbation is examined as soon as possible for the number, shape, and degree of motility of the sperm. A postcoital semen test may also be performed.

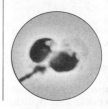

**Abnormal sperm**
The presence in the semen of large numbers of abnormally shaped sperm, such as the two-headed one (left), may reduce a man's fertility.

may refer to a drug (such as a local anesthetic) that has been injected into a tissue or to the buildup of a substance within an organ (such as of fat in the liver caused by excessive alcohol consumption). Radiologists use the term to refer to the presence of a tumor or pneumonia within a tissue (such as lung cancer or bronchopneumonia as seen on a chest X ray).

## Inflammation

Redness, swelling, heat, and pain in a tissue due to chemical or physical injury, or to infection.

When body tissues are damaged, specialized *mast cells* release a chemical called *histamine* (other substances are also involved in the inflammatory response, but histamine is believed to be responsible for most of the effects). Histamine increases blood flow to the damaged tissue, which causes the redness and heat. It also makes the blood capillaries more leaky, resulting in fluid oozing out of them and into the tissues, which causes localized swelling. The pain of inflammation is due to stimulation of nerve endings by the inflammatory chemicals.

Inflammation is usually accompanied by an accumulation of white blood cells, which are attracted by the inflammatory chemicals. These white cells help destroy invading microorganisms and are involved in repairing the damaged tissue. Thus, inflammation is an essential part of the body's response to injury and infection.

If inflammation is inappropriate (as in *rheumatoid arthritis* and some other *autoimmune disorders*), it may be suppressed by *corticosteroid drugs* or *nonsteroidal anti-inflammatory drugs*.

## Inflammatory bowel disease

A general term for a pair of chronic inflammatory disorders affecting the small and/or large intestine. The cause is unknown. Specific conditions within this group are *Crohn's disease* and nonspecific *ulcerative colitis*.

## Influenza

A viral infection of the respiratory tract (air passages) that causes fever, headache, muscle ache, and weakness. Popularly known as "the flu," it is spread by virus-infected droplets coughed or sneezed into the air. Influenza usually occurs in small outbreaks, or every few years in epidemics. Outbreaks tend to occur in winter; they spread particularly rapidly through schools and institutions for the elderly.

### CAUSES

There are three main types of influenza virus, called A, B, and C. A person who has had an attack with the type C virus acquires antibodies (proteins made by the *immune system*) that provide immunity against the type C virus for life. Anyone who has been infected with a certain strain of the type A or B viruses acquires immunity to that strain. Both the A- and B-type viruses occasionally alter to produce new strains that may be able to dodge or overcome immunity built up from a previous attack, thus leading to a new infection.

The type B virus is fairly stable, but it occasionally alters sufficiently to overcome resistance. The new strain often causes small outbreaks of infection. The type A virus is highly unstable; new strains arise constantly throughout the world. These are the strains that caused the influenza *pandemics* of this century, most notably Spanish flu in 1918, Asian flu in 1957, and Hong Kong flu in 1968.

### SYMPTOMS

The classic symptoms of flu (chills, fever, headache, muscular aches, loss of appetite, and fatigue) are brought on by types A and B. Type C causes only a mild illness that is indistinguishable from a common cold. In general, type A is more debilitating than type B.

The general symptoms described, which are more common in adults than in children, are usually followed by a cough (often accompanied by chest pain), a sore throat, and a runny nose. After two days, fever and other symptoms start to subside and, after five days, these symptoms have usually disappeared. Respiratory symptoms persist, however; the sufferer may feel weak and sometimes depressed. The illness usually clears up completely within seven to ten days. In rare cases, however, it takes a severe form, causing acute pneumonia that may be fatal within a day or two even in healthy young adults. The Spanish flu epidemic of 1918 killed millions of young adults in all countries of the world.

Type B infections in children sometimes mimic *appendicitis* and have been implicated in *Reye's syndrome*. In babies, the type A virus can cause febrile *seizures*.

Secondary bacterial infection is common, particularly in the elderly and in those with lung or heart disease; it may cause fatal *bronchitis*, *bronchiolitis*, or *pneumonia*.

### PREVENTION

Anti-influenza vaccines, containing killed strains of types A and B virus currently in circulation, are available, but have only a 60 to 70 percent success rate in preventing infection. In addition, any immunity provided is short-lived. Vaccination must be repeated each year just before the start of the influenza season. It is recommended that older people and sufferers of respiratory or circulatory disease be vaccinated, especially those living in institutions.

### TREATMENT

In all but the mildest cases, a person with influenza should rest in bed in a warm, well-ventilated room. Analgesics (painkillers) should be taken to relieve aches and pains and to reduce fever. Warm fluids soothe a sore throat and inhaling steam has a soothing effect on the lungs.

In the case of an elderly person or someone with a lung or heart disease, a physician should be called as soon as symptoms develop. The drug amantadine, which can reduce the severity of an attack if given within 24 hours of onset of symptoms, may be given. Antibiotics may also be used to combat secondary bacterial infection.

Once the fever has abated, the patient can get out of bed, but still needs rest. When he or she has started to regain strength, the return to normal activities should be gradual.

## Informed consent

Before a medical diagnostic procedure (or a surgical operation) a careful explanation is provided and the patient is asked to state that he or she understands the procedure and the risks involved, and that he or she consents to it. In most hospitals, the patient signs a consent form before an operation. (See also *Consent*.)

## Infrared

A term denoting the part of the electromagnetic spectrum immediately beyond the red end of the visible light spectrum. Directed onto the skin, infrared radiation heats the skin and the tissues immediately below it.

The infrared wave band includes heat waves; an infrared lamp is one means of giving *heat treatment*.

## Infusion, intravenous

See *Intravenous infusion*.

## Ingestion

The act of taking any substance (i.e., food, drink, or medications) into the body through the mouth. The term also refers to the process by which certain cells (e.g., some white blood cells) surround and engulf small particles.

## Ingrown toenail

A painful condition of the big toe in which one or both edges of the nail press into the adjacent skin, leading to infection and inflammation.

Infection is usually caused by poor personal hygiene, wearing tight-fitting shoes, or cutting the nail incorrectly. The nail should be cut straight across (not down the sides) to avoid exposing tender skin that easily becomes infected if a splinter of nail from the cut edge grows into it.

### TREATMENT

While waiting for medical treatment, pain can be relieved by bathing the foot in a strong, warm, salt solution once or twice a day and covering the nail with a dry gauze dressing.

The condition is usually treated by giving antibiotics to control infection and, if necessary, by removing the edge of the affected nail after applying a local anesthetic.

Unless preventive measures are taken, the problem is likely to recur.

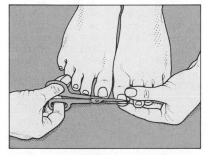

**Preventing ingrown toenails**
Cutting the toenails straight does not damage the skin at the corners of the nail and helps to prevent ingrown toenails.

## Inguinal

Relating to the groin (the area between the abdomen and thigh), as in inguinal *hernia*, the protrusion of part of the intestine into the muscles of the groin.

## Inhalation

The act of breathing in air (see *Breathing*). An inhalation is also a substance in gas, vapor, powder, or aerosol form to be breathed in.

## Inhaler

A device used for administering a drug in powder or vapor form. Inhalers are used principally in the treatment of various respiratory dis-

## HOW TO USE AN INHALER

With each type, the user puts the nozzle of the inhaler in the mouth, presses the end to release the drug, and simultaneously breathes in through the mouth. If the device is used correctly, the drug is dispersed to the bronchi. A *nebulizer* is a special type of inhaler that delivers the drug as a fine mist through a face mask.

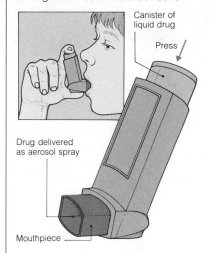

Canister of liquid drug
Press
Drug delivered as aerosol spray
Mouthpiece

**Aerosol inhaler**
This type of inhaler delivers the drug as an aerosol spray when the user presses the top of the canister.

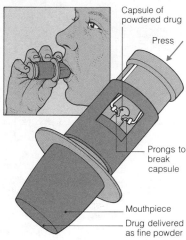

Capsule of powdered drug
Press
Prongs to break capsule
Mouthpiece
Drug delivered as fine powder

**Turbo-inhaler**
Here, a drug capsule is placed in the end chamber, the top of which is pressed to pierce the capsule and release the drug.

orders, including *asthma*, chronic *bronchitis*, and *alveolitis*. Among the medications administered in this way are *bronchodilator drugs* (to widen the airways) and *corticosteroid drugs* (to reduce inflammation).

## Inheritance

 The transmission of traits, characteristics, and disorders from parents to their children through the influence of *genes*. Genes are the units of DNA (deoxyribonucleic acid) in a person's cells; DNA controls all growth and body functioning. Half of a person's genes come from the mother, half from the father.

Children tend to resemble their parents, particularly in their physical characteristics. However, this resemblance may also apply to mental abilities, mannerisms, personality, and behavior. In addition, many disorders show a moderate to very notable tendency to "run in families."

Although there is a temptation to ascribe similarities in a family to inheritance, there are equally plausible alternative explanations for many family traits. For example, all the members of a family may be fat not through the influence of genes, but because they all eat the same fattening food and rarely exercise. Children may behave like their mother not because of inheritance, but because they imitate her. Certain abilities and behaviors (e.g., the language a person speaks) are clearly not inherited. Nevertheless, it is accepted that most physical characteristics, many disorders, and some mental abilities and aspects of personality are inherited.

### MECHANISMS OF INHERITANCE

Each of a person's cells contains exactly the same genes, which come originally from the egg and sperm cells from which he or she is derived.

The genes in a cell are organized into long strands of DNA called *chromosomes*. The genes controlling most characteristics come in pairs—one gene originating from the father, the other from the mother. Everyone has 22 pairs of chromosomes (called autosomes) bearing these paired genes. In addition, every individual has two more chromosomes called sex chromosomes. Women have two X chromosomes; men have an X chromosome and a Y chromosome.

The inheritance of normal traits and disorders can be divided into those

## INHERITANCE OF EYE COLOR

Eye color is determined by two main alleles (forms of a gene), one coding for brown eyes and the other for blue eyes. The brown allele is dominant to the blue one (which is therefore recessive).

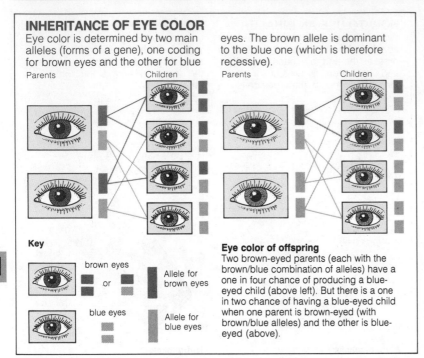

**Key**

brown eyes

or

blue eyes

Allele for brown eyes

Allele for blue eyes

**Eye color of offspring**
Two brown-eyed parents (each with the brown/blue combination of alleles) have a one in four chance of producing a blue-eyed child (above left). But there is a one in two chance of having a blue-eyed child when one parent is brown-eyed (with brown/blue alleles) and the other is blue-eyed (above).

controlled by a single pair of genes on the autosomal chromosomes (unifactorial inheritance); those controlled by genes on the sex chromosomes (sex-linked inheritance); and those controlled by the combination of many genes (multifactorial inheritance).

### UNIFACTORIAL INHERITANCE
A large number of variable traits, such as eye color, blood groups, and the ability to taste certain substances, is thought to be controlled by a single pair of genes. The ways in which these traits are inherited conform to laws first elucidated in the 19th century by the Austrian monk Gregor Mendel. Since then, they have been referred to as the laws of Mendelian inheritance.

Either of the pair of genes controlling a trait may take any of several forms, which are known as alleles. For example, the genes controlling eye color exist as two main alleles, coding for blue and brown eye color. Thus, an individual's gene pair for eye color may be blue/blue (giving blue eyes), brown/brown (giving brown eyes) or brown/blue (also giving brown eyes, because the brown allele is dominant, or "masks," the blue allele, which is called recessive to the brown allele).

When a couple has a child, only one of the pair of genes controlling a trait is passed to the child. For example, someone with the brown/blue combination for eye color has a 50 percent

chance of passing the blue gene, and a 50 percent chance of passing on the brown gene, to any child. This factor is combined with the gene coming from the other parent, according to dominant or recessive relationships, to determine the child's eye color. According to the combination of the parental genes, the numbers of brown- and blue-eyed offspring of a particular couple tend to conform to a certain ratio, in accordance with Mendelian laws (see illustration).

Similar laws and ratios apply to the inheritance of other traits controlled by single gene pairs, and also to the inheritance of certain *genetic disorders* (e.g., *cystic fibrosis* and *achondroplasia*).

### SEX-LINKED INHERITANCE
The most obvious example of sex-linked inheritance is gender itself. Male gender is caused by the existence in males of the genes on the Y chromosome, which is present only in males and is inherited by boys from their fathers. The genes on the Y chromosome almost certainly direct the development of the male primary sex organs (the testicles) and all male characteristics derive from the secretion of hormones by these organs.

The X chromosome, on the other hand, is less closely associated with the female sex because it is present in both males (in a single dose) and in females (in a double dose). It seems

that female gender is the natural course of development in the absence of the Y chromosome, does not require any extra genes to direct it, and that the X chromosome is concerned with general development.

Any faults in a male's genes on the X chromosome tend to be expressed outwardly, because such a fault cannot (as it can in females) be masked by the presence of a normal gene on a second X chromosome. Faults in the genes of the X chromosome include those responsible for *color vision deficiency*, *hemophilia*, and other sex-linked inherited disorders, which almost exclusively affect males.

### MULTIFACTORIAL INHERITANCE
A number of traits (such as height and build) are believed to be controlled by the combined effects of many genes, along with environmental effects. Using height as an example, a simple model proposes that there are several genes determining a person's stature, some of which are "tall" genes and others "short." A person's height depends on the relative number of tall to short genes.

When two people have children, a child may, in rare cases, inherit all the tall or all the short genes from both parents, and thus be exceptionally tall or short. The laws of chance dictate, however, that, in most cases, a child will inherit a mixture of tall and short genes and thus be in the range of average stature. Nevertheless, the child of tall parents tends to inherit more tall genes than the child of short parents. Dietary and other factors also affect growth so that a person with many short genes may still attain an average stature through good diet.

Multifactorial inheritance, along with the effects of environment, may also play a part in causing disorders, such as *diabetes mellitus* and *spina bifida* (see *Genetic disorders*).

## Inhibition
The process of preventing any mental or physical activity. Inhibition in the brain and spinal cord is carried out by special *neurons*, which damp down the action of other nerve cells to keep the brain's activity in balance.

In a psychological sense, certain mental activities can be described as inhibiting other thoughts or reflexes.

In *psychoanalysis*, an inhibition refers to the unconscious restraint of instinctual impulses. Such inhibition may cause symptoms, such as being temporarily unable to write because writing arouses forbidden ideas.

## Injection

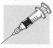

Introduction of a drug or vaccine into the body from a syringe through a needle. An injection may be intravenous (into a vein), intramuscular (into a muscle), subcutaneous (under the skin), or intra-articular (into a joint).

## Injury

Harm to any part of the body. Injury may arise from a wide variety of causes, including physical influences (such as force, heat, cold, electricity, vibration, and radiation), chemical causes (such as poisons and caustic substances), animal or human bites, or oxygen deprivation.

(See *Accidents*; *Bite, animal*; *Bite, human*; *Bleeding*; *Burns*; *Cold injury*; *Dislocation, joint*; *Electrical injury*; *First aid*; *Fractures*; *Head injury*; *Heat stroke*; *Insect bites*; *Poisoning*; *Radiation sickness*; *Snakebites*; *Soft-tissue injury*; *Spinal injury*; *Sports injuries*; *Sprains*; *Venomous bites and stings*; *Wounds*.)

## Ink blot test

A psychological test in which the subject is asked to interpret a number of ink blots. The most widely used example is the *Rorschach test*.

## Inlay, dental

A filling of porcelain or gold made outside the mouth and used to restore a badly decayed tooth. An inlay may be needed for back teeth or to provide protection for a weakened tooth.

The dentist first makes an angular cavity in the tooth to accept the inlay. A replica of the cavity is then made, generally using a wax *impression*; the inlay is constructed on the replica and cemented in place in the tooth.

## Inoculation

The act of introducing a small quantity of a foreign substance into the body, usually by injection, for the purpose of stimulating the *immune system* to produce *antibodies* (protective proteins) against the substance. Inoculation is usually done to protect against future infection by particular bacteria or viruses. (See *Immunization*.)

## Inoperable

A term applied to any condition that cannot be alleviated or cured by surgery, such as a very advanced cancer that has spread to many parts of the body or a brain tumor that is not surgically accessible.

## Inorganic

A term used to refer to any of the large group of substances that do not contain carbon (excepting certain simple carbon compounds such as *carbon dioxide* and *carbon monoxide*). Common examples of inorganic substances include table salt (sodium chloride) and bicarbonate of soda (sodium bicarbonate). See also *Organic*.

## Inpatient treatment

Medical care given to a patient who has been admitted to a hospital.

## Insanity

The common term for serious mental disorder. Today it has no technical meaning for psychiatrists, but is used in law to indicate a mental state that renders a person not legally responsible for his or her own actions. The "insanity defense" was introduced to ensure that people committing criminal acts as a result of mental illness or deficiency would not be imprisoned or given the death penalty, but would instead receive proper treatment. *Psychosis* now covers serious illnesses formerly denoted by insanity.

## Insect bites

Tiny puncture wounds in the skin inflicted by bloodsucking insects, such as mosquitoes, lice, midges, gnats, horseflies, sand flies, fleas, and bedbugs. Some small arachnids (eight-legged animals similar to insects), such as ticks and mites, can cause similar injuries.

Most bites cause only temporary pain (or itching for a day or two) although some people have severe skin reactions. In the tropics and subtropics, insect bites are potentially more serious because certain biting species can transmit disease (see *Insects and disease*).

### CAUSES

Insects that bite do so to obtain a blood meal. The mouthparts of biting insects are specially adapted for piercing skin and sucking blood. Insect bites are most common on exposed parts of the head, hands, arms, or legs.

Although mosquitoes (which attack mainly after dark) may be the most troublesome biting insects, many bites blamed on mosquitoes are in fact caused by cat or dog fleas. These fleas inhabit various domestic locations where the pet habitually rests (e.g., carpets, sleeping baskets, or sofas); when their normal host is absent, they may jump onto humans to feed.

Of the more easily visible insects, horseflies can produce a particularly painful bite, while gnats can be a menace if encountered in a swarm.

### SYMPTOMS

All insect bites provoke a reaction in the skin that is primarily an allergic response to substances in the insect's saliva or its feces, which are often deposited at or near the site of the bite and rubbed in by scratching. Reactions vary from innocuous red pimples to painful swellings (which may weep) or an intensely itching rash. People vary in their reactions to the same biting insect; in some people the reaction is extremely severe.

### AVOIDANCE

Avoiding insect bites can be particularly important for campers and hikers, anyone living in a mosquito-infested area, and travelers or residents in tropical countries.

Bites outdoors can be reduced by wearing trousers, socks, and long-sleeved shirts (especially after dark, when mosquitoes are most active), and by using insect repellents.

Indoors, bites can be reduced by using insect screens over open windows and by spraying bedrooms with aerosols containing pyrethroid insecticides before going to bed. If this fails, it may be necessary to use mosquito nets and slow-burning antimosquito coils that give off pyrethroids.

### TREATMENT

Bites or bitten areas should be thoroughly washed with soap and water, and a soothing ointment, such as calamine lotion, should be applied. Scratching should be avoided. If there is a severe reaction, a physician should be called; a cream containing an antihistamine may be required.

Severe itching on the scalp or in the pubic hair suggests the possibility of a louse infestation, which is treated with insecticidal lotions (see *Lice*). In the case of flea bites, the entire residence (not just the pet) may require treatment with insecticide to kill the flea population. (See also *Spider bites*; *Mites and disease*; *Ticks and disease*.)

## Insects and disease

Insects are six-legged animals with a pair of antennae, a firm exterior skeleton, and, in many cases, wings. They include such animals as ants, bees, cockroaches, fleas, flies, lice, and mosquitoes, but not mites, ticks, or spiders, which belong to another animal group, the arachnids. The insects and arachnids belong to a larger animal group, the arthropods.

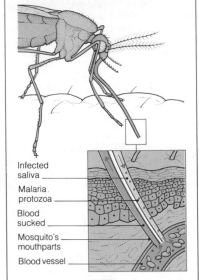

**INSECT-BORNE DISEASES**
Malaria is by far the most prevalent of the insect-borne diseases, affecting an estimated 200 to 300 million people worldwide.

Infected saliva

Malaria protozoa

Blood sucked

Mosquito's mouthparts

Blood vessel

**Transmission of malaria**
When an infected ANOPHELES mosquito feeds on a person's blood, it injects saliva through its mouthparts; the protozoa that cause malaria enter the blood via the insect's saliva.

**DISEASE CAUSED BY INSECTS**

There are about 1 million known species of insects; most are either harmless or positively beneficial to humans. The majority of the harmful species cause sickness by attacking crops or stored food, thus contributing to malnutrition and famine.

Other insects are a more direct cause of illness or disease. Certain insects directly parasitize humans, living underneath the skin or on the body surface (see *Lice*; *Chigoe*; *Myiasis*). Still others will sting if provoked, causing moderate discomfort (in most cases) to a severe life-threatening reaction (see *Insect stings*).

The most troublesome insects are flies and various biting insects. Many types of flies settle first on human or animal excrement and then on food to lay eggs or to feed. They can transmit disease organisms from excrement to food via their feet and legs. This is probably important in the spread of intestinal infections such as *typhoid fever* and *shigellosis*.

*Insect bites* are irritating in themselves, but the much more serious risk is of an insect spreading infectious organisms as a result of its bite. Serious diseases spread by biting insects include *malaria* and *filariasis* (transmitted by mosquitoes), *sleeping sickness* (tsetse flies), *leishmaniasis* (sand flies), epidemic *typhus* (lice), and *plague* (rat fleas). Also, various mosquitoes, sand flies, and ticks spread a group of viral illnesses called the arthropod-borne or arboviruses. They include *yellow fever*, *dengue*, and some types of viral *encephalitis*.

In each case, organisms picked up when an insect ingests blood from an infected animal or person are able to survive or multiply in the insect. Later, the organisms are either injected into a new human host via the insect's saliva or deposited in the feces at or near the site of the bite and later rubbed in by the victim.

Most of these diseases (of which malaria is by far the most important) are confined to the tropics and subtropics. However, some cases of plague and arthropod-borne encephalitis occur each year in the US. Leishmaniasis can be contracted by sand-fly bites in the Mediterranean.

**AVOIDANCE**

The avoidance of insect-borne disease is largely a matter of keeping flies off food, discouraging insect bites by the use of suitable clothing and insect repellents, and, in areas of the world where malaria is present, the use of mosquito nets and screens, *pesticides*, and antimalarial tablets.

## Insect stings

A fairly small number of insects (bees, wasps, hornets, and yellow jackets) are capable of stings. Insect venom contains inflammatory substances that cause local pain, redness, and swelling for about 48 hours. Normally, a very large number of stings (hundreds in the case of an adult) must be received for them to be life-threatening. However, about one person in 200 is allergic to insect venom. This means that, after the person's *immune system* has been sensitized by the venom from a sting, one subsequent sting (possibly months or years later) can provoke a severe allergic reaction leading to *anaphylactic shock*. The symptoms may include a severe itchy rash (hives), dizziness, facial and throat swellings, wheezing, vomiting, breathing difficulties, and collapse. About 50 to 100 people die of this cause annually in the US (more deaths than from snake bites).

*Immunotherapy*—a technique for reducing sensitivity to bee or wasp venom (and some other types of allergy)—is recommended for those known to suffer hypersensitivity.

**TREATMENT**

A bee often leaves its sting sac in the wound. The sac should be gently scraped out with a knife blade or fingernail, not by grasping with fingers or tweezers (which injects more venom). The stung area should be washed with soap and water, a cold compress applied, and analgesics taken to ease the discomfort.

If the symptoms of anaphylactic shock develop, obtain medical help immediately for emergency treatment, which initially consists of an injection of *epinephrine*. Any person known to be hypersensitive to bee or wasp venom should obtain and carry an emergency kit for self-injecting epinephrine. In severe cases, the victims of insect stings require *cardiopulmonary resuscitation*.

A sting in the mouth or throat may also be dangerous because swelling may obstruct breathing. Again, seek medical help immediately and give the victim ice cubes to suck. (See also *Scorpion stings*.)

## Insecurity

Lack of self-confidence and uncertainty about one's abilities, aims, and relationships with others. Repeated changes of environment (such as frequent moves of home or school) can lead to a sense of insecurity, especially in childhood. A feeling of insecurity may be a feature of *anxiety* and other neurotic mental disorders.

## Insight

Being aware of one's own mental state. In a general sense, this means knowing one's own strengths, weaknesses, and abilities.

The term insight also has the specific psychiatric meaning of knowing that one's symptoms are an illness. Some psychiatrists thus regard loss of insight as a sign of a *psychosis*, since it indicates being out of touch with reality. Others, however, point out that many people with psychotic illness know when they are ill and seek treatment, while those with neurotic and personality disorders often deny they are ill and fail to see the causes or results of their behavior.

In *psychoanalysis*, insight refers to a deep emotional understanding of one's inner feelings; it is regarded as essential to successful treatment.

## FIRST AID: INSECT STINGS AND TICK BITES

### INSECT STING

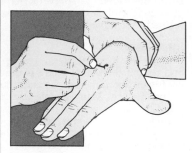

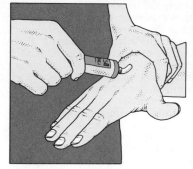

**1** Use a needle to remove the stinger and poison bag by dragging the stinger out of the skin's surface. Do not use tweezers because you may squeeze more poison into the wound.

**2** Apply some hydrocortisone cream or a weak solution of ammonia to the wound. An ice pack held on the wound will help reduce swelling.

### TICK BITE

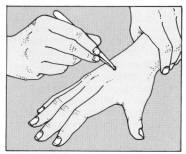

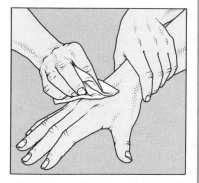

**1** If the tick is still clinging to the skin, remove it by grasping the tick with tweezers as close to its mouth as possible. Gently but firmly remove the whole tick.

**2** Use soap and warm water to wash the area thoroughly. Then rinse well and dry gently. Apply hydrocortisone cream.

## In situ

A Latin term meaning "in place." The phrase "carcinoma in situ" is used to describe tissue (particularly of the skin or cervix) that is cancerous only in its surface cells and is completely surrounded by normal cells without any signs of spread to deeper layers.

## Insomnia

Trouble sleeping. Insomnia is a common problem. A national survey has shown that one in every three US adults has some trouble sleeping and that hypnotic drugs are among the most widely used of all medicines. People with insomnia have difficulty falling asleep or staying asleep. Most insomnia sufferers also complain of increased daytime fatigue, irritability, and difficulty coping.

**CAUSES**

The most common cause of insomnia is worry about a problem (such as bad news received during the day or a difficult task to cope with the following morning), but other causes are implicated in about half of all cases.

Causes include physical disorders such as *sleep apnea* (a breathing problem), *restless legs*, environmental factors (such as noise and light), life-style factors (such as too much coffee in the evening, lack of exercise during the day, or keeping erratic hours), or misuse of hypnotic drugs (see *Anti-anxiety drugs; Barbiturate drugs*).

Insomnia also can be a symptom of a psychiatric illness. People with *anxiety* and/or *depression* may have difficulty getting to sleep; those suffering from depression typically wake early in the morning. Sleeping much less than usual is common in *mania*, in which the person is so full of drive and energy that he or she does not need much sleep. *Schizophrenia* often causes people to pace at night, aroused by "voices" or delusions. People with *dementia* or other brain disorders may be afraid in the dark and become restless and noisy, confused by the shadows and sounds of the night.

*Withdrawal syndrome* from hypnotic drugs, antidepressants, tranquilizers, and illicit drugs (such as heroin) may cause many weeks of insomnia.

People sometimes believe they have insomnia because of a misconception about the amount of sleep they need. In fact, sleep needs vary greatly, with some people requiring less than four hours and others needing more than 10. Some people who think they have insomnia are in fact "out of phase," lying awake for hours after going to bed, but sleeping normally if allowed to sleep late in the morning.

**INVESTIGATION AND TREATMENT**

If there is an obvious physical or psychological cause for insomnia, it is treated. For long-term insomnia with no obvious cause, *EEG* recordings of brain-wave patterns and an assessment of breathing, muscle activity, and other bodily functions during sleep may be useful in discovering the extent and pattern of the problem. Keeping a log of sleep patterns may also be helpful.

Studies have shown that many insomniacs sleep much more than they think they do. However, they also tend to wake more frequently than normal sleepers. It is the quality, more than the quantity, of sleep that is the problem in insomnia. People with insomnia should ensure they are active during the day and should establish a regular time and routine for going to bed each night and a regular time for waking in the morning. *Sleeping drugs* should be used only with a physician's advice.

## Instinct

An innate primitive urge. The needs for warmth, food, love, and sex are forms of instinct, although the instinct for survival is probably the most powerful. An instinct is distinguished from a reflex, which is an involuntary response to a stimulus (such as withdrawing one's hand from a fire).

In animals, instincts often take the form of specific inherited patterns of behavior. For example, ducks follow their mothers, birds fly, and beavers build dams—activities that do not appear to have been learned.

Humans have few of these set behaviors, and instincts may be more appropriately regarded as motivators of behavior. This idea was first developed as a central part of *Freudian theory*. Freud believed that instincts arose from energy aroused in the unconscious. The aim of the instinct was to calm the aroused state by directing the energy onto some outside object (e.g., sexual arousal leads to intercourse and orgasm).

Freud also described two "primal" (most important) instincts—Eros, the life instinct (which is positive, creative, and aimed at preserving life), and Thanatos, the death instinct (which is negative and destructive). Life was seen as a continual struggle between these two instincts.

## Institutionalization

The loss of personal independence that stems from living for long periods in a mental hospital, prison, or other large institution. Apathy, obeying orders unquestioningly, accepting a standard routine, and loss of interests are the main features. They are thought to be caused by a lack of rights and personal responsibility, the attitudes of controlling staff, and the effects of drugs.

Care of the long-term sick within the community (as an alternative to hospitalization) is designed to combat the institutionalization process.

## Insulin

A hormone produced by the *pancreas* in varying amounts depending on the level of blood glucose (sugar). Carbohydrate is absorbed as glucose, increasing the blood glucose level and stimulating the pancreas to produce insulin. Insulin promotes the absorption of glucose into the liver and into muscle cells (where it is converted into energy). In the liver, glucose is stored as glycogen, which is reconverted to glucose in response to stress or exercise. Insulin thus prevents a buildup of blood glucose and ensures that various tissues have sufficient amounts of glucose.

*Diabetes mellitus* occurs when the pancreas produces little or no insulin, causing *hyperglycemia* (abnormally high blood glucose). An *insulinoma* is a rare benign tumor that causes excessive production of insulin.

### INSULIN THERAPY

Insulin supplements have been used in the treatment of diabetes mellitus since 1922. Insulin preparations are produced from pig or ox pancreas (and now by *genetic engineering*). A variety of short-, intermediate-, or long-acting preparations is available.

Insulin is used in all cases of insulin-dependent diabetes mellitus (total absence of insulin production) and, occasionally, when oral *hypoglycemic* drugs are unable to control non-insulin-dependent diabetes mellitus (deficient production of insulin), such as during serious illness, surgery, or pregnancy. Insulin therapy is used to prevent hyperglycemia (high blood glucose) and *ketosis* (a buildup of certain acids in the blood), which, in severe cases, may cause coma.

Insulin is given to mimic the body's production of the natural hormone. Insulin may be self-injected before meals to act on the increase in blood glucose that occurs after eating. Alternatively, an insulin pump (see *Pump, insulin*) may be used to deliver insulin over 24 hours; the dose is increased before each meal.

Adjustment of the dose is often needed when there are variations in diet and exercise, and during illness (especially when there has been vomiting). Regular self-monitoring of the blood glucose level, either by blood or urine tests, is necessary to ensure adequate control.

### POSSIBLE ADVERSE EFFECTS

Insulin injections may cause irritation or dimpling of the skin. Too high a dose causes hypoglycemia with symptoms (such as dizziness, sweating, irritability, and a feeling of weakness) that are relieved by consuming food or a sugary drink. Severe hypoglycemia may cause coma, for which emergency treatment with an injection of glucose or *glucagon* (a hormone that opposes the effects of insulin) is necessary.

Allergic reactions to insulin, causing rash or breathing difficulty, are rare. Pig or ox insulin may make the body produce *antibodies* that reduce the effectiveness of the insulin preparation. If this occurs, an alternative preparation is taken.

## Insulinoma

A rare benign tumor of the insulin-producing cells of the pancreas. Such a tumor can produce abnormal quantities of *insulin* so that the amount of glucose in the blood (which is reduced by insulin) can fall to dangerously low levels. This is called *hypoglycemia* and, unless sugar is given immediately, can cause *coma* and death.

Blood insulin levels are normally low during fasting; insulinoma can be diagnosed by finding high levels after a period of fasting. A drug (diazoxide) is administered to prevent hypoglycemia until surgery can be performed to remove the tumor.

## Intelligence

The ability to understand concepts and reason them out. There is much confusion about the precise definition of intelligence. Many people use the word to mean a special degree of knowledge. The widespread use of *intelligence tests* has led to the idea that intelligence is a single quality.

Many scientists prefer to divide intelligence into various factors. Some see it as having three basic parts—speed of thought, learning, and problem-solving. Others argue that a general factor of intelligence exists, made up of seven special abilities—understanding the meaning of words, fluency with words, working with numbers, visualizing things in space, memory, speed of perception, and reasoning ability. Other researchers go further, dividing intelligence into more than 100 different factors.

Intelligence can also be considered as having three entirely separate forms—abstract intelligence (understanding ideas and symbols); practical intelligence (aptitude in dealing with practical problems, such as repairing machinery); and social intelligence (coping reasonably and wisely with human relationships). Personality plays an important role in this last type of intelligence.

### AGE AND INTELLIGENCE

Intelligence, however it is defined, increases up to the age of about 6 years and then stabilizes. Intelligence quotient (IQ), as measured by intelligence tests, continues to increase to about age 26, stays the same until about age 40, and then gradually declines (the drop occurring later in a person with an intellectually demanding job).

### HEREDITY AND INTELLIGENCE

The role of heredity in intelligence is much argued, but there is no doubt that intelligence is inherited in a fashion similar to height. Environment also plays a major part, as does physical health and personality. Intelligent parents tend to have intelligent children, but, even within one family, some children may be brighter than others. Adopted children from deprived social backgrounds, although having IQs closer to the biological than the adoptive parents, often score higher than would be expected had they been reared by their biological parents.

Whether or not some races are more intelligent than others is unknown since so many factors having to do with culture, health, and environment must be taken into account. People from different countries seem to excel at different sports, artistic activities, and occupations, but the reasons for these differences are unknown.

There are extremes of intelligence, as seen in *mental retardation* (defined by a low IQ) and the very gifted (defined by scores over 140). The latter are often very successful, but not always. Personality and social adjustment are equally important.

## Intelligence tests
Tests designed to provide an estimate of a person's mental abilities.
### TYPES
WECHSLER TESTS These are the most widely used of all tests today. There are two basic versions—the Wechsler Adult Intelligence Scale (WAIS) and the Wechsler Intelligence Scale for Children (WISC). Each is divided into verbal and performance sections, which can be used separately or combined to produce an overall score. The verbal sections are concerned with language skills and include measures of vocabulary, general knowledge, verbal reasoning, and verbal memory. The performance sections include measures of constructional ability and visual-spatial and perceptual ability (interpretation of shapes).

The performance sections of the test may be used separately for people with language problems. In this sense they can measure basic intellectual ability; verbal tests tend to be more culture-bound since they test skills that reflect social background.
### STANFORD-BINET TEST
This is a revised version of one of the oldest intelligence tests, devised by the Frenchman Alfred Binet (1857-1911). It is still widely used, mainly as a measure of scholastic ability.
### OTHER TESTS
Numerous tests that concentrate on testing one particular aspect of intelligence have been devised. The Goodenough-Harris test assesses performance by asking a child to make a picture of a man; scoring counts such items as details of the body, proportions, and clothing.
### SCORING
In most intelligence tests, scoring is based on the notion of mental age (MA) in relation to actual chronological age (CA), since intelligence normally increases with maturity. The intelligence quotient (IQ) is therefore MA divided by CA, multiplied by 100 to simplify the results. The tests are devised to ensure that three quarters of people have an IQ between 80 and 120. They are also standardized so that the score indicates the same relative ability at different age levels. Regardless of age group, an IQ of 65 indicates that a person is in the lower 1 percent of his or her age group; an IQ of 135 indicates the person is in the upper 1 percent of his or her age group.
### USES
Intelligence tests are useful in predicting whether a person has the ability to cope with certain jobs or pass certain exams; they may be used to assess school or job aptitude. However, intelligence tests have been criticized for their alleged bias regarding gender and race. The tests are also used to define the legal notion of *mental retardation* and to assess the effects of brain disease or dementia. In particular, a large difference in verbal and performance scores helps in assessing the degree of brain disease. Children with a particular difficulty (such as delayed reading) may be tested to assess the severity and nature of the problem so remedial teaching can be planned.

## Intensive care
The constant, close monitoring of seriously ill patients, which enables immediate treatment to be given if the patient's condition deteriorates. The intensive-care unit of a hospital contains electronic monitoring equipment

### A TYPICAL INTENSIVE-CARE UNIT
A modern intensive-care unit has a wide variety of sophisticated equipment so that the condition of seriously ill patients can be continuously monitored and any deterioration treated immediately.

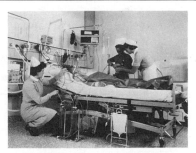

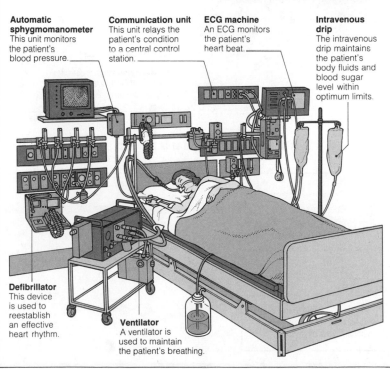

**Automatic sphygmomanometer** This unit monitors the patient's blood pressure.

**Communication unit** This unit relays the patient's condition to a central control station.

**ECG machine** An ECG monitors the patient's heart beat.

**Intravenous drip** The intravenous drip maintains the patient's body fluids and blood sugar level within optimum limits.

**Defibrillator** This device is used to reestablish an effective heart rhythm.

**Ventilator** A ventilator is used to maintain the patient's breathing.

that allows continuous assessment of vital body functions, such as blood pressure and heart and respiratory rate. Medical and nursing staff are in a high ratio to patients and are specially trained in the techniques of resuscitation. Most intensive-care units are under the supervision of hospital-employed specialists.

Intensive care is most often needed for patients who are on artificial *ventilation*; they may be unconscious and not breathing or may be suffering from a respiratory illness. Close monitoring in an intensive-care unit is also required for people recovering from a myocardial infarction or after

major surgery, for patients in *shock* who are not responding to emergency treatment, and for those with acute *renal failure* who require *dialysis*. (See also *Coronary care unit*.)

## Inter-
A prefix that means between, as in intercostal (between the ribs). See also *Intra-*.

## Intercostal
The medical term for between the ribs, as in the intercostal muscles, thin sheets of muscle between each rib that help expand and contract the chest during breathing.

## Intercourse, painful
Known as dyspareunia, pain during intercourse can affect both men and women. The pain may be superficial, occurring around the external genitals, or it may be experienced deep within the pelvis.

### CAUSES
Superficial pain is usually due to the condition of the external genitals. *Sexually transmitted diseases* (such as genital *herpes*, *gonorrhea*, or *chlamydial infections*) cause dyspareunia, with the pain being felt on the penis or around the vulval area. *Spermicides* sometimes cause a burning sensation in both men and women.

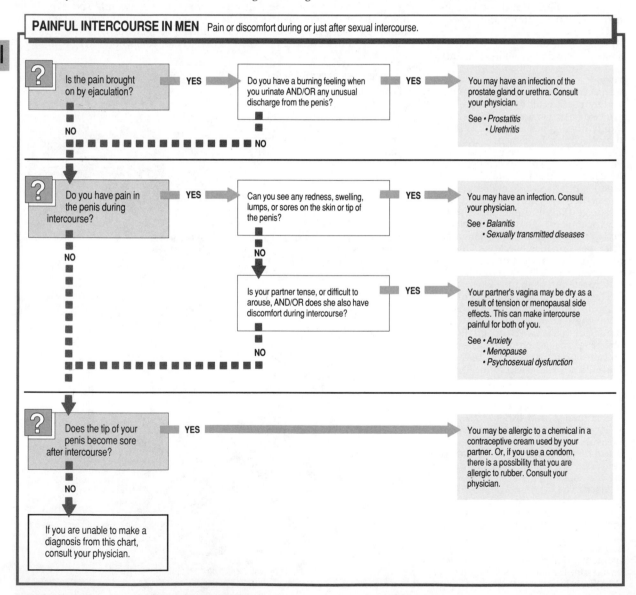

**PAINFUL INTERCOURSE IN MEN** Pain or discomfort during or just after sexual intercourse.

**I**

? Is the pain brought on by ejaculation? **YES** → Do you have a burning feeling when you urinate AND/OR any unusual discharge from the penis? **YES** → You may have an infection of the prostate gland or urethra. Consult your physician.

See • *Prostatitis*
• *Urethritis*

**NO** ····· **NO**

? Do you have pain in the penis during intercourse? **YES** → Can you see any redness, swelling, lumps, or sores on the skin or tip of the penis? **YES** → You may have an infection. Consult your physician.

See • *Balanitis*
• *Sexually transmitted diseases*

**NO**

Is your partner tense, or difficult to arouse, AND/OR does she also have discomfort during intercourse? **YES** → Your partner's vagina may be dry as a result of tension or menopausal side effects. This can make intercourse painful for both of you.

See • *Anxiety*
• *Menopause*
• *Psychosexual dysfunction*

**NO**

? Does the tip of your penis become sore after intercourse? **YES** → You may be allergic to a chemical in a contraceptive cream used by your partner. Or, if you use a condom, there is a possibility that you are allergic to rubber. Consult your physician.

**NO**

If you are unable to make a diagnosis from this chart, consult your physician.

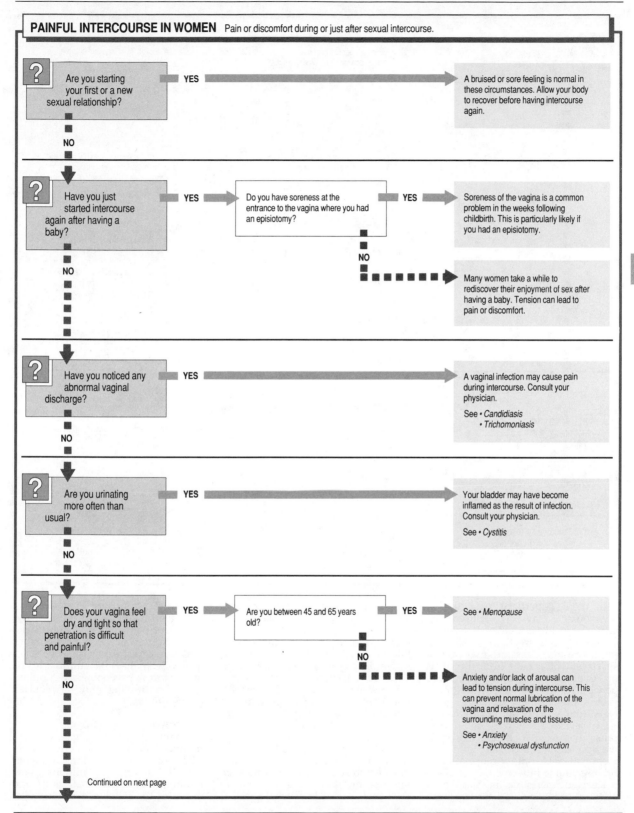

**PAINFUL INTERCOURSE IN WOMEN** Pain or discomfort during or just after sexual intercourse.

**Are you starting your first or a new sexual relationship?**

YES → A bruised or sore feeling is normal in these circumstances. Allow your body to recover before having intercourse again.

NO ↓

**Have you just started intercourse again after having a baby?**

YES → **Do you have soreness at the entrance to the vagina where you had an episiotomy?**

YES → Soreness of the vagina is a common problem in the weeks following childbirth. This is particularly likely if you had an episiotomy.

NO → Many women take a while to rediscover their enjoyment of sex after having a baby. Tension can lead to pain or discomfort.

NO ↓

**Have you noticed any abnormal vaginal discharge?**

YES → A vaginal infection may cause pain during intercourse. Consult your physician.

See • *Candidiasis*
• *Trichomoniasis*

NO ↓

**Are you urinating more often than usual?**

YES → Your bladder may have become inflamed as the result of infection. Consult your physician.

See • *Cystitis*

NO ↓

**Does your vagina feel dry and tight so that penetration is difficult and painful?**

YES → **Are you between 45 and 65 years old?**

YES → See • *Menopause*

NO → Anxiety and/or lack of arousal can lead to tension during intercourse. This can prevent normal lubrication of the vagina and relaxation of the surrounding muscles and tissues.

See • *Anxiety*
• *Psychosexual dysfunction*

NO ↓

Continued on next page

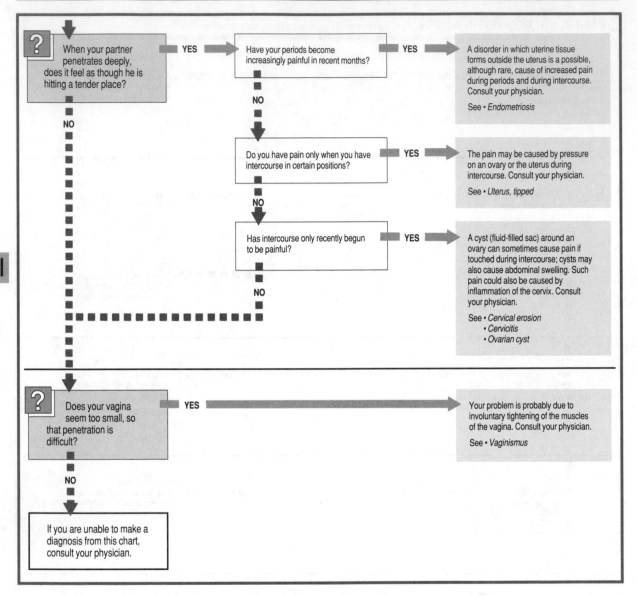

When your partner penetrates deeply, does it feel as though he is hitting a tender place?

**YES** → Have your periods become increasingly painful in recent months?

**YES** → A disorder in which uterine tissue forms outside the uterus is a possible, although rare, cause of increased pain during periods and during intercourse. Consult your physician.

See • *Endometriosis*

**NO** ↓

Do you have pain only when you have intercourse in certain positions?

**YES** → The pain may be caused by pressure on an ovary or the uterus during intercourse. Consult your physician.

See • *Uterus, tipped*

**NO** ↓

Has intercourse only recently begun to be painful?

**YES** → A cyst (fluid-filled sac) around an ovary can sometimes cause pain if touched during intercourse; cysts may also cause abdominal swelling. Such pain could also be caused by inflammation of the cervix. Consult your physician.

See • *Cervical erosion*
• *Cervicitis*
• *Ovarian cyst*

**NO**

**NO** ↓

Does your vagina seem too small, so that penetration is difficult?

**YES** → Your problem is probably due to involuntary tightening of the muscles of the vagina. Consult your physician.

See • *Vaginismus*

**NO** ↓

If you are unable to make a diagnosis from this chart, consult your physician.

---

In men, superficial pain during intercourse may be caused by anatomical abnormalities, such as *chordee* (bowed erection) or *phimosis* (tight foreskin). *Prostatitis* may cause a sharp, stabbing pain from the penis tip; there may also be a widespread pelvic ache or a burning sensation.

In some women, scarring (after tears from delivery or a poorly healed *episiotomy* repair, for example) may cause dyspareunia. Insufficient vaginal lubrication, especially after the menopause, is another cause of painful intercourse in women.

Deep dyspareunia in women is often caused by pelvic disorders (such

as *fibroids*, *ectopic pregnancy*, or *pelvic inflammatory disease*) or by disorders of the *ovary* (such as ovarian cysts or tumors). *Endometriosis* can cause thickening behind the uterus, resulting in deep pain during intercourse. Varicose veins in the pelvis and cervical disorders (such as tumors or infections) can also cause deep pain during intercourse. *Cystitis* commonly causes pain, primarily in women, as do other urinary tract infections.

*Psychosexual* problems may also cause painful intercourse. *Vaginismus*, in which the muscles of the vagina go into spasm, preventing insertion of the penis, is usually psychological.

**TREATMENT**
Treatment is directed at the underlying cause of the pain (for example, antibiotics for an infection or a lubricant for vaginal dryness). Analgesics (painkillers) may be helpful. If the discomfort is psychological in origin, special counseling may be required (see *Sex therapy*).

## Interferon
The name given to a group of proteins produced naturally by body cells in response to viral infections and other stimuli. Interferon inhibits viral multiplication (see illustration) and increases the activity of natural killer

## HOW INTERFERON FIGHTS VIRAL INFECTIONS

Interferon is part of the body's immune system, providing a defense against many different types of virally infected or tumor cells. It is produced naturally in the body during viral infections, but can also be given as a drug to enhance its natural actions.

### VIRAL MULTIPLICATION

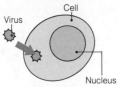

Cell

Virus

Nucleus

**1** A virus can multiply only by first invading one of its host's cells.

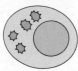

**2** The virus takes over the cell's chemical machinery to make copies of itself.

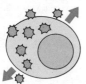

**3** The copies of the virus escape to invade more of the host's cells.

### HOW INTERFERON WORKS

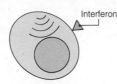

Interferon

Natural killer cell

**1** Interferon attaches to the membrane of host cells and stimulates them against viral attack.

**1** Interferon also causes natural killer cells to attack virally infected cells or tumor cells.

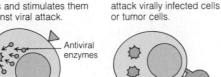

Antiviral enzymes

**2** If a virus invades a cell primed by interferon, enzymes are produced that impair viral copying.

**2** A natural killer cell attaches to the abnormal host cell and makes it disintegrate.

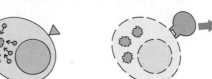

**3** Unable to copy itself, the virus is nullified, and the infection is stopped or shortened.

**3** The effect of this process is to help limit a viral infection or to slow tumor growth.

cells—types of *lymphocytes* that form part of the body's *immune system* (natural defenses).

### USE AS DRUG

Interferon has been approved for use in the treatment of hairy cell *leukemia*. It is currently under investigation for use in the treatment of various types of cancer, especially *Kaposi's sarcoma* (a skin cancer common in people with *AIDS*). Interferon is also being assessed as a treatment for life-threatening viral infections, particularly in people who have *immunodeficiency disorders*.

Interferon is produced from a culture of human cells exposed to a specific virus or is synthesized in the laboratory from specific nucleic acids (genetic material). It is given by injection or taken as a nasal spray. Possible adverse reactions include fever, headache, aching muscles, fatigue, nausea and vomiting, hair loss, and abnormal bleeding.

## Intern

A term for a medical graduate in the first year of hospital training.

## Internist

A specialist in the diagnosis and treatment of diseases in adults, particularly those related to the internal organs. Internists often provide a person's primary care.

## Intersex

A group of abnormalities in which the affected person has ambiguous genitalia (abnormal external sex organs that could be of either sex) or in which the external genitalia have the opposite appearance to the chromosomal sex of the individual. (See also *Sex determination*.)

## Interstitial pulmonary fibrosis

Scarring and thickening of the deep lung tissues, leading to shortness of breath; it is also known as IPF.

### TYPES AND CAUSES

The most important form of the disorder is known as idiopathic or diffuse interstitial pulmonary fibrosis, or fibrosing alveolitis. It is of unknown cause, but is probably an *autoimmune disorder* (caused by the body's *immune system* attacking its own tissues).

Less common causes include occupational exposure to mineral dusts and chemical fumes, radiation therapy, reactions to certain drugs, *lung cancer*, and allergic *alveolitis*.

### SYMPTOMS AND DIAGNOSIS

The symptoms are progressive shortness of breath, cough, chest pain, and finger clubbing, as well as symptoms of any underlying disease. The diagnosis is based on the patient's history and physical examination and is confirmed by *chest X ray* and lung *biopsy*.

### TREATMENT AND OUTLOOK

Treatment of idiopathic IPF often includes azathioprine and *corticosteroid drugs*, which suppress the immune system. In other cases, treatment of the disorder is directed to the underlying cause.

The outlook for recovery is generally poor for occupational dust diseases and idiopathic IPF, in which the lungs progressively stiffen. Progression of the disease may lead to heart failure and bronchopneumonia.

When IPF is caused by allergic alveolitis, the condition is more easily treated or reversible and the outlook may not be as gloomy.

## Interstitial radiation therapy

Treatment of a malignant tumor by inserting radioactive material into the growth (also called brachytherapy) or into neighboring tissue. With this method, radiation can be directed more accurately than is possible with X rays to the diseased area; there is also less risk of radiation harming healthy tissue.

### HOW IT IS DONE

The patient is given a general anesthetic. Radioactive material (usually artificial isotopes) contained in wires or small tubes is then implanted into or near the diseased tissue. If the tumor is in an easily accessible area (such as the mouth), the containers may be pushed in by means of a special needle; for a tumor deep in the body, a surgical procedure is necessary. The material is left in place for variable amounts of time (and sometimes permanently), depending on the radioactive substance and the tumor being treated. (See also *Intracavitary therapy; Radiation therapy*.)

# DISORDERS OF THE INTESTINE

The intestine is subject to various structural abnormalities and to the effects of many infective organisms and parasites; it may also be affected by tumors, impaired blood supply, and other disorders.

### CONGENITAL DEFECTS
Babies are sometimes born with an obstruction to the flow of the intestinal contents. This may be due to *atresia* (congenital closure), *stenosis* (narrowing), *volvulus* (twisting of loops of bowel), or blockage by meconium (fetal intestinal contents). Early surgery may be required.

### INFECTION AND INFLAMMATION
The general term for inflammation of the stomach and intestines is *gastroenteritis*. This is caused most commonly by viral or bacterial infections, which can range from the trivial to the life-threatening. They encompass many cases of *food poisoning* and travelers' diarrhea as well as serious diseases such as *typhoid fever* and *cholera*. Protozoal infections (caused by simple, single-celled parasites) include *giardiasis* and *amebiasis*.

Intestinal worm infestations are exceedingly common worldwide (see *Roundworms; Tapeworms*), although, in the US, only a few species of worms—including the *pinworm*—are prevalent.

Two important inflammatory conditions of the intestine, not caused by infection, are *ulcerative colitis* (mainly affecting the colon) and *Crohn's disease* (which may affect any part of the digestive tract but usually the small intestine). Sometimes, inflammation is confined to a localized area, such as in *appendicitis* and *diverticular disease*.

### TUMORS
Tumors of the small intestine are rare, but *lymphomas*, carcinoid tumors (producing *carcinoid syndrome*), and benign growths occur.

By contrast, tumors of the large intestine are very common (see *Intestine, cancer of*). Certain forms of familial *polyposis* (a disorder in which benign polyplike tumors grow in the colon) may progress to cancer.

### IMPAIRED BLOOD SUPPLY
Like other organs, the intestine is dependent on an adequate blood

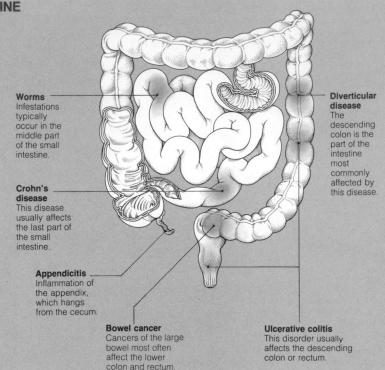

**Worms**
Infestations typically occur in the middle part of the small intestine.

**Crohn's disease**
This disease usually affects the last part of the small intestine.

**Appendicitis**
Inflammation of the appendix, which hangs from the cecum.

**Bowel cancer**
Cancers of the large bowel most often affect the lower colon and rectum.

**Diverticular disease**
The descending colon is the part of the intestine most commonly affected by this disease.

**Ulcerative colitis**
This disorder usually affects the descending colon or rectum.

supply. *Ischemia* (lack of blood) may result from several causes. Causes include partial or complete obstruction of the arteries in the abdominal wall (from disease such as *atherosclerosis*, *thrombosis*, or *embolism*) or from the blood vessels being compressed or trapped, as in *volvulus*, *intussusception*, or *hernias* (protrusion of intestines through the abdominal wall). Loss of blood supply to a segment of intestine may cause *gangrene* (tissue death) requiring immediate surgery.

### OBSTRUCTION
Intestinal obstruction may be caused by pressure from the outside, disease of the intestinal wall (such as cancer, Crohn's disease, or diverticular disease), or internal blockage (such as from *gallstones* or intussusception). One of the most common causes is paralytic *ileus,* in which intestinal contractions cease and the intestinal contents are no longer transported.

### OTHER DISORDERS
*Peptic ulcer* of the duodenum is a very common disorder, thought to affect 10 percent of the population. Ulceration of the small intestine occurs in typhoid and Crohn's

disease and may cause bleeding into the intestine or even perforation (hole formation). Ulceration of the large intestine occurs in amebiasis and in ulcerative colitis.

Diverticula are small outpouchings from the inside of the bowel. They are usually harmless, but, in diverticular disease, become inflamed. *Malabsorption* and *celiac sprue* result from changes to the intestinal lining. Finally, *irritable bowel syndrome* is associated with persistent abdominal pain and either constipation or diarrhea (or both) and is the most common intestinal disorder in Western societies.

### INVESTIGATION
Intestinal disorders are investigated by physical examination, and by techniques such as *barium X-ray examination*, *sigmoidoscopy*, or possibly *colonoscopy*, and by laboratory examination of the feces or of a *biopsy* specimen taken from the intestinal lining.

## Intertrigo

Inflammation of the skin caused by two surfaces rubbing together. Intertrigo is most common in obese people and usually occurs on the inner thighs, in the armpits, on the underside of the breasts, in folds of the abdomen, and between fingers and toes. The affected skin is red, moist, and may have an odor; there may be scales or blisters. The condition is made worse by sweating. It is sometimes accompanied by seborrheic *dermatitis* or *candidiasis* (thrush).

Treatment consists of weight reduction, keeping affected areas as clean and dry as possible, and, if dermatitis or candidiasis is present, applying a *corticosteroid* or *antifungal* cream.

## Intestinal imaging

See *Barium X-ray examinations*.

## Intestinal lipodystrophy

See *Whipple's disease*.

## Intestine

The major part of the digestive tract, extending from the exit of the stomach to the anus. The intestine forms a long tube divided into two main sections— the small intestine and the large intestine. The function of the intestine is to break down and absorb food and water into the bloodstream and carry away the waste products of digestion to be passed as feces.

### STRUCTURE

The small intestine is about 21 feet (6.5 m) in length and 1.5 inches (35 mm) in diameter. It has three sections—the duodenum (a short, curved segment fixed to the back wall of the abdomen) and the jejunum and ileum (two larger, coiled, and mobile segments). The bile and pancreatic ducts enter the duodenum (see *Biliary system*).

The walls of the intestine consist of circular and longitudinal muscles with an internal lining (the mucosa) and an external covering (the serosa). *Peristalsis* (the rhythmic contraction of the muscles) forces partially digested food along the intestine. The mucosa consists of many *villi* (small, fingerlike projections) covered with millions of fronds that create a large surface area to help the absorption of substances into the blood.

The large intestine is about 6 feet (1.8 m) in length and 2 inches (50 mm) in diameter; it frames the loops of the small intestine. Unlike the small intestine, much of it is fixed in position, the muscles run in bands rather than forming a continuous sheet along

**LOCATION OF THE INTESTINE**
Situated below the stomach and liver, the intestine occupies much of the central and lower parts of the abdomen.

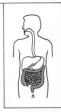

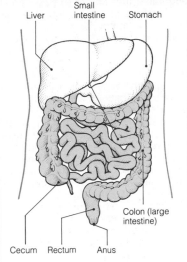

Liver — Small intestine — Stomach

Colon (large intestine)

Cecum — Rectum — Anus

its length, and there are no internal villi. The main section, the colon, is divided into an ascending, a transverse, a descending, and a pelvic portion (the sigmoid colon) that hangs down into the pelvis. The appendix hangs from a pouch (the cecum) between the small intestine and the colon. The final section of intestine, before the anus, is the rectum.

### FUNCTION

The small intestine is concerned with the digestion of food and the absorption of food into the bloodstream. Some digestion occurs in the stomach, but more digestive enzymes and bile are added to the partly digested food in the duodenum. Glands within the walls of each section of the small intestine produce mucus and more enzymes, all of which help to break down the food into easily absorbable chemical units. The numerous blood vessels in the intestinal walls then carry the digested food to the liver for distribution to the rest of the body.

Unabsorbed material leaves the small intestine in the form of liquid and fiber. As they pass through the large intestine, water, vitamins, and mineral salts are absorbed into the bloodstream, leaving feces made up of undigested food residue, small

amounts of fat, secretions from the stomach, liver, pancreas, and bowel wall, and various bacteria. The feces are gradually compressed and pass into the rectum. Distention of the rectum usually produces the desire to empty the bowel.

## Intestine, cancer of

Cancerous tumors in the small intestine are extremely rare, but the large intestine is the third most common cancer site (after the lung and breast). Colorectal cancer accounts for about 20 percent of all cancer deaths in the US.

Types found in both the small and large intestine include carcinoid tumors and lymphomas. Carcinoid tumors are very slow growing and usually symptomless (however, they may spread to the liver, leading to *carcinoid syndrome*). Lymphomas, which damage the wall of the intestine and nearby lymph nodes, cause malabsorption of food.

### CAUSES

Although there is no single cause of intestinal cancer, there are a number of possible contributory factors.

The higher incidence of cancer of the colon (by far the most common type of intestinal cancer) in Western countries suggests an environmental, probably dietary, factor. It is believed that a high-meat, high-fat, and low-fiber diet encourages the production and concentration of *carcinogens*.

There is also thought to be a genetic factor. Brothers, sisters, and children of people suffering from cancer of the colon are more likely than average to acquire the disease later in life.

Cancer of the colon frequently occurs in association with other diseases of the colon, such as *ulcerative colitis* and familial *polyposis*.

### SYMPTOMS

An inexplicable change in bowel movements (either constipation or diarrhea) lasting for 10 days or so may be one of the first symptoms of cancer of the large intestine.

Blood mixed in the feces (as opposed to the blood from *hemorrhoids*, which usually coats the feces) is another important warning signal, although, if the growth is high up in the colon, the blood can be detected only by chemical tests.

There may be pain and tenderness in the lower abdomen. Sometimes, however, there are no symptoms at all until the tumor grows so big that it causes an obstruction in the intestine or causes the intestine to rupture.

## DIAGNOSIS AND TREATMENT

Tests on feces, *barium X-ray examinations*, *sigmoidoscopy*, and *colonoscopy* may be carried out.

Treatment depends on the stage of development of the cancer, but, in most cases, a partial *colectomy* is performed. The diseased tissue and a small amount of surrounding normal tissue are removed and the cut ends are sewn together to reestablish the channel. If the disease is extensive, surgery may not be possible.

## OUTLOOK

The long-term prospects vary according to the stage the disease has reached when it is discovered. More than 50 percent of patients survive in good health for at least five years after a colectomy. Nonsurgical treatments merely arrest the growth and spread of the cancer and are not curative. The earlier the tumor is detected, the greater the chances of a full recovery after treatment. Anyone over the age of 50 who suddenly experiences a change in bowel movements should see a physician without delay. (See also *Rectum, cancer of*.)

## Intestine, obstruction of

A partial or complete blockage of the small or large intestine. Without treatment, complete obstruction of the intestine is usually fatal.

## CAUSES

The most common cause of intestinal obstruction is paralytic *ileus*, in which (for no medical reason) *peristalsis* (the rhythmic muscle contractions of the intestine) stops, the bowel dilates, and the intestinal contents are no longer moved along the digestive tract.

Other common causes, which have a mechanical basis, are strangulated *hernia*, *atresia* (congenital closure), *stenosis* (narrowing of the intestinal canal), *adhesions* (postoperative bands of scar tissue that bridge across the outer surface of segments of bowel, sometimes trapping another loop), *volvulus* (twisting or knotting of the bowel), and *intussusception*.

Intestinal obstruction also occurs in diseases (such as *Crohn's disease*, *diverticular disease*, and tumors) that affect the intestinal wall. Less commonly, internal blockage of the intestinal canal is caused by impacted food, feces, gallstones, or by some accidentally swallowed object.

## SYMPTOMS

The location and type of obstruction (partial or complete) dictate the symptoms. A blockage in the small intestine usually causes intermittent cramplike middle abdominal pain, which tends to be more severe the higher the obstruction. This is accompanied by increasingly frequent bouts of vomiting and by failure to pass gas or stools.

The symptoms of obstruction in the large intestine, particularly the colon, are pain, distention (swelling) of the abdomen, and failure to pass stools; the blockage may be so complete that even gas cannot be passed. Partial obstruction may be accompanied by diarrhea when the obstruction is intermittent. There is temporary relief when the liquid stool is able to pass through the remaining gap and the symptoms abate for a while.

## DIAGNOSIS AND TREATMENT

A careful history and physical examination are usually all the physician requires to make a diagnosis. Abdominal *X rays* are confirmatory. Most of the gas and intestinal contents are removed through a flexible tube inserted down the throat. Complete mechanical obstruction must be corrected by surgery, but the actual type of operation depends on the nature and site of the blockage to the flow of intestinal contents.

## OUTLOOK

The prospects for a full recovery after surgery are excellent, particularly if the underlying problem is a hernia, congenital atresia, or intussusception. However, if the problem is a tumor in the colon of an elderly patient, the risks of the operation are greater.

## Intestine, tumors of

Tumors of the intestine may be cancerous or benign (noncancerous). Cancers of the intestine include carcinoid tumors, lymphomas, cancer of the colon (see *Intestine, cancer of*), and cancer of the rectum (see *Rectum, cancer of*).

Noncancerous tumors are rare, but *polyps* in the colon, and *adenomas*, *leiomyomas*, *lipomas*, and *angiomas* in the small intestine are occasionally found. These tumors are usually symptomless and are often discovered only accidentally when *barium X-ray examinations* are being carried out for some other reason.

Very occasionally polyps undergo transformation and become cancerous, which is why they are usually removed at an early stage.

## Intoxication

A general term for a condition resulting from *poisoning*; it customarily refers to the effects of excessive drinking (see *Alcohol intoxication*), but also includes *drug poisoning* or poisoning from accumulation of metabolic substances in the body.

## Intra-

A prefix that means within, as in intramuscular (within a muscle). See also *Inter-*.

## Intracavitary therapy

Treatment of a malignant tumor in a body cavity by placing radioactive material within the cavity. The treatment is used mainly for cancer of the uterus, cervix (neck of the uterus), vagina, or rectum.

## HOW IT IS DONE

The radioactive material (usually in the form of artificial isotopes embedded in wires or small tubes) is introduced into the cavity and left there for a period of time, using a general or local anesthetic.

Sometimes *anticancer drugs* are introduced directly into the abdominal cavity or pleural cavity (the space around the lungs) to treat a malignant effusion (a fluid containing cancerous cells). A needle, sometimes with a catheter (fine tube) attached, is passed through the wall of the abdomen or chest into the cavity, using a local anesthetic. The needle is used to draw off the effusion and then to inject the drug. (See also *Interstitial radiation therapy*; *Radiation therapy*.)

## Intracerebral hemorrhage

Bleeding into the brain from a ruptured vessel. Intracerebral hemorrhage is one of the three main mechanisms by which a *stroke* can occur.

## INCIDENCE AND CAUSES

Each year in the US, about one person in 2,500 suffers an intracerebral hemorrhage. Most victims are middle-aged or elderly people with untreated *hypertension* (high blood pressure) or *atherosclerosis* (fatty deposits causing narrowing of the arteries) in the brain. Unlike most cases of *subdural* and *extradural hemorrhage* (bleeding between the surface of the brain and the skull), an intracerebral hemorrhage can occur without any injury or blow to the head.

The ruptured artery is usually in the cerebrum (the main mass of the brain), although sometimes it is in other brain structures (such as the cerebellum or the brain stem). The escaped blood seeps outward, forming a circular or oval mass up to a few inches in diameter, disrupting brain tissue in its path as bleeding continues and its volume increases. Adjacent brain tissues are displaced and compressed.

**SYMPTOMS**

The symptoms are sudden headache, weakness, and confusion, and often loss of consciousness. Usually the victim falls unconscious to the ground with no warning. Signs resulting from disruption of brain tissue (speech loss, facial paralysis, or one-sided weakness) may develop over periods of minutes or hours.

**DIAGNOSIS, TREATMENT, AND OUTLOOK**

Diagnosis is by *CT scanning*. Surgical treatment is usually impossible due to the inaccessibility of the rupture, so treatment is aimed at life-support and reduction of blood pressure.

Large hemorrhages are usually fatal, and, overall, only about 25 percent of patients survive. Recurrent bleeding from the same site is uncommon. For the survivor of an intracerebral hemorrhage, rehabilitation and outlook are as for stroke.

## Intractable

Any condition that does not respond to treatment.

## Intramuscular

A medical term meaning within a muscle, as in an intramuscular injection, in which a drug is injected deep within a muscle. Such injections are usually given into the upper, outer part of the buttock. The drug is absorbed from the muscle into the bloodstream, which distributes it throughout the body.

## Intraocular pressure

The balance between the rate of production and removal of aqueous humor within the eye, which maintains the shape of the eyeball. Aqueous humor enters the eye from the ciliary body, which constantly produces the fluid, and exits from the drainage angle (a network of tissue between the iris and cornea).

If drainage is impeded, intraocular pressure builds up and leads to *glaucoma*. Intraocular pressure is usually measured by *tonometry* during a routine eye examination.

## Intrauterine contraceptive device

See *IUD*.

## Intrauterine growth retardation

Poor fetal growth, usually due to a fetal defect or to failure of the placenta to provide adequate nutrients. Intrauterine growth retardation causes the fetus to be smaller than expected for the length of gestation.

**CAUSES**

Intrauterine growth retardation may be due to a chromosomal defect, such as *Down's syndrome*, which causes the fetus to be "small for dates." A maternal infection, such as *rubella* (German measles), in which the virus passes through the placenta, can also cause poor fetal growth.

Maternal factors may also be responsible, especially when the fetus is otherwise normal. Conditions such as *preeclampsia, hypertension*, or chronic *renal failure* can affect fetal growth, as can the mother's diet. Cigarette smoking is a major cause of intrauterine growth retardation, as are malnutrition and alcoholism.

**DIAGNOSIS AND TREATMENT**

The physician can check whether the uterus is smaller than expected during a prenatal examination; *ultrasound scanning* may be performed to estimate the fetal growth. The mother may be required to rest, and tests of placental function may be needed, including blood tests or electrical monitoring of the baby's heart.

If intrauterine growth retardation is diagnosed, the pregnancy is carefully monitored and the underlying cause of the placental insufficiency treated, if possible. If the baby's growth is slowing, *induction of labor* or a *cesarean section* may be necessary.

**OUTLOOK**

Because babies suffering intrauterine growth retardation have been chronically undernourished in the uterus, they are usually underweight and may be premature if labor has been induced. Because they are prone to low blood sugar, *hypothermia*, and infection, they are usually transferred to an *incubator* immediately after birth to provide them with special care.

## Intravenous

A term meaning within a vein, as in *intravenous infusion* (slow introduction of a substance into a vein) and intravenous *injection* (rapid introduction of a substance into a vein).

## Intravenous infusion

The slow introduction of a volume of fluid into the bloodstream. The fluid passes down from a plastic or glass container through tubing into a cannula (thin plastic tube) inserted into a vein, usually in the patient's forearm. The rate at which the fluid drips into the circulation is controlled by an adjustable valve.

An intravenous infusion, commonly known as a drip, is used to give blood (or plasma) to replace that lost in a serious accident or during an operation (see *Blood transfusion*). It is also used to replace or maintain body fluids in patients who are unable to drink or eat. In this case, the fluid is usually a mixture of glucose (sugar) and saline (salt solution). Other uses include providing more varied and concentrated nutrients to people unable to digest food normally (see *Feeding, artificial*) and administering certain drugs.

## Intravenous pyelography

See *Pyelography*.

## Introitus

A general term for the entrance to a body cavity or space, most commonly the vagina.

## Introvert

A person more concerned with his or her inner world. Introverts prefer to work alone, are shy, quiet, and withdrawn when under stress. (See also *Extrovert; Personality*.)

## Intubation

The process of passing an *endotracheal tube* (breathing tube) into the trachea (windpipe). Intubation is performed if a person needs mechanical ventilation to deliver oxygen to the lungs—for example, because he or she is in a coma, is anesthetized, or has severe respiratory disease.

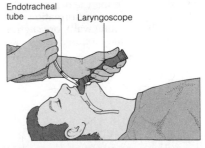

Endotracheal tube    Laryngoscope

**Endotracheal intubation**
Guided by an anesthesiologist, the endotracheal tube is passed through the patient's mouth and down the throat into the trachea.

**HOW IT IS DONE**

The anesthesiologist looks at the patient's throat with a laryngoscope (a viewing instrument) to identify the vocal cords. An endotracheal tube is passed through the patient's mouth and down the throat between the vocal cords into the trachea. Alternatively, the tube is passed through the nose. The external end of the tube is then secured by tape; an inflatable cuff may be used to hold the tube in place within the trachea.

Intubation also refers to the placement of a gastric or intestinal tube for purposes of suction or the giving of nutrients (see *Feeding, artificial*).

## Intussusception

A condition in which part of the intestine telescopes in on itself, forming a tube within a tube (like pulling a shirt sleeve partially inside out), usually resulting in intestinal obstruction (see *Intestine, obstruction of*). Intussusception occurs primarily in young children.

### CAUSES AND INCIDENCE

It is not known exactly why this condition occurs, but in some cases there is a definite association with a recent infection. In other instances it may start at the site of a *polyp* or *Meckel's diverticulum* (a small, pouchlike projection from the end section of the small intestine). An intussusception is the most common cause of intestinal obstruction in children under 2 years, affecting approximately two babies per 1,000.

### SYMPTOMS

Severe abdominal colic usually develops in the child, causing intermittent screaming attacks. Vomiting is a common feature, and blood and mucus are often found in the feces. In severe cases, the blood supply to the intestine becomes blocked and *peritonitis* (inflammation of the membrane covering the organs in the abdomen), *perforation* (formation of a hole in the intestine wall), or *gangrene* (tissue death) may follow.

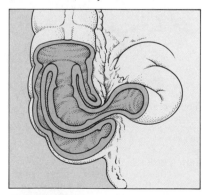

**Intussusception**
This disorder is characterized by part of the intestine telescoping in on itself. It usually affects parts of the small intestine and is most common in infants.

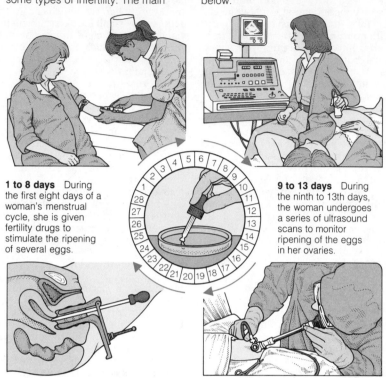

## PROCEDURE FOR IN VITRO FERTILIZATION

Fertilization of eggs outside a woman's body can be used to treat some types of infertility. The main stages involved in the procedure of in vitro fertilization are illustrated below.

**1 to 8 days** During the first eight days of a woman's menstrual cycle, she is given fertility drugs to stimulate the ripening of several eggs.

**9 to 13 days** During the ninth to 13th days, the woman undergoes a series of ultrasound scans to monitor ripening of the eggs in her ovaries.

**16 to 17 days** After about 40 hours, the eggs are examined to see if they have been fertilized and have started to develop into embryos. If they have, several embryos (usually at the two- or four-cell stage) are placed in the woman's uterus through the vagina.

**14 to 15 days** Immediately before ovulation (which may be induced with drugs), ripe eggs are removed by laparoscopy or by ultrasound-guided needle aspiration through the vagina or abdomen. The eggs are mixed with the man's sperm in a dish, which is then put in an incubator.

### DIAGNOSIS AND TREATMENT

A barium enema (see *Barium X-ray examinations*) is usually sufficient to reveal the obstruction. Sometimes the barium enema actually treats the condition; the pressure applied when the enema is introduced can force the prolapsed segment back into position. Otherwise, an operation is carried out. Usually, the intestine is gently squeezed to push out the inner segment, permitting surgery on the cause that led the segment of bowel to telescope. In rare cases, the prolapsed intestine must be cut out.

## Invasive

Having the tendency to spread throughout body tissues; the term is usually applied to malignant tumors or harmful microorganisms. An inva-

sive medical procedure is one in which body tissues are penetrated by an instrument. *Angiography* is an example. (See also *Noninvasive*.)

## In vitro

The performance of biological processes in the laboratory rather than in the body; in vitro literally means "in glass." Tests successfully carried out in vitro do not always work the same way in the body.

## In vitro fertilization

A method of treating *infertility* in which an egg is surgically removed from the ovary and fertilized outside the body. In vitro, which literally means "in glass," refers to the glass Petri dish that is used in the process.

The first successful birth as a result of in vitro fertilization (IVF) occurred in England in 1978.

**WHY IT IS DONE**

In vitro fertilization may be performed when the woman's *fallopian tubes* are permanently blocked or absent. IVF may also be done if the man's sperm count is very low or if it is thought that antibodies in the woman's cervical mucus are killing the sperm.

**HOW IT IS DONE**

Stages in the procedure are shown in the illustrated box.

After IVF, the woman's condition is monitored for a few days to determine if the fertilized eggs have become safely implanted in the uterine wall. Once this occurs, the pregnancy usually continues normally, although the early miscarriage rate is high, and multiple births may occur because more than one of the eggs "takes."

**OUTLOOK**

It is unlikely that in vitro fertilization will become a widespread treatment for infertility, at least in the near future. Currently, this highly specialized procedure is available only at a small number of clinics. It is expensive (costing about $5,000 per implantation attempt) and the success rate is limited.

Research into IVF has shown that half or more of all eggs have abnormal chromosomes and cannot develop into normal embryos; after fertilization, the eggs begin to divide, but the pregnancy miscarries. Only about 10 percent of couples achieve pregnancy on the first attempt, and many tries may be needed before a successful pregnancy is achieved. In addition, the legality of in vitro fertilization is still unclear. In the US, the procedure is prohibited in a number of states because of laws governing the rights of the embryo.

## In vivo

Biological processes occurring, or caused to occur, within the body.

## Involuntary movements

Uncontrollable movements of the body, usually affecting the face, head, limbs, and trunk. These movements occur spontaneously and may be slow and writhing (see *Athetosis*); rapid, jerky, and random (see *Chorea*); or predictable, stereotyped, and affecting one part of the body, usually the face (see *Tic*). They may be a feature of a disease (*Huntington's chorea*, for example) or a side effect of certain psychotherapeutic drugs.

## Iodine

An element essential for the formation of *thyroid hormones* (thyroxine and triiodothyronine). These hormones control the body's *metabolism* (internal chemistry), promote growth and development, burn excessive fat, improve mental processes, and promote the formation of healthy hair, skin, nails, and teeth.

Iodine is found in seafood (the best dietary source), dairy products, bread, and some table salt preparations. Adequate amounts are obtained from a well-balanced diet. Iodine deficiency may cause a *goiter* (enlarged thyroid gland), *hypothyroidism* (underactive thyroid gland), and, in babies, *cretinism*.

**MEDICAL USES**

Iodine is sometimes given to people to protect against the effects of consuming food or drink contaminated with radioactive iodine (see *Radiation hazards*). Saturation with radiation-free iodine prevents the thyroid gland from absorbing and being damaged by radioactive iodine.

Radioactive iodine is sometimes given to deliberately damage the thyroid gland to treat *thyrotoxicosis* (overactive thyroid gland).

Some iodine compounds are used as *antiseptics*; others are included in cough remedies. Iodine is also a constituent of the radiopaque contrast medium used in some X-ray procedures (see *Imaging techniques*).

**POSSIBLE ADVERSE EFFECTS**

Iodine supplements rarely cause an allergic reaction. Possible symptoms of allergy to iodine include rash, facial swelling, abdominal pain, vomiting, and headache.

## Ion

A particle (either an atom or a group of atoms) that carries an electrical charge; positively charged ions are called cations and negatively charged ions are called anions. Important cations in the body include sodium, potassium, hydrogen, and calcium. Important anions include bicarbonate, chloride, and phosphate.

**ROLE IN THE BODY**

Many vital body processes depend on the movement of ions across cell membranes. For example, the exchange of sodium for potassium across the membranes around nerve and muscle cells is the mechanism by which nerve impulses are transmitted and by which muscle contraction occurs. Calcium also plays an important role in muscle contraction, in addition to being involved in blood clotting and bone growth.

**IMPORTANT IONS AND THEIR ROLES**

| Cations (positively charged ions) | Major roles in body |
|---|---|
| Ammonium | Acid-base balance; produced by protein metabolism |
| Calcium | Nerve conduction; muscle contraction; blood clotting; bone and tooth formation; heart action |
| Hydrogen | Acid-base balance; component of stomach acid |
| Magnesium | Nerve conduction; muscle contraction; bone and tooth formation; enzyme activation; protein metabolism |
| Potassium | Nerve conduction; muscle contraction; water balance; acid-base balance |
| Sodium | Nerve conduction; muscle contraction; water balance; acid-base balance |
| **Anions** (negatively charged ions) | |
| Bicarbonate | Acid-base balance; neutralizes stomach acid |
| Chloride | Acid-base balance; water balance; component of stomach acid |
| Phosphate | Acid-base balance; bone and tooth formation; protein metabolism; energy metabolism; structure of cell membranes |

Sodium is the principal cation in extracellular fluid (which surrounds all cells in the body), where it affects the flow of water into and out of cells (see *Osmosis*) and thereby influences the concentration of body fluids.

The levels of sodium, potassium, and calcium are regulated by the kidneys, which control the amount lost from the body in the urine. The level of calcium is also affected by hormonal effects on bones.

The acidity of the blood and other body fluids depends on the level of hydrogen cations, which are produced by various metabolic processes. To prevent these fluids from becoming too acidic, hydrogen cations are neutralized by bicarbonate anions in the extracellular fluid and blood, and by phosphate anions inside cells (see *Acid-base balance*).

**ION DISTURBANCES**

For the body to function normally, the level of each ion must be maintained within narrow limits; any substantial deviation can cause symptoms, such as muscle weakness caused by hypokalemia (too low a level of potassium cations in the blood).

*Dehydration* caused by insufficient water intake or excessive water loss (from diarrhea, vomiting, or sweating) increases the concentration of all ions. This may cause thirst, muscle cramps, dizziness, and faintness.

## Ipecac

A drug used to induce vomiting in the treatment of *poisoning*. Ipecac (also known as ipecacuanha) is derived from a plant native to South and Central America. It is available over-the-counter in syrup form. It should not be used if poisoning has been caused by corrosive or petroleum-based substances, if the victim is not fully conscious, or if the victim is less than 1 year old.

## Ipratropium

An *anticholinergic drug* used as a *bronchodilator drug* in the treatment of *asthma* and chronic *bronchitis*. It is also used as a *decongestant drug* in the treatment of *rhinitis*.

## IQ

Abbreviation for intelligence quotient, an age-related measure of intelligence (see *Intelligence tests*).

## Iridectomy

Removal of part of the *iris*, usually to treat narrow-angle *glaucoma*. Iridectomy involves making a small opening near the root of the iris to form a channel through which aqueous humor can drain. Called a "peripheral iridectomy," the opening is made by laser or by operative surgery.

Iridectomy is sometimes performed to remove tumors and to improve the vision of children who have small central cataracts.

## Iridencleisis

A surgical procedure that was used in the 1940s and 1950s (to control chronic *glaucoma*) in which an artificial channel was created for the drainage of aqueous humor. Iridencleisis has been replaced by *trabeculectomy*, which is a more reliable procedure.

## Iridocyclitis

Inflammation of the *iris* and ciliary body. The term is rarely used today; the condition is now called anterior *uveitis*. (See also *Eye* disorders box.)

## Iris

The colored part of the eye that lies behind the cornea. The iris is connected at its outer edge to the ciliary body and has a central perforation called the *pupil* through which light enters the eye and falls on the retina. This loose framework of transparent *collagen* (a fibrous protein) and muscle fibers constantly contracts and dilates to alter the size of the pupil and control the amount of light that passes through the pupil. The color of the iris is mostly due to the amount and distribution of the pigment cells on the back of the iris.

## Iritis

An infrequently employed term for inflammation of the *iris*; the condition is now known as *uveitis*.

## Iron

A mineral essential for certain *enzymes* (proteins that stimulate chemical reactions) and for the formation of *hemoglobin* (red blood cell pigment) and *myoglobin* (muscle cell pigment).

Iron is contained in a variety of foods, such as liver, eggs, fish, green leafy vegetables, nuts, and beans. Adequate amounts are usually obtained from a well-balanced diet. During pregnancy, iron supplements may be necessary for the healthy development of the baby.

Iron deficiency leading to anemia (see *Anemia, iron-deficiency*) is usually caused by abnormal blood loss, such as that from *menorrhagia* (heavy periods) or a *peptic ulcer*.

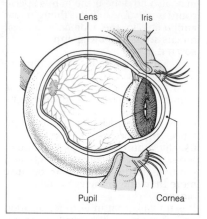

**LOCATION OF THE IRIS**
The iris lies behind the cornea and in front of the lens. The outer edge of the iris is connected to the ciliary body; at the center is an aperture called the pupil.

Lens     Iris

Pupil     Cornea

Iron supplements may cause nausea, abdominal pain, constipation, or diarrhea. They also color the feces black. Excessive intake of iron may cause *cirrhosis* of the liver.

## Iron-deficiency anemia

See *Anemia, iron-deficiency*.

## Irradiation

See *Radiation hazards*; *Radiation therapy*.

## Irrigation, wound

The cleansing of a deep wound by repeatedly washing it out with a medicated solution or sterile saline.

**WHY IT IS DONE**

A deep wound is often contaminated with infected foreign material, and, unless it is completely cleansed before repair, it may fail to heal, an abscess may form in it, or, in extreme cases, *gangrene* may result. If the wound contains soil, *tetanus* is a risk.

## Irritable bladder

Intermittent, uncontrolled contractions of the muscles in the bladder. Irritable bladder may cause urge incontinence (see *Incontinence, urinary*).

Irritability of the bladder is commonly due to a urinary tract infection (see *Cystitis*), the presence of a catheter within the bladder, a bladder stone (see *Calculus, urinary tract*), or obstruction to the outflow of urine by an enlarged *prostate gland*. In many cases of irritable bladder, however, no underlying cause for the muscular irritability and spasm is found.

Symptoms may be relieved by *antispasmodic drugs*; other treatment is directed at any underlying cause.

## Irritable bowel syndrome

A combination of intermittent abdominal pain and irregular bowel habit (i.e., constipation, diarrhea, or both, alternating) that occurs in the absence of demonstrable disease. Alternative names are irritable colon syndrome and spastic colon.

Although symptoms subside and even disappear for periods of time, the condition usually is recurrent throughout life and, without being life-threatening or leading to complications, can cause much distress.

**CAUSES AND INCIDENCE**
The cause is not fully understood, but the basic abnormality is a disturbance of involuntary muscle movement in the large intestine. However, there is no abnormality in the intestinal structure and people with irritable bowel syndrome neither lose weight nor become malnourished. It is the most common disorder of the intestine, accounting for more than half the patients seen by gastroenterologists.

The condition is twice as common in women as in men, usually beginning in early or middle adulthood. Sufferers are usually otherwise in good health and have had the condition for some time before seeking medical advice.

A psychological element, particularly anxiety, is believed by some physicians to be the main causative factor; emotional stress tends to exacerbate the condition. However, bowel upset is a normal reaction to stress in many people who do not suffer from the illness.

**SYMPTOMS**
The symptoms include intermittent cramplike pain in the abdomen, abdominal distention (swelling), often on the left side, transient relief of pain by bowel movement or passing gas, mucus in the feces, sense of incomplete evacuation of the bowels, excessive gas, and symptoms aggravated by food. Various other symptoms may also occur (which are not precisely part of the irritable bowel syndrome), such as heartburn, back pain, weakness, faintness, agitation, tendency to tire easily, reduced appetite, and palpitations.

**DIAGNOSIS**
Following a careful history and physical examination (which is valuable in both diagnosis and treatment), patients may have their feces tested and may be given a *barium X-ray examination* and a *sigmoidoscopy* (examination of the colon through an endoscope passed via the anus). These tests are intended to exclude conditions, such as cancer and inflammatory bowel disease, that may have similar symptoms.

**TREATMENT**
Bulk-forming agents, such as bran or methylcellulose, may be prescribed for constipation along with an *antispasmodic drug* to relieve some of the muscular spasm. *Antidiarrheal drugs* (such as loperamide) may be given briefly for prolonged diarrhea. A high-fiber diet is advised for certain types of irritable bowel syndrome. Although these treatments can alleviate the disorder's troublesome symptoms, there is no cure.

## Ischemia

Insufficient supply of blood to a specific organ or tissue. Ischemia is usually caused by a blood vessel disease, such as *atherosclerosis*, but may also result from injury to a vessel, constriction of a vessel due to spasm of the muscles in the vessel wall, or inadequate blood flow due to inefficient pumping action of the heart. The symptoms of ischemia depend on the part of the body affected.

Treatment may include *vasodilator drugs* to widen the blood vessels or, in more severe cases, an *angioplasty* or *bypass operation*.

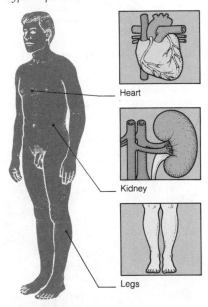

Heart

Kidney

Legs

**Symptoms of ischemia**
Ischemia (insufficient blood supply) of the heart causes the chest pain of angina pectoris; ischemia of blood vessels in the legs may cause a cramplike pain during exercise. Ischemia may also affect the kidneys (causing renal failure) or the brain (resulting in a stroke).

## Isocarboxazid

A monoamine oxidase inhibitor *antidepressant drug*. Like other monoamine oxidase inhibitors, isocarboxazid is not usually prescribed unless other antidepressant drugs are ineffective or the patient is intolerant of other antidepressant drugs.

Possible adverse effects of isocarboxazid include headache, dizziness, blurred vision, tremor, and constipation. If taken with foods containing tyramine (such as cheese and red wine) or certain other drugs, isocarboxazid may cause a dangerous rise in blood pressure.

---

**IRRIGATION TECHNIQUES**
After removal of contaminated tissue, a wound may be cleansed either by forced syringe (or catheter) irrigation or by using an irrigation chamber.

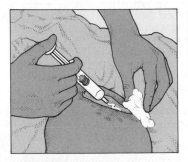

**Forced syringe irrigation**
A syringe (sometimes with a catheter attached) is used to flush irrigation fluid repeatedly into and out of the wound until the drained fluid is clear.

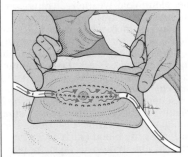

**Irrigation chamber**
A flexible, plastic irrigation chamber is sealed over the wound; irrigation fluid is then run through the chamber until the drained fluid is clear.

## Isolation

Nursing procedures designed to prevent a patient from infecting others or from being infected by them. In either case, the patient is usually isolated in an individual room.

**TYPES**

**COMPLETE ISOLATION** This is used if a patient has a contagious disease, such as *tuberculosis* or *Lassa fever*, that can be transmitted to others both by direct contact and by airborne germs. All nursing staff members wear masks, gowns, caps, and gloves, which afterward are incinerated or sterilized. Bed linen, eating utensils, bedpans, and any other items that come in contact with the patient are also sterilized and, even though they wear gloves, staff members wash their hands thoroughly after each nursing task.

**PARTIAL ISOLATION** This is carried out if the patient's disease is transmitted in a more limited way—for example, only by respiration (as in *pertussis*) or only by contact with infected skin (as in *impetigo*), blood (as in *AIDS*), or feces (as in *cholera*). In these cases, some of the precautions taken in complete isolation nursing are unnecessary.

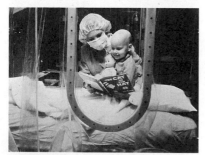

**Child being nursed in an isolator**
The plastic tent and strict sterilization procedures protect the patient from infection.

**REVERSE ISOLATION** This technique is used to protect a patient whose resistance to infection has been severely lowered. Air entering the room is first filtered. Visiting is drastically limited and all staff members and visitors wear caps, gowns, masks, and gloves. Bed linen and all items used by the patient are sterilized. When these measures do not give enough protection (such as after *bone marrow transplantation*), the patient is placed in an isolator (plastic tent) or in a room ventilated with specially purified air.

Occasionally, long-term reverse isolation is needed for patients with severe combined *immunodeficiency*; these people are born without normal defenses against infection.

## Isoniazid

An *antibacterial drug* used to prevent and treat *tuberculosis*. As a preventive measure, isoniazid may be given to close contacts of people suffering from tuberculosis. To treat the disease, isoniazid is given in combination with other antibacterial drugs, usually for at least nine months.

Adverse effects are rare and include nausea, fatigue, numbness, twitching, and insomnia. Because isoniazid may increase the amount of pyridoxine (vitamin $B_6$) lost from the body, vitamin $B_6$ supplements are usually given to prevent nerve damage.

## Isoproterenol

A *bronchodilator drug* used in the treatment of lung disorders (such as *asthma*, chronic *bronchitis*, and *emphysema*). Isoproterenol widens the airways in the lungs and thus improves air flow and relieves breathing difficulty. Isoproterenol is also given in the emergency treatment of *heart block* (abnormally slow heart beat) before a *pacemaker* is fitted.

Adverse effects are dry mouth, nervousness, dizziness, and palpitations.

## Isosorbide dinitrate

A long-acting form of nitroglycerin that acts as a *vasodilator drug*. It is used to reduce the severity and frequency of *angina pectoris* (chest pain due to impaired blood supply to heart muscle). Isosorbide dinitrate is also given to treat severe *heart failure* (reduced pumping efficiency).

Adverse effects include headache, hot flashes, and dizziness.

## Isotope scanning

See *Radionuclide scanning*.

## Isotretinoin

A drug derived from *vitamin A* used in the treatment of severe *acne* when other treatments have proved ineffective. Isotretinoin is also given to treat *ichthyosis* (a disorder characterized by thickening and scaling of the skin). It works by reducing the formation of sebum (natural skin oils) and keratin (the tough, outer layer of skin).

**POSSIBLE ADVERSE EFFECTS**

Isotretinoin may cause itching, dryness, and flaking of the skin. Rarely, it may cause liver damage and an increased risk of *coronary heart disease* and *peripheral vascular disease*. Isotretinoin may damage a developing fetus; pregnancy should be avoided during treatment and for at least three months after taking the drug.

## Isoxsuprine

A *vasodilator drug* used in the treatment of *peripheral vascular disease*, *transient ischemic attacks* (symptoms of *stroke* lasting less than 24 hours), and *dementia* caused by reduced blood supply to the brain. Its efficacy in the treatment of these disorders is questioned by many physicians.

Isoxsuprine also relaxes muscles in the uterus and is given to suppress contractions in premature labor.

Adverse effects of isoxsuprine include dizziness and palpitations.

## Itching

Intense, distracting irritation or tickling sensation in the skin that may be generalized (felt all over the skin's surface) or local (confined to one area). The reason for the sensation is not fully understood.

Itching is the most prominent symptom in skin disease, but does not itself necessarily indicate an underlying skin disorder. People differ in their tolerance to itching, and a person's threshold can be altered by stress, emotions, or other factors. Itching is worse when the skin is warm and when there are few distractions, making it more noticeable at night.

**CAUSES**

**GENERALIZED ITCHING** Excessive bathing, which removes the skin's natural oils and may leave the skin excessively dry and scaly, is a common cause of itching. Some people experience itching after taking certain drugs, such as cocaine, codeine, and some antibiotics. Soap, detergents, and roughly textured clothing (e.g., made of wool) also produce itching in some people.

Many elderly people suffer for no apparent reason from dry, itchy skin, especially on their backs. A similar condition affects some younger people in cold weather. Itching commonly occurs during pregnancy.

Many skin conditions produce an itchy rash—for example, *chickenpox*, *urticaria* (hives), *eczema*, and fungal infections (see *Tinea*). Less common causes include *psoriasis* or *dermatitis herpetiformis*.

Generalized skin itchiness can be a result of *diabetes mellitus*, *renal failure*, *jaundice*, and thyroid disorders. Disorders of the blood (such as *leukemia*) and of the lymphatic system (e.g., *Hodgkin's disease*) may occasionally cause itching.

**LOCAL ITCHING** Pruritus ani (itching around the anal region) occurs in adults, particularly those with such problems as *hemorrhoids*, *anal fissure*, and persistent diarrhea. Pruritus ani often results from irritation caused by overzealous cleansing after defecation. Worm infestation is the most likely cause of itching in children.

Another form of intense skin irritation confined to one area occurs with pruritus vulvae; it affects the external genitalia in women. The condition may be due to *candidiasis*, hormonal changes (at puberty, pregnancy, and the menopause), or to use of spermicides or vaginal suppositories, ointments, and deodorants.

Lice and scabies infestations cause notable itching. Insect bites, too, can produce intense skin irritation.

### TREATMENT
Specific treatment depends on the underlying cause, if known. Cooling lotions, such as calamine, relieve irritation; *emollients* reduce dryness.

Soaps often irritate itchy skin, especially if a rash is visible. They should be used only when necessary. Often, extremely mild cleansing lotions or water alone is sufficient to keep most of the skin adequately clean. Itchy skin should be handled very gently. Scratching temporarily relieves itching, but makes the itching worse in the long run. The scratching habit can be suppressed by applying a soothing lotion, salve, or wet compress to the affected areas when the urge to scratch occurs.

## -itis
A suffix meaning "inflammation of." Virtually every organ or tissue in the body can suffer inflammation (the most common form of tissue disorder), so "-itis" is by far the most common word ending in medicine. An example of its use is *bronchitis* (inflammation of the bronchi).

The term -itis is applied strictly to cases of inflammation with redness, pain, heat, and swelling. The term should not be used loosely to imply general disorder, for which the ending "-opathy" is appropriate.

## IUCD
Abbreviation for intrauterine contraceptive device. (See *IUD*.)

## IUD
A mechanical device inserted into the uterus for the purposes of *contraception*. IUDs (intrauterine contraceptive devices) became widely used in the 1960s and 1970s; except for two types, they are no longer being manufactured or sold in the US.

### TYPES
Most types of IUD are made of plastic molded into various forms and shapes. They have a plastic string that, once inserted, comes through the cervix into the vagina. The string makes removal easier and indicates the presence of the IUD.

Some IUDs are inert; others contain bioactive substances. Because of their larger size, inert IUDs are more suitable for women who have had at least one child. They must be replaced about every five years.

The bioactive (progesterone-containing) IUDs are much smaller than inert IUDs and may be used by women who have never had children, although most physicians recommend their use only by women who do not plan to have children in the future. Devices containing copper need replacing every two to three years; the progesterone-containing types should be replaced once a year.

### HOW THEY WORK
IUDs are about 97 to 98 percent effective, though it is still not certain exactly how they work. It is thought that a foreign body in the uterus prevents pregnancy by creating an inflammation in the uterine lining that destroys sperm as they pass through the uterus. It is also thought that the presence of an IUD may inhibit implantation of the fertilized egg in the uterine wall (see *Implantation, egg*).

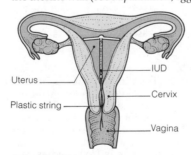

**Site of an IUD**
An IUD is inserted into the uterus; it has a plastic string that hangs down through the cervix and into the vagina.

### HOW THEY ARE USED
An IUD is usually inserted by the woman's gynecologist or family practitioner. It can be inserted any time during the menstrual cycle, but the preferred time is during or just after menstruation (because it is unlikely that the woman is pregnant and because the cervix is easier to handle). After a full-term pregnancy, a woman should wait six weeks before having an IUD inserted.

An IUD is inserted through the vagina and cervix into the uterine cavity. Most IUDs are loaded in a small plastic tube that is inserted through the cervical canal; the device is gently pushed out by means of a plunger. Once an IUD is in place, it provides immediate protection. The woman should check once or twice a week that the string is present. If it is not, the string has probably curled up into the uterus, but it is possible that the IUD has been expelled.

### WHO SHOULD NOT USE IUDS
Women who have never been pregnant are more likely to have serious complications than women who have had children. Women with no previous pregnancies usually have more pain on insertion, higher expulsion rates, and a heavier menstrual flow. A woman with *fibroids* may be advised not to have an IUD. Any woman with a history of pelvic disease or tubal infection should not use an IUD. Women with multiple partners (or whose partner has other sexual partners) are at increased risk of *pelvic inflammatory disease* (PID) and should probably avoid IUDs. Young women have a higher infection rate than older women. Women with heavy or painful periods may find the IUD makes the symptoms worse.

### COMPLICATIONS
Immediately after insertion, there may be heavy bleeding, pain, or vaginal discharge. Menstrual periods after insertion may become irregular, heavier, and more painful.

Women with IUDs also have a higher rate of *ectopic pregnancy*, especially if the pregnancy occurred with the IUD still in place. Pelvic inflammatory disease may be severe and lead to permanent infertility. A rare complication of IUD use is a perforated uterus, in which the device works its way through the wall of the uterus into the abdominal cavity, causing infection.

### OUTLOOK
Most pharmaceutical companies have discontinued the manufacture and sale of IUDs in the US because of economic factors. The cost of the large number of lawsuits claiming that IUDs have caused serious complications has been enormous.

## IVF
See *In vitro fertilization*.

## IVP
The abbreviation for intravenous *pyelography*.

# J

## Jakob-Creutzfeldt disease
See *Creutzfeldt-Jakob syndrome*.

## Jaundice
Yellowing of the skin and the whites of the eyes caused by an accumulation of the yellow-brown bile pigment bilirubin in the blood. Jaundice is the chief sign of many disorders of the liver and biliary system.

### TYPES AND CAUSES
Bilirubin is formed from *hemoglobin* (the oxygen-carrying substance in red blood cells) when old red cells are broken down, mainly by the spleen. The pigment is absorbed from the blood by the liver, where it is made soluble in water and is excreted in bile. The process can be upset in any of three ways, causing the main types of jaundice: hemolytic, hepatocellular, and obstructive.

In hemolytic jaundice, the amount of bilirubin produced is too great for the liver to process. This is caused by excessive *hemolysis* (breakdown of red cells), which can have many causes (see *Anemia, hemolytic*). Similar types of jaundice can develop in the newborn as a result of an insufficiently developed capacity of the liver to take up bilirubin. In adults, a type of jaundice similar to hemolytic jaundice can develop as a result of a mild liver disorder called *Gilbert's disease*.

In hepatocellular jaundice, bilirubin builds up in the blood because its transfer from liver cells to bile is prevented, usually as the result of acute *hepatitis* (inflammation of the liver) or *liver failure*.

In obstructive jaundice, bile is prevented from flowing out of the liver because of disorders causing blockage of the bile ducts (see *Bile duct obstruction*) such as *gallstones* or a tumor. Obstructive jaundice can also occur if the bile ducts are not present (as in *biliary atresia*) or have been destroyed within the liver (for example, in primary *biliary cirrhosis*). As a result, bile stagnates in the liver (a condition called *cholestasis*) and bilirubin is forced back into the blood.

### SYMPTOMS AND SIGNS
Sometimes (as in acute hepatitis) jaundice is only one of several signs and symptoms. In other cases (such as Gilbert's disease) it may be the sole sign of a disorder.

Obstructive or cholestatic jaundice is usually accompanied by two other characteristic features: pale feces and dark urine. The feces are pale because bilirubin, which normally colors feces brown, does not reach the intestine; the urine is dark due to large amounts of water-soluble bilirubin being filtered into it from the blood. Bilirubin may also be deposited in the skin, causing itching.

In hemolytic jaundice, both urine and feces color are normal. In hepatocellular jaundice, the feces are normal but the urine may be dark.

### DIAGNOSIS AND TREATMENT
If excessive hemolysis is suspected, *blood tests* are carried out to determine the amount of water-insoluble bilirubin. A *blood smear* indicates whether large numbers of immature red cells are present; if they are, hemolysis is the suspected cause of the jaundice.

To diagnose hepatocellular jaundice, the blood is tested and a *liver biopsy* (removal of a small sample of tissue for analysis) may be performed.

If the physician suspects obstructive jaundice, *ultrasound scanning*, *liver function tests*, and *cholangiography* may be carried out to determine if the bile ducts are diseased or blocked.

In all cases, treatment is for the underlying cause.

## Jaw
The lowest and only mobile bone of the face, also known as the mandible. The term jaw sometimes includes the bone that extends from the inner rims of the eyes to the mouth, more commonly known as the *maxilla*.

The mandible is U-shaped as seen from above and bears the lower teeth on its upper surface. It is connected to the base of the skull at the temporomandibular joints, which can be felt in the cheek just in front of the earlobe. Powerful muscles, arising from the temple on either side, attach to the jaw for movements needed in chewing and biting; other muscles allow side-to-side and downward movement.

## Jaw, dislocated
Displacement of the lower jaw from one or both of the temporomandibular joints (the joints between the jaw and the base of the skull). A dislocated jaw is usually caused by a blow or by yawning. The jaw is the most commonly dislocated joint because it is very unstable. Once dislocation has happened, it tends to recur.

### SYMPTOMS
There is pain in front of the ear on the affected side or sides and the jaw projects forward. The mouth cannot be fully closed and, as a result, the victim drools and has difficulty speaking.

### TREATMENT
A second person can easily correct the dislocation. He or she should stand in front of the victim, place a thumb on the lower back teeth at each side, and press downward. The lower jaw should then click back into position. To avoid causing injury when the teeth snap shut, the thumbs should be wrapped in cloth.

Recurrent dislocation requires an operation to stabilize the joint, such as strengthening the ligaments with stitches. However, surgery is rarely successful in curing the problem.

## Jaw, fractured
Fractures of the jaw are most often caused by a direct blow to the face. Because of the shape of the jaw, fracture often occurs not only at the site of the blow, but also on the other side of the jaw.

### SYMPTOMS
If the fracture is minor, the only symptoms may be some tenderness, pain on biting, and slight stiffness of

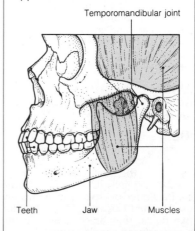

**ANATOMY OF THE JAW**
The U-shaped, mobile bone of the face that meets the skull in front of the ears at the temporomandibular joint. The jaw bears teeth on its upper surface.

Temporomandibular joint

Teeth          Jaw          Muscles

the jaw. In more severe injuries, teeth may be loosened or damaged, movement of the jaw may be severely limited, and there may be loss of feeling in the lower lip.

### DIAGNOSIS AND TREATMENT

If a fracture is suspected, X rays of the area are taken. Minor fractures are normally left to heal on their own.

For severe fractures in which the bones have become displaced, surgical treatment is required. The bone fragments are first manipulated back into the correct position. Teeth too badly damaged to be saved may require extraction. The jaw is immobilized to allow healing to occur, usually by wiring the upper and lower teeth together. If the patient has no teeth, special dentures can be constructed to hold the wires.

Some fractures cannot be adequately immobilized by this method. In such cases, an incision is made in the skin to expose the jaw bone, holes are drilled in each bone fragment, and wires are inserted and twisted together. The skin incision is sewn up with the wires in position.

### RECOVERY PERIOD

If the teeth have been wired together, the patient is given a liquid diet. The wires are usually removed after about six weeks.

## Jealousy, morbid

Preoccupation with the sexual infidelity of one's partner. The sufferer, usually a man, becomes convinced that his partner is having an affair; he constantly spies on her and often resorts to physical violence.

Morbid jealousy is usually due to *personality disorder*, *depression*, or *paranoia*, but may also occur in those suffering from *alcohol dependence* or organic *brain syndrome*.

Treatment of the underlying disorder may improve the condition, but the outlook is generally poor. Psychiatrists usually recommend separation of the partners, since morbid jealousy is a significant cause of murder within established relationships.

## Jejunal biopsy

A diagnostic test in which a small piece of tissue is removed from the lining of the *jejunum* (the middle, coiled section of the small intestine) for laboratory examination under the microscope.

### WHY IT IS DONE

The procedure is especially useful in the diagnosis of *Crohn's disease, celiac sprue, lymphoma*, and all other causes of *malabsorption* because these conditions are associated with recognizable changes in the small intestine.

### HOW IT IS DONE

The patient may be sedated slightly before the procedure is started. A small device called a Crosby capsule is attached to a length of fine tubing; both are well lubricated and the patient is asked to swallow the capsule. The tube is guided down the esophagus through the stomach and duodenum until the capsule reaches the jejunum. An X ray is then performed to ensure that the capsule is in the correct position. A syringe is used to withdraw air from the tube, causing a minute piece of tissue to be sucked into the capsule, where it is sheared off. The tube and capsule are then withdrawn and the tissue is taken from the capsule for examination.

## Jejunum

The middle, coiled section of the small *intestine*, joining the *duodenum* to the *ileum*. It is wider than the ileum and has a thicker wall, but its function is the same—the digestion of food and the absorption of nutrients from it. Among the few disorders that affect the jejunum are *celiac sprue, Crohn's disease*, and *lymphoma*.

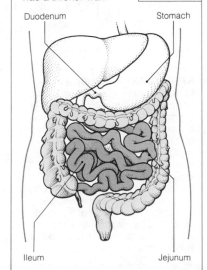

**ANATOMY OF THE JEJUNUM**
This section of the small intestine joins the duodenum to the ileum. It is wider than the ileum and has a thicker wall.

Duodenum

Stomach

Ileum

Jejunum

## Jellyfish stings

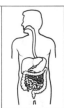

Jellyfish, together with corals, sea anemones, and Portuguese men-of-war, belong to a group of marine animals called the coelenterates. These animals have tentacles armed with stinging capsules that discharge when touched. Usually, the result of a sting is no more than an itchy or mildly painful rash, but some jellyfish and Portuguese men-of-war can cause a severe sting. In rare cases, venom entering the bloodstream may cause vomiting, sweating, shock, breathing difficulties, convulsions, and collapse. Dangerous species live mainly in tropical waters.

### TREATMENT

If fragments of jellyfish tentacle remain attached to the skin after a sting, vinegar should be applied to inactivate the stinging capsules; the tentacle fragments should then be scraped off. Analgesics (painkillers) may be taken. A severe reaction requires hospitalization and sometimes *cardiopulmonary resuscitation*. Antivenoms effective against the more dangerous species of jellyfish may be available in areas where these species are common.

## Jet lag

Interruption of the sleep/wake cycle, fatigue, and other symptoms caused by disturbance of normal body rhythms as a result of flying across different time zones.

### CAUSES

Each person has an "internal clock" that determines when the desire to sleep, wake, and eat, the release of various hormones, and many other bodily functions take place in every 24-hour period. The near 24-hour cycle of each activity is called a circadian rhythm. When an air traveler crosses several time zones, his or her day (as timed by an external clock) is longer or shorter than 24 hours, depending on the direction of the flight. Most of the traveler's circadian rhythms are unable to adjust to this shorter or longer day, resulting in jet lag when the flight is over. Jet lag is the desire to sleep during the local day, wakefulness at night, general fatigue, reduced physical and mental activity, and poor memory.

Jet lag tends to be worse after an eastward flight (which shortens the traveler's day) than after a westward one. It is most likely to affect people over 30 who normally follow an established daily routine.

J

# TYPES OF JOINTS

Some joints are fixed (e.g., the skull) and some allow a little movement (e.g., the vertebrae). Of the mobile joints, the hinge joint is the simplest. Pivot joints allow rotation only, while ellipsoidal joints allow all types of movement except pivotal. Ball-and-socket joints allow the widest range of movement.

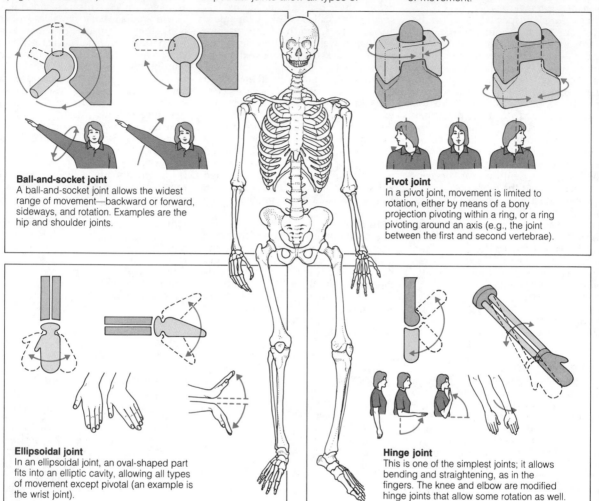

### Ball-and-socket joint
A ball-and-socket joint allows the widest range of movement—backward or forward, sideways, and rotation. Examples are the hip and shoulder joints.

### Pivot joint
In a pivot joint, movement is limited to rotation, either by means of a bony projection pivoting within a ring, or a ring pivoting around an axis (e.g., the joint between the first and second vertebrae).

### Ellipsoidal joint
In an ellipsoidal joint, an oval-shaped part fits into an elliptic cavity, allowing all types of movement except pivotal (an example is the wrist joint).

### Hinge joint
This is one of the simplest joints; it allows bending and straightening, as in the fingers. The knee and elbow are modified hinge joints that allow some rotation as well.

### STRUCTURE OF A FIXED JOINT
Fixed joints are firmly secured by fibrous tissue. The joints between the bones of the skull are an example.

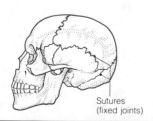

Sutures
(fixed joints)

### STRUCTURE OF A MOBILE JOINT
In mobile joints, the surfaces of the bones are coated with smooth and slippery cartilage to reduce friction during movement. The joint is sealed within a tough fibrous capsule lined with synovial membrane, which produces a clear, sticky fluid that lubricates the joint. Each joint is surrounded by strong ligaments that support it and prevent excessive movement. Movement of the joints is controlled by muscles that are attached to bone by tendons on either side of the joint.

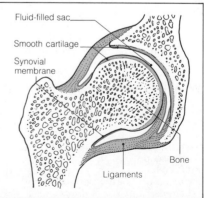

Fluid-filled sac

Smooth cartilage

Synovial membrane

Bone

Ligaments

J

PREVENTIVE MEASURES

The symptoms of jet lag can be minimized by drinking plenty of nonalcoholic fluids during the flight and avoiding heavy meals. Also, people flying east should go to bed earlier than usual for a few days before the journey; people flying west should do the opposite. If possible, try to arrive in the new time zone in the early evening and go to bed early.

It may take several days to adjust to a new time zone (about half a day to one day for each time zone crossed). The adjustment can be eased by breaking up a long journey with a stopover and by resting after the flight.

## Jigger flea
See *Chigoe*.

## Jock itch
See *Tinea*.

## Joggers' nipple
Soreness of the nipple caused by the rubbing of clothing against it, usually during sports such as jogging or long-distance running. Joggers' nipple, which affects both men and women, can be prevented by applying petroleum jelly to the nipple before prolonged running. Wearing a clean shirt also helps because sweat can aggravate the condition. Treatment involves covering the nipple with a bandage to reduce rubbing.

## Joint
The point at which two bones meet. At these junctions, the surfaces of the ends of the bones are covered with cartilage and the joint lined with a synovial membrane. Some joints are fixed (such as those between bones of the skull) and some allow a small amount of movement (those between the bodies—central areas—of the vertebrae, for example). Highly mobile joints are far more common; there are several types capable of different types of movement.

DISORDERS

Common joint injuries include *sprains*, ligament tears, cartilage damage, and tears of the joint capsule.

*Dislocation* of a joint is usually the result of injury, but is occasionally congenital. A less severe injury may cause *subluxation* (partial dislocation). Rarely, the bone ends are fractured, sometimes leading to *hemarthrosis* (bleeding into the joint) or *effusion* (accumulation of fluid in a joint) due to *synovitis* (inflammation of the lining of the joint).

Joints are commonly affected by forms of *arthritis* (inflammation of a joint). *Bursitis* (inflammation of a bursa) may occur as a result of local irritation or strain.

Permanent joint deformities may be caused by severe injury or arthritis. Temporary deformities may occur in childhood, usually affecting a joint in the legs; they resolve later in life as growth continues. Surgery may be required to relieve certain deformities.

## Joint replacement
See *Arthroplasty*.

## Joule
The international unit of *energy*, work, and heat. Approximately 4,200 joules (symbol J), or 4.2 kilojoules (kJ), equal one kilocalorie (1,000 calories, or 1 C); 1 kJ equals about 240 C.

## Jugular vein
One of three veins on each side of the neck that return deoxygenated blood from the head to the heart. Of the three (internal, external, and superficial) by far the largest is the internal jugular, which arises at the base of the skull, travels down the neck alongside the carotid arteries, and passes behind

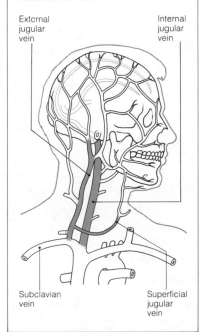

**ANATOMY OF THE JUGULAR VEIN**
These three veins on each side of the neck return blood from the head to the heart.

External jugular vein

Internal jugular vein

Subclavian vein

Superficial jugular vein

the clavicle (collarbone), where it joins the subclavian vein (the large vein that drains blood from the arms). The jugular is rarely injured because it lies deep in the structures of the neck.

## Jumpers' knee
Inflammation of the tendon below the patella (kneecap) usually caused by repetitive exercise such as long-distance running (see *Overuse injury*). Jumpers' knee can also be caused by exercise that strains the kneecap.

## Jungian theory
Ideas put forward by the Swiss psychiatrist Carl Gustav Jung (1875-1961). Originally an associate of Sigmund Freud, Jung broke away in 1913 to form his own school of analytical psychology, mainly because he did not believe that sexual drive was the only force behind all human activity. Instead, he theorized that certain ideas (called archetypes) inherited from experiences in our distant past were present in each person's unconscious and controlled the way in which each person viewed the world. Jung called these shared ideas the "collective unconscious."

Although Jung believed that each individual also had a "personal unconscious" containing experiences from his or her life, he regarded the collective unconscious as superior. Therapy was therefore aimed at putting people in touch with this source of profound ideas, particularly through interpretation of dreams.

Jung's therapeutic approach was also based on his theory of personality, which postulated two basic types, the *extrovert* and the *introvert*. He believed that one of these types dominates a person's consciousness and that the other must be brought into consciousness and reconciled with its opposite.

## Junk food

The name commonly applied to refined or processed foods, such as candy, potato chips, and sweetened carbonated beverages. Junk food provides *calories* but few of the other *nutrients* needed for a healthy diet. Small amounts of junk food are not harmful, but people who consume large quantities may not eat enough other foods to provide a well-balanced diet. (See also *Nutrition*.)

## Juvenile arthritis
See *Rheumatoid arthritis, juvenile*.

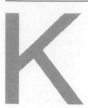

# K

## Kala-azar
A form of the insect-spread parasitic disease *leishmaniasis*. Kala-azar occurs in many parts of Africa, the Mediterranean area, and India.

## Kaolin
An *aluminum* compound used as an ingredient in some *antidiarrheal drugs*. It is thought that kaolin helps treat *diarrhea* by adsorbing *bacteria*, *viruses*, and toxins (poisons) from the intestine and eliminating them from the body when the drug is excreted in the feces.

## Kaposi's sarcoma
A condition, characterized by malignant skin tumors, that is a prominent feature of *AIDS*. In the past, Kaposi's sarcoma developed slowly and was seen almost exclusively in elderly Italian and Jewish men. In patients with AIDS, it is highly aggressive and tumors soon become widespread.

The tumors, consisting of blue-red nodules, usually start on the feet and ankles, spread further up the legs, and then appear on the hands and arms. In people with AIDS, tumors also commonly affect the gastrointestinal and respiratory tracts, where they may cause severe internal bleeding.

For mild cases of Kaposi's sarcoma, low-dose *radiation therapy* is usually effective. For more severe cases, *anticancer drugs* may be necessary to slow the spread of the tumors.

## Kawasaki disease
An acute childhood illness that affects many systems in the body. It is also called mucocutaneous lymph node syndrome. The condition was first observed in Japan in the 1960s. It is becoming increasingly common in the US in all children, not only those of Japanese ethnic origin. It usually occurs in the first two years of life. The cause is unknown.

### SYMPTOMS
Fever is the first symptom; it usually persists for one or two weeks. Other characteristic symptoms are *conjunc-tivitis*, dryness and cracking of the lips, and swollen lymph nodes in the neck. Toward the end of the first week of illness, the palms and soles become red, the hands and feet swell, and a rash similar to that of measles appears over the body. By the end of the second week, the skin at the tips of the fingers and toes peels and the other symptoms subside.

### TREATMENT AND OUTLOOK
There is no cure, but *aspirin* may help prevent possible heart complications. Most children make a complete recovery. In about 1 to 2 percent of cases, however, sudden death occurs after the acute phase of the illness, usually due to *coronary thrombosis*.

## Keloid
A raised, hard, irregularly shaped, itchy scar on the skin. A keloid occurs because of a defective healing process in which an excess of *collagen* forms at the site of a healing scar. Keloids are more common in black people than in white people.

Keloids can occur anywhere on the body, but are most common over the sternum (breastbone) and over the shoulder. They often enlarge after developing and may be unsightly; after some months most flatten and cease to be itchy.

Injections of *corticosteroid drugs* directly into the keloid may reduce itchiness and cause some shrinkage. Surgical removal is of little use since the new scar that forms is almost always a keloid.

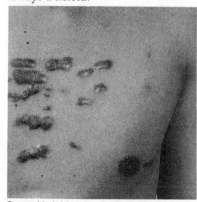

**Crop of keloids over the breastbone**
These overgrowths of scar tissue usually flatten out and become less noticeable over a period of months or years.

## Keratin
 A fibrous protein that is the main constituent of the outermost layer of the *skin*, *nails*, and *hair*. Keratin is a tough substance that is resistant to damage from a wide range of chemical and physical agents.

## Keratitis
Inflammation of the *cornea* (the front part of the eyeball). The term is often used loosely to refer to corneal disorders that do not meet the strict definition of inflammation (since inflammation involves blood vessels and the normal cornea has none). A better general term for disorders of the cornea is *keratopathy*.

True keratitis is rare. One form is interstitial keratitis, which affects about 70 percent of children with congenital *syphilis*. Symptoms include eye pain, excessive watering, and photophobia (sensitivity to bright light); blood vessels grow into the cornea. Treatment with antibiotics usually restores vision.

## Keratoacanthoma
A harmless skin nodule that generally occurs singly on the face or arm of elderly people. Initially resembling a small, round wart with a soft center, the keratoacanthoma grows rapidly over a period of about eight weeks. At this point it reaches its maximum size of about 0.8 inch (2 cm) across. The mature nodule has bulging sides and its center may have a whitish appearance. Without treatment, the keratoacanthoma slowly disappears after reaching its mature state.

The cause of the growth is unknown, but it tends to be more common in people who have had years of exposure to strong sunlight and in people taking long-term *immunosuppressant drugs*.

A *biopsy* (removal of a small piece of tissue for analysis) may be necessary to distinguish a keratoacanthoma from a *squamous cell carcinoma*, a form of skin cancer.

## Keratoconjunctivitis
A disorder of the cornea associated with *conjunctivitis*. The most common form is epidemic keratoconjunctivitis, caused by a virus that usually causes painful swelling of a small lymph gland in front of the ear. It is highly infectious and is spread mainly by sharing towels or by unsterile instruments and eye drops.

The conjunctivitis is often severe, with notable redness, swelling, or destruction of the surface layer of the conjunctiva, leaving a whitish membrane. Seven to ten days after the onset, tiny opaque spots resembling snowflakes develop in the cornea. The spots may persist for many months and sometimes interfere with vision.

There is no specific treatment for epidemic keratoconjunctivitis. The corneal opacities can sometimes be minimized with *corticosteroid drugs* in eye-drop form. (See also *Keratoconjunctivitis sicca*.)

## Keratoconjunctivitis sicca

A condition of persistent corneal and conjunctival dryness caused by deficiency in tear production. Commonly referred to as "dry eye," keratoconjunctivitis sicca occurs in *autoimmune disorders* such as *rheumatoid arthritis*, *Sjögren's syndrome*, and systemic *lupus erythematosus*; all of these conditions can damage the tear-producing glands. Prolonged dryness may cause blurred vision, burning, itching, and grittiness. In severe cases, opacification or ulceration of the cornea may occur. The most effective treatment for dry eyes is artificial tears, which may require frequent use.

## Keratoconus

A condition of abnormal corneal growth in which both corneas gradually become thinned and conical.

Keratoconus usually starts around puberty and affects more females than males. It causes increasing *myopia* (nearsightedness) and a progressive distortion of vision that cannot be fully corrected by glasses. Hard contact lenses improve vision in the early stages but are less effective as the condition progresses.

A *corneal graft* is usually performed when vision has seriously deteriorated and contact lenses no longer are helpful. The results of corneal grafting are generally excellent.

## Keratolytic drugs

Drugs that loosen and remove keratin (the tough, outer layer of the skin). Keratolytic drugs, which include preparations of *sulfur* and *salicylic acid*, are used in the treatment of skin and scalp disorders, such as *warts*, callosities (see *Callus, skin*), *acne*, *dandruff*, and *psoriasis*.

## Keratomalacia

The last stage of corneal damage due to *vitamin A* deficiency. Keratomalacia usually occurs only in severely malnourished children; it is very rare in developed countries.

Prolonged lack of vitamin A causes severe dryness of the eyes with a characteristic foamy patch on the cor-

ners of the conjunctiva. There may also be a gritty feeling in the eyelids and sensitivity to bright light. Until this point, the condition is easily reversible by taking large doses of vitamin A. If the deficiency is not treated, keratomalacia develops and the cornea becomes opaque and ulcerated. Perforation of the cornea is common, usually leading to loss of the eye from infection.

## Keratopathy

A general term used to describe a wide variety of disorders of the *cornea* (the front part of the eyeball). The word also forms part of the name of certain specific disorders.

Actinic keratopathy is damage to the outer layer of the cornea by ultraviolet light, either from the sun or from artificial sources, such as sunlamps or arc welding torches. The corneal layer tends to strip off, exposing the nerve endings and causing severe pain. Skiers or mountaineers may suffer a similar effect known as snow blindness.

Exposure keratopathy is damage to the cornea caused by loss of the normal protection afforded by the tear film and the blink reflex. It may occur in a variety of conditions in which the lids cannot cover the cornea, including severe *exophthalmos*, *facial palsy*, and *ectropion*.

## Keratoplasty

See *Corneal graft*.

## Keratosis

A skin growth caused by an overproduction of *keratin* (the main skin protein). Keratoses occur mainly in the elderly.

### TYPES

**SEBORRHEIC KERATOSES** Often called seborrheic warts, they range from flat, dark brown, rough patches to small, wartlike protrusions and are covered with a greasy, removable crust. Seborrheic keratoses are completely harmless, but can be unsightly.

**SOLAR KERATOSES** Small, wartlike, red or flesh-colored growths that appear on exposed parts of the body as a result of overexposure to sun over a period of years. Solar keratoses may rarely develop into skin cancer, usually a *squamous cell carcinoma*.

### TREATMENT

Unless they are large and unsightly, seborrheic keratoses require no treatment. However, solar keratoses must always be removed because of the risk of skin cancer. Removal is usually

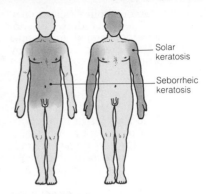

**Sites of keratoses**
Seborrheic keratoses occur mainly on the trunk; solar keratoses usually affect the face, arms, and hands.

done as an outpatient procedure by *cryosurgery* (the destruction of tissue by extreme cold).

## Keratosis pilaris

A very common skin condition in which patches of raised, rough skin appear on the upper arms, thighs, and buttocks. The openings of the hair follicles become distended with hard plugs of *keratin* (the main skin protein) and the hairs that grow in them may be distorted.

The condition occurs most commonly in older children, adolescents, and obese people, and is often worse in winter. It is not serious and usually clears up on its own. In severe cases, symptoms can be improved by rubbing a mixture of salicylic acid and soft paraffin into the affected areas; scrubbing these areas with a loofah may also help.

## Keratotomy, radial

A relatively new surgical procedure to reduce *myopia* (nearsightedness).

The results of radial keratotomy vary and the effect is not always per-

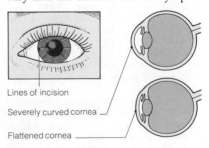

Lines of incision
Severely curved cornea
Flattened cornea

**Procedure for keratotomy**
Eight or more radial cuts are made in the cornea, avoiding the central zone. During healing, the scars contract, causing the cornea to become flatter and less powerful.

manent. Serious complications may develop. The procedure is not generally recommended for people whose vision can be corrected by glasses or contact lenses.

## Kerion

 A red, pustular swelling that develops as a reaction to a fungal infection, usually scalp ringworm (see *Tinea*). The inflammation gradually subsides over six to eight weeks but, if severe, may leave a scar and permanent loss of hair from the affected area. It is treated by applying ichthammol paste to the swelling and by taking the antibiotic griseofulvin.

## Kernicterus

A rare disorder in which excess bilirubin (a pigment derived from the breakdown of red blood cells) causes brain damage in newborn (especially premature) infants, resulting in a form of mental retardation.

### SYMPTOMS AND SIGNS

Excess bilirubin produces signs of *jaundice* in the first few days of life. In addition, the baby becomes more and more listless, sometimes adopting a characteristic posture with arched back and neck. Without treatment, the baby is likely to die at the end of the first week of life. Survivors may be deaf and may suffer from *athetosis* (uncontrollable, writhing movements) and *spasticity* (abnormal muscle stiffness). Mental retardation, bizarre eye movements, difficulty speaking, and a proneness to seizures may follow.

### PREVENTION AND TREATMENT

Kernicterus is completely preventable if jaundice is treated promptly; there is no cure for the brain damage if kernicterus has occurred.

## Ketoconazole

An *antifungal drug* used in the treatment of severe fungal infections of the lungs, brain, kidney, and lymph glands (see *Fungi*). Ketoconazole is also given to treat *candidiasis* (thrush) of the skin, mouth, or vagina when other antifungal preparations have proved ineffective.

Ketoconazole may cause nausea but it can sometimes be avoided if the drug is taken with food. Other possible adverse effects include rash and, rarely, liver damage.

## Ketoprofen

A *nonsteroidal anti-inflammatory drug* (NSAID) prescribed as an *analgesic* (painkiller) in the treatment of injury to soft tissues, such as muscles and ligaments. Ketoprofen is also given to reduce joint pain and stiffness in people with types of arthritis, including *rheumatoid arthritis*, *osteoarthritis*, and *ankylosing spondylitis*.

Ketoprofen may cause abdominal pain, nausea, indigestion, and an increased risk of *peptic ulcer*.

## Ketosis

A potentially serious condition in which excessive amounts of ketones accumulate in the body. Ketones are substances chemically related to acetone, which is found in solvents such as nail polish remover. Ketosis results whenever glucose is not available to use as a source of energy, which forces the body to use fats instead. This, in turn, leads to fatty acids being released into the blood; they are then converted to ketones.

The underlying causes of ketosis include fasting or starvation, and untreated or inadequately controlled *diabetes mellitus*, in which the lack of insulin prevents glucose from being used as fuel.

Symptoms and signs may include sweet, "fruity-smelling" breath, loss of appetite, nausea, vomiting, and abdominal pain. If the condition is not treated, confusion, unconsciousness, and death may follow.

Ketosis can be diagnosed by a test to detect ketones in the urine. Treatment is the same as for diabetes unless the cause is fasting or starvation, in which case gradual reintroduction of a nutritious diet is usually effective.

## Kidney

The organ responsible for filtering the blood and excreting waste products and excess water in the form of urine. The kidney, ureter, bladder, and urethra make up the *urinary tract*.

### STRUCTURE

There are two kidneys, each about 4 to 5 inches long and about 6 ounces in weight. They lie in the abdomen underneath the liver on the right and the spleen on the left. The arteries that supply the kidneys arise directly from the aorta (the main artery of the body leading from the heart). Once within the kidneys, the renal arteries divide into smaller and smaller branches, ending in capillaries in the glomeruli (the kidney's primary filtering units). Each kidney contains about 1 million glomeruli, which pass the filtered blood through long tubules into the medulla (the central collecting

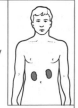

### LOCATION OF THE KIDNEYS

The kidneys are situated at the back of the abdominal cavity, just above the waist, on either side of the spinal column. The kidney on the right lies below the liver, while the kidney on the left is situated below the spleen. The arteries that supply the kidneys arise directly from the aorta.

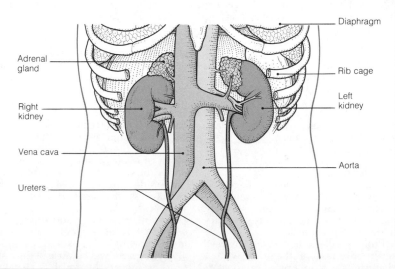

Diaphragm

Rib cage

Left kidney

Aorta

Adrenal gland

Right kidney

Vena cava

Ureters

region of the kidney). The glomeruli and tubules make up the nephrons, the functioning units of the kidney. As people age, the number of functioning nephrons is reduced; this process may be speeded up by disease.

**FUNCTION**

The main functions of the kidney are to regulate blood and electrolytes and to eliminate waste products. The most important waste products are those generated by the breakdown of proteins. The kidneys also control the body's acid-base balance. When blood and body fluids become too acid or too alkaline, the urine acidity is altered to restore the balance. When excess water is ingested, the kidney excretes it; when water is lost (as a result of diarrhea or sweating), the kidney conserves it (see *ADH*).

The kidney also produces several hormones, including erythropoietin, which regulates the production and release of red blood cells from the bone marrow. *Vitamin D* is converted into active hormonal form by the kidney. Renin, an enzyme released by the kidney when blood pressure falls, acts on a protein in the blood to produce *angiotensin* (a powerful constrictor of small arteries that helps regulate blood pressure). Angiotensin also controls the release of *aldosterone*, an adrenal hormone that acts on the tubules to promote reabsorption of sodium and excretion of potassium.

## Kidney cancer

Cancers that have their origins in the kidneys themselves are not rare. Cancer that starts in other organs rarely spreads to the kidneys.

**TYPES**

There are three main types of cancer arising in the kidneys.

**RENAL CELL CARCINOMA** This is the most common type of kidney cancer, accounting for about 75 percent of all kidney growths. The tumor usually occurs after the age of 40 and affects twice as many men as women. The most common symptom is *hematuria* (blood in the urine). There may be pain in the loins, a lump in the abdomen, fever, or weight loss. About 25 percent of patients survive five years or more because the tumor often has spread to the lungs, bone, liver, and brain by the time treatment is started.

**NEPHROBLASTOMA** Also called Wilms' tumor, this cancer accounts for about 20 percent of all cancers in children. It is found mainly in children under the age of 4 years and occurs almost twice as often in males. Nephroblastoma

## THE FUNCTION OF THE KIDNEY

The kidney is essential to the regulation of the body's fluid balance and acid-base balance. The kidney contains about 1 million nephrons, each of which consists of a glomerulus and a tubule that drain urine into the renal pelvis. Capillaries feed each glomerulus and surround each tubule.

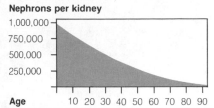

### RENAL FUNCTION AND AGE

The efficiency of the kidney diminishes with age as the number of functional nephrons is reduced.

**Nephrons per kidney**

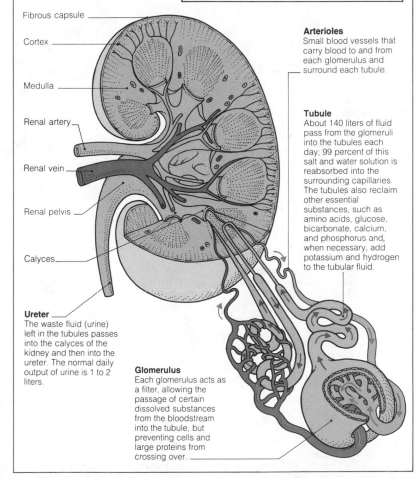

Fibrous capsule

Cortex

Medulla

Renal artery

Renal vein

Renal pelvis

Calyces

**Ureter**
The waste fluid (urine) left in the tubules passes into the calyces of the kidney and then into the ureter. The normal daily output of urine is 1 to 2 liters.

**Arterioles**
Small blood vessels that carry blood to and from each glomerulus and surround each tubule.

**Tubule**
About 140 liters of fluid pass from the glomeruli into the tubules each day; 99 percent of this salt and water solution is reabsorbed into the surrounding capillaries. The tubules also reclaim other essential substances, such as amino acids, glucose, bicarbonate, calcium, and phosphorus and, when necessary, add potassium and hydrogen to the tubular fluid.

**Glomerulus**
Each glomerulus acts as a filter, allowing the passage of certain dissolved substances from the bloodstream into the tubule, but preventing cells and large proteins from crossing over.

grows rapidly and is often felt as a lump in the abdomen. This cancer occasionally causes abdominal pain. Nephroblastoma frequently spreads to the lungs, liver, and brain. If treatment is started early, about 50 to 80 percent of children survive.

**TRANSITIONAL CELL CARCINOMA** This type arises from cells lining the renal pelvis. It develops in tobacco smokers and in people who have consumed very large quantities of analgesics (painkillers) over the course of many years. Hematuria is a common symptom; *hydronephrosis* (distention of the kidney with urine) may occur due to blockage of the ureter. Survival rates vary greatly, depending in part on early detection and treatment of the tumor.

K

## DISORDERS OF THE KIDNEY

The kidneys are susceptible to a wide range of disorders. However, only one normal kidney is needed for good health, so disease is rarely life-threatening unless it affects both kidneys and has reached an advanced stage.

*Hypertension* (high blood pressure) can be both a cause and effect of kidney damage. Other effects of serious disease or damage include the *nephrotic syndrome* (in which large amounts of protein are lost in the urine and fluid collects in body tissues) and acute or chronic *renal failure*.

### CONGENITAL AND GENETIC DISORDERS

Congenital abnormalities of the kidneys are fairly common. In *horseshoe kidney*, the two kidneys are joined at their base. Some people are born with one kidney missing, both kidneys on one side, or a kidney that is partially duplicated and gives rise to two ureters (duplex kidney). These conditions seldom cause problems. In rare cases, a baby is born with kidneys that are so underdeveloped that they are barely functional.

Polycystic disease of the kidneys is a serious inherited disorder in which multiple cysts develop on both kidneys (see *Kidney, polycystic*). In *Fanconi's syndrome* and *renal tubular acidosis* (which are rare), there are subtle abnormalities in the functioning of the kidney tubules, so that certain substances are inappropriately lost in the urine.

### IMPAIRED BLOOD SUPPLY

Various diseases may cause damage to, or lead to obstruction of, the small blood vessels within the kidneys, impairing blood flow. *Diabetes mellitus* and *hemolytic-uremic syndrome* are examples. In physiological *shock*, blood pressure and flow through the kidneys are seriously reduced; this can cause a type of damage known as acute tubular necrosis. The larger blood vessels in the kidney may be affected by *periarteritis nodosa* and systemic *lupus erythematosus*. In rare cases, there is a defect of the renal artery supplying a kidney, which may lead to hypertension and tissue damage.

### AUTOIMMUNE DISORDERS

*Glomerulonephritis* refers to an important group of autoimmune disorders in which the glomerular filtering units of the kidneys become inflamed. It sometimes develops after infection with streptococcal bacteria.

### TUMORS

Benign *kidney tumors* are rare. They may cause *hematuria* (blood in the urine), although most cause no symptoms. Malignant tumors are also rare. Renal cell carcinoma, the most common type, occurs mostly in adults over 40; nephroblastoma (Wilms' tumor) affects mainly children under 4 (see *Kidney cancer*).

### METABOLIC DISORDERS

Kidney stones are common in middle age. They are usually caused by excessive concentrations of various substances (such as calcium) or lack of inhibitors of crystallization in the urine. In *hyperuricemia*, there is a tendency for uric acid stones to form (see *Calculi, urinary tract*).

### INFECTION

Infection of a kidney is called *pyelonephritis*. An important predisposing factor is obstruction of the flow of urine through the urinary tract, leading to stagnation and subsequent infection spreading up from the bladder. The cause of the obstruction may be a congenital defect of the kidney or ureter, a kidney or ureteral stone, a bladder tumor, or, in a man, enlargement of the prostate gland.

Tuberculosis of the kidney is caused by infection carried by the blood from elsewhere in the body, usually the lungs.

### DRUGS

Allergic reactions to certain drugs can cause an acute kidney disease, with most of the damage affecting the kidney tubules. Other drugs may directly damage the kidneys if taken in large amounts for prolonged periods. For example, renal failure can develop after many years of taking excessive amounts of analgesics. Some potent antibiotics can damage the kidney tubules, producing acute tubular necrosis.

### OTHER DISORDERS

*Hydronephrosis* refers to a kidney swollen with urine as a result of obstruction further down the urinary tract. In the *crush syndrome*, kidney function is disrupted by proteins (released into the blood from severely damaged muscles) that block the filtering mechanisms.

---

### INVESTIGATION

Kidney disorders are investigated by *kidney imaging* techniques such as *ultrasound scanning*, intravenous or retrograde *pyelography*, *angiography*, and *CT scanning*; by *renal biopsy* (removal of a small amount of tissue for analysis); by *blood tests*; and by *kidney function tests*, such as *urinalysis*.

---

### DIAGNOSIS AND TREATMENT

Diagnosis is made by intravenous *pyelography* or by renal *angiography*. Treatment consists of *nephrectomy* (removal of the kidney) and sometimes removal of the ureter as well. In the case of a nephroblastoma, nephrectomy is followed by *radiation therapy* and *chemotherapy*.

## Kidney cyst

A fluid-filled sac within the kidney. Most are noncancerous.

Simple kidney cysts are found in about half the people over 50; most of them develop for no known reason. The cyst usually produces no symptoms unless it becomes large enough to cause pain in the lower back due to pressure from a buildup of fluid. Multiple cysts sometimes occur in one or both kidneys.

Kidney cysts also occur in polycystic kidney disease (see *Kidney, polycystic*), a hereditary condition that often leads to *renal failure* before the age of 50.

### DIAGNOSIS AND TREATMENT

Cysts are frequently discovered only when the person is being examined for some other reason. Treatment is not usually necessary. *Aspiration* of the cyst may be performed to ensure that there is no malignancy or to relieve severe pain. When the cyst is large, fluid often reaccumulates, requiring excision.

## Kidney failure

See *Renal failure*.

## Kidney function tests

Tests performed to investigate urinary symptoms and kidney disorders. Kidney function tests may also be performed as part of a routine investigation before major surgery, or before prescribing drugs that are eliminated by the kidney. The tests are also performed to determine the function of a transplanted kidney.

### TYPES

*Urinalysis* is a simple kidney function test. Collected urine is examined under the microscope for blood cells, pus cells, and casts (cells and mucuslike material that accumulate within the tubules and pass into the urine). Urine may also be cultured to confirm the presence of infection. It also may be tested for substances that are present only when the kidneys are diseased or damaged.

Kidney function can be assessed by measuring the concentration of substances in the blood (such as *urea* and creatinine) normally eliminated from the body via healthy kidneys. The creatinine clearance test provides an assessment of kidney function by comparing the amount of creatinine in the blood with the amount excreted in the urine over a timed interval, usually 24 hours.

Kidney function may also be assessed by *kidney imaging* techniques, which can help identify whether one or both kidneys are diseased.

## Kidney imaging

Techniques for visualizing the kidneys, usually performed for diagnostic purposes.

### TYPES

*Ultrasound scanning* provides remarkably clear pictures of the kidney. It can show an enlarged kidney, indicate the site of any blockage, and show the presence of a cyst or other tumor.

Conventional *X rays* show the outlines of the kidney and most kidney stones. Intravenous *pyelography* (in which a radiopaque contrast material is injected into a vein) gives a good picture of the internal anatomy of the kidney and ureters, as well as the presence of stones. *Angiography* involves injecting a material similar to that used in intravenous pyelograms into the renal arteries or veins to demonstrate the blood supply of the kidneys. When the material is injected into the arteries, it is known as arteriography. Digital subtraction angiography permits imaging of the renal circulation with less contrast material and greater safety.

*CT scanning* provides a complete cross section of the kidney displayed as computerized X-ray pictures. It is particularly useful for showing abscesses or tumors.

*Radionuclide scanning* is cheaper than conventional X rays and exposes the patient to less radiation. The two types usually used for the kidney are the DMSA scan and DTPA scan. DMSA is a substance given by intravenous injection that binds to the cells of the kidney tubules and gives a single static picture of the kidneys, indicating their relative size, shape, position, and function. DTPA, also given intravenously, is filtered by the glomeruli and passes out in the urine. Pictures are taken at intervals to record its passage through the renal tract. DTPA provides similar information to that provided by the intravenous pyelogram, although the anatomical details are less clear.

## Kidney, polycystic

An inherited disorder in which there are numerous cysts in both kidneys. The cysts gradually increase in size until most of the normal kidney tissue is destroyed; cysts may also occur in the liver and, rarely, in other organs. Polycystic kidney disease is distinguished from multiple simple cysts of the kidneys, which occur commonly with age (see *Kidney cyst*).

### TYPES

**ADULT POLYCYSTIC DISEASE** This disorder shows an autosomal dominant pattern of inheritance (see *Genetic disorders*). Symptoms, which may appear at any time (but usually appear in middle age) include abdominal swelling, pain, *hematuria* (blood in the urine), and frequent *urinary tract infections*. As the disease progresses, *hypertension* and *renal failure* may result.

**JUVENILE POLYCYSTIC DISEASE** This rare disorder causes *renal failure* in infants and young children. It is usually diagnosed at birth because of massive enlargement of the kidneys.

### TREATMENT

There is no effective treatment for preserving kidney function in polycystic kidney disease. Symptoms of renal failure can be treated by *dialysis* (artificial purification of the blood) and *kidney transplant*.

## Kidney stone

See *Calculus, urinary tract*.

## Kidney transplant

A transplant operation in which the diseased kidney of a person who has chronic *renal failure* is replaced by a transplanted healthy kidney, either from a living donor or a cadaver. One healthy donor kidney is sufficient to maintain the health of the recipient.

Kidney transplantation is more straightforward than the transplantation of any other major organ and is by far the most commonly performed. In addition, the failure of a kidney transplant is far less serious than an unsuccessful heart, liver, or lung transplant because kidney function can be taken over by *dialysis*.

### HOW IT IS DONE

For a description of a kidney transplant, see box (next page).

### OUTLOOK

Kidney transplants are successful in more than 80 percent of cases. This figure climbs to more than 90 percent if the donor is a close blood relative. The primary danger is rejection of the donated kidney within the first month or two after transplantation. If the kidney is rejected, the patient returns to dialysis (artificial purification of the blood). However, more transplants may be attempted if the patient is in good health otherwise. All kidney transplant patients must take a lifelong course of *immunosuppressant drugs* to prevent rejection.

## Kidney tumors

Growths of the kidney. Kidney tumors may be malignant (see *Kidney cancer*) or benign.

*Fibromas*, *lipomas*, and *leiomyomas* (which are benign) often cause no symptoms and may be discovered only during surgery on the kidney. Occasionally, a *hemangioma* grows very large and is mistaken for a cancer; it may also cause *hematuria* (blood in the urine).

No treatment is necessary for benign tumors unless they are very large or cause pain or bleeding.

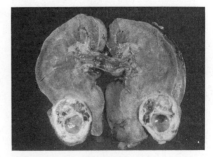

**Example of a kidney tumor**
A malignant tumor of one kidney (sliced in half). Surgical removal of a kidney tumor is always necessary.

K

## PROCEDURE FOR A KIDNEY TRANSPLANT

The donated kidney comes from a close (living) blood relative of the patient or from any person who consented to medical use of organs after death (cadaver transplant). To prevent rejection of the kidney by the recipient's *immune system,* the tissue type and blood group of recipient and donor must be a close match (see *Transplant surgery*).

### HOW IT IS DONE

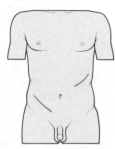

**Removal**
The kidney is removed via an incision under the ribs.

**Insertion**
The donor kidney is in-serted low in the pelvis.

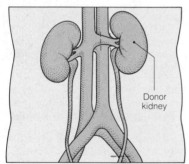

Donor kidney

**1** Usually the left kidney is removed from living donors because it has a longer vein than the right and is easier to remove safely. After removal, the kidney is flushed with saline solution.

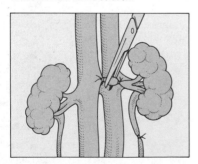

**2** The surgeon may remove one or both of the patient's kidneys. Before removing a kidney, it is necessary first to clamp and cut the renal blood vessels that supply the kidney. The ureter must also be clamped and cut.

### DIALYSIS AND TRANSPLANTATION IN THE US

About one third to one half of new patients with end-stage kidney failure are suitable for a transplant, but many have to wait some time for a suitable donor kidney to become available; in the meantime they add to the growing number of patients undergoing dialysis.

**Year**

| Year | Transplants | Patients on dialysis |
|------|-------------|----------------------|
| 1986 | 8,976 | 90,886 |
| 1984 | 6,968 | 78,483 |
| 1982 | 5,358 | 65,765 |
| 1980 | 4,697 | 52,364 |

**Key**
Patients on dialysis
Transplants

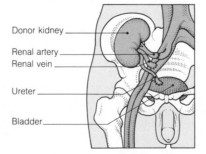

**Maintaining the kidneys**
Kidneys from a cadaver can be maintained for transplantation by a simple machine that passes a cooling saline solution through them.

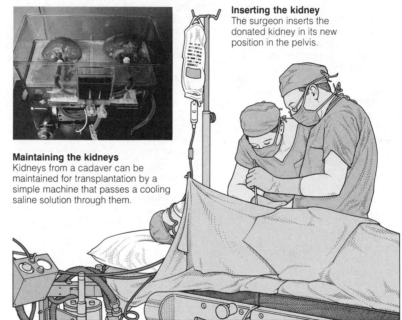

**Inserting the kidney**
The surgeon inserts the donated kidney in its new position in the pelvis.

Donor kidney
Renal artery
Renal vein
Ureter
Bladder

**3** The donor kidney is usually placed in the pelvis. The renal artery and vein of the donor kidney are joined to the recipient's artery and vein and the lower end of the donor ureter is connected to the recipient's bladder. The clamps are then removed.

### THE DONOR (AFTER THE OPERATION)

The health of the donor is not affected by losing one kidney; the remaining kidney enlarges to take over full function.

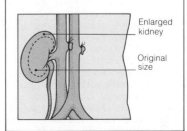

Enlarged kidney
Original size

## Kilocalorie

The unit of energy equal to 1,000 *calories*. In dietetics, a kilocalorie is often called simply a Calorie.

## Kilojoule

The unit of energy equal to 1,000 *joules*, abbreviated kJ.

## Kleptomania

A recurring inability to resist the impulse to steal objects that are not necessarily wanted or needed. The condition is rare, although it is often used by shoplifters and other thieves as an excuse.

In true kleptomania, the person experiences an increasing sense of tension before committing the act of theft and a sense of relief or pleasure while carrying it out. The act is not preplanned and little thought is given to the consequences, but later there may be anxiety and depression caused by the fear of being caught.

Kleptomania is usually a sign of an immature personality. It may also be caused by *dementia* and be the result of some forms of brain damage.

## Klinefelter's syndrome

A *chromosomal abnormality* in which a male has one or more extra X *chromosomes* in his cells, giving him a chromosome complement of XXY or, more rarely, XXXY, XXXXY, and so on (instead of XY). About one in every 500 male infants born has the syndrome. The chances of a baby having the condition increase with age of the mother.

**SYMPTOMS AND SIGNS**
The features of Klinefelter's syndrome may pass unnoticed until puberty, when *gynecomastia* (breast enlargement) occurs and the testes remain small. Affected males are infertile due to *azoospermia* (absence of sperm production). They are usually tall and thin, and the body shape looks female rather than male. The incidence of mental retardation is higher in people with Klinefelter's syndrome than in the general population.

**DIAGNOSIS AND TREATMENT**
Diagnosis is confirmed by *chromosome analysis*. There is no treatment, although mastectomy may be performed if gynecomastia causes psychological distress; hormonal treatment may be used to induce secondary sexual characteristics, such as growth of facial hair. Parents who have had an affected child should receive *genetic counseling*.

## Klumpke's paralysis

Paralysis of the lower arm, with wasting of the small muscles in the hand and numbness of the fingers (excluding the thumb) and of the inside of the forearm.

Klumpke's paralysis is caused by injury to the first thoracic nerve (one of the *spinal nerves*) in the brachial plexus (the network of nerves behind the shoulder blade); injury to this nerve is usually the result of dislocation of the shoulder.

In some cases, there may also be drooping of the upper eyelid, constriction of the pupil, and loss of sweating on one side of the face and neck (a collection of symptoms known as *Horner's syndrome*).

The condition is usually permanent. The only treatment consists of exercises to maintain mobility of the joints.

## Knee

The joint between the femur (thigh bone) and tibia (shin); the patella (kneecap) lies across the front of the joint. The knee is a modified hinge joint, capable of bending and straightening, and capable of slight rotation in the bent position.

**STRUCTURE**
Two disks of protective cartilage called menisci (see *Meniscus*) cover the surfaces of the femur and tibia; they reduce friction between the bones during movement. The joint is partly surrounded by a fibrous capsule lined with synovial membrane, which secretes a lubricating fluid that allows the cartilage to move freely.

Strong ligaments on each side of the joint provide support and limit side-to-side movement. *Cruciate ligaments* within the joint, which cross over each other as they run diagonally between the femur and tibia, provide additional support, prevent overbending and overstraightening of the knee, and limit sliding movement between the bones.

Bursas (fluid-filled sacs) are present above and below the patella and behind the knee. The *quadriceps muscles* (which run along the front of the thigh) straighten the knee; the *hamstring muscles* at the back of the thigh bend the knee.

**DISORDERS**
Sudden twisting of the knee may cause a ligament sprain or tear a meniscus. If a meniscus is torn and a fragment of the cartilage catches between the surfaces of the joint, the knee may become temporarily locked in one position.

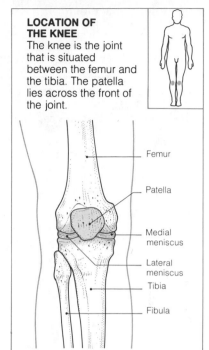

**LOCATION OF THE KNEE**
The knee is the joint that is situated between the femur and the tibia. The patella lies across the front of the joint.

Femur

Patella

Medial meniscus

Lateral meniscus

Tibia

Fibula

K

Severe damage to a joint, often as the result of a sports injury, may cause *hemarthrosis* (bleeding into the joint); minor injuries may lead to *synovitis* (inflammation of the joint lining). Repetitive activity, such as running, may cause inflammation of the tendon below the patella. In children, inflammation of the tibial tubercle (the bony prominence beneath the knee) may occur temporarily (see *Osgood-Schlatter disease*).

*Bursitis* (inflammation of a bursa) usually occurs in response to local pressure on the front of the knee. Fluid escaping from a bursa behind the knee causes a *Baker's cyst*.

Arthritic conditions most likely to affect the knee are *osteoarthritis*, *rheumatoid arthritis*, and retropatellar arthritis (inflammation of the undersurface of the patella). A condition similar to retropatellar arthritis, known as *chondromalacia patellae*, is common in adolescents.

Fractures of the lower femur, upper tibia, or the patella disrupt normal movement of the knee. A sharp blow to the knee may result in dislocation of the patella.

*Knock-knee* and *bowleg* are common in childhood as temporary deformities that resolve as growth continues; in adults, they may be caused by injury or disease.

## Knee joint replacement

A surgical procedure to replace a diseased knee joint with an artificial substitute. Early replacement knees were simply large hinges. Today, most artificial knees take the form of metal and plastic implants that cover the worn cartilage. The aim is generally to preserve as much of the original joint as possible.

### PROCEDURE FOR A KNEE REPLACEMENT

The surgeon usually makes one long incision, cuts through the joint capsule and synovial membrane, and then pushes aside the patella to reach the joint. Special instruments are used to make precise measurements and to cut away areas of bone so that the artificial components will fit and move correctly.

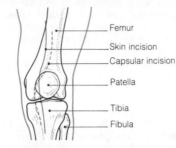

Femur
Skin incision
Capsular incision
Patella
Tibia
Fibula

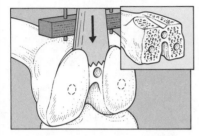

**1** The lower end of the femur is shaped and holes are drilled into it to accept the femoral component of the prosthesis. Cutting and drilling are done using special instruments.

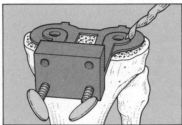

**2** The upper end of the tibia is shaped and holes are drilled into it to accept the tibial component. The cutting and drilling are again carried out using special precision instruments.

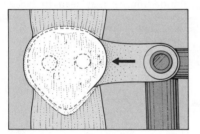

**3** The back part of the patella is cut away to leave a flat surface. Small holes are then drilled into this surface to accept the patellar component of the artificial joint.

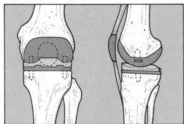

**4** Having achieved a satisfactory fit using trial components, the final prosthesis is cemented in place. Excess cement is then removed and a final check is made of the joint movements.

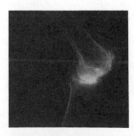

**X ray of arthritic knee**
Severe wear and tear of the bone and cartilage can easily be seen.

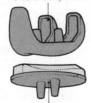

Femoral component

Tibial component

**Knee prosthesis**
The two main components fit over the femur and tibia.

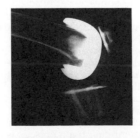

**X ray of artificial knee**
The X ray shows the components of the prosthesis in position.

### WHY IT IS DONE

Knee joint replacement is most often carried out in older people whose knees are severely affected by pain and impaired motion due to *osteoarthritis* or *rheumatoid arthritis*. An artificial knee is not normally recommended for younger patients because it does not restore the full range of movements and is unlikely to withstand vigorous activity.

### RECOVERY PERIOD

The plaster cast fitted after the operation is usually removed after five days and exercises are started to strengthen the quadriceps. The patient can normally put weight on the leg after two or three weeks.

### OUTLOOK

Although knee replacements can relieve pain and restore a degree of movement, results are often uncertain and the durability of the artificial parts is limited. However, research continues into the development of stronger materials, better cements (glues), and joint designs that more closely resemble natural joints.

## Knock-knee

Inward curving of the legs so that the knees touch, causing the feet to be kept farther apart.

### CAUSES

Knock-knee is a part of normal development in some children and is common between the ages of 3 and 5 years. It may also be the result of injury or disease. Among the common causes are diseases that soften the bones (such as *rickets* or *osteomalacia*), *rheumatoid arthritis* or *osteoarthritis* of the knee, or a fracture of the lower femur (thigh bone) or upper tibia

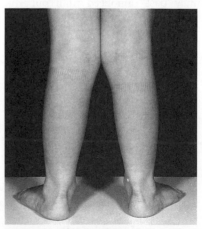

**The appearance of knock-knee**
This condition is common in toddlers but nearly always disappears by age 7.

K

(shin) that has not healed in a straight, vertical line.

**TREATMENT**

In children, the condition usually requires no treatment unless it persists after the age of 10, when it may start to strain the joints of the lower leg. Wearing heel wedges in the shoes may help correct the line of the leg, but most people require *osteotomy* (an operation in which the tibia is cut and realigned to straighten the leg).

In adults, treatment consists of osteotomy, or, when the condition has been present for a considerable time, *knee joint replacement*.

## Knuckle

The common name for a *finger* joint.

## Koilonychia

A condition in which the nails are dry, brittle, and thin, eventually becoming concave (spoon shaped). Koilonychia may be caused by injury to the nail. Other causes include iron-deficiency *anemia* and *lichen planus*; rarely, the condition is inherited.

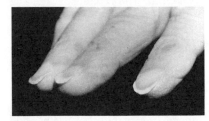

**The appearance of koilonychia**
In koilonychia, the nails are flattened and look fragile, bending where they protrude past the finger ends.

## Koplik's spots

Tiny, gray-white spots within the mouth (on the inner lining of the cheeks) that appear during the incubation period of *measles*.

## Korsakoff's psychosis

See *Wernicke-Korsakoff syndrome*.

## Kraurosis vulvae

See *Vulvitis*.

## Kuru

A progressive and fatal infection of the brain that affects some natives of the highlands of New Guinea. Kuru is caused by a virus spread by cannibalism. The condition is now rare.

The disease is caused by a "slow" virus (which causes no signs of disease until many months or years after entry into the body) and the incubation period may be as long as 30 years. Symptoms include progressive difficulty in controlling movements and, eventually, *dementia*.

Kuru has aroused special interest recently because of certain similarities between the causative virus and *HIV* (human immunodeficiency virus), which causes *AIDS*. It is known that HIV can cause brain changes similar to those in kuru.

## Kwashiorkor

A severe type of malnutrition in young children, occurring mainly in poor rural areas in the tropics. It is chiefly confined to children between 1 and 3 years old. The term kwashiorkor is derived from a Ghanaian word meaning "disease suffered by a child displaced from the breast."

**CAUSES**

The illness starts when the child is suddenly weaned onto a poor diet low in calories, protein, and certain essential micronutrients such as zinc, selenium, and vitamins A and E. To obtain enough nutrients from the food that is available, the child would need to eat a larger amount than he or she is capable of taking in. The problem is often exacerbated by a poor appetite due to illness. In addition, the lacking micronutrients provide protection against certain chemicals that are produced during infections and which also lead to *edema* (accumulation of fluid in the tissues). Measles and other infections common in the tropics precipitate kwashiorkor in undernourished children.

**SYMPTOMS AND SIGNS**

Growth is stunted, but edema makes the child look puffy and generally less emaciated than a child with *marasmus*, another form of malnutrition. Affected children are apathetic, weak, irritable, and inactive. Their skin sometimes flakes off, leaving a raw, weeping area beneath, and their hair may lose its curliness, become sparse and brittle, and turn from dark to fair.

The liver often enlarges, dehydration may develop (despite the simultaneous presence of edema), and the child loses resistance against severe infection, which may be fatal. In its severe, advanced stage, the illness is often marked by jaundice, drowsiness, and a fall in body temperature.

**DIAGNOSIS AND TREATMENT**

Diagnosis is based on a physical examination and the child's medical and dietary history.

The priorities in severe cases are to keep the child warm, replace lost fluids, and treat any infection. Initially, the child is fed milk (in frequent small amounts) and vitamin and mineral tablets, if possible. Zinc is given to prevent more flaking of the skin. When the edema has disappeared and the child's appetite has returned, a high-calorie, protein-rich diet is given.

**OUTLOOK**

Most children treated for kwashiorkor recover, but those less than 2 years old are likely to suffer permanent stunting of growth. Of the children ill enough to be admitted to a hospital, about 85 percent survive.

## Kyphoscoliosis

A combination of *kyphosis* (abnormal backward curvature of the spine) and *scoliosis* (curvature of the spine to one side or the other).

## Kyphosis

The medical term for excessive backward curvature of the spine. Kyphosis usually affects the spine at the top of the back, resulting in either a hump or a more gradually rounded back. Less commonly, it affects normally forward-curving parts of the spine at the neck and lower back.

Kyphosis may be caused by any of a variety of spinal disorders, including *osteoporosis* (bone degeneration from softening due to calcium loss), fracture of a vertebra, or a tumor of a vertebra (see *Spine* disorders box). In the past, the main cause of kyphosis was spinal tuberculosis. Treatment, which is rarely successful, is of the underlying disorder.

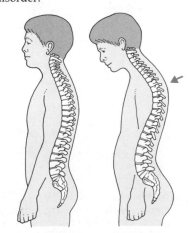

Normal curvature    Kyphosis of the thoracic spine

**The appearance of kyphosis**
In kyphosis, the thoracic part of the spine is excessively curved, producing a humped (rounded) appearance.

# L

## Labetalol

A *beta-blocker drug* used to treat *hypertension* (high blood pressure) and *angina pectoris* (chest pain caused by impaired blood supply to the heart).

Possible adverse effects include indigestion, nausea, and, in rare cases, depression and temporary impotence. Labetalol is less likely than some other beta-blocker drugs to cause cramping of the legs or coldness of the hands and feet.

## Labia

The lips of the *vulva* (the female external genitalia) that protect the vaginal and urethral openings. There are two pairs of labia. The outer pair, called the labia majora, are fleshy folds that bear hair and contain sweat glands. They cover the smaller, hairless inner folds, the labia minora, which meet to form the hood of the *clitoris*.

---

### LOCATION OF LABIA
The labia majora extend forward from the perineum and fuse at the front at the mons pubis. The labia minora lie within.

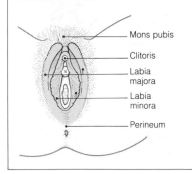

- Mons pubis
- Clitoris
- Labia majora
- Labia minora
- Perineum

---

## Labile

Unstable; likely to undergo change. Vitamins are labile because they are broken down easily by such factors as heat and excess acidity. Blood pressure that has a tendency to fluctuate may be described as labile. In psychiatry, the term is sometimes used to mean emotional instability.

## Labor

See *Childbirth*.

## Labyrinthitis

Inflammation of the labyrinth (the fluid-filled chambers in the inner ear that sense balance) that results in *vertigo*, a sensation that oneself or one's surroundings are spinning around.

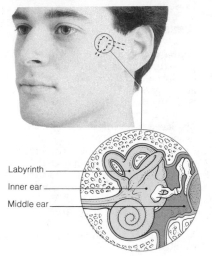

- Labyrinth
- Inner ear
- Middle ear

**Mechanism of labyrinthitis**
In labyrinthitis, inflammation of the fluid-filled chambers (labyrinth) of the inner ear causes disruption of the individual's sense of balance. The inflammation is usually caused by viral or bacterial infection.

### CAUSES

Labyrinthitis is almost always caused by bacterial or viral infection. Viral labyrinthitis may occur during a flulike illness or during illnesses such as measles or mumps. Bacterial labyrinthitis is commonly caused by inadequately treated *otitis media* (infection of the middle ear), particularly if a *cholesteatoma* (an infected collection of debris in the middle ear) has developed and eroded a pathway into the inner ear. Infection may also reach the inner ear (via the bloodstream) from elsewhere in the body. Less commonly, bacterial labyrinthitis results from a head injury.

### SYMPTOMS AND TREATMENT

Apart from vertigo, labyrinthitis can cause nausea, vomiting, *nystagmus* (jerky eye movements), *tinnitus* (ringing in the ears), and deafness.

Viral labyrinthitis clears up on its own, but symptoms are relieved by antihistamines such as meclizine. Bacterial labyrinthitis requires immediate treatment with *antibiotic drugs* to eradicate the infection. Otherwise, the

infection may lead to permanent deafness or may spread to the tissue covering the brain, causing *meningitis*.

Surgery may be necessary to drain pus from the ear or to remove any cholesteatoma.

## Laceration

A torn, irregular wound, as opposed to a straight cut, or *incision*. One example of a laceration is the tearing of the perineum (the area between the vagina and anus) that sometimes occurs during childbirth.

## Lacrimal apparatus

The system that produces and drains tears. The lacrimal apparatus includes the main and accessory lacrimal glands and the nasolacrimal drainage ducts. The main glands secrete *tears* during crying and when the eye is irritated; the accessory glands maintain the normal tear film.

### STRUCTURE

The main lacrimal glands lie just within the upper and outer margin of the orbit (socket) and drain into the *conjunctiva*. The accessory glands lie within the conjunctiva, secreting directly onto its surface.

Tears drain through the lacrimal puncta, tiny openings toward the inner end of each eyelid. The puncta are connected by narrow tubes to the lacrimal sacs, which lie in shallow hollows in the lacrimal bones. These bones are situated just within the inner margin of the orbit on either side of the nose. Overlying the lacrimal sacs are flat muscles that compress the sacs during blinking. Leading from the sacs are the nasolacrimal ducts, which run down through the bone to open inside the nose.

The action of blinking provides a suction effect to draw away excess fluid by compressing and releasing the lacrimal sacs.

### FUNCTION

The principal function of tears is to keep the *cornea* and conjunctiva constantly moist. Moisture is essential to maintain transparency of the cornea and to prevent ulceration. By lubricating the surface of the eye, tears aid movement of the eyelid in blinking. Tears also wash away small foreign bodies and contain a natural antibiotic called lysozyme. Another function is their role in expressing emotion.

## Lactase deficiency

A condition in which lactase, an enzyme that breaks down the lactose (milk sugar) present in the cells of the

## FUNCTIONS OF THE LACRIMAL APPARATUS

Tear production must be sufficient to compensate for evaporation and maintain the tear film. Accessory lacrimal glands in the conjunctiva perform this function. The main lacrimal glands secrete when excess fluid is required. Surplus tears drain into the nose.

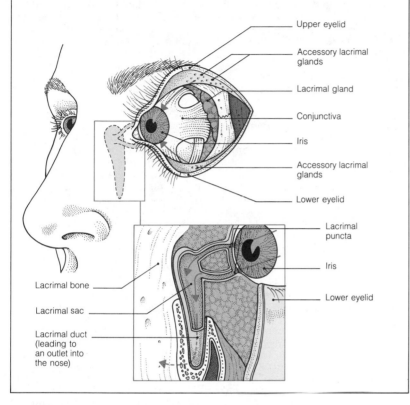

- Upper eyelid
- Accessory lacrimal glands
- Lacrimal gland
- Conjunctiva
- Iris
- Accessory lacrimal glands
- Lower eyelid
- Lacrimal puncta
- Iris
- Lower eyelid
- Lacrimal bone
- Lacrimal sac
- Lacrimal duct (leading to an outlet into the nose)

small intestine, is missing. Lactase deficiency causes lactose intolerance, an inability to digest lactose.

### TYPES, INCIDENCE, AND SYMPTOMS

Lactase deficiency may be present at birth, may develop immediately after weaning, or may not become evident until puberty or later.

Congenital lactase deficiency is sometimes permanent, but is more often temporary. This type is caused by delayed enzyme maturation, especially in premature babies.

Permanent lactase deficiency develops in about 80 to 90 percent of blacks and Orientals and in about 5 to 15 percent of whites. Lactase deficiency may also occur as a complication of intestinal diseases (such as *celiac sprue* and *gastroenteritis*). In these cases, the deficiency frequently disappears as the disease improves.

Undigested lactose ferments in the intestine and causes severe abdominal cramps, bloating, flatulence, and diarrhea; weight loss and malnutrition may also occur.

### DIAGNOSIS AND TREATMENT

The diagnosis can be confirmed by tests on blood and feces. Treatment is a lactose-free diet; milk must be avoided but fermented milk products, such as yogurt, can be eaten. Enzyme replacements (which partially or fully break down lactose) may be used.

## Lactation

The production and secretion of milk after childbirth. (See *Breast-feeding.*)

## Lactic acid

A weak acid produced by cells when they break down glucose to produce energy by anaerobic metabolism (chemical processes that do not require oxygen). This process occurs only when there is too little oxygen for the more usual aerobic metabolism. For example, lactic acid is produced by muscles during vigorous exercise and is one of the factors that contributes to *cramp*. Lactic acid is also produced in tissues when their blood supply (oxygen) fails due to a *myocardial infarction* (heart attack) or *shock*.

Normally, lactic acid is removed from the blood by the liver; if lactic acid accumulates, a condition called *acidosis* results.

## Lactose

One of the sugars present in milk. Chemically, lactose is a disaccharide *carbohydrate*, a sugar made up of two monosaccharide (simple sugar) units.

Lactose is broken down by lactase (an enzyme released by the lining of the small intestine) into the monosaccharides glucose and galactose, which are then absorbed into the bloodstream. *Lactase deficiency* results in a reduced ability to digest lactose. If the diet contains milk, lactose accumulates and ferments in the feces, sometimes causing diarrhea.

## Lactose intolerance

The inability to digest lactose, a sugar found in milk. It is usually caused by a deficiency of lactase, an enzyme found in the small intestine (see *Lactase deficiency*). Rarely, it occurs in a person who is not deficient in lactase.

## Lactulose

A *laxative drug* used to treat *constipation* and *liver failure*. Lactulose causes water to be absorbed into the feces from the intestinal blood vessels, making the feces softer and easier to pass. It is used to treat liver failure because it helps eliminate ammonia from the bloodstream into the feces.

## Lambliasis

Another name for *giardiasis*.

## Laminectomy

Surgical removal of part or all of one or more laminae (the bony arches of the vertebrae that surround the spinal cord) to expose the spinal cord. Laminectomy is performed as the first stage of spinal canal decompression, an operation carried out to relieve pressure on the spinal cord or on a nerve root leading from it (see *Decompression, spinal canal*).

### HOW IT IS DONE

An incision is made in the patient's back and the laminae are exposed. Enough of one or more adjacent laminae is then chipped away to give the surgeon access to the cord. Rarely, several complete laminae must be removed. In this case, *spinal fusion*

L

L

(immobilization of the spine with metal rods or bone grafts) is then necessary to prevent subsequent instability of the spine.

## Lance

To incise (cut) using a *lancet* or a surgical scalpel.

## Lancet

A small, pointed, double-edged knife used to open and drain lesions such as boils and abscesses.

## Lanolin

A mixture of a yellow, oily substance obtained from sheep's wool and purified water, used as an *emollient* in the treatment of dry skin. Lanolin is a common ingredient in bath oils and hand creams; it is also used to treat mild *dermatitis*. Occasionally, lanolin may irritate the skin.

## Lanugo hair

Fine, soft, downy hair that covers a fetus. Lanugo hair first appears in the fourth or fifth month and usually disappears by the ninth month. It can still be seen in some premature babies.

Lanugo hair sometimes reappears in adults who have cancer, particularly of the breast, bladder, lung, or large intestine. It may also occur with *anorexia nervosa* or be a side effect of drugs (especially *cyclosporine*).

## Laparoscopy

A method of examining the abdominal cavity by means of a laparoscope, a type of *endoscope* (viewing tube).

**WHY IT IS DONE**
Laparoscopy is usually performed to determine the cause of pelvic pain or gynecological symptoms (such as *ectopic pregnancy* or *pelvic inflammatory disease*) that cannot be confirmed by physical examination. It is frequently used to examine the condition of the fallopian tubes when investigating cases of *infertility*. Laparoscopy can also be used to examine the appendix, gallbladder, and liver.

## Laparotomy, exploratory

An operation in which the abdomen is opened to look for the cause of an undiagnosed illness. Laparotomy strictly describes any abdominal surgery because, even when the surgeon is operating to treat a known disorder, a thorough examination of the entire abdomen is carried out.

**WHY IT IS DONE**
The primary reason for a laparotomy is to investigate symptoms and signs whose cause other tests have failed to discover. Common examples include recurrent abdominal pain and *peritonitis* (infection within the abdominal cavity). The operation may also be performed as an emergency procedure if the abdomen has been seriously injured in an accident.

**HOW IT IS DONE**
A vertical (or, less commonly, a crosswise or oblique) incision is made in the abdomen and the abdominal cavity is opened and explored for signs of disease. Any diseased organ is repaired or removed, after which the incision is sewn up.

The recovery period depends upon the nature and extent of the disease discovered and treated.

## Larva migrans

 Infections characterized by the presence of the larval (immature) forms of certain worms in the body and by the symptoms caused by movement of the worms.

Visceral larva migrans, better known as *toxocariasis*, is caused by a type of worm that normally parasitizes dogs. Cutaneous larva migrans is caused by hookworm larvae that normally parasitize dogs, cats, or other animals. Also known as creeping eruption, it is contracted by walking barefoot on soil or beaches contaminated with animal feces. The larvae penetrate the skin of the feet and move randomly, leaving intensely itchy red lines sometimes accompanied by blistering.

Both types of larva migrans can be treated with *antihelmintic drugs*, such as thiabendazole.

## Laryngeal nerve

One of a pair of nerves that carries instructions from the brain to the larynx (voice box) and sends sensations from the larynx to the brain. Each nerve leaves the brain through a hole in the base of the skull and passes down the neck. The right-hand nerve then hooks around an artery behind the clavicle (collarbone) before returning to the larynx. The other nerve travels farther, hooking around the

---

### PROCEDURE FOR LAPAROSCOPY

A hollow needle is inserted into the abdomen just below the navel (using anesthesia), and carbon dioxide gas is pumped through the needle to expand the abdominal cavity. The laparoscope (see below) is then inserted through another incision to view the internal organs. The gas in the abdomen may cause discomfort for a day or two afterward.

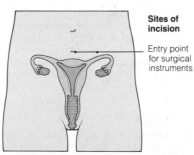

Sites of incision

Entry point for surgical instruments

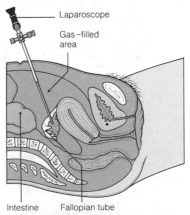

Laparoscope

Gas–filled area

Intestine    Fallopian tube

**Gynecological laparoscopy**
Laparoscopy is used in diagnosis and for removing ova for in vitro fertilization. Laparoscopic sterilization is a common sterilization procedure for women.

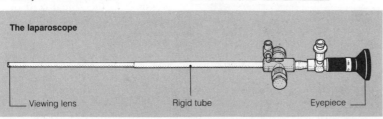

**The laparoscope**

Viewing lens          Rigid tube          Eyepiece

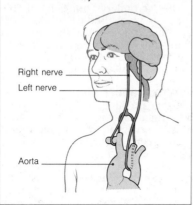
aorta (the major artery leaving the heart) before passing back to the larynx. Damage to one or both nerves causes *vocal cord* paralysis, resulting in loss of voice and sometimes obstruction to breathing.

## Laryngectomy
Surgical removal of all or part of the larynx (voice box) to treat advanced cancer of the larynx (see *Larynx, cancer of*). After the operation, the patient is no longer able to speak in the usual fashion.

#### WHY IT IS DONE
If cancer of the larynx is detected early, the prospects of curing it with *radiation therapy* are good. However, tumors that have grown to a considerable size, and those that are not responding to radiation therapy, require surgical removal.

#### HOW IT IS DONE
An incision is made in the neck and the larynx is removed, using general anesthesia. The top of the trachea (windpipe) immediately below the larynx is then sewn to the skin around the surgical wound in the neck to form a permanent opening called a stoma, through which the patient will breathe from then on.

#### RECOVERY PERIOD
Immediately after the operation, a bell or buzzer and pen and paper are given to the patient so that he or she can communicate. A tube is left in the stoma for a few days so that, as the surrounding tissues heal, they do not close the opening. The air in the patient's room is humidified to reduce the production of mucus in the stoma, and any excess mucus is sucked away.

Initially, all food is passed through a thin tube running from the nose to the stomach. After about 10 days the feeding tube is removed and food (fluid or semisolid at first) can be taken normally again. Speed of recovery depends partly on age and health.

#### OUTLOOK
With persistence, the patient can learn from a speech therapist a new way of speaking (called esophageal speech). Air is swallowed, then expelled in a controlled way; this noise is modulated by the tongue, palate, and lips to form gruff, though distinguishable, words. The technique requires painstaking practice. Alternatively, patients may use an electronic larynx, a device that emits a buzzing noise and is held against the top of the throat. By mouthing words, the person converts the buzz to speech.

Swimming is not possible, and care must be taken when bathing.

## Laryngitis
Inflammation of the larynx (voice box) usually caused by infection and resulting in *hoarseness*. Laryngitis may be acute, lasting only a few days, or chronic, persisting over a long period.

#### CAUSES
Acute laryngitis is usually caused by a viral infection, such as a cold, but it can also be due to an allergy to a drug, pollen, or some other substance.

Chronic laryngitis may be caused by overuse of the voice, by violent coughing, by irritation due to tobacco smoke, alcohol, or fumes, or by damage during surgery.

#### SYMPTOMS AND SIGNS
Hoarseness is the most common symptom, and it may progress to loss of voice. There may also be pain or a feeling of discomfort in the throat (especially during swallowing) and a dry, irritating cough. Laryngitis caused by a viral infection is often accompanied by fever and a general sick feeling.

#### TREATMENT
A person with laryngitis should rest in bed, avoid tobacco and alcohol, keep the throat lining moist with humidifiers, and take *antipyretic drugs* to reduce fever and *analgesic drugs* to relieve pain.

If the symptoms do not subside within four or five days, if sputum (phlegm) is coughed up, or if hoarseness persists for several weeks, a physician should be consulted. Antibiotic drugs will be prescribed if there is a bacterial infection. If the physician suspects a cause other than infection, diagnostic tests may be required, possibly to check for signs of cancer (see *Larynx, cancer of*), which can be cured if treated at an early stage.

## Laryngoscopy
Examination of the larynx (voice box) using a mirror held against the back of the palate (indirect laryngoscopy), or a viewing tube called a laryngoscope (direct laryngoscopy). Either a rigid or a flexible laryngoscope may be required.

#### WHY IT IS DONE
The larynx is inspected when a person complains of persistent hoarseness or has other change in the voice, when there is persistent stridor (a harsh noise when breathing in), or when someone experiences difficulty inhaling. Laryngoscopy is also useful in examining people who have throat pain or difficulty swallowing.

**INDIRECT LARYNGOSCOPY** This technique is used to detect *epiglottiditis* (in adults), *laryngitis*, benign or malignant laryngeal tumors, and any reduction of movement in the vocal cords.

**DIRECT LARYNGOSCOPY** This procedure is used when a biopsy or more careful evaluation is needed (e.g., assessing the extent of a tumor). The laryngoscope also allows more elaborate procedures, such as complete excision of a benign *lesion*, foreign body removal, laser surgery, or injection of polytef into paralyzed vocal cords. Often, a microscope is used with the laryngoscope. Direct laryngoscopy is also done before *intubation*.

#### HOW IT IS DONE
Indirect and direct laryngoscopy procedures are shown in the illustrated box, next page.

## Laryngotracheobronchitis
Inflammation of the larynx, trachea, and bronchi. It is the most common cause of *croup*.

## Larynx
The organ in the throat responsible for voice production and for preventing food from entering the airway during swallowing. Its common name is the voice box.

#### STRUCTURE
The larynx, which lies between the *pharynx* (upper part of the airway) and the *trachea* (windpipe), forms part of the tube in the throat that carries air to and from the lungs. It consists of areas

## PROCEDURE FOR LARYNGOSCOPY

There are two techniques. In indirect laryngoscopy, the patient's throat is examined with the use of a mirror. In direct laryngoscopy, the patient's throat is viewed with an instrument called a laryngoscope. If a rigid laryngoscope is used, general anesthesia is required. Only mild sedation is needed if a flexible laryngoscope is used.

### INDIRECT LARYNGOSCOPY

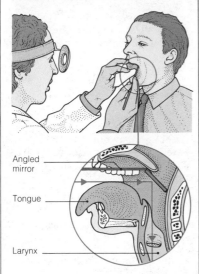

Angled mirror

Tongue

Larynx

The patient sticks out his or her tongue and the physician rests an angled mirror on the soft palate. A lamp or mirror on the physician's head illuminates the larynx, which is reflected in the mirror.

### DIRECT LARYNGOSCOPY

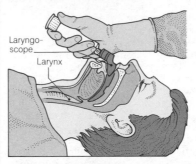

Laryngo-scope

Larynx

A rigid laryngoscope is passed down the throat via the mouth; a flexible laryngoscope is passed via the nostril.

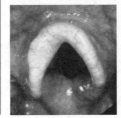

**View of larynx**
This view was obtained with a laryngoscope. The vocal cords are at the center and the epiglottis forms the arc at the top.

larynx open as part of the airway to the lungs; as soon as swallowing begins, the epiglottis drops like a lid over the larynx, directing food to either side. Closure of the true vocal cords and the false vocal cords just above them also helps protect the airway. The food or drink then passes down the *esophagus* to the stomach.

The secondary function of the larynx is voice production. Air from the lungs passes over the stretched vocal cords. The resultant vibrations are modified by the tongue, palate, and lips to produce *speech*.

## Larynx, cancer of

A malignant tumor of the larynx (voice box), often causing persistent hoarseness. Laryngeal cancer represents about 2 percent of all cancers.

### CAUSES AND INCIDENCE

The exact causes of this type of cancer are not known, but it occurs most commonly in heavy smokers. Laryngeal cancer is also associated with high alcohol consumption.

In the US, laryngeal cancer primarily affects people over age 60; it is more common in men than in women.

### SYMPTOMS

Hoarseness is the main symptom, particularly when the tumor originates on the vocal cords. A tumor that develops elsewhere in the larynx often passes unnoticed until an advanced stage of the disease, when the tumor causes discomfort in the throat, difficulty breathing and swallowing, and coughing up blood.

### DIAGNOSIS

*Laryngoscopy* (examination of the larynx indirectly with a mirror, or directly with an endoscope) reveals any tumor on the larynx. A *biopsy* (removal of a sample of tissue) is carried out in the hospital using local or general anesthesia to determine whether the growth is benign or malignant, and whether the lining of the larynx shows any signs of early cancerous change.

### TREATMENT

If the tumor is discovered when it is still small, the outcome is usually favorable. A small cancer of the true vocal cords has about a 95 percent chance of cure, usually by *radiation therapy* alone.

For larger tumors (and for those that do not respond to radiation therapy) partial or total *laryngectomy* (removal of the larynx) is considered for all but frail or elderly patients. The cure rate of surgery varies according to the site and extent of the tumor. In all cases

of cartilage (tough but flexible tissue), the largest of which is the thyroid cartilage, which projects at the front to form the Adam's apple. Below it, connecting the thyroid cartilage to the trachea, is the cricoid cartilage, which is shaped like a signet ring with the seal at the back. Situated on top of the seal are the two pyramid-shaped arytenoid cartilages. Between these two cartilages and the interior surface of the Adam's apple stretch two fibrous sheets of tissue, the *vocal cords*, which are responsible for voice production.

Attached to the top of the thyroid cartilage at the entrance to the larynx is the *epiglottis*, a leaf-shaped flap of cartilage that prevents food from entering the larynx during swallowing. The entire larynx is lined with *mucous membrane*, which is of the squamous cell type.

### FUNCTION

The most important function of the larynx is to prevent *choking*. When a person is not eating or drinking, the epiglottis stays upright, keeping the

## LOCATION OF LARYNX

The larynx, commonly called the voice box, is situated deep in the throat between the pharynx and the trachea (windpipe).

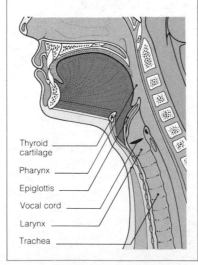

Thyroid cartilage

Pharynx

Epiglottis

Vocal cord

Larynx

Trachea

L

## DISORDERS OF THE LARYNX

Disorders affecting the larynx (voice box) are common. They usually cause *hoarseness* because they interfere with the functioning of the vocal cords. Other symptoms include difficulty breathing, stridor (a harsh noise on breathing in), a painful throat, and coughing. Persistent hoarseness should be reported to a physician.

### CONGENITAL DEFECTS

Rarely, a baby is born with a soft, limp larynx, a condition called laryngomalacia. The main signs are stridor and noisy breathing when feeding. The larynx usually attains a normal firmness by age 2.

### INFLAMMATION

*Laryngitis* (inflammation of the larynx) is the most common laryngeal disorder in adults; symptoms are hoarseness, fever, and discomfort in the throat. In children, *croup* (inflammation and narrowing of the air passages) is very common up to age 4. Much rarer is *epiglottiditis* (inflammation of the epiglottis, the flap of cartilage that closes the larynx during swallowing). This is a life-threatening disorder in young children.

### TUMORS

Various kinds of benign growth may develop on the vocal cords. The most common is a polyp, a smooth swelling usually caused by smoking, by an infection such as influenza, or by straining the voice. Warts occasionally develop on a child's vocal cords. Both polyps and warts require removal and microscopic analysis to exclude cancer. *Singers' nodes* are small benign growths that can occur on the vocal cords of people who strain their voices. They give the voice a hoarse tone.

Malignant tumors, which cause persistent hoarseness, are usually caused by smoking and/or alcohol use (see *Larynx, cancer of*).

### OTHER DISORDERS

A tumor, an infection, or, rarely, throat surgery can damage one or both of the nerves supplying the larynx, causing *vocal cord* paralysis, which results in loss of voice and may interfere with breathing.

### INVESTIGATION

Disorders of the larynx are investigated by *laryngoscopy*. Sometimes a *biopsy* sample is taken for pathologic analysis; X rays, especially *tomography*, may provide more information.

---

after losing part or all of the larynx, the patient must master new techniques for producing speech.

If the tumor has spread throughout the larynx, or to other parts of the throat (or, rarely, other parts of the body), the patient is treated with radiation therapy and *anticancer drugs*. This combination relieves symptoms and often temporarily arrests the progress of the disease.

## Laser

A device that produces a concentrated beam of light radiation; laser is an acronym for light amplification by stimulated emission of radiation. A laser beam is parallel, of a single specific wavelength (or sometimes of a narrow band of wavelengths), and coherent (that is, all the crests of the individual waves coincide).

## Laser treatment

The use of a *laser* beam in a variety of medical procedures.

### LOW-INTENSITY TREATMENT

Treatment with low-intensity beams stimulates tissue healing and reduces pain, inflammation, and swelling. It works by improving blood and lymph flow and by reducing the production of *prostaglandins* (hormonelike substances that stimulate inflammation and cause pain). Low-intensity beams are used in the treatment of muscle tears, ligament sprains, and inflamed tendons and joints.

### HIGH-INTENSITY TREATMENT

High-intensity treatment destroys cells directly under the beam while leaving adjacent cells undamaged, making it useful in the treatment of some tumors. The beam cuts through tissue and, simultaneously, causes blood clotting, making it a useful surgical tool.

**LASERS IN OPHTHALMOLOGY** Lasers are used in the treatment of diabetic *retinopathy* (to prevent bleeding from abnormal blood vessels), to prevent and treat retinal detachment (by sealing small tears or areas of degeneration), and to destroy small tumors of the retina. The laser can also be used to make a central hole to restore vision if the lens capsule becomes opaque after *cataract surgery*.

**LASERS IN GYNECOLOGY** Laser beams are sometimes used to unblock fallopian tubes by removing scar tissue formed after an infection or a *sterilization* procedure. Lasers are used to destroy abnormal cells in the *cervix*.

**OTHER USES** Lasers are commonly used to remove small birthmarks and tattoos; the results are variable. Early malignant tumors of the larynx can be successfully removed without damaging the vocal cords.

Many new applications are being investigated. Potential uses include the removal of atherosclerotic *plaque* from inside arteries. It may also be possible to use lasers to disintegrate bladder and kidney stones, and to remove otherwise inaccessible tumors of the brain and spinal cord. (See also illustrated box, overleaf.)

## Lassa fever

 A dangerous infectious disease, caused by a virus, that was first reported in 1969. The disease occurs in occasional outbreaks in West Africa; a small number of cases have been imported into the US and Europe.

In Africa, where the virus is harbored by a type of rat, infection may be acquired by inhaling droplets of the rat's urine. Medical and nursing staff are at risk of acquiring the virus from the blood of an infected person or from droplets coughed into the air. No one in the US has ever acquired the disease from an infected person.

### SYMPTOMS AND TREATMENT

After an incubation period of three to 17 days, the illness starts with fever, headache, muscular aches, and a sore throat. Later, severe diarrhea and vomiting develop. In extreme cases, the patient's condition deteriorates rapidly in the second week. About one quarter to one third of hospitalized patients die from the illness.

Lassa fever can be diagnosed by a blood test. Infected people must be isolated; they are treated by relief of symptoms and injections of the *antiviral drug* ribavirin and of serum containing *antibodies* that are active against the virus.

## USE OF A LASER

The concentrated beam of light released by a laser has a variety of medical purposes. When set to low intensity, the laser works to stimulate tissue healing and reduces pain, inflammation, and swelling. At high intensity, the beam destroys cells on which it is focused while leaving adjacent tissue unharmed. It can also cut through tissues without causing bleeding.

### Argon laser

Photocoagulation of blood vessels occurs when the blue-green light from this laser is absorbed by hemoglobin.

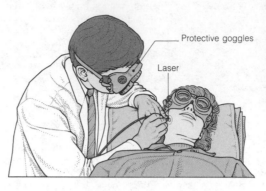

Protective goggles

Laser

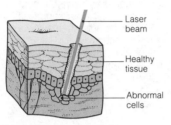

Laser beam

Healthy tissue

Abnormal cells

### Focused carbon dioxide laser

This laser is ideal for precision cutting or for destroying abnormal cells because its focused beam leaves surrounding areas of tissue intact.

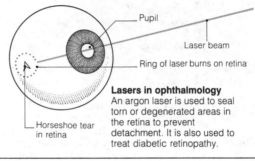

Pupil

Laser beam

Ring of laser burns on retina

Horseshoe tear in retina

### Lasers in ophthalmology

An argon laser is used to seal torn or degenerated areas in the retina to prevent detachment. It is also used to treat diabetic retinopathy.

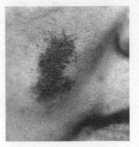

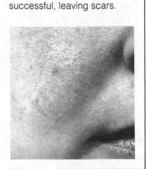

### Removing skin blemishes

These photographs, taken before and after laser treatment, show removal of a port-wine stain. In some cases, treatment is less successful, leaving scars.

## Lassitude

A term describing a feeling of *tiredness*, weakness, or exhaustion.

## Lateral

Relating to, or situated on, one side. Bilateral means on both sides.

## Laudanum

A solution of *opium* once used as a sedative and painkiller and in the treatment of diarrhea.

## Laughing gas

The popular name for *nitrous oxide*, a gas inhaled in combination with oxygen to produce general *anesthesia*. Laughing gas is so called because of the euphoric effects it produces.

## Laurence-Moon-Biedl syndrome

A very rare inherited disorder characterized by increasing *obesity*, *retinitis pigmentosa* that may lead to blindness, mild to moderate *mental retardation*, *polydactyly*, and *hypogonadism*.

The condition is probably caused by a disorder of the hypothalamus (part of the brain that controls the hormone balance). There is no treatment; parents should seek *genetic counseling*.

## LAV

Lymphadenopathy-associated virus, a name formerly given to the virus responsible for *AIDS*. The virus was renamed *HIV* (human immunodeficiency virus) in 1986.

## Lavage, gastric

Washing out the stomach with water, usually to remove poisons.

HOW IT IS DONE

The patient is placed face down with his or her head below the level of the stomach and turned to one side. A lubricated tube is passed down the esophagus into the stomach and a funnel is attached to the top. (If the patient is not fully conscious, a tube is also passed down the throat into the windpipe to prevent regurgitated water and stomach contents from entering the lungs.) Water is poured into the funnel until the stomach is filled. The top of the tube is then lowered, allowing the fluid in the stomach to drain into a bucket. This process is repeated until the water returns clear. An early sample of fluid from the stomach is kept so that the poison can be analyzed. In certain cases, an antidote to the poison (or a substance that neutralizes the poison)

is added to the water or is passed into the stomach after lavage is finished.

Lavage is not used if a corrosive poison has been swallowed because of the risk of the tube perforating tissues. Corrosive acids or alkalis may be diluted by giving large amounts of water or milk (see *Poisoning*).

## Laxative drugs

| COMMON DRUGS |
|---|
| Bulk-forming<br>*Methylcellulose Psyllium* |
| Lubricant<br>*Mineral oil* |
| Saline<br>*Magnesium sulfate Sodium phosphate* |
| Stimulant<br>*Bisacodyl Senna* |
| Others<br>*Lactulose* |

> **WARNING**
> If constipation lasts for more than a week, consult your physician; you may have a serious underlying disorder.

A group of drugs used to treat *constipation*. A high-fiber diet, plenty of liquids, and proper toilet habits may relieve constipation without use of laxative drugs. They may be given to prevent constipation when straining should be avoided (e.g., following childbirth, abdominal surgery, or a *myocardial infarction*). Laxatives are sometimes used to clear feces from the intestine before surgical or investigational procedures.

### TYPES

**BULK-FORMING LAXATIVES** These drugs retain fluid drunk with the laxative, increasing bulk and stimulating propulsion. They increase the volume of feces, making them softer and easier to pass.

**STIMULANT LAXATIVES** These drugs stimulate the intestinal wall to contract and thus speed up the elimination of feces. Because the feces spend less time in the intestine, less water is reabsorbed into the blood vessels, which helps keep the feces soft.

**LUBRICANT LAXATIVES** These substances soften and thus facilitate the passage of feces.

**SALINE LAXATIVES** These drugs increase the concentration of salts within the feces, an action that draws fluids into the intestine from the surrounding blood vessels.

### POSSIBLE ADVERSE EFFECTS

Used in excess, laxative drugs may cause diarrhea. Since prolonged treatment may cause dependence on the laxative drug for normal bowel action, laxative use should be stopped as soon as normal habits are reestablished.

Stimulant laxatives and lactulose may cause abdominal cramps and flatulence. Prolonged use of saline laxatives is likely to cause a chemical imbalance in the blood. Lubricant laxatives may coat the intestine and prevent vitamin absorption.

## Lazy eye

An ambiguous name for the visual defect that commonly results from *strabismus*. (See *Amblyopia*.)

## LD$_{50}$

The abbreviation for median lethal dose, the amount of a drug needed to kill 50 percent of a group of animals. This dose is determined during experiments carried out to assess the toxicity of new drugs.

## Lead poisoning

Swallowing or inhaling lead or lead salts can damage the brain, nerves, red blood cells, and digestive system. Acute poisoning, which is relatively rare but sometimes fatal, occurs when a large amount of lead is taken into the body over a short period. Chronic poisoning results from small amounts of lead being taken in over a longer period. The body excretes lead very slowly, so it accumulates in body tissues (primarily in the bones). There is evidence that lead poisoning may produce no detectable physical effects but can cause mental impairment, particularly in children.

### CAUSES AND INCIDENCE

Lead poisoning is most common in children who have licked or eaten old paint that contains high levels of lead. Adults most at risk include workers in industries such as lead mining and smelting, soldering, demolition, and pottery glazing. Drinking liquor from illicit stills with lead piping or inhaling the fumes from burning battery casings containing lead may also cause lead poisoning. So, too, can eating acidic food or drink that is stored or cooked in lead-glazed or lead-soldered containers.

Almost everybody is exposed to lead from exhaust fumes. In recent years, atmospheric lead levels have decreased as a result of legislation requiring vehicles manufactured after 1975 to run on unleaded gasoline. There is also a legal limit to the amount of lead that paint may contain.

### SYMPTOMS AND SIGNS

Acute lead poisoning causes severe, colicky, abdominal pain, diarrhea, vomiting, weakness or paralysis of the limbs, seizures, and sometimes death.

In addition to the symptoms of acute poisoning, chronic poisoning may cause mental disturbances ranging from loss of memory, emotional instability, abnormal behavior, incoordination, and headaches to hallucinations, seizures, blindness, and coma. Seizures, behavioral abnormalities, and coma occur chiefly in children. There may also be *anemia*, loss of appetite, and a blue, black, or gray line along the gum margins.

If symptoms progress as far as seizures and coma, the risk of death is high. Even if the person survives, there is a high probability of permanent brain damage.

### DIAGNOSIS

Lead poisoning is diagnosed from the patient's condition and history, and from blood tests to measure lead levels, X rays of the bones and abdomen to reveal lead deposits, and urine tests to measure the level of lead breakdown products.

### TREATMENT

Treatment consists of avoiding further exposure to lead. The physician will prescribe *chelating agents* to bind to the lead and help the body excrete it at a faster rate. In mild cases, the chelating agent penicillamine may be used alone. In more severe cases, it may be used in combination with other chelating agents, such as edetate calcium disodium (calcium EDTA) and dimercaprol (BAL).

## Learning

A change in behavior as a result of experience. Committing facts to memory, often termed "learning by heart," is a separate process. True learning may not be immediately obvious. Whether or not a person has learned a skill or a fact can be judged only on the basis of his or her performance in a real-life situation.

### THEORIES OF LEARNING

According to behavioral theories, all learning in humans and animals occurs by *conditioning*. The simplest form (as described by Ivan Pavlov) is classical conditioning, in which a particular stimulus becomes associated with a particular response. In Pavlov's experiments, a bell was rung every time dogs were presented with food; eventually the dogs salivated in response to the bell alone.

A more sophisticated version of learning, termed operant conditioning by B.F. Skinner, relies on a system of rewards, known as reinforcements. Skinner observed that, if a hungry rat wandering about a cage accidentally bumped into a lever that released a food pellet, it learned to press the lever purposefully. The reinforcement need not appear every time for the rat to continue trying. In the same way, an occasional win on a slot machine is often enough to make people continue to play the game.

Rewards can also be used to encourage the development of new forms of behavior. Behavior "shaping" is the basis of animal training, and is used in dealing with behavioral problems in children and the mentally retarded. It can also apply to family and marital difficulties; partners or family members give each other rewards for desirable behavior. (See *Behavior therapy*.)

Another theory of learning proposes that, with experience, an abstract "cognitive" structure is built on which future decisions and behavior is based. Cognitive theorists believe that the simple responses of

L

conditioning are not sufficient to explain the ability to cope with new situations or solve new problems. For these processes, the more abstract mental qualities of *memory*, insight, and understanding are necessary.

The behavioral and cognitive approaches are combined in the "social learning theory," which proposes that learning occurs as a result of observation and imitation of the behavior of others.

No one theory can account for the complexities of learning. It is probable that some things are learned automatically, by conditioning, and others by complex thought processes that take account of many facts. Different factors may be more important at different times in a person's life; trial and error and observational learning are particularly important in young children. The ability to learn is also affected by personal interest in a task or subject, past experiences, and anxiety levels. In general, people learn faster when they are given a little at a time to learn; learning slows down as skill improves.

## Learning disabilities

A range of physical and psychological disorders that interferes with learning. Learning disabilities include problems in learning caused by defects in mental activities (such as speech, hearing, and memory), but do not include those due to emotional or environmental deprivation or to poor teaching.

Children of borderline or retarded intelligence have general difficulty learning. So, too, do those with *hyperactivity*, which lowers the attention span. Others have specific problems, such as *dyslexia* (difficulty reading), dyscalculia (inability to perform mathematical problems), or dysgraphia (writing disorders). Some psychologists believe that specific learning difficulties in children of normal intelligence may be caused by forms of *minimal brain dysfunction*, which may be inherited. Attempts to assess and treat such children have so far not been very successful.

## Leech

A type of blood-sucking worm with a flattened body and a sucker at each of its ends. Different types live on land or in water. Land leeches inhabit tropical forests. They can work their way through clothing and attach themselves to the ankles and lower legs. Aquatic, blood-sucking leeches live in warm water and attach themselves to swimmers, sometimes penetrating to the bronchi and the esophagus.

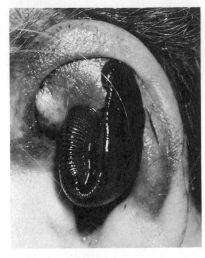

**Use of a leech to drain blood**
Leeches bite painlessly, introducing saliva into the wound before sucking blood. When they are satiated, they drop off. Here, a leech is being used to drain a hematoma (collection of blood) from a person's outer ear following an injury.

### TREATMENT OF BITES

Attached leeches should be startled by applying a lighted match, alcohol, salt, or vinegar. They can then be pulled off gently to prevent the mouth parts from staying attached and becoming infected. A styptic pencil helps stop the bleeding after the leech has been removed. *Endoscopy* (use of an internal viewing tube) may be necessary to remove leeches from inside the body.

### MEDICAL USES

Leeches were once attached to a patient's skin to "treat" many illnesses ascribed to excess blood. Today, leeches are sometimes used to drain a *hematoma* (a collection of partially clotted blood) from a wound.

## Leg, broken

See *Femur, fracture of; Fibula; Tibia.*

## Legionnaires' disease

A form of pneumonia (infection of the lungs) named after an outbreak that caused the death of 29 members of the American Legion who were attending a convention in a Philadelphia hotel in 1976. The bacterium responsible was isolated and the genus named *LEGIONELLA*. Tests identified the causatine organism as a common contaminant of water systems that had been responsible for earlier epidemics of pneumonia (the cause of which had not been understood at the time).

### CAUSES AND INCIDENCE

The bacterium breeds most readily in warm, moist conditions; in most outbreaks the source of infection has been the water or air-conditioning system in a large public building. Infection follows the inhalation of droplets of heavily contaminated water (from air-conditioning outlets and showers, for example). Elderly people, especially heavy smokers or drinkers, are particularly at risk.

The disease occurs both in localized outbreaks and as isolated cases. Over 700 diagnosed cases are reported in the US each year, but the true incidence is probably much higher. One to 2 percent of hospital cases of pneumonia may be caused by legionnaires' disease.

Control of the disease relies on the disinfection of water systems by chlorination or other means.

### SYMPTOMS AND SIGNS

The first symptoms develop within a week of infection; they include headache, muscular and abdominal pain, diarrhea, and a dry cough. Over the next few days pneumonia develops, resulting in a high fever, shaking chills, the coughing up of thick sputum (phlegm), drowsiness, and sometimes delirium. Like other types of pneumonia, the illness usually becomes more severe unless treated. This phase lasts about a week, after which either a gradual recovery takes place or progressively serious breathing problems develop.

### DIAGNOSIS AND TREATMENT

The patient is admitted to the hospital, where analysis of a sample of sputum (cultured on special media) or a lung biopsy reveals the microorganism responsible for the pneumonia. If it is *LEGIONELLA PNEUMOPHILA*, the patient is given the antibiotic erythromycin, often intravenously, which usually relieves symptoms quickly. Occasionally another antibiotic drug, rifampin, may be required.

### OUTLOOK

The outcome of the disease depends on the age and general health of the patient. Younger people generally recover fully, but a substantial proportion of elderly, unfit people die from the illness. Death is usually due to irreversible lung damage.

## Leg, shortening of

Shortening of the leg is usually caused by faulty healing of a fractured femur (thigh bone) or tibia (shin). Other causes are an abnormality present from birth, surgery on the leg, or muscle weakness associated with *poliomyelitis* or some other neurological disorder. Also, a deformity of the hip, knee, or spine may make one leg effectively shorter than the other even if the two are in fact of equal length.

If the difference in leg length exceeds 1.5 inches (4 cm), there is usually a noticeable limp; the resultant stress on the lower spine often causes *back pain*. Placing a raised heel on the shoe of the shortened side is a common remedy for a shortened leg.

## Leg ulcer

An open sore on the leg that fails to heal, usually resulting from an inadequate arterial blood supply to or insufficient venous drainage from the area. Elderly people are most commonly affected.

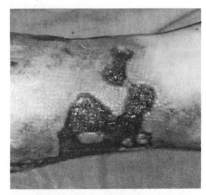

**Venous ulcer on leg**
This type of ulcer, also known as a stasis ulcer, is caused by impaired drainage of blood from the leg by the veins. It is usually accompanied by edema (fluid accumulation) in the lower leg.

### TYPES

Varicose ulcers, which occur mainly on the ankles and lower legs, are caused by valve failure in veins ; these ulcers usually appear in conjunction with *varicose veins*.

*Bedsores* (also called decubitus ulcers) develop on pressure spots on the legs as a result of a combination of poor circulation, pressure, and immobility over a long period.

Leg ulcers may also be due to *peripheral vascular disease*, in which fatty deposits on or thickening of the walls of arteries restricts blood supply to the extremities.

*Diabetes mellitus*, which increases susceptibility to blood vessel disease and skin infection and impairs sensation, may lead to ulcers.

Ulcers may also develop through neglect of an infected small wound. In the tropics, infection with microorganisms can cause *tropical ulcers*.

### PREVENTION AND TREATMENT

Prevention is always easier than cure. In general, anyone susceptible to leg ulcers should attempt to avoid obesity, leg injury, and immobility.

Treatment of leg ulcers, which depends on the cause, should be sought at the earliest sign of trouble. If an ulcer is exuding pus, a wet dressing may be applied under a bandage. This dressing should be changed only every three to seven days to avoid removing new skin from the area.

## Leiomyoma

A benign tumor of smooth muscle (a type of muscle not under voluntary control). Leiomyomas usually occur in the smooth muscle of the uterus, where they gradually become replaced with fibrous tissue (hence their popular name, *fibroids*). More rarely, leiomyomas develop from smooth muscle in the wall of blood vessels in the skin, where they form tender lumps.

Leiomyomas are usually multiple and, although they are not malignant (cancerous), they may require surgical removal if they cause symptoms.

## Leishmaniasis

Any of a variety of diseases affecting the skin, mucous membranes, and internal organs, caused by infection with single-celled parasites called leishmania. The parasites are harbored by dogs and rodents in various parts of the world, and are transmitted from infected animals or people to new hosts by the bites of sand flies.

About 12 million people worldwide are thought to be affected. Leishmaniasis is not contracted in the US, but travelers occasionally contract an infection abroad.

### TYPES AND INCIDENCE

The most serious form of leishmaniasis, mainly affecting the internal organs, is called kala-azar or visceral leishmaniasis. It is prevalent in some parts of Asia, Africa, and South America, and also occurs in some Mediterranean countries.

In addition, there are at least three varieties of cutaneous leishmaniasis (mainly affecting the skin), one of which is prevalent in the Middle East, North Africa, and in the Mediterranean; the others occur only in parts of Central and South America.

Travelers can minimize the risk of infection by taking common-sense measures to discourage sand-fly bites (see *Insect bites*).

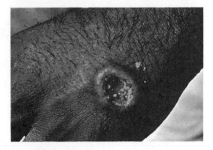

**Leishmaniasis ulcer**
This skin ulcer, which developed at the site of a sand-fly bite, is typical of the lesions found on the skin of people who are suffering from cutaneous leishmaniasis.

### SYMPTOMS

Kala-azar causes a persistent fever, enlargement of the spleen, anemia, and, in the later stages, darkening of the skin. The illness may develop anytime up to two years after the initial infection, and, unless treated, is sometimes fatal.

The cutaneous forms cause the appearance of a persistent ulcer at the site of the sand-fly bite. The ulcer may eventually heal, but can leave an ugly scar. With the South American forms, more extensive tissue damage may occur, often on the face, causing severe disfigurement.

### DIAGNOSIS AND TREATMENT

Kala-azar is diagnosed by a *bone marrow biopsy* and a blood test. The cutaneous forms are diagnosed by identifying parasites in scrapings taken from the edge of affected skin patches. All types of leishmaniasis are treated effectively with drugs, such as sodium stibogluconate, which are given by injection into a muscle or into a vein.

## Lens

The internal optical component of the eye. Also called the crystalline lens, it is responsible for adjusting focus. This lens is one of two lenses in each eye; the other is the *cornea*, which provides most of the power needed to form an image on the *retina*.

The crystalline lens is situated behind the iris and is suspended on delicate fibers from the ciliary body. It is elastic, transparent, and slightly less

## LOCATION OF THE LENS

This elastic and transparent organ is situated behind the iris and is suspended on delicate fibers from the ciliary body. Its full name—the crystalline lens—differentiates it from the cornea (another lens).

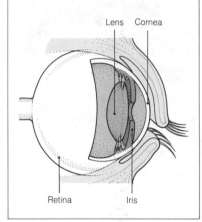

convex on the front surface than on the back. Changing degrees of curvature alter the focus of the eye so that an image remains sharp whether a near or a distant object is being viewed (see *Accommodation*).

Opacification of the crystalline lens, from any cause, is called *cataract*. (See also *Lens dislocation*.)

## Lens dislocation

Displacement of the eye's crystalline *lens* from its normal position. Lens dislocation is almost always caused by an injury that ruptures some or all of the fibers that connect the lens to the ciliary body. In *Marfan's syndrome*, the fibers are particularly weak and lens dislocation is common.

A dislocated lens may slide downward, causing severe visual distortion or double vision in the affected eye, or it may slip backward into the vitreous humor. A lens dislocated forward usually causes a form of *glaucoma* because of closure of the drainage angle of the eye. If the glaucoma is severe, the lens may be removed. (See also *Aphakia*.)

## Lens implant

A plastic prosthesis used to replace the removed opaque lens in *cataract surgery*. There are many different designs, which may be positioned in front of the iris, clipped to the pupil, or held in place behind the pupil by delicate plastic loops.

A lens implant usually provides excellent distance vision without glasses. However, most people need reading glasses or bifocal lenses for close vision after the implant.

## Lentigo

A flat, discolored area of skin similar to a freckle. Lentigines (the plural of lentigo) are usually light brown and may occur singly or in groups. Unlike freckles they are as common on covered as on exposed parts of the body, and they do not fade in winter. Lentigines are more common in middle-aged and elderly people, especially those who have been exposed to a lot of sun.

Lentigines are harmless and no treatment is necessary. If raised, darker brown areas appear within them, a physician should be consulted; there is a danger that these areas could develop into malignant melanomas (see *Melanoma, malignant*).

## Leprechaunism

A very rare congenital disorder in which affected infants have elfin faces, with wide-set eyes, large lips, and large, low-set ears; they also have large hands and feet. Hormonal imbalances cause enlargement of the penis in males and the clitoris and breasts in females, as well as hirsutism (hairiness). Most babies who have leprechaunism die in the first weeks or months of life.

## Leprosy

A chronic bacterial infection, also known as Hansen's disease, that damages nerves, mainly in the limbs and facial area, and may also lead to skin damage. Untreated leprosy can have severe complications, which include blindness and disfigurement. Contrary to popular belief, it is not highly contagious.

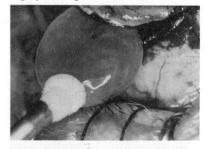

**Surgery on the lens**
The photograph shows an operation in which the lens is being extracted from behind the iris prior to the insertion of a plastic implant.

### CAUSES

Leprosy is caused by a bacterium, *MYCOBACTERIUM LEPRAE*, spread in droplets of nasal mucus. A person is infectious to others only during the first stages of the disease. Only people living in prolonged close contact with the infected person are at risk of infection. This, along with the fact that only 3 percent of the population is susceptible to leprosy, means that there is no justification for the practice (still prevalent in some countries) of isolating people with the disease.

### INCIDENCE

Worldwide, there are about 20 million sufferers from leprosy, mostly in Asia, Central and South America, and Africa. Probably fewer than 20 percent of these have access to treatment. In the US, there are now more than 4,000 known cases, mainly in California, Florida, Hawaii, Louisiana, New York, and Texas; three quarters of the people affected were born outside the US.

### SYMPTOMS AND SIGNS

Leprosy has a very long incubation period—about three to five years. Most of the destructive effects of the bacteria on nervous tissue are caused not by bacterial growth but by a reaction of the body's *immune system* to the organisms as they die. There are two main types of the disease. In lepromatous leprosy, damage is widespread, progressive, and severe. Tuberculoid leprosy is milder.

Initially, damage is confined to the peripheral nerves (those supplying the skin and muscles). There is lightening or darkening of skin areas, with associated reduced sensation and reduced sweating. As the disease progresses, the peripheral nerves swell and become tender. Hands, feet, and facial skin eventually become numb and muscles become paralyzed.

Complications include loss of all sensation in the hands and feet, so that accidental burns or injuries are not noticed, leading to extensive scarring or even to loss of fingers or toes. Muscle paralysis can lead to further deformity. Damage to the facial nerve means that the eyelids cannot be closed; the cornea dries and ulcerates, leading to blindness. Alternatively, direct invasion by bacteria may lead to inflammation of the eyeball, again leading to blindness. The disability caused by the combined effects of blindness and loss of touch sensation is extremely severe.

Cartilage and bone in the nose are often eroded, and bones elsewhere in the body may be destroyed. In addition, the testes may atrophy, leading to sterility.

### DIAGNOSIS AND TREATMENT

Early diagnosis of the disease is essential to prevent permanent disfigurement and disability. A provisional diagnosis is made from a physical examination of the patient; the presence of the bacteria is confirmed by a skin *biopsy* (removal of a sample of tissue for analysis).

Treatment is with the drug dapsone, which kills most of the causative bacteria within a few days. Any damage that has already occurred, however, is irreversible. Patients cease to be infectious soon after treatment starts. To prevent a relapse, use of the drug needs to be continued for at least two years after the last signs have disappeared.

Prevention of damage to the feet and other insensitive areas—through the use of proper footwear and health education—is very important. Plastic surgery may be helpful for facial deformities. Nerve and tendon transplants may improve the function of damaged limbs.

In the US, patients are eligible for treatment by the Public Health Service. There are special clinics and hospitals in different areas.

### OUTLOOK

Resistance to dapsone is becoming more common worldwide; other curative drugs, such as rifampin and clofazimine, are much more expensive. With no vaccine and so many sufferers in poor countries, the battle against leprosy has only just begun.

## Leptospirosis

 A rare disease caused by a spirochete (spiral-shaped) bacterium harbored by rodents and excreted in their urine. It is also known as Weil's disease. About 100 cases of leptospirosis, leading to a few deaths, are reported in the US each year.

### SYMPTOMS

After an incubation period of one to three weeks, there is an acute illness with fever, chills, an intense throbbing headache, severe muscle aches, eye inflammation, and a skin rash. In most cases, the kidneys are affected, often severely. Liver damage leading to jaundice is also common.

### TREATMENT

Antibiotics are effective against the spirochetes. In about one third of all cases the condition improves promptly. However, many patients

suffer a more persistent illness in which kidney and liver function recover only slowly. In these cases, the nervous system may also be affected, often producing signs of *meningitis* (inflammation of the membranes covering the brain and spinal cord).

## Lesbianism

Female homosexuality. According to Alfred Kinsey's studies carried out in the 1940s, about 5 percent of women are entirely lesbian in their sexual activity, although some 15 percent have had, by the age of 45, a homosexual experience. Lesbianism is less common than male homosexuality (see *Homosexuality, male*), but relationships tend to be more stable and often are lifelong. Masturbation, oral sex, and mutual rubbing of the clitoris are the usual means of reaching orgasm.

## Lesion

An all-encompassing term for any abnormality of structure or function in any part of the body. The term may refer to a wound, infection, tumor, abscess, or chemical abnormality.

## Lethargy

A feeling of *tiredness*, drowsiness, or lack of energy.

## Leukemia

Any of several types of cancer in which there is usually a disorganized proliferation of white *blood cells* in the bone marrow (from which all blood cells originate). The production of red blood cells, platelets, and normal white blood cells is impaired as they are crowded out from the marrow by the leukemic cells.

Other organs, such as the liver, spleen, lymph nodes, testes, or brain, may cease to function properly as they become infiltrated by the leukemic cells. The number of leukemic cells circulating in the blood may be high.

Leukemias are classified into acute and chronic types; acute leukemia generally develops more rapidly than chronic leukemia. They are also classified according to the type of white cell that is proliferating abnormally. If the abnormal cells are derived from lymphocytes or their immature precursors (lymphoblasts), the leukemia is called lymphocytic or lymphoblastic leukemia. If the abnormal cells are derived from other types of white blood cells or their precursors, it is called myeloid, myeloblastic, or granulocytic leukemia.

There are about 13 new cases of leukemia per 100,000 annually in the US, leading to about six to seven deaths per 100,000. (See also *Leukemia, acute; Leukemia, chronic lymphocytic; Leukemia, chronic myeloid.*)

## Leukemia, acute

A type of leukemia in which the white blood cells produced in excess within the bone marrow are immature cells called blasts. Untreated, acute leukemia can be fatal within a few weeks to months. Treatment today can often prolong life and may even provide a complete cure.

The abnormal cells may be of two types: lymphoblasts (immature *lymphocytes*) in acute lymphoblastic leukemia, and myeloblasts (immature forms of other types of white cell) in acute myeloblastic leukemia. Various subtypes are recognized according to the nature of the abnormal cells.

### INCIDENCE AND CAUSES

About six or seven new cases of acute leukemia are diagnosed annually per 100,000 people in the US. The incidences of the two main types (acute lymphoblastic leukemia and acute myeloblastic leukemia) at different ages are shown on the next page.

Both types seem to result from a single white cell mutating (altering in its genetic structure). The cell undergoes an uncontrolled series of divisions until billions of copies of the abnormal cell are present in the bone marrow, blood, and other tissues.

There are a number of possible causes for the original mutation. One type of acute lymphoblastic leukemia is thought to be caused by a virus similar to the one that causes *AIDS*. Exposure to certain chemicals (such as benzene and some anticancer drugs) and to atomic radiation or radioactive leaks from nuclear reactors can be a cause. Inherited factors may play a part; there is an increased incidence in people with certain genetic disorders (such as *Fanconi's anemia*) and chromosomal abnormalities (such as *Down's syndrome*). People with certain other blood disorders, such as chronic myeloid leukemia and primary *polycythemia*, are also at increased risk.

### SYMPTOMS AND SIGNS

The symptoms and signs of both types of acute leukemia are caused by overcrowding of the bone marrow by blasts and by infiltration of various organs by the abnormal cells. The overcrowding causes the marrow's failure to produce normal blood cells of all types (see box, next page).

L

# LEUKEMIA

In all forms of leukemia, abnormal white cells proliferate in the bone marrow. There are four main types—acute lymphoblastic leukemia (ALL), acute myeloblastic leukemia (AML), chronic lymphocytic leukemia (CLL), and chronic myeloid leukemia (CML). Their incidence varies with age (see right). The acute types have a rapid onset. There is a risk of death from overwhelming infection or blood loss, but modern treatment has greatly improved survival rates (below) and may bring a cure.

The chronic forms of leukemia progress much more gradually but are essentially incurable.

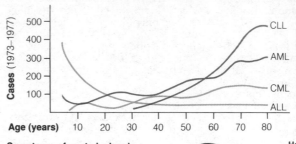

**Incidence**
The graphs show how the four main types of leukemia vary in incidence with age. Acute lymphoblastic leukemia (ALL) is the common type in children, chronic lymphocytic leukemia (CLL) is the most common after 40.

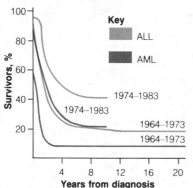

**Survival rates for acute leukemia**
The graphs show survival rates for acute lymphoblastic leukemia (ALL) and acute myeloblastic leukemia (AML) for cases diagnosed in the years 1964 to 1973 and 1974 to 1983. The improved survival rates are the result of better treatment.

**Symptoms of acute leukemia**
Symptoms are caused partly by the abnormal white cells crowding out the bone marrow (so that it fails to produce sufficient normal blood cells of all types) and partly by the invasion of other body organs by abnormal cells.

**Gum bleeding**
This results from insufficient production of platelet cells by the bone marrow; platelets are needed for the arrest of bleeding.

**Bone tenderness**
This may be felt as the bone marrow becomes packed with immature white cells.

**Frequent bruising**
Reduced numbers of platelets may lead to bleeding points in the skin and bruising after mild trauma.

**Headache**
Headache may be caused by anemia or by abnormal white cells affecting the nervous system.

**Enlarged lymph nodes**
The lymph nodes in the neck, armpits, and groin may be swollen with huge numbers of immature white cells. The liver, spleen, and testes may also be swollen.

**Anemia**
Anemia develops if there is insufficient production of red blood cells by the bone marrow. Anemia causes tiredness, breathlessness on exertion, and pallor.

**Infections**
White blood cells play a major part in the defense against infection. However, in acute leukemia, only immature, nonfunctioning white cells are made, so the patient may suffer from repeated chest or throat infections, herpes zóster, or skin and other infections.

## HOW LEUKEMIA ATTACKS THE BODY

Leukemia is a form of cancer, but with the abnormally growing cells—mutated white blood cells—scattered throughout the body in bone marrow, rather than grouped into a single tumor. The abnormal cells may spill into the blood and may infiltrate and interfere with the function of other organs. But worse, the abnormal cells "take over" the marrow and prevent it from making enough normal blood cells—including normal white cells, red cells, and platelets. This leaves the sufferer highly susceptible to serious infections, anemia, and bleeding episodes.

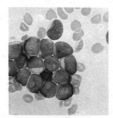

**Cell photograph**
Shown is blood in acute leukemia. The large cells are abnormal, immature white cells; the smaller, paler cells are red blood cells.

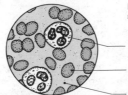

**Normal blood smear**

White cells fight infection

Red cells transport oxygen

Platelets help blood clot

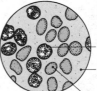

**Blood smear in leukemia**

Abnormal white cells—susceptibility to infection

Fewer platelets—bleeding tendency

Fewer red cells—anemia

**Appearance of blood in leukemia**
In leukemia (above), the blood usually contains many abnormal white cells, and fewer red cells and platelets.

**Normal appearance of blood**
In a normal blood smear (left), there are large numbers of red cells, many platelets, and a few white cells.

L

## DIAGNOSIS

The diagnosis of acute leukemia is based on a *bone marrow biopsy* that confirms an abnormal number of blast cells. The blast cells are sometimes also seen in the blood. When acute lymphoblastic leukemia is diagnosed, a *lumbar puncture* is usually performed to examine the cerebrospinal fluid for the presence of blast cells.

## TREATMENT

Treatment includes giving the patient transfusions of blood and platelets, and the use of *anticancer drugs* to kill the leukemic cells. These drugs tend to make the patient even more susceptible to infection, so powerful antibiotics may also be given.

From the beginning of treatment, it is common for the patient to have inserted into a large vein near the heart a catheter (tube) through which all drugs and transfusions are given. Treatment of leukemic cells in the cerebrospinal fluid is accomplished by the direct injection of drugs into the fluid and by subsequent *radiation therapy* to the head and spinal cord. Radiation therapy is more commonly given in the treatment of acute lymphoblastic leukemia than for acute myeloblastic leukemia.

The course of drug treatment may last for many weeks. When there is no evidence of leukemic cells in the blood or bone marrow, a state of remission is said to have been achieved. However, without repeated courses of treatment, the leukemia often relapses (returns). For this reason, the use of drugs is usually continued for many weeks after remission.

If the leukemia relapses after the first remission, *bone marrow transplantation* may be considered.

## OUTLOOK

The outlook for people with acute lymphoblastic leukemia is generally better than it is for acute myeloblastic leukemia, and it is better for children than for adults. Survival rates are shown in the illustrated box.

## Leukemia, chronic lymphocytic

A type of leukemia caused by proliferation of mature-looking *lymphocytes* (a type of white *blood cell* important in the body's *immune system*). Although incurable, the disease is not invariably fatal.

## INCIDENCE AND CAUSES

There are about four new cases of chronic lymphocytic leukemia annually per 100,000 people in the US. Nearly all patients are over 50. The cause of the disorder is unknown.

## SYMPTOMS AND SIGNS

Symptoms develop slowly, often over many years. Many cases are discovered by chance when a blood test is performed. In addition to features common to acute forms of leukemia (see opposite), symptoms and signs may include an enlarged liver and spleen, persistent raised temperature, and night sweats.

## DIAGNOSIS AND TREATMENT

Chronic lymphocytic leukemia is diagnosed by finding large numbers of lymphocytes, all of the same type, in the blood and on a *bone marrow biopsy*. The severity of the disease is assessed by the degree of liver and spleen enlargement, anemia, and lack of platelet cells in the blood. Often, no treatment is required if the disease is mild. If more severe, *anticancer drugs* are given by mouth, sometimes combined with *radiation therapy*. Other measures include transfusions of blood and platelets, antibiotics to combat infection, and injections of *immunoglobulins* to boost the patient's immune system.

## OUTLOOK

The progression of chronic lymphocytic leukemia is slow. More than half of the patients survive for five years from the time of diagnosis. Eventually, death usually results from overwhelming infection.

## Leukemia, chronic myeloid

Also known as chronic granulocytic leukemia, chronic myeloid leukemia results from uncontrolled proliferation of the class of white *blood cell* called granulocytes. Large numbers of these cells, in various stages of maturity, appear in the blood.

## INCIDENCE AND CAUSES

There are about two new cases of chronic myeloid leukemia diagnosed per 100,000 people in the US each year. Cases occur mainly among middle-aged to elderly people.

The cause of chronic myeloid leukemia is not known. However, in most cases, the patient's cells contain a specific *chromosomal abnormality* known as the Philadelphia chromosome. Part of one chromosome is attached to another chromosome.

## SYMPTOMS

The disease usually has two phases—a chronic phase that may last several years and a more malignant phase in which large numbers of immature granulocytes are produced.

During the chronic phase, symptoms develop slowly; they may include tiredness, fever, night sweats,

and weight loss. If the number of white cells in the blood rises very high, the blood may become excessively viscous (sticky), impairing the supply of oxygen to various organs. The effects can include visual disturbances and abdominal pain due to death of tissues within the spleen. *Priapism* (persistent, painful erection of the penis) is sometimes a feature.

The symptoms of the second phase are like those of acute forms of leukemia (see opposite).

## DIAGNOSIS AND TREATMENT

The disease is sometimes not apparent until the patient has a blood test for some other reason. The diagnosis is made from the increased numbers of granulocytes in the blood and in the bone marrow (as detected by *bone marrow biopsy*). The presence of the Philadelphia chromosome, found by *chromosome analysis*, may help establish the diagnosis.

Treatment of the chronic phase includes the use of *anticancer drugs*. When the disease transforms into the acute phase, treatment is similar to that given for acute leukemia. If the number of white cells rises very high, the cells may be removed from the patient using a machine known as an apheresis machine.

Treatment of the acute phase is seldom successful; the patient usually dies of bleeding or infection. *Bone marrow transplantation* is now being used in an attempt to cure patients while the condition is still in the chronic phase.

## OUTLOOK

The average survival time from first diagnosis is about three years. However, about one fifth of patients survive for 10 years or more. A successful bone marrow transplantation may improve the outlook, but is not without its own risks.

## Leukocyte

Any type of white *blood cell*.

## Leukodystrophies

A rare group of inherited childhood diseases in which the *myelin* sheaths that form a protective covering around many nerves are destroyed.

Diseases included in this group are metachromatic leukodystrophy (which causes impaired speech, blindness, paralysis, dementia, and death within a few years), Krabbe's disease (which results in blindness, deafness, seizures, paralysis, and death within one year), and Merzbacher-Pelizaeus disease (which causes progressive incoordination, speech difficulties, paralysis, and mental deterioration from infancy until death, which occurs in early childhood).

## Leukoplakia

Raised, white patches on the mucous membranes of the mouth or the vulva (the area around the opening to the vagina). Leukoplakia is due to the thickening of tissue and is most common in elderly people.

### CAUSES

Leukoplakia in the mouth, which is most common on the tongue, is usually due to tobacco-smoking (particularly pipe-smoking) or to the rubbing of a rough tooth or denture. It is not known what causes the condition to develop on the vulva.

### SYMPTOMS AND TREATMENT

The patches, which develop slowly, cause no discomfort and are usually harmless. Occasionally, they result from a malignant change in the affected tissue. For this reason, leukoplakia should always be reported to a physician.

Leukoplakia in the mouth may clear up once the cause has been treated. If the condition persists, the patches are removed using a local anesthetic. Leukoplakia of the vulva is treated in the same way. The removed tissue is examined microscopically for any signs of malignant change. (See also *Mouth cancer; Vulva, cancer of.*)

## Leukorrhea

See *Vaginal discharge.*

## Levodopa

A drug used in the treatment of *Parkinson's disease*, a neurological disorder caused by deficiency of the chemical dopamine in part of the brain.

### HOW IT WORKS

Levodopa is absorbed into the brain and converted into dopamine. The drug is usually given with an enzyme (such as carbidopa) that reduces the amount of levodopa broken down by the liver before it can reach the brain. This allows a lower dose of levodopa to be given and thereby reduces the risk of adverse effects.

### POSSIBLE ADVERSE EFFECTS

Adverse effects include nausea, vomiting, nervousness, and agitation. Prolonged use often impairs the effectiveness of treatment or increases the severity of adverse effects.

## Levonorgestrel

A *progesterone drug* used in some *oral contraceptive* preparations.

## Levothyroxine

A synthetic drug preparation related to thyroxine, the most important of the *thyroid hormones.*

## LH

The abbreviation for luteinizing hormone—a *gonadotropin hormone* produced by the *pituitary gland.*

## LH-RH

The abbreviation for *luteinizing hormone-releasing hormone.* This hormone is released by the *hypothalamus.*

## Liability insurance, professional

A protection against lawsuits, traditionally purchased by physicians. As a result of the tremendous growth in the number of suits and size of awards in the 1970s and 1980s, coupled with less stringent interpretation of negligence, insurance companies have dramatically raised premiums, restricted policies to low-risk medical specialties, and, in some cases, stopped providing liability insurance.

## Libido

Sexual desire. Libido is a healthy, normal feeling, especially strong in youth and gradually fading with age. Loss of libido is a symptom of numerous physical illnesses, and of *depression, drug abuse,* and *alcohol dependence.*

The libido theory of Sigmund Freud describes sexual development in childhood in terms of oral, anal, and genital stages (representing the areas of the body toward which a child's attention is directed at different ages). Freud believed that certain neurotic disorders and abnormal sexual behaviors were due to fixation of libido at one of these stages. By contrast, directing the libido (or "love energy") away from oneself to other people or objects was seen as a sign of maturity. (See also *Narcissism; Sexual desire, inhibited.*)

## Lice

Small, wingless insects that feed on human blood. There are three species: PEDICULUS HUMANUS CAPITIS (the head louse), PEDICULUS HUMANUS CORPORIS (the body louse), and PHTHIRUS PUBIS (the crab, or pubic, louse). All lice have flattened bodies and measure up to one eighth of an inch (3 mm) across.

### HEAD LICE

These lice live on and suck blood from the scalp. They leave red spots that itch intensely, leading to scratching,

*dermatitis* (skin inflammation), and *impetigo* (a bacterial infection of the skin). The females lay a daily batch of tiny, pale eggs (nits) that are attached to hairs close to the scalp; the nits hatch in about seven days. The adults may live for several weeks.

Head lice affect all social classes. Children are most affected, women occasionally, and men rarely. The lice are spread by direct (although not necessarily head-to-head) contact.

Lotions containing malathion or carbaryl kill lice and nits rapidly. The lotion should be washed off 12 hours after application, and a fine-toothed comb run through the hair to remove dead lice and nits. Shampoos containing malathion or carbaryl are also effective if used repeatedly over several days. Combs and hairbrushes should be treated with very hot water to kill any attached eggs.

### BODY LICE

These lice live, and lay eggs, on clothing next to the skin. The lice visit the body only to feed. Body lice transmit epidemic *typhus* and *relapsing fever,* which are rare today, but, in the past, were common in areas affected by war or natural disaster.

Body lice affect only people who rarely change their clothes. These lice can be killed by placing infested clothes in a hot dryer for five minutes, by washing them in very hot water, or by burning them.

### CRAB LICE

These lice live in pubic hair or, more rarely, armpits or beards. They are usually passed from one person to another during sexual contact. (See *Pubic lice.*)

## Licensure

Physicians must be licensed by the state in which they practice. The qualifications for licensure vary from state to state. In general, however, a physician must graduate from an accredited medical or osteopathic school, complete one year of residency training (internship), and pass a state's licensing examination. Graduates of foreign medical schools may be licensed if they meet the state's requirements for residency training and pass its licensing examination. Only a state licensing board has the legal power to restrict or suspend a physician's license to practice.

## Lichenification

Thickening and hardening of the skin caused by repeated scratching. Lichenification is often the result of trying to relieve the intense itching of disorders such as atopic *eczema* or *lichen simplex*.

## Lichen planus

A common skin disease of unknown cause that usually affects middle-aged people. Small, shiny, extremely itchy, pink or purple raised spots appear on the skin of the wrists, forearms, or lower legs. There is often a lacy network of white spots covering the inside lining of the cheeks.

Treatment is with *corticosteroid drugs*. Creams, sometimes supplemented by injections in severe cases, are used to treat the skin rash and tablets are used to treat lichen planus in the mouth. Most cases clear up within 18 months.

## Lichen simplex

Patches of thickened, itchy, and sometimes discolored skin caused by repeated scratching. Typical sites are the neck, wrist, arm near the elbow,

and ankles. Lichen simplex is most common in women and is psychological in origin; sufferers often rub the patches (without being aware of what they are doing) when agitated or under stressful circumstances.

A cycle is established in which repeated scratching to relieve itching leads to more skin thickening and itching, which in turn requires yet more scratching.

Treatment is with *antihistamine* tablets and *corticosteroid* creams to relieve the itching and thus break the cycle. This permits the disorder to subside and the drug treatment to be effective.

## Lid lag

A momentary delay in the normal downward movement of the upper eyelids that occurs when the eye looks down. A characteristic feature of *thyrotoxicosis*, lid lag usually occurs in conjunction with *exophthalmos* (protrusion of the eyeball).

## Lidocaine

ANTIARRHYTHMIC LOCAL ANESTHETIC

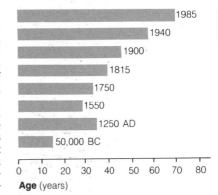

Liquid Injection Cream Ointment

Ointment available over-the-counter

Available as generic

A local anesthetic (see *Anesthesia, local*). Lidocaine is used to relieve the pain and irritation caused by *sunburn* or *hemorrhoids*. It is given to numb tissues before minor surgical procedures and as a *nerve block* (to numb the area supplied by a particular nerve). Lidocaine is also used topically to relieve discomfort during the insertion of a *catheter* or an *endoscope*.

Lidocaine is given by intravenous injection after *myocardial infarction* to reduce the risk of *ventricular fibrillation* (an irregularity of the heart beat).

POSSIBLE ADVERSE EFFECTS
High doses given by injection occasionally cause nausea and vomiting.

## Life expectancy

The number of years a person can expect to live. In most Western countries, life expectancy at birth is about 70 years for men and 75 years for women. This sex difference is thought to be due to the fact that many more men than women smoked in the first half of this century. However, since then, the smoking sex ratio has evened out and there has been an increase in deaths from lung cancer in women. As a result, the sex difference in life expectancy is narrowing.

The expected age of death becomes greater the longer a person lives, so someone aged 70 may have a life expectancy of 15 years; even a 100 year old can expect to live a year or two.

**LIFE EXPECTANCY AND LIFE SPAN**
Life expectancy should be distinguished from life span. Since records began, some old people have lived well beyond 70 years. Gerontologists agree that, in the absence of disease, the average normal life span is about 85 years (see *Aging*).

The natural life span is determined largely by genetic factors. People whose parents and grandparents lived to be 90 are likely to live to about this age. However, the extent to which individuals fulfill their genetic potential is affected by environmental factors, such as nutrition and accidents, as well as by disease.

The proportion of the population that attains its natural life span

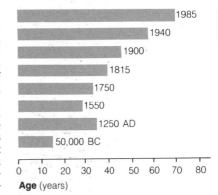

Age (years)

**Life expectancy through history**
Advances in medicine have dramatically increased life expectancy at birth. Life expectancies in England fluctuated around age 30 to 35 for many centuries, before reaching 40 in the early 19th century and climbing to over 70 in recent decades. Most developed countries follow a similar pattern.

L

depends on the general health of that population, so life expectancy is a good means of comparing the state of health in different countries or in different parts of the same country.

Life expectancy at birth may be as low as 35 years in some developing countries. However, although statistically accurate, this figure is misleading because it reflects the high mortality during infancy in these countries. Records show that life expectancy at age 40 is not greatly different around the world.

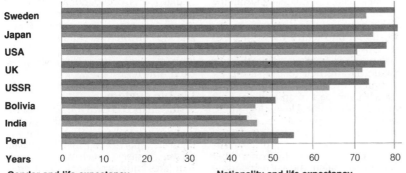

**Gender and life expectancy**
In rich and poor countries, life expectancy at birth is generally higher for females (gray bars) than males (red). India is an exception.

**Nationality and life expectancy**
Average life expectancy at birth in most developed countries is now 70 or more; in developing countries it is 40 to 55.

L

## Life support
The process of keeping a person alive by artificially inflating the lungs (see *Ventilation*) and, if necessary, maintaining the heart beat with a *pacemaker*.

## Ligament
A tough band of white, fibrous, slightly elastic tissue. Ligaments are important components of joints, binding together the bone ends and preventing excessive movement of the joint. Ligaments also support various organs, including the uterus, bladder, liver, and diaphragm, and help maintain the shape of the breasts.

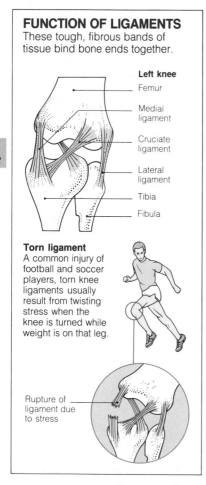

### FUNCTION OF LIGAMENTS
These tough, fibrous bands of tissue bind bone ends together.

**Left knee**
- Femur
- Medial ligament
- Cruciate ligament
- Lateral ligament
- Tibia
- Fibula

**Torn ligament**
A common injury of football and soccer players, torn knee ligaments usually result from twisting stress when the knee is turned while weight is on that leg.

Rupture of ligament due to stress

INJURY
Ligaments, especially those in the *ankle joint* and *knee*, are sometimes damaged by injury. Minor sprains are treated with ice, bandaging, and sometimes physical therapy. If the ligament is torn, the joint is either immobilized by a plaster cast to allow healing or repaired surgically.

## Ligation
The surgical process of ligating (tying off) a blood vessel to prevent bleeding, or a duct to close it, with a length of thread or other material. The term is used in *tubal ligation*, a form of sterilization in which the fallopian tubes are tied off.

## Ligature
A length of thread or other material used for *ligation* (tying off) of a blood vessel or duct.

## Lightening
A feeling experienced by many pregnant women when the baby's head drops into the pelvic cavity. Lightening usually occurs in the last three weeks of pregnancy, leaving more space in the upper abdomen and relieving pressure under the ribs, making breathing easier.

## Light treatment
See *Phototherapy*.

## Limb, artificial
Most artificial legs and arms, known medically as limb prostheses, are fitted to replace all or part of a limb amputated because of disease or severe injury (see *Amputation*). In some cases, however, they are required as a substitute for limbs missing from birth (see *Limb defects*).

To be acceptable, an artificial limb must restore as much as possible the function of the lost limb, be light enough to be worn comfortably, be easy to put on and take off, and look as natural as possible.

CONSTRUCTION AND MATERIALS
Artificial limbs can be obtained ready-made. However, for the best results, they should be constructed by a prosthetist (a specialist in making and fitting artificial limbs) to suit the individual's needs. A mold taken from the stump of the missing limb is used to make a socket for the top of the prosthesis into which the stump can fit closely and comfortably. The socket, made from wood, leather, or plastic, is attached to the stump by suction or by straps.

Each main part of an artificial limb replacing the natural lower leg, thigh, forearm, or upper arm is called an extension. The extension consists of an inner strut made of various materials; it is covered by foam rubber shaped to match the corresponding part of the natural limb. This unit is enclosed by an outer shell of metal, wood, or leather.

Artificial joints are usually made of plastic and metal and today incorporate sophisticated mechanisms that rotate the wrist, stabilize the knee joint, and control the length of stride.

Generally, artificial legs are more useful than artificial arms because the straightforward movements of the natural leg are easier to duplicate than the wide-ranging, often intricate, movements of the arm (especially the hand). Even so, the design of artificial hands is now extremely advanced. Electronic circuitry has been developed to pick up muscle and nerve impulses reaching the stump from the spinal cord. The circuitry transforms the impulses into movements of the prosthesis. People with an artificial arm or hand may have several prostheses (e.g., one with a glove for social use and others with a claw or powered attachments for working).

## Limb defects
Incomplete development of one or more limbs at birth. Sometimes an entire limb is missing, sometimes only the hand or foot, or the upper or lower half of a limb, is missing. In other people, hands, feet, or tiny fingers or toe buds are attached to limb stumps or grow directly from the trunk (a condition called phocomelia). Any combination of limbs may be affected.

Limb defects are rare; the incidence in the US is only about one in every 2,000 live births. The sedative drug *thalidomide* is known to have caused phocomelia when taken during pregnancy. (This drug was never sold in the US.) Otherwise, apart from those cases in which limb defects are inherited or part of a syndrome, their cause remains unknown.

MANAGEMENT
A child with a limb defect usually needs to attend a specialized center. Pediatricians, occupational therapists, psychologists, social workers, and other experts will treat the condition and advise on the child's development. A prosthetist will fit an artificial limb (see *Limb, artificial*) and teach the child how to use it.

## Limbic system
A ring-shaped area in the center of the brain that consists of a number of connected clusters of nerve cells. The limbic system plays a role in the *autonomic nervous system* (which automatically regulates body functions), in the emotions, and in the sense of smell. The limbic system is extensive, and the different substructures within it

## TYPES OF ARTIFICIAL LIMBS

Different types of artificial limbs must restore as much as possible the function of the lost limb, be light enough to be worn comfortably, be easy to put on and take off, and look as normal as possible. Although ready-made prostheses are available and can be quite effective, the best artificial limbs are constructed by specialists and specially adapted to meet an individual's particular needs.

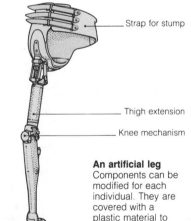

**Initiating movement**
The nerve impulses that move the prosthesis originate in the brain and pass via the spinal cord to the stump.

**Prosthetic movement**
Electronic circuitry in the prosthesis picks up nerve impulses in the stump and causes the prosthesis to move in a near-normal way.

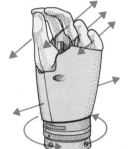
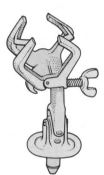

**Artificial hands**
Many devices are available. The prosthesis on the left is servo-mechanism-controlled and battery-operated; it allows finger and wrist movements. The shovel grip is a prosthesis designed to meet a specific need, as are precision tweezers and golf-club grips.

Strap for stump

Thigh extension

Knee mechanism

**An artificial leg**
Components can be modified for each individual. They are covered with a plastic material to give the limb a natural appearance.

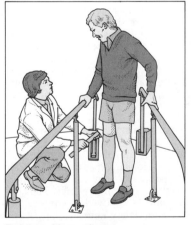

**Training with prostheses**
Special walking classes enable patients to adjust to their new limbs.

have been named (for example, the hippocampus, the cingulate gyrus, and the amygdala).

Much of our knowledge of the limbic system comes from the observation and investigation of the behavior of animals and people known to have damage to or disease in the limbic area of the brain. The most commonly observed effects are abnormalities of emotional response, such as inappropriate crying or laughing, easily provoked rage, unwarranted fear, anxiety and depression, and excessive sexual interest.

## Limp

An abnormal, uneven pattern of *walking* in which the movements of one leg (or of the pelvis on one side of the body) are different from those of the other. A limp may involve dipping of the pelvis to one side, or failure to straighten the leg fully when the foot is placed on the ground.

## Lincomycin

An *antibiotic drug* used to treat serious infections of the lungs, skin, bones, joints, and pelvis that are resistant to commonly prescribed antibiotic drugs such as *penicillin*. Lincomycin may rarely cause a type of *colitis* (inflammation of the intestine) called pseudomembranous enterocolitis.

## Lindane

A drug used to treat infestation by *scabies* or *lice* and available in the form of a lotion, cream, or shampoo. Lindane sometimes irritates the skin and scalp and causes itching.

## Linear accelerator

A device for accelerating subatomic particles, such as electrons, to a speed approaching that of light so that they have extremely high energies. A linear accelerator can also be used to generate high-energy X rays.

In medicine, high-energy electrons or X rays are used in *radiation therapy* to treat certain cancers. This method causes less damage to the healthy tissue around a tumor than does low-energy radiation therapy.

## Lip

One of two fleshy folds around the entrance to the mouth. Externally the lips are covered with skin and internally with mucous membrane, the relative transparency of which allows the red-pink of the underlying capillaries to show through.

The main substructure of the lips is a ring of muscle; its functions include keeping food in the mouth, helping to produce speech and other sounds (like whistling), and kissing. Smaller muscles at the corners of the lips are responsible for facial expression.

### DISORDERS

These include chapping (see *Chapped skin*), *cheilitis* (inflammation, cracking, and dryness), *cold sores* (blisters on the lips), syphilitic ulcers (see *Chancre, hard*), and *lip cancer*.

L

## Lip cancer

A tumor, usually on the lower lip. Lip cancer is largely confined to older people, especially those exposed to a lot of sunlight through working outdoors and those who have smoked cigarettes or a pipe for many years. Lip cancer is the most common form of mouth cancer, but represents only about 1 percent of all cancers.

### SYMPTOMS

A white patch develops on the lip and soon becomes scaly and cracked with a yellow crust. The affected area grows, eventually becoming ulcerous; the cancer may spread to the lymph nodes in the jaw and then the neck.

### DIAGNOSIS AND TREATMENT

Any lip sore that persists for longer than a month should be seen by a physician. Lip cancer (usually a *squamous cell carcinoma*) is diagnosed by *biopsy* (microscopic examination).

Treatment is surgical removal, *radiation therapy*, or a combination of both. If the tumor has spread to the lymph nodes in the neck, *neck dissection* and more radiation may be necessary.

## Lipectomy, suction

A type of *body contour surgery* in which excess fat is suctioned out through a small incision made in the skin.

## Lipid disorders

Disorders of metabolism that cause abnormal amounts of *lipids* in the body. The most common of these disorders are the *hyperlipidemias*, which may be inherited or brought on or aggravated by diet or a disorder. In addition, there are also some very rare lipid disorders that are due solely to heredity, such as *Tay-Sachs disease*.

## Lipid-lowering drugs

| COMMON DRUGS |
| --- |
| Drugs that act on the liver<br>*Clofibrate Gemfibrozil Lovastatin* |
| Drugs that act on bile salts<br>*Cholestyramine Colestipol Neomycin* |

A group of drugs used to treat *hyperlipidemia* (abnormally high levels of one or more types of *lipid*, such as *cholesterol*, in the blood). Lipid-lowering drugs are given to reduce the risk of severe *atherosclerosis* (narrowing of the arteries causing impaired blood flow), usually when dietary measures have not worked.

### HOW THEY WORK

Some lipid-lowering drugs alter enzyme activity in the liver to prevent the production of one or more types of lipid from fatty acids. This action reduces the level of lipids in the blood.

Other lipid-lowering drugs interfere with the absorption of bile salts from the intestine into the blood. Bile salts contain large amounts of cholesterol; a decrease in their concentration in the blood stimulates the liver to convert more cholesterol into bile salts, thus reducing the amount of cholesterol in the blood.

### POSSIBLE ADVERSE EFFECTS

Lipid-lowering drugs that act on the liver cause increased susceptibility to gallstones. Those that act on bile salts may cause nausea and diarrhea.

## Lipids

Often called structural *fats*, lipids are a group of fatty substances that includes triglycerides (the principal forms of fat in body fat), phospholipids (important constituents of cell membranes), and sterols such as *cholesterol*.

## Lipoatrophy

Loss of *adipose tissue* (body fat). Patchy lipoatrophy may be caused in diabetics by repeated injections of insulin into one area of skin. Other causes include *malabsorption* of fat from the intestine and lipodystrophies (disorders of fat metabolism).

## Lipoma

A common benign tumor of fatty tissue. Lipomas give rise to soft swellings that are slow-growing and often occur in multiples. They may develop anywhere in the body, but occur most commonly on the thigh, trunk, or shoulder. Lipomas are painless and harmless and do not need treatment, although they may be surgically removed for cosmetic reasons.

## Liposarcoma

A rare malignant tumor of fatty tissue that usually develops during late middle age. Liposarcomas usually occur in the abdomen or on the thigh, where they produce firm swellings. They can generally be removed by surgery, but have a tendency to recur.

## Lipreading

A way of understanding words or conversation through the use of visual clues rather than hearing. Lipreading is invaluable in helping people who are deaf understand more of what is said to them (see *Deafness*).

### HOW IT IS DONE

The basis of lipreading is that certain speech sounds are produced by characteristic movements, positions, and relationships of the jaw, lips, and tongue. Because there are more than 40 clearly distinct sounds in the English language, facial expression and context are also important. However, many of the language sounds are produced by similar mouth patterns ("p," "b," and "m" all share the same pattern). There are only about 14 visibly distinguishable mouth patterns; of these, only four or five can be consistently recognized under normal viewing conditions.

### EFFECTIVENESS

Tests have shown that the proportion of identified words can rise from 20 to 60 percent after training. Anyone speaking to a deaf person can help improve the effectiveness of lipreading by speaking slightly more slowly than usual, by not covering the mouth when speaking, and by looking directly at the deaf person.

## Liquid petrolatum

See *Mineral oil*.

## Lisp

The most common form of *speech disorder*. A lisp is due to protrusion of the tongue between the teeth so that the "s" sound is replaced by "th." Most children with a lisp have completely normal structures of the mouth and lips. However, sometimes the speech defect is caused by a cleft palate (see *Cleft lip and palate*).

In most children, lisping disappears without treatment. If it persists after the age of about 4, *speech therapy* may be considered.

## Listeriosis

An infection common in animals, including cattle, pigs, and poultry, that also occurs very rarely in humans. It is caused by the bacterium LISTERIA MONOCYTOGENES. Possible causes include eating improperly cooked, infected meat or direct spread of the bacteria from an infected live animal.

A fever and generalized aches and pains are the only symptoms that most affected adults develop, but, in the elderly or infirm, the disease can be life-threatening. If an unborn child is infected through its mother's blood, it may be stillborn. *Pneumonia*, *septicemia*, and *meningitis* may develop in a newborn with the disease.

Listeriosis is diagnosed from blood tests and cultures of other fluids obtained from the infected person. Treatment with antibiotics usually clears up the infection.

## Lithium

A drug used in the long-term treatment of *mania* and *manic-depressive illness*. Lithium helps prevent mood swings in mania and reduces their frequency and their severity in manic-depressive illness.

### HOW IT WORKS

Lithium reduces excessive nerve activity in the brain. It is thought to work by altering the chemical balance within certain nerve cells.

### POSSIBLE ADVERSE EFFECTS

High levels of lithium in the blood may cause nausea, vomiting, diarrhea, blurred vision, tremor, drowsiness, rash, and, in rare cases, kidney damage. Regular blood tests are carried out to monitor the level of lithium in the body.

Too much tea and coffee increases the risk of adverse effects. Too much sodium in the diet reduces the effectiveness of treatment.

## Lithotomy

Surgical removal of a *calculus* (stone) from the urinary tract, especially from the bladder.

The operation of "cutting for stone" is one of the oldest known surgical procedures. Until the discovery of antiseptic surgical techniques, bladder stones were removed by approaching the organ through incisions between the thighs rather than via the abdomen. The patient would lie back with hips and knees bent and the legs open. Today, this *lithotomy position* is used primarily for gynecological examinations.

The operations of ureterolithotomy and *pyelolithotomy* (removal of ureteral and kidney stones, respectively, by incision) are still occasionally performed. In developed countries, surgical removal of bladder stones is rarely performed, and then only for large stones. Today, bladder stones are usually crushed and dissolved by use of a cystoscope (see *Cystoscopy*) or by *lithotripsy*.

## Lithotomy position

Position in which a patient lies on his or her back with knees bent and wide apart. Originally used for *lithotomy* (surgical removal of stones), the position is still used for *pelvic examinations*, childbirth, and many types of pelvic surgery. Stirrups are usually used to support the feet and legs.

## Lithotripsy

The process of using shock waves or ultrasonic waves to break up *calculi*

## LITHOTRIPSY PROCEDURES

Calculi can sometimes be removed without major surgery. Lithotripsy uses ultrasonic or shock waves to break up the calculi. In percutaneous lithotripsy, the stones are easily removed through a small incision. After extracorporeal shock-wave lithotripsy (ESWL), stone fragments are passed in the urine.

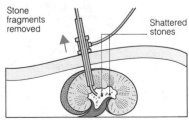

**Abdominal calculi**
This X ray shows two staghorn calculi in the kidneys. Before lithotripsy, stones such as these could be removed only by major surgery.

### PERCUTANEOUS LITHOTRIPSY

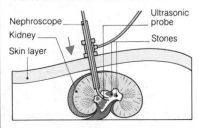

**1** The surgeon first makes a small incision in the flank and inserts a nephroscope (a type of viewing tube) into the kidney.

**2** A probe is passed through the nephroscope to direct ultrasound waves at the stones, causing them to shatter. Stone fragments are then removed.

### EXTRACORPOREAL SHOCK-WAVE LITHOTRIPSY (ESWL)

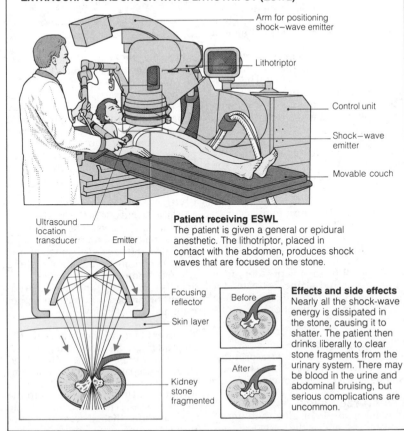

**Patient receiving ESWL**
The patient is given a general or epidural anesthetic. The lithotriptor, placed in contact with the abdomen, produces shock waves that are focused on the stone.

**Effects and side effects**
Nearly all the shock-wave energy is dissipated in the stone, causing it to shatter. The patient then drinks liberally to clear stone fragments from the urinary system. There may be blood in the urine and abdominal bruising, but serious complications are uncommon.

(stones) for excretion. There are two different procedures—extracorporeal shock wave lithotripsy (ESWL) and percutaneous lithotripsy.

### WHY IT IS DONE

Lithotripsy is used to break up kidney and upper ureteral stones (see *Calculus, urinary tract*) into tiny pieces so that they can be excreted in the urine. It is also being investigated as a treatment for gallstones.

ESWL is used to break up smaller stones; percutaneous lithotripsy is used to break up larger stones. Very large stones may be treated with a combination of the two.

### HOW IT IS DONE

Both procedures are performed using a general or epidural anesthetic. In some cases, more than one treatment is required.

**ESWL** This technique uses a machine called a *lithotriptor* to produce external shock waves to break up stones. X-ray imaging systems are used to show the position of the stone and to monitor its destruction into a fine sand, which is passed out of the body in the urine or the bile over the following few weeks. ESWL has radically changed the treatment of kidney stones by eliminating the need for most surgery. The technique may also change the treatment of gallstones.

**PERCUTANEOUS LITHOTRIPSY** A nephroscope (type of *endoscope*) is inserted into the kidney via a small flank incision. An ultrasonic probe is directed through the nephroscope to break up the stone; fragments are removed through the nephroscope.

### RECOVERY PERIOD

There may be hematuria (blood in the urine) for about 12 hours after the treatment. After ESWL there may be some bruising of the skin at the entry and exit points of the shock wave. Most people can return to full activity within a week.

### COMPLICATIONS

*Renal colic*, a sudden, severe pain in the side due to obstruction of the ureter by small fragments of stone, may occur after ESWL. Patients treated for gallstones may need drug treatment to aid the final elimination of stone residue.

## Lithotriptor

The machine used in extracorporeal shock wave *lithotripsy* (ESWL) to disintegrate small *calculi* (stones).

## Livedo reticularis

A netlike purple or blue mottling of the skin, usually on the lower legs. It is

## LOCATION OF THE LIVER

The liver is a roughly cone-shaped, red-brown organ that occupies the upper right-hand portion of the abdominal cavity. It lies immediately beneath the diaphragm, to which its upper side is attached. Its base is in contact with the stomach, right kidney, and intestines. Tucked within a depression on the underside of the liver is the gallbladder.

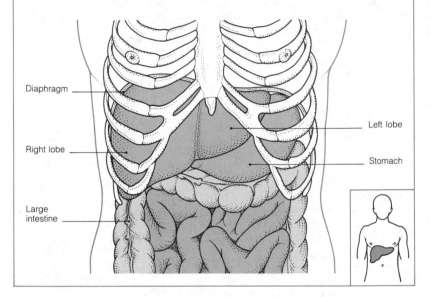

caused by the enlargement of blood vessels beneath the skin and tends to be worse in cold weather.

Though harmless, the condition is present for life. Livedo reticularis may appear in healthy people, but is more common in those who are abnormally sensitive to cold or in people who have suffered damage to blood vessels just beneath the skin (see *Vasculitis*).

## Liver

The largest and one of the most important internal organs, which functions as the body's chemical factory and regulates the levels of most of the main chemicals in blood. Weighing 2.5 to 3.3 pounds (1.1 to 1.5 kg), the liver is a roughly cone-shaped, red-brown organ that occupies the upper right abdominal cavity.

### STRUCTURE

The liver lies immediately beneath the diaphragm; it has two main lobes.

The liver receives oxygenated blood from the hepatic artery and nutrient-rich blood via the portal vein (see illustration). The blood drains into the hepatic veins. The liver cells secrete *bile*, a fluid that leaves the liver through a network of ducts, the bile

ducts. Within the liver, the small bile ducts and branches of the hepatic artery and the portal vein form a kind of conduit system known as the portal tracts.

### FUNCTION

The liver has many functions vital to the body. One is to produce important proteins for blood plasma. They include albumin (which regulates the exchange of water between blood and tissues), complement (a group of proteins that plays a part in the *immune system's* defenses against infection), coagulation factors (which enable blood to clot when a blood vessel wall is damaged), and globin (a constituent of the oxygen-carrying pigment *hemoglobin*. The liver also produces *cholesterol* and special proteins that help carry fats around the body.

Another function of the liver is to take up glucose that is not required immediately by the body's cells, and store it as glycogen. When the body needs to generate more energy and heat, the liver (under the stimulation of hormones) converts the glycogen back to glucose and releases it into the bloodstream.

The liver also regulates the blood level of amino acids, chemicals that

L

form the building blocks of proteins. When the blood contains too high a level of amino acids (such as after a meal), the liver converts some of them into glucose, some into proteins, some into other amino acids, and some into urea, which is passed to the kidney for excretion in the urine.

Along with the kidneys, the liver acts to clear the blood of drugs and poisonous substances that would otherwise accumulate in the blood-stream. The liver absorbs the substances to be removed from the blood, alters their chemical structure, makes them water soluble, and excretes them in the bile.

Bile carries waste products away from the liver and helps in the break-down and absorption of fats in the small intestine (see *Biliary system*).

Although extremely complex in its functions, the liver is a remarkably resilient organ. Up to three quarters of its cells can be destroyed or surgically removed before it ceases to function.

## Liver abscess

A localized collection of pus in the liver. The most common causes are a spread of bacteria from intestines inflamed by *diverticular disease* or *appendicitis* and invasion of the liver by amebae (single-celled animal parasites) in people infected with *amebiasis*. In some cases, the source of infection cannot be identified.

An affected person is obviously sick, has a high fever and pain in the upper right abdomen, and (especially if elderly) may be confused.

### DIAGNOSIS AND TREATMENT

*Ultrasound scanning* usually shows the abscess. The responsible microorganisms can sometimes be grown in *culture* from a blood sample or direct needle aspiration of the liver.

If possible, the abscess may be drained through a needle inserted through the abdominal wall and guided by ultrasound. Otherwise, abdominal surgery is needed.

## Liver biopsy

A diagnostic test in which a small sample of tissue is removed from the liver. The procedure is relatively safe, and complications are rare.

### WHY IT IS DONE

The main function of the test is to diagnose liver diseases, such as *cirrhosis* and different types of *hepatitis*. A liver biopsy can also help diagnose diseases such as tumors and *lymphomas*, which spread throughout the body and affect many organs. In addition, the test can provide an important check on the efficacy of treatment of diseases such as chronic active hepatitis.

### HOW IT IS DONE

Most liver biopsies are performed using a local anesthetic. While the patient holds his or her breath, a slim needle is inserted into the liver via a very small incision made over the right lower ribs. The needle is removed with a small sample of liver tissue, the structure and cells of which are examined by a pathologist.

A liver biopsy is sometimes performed during the course of another abdominal operation.

## LIVER STRUCTURE AND FUNCTION

The liver is a large organ with numerous functions. It absorbs oxygen and nutrients from the blood, and regulates the blood's glucose and amino-acid levels. It helps break down drugs and various toxins, and manufactures important proteins, such as albumin and blood coagulation factors. The liver also produces bile, which removes waste products and helps process fats in the small intestine.

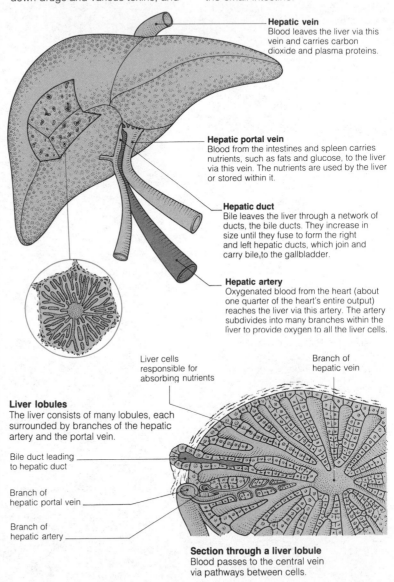

**Hepatic vein**
Blood leaves the liver via this vein and carries carbon dioxide and plasma proteins.

**Hepatic portal vein**
Blood from the intestines and spleen carries nutrients, such as fats and glucose, to the liver via this vein. The nutrients are used by the liver or stored within it.

**Hepatic duct**
Bile leaves the liver through a network of ducts, the bile ducts. They increase in size until they fuse to form the right and left hepatic ducts, which join and carry bile to the gallbladder.

**Hepatic artery**
Oxygenated blood from the heart (about one quarter of the heart's entire output) reaches the liver via this artery. The artery subdivides into many branches within the liver to provide oxygen to all the liver cells.

Liver cells responsible for absorbing nutrients

Branch of hepatic vein

**Liver lobules**
The liver consists of many lobules, each surrounded by branches of the hepatic artery and the portal vein.

Bile duct leading to hepatic duct

Branch of hepatic portal vein

Branch of hepatic artery

**Section through a liver lobule**
Blood passes to the central vein via pathways between cells.

L

# DISORDERS OF THE LIVER

By far the most common cause of liver disease in the US and other developed countries is excessive consumption of alcohol (see *Liver disease, alcoholic*). Alcohol-related disorders, which include alcoholic *hepatitis* and *cirrhosis*, outnumber all other types of liver disorder by at least five to one.

Worldwide, the pattern of liver disease is different. In parts of Africa and Asia, up to 20 percent of the population are carriers of the *hepatitis B* virus; in these parts of the world, the most important liver disorders are virus-induced cirrhosis and primary *liver cancer*.

Apart from alcohol- and virus-induced liver disease, the liver may be affected by congenital defects, bacterial and parasitic infection, circulatory disturbance, metabolic disorders, poisoning, and autoimmune processes.

*Liver failure* (complete loss of liver function) may occur as a result of acute hepatitis, poisoning, or cirrhosis. Enlargement of the liver (hepatomegaly) and *jaundice* are two common signs of liver disease.

## CONGENITAL DEFECTS

Defects of liver structure at birth principally affect the bile ducts. A choledochal cyst is a malformation of the hepatic duct (formed from the union of all the small bile ducts in the liver) that may obstruct the flow of bile in infants (causing jaundice); it requires removal. In *biliary atresia*, the bile ducts are absent, again causing jaundice.

## INFECTION AND INFLAMMATION

*Hepatitis* is a general term for inflammation in the liver; it may be caused by viruses such as the hepatitis A, B, and non A, non B viruses (see *Hepatitis, viral*). Bacteria may spread up the biliary system toward the liver to cause *cholangitis* or *liver abscess*. Parasitic diseases that may affect the liver include *schistosomiasis*, *liver fluke*, and *hydatid disease* (caused by various types of worm or fluke) and *amebiasis* (caused by a single-celled parasite).

## POISONING AND DRUGS

Apart from alcohol, many drugs and toxins are broken down by the liver, damaging liver cells in the process.

**Hepatitis** Inflammation of the liver may be caused by one of the hepatitis viruses, alcohol, or various poisons.

**Amebiasis** Infection by amebic parasites can cause painful abscesses in the liver.

**Liver cancer** Malignant tumors may arise from the liver itself or may spread from cancer elsewhere in the body.

**Choledochal cyst** This congenital malformation blocks the flow of bile through the hepatic duct.

Suicidal overdose with the painkilling drug acetaminophen causes severe liver damage, which may not be obvious until up to two days after the overdose. Some medications, even in normal doses, can cause acute or chronic hepatitis by a direct toxic effect or through drug allergy.

Poisoning by certain types of mushrooms can cause acute liver failure (see *Mushroom poisoning*).

## AUTOIMMUNE DISORDERS

Liver cells and bile ducts can be targets for autoimmune reactions (in which the body's immune system attacks its own tissues). A gradual destruction of liver cells is the main problem in autoimmune chronic active hepatitis (see *Hepatitis, chronic active*). The slowly progressive bile duct damage that occurs in primary *biliary cirrhosis* and sclerosing cholangitis possibly also has an autoimmune basis.

## METABOLIC DISORDERS

The two main metabolic disorders affecting the liver are *hemochromatosis* (in which there is too much iron in the body) and *Wilson's disease* (in which there is too much copper).

## TUMORS

The liver is a common site of malignant tumors that have spread from cancers of the stomach, pancreas, or large intestine. Enlargement of the liver and spleen is a common feature of *leukemias* and *lymphomas*. Primary tumors of the liver are much less common. (See *Liver cancer*.)

## OTHER DISORDERS

In *Budd-Chiari syndrome*, the veins draining the liver become blocked by blood clots, causing painful swelling of the liver and severe *ascites* (collection of fluid in the abdomen). Obstruction of the portal vein is one cause of *portal hypertension* (high blood pressure in the portal vein), which can lead to *esophageal varices* (swollen veins in the esophagus) and ascites. Portal hypertension is also one of the usual complications of cirrhosis.

### INVESTIGATION

Disorders of the liver may be investigated by physical examination, *liver biopsy, liver function tests, ultrasound scanning,* and *CT scanning.*

# Liver cancer

A malignant tumor in the liver. The tumor may be primary (originating within the liver itself) or secondary (spread from elsewhere). There are two main types of primary tumor—a hepatoma, which develops in the liver cells, and a *cholangiocarcinoma*, which arises from cells lining the bile ducts.

### CAUSES AND INCIDENCE

Hepatomas are the most common form of cancer worldwide. They are closely linked to hepatitis B (see *Hepatitis, viral*), common throughout Africa, the Middle East, and the Far East. In the US, hepatitis B is a relatively uncommon infection, so hepatomas are rare. There are only about three or four new cases per 100,000 people annually. When a hepatoma does occur, it is usually a complication of *cirrhosis* of the liver.

Secondary liver cancer is relatively common in the US (about 20 times more common than primary cancer); it often originates from cancers in the stomach, pancreas, or large intestine, where the primary tumor may have been small and caused no symptoms.

### SYMPTOMS AND SIGNS

The most common symptoms of any liver cancer are weight loss, loss of appetite, and lethargy. In addition, there is often pain in the upper right abdomen. The later stages of the disease are marked by *jaundice* and *ascites* (fluid in the abdomen).

### DIAGNOSIS

Liver tumors are usually detected as a result of *ultrasound scanning* that reveals abnormal areas in the liver. The diagnosis is confirmed by *liver biopsy* (removal of a small sample of liver for analysis).

About 80 percent of hepatomas raise the production by the liver of a substance called *alpha-fetoprotein*; measurement of the blood level of this protein is used as a screening test in areas where the cancer is common. *Angiography* is also used to detect hepatomas too small to be seen by other imaging techniques.

### TREATMENT

A hepatoma usually remains confined to the liver for a long time. In cases where cirrhosis is not also present (which is rare in the US), complete removal of the tumor, leading to cure, is sometimes possible. In other cases, *anticancer drugs* can help the patient survive longer. A *liver transplant* may occasionally be considered.

There is no cure for secondary liver cancer, but anticancer drugs can help slow the progress of the disease.

Tying off or blocking the hepatic artery or one of its branches to deprive the tumor of its blood supply has been attempted, as has placing a catheter into the artery for continuous administration of anticancer drugs.

# Liver, cirrhosis of

See *Cirrhosis*.

# Liver disease, alcoholic

Damage to the liver caused by persistent heavy alcohol consumption, with progression to *cirrhosis* (severe structural damage and loss of liver function) and death.

### TYPES

Excess fat accumulation in the liver affects almost everyone with a moderate to high alcohol consumption. It is completely reversible through abstinence and, with the reversal, carries a low risk of progression to cirrhosis.

Acute or chronic *hepatitis* can sometimes develop in the persistent drinker. Individual liver cells are destroyed and there is inflammation of the liver with scarring. In people who continue to drink, there is a high risk (about 90 percent) of progression to cirrhosis; in most of those who stop drinking the liver returns to normal. Cirrhosis is irreversible, but abstinence often leads to a notable improvement in liver function.

### CAUSES AND INCIDENCE

Until the 1960s, alcoholic liver damage was thought to be caused mainly by the malnutrition associated with alcohol dependence rather than by alcohol itself. It is now accepted that alcohol is directly toxic to the liver.

There is a clear relationship between the total amount of alcohol consumed in a population and the *incidence* of cirrhosis. The *prevalence* of alcoholic liver disease has been rising rapidly in most developed countries since about 1960, and the increase has been particularly steep in women. In the US, the death rate from cirrhosis has risen by about 70 percent since 1960. In New York, alcoholic cirrhosis is now one of the most common causes of death in people 25 to 44.

A person who consumes 7 ounces of alcohol on average per day (contained in about three quarters of a bottle of whisky or two and a half bottles of wine) has a 50 percent chance of cirrhosis within 20 years. A much lower average daily intake of 1.5 ounces (contained in two double shots of whiskey or four glasses of wine) in a man, or half that consumption in a woman, still carries a substantial risk.

### SYMPTOMS AND DIAGNOSIS

The first symptoms or signs of liver damage are the same as those of hepatitis or cirrhosis. *Liver function tests* show a characteristic pattern of abnormalities, and *liver biopsy* may be recommended to define the type of damage precisely.

### TREATMENT AND OUTLOOK

Abstinence from alcohol is the only method of returning the liver to normal or improving its function and prolonging life expectancy. Treatment methods are as for *alcohol dependence*.

# Liver failure

A complication of acute *hepatitis* (inflammation of the liver) in which there is such a severe impairment of liver function that it affects other organs, particularly the brain. Liver failure may also refer to a critical stage in *cirrhosis* of the liver.

### SYMPTOMS

The principal symptoms of acute liver failure are those of the underlying hepatitis; later, symptoms of brain dysfunction develop. The brain dysfunction probably occurs because the liver fails to break down certain substances that build up in the blood (such as ammonia), which then poison or alter the transmission of nerve messages in the brain. The symptoms may include agitation and restlessness, followed by drowsiness, confusion, and coma—a condition known as hepatic *encephalopathy*.

When liver failure accompanies cirrhosis, other complications, such as *ascites* (fluid collection in the abdomen) and internal bleeding, may develop in addition to hepatic encephalopathy. The symptoms of brain dysfunction develop more slowly, with recurrent episodes of drowsiness or confusion. These episodes are frequently precipitated by bacterial infections or changes in drug treatment or diet.

### DIAGNOSIS AND TREATMENT

A diagnosis is made from the patient's history, physical examination, *liver function tests*, and tests for viruses that can cause acute hepatitis.

Treatment of acute liver failure consists of skilled intensive care. There is no specific cure, although the use of antibiotics and enemas can reduce the number of intestinal bacteria, which are one of the main sources of toxic ammonia entering the bloodstream. A *liver transplant* is occasionally possible and suitable for certain patients. Only about one quarter of patients survive acute liver failure.

When brain dysfunction complicates cirrhosis, treatment of precipitating causes (such as infection) often leads to an improvement.

## Liver fluke

 Any of various species of flukes (small, flattened, worms) that infest the bile ducts within the liver. The only fluke of any importance in the US is *FASCIOLA HEPATICA*, which causes the disease fascioliasis. The adult flukes normally infest sheep and produce eggs that are passed in the sheep's feces. The eggs are eaten by snails, from which immature forms of the fluke emerge. They then become encysted (enclosed in a sac) on aquatic vegetation, particularly watercress. In the US the disease is confined to some western and southern states.

The disease has two stages. During the first stage, young flukes migrate through the liver, causing liver tenderness and enlargement, fever, night sweats, and sometimes a rash. In the second stage, adult worms are present in the bile ducts. This may lead to *cholangitis* (inflammation of the bile ducts) and *bile duct obstruction*, which can cause *jaundice*. In light infections, there may be no symptoms.

The disease is diagnosed from the presence of fluke eggs in the patient's feces. Treatment with the antihelmintic drug praziquantel may be effective.

A different species, *CLONORCHIS SINENSIS*, is common in the Far East. Infection is acquired from eating raw or uncooked freshwater fish. The symptoms and treatment are broadly similar to those for fascioliasis.

## Liver function tests

A series of tests of blood chemistry that can detect changes in the way the liver is making new substances, breaking down and/or excreting old ones, and whether liver cells are healthy or being damaged. The tests are widely used to help in the diagnosis of liver disease, and to assess responses to treatment. They are particularly useful in distinguishing between acute and chronic liver disorders and between *hepatitis* (liver inflammation) and *cholestasis* (failure of bile flow). The most commonly performed tests are shown in the table.

## Liver imaging

A technique that produces images of the liver, gallbladder, bile ducts, and blood vessels supplying the liver to detect abnormality or disease.

### TABLE OF LIVER FUNCTION TESTS

| Test | Significance |
|---|---|
| Serum bilirubin | Bilirubin is the yellow breakdown product of red blood cells that is passed to the liver and excreted in bile. It is the substance that gives the yellow color to the skin in jaundice. A high bilirubin level in the blood may indicate defective processing of bile by the liver or obstruction to bile flow |
| Serum albumin | Albumin is one of the main proteins in blood. Made by the liver, one of its actions is to hold fluid inside the blood vessels. A low level is found in many chronic liver disorders and is often associated with ascites and ankle edema (fluid collection in the abdomen and around the ankles). |
| Serum alkaline phosphatase | Alkaline phosphatase is an enzyme found in bile. The blood level of this enzyme rises when there is obstruction to the flow of bile (cholestasis). |
| Serum aminotransferases (transaminases) | The aminotransferases are enzymes released from liver cells into the blood when the liver cells are damaged. The levels will be raised in acute and chronic hepatitis. |
| Prothrombin time | A normal result in this test of blood clotting depends on the presence in the blood of a protein made by the liver from a fat-soluble vitamin, vitamin K. The test result can be abnormal in two kinds of disorders—when the protein is not made because of liver cell damage, and when there is a blockage to bile flow in the liver, causing a lack of bile in the intestines (which interferes with fat and vitamin K absorption). |

### TYPES

**CONVENTIONAL X-RAY TECHNIQUES** *Cholecystography* and *cholangiography* are techniques in which a contrast medium (iodine-containing substance opaque to X rays) is introduced to show up gallstones, tumors, and blockages. *ERCP* (endoscopic retrograde cholangiopancreatography) is an alternative method of examining the biliary system by means of a contrast medium; it is especially useful in detecting blockage or narrowing of a bile duct or a pancreatic duct by a stone or tumor.

*Angiography* shows up the blood vessels within the liver that supply the liver. It also may be used to confirm the diagnosis of a hemangioma or to plan the treatment of liver tumors and other disorders.

**SCANNING TECHNIQUES** *Ultrasound scanning* is the most widely used of all liver imaging techniques. It is simple, safe, noninvasive, and produces excellent images, particularly of gallstones. *CT scanning* also provides good images and may be used if ultrasound has proved inconclusive.

*Radionuclide scanning* can indicate the presence of a cyst or a tumor. It is also useful in recording the progress of radioactive isotopes as they are excreted from the liver in bile.

## Liver transplant

Replacement of a diseased liver with a healthy organ removed from a donor who has been declared brain dead. Liver transplantation is a technically difficult procedure, but is now accepted as a feasible and appropriate treatment for some types of advanced liver disease. The chances of surviving for many years with a transplanted liver are improving, but they are not yet as high as the chances of surviving with a kidney transplant.

### WHY IT IS DONE

Transplantation is worth considering only for people with life-threatening or severely debilitating liver disease. However, if the disease process is too advanced, the person is unlikely to survive the operation. An assessment must be made of the likely length of survival and the quality of life with and without the operation.

In adults, the best results are obtained in the treatment of advanced liver *cirrhosis* in people with long-standing chronic active *hepatitis* or primary *biliary cirrhosis*. In acute *liver failure*, there can be difficulty in obtaining donor organs at an appropriate time, but people with a slightly less acute illness and those with *Budd-Chiari syndrome* have been successfully treated. People with primary *liver cancer* are rarely considered for transplantation because there is a high risk that the tumor will recur.

In children, congenital *biliary atresia* is the most common reason for transplantation.

**HOW IT IS DONE**

The donor organ is obtained from someone who has suffered *brain death* but whose liver is still healthy. The organ can be stored in cold salt solutions for a few hours.

A general anesthetic is given and the recipient's abdomen is opened. The diseased liver is removed, the donor organ is inserted in its place, and the major blood vessels and common bile duct are reconnected.

**RECOVERY PERIOD**

The first few days after the operation are spent in an *intensive-care* unit. *Immunosuppressant drugs* (particularly cyclosporine) are given to reduce the risk of rejection.

**OUTLOOK**

In some cases rejection occurs and a second transplant operation provides the only hope. There is now a 60 to 80 percent chance of surviving one year, which may mean that more than half of the people now receiving liver transplants will survive for five years. The quality of life is generally excellent, with most people returning to near normal activity within a few weeks of the operation.

## Living will
See *Will, living*.

## Lobe
One of the clearly defined parts into which certain organs, such as the brain, liver, lungs, and thyroid gland, are divided. The term may also be used to describe any projecting, flat, pendulous part of the body, such as the earlobe.

## Lobectomy
An operation to cut out a lobe in the brain (see *Lobotomy, prefrontal*), liver (see *Hepatectomy, partial*), lungs (see *Lobectomy, lung*), or thyroid gland (see *Thyroidectomy*).

## Lobectomy, lung
An operation to remove one of the lobes of the lung. Lobectomy is usually performed to remove a malignant tumor, but may also be used to treat localized *bronchiectasis* that has not responded to medical treatment. In the past, lobectomy was carried out to treat tuberculosis, which is treated today by drugs.

After lobectomy, the remaining lobes expand to fill the pleural space.

**HOW IT IS DONE**

A curved incision is made (using a general anesthetic), starting under the armpit and extending across the back, following the line of the lower edge of the shoulder blade. The muscles are cut through and the ribs are gently spread apart (or one is removed) to expose the lung. The blood vessels and bronchus (air passage) leading to the diseased lobe are then tied off and divided, and the lobe is removed. Before the incision is sewn up, a tube is inserted into the pleural space surrounding the lung to drain off fluid. It is usually removed after 24 hours.

## Lobotomy, prefrontal
The cutting of some of the fibers linking the frontal lobes to the rest of the brain. Prefrontal lobotomy was widely used in the 1940s and 1950s to treat serious psychiatric disorders. However, the operation often resulted in harmful personality changes and is now used only as a last resort to treat people with severe, chronic depression. (See also *Psychosurgery*.)

## Lochia
The discharge after childbirth of blood and fragments of the lining of the uterus where the placenta was attached. Lochia is bright red for the first three or four days and then becomes paler. The discharge decreases as the placental site heals and usually ceases within six weeks.

## Locked knee
See *Knee*.

## Lockjaw
A painful spasm of the jaw muscles that makes it difficult or impossible to open the mouth. Lockjaw is the most common symptom of *tetanus*.

## Locomotor
Relating to movement of the extremities, as in locomotor *ataxia*, the incoordinated movements and lurching gait that occur in the later stages of untreated syphilis.

## Loiasis
 A form of the tropical parasitic disease *filariasis* that is caused by an infestation by the worm *LOA LOA*. The worm travels beneath the skin, producing areas of inflammation known as Calabar swellings.

## Loin
The part of the back on each side of the spine between the lowest pair of ribs and the top of the pelvis.

## Loose bodies
Fragments of bone, cartilage, or capsule linings that are free to move within a joint. They may occur whenever there is any damage to a joint, as in *osteoarthritis* (degeneration due to wear and tear), fracture, or *osteochondritis dissecans* (inflammation of bone and cartilage due to disrupted blood supply).

**SYMPTOMS AND SIGNS**

Loose bodies can sometimes be felt. They are troublesome only if they lodge between joint surfaces, where they cause the joint to lock (usually only briefly), resulting in severe pain. The joint usually swells several hours later. Though the swelling subsides, further locking and swelling can recur at any time.

**DIAGNOSIS AND TREATMENT**

X rays or *arthroscopy* (examination of the interior of the joint through a viewing tube) show whether loose bodies are present.

Occasionally, gentle manipulation of the joint is required to unlock it. If locking occurs frequently, the loose bodies are removed during arthroscopy or by an open operation.

## Loperamide
An *antidiarrheal drug* used in the treatment of recurrent and sudden bouts of diarrhea. Loperamide is also given to help regulate bowel action in people who have had an *ileostomy*.

**POSSIBLE ADVERSE EFFECTS**

Loperamide occasionally produces a rash. Other rare adverse effects, such as fever, abdominal cramps, and bloating, are often difficult to distinguish from symptoms of the disorder causing the diarrhea.

## Lorazepam
A *benzodiazepine drug* used to treat *insomnia* and *anxiety*. If use of lorazepam is suddenly stopped after it has been taken regularly for more than three weeks, there may be withdrawal symptoms (see *Drug dependence*).

**L**

## Lordosis

Inward curvature of the spine, which is normally present to a minor degree in the lower back. Lordosis in the lower back can become exaggerated by poor posture (especially in someone who is overweight and has weak abdominal muscles) or by *kyphosis* (backward curvature of the spine) above the lower back.

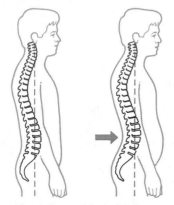

**Normal and abnormal lordosis**
The normal inward curvature of the spine (left) is exaggerated in abnormal lordosis (right).

Once pronounced lordosis has developed, it is usually a permanent condition and can lead to *disk prolapse* or *osteoarthritis* of the spine.

Loss of normal lordosis in the lower back or neck can occur when the back or neck muscles are in spasm. The condition corrects itself once the cause is successfully treated.

## Lotion

A liquid drug preparation applied to the skin. Lotions have a cooling, soothing effect and are useful for covering large areas. Examples of drugs prepared as a lotion include *calamine* (used to treat skin inflammation) and *lindane* (used in the treatment of scabies and lice infestations).

## Lou Gehrig's disease

A name used commonly by the public for amyotrophic lateral sclerosis (see *Motor neuron disease*).

## Lovastatin

A lipid-lowering drug approved in 1987 that lowers serum cholesterol levels by inhibiting cholesterol-producing enzymes. Lovastatin should not replace standard diet therapy; it is recommended when dietary measures and other nondrug therapy have been ineffective. Long-term effects are yet to be ascertained.

## LSD

A synthetic *hallucinogenic drug* (drug that produces hallucinations) derived from ergot (a type of fungus). LSD is the abbreviation for lysergic acid diethylamide. The drug has no medical role. Its distribution and manufacture are governed by the Controlled Substance Act because of the drug's high potential for abuse.

LSD sometimes produces "bad trips" in which a person experiences panic, fear, and physical symptoms, such as nausea, dizziness, and weakness. In severe cases, sedation in the hospital may be necessary for several days. There may also be "flashbacks" to previous trips months or years afterward. Although there is no evidence that LSD causes *psychosis* (mental illness characterized by a loss of contact with reality), it may act as a trigger in a person predisposed to mental illness. There is evidence that LSD damages chromosomes.

## Ludwig's angina

A bacterial infection of the floor of the mouth that becomes life-threatening as it spreads to the throat. The tissues become inflamed, swell, and harden.

The disorder is usually caused by an infected tooth or gum and is most common in people with poor *oral hygiene*. It generally results in fever, pain in the mouth and neck, and difficulty opening the mouth and swallowing. If not treated immediately with antibiotics, the swollen tissues of the throat may cause difficulty breathing. *Tracheostomy* (making a hole in the windpipe and inserting a tube through it) may be necessary to prevent asphyxiation.

## Lumbar

Relating to the part of the back between the lowest pair of ribs and the top of the pelvis. The lumbar region of the spine consists of the five lumbar vertebrae between the lowest (12th) thoracic vertebra and the sacrum.

## Lumbar puncture

A procedure in which a hollow needle is inserted into the lower part of the spinal canal to withdraw *cerebrospinal fluid* (the watery liquid that surrounds the brain and spinal cord) or to inject drugs or other substances.

**WHY IT IS DONE**
The main use of the lumbar puncture is to examine cerebrospinal fluid to diagnose and investigate disorders of the brain and spinal cord (such as *meningitis* and *subarachnoid hemor-*

*rhage*). The procedure is also used to inject drugs into the fluid (such as *anticancer drugs* to treat *leukemia* and other malignant diseases of the central nervous system). Another use of lumbar puncture is to inject a dye that will show up on X ray (see *Myelography*) to produce images of the spinal cord. Finally, lumbar puncture can be used to inject a local anesthetic to achieve extensive anesthesia without causing loss of consciousness.

**HOW IT IS DONE**
The patient lies on his or her side, chin on chest and knees drawn up, to pull the vertebrae (bones of the spine) apart; the area of skin overlying the lumbar vertebrae at the base of the spine is anesthetized with a local anesthetic. A hollow needle is then inserted between two of the vertebrae and into the spinal canal and is used to withdraw cerebrospinal fluid or to inject drugs, dye, or anesthetic.

After the needle is removed, the puncture site is covered with sterile tape. The procedure takes less than 20 minutes. It usually causes no discomfort; a headache that soon wears off may occur in some people.

## Lumbosacral spasm

Prolonged, excessive tightening of the muscles that surround and support the lower part of the spine. Lumbosacral spasm is a cause of *back pain* and may occasionally result in temporary *scoliosis* (curvature of the spine to one side). Treatment may include bed rest, *analgesic drugs* (painkillers), and *muscle-relaxant drugs*.

## Lumen

The space within a tubular organ. The term is most commonly used to refer to the cavity of the intestine.

## Lumpectomy

An operation to treat breast cancer (see *Mastectomy*).

## Lunacy

An outdated term for insanity. It was coined because of the belief that phases of the moon ("luna" in Latin) could bring on mental illnesses, especially illnesses that seemed to come and go. Patients were called lunatics and mental hospitals were known as lunatic asylums.

## Lung

The main organ of the *respiratory system*. The two lungs supply the body with oxygen and eliminate carbon dioxide from the blood.

L

## STRUCTURE

The *trachea* (windpipe) branches in the chest into two main *bronchi* (air passages), which supply the left and right lungs. The main bronchi divide again into smaller bronchi and then into bronchioles, which lead to air passages that open out into grapelike air sacs called alveoli. It is through the thin walls of the alveoli that gases diffuse into or out of the blood.

Each lung is enclosed in a double membrane called the *pleura*, which allows the lungs to slide freely as they expand and contract during *breathing*. (See also *Respiration*.)

# Lung cancer

One of the most common forms of *cancer* in the US, lung cancer is the leading cause of cancer deaths in men and the second most common cause (after breast cancer) in women. There were about 160,000 deaths from lung cancer in 1986 in the US. The peak age for lung cancer is 65 years for men and 70 years for women. The disease is uncommon before age 40.

## CAUSES

Cigarette smoking is the main cause of lung cancer. The more cigarettes smoked per day and the lower the age at which smoking started, the greater the risk of lung cancer. Cigar or pipe smokers have a lower risk of having lung cancer than cigarette smokers, but still have a significantly higher risk than nonsmokers (see *Tobacco smoking*). Passive smoking (the inhalation of tobacco smoke by nonsmokers) has been shown to increase the risk.

Living in an environment with a high level of air pollution or working with radioactive minerals or asbestos may cause some cases of lung cancer.

## TYPES

There are several types of lung cancer, the most common being squamous cell carcinoma, small (oat) cell carcinoma, adenocarcinoma, and large cell carcinoma; each has a different natural history (growth pattern) and response to treatment. The squamous cell, small cell, and large cell types are all strongly associated with tobacco abuse; the relation between adenocarcinoma and tobacco use is less clear.

## SYMPTOMS AND SIGNS

The first and most common symptom is a cough, occurring in about 80 percent of people with lung cancer. About half of all people with lung cancer have a chronic cough from *bronchitis*. Other symptoms include coughing up blood, shortness of breath, chest pain, and wheezing.

## LOCATION AND STRUCTURE OF THE LUNGS

The lungs lie in the chest within the rib cage. Air entering the body via the nose and mouth travels down the trachea to the main bronchi, which divide into smaller bronchi and then into bronchioles. These in turn lead to alveoli, where the oxygen/carbon dioxide exchange takes place. During expiration (breathing out), air leaves the body by the same routes.

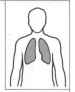

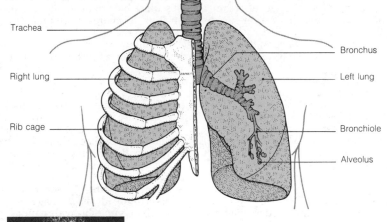

Trachea

Right lung

Rib cage

Bronchus

Left lung

Bronchiole

Alveolus

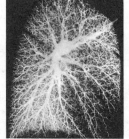

**Blood vessels in a lung**
The tiniest "twigs" of this extensive blood vessel "tree" form into capillaries that surround the alveoli (air sacs) in the lung. Oxygen and carbon dioxide are exchanged between the alveoli and the capillaries.

Lung cancer can spread locally to affect tissues immediately surrounding the lungs, or can spread to other parts of the body, especially the liver, brain, and bones. Pain may occur in these sites, and weight loss is a frequent symptom. Local spread may cause the collapse of a lung or *pneumonia*, or affect the pleura (membrane covering the lung), causing *pleural effusion* (a collection of fluid between the lung and the chest wall).

## DIAGNOSIS

Lung cancer may be suspected during *history-taking* or a physical examination but, most often, it is discovered when a chest X ray shows a characteristic shadow on the lung.

To confirm the diagnosis, tissue must be examined cytologically for the presence of cancerous cells (see *Cytology*). The simplest test is to examine samples of sputum (phlegm), because cancer cells may have been shed into the airways and occur in the sputum.

A *bronchoscopy* may be performed to examine the condition of the lungs or to take a biopsy (small sample of tissue) for analysis or examination. Sometimes biopsy of the suspected tumor is necessary. Cells are obtained through a needle inserted into the chest or by performing an operation to expose the tumor for a direct biopsy (excision of part of the tumor).

## TREATMENT

If lung cancer is diagnosed at an early stage, *pneumonectomy* (surgical removal of the lung) or *lobectomy* (removal of part of the lung) may be performed. Surgery is usually possible only when the cancer is still fairly small and confined to one lung, and when the patient's general condition enables a major operation to be performed. *Anticancer drugs* and *radiation therapy* may be used to contain the spread of the tumor or destroy cancerous cells; they are the usual treatment for small cell lung cancer.

L

## OUTLOOK

Overall, less than 10 percent of lung cancer patients survive for five years after the disease is diagnosed. After surgery, the five-year survival rate is between 15 and 30 percent; there have been cases of long-term survival in patients treated with chemotherapy for small cell carcinoma.

The highest chance of cure is obtained when the cancer is discovered and treated early. If the cancer has spread beyond the chest, a cure is highly unlikely.

## Lung, collapse of

See *Atelectasis*; *Pneumothorax*.

## Lung disease, chronic obstructive

The combination of chronic *bronchitis* and *emphysema*, in which there is persistent disruption of airflow into or out of the lungs.

## Lung imaging

A technique that provides images of the lungs to aid in the diagnosis of abnormalities or disease.

### TYPES

**CONVENTIONAL X-RAY TECHNIQUES** A *chest X ray* provides an excellent image of the lungs, from which almost every type of lung disorder can be detected. *Tomography* produces a sharp image of a cross section of an organ at a particular depth and is sometimes used to visualize the interior of a lung that is obscured by an overlying diseased area or to more clearly identify a nodule in the lung.

In pulmonary *angiography*, a contrast medium (a substance opaque to X rays) is injected into the pulmonary artery to detect *pulmonary embolism* (blockage by a blood clot). *Bronchography* (in which the contrast medium is injected into the bronchi) was once widely used to examine bronchi damaged by chronic infections; it has now been largely replaced by *bronchoscopy*. Other imaging techniques are also used.

**SCANNING TECHNIQUES** *CT scanning* provides a more detailed image of the lungs than is possible with standard X rays and plays an important role in detecting the presence and spread of *lung tumors*. *Ultrasound scanning* is sometimes used to reveal *pleural effusion* (fluid around a lung).

Other less commonly employed imaging techniques involve the use of *radionuclide scanning* to aid in detecting pulmonary embolism. Digital radiography uses a computer to process a standard X-ray film. The computer removes all unwanted elements (such as the bones of the chest) from the image, leaving a clearer view of the structures to be examined.

## Lung tumors

Growths in the lung that may be malignant (see *Lung cancer*) or benign. Benign lung tumors are less common than malignant tumors and, unlike malignant tumors, typically affect younger adults and are unrelated to cigarette smoking.

The most common benign tumor is a bronchial *adenoma*, which arises in the lining of a bronchiole. Adenomas often cause partial bronchial obstruction; hemoptysis (coughing up blood) may also occur. Treatment involves surgical removal of the tumor.

L

## DISORDERS OF THE LUNG

The lungs are continuously exposed to airborne particles, such as bacteria, viruses, and allergens, all of which can cause lung disorders. Most of these disorders do not interfere with oxygen supply; those that do are a major threat to health.

### INFECTION

Infective disorders are common, especially *tracheitis* (inflammation of the lining of the windpipe) and *croup* (a virus infection of young children). *Bronchitis* (inflammation of the bronchi), *bronchiectasis* (swelling of the bronchi), and *bronchiolitis* (inflammation of the bronchioles) commonly follow colds or *influenza*. *Pneumonia* (inflammation of the lung) is usually caused by infection by viruses or bacteria. Fungal infections of the lungs, such as *aspergillosis*, *actinomycosis*, *histoplasmosis*, and *candidiasis*, are relatively uncommon.

### ALLERGIES

Bronchial *asthma*, in which the muscles of the bronchi contract and obstruct the free passage of air, often occurs in sensitized people exposed to pollens, house mites, fungal spores, animal dander, and many other agents. Allergic *alveolitis* (inflammation of the alveoli) may be caused by many organic dusts, such as moldy hay.

### TUMORS

*Lung cancer* is one of the most common of all malignant tumors; in most cases it is associated with cigarette smoking. Secondary malignant tumors, which have spread from other parts of the body to the lungs, are common. However, benign tumors affecting the lung are uncommon.

### INJURY

Lung injury usually results from penetration of the chest wall. *Pneumothorax* (air in the pleural cavity) and *hemothorax* (blood in the pleural cavity) are usually caused by a penetrating injury; either may cause collapse of the lung. Injury can also occur from the inhalation of poisonous dusts, gases, or toxic substances. *Silicosis* and *asbestosis* are caused by inhalation of silica and asbestos, respectively; they may lead to progressive *fibrosis* of the lung.

### IMPAIRED BLOOD AND OXYGEN SUPPLY

The most serious disorder is *pulmonary embolism*, in which a blood clot formed in one of the major veins breaks free and is carried to the lungs. The clot may block the pulmonary arteries and cause death. Heart failure may cause pulmonary *edema*, in which the lungs become filled with fluid. *Respiratory distress syndrome*, which may affect newborn babies or adults, has many causes. In this condition, leakage of fluid into the alveoli seriously interferes with oxygen supply. *Emphysema*, in which the walls of the alveoli break down so that the area for oxygen exchange is reduced, is frequently seen in people suffering from chronic bronchitis and asthma.

### INVESTIGATION

Lung disorders are investigated by *chest X ray*, *bronchoscopy*, *pulmonary function tests*, *sputum* analysis, *blood tests*, and physical examination. Sometimes a biopsy of lung tissue is taken for analysis.

Other rare benign tumors include *fibromas* (made up of fibrous tissue) and *lipomas* (made up of fatty tissue). No treatment is necessary unless the tumors are causing problems.

## Lupus erythematosus

A chronic disease that causes inflammation of *connective tissue*. The more common type, discoid lupus erythematosus (DLE), affects exposed areas of the skin. The more serious and potentially fatal form, systemic lupus erythematosus (SLE), affects many systems of the body, including the joints and the kidneys.

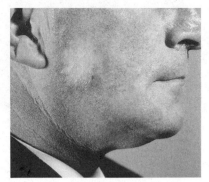

**Discoid lupus erythematosus on cheek**
The disease causes circular, reddened areas of skin. The patch shown here is healing at its center to form white scar tissue.

### CAUSES
Lupus erythematosus is an *autoimmune disorder* in which the body's *immune system*, for unknown reasons, attacks the connective tissue as though it were foreign, causing inflammation. It is probable that the disease can be inherited and that hormonal factors play a part. Sometimes the agent that triggers the immune response (e.g., a viral infection) can be inferred. Certain drugs can induce some of the symptoms of SLE, particularly in elderly people; drugs most frequently responsible are hydralazine, procainamide, and isoniazid.

### INCIDENCE
Lupus erythematosus affects nine times as many women as men, usually those of childbearing age. It occurs worldwide, although its incidence is higher in certain ethnic groups, such as blacks in the US, West Indians, and Chinese in the Far East. In high-risk groups the incidence may be as high as one in 250 women.

### SYMPTOMS
The symptoms of both varieties of lupus erythematosus periodically subside and recur with varying severity.

In DLE the rash starts as one or more red, circular, thickened areas of skin that later scar. They may occur on the face, behind the ears, and on the scalp, sometimes causing permanent hair loss in affected areas.

SLE causes a characteristic red, blotchy, almost butterfly-shaped rash over the cheeks and bridge of the nose. There is no scarring and the hair grows back between attacks. Most sufferers feel sick, with malaise, fatigue, fever, loss of appetite, nausea, joint pain, and weight loss. There may be iron-deficiency *anemia*, neurological or psychiatric problems, *renal failure*, *pleurisy* (inflammation of the lining of the lungs), *arthritis*, and *pericarditis* (inflammation of the membrane surrounding the heart).

### DIAGNOSIS
Blood tests and sometimes a skin *biopsy* (removal of tissue for microscopic examination) are performed to look for specific *antibodies* that occur when the disease is active.

### TREATMENT
Treatment aims to reduce inflammation and alleviate symptoms; there is no cure. *Nonsteroidal anti-inflammatory drugs* may be prescribed for joint pain, antimalarial drugs for the skin rash, and *corticosteroid drugs* for fever, pleurisy, and neurological symptoms. Sufferers whose symptoms are made worse by sunlight should avoid sun exposure and use *sunscreens*.

### OUTLOOK
The future for patients with SLE has improved dramatically over the past 20 years, although the disease may be life-threatening if the kidneys are affected. Today, many people who have SLE survive for more than 10 years after diagnosis of the disease. This improvement may be due to earlier diagnosis, especially of mild cases, and to more effective treatment of kidney problems.

## Lupus pernio

A variant of the disease *sarcoidosis* in which purple swellings appear on the nose, cheeks, or ears. It more commonly affects women than men.

## Lupus vulgaris

A form of *tuberculosis* affecting the skin, especially of the head and neck. Painless, clear, red-brown nodules appear and ulcerate; they eventually heal, leaving deep scars.

## Luteinizing hormone

A *gonadotropin hormone*, also known as LH, produced by the *pituitary gland*.

## Luteinizing hormone-releasing hormone

A naturally occurring hormone released by the hypothalamus in the brain, also prepared synthetically as a drug. Natural luteinizing hormone-releasing hormone (LH-RH) stimulates the release of *gonadotropin hormones* from the *pituitary gland*. Gonadotropin hormones, in turn, control the production of *estrogen hormones* and *androgen hormones*.

### WHY IT IS USED
Synthetic LH-RH is given to treat abnormally early onset of puberty. It is also currently under investigation as a male contraceptive and as a treatment for uterine *fibroids*, prostatic cancer (see *Prostate, cancer of*), and certain types of *breast cancer*.

### HOW IT WORKS
Synthetic LH-RH reduces the amount of natural gonadotropins released from the pituitary gland and thus the amount of *estrogen hormones* and *androgen hormones* produced by the ovary and testes. This action reduces the level of cell activity in organs stimulated by these sex hormones, such as the uterus, breasts, testes, ovaries, and prostate gland.

### POSSIBLE ADVERSE EFFECTS
LH-RH may cause headache, nausea, hot flashes, vaginal dryness, and irregular periods.

## Luxated tooth

A tooth displaced in its socket as the result of an accident. The upper front teeth are the most vulnerable. The tooth may be depressed deep into the gum, tilted backward or forward, and loosened. A dentist can usually manipulate a luxated tooth back into position, after which it is usually immobilized with a splint (see *Splinting, dental*). If the tooth's blood vessels are torn and the pulp dies, the tooth requires *root-canal treatment*.

## Lyme disease

 A disease characterized by skin changes, flulike symptoms, and joint inflammation. It was first described in the community of Old Lyme, Connecticut, in 1975.

### CAUSES AND INCIDENCE
Lyme disease is caused by the bacterium *BORRELIA BURGDORFERI*, which is transmitted by the bite of a tick that usually lives on deer but can infest dogs. Most cases have occurred in the northeastern US, but the disease has also been reported in other parts of the US and in other countries.

**SYMPTOMS AND COMPLICATIONS**

At the site of the tick bite, a red dot may appear and gradually expand into a reddened area several inches across (although in some cases the bite passes unnoticed). Symptoms such as fever, headache, lethargy, and muscle pains usually develop, followed by a characteristic joint inflammation, with redness and swelling typically affecting the knees and other large joints.

The symptoms may vary in severity and occur in cycles lasting a week or so. Unless the disease is diagnosed and treated, symptoms may continue for several years, gradually declining in severity. There is usually no permanent damage to joints.

Complications affecting the heart (such as *myocarditis* and *heart block*) or nervous system (such as *meningitis*) occur in some cases.

**DIAGNOSIS AND TREATMENT**

Anyone in whom the above symptoms develop, particularly after a tick bite, should consult a physician. The diagnosis of Lyme disease can be confirmed by blood tests.

If diagnosed before joint inflammation occurs, the disease can be quickly cleared up with antibiotics. If the disease is more advanced, *nonsteroidal anti-inflammatory drugs* and sometimes *corticosteroid drugs* are given and a cure may take longer.

## Lymph

A milky body fluid that contains lymphocytes (a type of white blood cell), proteins, and fats. Lymph accumulates outside the blood vessels in the intercellular spaces of body tissues and is collected into the *lymphatic system* to flow back into the bloodstream. Lymph plays an important part in the *immune system* and in absorbing fats from the intestine.

## Lymphadenitis

A little-used medical term for inflammation of the lymph nodes, a common cause of lymphadenopathy (swollen glands). See *Glands, swollen.*

## Lymphadenopathy

The medical term for swollen lymph nodes (see *Glands, swollen*). A condition called persistent generalized lymphadenopathy, which causes generalized swelling of the lymph nodes, develops in some people infected with HIV (the *AIDS* virus).

## Lymphangiography

A diagnostic procedure that enables lymph vessels and lymph nodes to be

---

## PROCEDURE FOR LYMPHANGIOGRAPHY

To plan and monitor the progress of treatment for certain types of cancer, such as of the testis or cervix, X-ray pictures of the lymph vessels and nodes can be taken to reveal the spread of the cancer throughout the body. A contrast medium is injected into the foot, from where it travels throughout the lymphatic system. The procedure takes about two and a half hours.

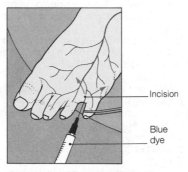

**1** A blue dye is injected through a needle into the web spaces between the toes of each foot, and into the outside of the little toes. The dye spreads rapidly into the tiny lymphatic vessels along the top of the foot, and makes them visible.

Incision

Blue dye

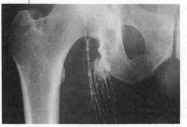

**2** After the use of a local anesthetic, an incision is made over a stained lymphatic vessel in each foot. Contrast medium is injected through a needle into the vessels and passes up the legs, into the groin and abdomen. When the limit of diffusion is reached, the needles are removed and the incisions sewn.

Contrast medium spreading through lymphatic system

**3** The lymph vessels and nodes containing the contrast medium show up clearly on the X-ray pictures. More lymphangiograms are taken after 24 hours.

---

seen on X-ray film after a contrast medium (a substance opaque to X rays) has been injected into them.

**WHY IT IS DONE**

Until recently, lymphangiography was frequently used to determine the extent to which a cancer had spread throughout the body (because lymph nodes trap cancer cells). However, the more straightforward techniques of *CT scanning* and *MRI* also clearly reveal abnormal lymph nodes and have largely superseded lymphangiography. Even so, in certain types of cancer (such as cancer of the testis or cervix), the additional information provided by lymphangiography is useful in planning treatment and monitoring progress.

**HOW IT IS DONE**

A blue dye is injected into the web spaces between all the toes. This dye quickly finds its way into the tiny, usually invisible, lymphatic vessels, allowing the radiologist to see them and select suitable vessels for further examination (see box).

Lymphangiography is sometimes performed on the arms to reveal lymph nodes in the upper body.

## Lymphangioma

A rare benign tumor of the skin or tongue consisting of a collection of abnormal lymph vessels. It is usually present from birth.

There are two types of lymphangioma. One consists of a group of clear blisters that may be inconspicuous at birth but are usually obvious by the age of about 2. If the blisters are damaged they fill with blood, giving a red and white appearance to the lymphangioma. The growth often disappears on its own, but some cases require removal.

The other type, known as a cystic hygroma, is a soft swelling that resembles a bunch of small white grapes. It grows just beneath the skin (commonly in the neck), and may become very large and unsightly. It is usually removed at about age 5.

## Lymphangitis

Inflammation of the lymphatic vessels as a result of the spread of bacteria (commonly streptococci) from an infected wound. The inflammation is so severe that it causes tender red streaks to appear on the skin overlying the lymphatic vessels. These streaks extend progressively from the site of infection toward the nearest lymph nodes (for example, from an infected finger up the arm toward the lymph nodes in the armpits). The affected nodes become swollen and tender. There is usually fever and a general feeling of illness.

Lymphangitis is a clear indication of a serious infection and requires urgent treatment with *antibiotic drugs*. Upon treatment, the condition usually clears up quickly without complications. (See also *Lymphadenitis*.)

## Lymphatic system

A system of vessels (lymphatics) that drains *lymph* from all over the body back into the bloodstream. This system is part of the *immune system*, playing a major part in the body's defenses against infection and cancer.

### STRUCTURE AND FUNCTION

All body tissues are bathed in a watery fluid derived from the bloodstream. Much of this fluid returns to the bloodstream through the walls of the capillaries, but the remainder (along with cells and small particles such as bacteria) is transported to the heart through the lymphatic system (see box, next page).

Throughout the course of the lymphatics lie *lymph nodes*, through which the lymph flows. These nodes are, in effect, filters that trap microorganisms and other foreign bodies in the lymph. The nodes contain many lymphocytes (a type of white blood cell), which can neutralize or destroy invading bacteria and viruses. If part of the body is inflamed or otherwise diseased, the nearby lymph nodes become swollen and tender as they limit the spread of the disease (see *Glands, swollen*). If an infection is particularly virulent, the lymphatics may also be inflamed, becoming visible as thin red lines running along a limb (see *Lymphangitis*).

The lymphatic system also plays a part in the absorption of fats from the intestine. While the products of carbohydrate and protein digestion pass directly into the bloodstream, fats pass into the intestinal lymphatics (lacteals); the lymph in them is so rich in fat that it appears milky.

### DISORDERS

In some conditions, such as after radical breast surgery (which is rarely performed today), the lymphatics to a limb become obstructed and the limb becomes hard and swollen as a result, a condition known as *lymphedema*.

Cancer commonly spreads via the lymphatic system. A primary tumor invades the lymphatics and fragments (metastases) break off and travel to the local group of lymph nodes, where the metastases continue to grow and produce a secondary tumor. This is particularly evident in *breast cancer*, which tends to spread early to the lymph nodes in the armpit.

## Lymphedema

An abnormal accumulation of *lymph* in the tissues, causing swelling of a limb. Lymphedema occurs if lymphatic vessels are blocked, damaged, or removed, resulting in disruption of the normal drainage of lymph (see *Lymphatic system*).

### CAUSES

There are various causes. In the tropical disease *filariasis*, for example, the lymphatic vessels may be blocked by parasitic worms. Blockage may also occur if cancer spreads through the lymphatic system and deposits cancer cells in the lymph vessels.

Surgical removal of lymph nodes under the arm or in the groin or radiation therapy for a tumor destroys lymph nodes and vessels, sometimes resulting in lymphedema.

Lymphedema may also occur for no known cause. It may be present from birth or may develop later in life. Lymphedema of unknown cause affects twice as many women as men.

### SYMPTOMS AND SIGNS

In about 10 percent of women who have had a radical mastectomy, lymphedema develops in the arm (but not usually in the hand) on the same side as the breast removed. In some such cases, the arm becomes disablingly heavy and cumbersome. The incidence of lymphedema is much lower with newer surgical techniques.

Other than following mastectomy, lymphedema usually causes swelling of one or both legs. Starting with only a slight, intermittent puffiness around one ankle, the swelling gradually extends up the leg. In about half of all cases, the other leg also becomes affected. The swelling is usually painless, but the leg feels heavy.

In some people the legs enlarge to an unsightly and incapacitating degree, but in others the swelling may be only minimal even 40 or more years after the onset of the condition.

### TREATMENT

There is no known cure for lymphedema. Treatment consists of taking *diuretic drugs*, massaging the affected limb, wearing an elastic bandage or compression sleeve, and performing exercises with the leg or arm elevated. However, these measures usually produce only a slight improvement. If the leg or arm is so large that it causes disability, the swollen tissue and some of the overlying skin may be removed surgically.

## Lymph gland

A popular name for a *lymph node*. (See also *Lymphatic system*.)

## Lymph node

Popularly known as a lymph gland, a small organ lying along the course of a lymphatic vessel.

### STRUCTURE AND FUNCTION

Lymph nodes vary considerably in size from microscopic to about 1 inch (2.5 cm) in diameter. Each node consists of a thin, fibrous outer capsule and an inner mass of lymphoid tissue. Penetrating the capsule are several small lymphatic vessels (which carry lymph into the gland) and a single, larger vessel (which carries it out).

Lymphoid tissue forms *antibodies* and houses *lymphocytes*, both of which play a very important role in fighting infection. Lymph nodes also contain macrophages, large cells that engulf bacteria and other foreign particles. The nodes act as a barrier to the spread of infection, destroying or filtering out bacteria before they can pass into the bloodstream. (See also *Glands, swollen*; *Lymphatic system*.)

## Lymphocyte

Any of a group of white *blood cells* of crucial importance to the adaptive part of the body's *immune system*. The adaptive portion of the immune system mounts a tailor-made defense when dangerous invading organisms penetrate the body's general defenses (such as those provided by other types of white blood cell).

Some lymphocytes retain a memory of invading microorganisms so that the invaders can be dealt with more rapidly when next encountered. It is this memory function that is stimulated by vaccines. Lymphocytes protect against the development of tumors and cause rejection of tissue in organ transplants.

### TYPES

There are two principal types of lymphocytes. They are called B- and T-lymphocytes.

**B-LYMPHOCYTES** This type accounts for about 10 percent of circulating lymphocytes. When a particular *antigen* (foreign protein), such as a

L

# STRUCTURE AND FUNCTION OF THE LYMPHATIC SYSTEM

The lymphatic system is a collection of organs, ducts, and tissues that has the dual role of draining tissue fluid (lymph) back into the bloodstream and of fighting infection. Lymph is drained by a system of channels (the lymphatic vessels). White cells produced by the bone marrow, thymus, and spleen are present in lymph nodes or circulate through the lymphatic system, providing defenses against infection.

## The lymphatic network

The lymphatic system consists of a network of lymph nodes connected by lymphatic vessels. The nodes generally occur in clusters, mainly around the neck, armpits, and groin.

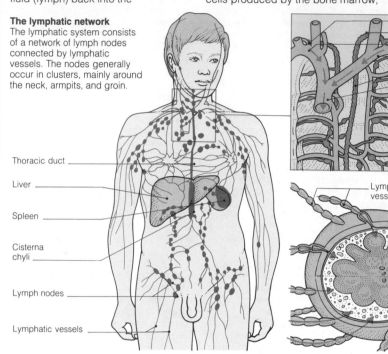

Thoracic duct

Liver

Spleen

Cisterna chyli

Lymph nodes

Lymphatic vessels

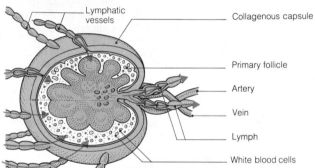

Right lymphatic duct
Thoracic duct
Right subclavian vein
Left subclavian vein
Lymph
Superior vena cava

## Lymphatic drainage

Just below the neck, the thoracic duct and the right lymphatic duct drain into the two subclavian veins. These veins unite to form the inferior vena cava, which passes into the heart; in this way, the lymph fluids rejoin the circulation.

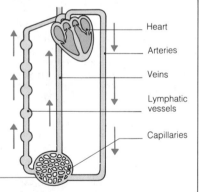

Lymphatic vessels

Collagenous capsule

Primary follicle

Artery

Vein

Lymph

White blood cells

## Structure of a lymph node

Any fluid absorbed into the lymphatic system passes across at least one lymph node before it returns to the circulation. The fluid filters through a mesh of tightly packed white blood cells—some of which are grouped into primary follicles consisting of similar cells—which attack and destroy harmful organisms. Every lymph node is supplied by its own tiny artery and vein.

# MOVEMENTS OF BODY FLUIDS

Lymph is constantly moving around the body, but the lymphatic system has no central pump equivalent to the heart. Lymph is circulated by the movement of the body's muscles; a system of one-way valves in the lymphatic vessels ensures that it moves in the right direction. Exertion also pushes fluid from body tissues into the bloodstream.

Heart

Arteries

Veins

Lymphatic vessels

Capillaries

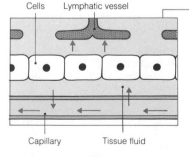

Cells    Lymphatic vessel

Capillary    Tissue fluid

## Fluid exchange

During a 24-hour period, approximately 42 pints of serumlike fluid pass from the bloodstream to the body's tissues. This fluid bathes the cells and provides them with oxygen and nutrients. During the same period of time, approximately 36 pints of fluid pass back from the tissues to the bloodstream, carrying carbon dioxide and other waste products. The remaining 6 pints pass from the tissues to the lymphatic system and return eventually to the circulation from there.

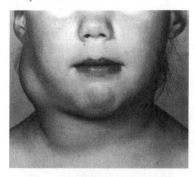

## Enlarged lymph nodes

This photograph shows a girl with marked enlargement of the lymph nodes in her neck. In this case, the appearance is due to Hodgkin's disease, a rare cancer that affects the lymph nodes. Enlargement of the lymph nodes may also be due to infection.

L

substance on the surface of a bacterium, is encountered by the immune system, certain B-lymphocytes are stimulated to enlarge and undergo cell division, transforming into cells called plasma cells. The plasma cells secrete into the blood vast numbers of tailor-made *immunoglobulins* or *antibodies* that attach to the antigen on the surface of the microorganism. This starts a process that leads to the destruction of the microorganism. The protective effect of immunoglobulins is called humoral immunity.

**T-LYMPHOCYTES** This type accounts for more than 80 percent of circulating lymphocytes. T-lymphocytes are derived from white cells that have at some stage entered the thymus gland, where they were "educated" to fulfill a particular function.

There are two main groups of T-lymphocytes: killer (cytotoxic) and helper cells. The killer T-lymphocytes (like B-lymphocytes) are sensitized and stimulated to multiply by the presence of antigens, in this case by antigens present on abnormal body cells (e.g., cells that have been invaded by viruses, cells in transplanted tissue, and tumor cells). Unlike the B-lymphocytes, the killer cells do not produce antibodies; instead, they travel to and attach to the cells recognized as abnormal. The killer cells then release chemicals known as lymphokines, which help destroy the abnormal cells. This is called cell-mediated immunity.

Helper T cells enhance the activities of the cytotoxic cells and control other aspects of the immune response. In people infected with HIV (the *AIDS* virus) these helper T cells are reduced in number, thus impairing the body's ability to fight certain types of infections and tumors.

**MEMORY FUNCTION**
Some lymphocytes do not participate directly in immune responses; instead, they serve as a memory bank for the different antigens that have been encountered in the past. These cells may survive for many years.

## Lymphogranuloma venereum
A sexually transmitted disease, common in tropical countries. It is caused by a *chlamydial infection* that is common in tropical countries.

The first sign of infection is a small genital blister that appears three to 21 days after infection; this blister heals in a few days without leaving a scar. There may also be fever, headache, muscle and joint pains, and a rash.

The lymph glands, particularly in the groin, become painfully enlarged and inflamed. Abscesses may form and ulcers may develop on the skin over the affected glands; the ulcers take several months to heal.

Treatment of lymphogranuloma venereum is with *antibiotic drugs*.

## Lymphoma
Any of a group of cancers in which the cells of lymphoid tissue (found mainly in the lymph nodes and spleen) multiply unchecked.

Lymphomas fall into two categories. If characteristic abnormal cells (Reed-Sternberg cells) are present, the disease is called Hodgkin's lymphoma. All other types are called non-Hodgkin's. (See *Hodgkin's disease; Lymphoma, non-Hodgkin's*.)

## Lymphoma, non-Hodgkin's
Any cancer of lymphoid tissue (found mainly in the lymph nodes and spleen) other than *Hodgkin's disease*.

Non-Hodgkin's lymphomas vary in their malignancy according to the nature and activity of the abnormal cells. Lymphomas are most malignant when the cells are primitive or are poorly differentiated (unspecialized). These cells tend to take over entire lymph nodes quickly. Low-grade lymphomas consist of cells that are better-differentiated.

**CAUSES AND INCIDENCE**
In most cases of non-Hodgkin's lymphoma, the cause is unknown. Occasionally, the disease is associated with suppression of the *immune system*, particularly after organ transplantation. One type of non-Hodgkin's lymphoma, called *Burkitt's lymphoma* (common only in the tropics), is thought to be caused by the Epstein-Barr virus. It is suspected that *HIV* (the *AIDS* virus) permits other viruses to cause lymphomas.

About eight new cases of non-Hodgkin's lymphoma are diagnosed annually per 100,000 people in the US. Most sufferers are over 50.

**SYMPTOMS AND SIGNS**
In most patients, there is painless swelling of one or more groups of lymph nodes in the neck or groin. The liver and spleen may enlarge and lymphoid tissue in the abdomen may be affected, in rare cases causing abdominal pain and bleeding from the intestines, which is revealed as tarry-looking feces or vomiting of blood. Many other organs may also become involved, leading to diverse symptoms ranging from headache to

skin ulceration. Unless it is controlled, spread of the disease (often marked by fever) progressively impairs the immune system, leading to death from infections. The patient may also die of an uncontrolled spread of cancer.

**DIAGNOSIS**
Diagnosis is based on a *biopsy* (removal of a sample for analysis) of lymphoid tissue, usually from a lymph node. The extent of the disease is assessed by a process called staging. A *chest X ray, CT scanning, bone marrow biopsy,* and *lymphangiography* (X rays of the lymph glands) of the abdomen may be required.

**TREATMENT AND OUTLOOK**
If the lymphoma is confined to a single group of lymph nodes, treatment consists of *radiation therapy*. If the disease is more extensive, *anticancer drugs* are given. In some cases both forms of treatment are used. When all else fails, autologous *bone marrow transplantation* and high doses of chemotherapy and/or radiation may be used.

About three quarters of patients with a low-grade localized non-Hodgkin's lymphoma survive at least five years. In more severe types of lymphoma that have spread, 40 to 50 percent of patients survive for two years or more.

## Lymphosarcoma
A now uncommonly used name for non-Hodgkin's lymphoma (see *Lymphoma, non-Hodgkin's*).

## Lypressin
A synthetic preparation of *ADH* (antidiuretic hormone), a hormone that controls the volume of water excreted in the urine. Lypressin is used as a nasal spray to treat *diabetes insipidus* (a deficiency of ADH causing excessive urination and thirst).

Possible adverse effects are abdominal cramps, an urge to pass bowel movements, and nasal congestion that, if severe, may impair the efficiency of treatment.

## Lysis
A medical term for the destruction of a cell by damage to its outer membrane. A common example is *hemolysis*, the breakdown of red blood cells. Lysis may be caused by chemical action, such as that of an *enzyme* (a protein that controls a chemical reaction), or by physical action, such as heat or cold. The term lysis is also occasionally used to refer to a sudden recovery from a fever.

L

# M

## Macro-

A prefix meaning large, as in macrophage (a large cell that plays an important part in the body's defense system by engulfing bacteria and other foreign particles) or macroglossia (enlargement of the tongue).

## Macrobiotics

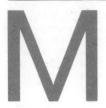 A diet based on the oriental belief that all foods are either yin or yang (possessed of negative or positive energy), and that a balance of yin and yang must be maintained for health. Foods are classified yin or yang according to many factors, including where they are grown, their color, texture, and taste. There are several levels of macrobiotic diet; the most advanced consists mainly of whole grains. Eating such a diet may lead to severe malnutrition, scurvy, or anemia due to the lack of protein, vitamins, and minerals.

## Macroglossia

Abnormal enlargement of the tongue. Macroglossia is a feature of *Down's syndrome*, of *hypothyroidism*, and of *acromegaly*. Tumors of the tongue, such as a *hemangioma* or *lymphangioma*, also cause macroglossia; *amyloidosis* is another possible cause.

In addition to being unsightly, an abnormally large tongue can cause snoring and is sometimes responsible for *sleep apnea*. Treatment is limited and depends on the underlying cause.

## Macular degeneration

A progressive disorder that affects the central part of the *retina*, causing gradual loss of vision. Macular degeneration is a painless condition that is common in the elderly. It usually affects both eyes, either simultaneously or one after the other.

The macula is the part of the retina that distinguishes fine detail at the center of the field of vision. Degeneration begins with partial breakdown of an insulating layer between the retina and the *choroid* (layer of blood vessels behind the retina). Fluid leakage occurs, and new blood vessels growing from the choroid destroy the retinal nerve tissue and replace it with scar tissue. The effect is a roughly circular area of blindness, increasing in size until it is large enough to obliterate two or three words at normal reading distance.

With early diagnosis, it is sometimes possible to seal off the leakage with a *laser*. In most cases, however, the disorder is untreatable.

## Macule

A spot on the skin (level with the surface) discernible only by difference in color or texture.

## Magnesium

A metallic element that plays several vital roles in the body. Magnesium is essential for the formation of bones and teeth, for muscle contraction, for the transmission of nerve impulses, and for the activation of many *enzymes* (substances that promote biochemical reactions in the body). There are about 1.25 ounces (35 g) of magnesium in an average-sized person, much of it in the bones and teeth.

The recommended daily intake of magnesium varies from 50 mg in the newborn to 400 mg in young men. Women require slightly less than men, except during pregnancy and breast-feeding. Dietary sources are green, leafy vegetables, nuts, whole grains, soybeans, milk, and seafood.

**MAGNESIUM-CONTAINING DRUGS**

Magnesium compounds are used in *antacid drugs* and *laxatives*. Magnesium carbonate and magnesium oxide are common ingredients of antacids; magnesium sulfate is used in laxatives. Magnesium is also a constituent of some mineral supplements.

**DEFICIENCY AND EXCESS**

A normal diet contains sufficient magnesium. Deficiency (which is rare) usually occurs as a result of an intestinal disorder that impairs absorption of both calcium and of magnesium, a severe kidney disease, alcoholism, or prolonged treatment with *diuretic drugs* or *digitalis drugs*. Symptoms of deficiency include anxiety, restlessness, tremors, palpitations, and depression. There is also thought to be an increased risk of kidney stones or coronary heart disease. Deficiency is treated with supplements.

Magnesium excess is usually caused by taking too much of a magnesium-containing antacid or laxative. Too much magnesium may cause nausea, vomiting, diarrhea, dizziness, and muscle weakness. Very large amounts may lead to heart damage or respiratory failure, especially in people with kidney disease. Mild magnesium excess does not usually require treatment. However, anyone who has taken a substantial overdose may require hospitalization so that breathing and heart activity can be monitored (and supported, if necessary) and drugs can be given to help the body excrete the excess.

## Magnetic resonance imaging

See *MRI*.

## Malabsorption

Impaired absorption of nutrients, vitamins, or minerals from the diet by the lining of the small intestine.

**CAUSES**

Malabsorption is caused by many conditions. In *lactose intolerance*, deficiency of the enzyme lactase in the intestine prevents the breakdown and absorption of lactose (sugar found in milk). In *cystic fibrosis* and chronic *pancreatitis*, damage to the pancreas prevents the production of enzymes required for the digestion and absorption of fats and other nutrients.

In *celiac sprue*, many nutrients cannot be absorbed because of damage to the small intestine by sensitivity to the protein gluten. Uncommon diseases in which the intestinal lining is damaged include *Crohn's disease*, *amyloidosis*, *giardiasis*, *Whipple's disease*, and *lymphoma*.

Removal of portions of the small intestine can cause malabsorption, as can stomach operations that cause food to pass through the digestive tract more quickly than normal.

There are also some disorders that interfere with the passage of bile salts to the small intestine or that interfere with their uptake, thus preventing the breakdown and absorption of fats. These disorders include *bile duct obstruction*, primary *biliary cirrhosis*, and Crohn's disease.

**SYMPTOMS AND DIAGNOSIS**

Common effects are diarrhea and weight loss; in severe cases, there may also be malnutrition (see *Nutritional disorders*), *vitamin* deficiency, *mineral* deficiency, or *anemia*.

The diagnosis is confirmed by examining feces for unabsorbed fat and by blood tests to detect anemia and deficiencies of nutrients, vitamins, and minerals. To determine the cause of malabsorption, tests may be carried out, including *barium X-ray examination* of the small intestine and *jejunal biopsy* (removal of tissue from the jejunum for examination).

**TREATMENT AND OUTLOOK**

Treatment depends on the underlying cause. In most cases, modifications or supplements to the diet restore the affected person to health. However, if there is severe, irreversible damage to the lining of the intestine, infusion of nutrients into a vein may be necessary (see *Feeding, artificial*).

## Maladjustment

Failure to adapt to a change in one's environment, resulting in an inability to cope with work or social activities. Maladjustment is common and can occur at any age as a reaction to stressful situations (such as starting school, changing residence, divorce, physical illness, or retirement). It may be expressed by feelings of *depression* or *anxiety*, or by *behavioral problems in children* and adolescents.

Maladjustment is usually temporary, clearing up when the person is removed from the stressful situation or learns to adapt to it.

## Malaise

A vague feeling of being sick or of physical discomfort. It is a general symptom of little value in diagnosis.

## Malalignment

Positioning of teeth in the jaw so that they do not form a smooth arch shape when viewed from above or below (see *Malocclusion*). The term is also used to refer to a *fracture* in which the bone ends are not in a straight line. These fractures must be manipulated back into position so that the bone is not deformed when it heals.

## Malar flush

A high color over the cheekbones, with a bluish tinge caused by reduced oxygen concentration in the blood. Malar flush is considered to be a sign of *mitral stenosis* (narrowing of one of the heart valves), usually following *rheumatic fever*. However, malar flush is not always present in mitral stenosis, and many people with this coloring do not have heart disease.

## Malaria

 A serious parasitic disease, spread by the bites of *ANOPHELES* mosquitoes. The disease produces severe fever and, in some cases, complications affecting the kidneys, liver, brain, and blood that can be fatal.

Malaria is prevalent throughout the tropics, affecting up to 300 million people worldwide each year. It is the single most important disease hazard for travelers to warm climates.

**CAUSES**

The parasites responsible for malaria are single-celled (protozoal) organisms called plasmodia. Four different species can cause disease in humans: *PLASMODIUM FALCIPARUM*, *PLASMODIUM VIVAX*, *PLASMODIUM OVALE*, and *PLASMODIUM MALARIAE*. Each of these species spends part of its life cycle in humans and part in *ANOPHELES* mosquitoes (see diagram, overleaf).

Symptoms, including shaking, chills, and fever, appear only when red blood cells, infected with parasites, rupture to release more parasites into the bloodstream.

**INCIDENCE**

Malaria occurs in much of the tropics, where it is a major health problem (see map). Children in affected countries suffer repeated infections, and many die. Malaria kills about 1 million infants and children every year in Africa alone; those who survive gradually build up immunity. The World Health Organization has undertaken a massive program of malaria control, but little progress has been made in the past 20 years. Mosquitoes have developed resistance to insecticides and, in many areas, the parasites have developed resistance to drugs.

The number of cases diagnosed in the US has increased significantly over the last 15 years, from a few hundred cases annually in the early 1970s to about 1,000 cases in both 1984 and 1985. Part of this rise is attributable to increased travel; about 40 percent of cases occur in people recently returned from the tropics. The risk of contracting the disease in Africa seems particularly high. The remaining 60 percent of cases affect foreign immigrants to the US.

The chance of contracting malaria within the US is very small. Cases have occurred among drug users who have shared needles with an infected person, and in people who have received infected blood transfusions.

**SYMPTOMS**

The period between the mosquito bite and the appearance of symptoms is usually a week or two, but can be as long as a year if the person has been taking antimalarial drugs (which suppress rather than cure malaria).

The prime symptom of infection is the classic malarial ague (fever). Except for most *P. FALCIPARUM* infec-

tions, this fever has three stages: a cold stage of uncontrollable shivering (rigors), a hot stage in which the temperature may reach 105°F, and finally a sweating stage that drenches the bedding and brings down the temperature. A severe headache, general malaise, and vomiting may accompany the attack. At the end of an attack, the patient is left weak and tired, and sleeps. In many cases, the parasitized red blood cells rupture at the same time in each cycle and the fever develops cyclically, occurring every other day (with *P. VIVAX* and *P. OVALE* infections) or every third day (with *P. MALARIAE*).

*P. FALCIPARUM* infects all ages of red blood cells, whereas the other varieties attack only young or old cells. Falciparum malaria thus affects a greater proportion of the blood cells and is therefore more severe. It can be fatal within a few hours of the first symptoms. The fever is prolonged and irregular. So many blood cells may be destroyed that they block blood vessels in vital organs, especially the kidneys. The spleen becomes enlarged and the brain may be affected, leading to coma and convulsions. Destruction of blood cells leads to hemolytic *anemia*. Kidney and liver failure are common complications of falciparum malaria.

**DIAGNOSIS**

Malaria is diagnosed from studying *blood smears* in the laboratory at six- to 12-hour intervals; the parasites are clearly visible under the microscope.

**TREATMENT**

Malaria, especially falciparum malaria, is a medical emergency that is treated in the hospital.

The antimalarial drug chloroquine, which eradicates the parasites from the blood, is the usual treatment for all types of malaria. However, chloroquine-resistant falciparum malaria is now widespread in many tropical areas. If a chloroquine-resistant form is suspected, or if the number of parasites does not diminish over 24 hours, other drugs, such as quinine or the combination of pyrimethamine and sulfadoxine, may be given.

In serious illness, exchange blood transfusions have been investigated as a lifesaving effort.

For any type other than falciparum malaria, another drug, primaquine, must be taken for another two weeks to eradicate parasites in the liver. Primaquine may cause hemolytic anemia in people who have a disorder called *G6PD deficiency*.

M

### PREVENTION

In countries where malaria is common, most people have acquired some immunity to the disease. However, this does not apply to visitors to the tropics, who should take preventive antimalarial drugs. These drugs should be taken a day or two before entering a malarious area and use should be continued for at least four weeks after leaving it.

The physician will want to know what countries are to be visited before prescribing a drug. For areas where there is no resistance to chloroquine, this drug is recommended; proguanil is recommended for longer term use because it has fewer side effects. For chloroquine-resistant areas there are various possibilities, such as a combination of chloroquine and proguanil, or the combination of pyrimethamine with either sulfadoxine or dapsone. These drugs may then be followed by a course of primaquine, which provides a radical cure of the forms of malaria found in the liver.

Antimalarial drugs should be taken even by pregnant women in highly malarious areas (proguanil or chloroquine are the recommended drugs in this case). Although the drugs present a slight risk to the fetus, it is less than the risk to the fetus if the mother contracts malaria.

In addition, visitors to the tropics should avoid mosquito bites by wearing protective clothing over the arms and legs in the evening; other preventive measures include screens over windows, insecticide sprays, and, if necessary, mosquito nets. People should also avoid entering jungle areas at night.

Even people who take antimalarial drugs and precautions against bites may contract malaria. Anyone in whom a fever and headache develops after returning from the tropics should see a physician as soon as possible and mention the trip abroad so that appropriate blood smears can be arranged to diagnose malaria.

## Malformation

A deformity, particularly one resulting from faulty development.

## Malignant

A term used to describe a condition that tends to become progressively worse and to result in death. By contrast, a *benign* disorder remains relatively mild and is not usually fatal. The term malignant is primarily used to refer to a *tumor* that spreads from its original location to affect other parts of the body, with potentially life-threatening results.

## Malignant melanoma

See *Melanoma, malignant.*

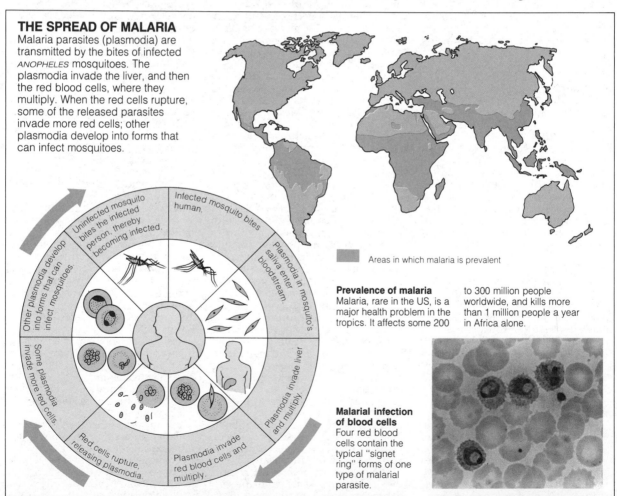

## THE SPREAD OF MALARIA

Malaria parasites (plasmodia) are transmitted by the bites of infected *ANOPHELES* mosquitoes. The plasmodia invade the liver, and then the red blood cells, where they multiply. When the red cells rupture, some of the released parasites invade more red cells; other plasmodia develop into forms that can infect mosquitoes.

Uninfected mosquito bites the infected person, thereby becoming infected.

Infected mosquito bites human.

Plasmodia in mosquito's saliva enter bloodstream.

Plasmodia invade liver and multiply.

Plasmodia invade red blood cells and multiply.

Red cells rupture, releasing plasmodia.

Some plasmodia invade more red cells.

Other plasmodia develop into forms that can infect mosquitoes.

Areas in which malaria is prevalent

**Prevalence of malaria**
Malaria, rare in the US, is a major health problem in the tropics. It affects some 200 to 300 million people worldwide, and kills more than 1 million people a year in Africa alone.

**Malarial infection of blood cells**
Four red blood cells contain the typical "signet ring" forms of one type of malarial parasite.

## Malingering

Deliberate simulation of physical or psychological symptoms for a particular purpose, such as obtaining time off work, avoiding military service, or obtaining compensation. Malingering differs from *factitious disorders*, in which the person feigns illness for no reason other than a wish to gain the attention associated with illness and being a patient. Malingering is also distinguished from a *somatization disorder* (such as *hypochondriasis*), in which symptoms are not under the voluntary control of the person.

## Mallet finger

See *Baseball finger.*

## Mallet toe

A deformity of one or more toes (excluding the big toe) in one or both feet. The end of the affected toe bends downward so that the toe curls under itself. The cause is unknown. A painful corn may develop on the tip of the toe or over the top of the bent joint. Protective pads can sometimes relieve excessive pressure from footwear; if not, surgical treatment of the toe may be needed. (See also *Clawfoot.*)

## Mallory-Weiss syndrome

A condition in which a tear at the lower end of the esophagus causes vomiting of blood. Mallory-Weiss syndrome is particularly common in alcoholics after a bout of excessive drinking accompanied by retching and vomiting. Occasionally, the tear may be produced by violent coughing, a severe asthma attack, or epileptic convulsions. The damage is thought usually to result from violent contractions of the diaphragm during prolonged retching and vomiting.

**DIAGNOSIS AND TREATMENT**

Diagnosis is made by passing an *endoscope* (a tubelike instrument with a light source and lens attachment) down the esophagus. The tear usually heals within 10 days and no special treatment is required unless the person has lost a considerable amount of blood, in which case blood transfusions may be necessary.

## Malnutrition

See *Nutritional disorders.*

## Malocclusion

An abnormal relationship between the upper and lower sets of teeth when they are closed. In ideal occlusion the upper incisors and canines (front teeth) slightly overlap the lower ones, the outer ridges of the lower premolars and molars (back teeth) fit into the hollows in the corresponding upper teeth, and, except for the four frontmost incisors, the other upper and lower teeth alternate. This arrangement enables food to be bitten and chewed efficiently.

---

**TYPES OF MALOCCLUSION**

Unsatisfactory contact between the upper and lower teeth (malocclusion) is of three main types, shown below.

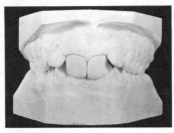

**Type 1 malocclusion**
In this (the most common) type, the jaw relationship is normal, but, because the teeth are poorly spaced, tilted, or rotated, the upper and lower set do not meet properly.

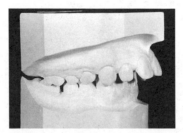

**Type 2 malocclusion**
In this type—called retrognathism—the lower jaw is too far back; the normal small overbite of the upper incisors is greatly increased, and the molar bite is displaced backward.

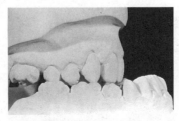

**Type 3 malocclusion**
In this (the least common) type (called prognathism), the lower jaw is too far forward; the lower incisors meet, or lie in front of, the upper ones, and the molar bite is displaced forward.

---

Ideal occlusion is uncommon; most people have some teeth slightly out of position. Only severe malocclusion usually requires treatment.

**CAUSES**

Malocclusion usually develops in childhood, when the teeth and jaws are growing. Most malocclusion is the result of *heredity*. Other cases may result from *thumb-sucking* beyond a certain age or from a mismatch between the teeth and the jaws (for example, large teeth in a small mouth, leading to *overcrowding*).

**TREATMENT**

Malocclusion may require treatment to improve appearance, to prevent strain from the abnormal bite (which causes pain, stiffness, and sometimes *arthritis* in the jaw joints), or to facilitate teeth cleaning and thus help prevent *periodontal disease* and decay (see *Caries, dental*).

The dentist may be able to correct uneven contacts between teeth by recontouring opposing tooth surfaces or by fitting an onlay restoration (see *Onlay, dental*) to alter the shape of a tooth. However, most serious abnormalities require orthodontic treatment, which consists mainly of using *orthodontic appliances* (braces) to train teeth to grow into the proper position. In cases of tooth crowding, some teeth may need to be extracted. *Orthognathic surgery* is used to treat recession or protrusion of the lower jaw.

Treatment is best carried out in childhood or adolescence, when the teeth and bones of the jaw are still developing. Problems left until adulthood can be treated successfully, but may take longer to correct than when treated earlier.

## Malpractice

See *Liability insurance, professional.*

## Malpresentation

A condition in which a baby is not in the usual face downward, head first position during *childbirth*. Only 5 percent of babies enter labor malpresented. Most malpresentations are bottom first (breech position) or head first but face upward (occipital posterior position); some lie transversely across the uterus.

A baby lying bottom first may be delivered by *breech delivery* or *cesarean section*. A baby lying transversely usually is delivered by cesarean section. A baby in the occipital posterior position usually rotates into a normal position during labor; sometimes a cesarean is necessary.

**M**

# Mammary gland
See *Breast*.

# Mammography
An X-ray procedure for detecting *breast cancer* at an early stage.

### WHY IT IS DONE
Successful treatment of breast cancer depends on early diagnosis (detection of tumors less than about one half inch across). Growths this small may not be discernible on physical examination (see *Breast self-examination*) and can be effectively detected only by mammography. Screening tests using mammography have reduced death rates from breast cancer in women over the age of 50 by 30 percent.

Mammography is also used to aid diagnosis of established breast disease and to help plan treatment.

# Mammoplasty
A cosmetic operation to reduce the size of extremely large or pendulous breasts, to enlarge small breasts, or to reconstruct a breast after it has been removed to treat cancer.

### BREAST REDUCTION
This operation is performed using a general anesthetic. Incisions are inconspicuous and positioned so that unwanted tissue is easily removed. This procedure reduces the size of the breast and raises its position to correct any drooping.

Most patients are pleased with the results. The nipple scar and the scar beneath the breast are usually well hidden, but the vertical scar is usually evident and may need to be made less obvious at a second, minor operation.

### BREAST ENLARGEMENT
This procedure is usually performed using a short-acting general anesthetic. A small opening at the side or below the breast allows a pocket to be made to accommodate the implant.

The immediate results are usually excellent, but internal scar tissue often eventually forms around the implant, altering its shape and making the breast harder. External pressure on the implant to restore its shape or sometimes another minor operation may be necessary.

### BREAST RECONSTRUCTION
This operation is carried out either at the same time as a *mastectomy* (breast removal) or at a later date, again using a general anesthetic. Depending on the type of mastectomy, reconstruction takes one of two forms.

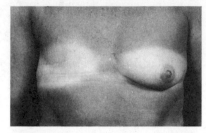

**Before**

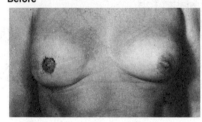

**After**

**Reconstruction of a breast**
A breast removed at an earlier mastectomy operation can be reconstructed later using a silicone rubber implant.

If the entire breast is removed, a portion of skin and underlying fat and muscle is transplanted from a site near the breast; a silicone rubber implant is incorporated at the same time. In this case, scarring is extensive.

Increasingly often, surgeons remove only the tumor and surrounding tissue, leaving the overlying skin in place; the implant can then be inserted with minimal scarring.

In both operations the size of the other breast may be reduced to make the breasts look balanced.

# Mandible
The lower *jaw*.

# Mandibular orthopedic repositioning appliance
A device used by some dentists to treat conditions claimed to result from misalignment of the jaw, such as headaches, temporomandibular disorders, scoliosis (curvature of the spine), and loss of balance. A mandibular orthopedic repositioning appliance (MORA) is often mistaken for a mouth protector, but does not perform the same function.

M

## PROCEDURE FOR MAMMOGRAPHY
Mammography is simple, safe, and causes minimal discomfort. Only low-dose X rays are used. The breast may be X-rayed from above, the side, or both; sometimes an oblique (angled) view is taken.

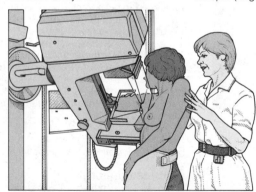

**How mammography is done**
In the method shown here, the breast is placed on the machine and gently compressed between the X-ray plate below and a plastic cover above. This flattens the breast so that as much tissue as possible can be imaged. Several views may be taken. In another method, the breast hangs freely and is X-rayed from the side.

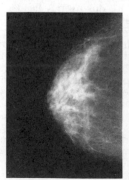 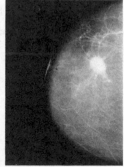

**Mammograms**
The normal mammogram (far left) shows a side view of a healthy breast, with the milk ducts appearing as denser areas. In the abnormal mammogram (left), an irregular, dense mass in the upper part of the breast indicates a tumor. A biopsy (removal of a tissue sample for analysis) is necessary to determine whether a tumor is cancerous.

## PROCEDURE FOR MAMMOPLASTY

One of the most common cosmetic operations, mammoplasty is done to improve the appearance of the breasts by removal of excess fat and skin or by using an implant to increase their size.

### BREAST REDUCTION

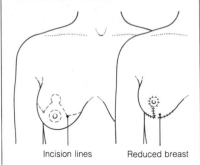

Incision lines          Reduced breast

Incisions are made around the edge of the nipple and in the crease below the breast. These are joined by a third vertical cut. Excess tissue and skin are removed, and the incisions are closed with stitches.

### BREAST ENLARGEMENT

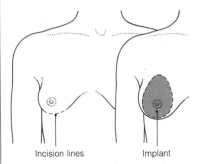

Incision lines          Implant

An incision is made in the armpit or along the crease under the breast, and a pocket is created behind the breast to receive the implant. After the implant has been inserted, the incision is stitched.

---

Much controversy exists over whether a MORA can improve athletic performance by building strength and endurance. Such claims have not been scientifically proved. In fact, there is evidence that continued use of a MORA may result in severe malocclusion that requires extensive orthodontic or reconstructive treatment.

## Mania

A mental disorder characterized by episodes of overactivity, elation, or irritability. Mania usually occurs as part of a *manic-depressive illness*.

### SYMPTOMS

The primary symptom of mania is an abnormal increase in activity (for example, the sufferer may make elaborate plans for a constant round of social activity). Other symptoms may include extravagant spending, repeatedly starting new tasks, less need to sleep, increased appetite for food, alcohol, sex, and energetic exercise, outbursts of inappropriate anger, laughter, or sudden socializing, and a grandiose sense of knowing better than others. This may extend to delusions of grandeur (for example, believing oneself to be God). When symptoms are relatively mild, the condition is called hypomania.

Manic attacks usually first appear before the age of 30, and may last for a few days or several months. If attacks begin after age 40, they are frequently more prolonged.

### TREATMENT

Severe mania often leads to marked social disruption or even violence; hospital admission is usually required. Treatment is generally by means of *antipsychotic drugs* and relapses are prevented by giving *lithium*. Carbamazepine is sometimes used to augment the effect of lithium.

## Manic-depressive illness

A mental disorder in which a disturbance of mood is the major symptom. This disturbance may consist of *depression* or of *mania* (unipolar) or of a swing between the two states (bipolar).

### CAUSES

A number of physical illnesses (especially brain disorders), certain drugs, and a clear inherited tendency are all established factors. Research has located at least one of the defective genes responsible on chromosome 11.

Overactivity seems due largely to extra amounts of the neurochemical dopamine in parts of the brain; this may simply represent a manic reaction to an underlying depression caused by loss or grief.

### PREVALENCE

Depression is very common, affecting about one in 10 men and one in five women at some time in their lives. About a third of these illnesses are severe. By contrast, mania (unipolar or bipolar) is rare, affecting only about eight per 1,000 people, men and women equally.

### TREATMENT

Admission to the hospital is often required for severe manic-depressive illness. *Antidepressant drugs* and/or *ECT* (electroconvulsive therapy) are effective in treating depression. *Antipsychotic drugs* (e.g., chlorpromazine and haloperidol) are used to control manic symptoms. *Lithium* alone or, when inadequate, with carbamazepine may be used during remission to prevent relapse.

Group, family, and individual therapy are useful in treating neurotic disorders and in aiding recovery after a severe episode. *Cognitive-behavioral therapy* may also be helpful.

### OUTLOOK

Though often crippling in the acute phase, manic-depressive illnesses have a good prognosis. Abilities are not affected, and more than 80 percent of patients recover.

Repeated, severe illnesses, however, or persistent depression, can seriously disrupt life. A significant number of depressed people commit, or attempt, *suicide*. Others suffer from social isolation, poverty, and problems caused by alcohol dependence. Nevertheless, the widescale use of maintenance treatment with lithium has restored many people who have manic-depressive illness to near normal health.

## Manipulation

As a therapy, the skillful use of the hands to move a part of the body or a specific joint or muscle to treat certain disorders. Manipulation at times is carried out by a physician, sometimes using a general anesthetic. The technique of manipulation is widely practiced by physical therapists, osteopaths, and chiropractors.

Manipulation is used to correct deformity by aligning the bones of a displaced *fracture*, putting a joint back into position following *dislocation*, or stretching a *contracture* (shortened muscle or tendon). It may also be used to increase the range of movement of a stiff joint, usually following injury. Occasionally, it is helpful in treating *frozen shoulder*, but does not usually relieve stiffness caused by *arthritis* (inflammation of a joint).

## Mannitol

An osmotic *diuretic drug*. Mannitol is used as a short-term treatment for *glaucoma* (raised pressure in the eyeball) before corrective surgery. It is also given to reduce *edema* (fluid retention) in the brain before and after

**M**

surgical treatment of a *brain tumor* or an intracerebral *hematoma* (blood clot on the brain).

Mannitol is occasionally used to prevent *renal failure* following severe shock. In some cases of drug overdose, mannitol is given to increase urine production and thus the amount of the drug excreted from the body.

Possible adverse effects include headache, nausea, vomiting, dizziness, and confusion.

## Manometry

The measuring of pressure (of either liquid or gas) by means of a manometer. The simplest type of manometer is a glass U-shaped tube containing mercury, oil, or water. One limb of the tube is connected by flexible tubing to the pressure source; the other limb is either open to the atmosphere or closed. Increased pressure forces the liquid down in one limb and up in the other; the change in height represents a measure of the pressure. This form of manometer is used to measure blood pressure (see *Sphygmomanometer*) and cerebrospinal fluid pressure.

There are also more sophisticated manometers that measure pressure by a coiled spring, a diaphragm, or an electrical transducer.

## Mantoux test

A type of skin test for tuberculosis (see *Tuberculin tests*).

## Maprotiline

An *antidepressant drug.* Because maprotiline has a sedative effect, it is useful in the treatment of *depression* accompanied by anxiety or difficulty sleeping. Maprotiline usually takes about six weeks to become fully effective. Possible adverse effects include dizziness, drowsiness, palpitations, and rash.

## Marasmus

A severe form of protein and calorie malnutrition (see *Nutritional disorders*) that occurs principally in famine or semistarvation conditions. In developing countries, marasmus is widespread in children under 3 years of age, usually because they have been weaned too early onto an inadequate diet or kept too long on unsupplemented breast milk.

Children with marasmus are stunted and emaciated; they have loose folds of skin on the limbs and buttocks due to loss of muscle and fat. Other signs include sparse, brittle hair, diarrhea, and dehydration.

### DIAGNOSIS AND TREATMENT
Marasmus is diagnosed from a physical examination and the child's dietary history. Treatment consists of keeping the child warm and giving a high-calorie, protein-rich diet. Persistent marasmus can cause permanent mental retardation and impairment of growth. (See also *Kwashiorkor*.)

## Marble bone disease
See *Osteopetrosis*.

## March fracture

A break in one of the *metatarsal bones* (long bones in the foot) caused by repeated jarring. Usually affecting the second or third metatarsal, march fracture is caused by running or walking long distances on a hard surface. The name is derived from the high incidence of this fracture in soldiers after long marches.

Pain, tenderness, and swelling occur around the site of the fracture. However, X rays may not show the fracture until healing has begun, when callus (new bone) appears as a white shadow. Treatment is rest and, occasionally, immobilization in a plaster cast. (See also *Stress fracture*.)

## Marfan's syndrome

A rare, inherited disorder of connective tissue that results in abnormalities of the skeleton, heart, and eyes. The incidence of Marfan's syndrome is about two cases per 100,000 people. The precise cause is unknown.

### SYMPTOMS AND SIGNS
The features of Marfan's syndrome usually appear after age 10. Affected people grow very tall and thin, the fingers are long and spidery, the chest and spine are often deformed, and the tendons, ligaments, and joint capsules are weak, leaving the sufferer "double-jointed" and prone to joint

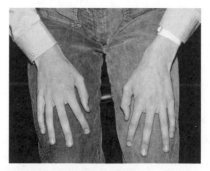

**Features of Marfan's syndrome**
One of the characteristic features of Marfan's syndrome is long, thin, "spider" fingers (arachnodactyly).

dislocation. In 90 percent of cases, the heart or aorta (major blood vessel leading from the heart) is abnormal; in over 60 percent of sufferers, the lens of the eye is dislocated.

### DIAGNOSIS
There are no specific diagnostic tests for the syndrome; *echocardiography* may be used to examine the valve deformities in the heart. An eye examination may also be performed.

### TREATMENT AND OUTLOOK
Orthopedic braces or surgery may be required to correct spinal deformity. Beta-blockers (such as propranolol) may help control heart problems, but heart surgery is sometimes necessary.

Affected people should receive genetic counseling; there is a 50 percent chance that their offspring will inherit the disease. Women with Marfan's syndrome risk heart complications if they become pregnant.

Sufferers usually do not live beyond 50, with death often caused by heart failure or rupture of the aorta.

## Marijuana

The dried leaves and flowering tops of the Indian hemp plant *CANNABIS SATIVA.* Marijuana contains the active ingredient *THC* (tetrahydrocannabinol), which is also found in cannabis resin (hashish). The chopped leaves are usually smoked alone as a joint, or "reefer," but can be taken as tea or in food.

### EFFECTS
When marijuana is smoked, effects occur within minutes and last for an hour or more. When eaten, one half to one hour usually elapses before effects are felt, and they may last for three to five hours.

Physical effects include a dry mouth, mild reddening of the eyes, slight clumsiness, and increased appetite. The main subjective feelings are usually of well-being and calmness, although depression occasionally occurs. Users become dreamy and relaxed, laughing readily and experiencing time as passing very slowly. Sights and sounds become more vivid, imagination increases, and random connections between things seem more relevant.

Large doses may result in panicky states, fear of death, and illusions. Rarely, true psychosis (loss of contact with reality) occurs, producing paranoid delusions, confusion, and other symptoms. These symptoms usually disappear within several days if triggered by the drug, which may

M

merely be acting on an underlying illness. A more permanent state of apathy and loss of concern—the amotivational syndrome—has been attributed to prolonged, regular use.

There is evidence that regular users of marijuana can become physically dependent on its effects. Whether the drug causes brain or other physical damage is much debated. Possession and use of marijuana is subject to legal controls, which vary from state to state.

## Marital counseling
Professional therapy for married couples or established partners that is aimed at resolving problems in relationships. Usually the partners attend sessions together on a regular basis. The counselor promotes communication and sorts out differences between the partners.

### HOW IT IS DONE
Marital therapy today is largely based on the ideas and methods of *behavior therapy*. It assumes that behavior in a relationship is learned; it also is based on the idea that both people are responsible for problems because they have either failed to reinforce desirable behavior in the partner or have failed to respond themselves with appropriate behavior.

Therapy starts by analyzing the good and bad aspects of the relationship, and then by detailing clearly how each partner would like the other to behave. A contract may be drawn up in which each person agrees to do something that the other wants. Alternatively, each person may be given a supply of tokens, which are used to reward the partner for pleasing or helpful behavior.

### EFFECTIVENESS
Although behavioral marital therapy may seem superficial and ineffective, it has radically altered behavior and marital happiness. Research evidence shows that it may be more effective than lengthy personal analysis.

## Marrow, bone
See *Bone marrow*.

## Marsupialization
A surgical procedure used to drain an abscess of a *Bartholin's gland* (glands on either side of the entrance to the vagina) and to prevent further abscesses from developing. Marsupialization involves cutting out part of the abscess wall and a small piece of vaginal tissue, then stitching the opened abscess wall to the vaginal

wall, forming a pouch. This maneuver is also used to drain certain pancreatic cysts into the bowel.

## Masculinization
See *Virilization*.

## Masochism
A desire to be physically, mentally, or emotionally abused. The term is derived from the name of the 19th century Austrian novelist Leopold von Sacher-Masoch.

Masochism is often used specifically to refer to the achievement of sexual excitement exclusively or preferably by means of one's own suffering. Activities include bondage, flagellation, and verbal abuse. The condition is usually chronic, and may be life-threatening when people increase the severity of their masochistic acts.

Masochists rarely seek professional treatment; when they do, it is usually at the instigation of a spouse who threatens to leave. (See also *Sadism*; *Sadomasochism*.)

## Massage
Rubbing and kneading areas of the body, usually using the hands. Massage is used to relieve painful muscle spasm, treat muscle injury, reduce edema (fluid retention in tissue), and, in the treatment of scars, to prevent tethering of skin and underlying tissue. Massage increases blood flow, reduces pain by counter-irritation (alleviation of deep-seated pain by irritation of nerve endings in the skin), relaxes muscles, and increases the suppleness of the skin.

## Mast cell
 A type of cell that plays an important part in the body's allergic response (see *Allergy*). Mast cells are present in most body tissues, but are particularly numerous in connective tissue, such as the dermis (innermost layer) of the skin.

In an allergic response, an allergen stimulates the release of antibodies, which attach themselves to mast cells.

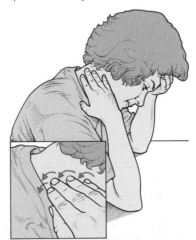

**SELF-MASSAGE**
Although massage is most effective when carried out by another person, self-massage can still be useful; for example, it may help to alleviate pain caused by muscular tension.

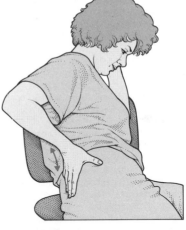

**Kneading the lower back**
For self-massage of the lower back, the hands should be placed with the thumbs pointing forward, and the fingertips close together at the back. Firm finger pressure is required to massage this area.

**Finger kneading of the neck and foot**
For neck massage, the elbows are rested on a firm surface, such as a table, and the head is supported with one hand while the fingertips of the other hand knead the back and side of the neck. After one side of the neck has been massaged, switch hands and massage the other side. The foot contains few muscles, but many nerve endings, so foot massage is often very soothing.

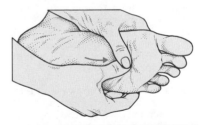

As a result, the mast cells release substances such as *histamine* (a chemical responsible for allergic symptoms) into the tissue.

## Mastectomy

Surgical removal of all or part of the breast. Mastectomy is usually performed to treat *breast cancer* and is often followed by a course of *radiation therapy* or *anticancer drugs*.

The amount of breast and surrounding tissue that is removed depends on the size and location of the tumor, how much the cancer has spread, and the age and health of the patient. The final choice of treatment should be a matter for discussion between the woman and her physician.

### TYPES

Until the late 1960s, the standard operation was the radical mastectomy, which involves removal of the affected breast, the chest muscles, all chest and underarm lymph nodes, and additional fat and skin from the chest. When certain chest muscles are left intact, the operation is known as a modified radical mastectomy.

Today, surgeons more often recommend lumpectomy (in which only cancerous tissue is removed) or a quadrantectomy (in which one quadrant of the breast is removed). Another alternative is simple mastectomy, which consists of removing the affected breast and sometimes a portion of the underarm lymph nodes. If possible, surgeons leave the overlying skin intact, or leave plenty of surrounding skin, to allow the breast to be reconstructed.

### HOW IT IS DONE

Each of the operations is performed using general anesthesia. For lumpectomy and quadrantectomy, an incision is made over the breast lump, which is cut free and removed (with or without surrounding tissue).

For subcutaneous mastectomy, a surgical incision is made along the perimeter of the breast closest to the tumor. For more extensive operations, the incision extends from the armpit to encompass the entire breast. Underlying tissue is then cut free and removed, and a drainage tube is inserted. In all cases, the skin is closed with stitches or clips, which are usually removed after a week. A skin graft is sometimes needed.

### RECOVERY PERIOD

Patients can usually go home one to two days after lumpectomy and quadrantectomy, and can resume most activities within two weeks.

## TYPES OF MASTECTOMY

The type of operation depends on many factors, including the location of the tumor and the woman's health.

A small tumor may be treated by lumpectomy; other cases may require more extensive surgery.

### LUMPECTOMY

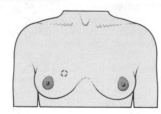

Only the area of cancerous tissue is removed. Lumpectomy is the least invasive procedure and leaves the breast looking normal.

### QUADRANTECTOMY

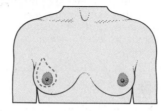

The cancerous tissue plus a wedge of surrounding tissue is removed. The lymph nodes in the armpit may also be removed. The breast is slightly smaller after the operation.

### SUBCUTANEOUS MASTECTOMY

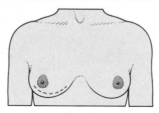

An incision is made under the breast and internal breast tissue is removed, leaving most of the skin intact. The nipple is not involved, but the milk ducts leading to it are cut. In some cases, the appearance of the breast is restored by immediate insertion of a silicone rubber implant. More often, however, this is done later.

### TOTAL MASTECTOMY

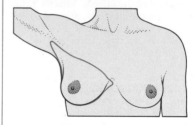

**1** A large elliptical incision, encompassing the nipple and sometimes the entire breast, is made. The incision extends into the armpit.

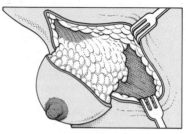

**2** All the breast tissue, including the skin and some of the fat, is dissected (cut out) down to the chest muscles. The dissection is continued under the skin into the armpit, to free the upper and outer "tail" of breast tissue with its lymph nodes. All bleeding vessels are tied off before inserting a drainage tube and closing the skin with stitches or clips.

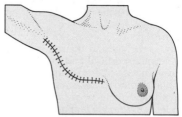

**3** The scar after the operation. The woman may wear a prosthesis or may have a silicone implant inserted later.

After other operations, the hospital stay is usually several days, with the drainage tube being removed on the second or third day. Analgesics (painkillers) may be necessary for the first week.

### OUTLOOK

Healing is usually very good after lumpectomy and quadrantectomy, with no noticeable scarring. Wound infection is uncommon. Skin scars after more radical procedures may be extensive, but usually fade within a year. Possible long-term complications, particularly of radical mastectomy, include *lymphedema* (accumulation of fluid under the skin) and stiffness of the arm and shoulder.

M

If the entire breast has been removed, the woman may decide to be fitted with a prosthesis (artificial breast). A temporary prosthesis may be worn until the chest scars have healed, when a more permanent prosthesis can be fitted. Alternatively, a plastic silicone implant can be inserted either at the end of the mastectomy operation or at a later operation (see *Mammoplasty*).

## Mastication

The process of chewing food. Mastication consists of two stages. In the first, the canines and incisors (front teeth) shear the food. In the second, the tongue pushes the food between the upper and lower premolars and molars (back teeth) to be ground by side-to-side and circular movements of the lower jaws. At the same time, saliva is mixed with the food to help break it down for swallowing.

Any food that spills over between the gums and cheeks is scooped up by rhythmic contractions of the cheeks and lips. The muscles of mastication, which attach the lower jaw to the rest of the skull, are controlled by signals from sensory nerves in the mouth to prevent undue stress on tooth-supporting tissues.

Only gross irregularities in the positional relationship of upper to lower teeth (see *Malocclusion*) prevent normal mastication.

## Mastitis

Inflammation of breast tissue often caused by bacterial infection.
### CAUSES
Mastitis usually occurs during breast-feeding when bacteria enter the breast through the nipple (especially if it is cracked). Infection with the *mumps* virus is another cause of mastitis.

Changes in levels of sex hormones can cause mastitis in the newborn (due to high levels of hormones from the mother's circulation) and at the start of puberty. Hormonal variations may also be the cause of chronic mastitis in women who are prone to lumpy breasts. This common disorder is known as fibrocystic disease of the breast, fibroadenosis, cystic mastitis, benign mammary dysplasia, or benign breast disease.
### SYMPTOMS
Pain, tenderness, and swelling occur in all types of mastitis and may be present in one or both breasts.

In mastitis caused by bacterial infection during breast-feeding, the breasts become red and engorged. The problem tends to occur during the first month of breast-feeding and may result in a breast abscess.

Symptoms of acute mastitis in babies and at puberty usually last for only a few weeks and clear up without specific treatment.

In chronic mastitis, there may be diffuse lumpiness of the breasts or a single breast lump caused by an overgrowth of glandular and fibrous tissue and sometimes resulting in cysts. There may also be a feeling of heaviness in the breast and, occasionally, a discharge from the nipple. The symptoms are worse during the second half of the menstrual cycle and usually affect the upper, outer part of the breast.
### DIAGNOSIS AND TREATMENT
If the cause of mastitis is unknown, *mammography* may be performed or a *biopsy* (removal of a small piece of tissue for examination) of a breast lump carried out to exclude the possibility of cancer.

Acute mastitis caused by infection is treated with *antibiotic drugs*, *analgesics* (painkillers), and *expressing milk* to relieve engorgement. Breast-feeding should be continued unless pus begins to drain from the nipple. If a breast abscess develops, it requires surgical drainage.

Breast tenderness caused by chronic mastitis generally requires no specific treatment, although *diuretic drugs* may relieve symptoms. If symptoms are severe, progesterone, danazol, or bromocriptine may be prescribed. Any cysts in the breast may be aspirated (drained by a needle and syringe).

## Mastocytosis

An unusual condition, also called urticaria pigmentosa, characterized by numerous itchy, irregular, yellow or orange-brown swellings on the skin. Mastocytosis may affect any part of the body but is most commonly found on the trunk; it is worse after bathing or scratching.

Mastocytosis usually begins in the first year of life and disappears by adolescence. Treatment is difficult, although *antihistamine drugs* sometimes help.

## Mastoid bone

The prominent bone behind the ear. Projecting from the temporal bone of the skull, it is honeycombed with air cells, which are connected to a cavity in the upper part of the bone called the mastoid antrum. This bone, in turn, is connected to the middle ear. As a result, infections of the middle ear (see *Otitis media*) occasionally spread through the mastoid bone to cause acute *mastoiditis*.

## Mastoiditis

Inflammation of the *mastoid bone*, the prominent bone behind the ear.
### CAUSE AND INCIDENCE
The disease is caused by the spread of infection from the middle ear (see *Otitis media*) to the antrum (a cavity in the mastoid bone), and from there to a honeycomb of air cells in the bone.

Mastoiditis has been uncommon since the advent of antibiotic drugs, which control middle-ear infection.
### SYMPTOMS AND SIGNS
Mastoiditis causes severe pain, swelling, and tenderness behind the ear, as well as pain within the ear. These symptoms are usually accompanied by fever, a creamy discharge from the ear, progressive hearing loss, and some displacement of the outer ear.
### COMPLICATIONS
There is always a risk that the infection may spread to inside the skull, causing *meningitis*, *brain abscess*, or blood clotting in veins within the brain. The infection may also spread outward to damage the facial nerve and cause *facial palsy*.
### DIAGNOSIS AND TREATMENT
Prompt diagnosis, based on a physical examination, is essential because of the possible complications.

Treatment is with antibiotics, which usually clear up the infection. If the infection persists, an operation known as a mastoidectomy may be necessary. This procedure involves

**M**

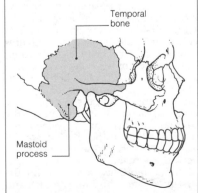

**LOCATION OF MASTOID BONE**
Forming the prominence behind the ear, the mastoid process (bone) is not a separate bone but is part of the temporal bone.

Temporal bone

Mastoid process

making an incision behind the ear, opening up the mastoid bone, and removing the infected air cells. The wound is stitched up around a drainage tube, which is removed a day or two later.

## Masturbation

Sexual self-stimulation, usually to orgasm. It is now accepted as a normal behavior, particularly among teenagers and young adults. Over 90 percent of men and about 65 percent of women masturbate at some time during their lives. Massaging the penis or clitoris with the hand is the usual method.

There is no evidence that masturbation causes any physical or psychological harm, despite the 19th-century belief that it caused insanity, blindness, or other disorders. This notion may have been based on the observation that people who are severely retarded or suffering from *schizophrenia* sometimes masturbate publicly. Such behavior is a sign, not a cause, of mental illness that also occurs in *dementia* and other forms of brain damage.

## Maternal mortality

The death of a woman during pregnancy or within 42 days of *childbirth*, *miscarriage*, or elective *abortion* from any cause related to, or made worse by, pregnancy. Maternal mortality is the number of such deaths per year per 100,000 (or sometimes per 1,000 or 10,000) pregnancies.

**CAUSES**
Maternal deaths may occur as a direct result of complications of pregnancy, or as an indirect result of a medical condition that has been aggravated by pregnancy. The principal direct causes include *pulmonary embolism* (blood clots in the lungs), *hypertension* (high blood pressure), *antepartum hemorrhage* or *postpartum hemorrhage*, *ectopic pregnancy* (development of the fetus outside the uterus), *eclampsia* (a condition characterized by seizures during late pregnancy), abortion, miscarriage, or *cesarean section*, and *puerperal sepsis* (infection of the uterus after childbirth). Important indirect causes are heart disease, *anemia*, *hyperthyroidism* (overactivity of the thyroid gland) or *hypothyroidism* (underactivity of the thyroid gland), *diabetes mellitus*, and some cancers.

**RELATED FACTORS**
Maternal mortality is highest for the first pregnancy, and for the fifth and subsequent pregnancies. It is also greater in women who are younger than 20 or older than 30. Statistically, it is safest for a woman to have her first baby when she is between 20 and 25 years old; it becomes increasingly less safe after age 30.

Social factors also play a part. Maternal mortality is higher among poor, less well-educated women, and is greater in blacks than in whites. Maternal mortality generally is greater among women who do not receive adequate prenatal care.

**TRENDS**
Maternal mortality has decreased considerably since about the 1940s. In the US, the death rate has fallen from 74 per 100,000 pregnancies in 1950, to eight per 100,000 in 1983. This dramatic decline is due largely to social improvements, better obstetric care, the development of antibiotics and other drugs to combat infection, and the availability of blood transfusions. In addition, because of the ready availability of contraception, fewer women than formerly have a large number of pregnancies.

## Maxilla

One of a pair of bones that forms the upper jaw. At their base the maxillas carry the upper teeth and form the roof of the mouth; at the top they form the floor of the orbits (the sockets that contain the eyes). Each bone contains a large air-filled cavity (called the maxillary sinus) that is connected to the nasal cavity.

---

**LOCATION OF THE MAXILLA**
The maxilla is one of a pair of bones that together form the center of the face, the upper jaw, and the roof of the mouth.

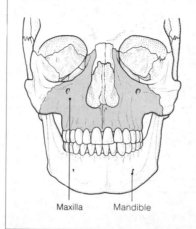

Maxilla          Mandible

---

**DISORDERS**
The most common disorder affecting the maxilla is *sinusitis* (inflammation of the mucous membrane that lines the maxillary sinuses), usually caused by infection spreading from the nose. Severe sinusitis occasionally leads to *osteomyelitis* (bone infection).

The maxilla is often fractured in motor vehicle accidents, causing a variety of facial deformities, such as backward displacement of the teeth or caving in of the center of the face. Immediate surgery to reposition and secure the bones is necessary to prevent permanent disfigurement.

Various kinds of tumors may develop in the maxillary sinus; 80 percent of them are malignant, and they may eventually alter the shape of the jaw, loosen the teeth, block one of the nasolacrimal ducts (causing the eye to water), push the eyeball upward or outward, or block the nose and cause a bloody, offensive-smelling discharge. Treatment is by *radiation therapy*, followed by surgical removal of the maxilla. About one third of sufferers survive for five years.

## McArdle's disease

A rare genetic disorder characterized by muscular stiffness and painful cramps that increase during and after exertion. McArdle's disease is caused by a deficiency of the enzyme in muscle cells that stimulates the breakdown of *glycogen* (a complex carbohydrate) to glucose (a type of sugar). This deficiency results in a build up of glycogen within the muscle tissue and prevents the release of glucose as an essential source of energy during exercise.

Symptoms usually start between the ages of 20 and 30. Myoglobinuria (muscle cell pigment in the urine) occurs because of the damage to muscle cells; rarely, it is severe enough to cause *renal failure*. Affected people are usually healthy apart from the need to restrict their exercise.

There is no treatment, although symptoms may be helped by eating glucose or fructose before exercise.

## Measles

A distressing viral illness that causes a characteristic rash and a fever. Measles mainly affects children but can occur at any age. One attack usually confers lifelong immunity.

**CAUSES AND INCIDENCE**
The measles virus is highly infective and is spread primarily by airborne droplets of nasal secretions. There is

an incubation period of nine to 11 days before symptoms appear. Infected children can transmit the virus from shortly after the start of this period up to one week following the development of symptoms. Infants under 8 months old are rarely affected because they have acquired some immunity from their mothers.

Measles was once very common throughout the world, occurring in epidemics. It is now less common in developed countries due to immunization. In the US, where proof of immunization is required before a child can attend school, there are several thousand cases reported annually. Prevention of the illness is important because it can have rare but serious complications. It may also be serious, or fatal, in children with impaired immunity (e.g., those being treated for leukemia).

In developing countries, measles is still common, accounting for more than 1 million deaths a year, especially in malnourished children whose defenses against infection are seriously impaired.

### SYMPTOMS AND SIGNS
The illness starts with a fever, runny nose, sore eyes, and cough, and the sufferer is sick. After three to four days a red rash appears, usually starting on the head and neck and spreading downward to cover the whole body. The spots sometimes join to produce large red blotchy areas, and the lymph glands may be enlarged. After three days the rash starts to fade and symptoms subside.

The most common complications are ear and chest infections, which usually occur with a return of fever two to three days after appearance of the rash. Diarrhea, vomiting, and abdominal pain also occur. A more serious complication, occurring in about one in 1,000 cases, is *encephalitis* (inflammation of the brain). It causes headache, drowsiness, and vomiting, starting seven to 10 days after the rash appears. Seizures and coma may follow, sometimes leading to mental retardation or death (however, seizures are common with measles and do not necessarily indicate encephalitis).

Very rarely (in about one in a million cases) a progressive brain disorder (subacute sclerosing panencephalitis) develops years after the acute illness. Measles during pregnancy results in death of the fetus in about one fifth of cases. There is no evidence that measles causes birth defects.

### TREATMENT
Plenty of fluids should be given and acetaminophen taken to treat the fever. Antibiotics are not routinely required but may be needed to treat secondary infections.

### IMMUNIZATION
In the US, children are routinely immunized early in the second year of life. The vaccine is given by injection (usually combined with mumps and rubella vaccine), producing immunity in 97 percent of people. Side effects of the vaccine are generally mild. There may be a low fever, slight cold, and rash about one week after vaccination.

The vaccine should not be given to children under age 1 or to those with any of the usual risk factors for vaccination (see *Immunization*). The vaccine may induce a seizure in children who have had one before and if there is a history of epilepsy in the family. In these cases simultaneous injection of measles-specific immunoglobulin (which contains antibodies against the virus) should be given.

A pregnant woman who has never had measles or been immunized against the disease should avoid people with measles. If she does come into contact with an infected person, she should be passively immunized against measles with *immunoglobulin* within five days.

## Meatus
A canal or passageway through part of the body. The term usually refers to the external auditory meatus, the canal in the outer *ear* that leads from the outside to the eardrum.

## Mebendazole
An *antihelmintic drug* used to treat *worm infestations* of the intestine. Mebendazole is under investigation as a treatment for worms that infest other areas, such as the lungs and liver (as in *hydatid disease*).

Possible adverse effects include abdominal pain and diarrhea.

## Meckel's diverticulum
A common congenital anomaly of the digestive tract in which a small, hollow, wide-mouthed sac protrudes from the *ileum* (the final section of the small intestine). Meckel's diverticulum occurs in 2 percent of people.

There are usually no symptoms unless the diverticulum is affected by infection, obstruction, or ulceration. The most common symptom is painless bleeding, which may be sudden and severe, making immediate blood

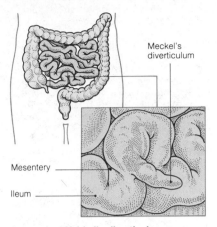

**Anatomy of Meckel's diverticulum**
In this birth defect, an appendixlike sac protrudes from the ileum (the last part of the small intestine).

transfusion necessary. Sometimes, inflammation causes symptoms so similar to those of acute *appendicitis* that the disorder is diagnosed only when abdominal surgery is carried out. A Meckel's diverticulum occasionally causes *intussusception* (telescoping) or *volvulus* (twisting) of the small intestine.

Disorders are treated by removal of the diverticulum.

## Meclizine
An *antihistamine drug* used as an *antiemetic drug*. Meclizine is given to treat nausea, vomiting, and *vertigo* in *motion sickness* and *Meniere's disease* and when these symptoms are due to *anticancer drugs* or *radiation therapy*. Meclizine may cause drowsiness, dry mouth, and blurred vision.

## Meclofenamate
A *nonsteroidal anti-inflammatory drug* (NSAID) used to relieve joint pain and stiffness in types of arthritis, such as *osteoarthritis* and *rheumatoid arthritis*. Meclofenamate produces adverse effects, such as diarrhea and nausea, and is normally prescribed only when similar drugs have proved ineffective.

## Meconium
The thick, sticky, greenish-black feces passed by infants during the first day or two after birth. Meconium consists of bile, mucus, and sloughed intestinal cells. After the baby starts feeding, the feces gradually change in color and consistency.

Occasionally, the fetus passes meconium into the amniotic fluid in the uterus. This is more common in

M

babies who experience *fetal distress* during labor or who are postmature (that is, over 40 weeks' gestation). Meconium in the amniotic fluid may be inhaled when the baby starts to breathe, sometimes blocking the airways and damaging the lungs.

In some babies with *cystic fibrosis*, the meconium is so thick and sticky that it blocks the intestine and causes intestinal obstruction.

## Medial

A medical term meaning situated toward the midline of the body. Less commonly, the word is used to refer to the middle layer of a body structure, particularly of a blood vessel wall.

## Median nerve

A branch of the *brachial plexus*; one of the main nerves of the arm that runs down the arm's full length into the hand. The median nerve controls the muscles of the forearm and hand, which carry out bending movements of the wrist, fingers, and thumb, and which rotate the forearm palm-inward. This nerve also conveys sensations from the thumb, index finger, middle finger, part of the ring finger, and the region of the palm at the base of these digits.

### DISORDERS

The nerve may be damaged where it originates from the brachial plexus as a result of injury to the shoulder, just above the wrist by a *Colles' fracture*, or by pressure on the nerve where it passes through the wrist (see *Carpal tunnel syndrome*). The principal symptoms of any damage are numbness and muscle weakness in the areas controlled by the nerve.

## Mediastinoscopy

Investigation of the right side of the *mediastinum* (the central compartment of the chest containing the heart, esophagus, and trachea) by means of an *endoscope* (a viewing tube with a light and lens) inserted into the cavity through an incision in the neck. Because more of the heart occupies the left side of the mediastinal cavity, endoscopic investigation of this area is difficult and dangerous; *imaging techniques* are preferred.

Mediastinoscopy is used mainly to perform a *biopsy* (removal of a small sample of tissue for analysis) of a lymph gland to look for disease. Using a general anesthetic, an incision is made in the base of the neck and an endoscope is passed through it into the mediastinum. A tissue sample is

removed by minute blades at the end of the endoscope. After the instrument has been withdrawn, the incision is closed with stitches.

## Mediastinum

The space between the lungs and the structures within that space. The mediastinum extends from the sternum (breastbone) in front to the spine behind, and from the inlet of the thoracic duct (one of the main lymphatic vessels) at the top to the diaphragm at the bottom.

It contains the *heart*, *trachea* (windpipe), *esophagus*, *thymus* gland, the major blood vessels entering and leaving the heart, *lymph nodes* and lymphatic vessels, and nerves (including the *vagus nerve* and *phrenic nerve*).

## Medicaid

A term applied (in some states) to a federal program that provides funds to support state programs of medical assistance to people receiving or eligible for welfare. Programs vary widely from state to state. (See also *Medicare*.)

## Medical examiner

A public official and physician (often a pathologist) who is responsible for determining causes of death not obviously due to natural causes. The medical examiner (a county office in most cases) has largely replaced the office of *coroner*.

## Medicare

A federal program that finances medical care for certain dependents. Part A of the program covers many hospital services. Part B helps with physician charges, assuming a retired person elects to pay a monthly insurance premium. (See also *Medicaid*.)

## Medication

A term used to describe any substance prescribed to treat illness. (See also *Drug*; *Medicine*.)

## Medicine

The study of human diseases, including their causes, frequency, treatment, and prevention. The term is also applied to any substance prescribed to treat illness.

### EARLY HISTORY

In many early cultures, medicine was closely associated with religion because disease was regarded as a punishment from the gods. As a result, the victim would turn for help to a priest, who took on the additional function of a medicine man. Medicine

probably became separated from religion with the emergence of people skilled in treating injuries such as broken bones and dislocated joints. These healers attracted patients and, in time, apprentices who wanted to learn the same skills.

By the fifth century BC, the Greek physician Hippocrates had established medicine as a profession with a body of learning and a code of ethics to be passed on to each new generation of physicians (the Hippocratic oath is still used as an ethical guide for the medical profession). The dominant figure after Hippocrates was the second-century, Greek-born Roman physician Galen, who made valuable contributions but whose many false theories about anatomy and physiology were uncritically accepted for more than 13 centuries; these theories effectively held back advances in medical knowledge.

### RENAISSANCE DISCOVERIES

With the Renaissance, medicine began to emerge from its long period of stagnation. In 1543 the Flemish anatomist and physician Andreas Vesalius (1514-1564) produced the first truly accurate anatomical text; in 1628 the English physician William Harvey (1578-1657) first demonstrated how blood circulates through the body. Also in the 17th century, the Dutch microscopist Antonj van Leeuwenhoek (1632-1723) became the first to observe and describe microorganisms and the detailed structure of blood, muscles, and sperm.

### MODERN MEDICINE

Despite the medical achievements of the Renaissance—and some notable later achievements, such as the English physician Edward Jenner's (1749-1823) discovery of the principle of vaccination in the late 18th century—it was not until the 19th century that the foundations of modern scientific medicine were laid. This was the result of a growing realization that medicine needed to become a true science, systematic in its approach and based on scrupulous observation and experimentation. Significant advances in other disciplines also played an important role. For example, the first practical high-powered microscope was developed during the 19th century; the ophthalmoscope (an instrument for examining the retina of the eye) was invented in 1851; the first practical thermometer was introduced in the 1860s; and X rays were discovered in 1896, an occurrence that revolutionized medical diagnosis. These developments, along with the French scientist Louis Pasteur's (1822-1895) work on the germ theory of disease, brought about an enormous advance in the understanding of a large number of diseases.

Curing and controlling disease was not a reality until the 20th century, however, when vaccines were developed against many serious diseases (including typhoid, cholera, and diphtheria); insecticides and improved sanitation helped control diseases such as malaria, yellow fever, and sleeping sickness.

The early 20th century was also marked by the development of safe anesthesia, effective surgery, and a steady growth in the number of new drugs. In the late 1930s, the first effective antibacterial drugs (the sulfonamides) were produced, followed in the 1940s by penicillin, streptomycin, and the tetracyclines; these drugs saved millions of lives.

Among the important recent developments are the introduction of sophisticated diagnostic techniques, such as MRI, CT scanning, and ultrasound scanning; more effective drugs and other treatments (such as radiation therapy) to treat a wider range of diseases and disorders; and developments in surgical techniques that have made it possible to transplant organs and rejoin severed nerves.

Today, the boundaries between medicine and other sciences are becoming progressively less distinct; medical research is being increasingly undertaken by scientists who have little or no formal medical training. (See also entries for individual medical, surgical, and scientific specialties.)

## Medicolegal

Relating to aspects of medicine and law that overlap, particularly to medical matters that come before the courts. Among the matters on which medicolegal experts advise are the laws concerning damages for injuries due to medical negligence or malpractice, medical evidence concerning the extent of injury in a civil action, the use of tests in determining paternity, the mental competence of people who have drawn up wills, and restrictions on the liberty of the mentally ill.

In recent years, new areas of medicolegal study have emerged, notably an individual's right to die (see *Brain death; Euthanasia; Will, living*); the necessity for informed consent to any surgical procedure; the

legal aspects of *artificial insemination, in vitro fertilization, sterilization*, and *surrogacy*; and a person's right to confidentiality concerning his or her illness, particularly in the context of AIDS. (For medical aspects of criminal law, see *Forensic medicine*.)

## Meditation

Concentration on an object, a word, or an idea with the intention of inducing an altered state of consciousness. Meditation of different kinds has traditionally been a feature of many religions, particularly Eastern ones.

At its deepest level, meditation can resemble a trance or be an all-engrossing spiritual experience. More commonly, it is a physically calming therapy for body and mind. Some clinical trials have shown that meditation can be a valuable therapy for reducing stress levels and in helping treat stress-related disorders. The most common form of meditation practiced in the west is transcendental meditation (TM), introduced by the Maharishi Mahesh Yogi in the 1960s.

## Medroxyprogesterone

A *progesterone drug* used in the treatment of *endometriosis* and certain types of *breast cancer* and uterine cancer (see *Uterus, cancer of*). Medroxyprogesterone is occasionally given to treat menstrual disorders such as mid-cycle bleeding and *amenorrhea* (absence of menstruation). It is also given with an estrogen drug in *hormone replacement therapy* to reduce the risk of cancer of the uterus.

Injections of medroxyprogesterone are widely used as a contraceptive (see *Contraception, hormonal methods*) in developing countries; this use is not permitted in the US.

Possible adverse effects include weight gain, swollen ankles, and breast tenderness.

## Medulla

The innermost part of an organ or body structure; the adrenal medulla is the central region of an adrenal gland, and the medulla of bone is the bone marrow. The term medulla is also sometimes used to refer to the medulla oblongata (part of the *brain stem* joining the spinal cord).

## Medulla oblongata

Also known as the medulla, the medulla oblongata is the lowest part of the *brain stem*; it is situated in the skull between the pons (above) and the spinal cord (below).

## Medulloblastoma

A type of malignant *brain tumor* that occurs mainly in children (in whom it is the most common type of brain tumor). The tumor usually arises from the cerebellum (the organ at the back of the brain concerned with posture and balance). It grows rapidly and may spread to other parts of the brain and spinal cord.

Several hundred cases of medulloblastoma are diagnosed each year in the US. Typically, a morning headache, repeated vomiting, and a clumsy gait develop, with frequent falls caused by disturbance of the function of the cerebellum. The tumor is diagnosed by *CT scanning* or *MRI* and often responds to *radiation therapy*. This, combined with surgery and the use of *anticancer drugs*, often allows survival for five years or more.

## Mefenamic acid

A *nonsteroidal anti-inflammatory drug* (NSAID) used to relieve pain after a minor operation, injury to soft tissues (such as muscles and ligaments), or joint pain and stiffness caused by types of arthritis (including *osteoarthritis* and *rheumatoid arthritis*). It is also used to relieve the pain that can occur with menstruation.

Possible adverse effects include abdominal pain, nausea, vomiting, and, after prolonged use, a *peptic ulcer*.

## Mega-

A prefix meaning very large, as in *megacolon*, a condition in which the colon (part of the large intestine) is greatly enlarged. The prefix megalo- is synonymous with mega-.

## Megacolon

A grossly distended colon usually accompanied by severe, chronic constipation. Megacolon may be present at birth or may develop later in life; it occurs in all age groups.

**CAUSES**

In children, the main causes are *Hirschsprung's disease* (congenital absence of nerve cells in part of the colon), *anal fissures*, and psychological factors that may have developed at the time of toilet-training.

In the elderly, megacolon may be caused by long-term use of powerful laxatives, particularly those containing senna, rhubarb, or cascara.

People suffering from chronic depression or schizophrenia, particularly if they live in an institution, often suffer from megacolon. Other rarer causes include *Chagas' disease*,

M

*hypothyroidism*, neurological disorders (for example, spinal cord injury), and certain drugs (notably the narcotics morphine and codeine).

### SYMPTOMS
The symptoms are severe constipation and abdominal bloating; some sufferers lose their appetite, which may result in weight loss. Occasionally there is diarrhea, caused by a leakage of semiliquid feces around the obstructing hard stools.

### DIAGNOSIS
The condition is diagnosed by proctoscopic examination of the rectum (see *Proctoscopy*), *barium X-ray examination*, tests of bowel muscle function, and, if Hirschsprung's disease is suspected, *biopsy* (removal of a small sample of tissue for examination) of the large intestine.

### TREATMENT
In severe cases, impacted feces are removed manually. Often, however, the large intestine can be emptied by saline enemas.

## Megalomania
An exaggerated sense of one's own importance or ability. It may take the form of a *delusion* of grandeur (such as believing oneself to be Napoleon) or of a desire to organize activities that are expensive, large in scale, and involving many people (for example, leasing an ocean liner for a party). Megalomania is not a formal category of psychiatric illness, although such bizarre ideas and behavior often occur in *mania*.

## -megaly
A suffix meaning enlargement, as in *acromegaly*, a condition in which there is enlargement of the skull, jaw, hands, and feet during adulthood as a result of excessive production of growth hormone in the fore part of the pituitary gland.

## Megestrol
A *progesterone drug* used to treat certain types of *breast cancer* and uterine cancer (see *Uterus, cancer of*). Megestrol is usually prescribed when a tumor cannot be removed by surgery, if a tumor has recurred after surgery, or when other *anticancer drugs* or *radiation therapy* is ineffective.

Possible adverse effects include swollen ankles, loss of appetite, headache, dizziness, rash, and elevation of the blood's calcium level.

## Meibomian cyst
See *Chalazion*.

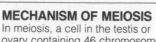

## MECHANISM OF MEIOSIS
In meiosis, a cell in the testis or ovary containing 46 chromosomes divides to form four germ cells (sperm or eggs), each with 23 chromosomes. Germ cells have only half the usual chromosome content because a child can receive only half the genes of each parent.

**Key**
Maternal chromosomes
Paternal chromosomes

Original cell

**1** The 46 chromosomes in the original cell form 23 pairs (only 10 of the pairs are shown in this sequence). During meiosis, there is exchange of material between pair members, so that each of the germ cells formed receives a unique mix of the parental genes.

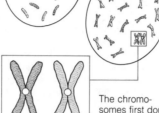

The chromosomes first double up and then form into pairs.

Exchange occurs between pair members.

**2** After exchange, the cell divides, the two members of each chromosome pair going into separate daughter cells.

First division

Each cell now has one doubled-up chromosome from each of the pairs.

Second division

**3** The daughter cells now divide into four germ cells. The doubled-up chromosomes are pulled apart so that each germ cell receives a single (nondoubled-up) chromosome from each of the original pairs.

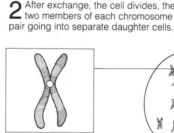

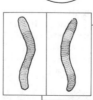

Separate germ cells receive chromosomes containing different genetic mixes.

Germ cells (sperm or eggs)

M

## Meibomianitis

An inflammation of the glands on the eyelid, which causes the normal, oily secretion to thicken. Meibomianitis usually affects middle-aged people, often those with *blepharitis* (inflammation of the eyelid), and frequently leads to recurrent meibomian cysts (see *Chalazion*).

## Meigs' syndrome

A rare condition in which *ascites* (fluid in the abdominal cavity) or a *pleural effusion* (fluid around one of the lungs) accompanies a tumor of the ovary. The fluid usually disappears with removal of the tumor.

## Meiosis

A special type of cell division that occurs only within the ovaries and testes. The cells that undergo meiotic division are the forerunners of egg and sperm cells.

In meiosis, the *chromosomes* (inherited genetic material) within the nucleus of a cell are first duplicated. In the course of two successive cell divisions, the chromosomal material is then divided into four parts, each part going into one of four daughter cells. The four daughter cells each acquire only half of the original cell's chromosomal material, and each daughter cell acquires a different "selection" of this material. Consequently, every egg and sperm formed in the ovary or testis is different in its chromosomal content. As a result of meiosis, parents contribute exactly half of their chromosomal material (genes) to each child, and the selection that each child receives is unique.

Meiosis differs fundamentally from *mitosis*, the more common and simpler method of cell division, in which a cell's chromosomes are exactly duplicated in one division into two daughter cells.

## Melancholia

An old term for *depression* derived from the Greek word for black bile, an excess of which was believed to be the cause of low spirits. Melancholia is used today to refer to certain symptoms that occur in severe depression. These include loss of pleasure in most activities, lack of reaction to pleasurable stimuli, and inappropriate guilt feelings.

## Melanin

The yellow, brown, or black pigment that gives skin, hair, and the iris of the eyes their coloring. The amount of melanin present in a person depends on race and on exposure to sunlight. The pigment is produced by cells called melanocytes, whose activity is controlled by a hormone secreted by the pituitary gland in the brain.

Exposure to sunlight increases the production of melanin, protecting the skin against the harmful effects of ultraviolet rays and darkening skin color in the process.

Localized overproduction of melanin in the skin can result in a pigmented spot called a *nevus*, of which moles and freckles are the most common examples.

## Melanoma, juvenile

A raised, reddish-brown skin blemish that sometimes appears on the face or legs in early childhood. A juvenile melanoma is a form of *nevus* that grows rapidly up to almost 1 inch (about 2 cm) across. Most juvenile melanomas are harmless. However, if the growth is unsightly, or if the physician suspects skin cancer, the melanoma can be removed surgically.

## Melanoma, malignant

The most serious of the three types of skin cancer (the other two being *basal cell carcinoma* and *squamous cell carcinoma*). Malignant melanoma occurs in the melanocytes, the cells that produce *melanin* (the pigment that colors the skin, hair, and the iris of the eyes).

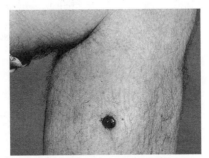

**Development of malignant melanoma**
Only one mole in a million becomes malignant, but change of shape, darkening, tenderness, pain, itching, or ulceration are warning signs.

### CAUSES AND INCIDENCE

Malignant melanomas account for 2 percent of all cancers that occur and are most common in middle-aged and elderly people with pale skin who have been exposed to strong sunlight for many years.

In the US, the incidence varies with latitude from 22,500 cases per year in the northern states to 65,000 cases in the south. This incidence appears to be rising, probably due to increased recreational exposure to sunlight.

### SYMPTOMS AND SIGNS

The growth usually develops on exposed areas of skin, but may occur anywhere on the body, including under the nails and in the eye (see *Eye tumors*). The melanoma usually grows from an existing mole, which may enlarge, become lumpy, bleed, change color, develop a spreading black edge, turn into a scab, or begin to itch. Occasionally, a tumor may develop on normal skin.

### DIAGNOSIS AND TREATMENT

Because the tumor is highly malignant and often spreads to other parts of the body, early diagnosis is essential. The diagnosis is made by a skin *biopsy* (removal of a small sample of tissue for microscopic analysis).

Treatment consists of excising (cutting out) the melanoma. To avoid an unsightly scar on exposed areas, a *skin graft* may be carried out at the same time. *Radiation therapy* or *anticancer drugs* may also be necessary.

## Melanosis coli

Black or brown discoloration of the lining of the colon, associated with chronic constipation and the use of certain laxatives (e.g., senna, rhubarb, and cascara) in chronic constipation.

Melanosis coli is most common in the elderly and usually produces no symptoms. The discoloration disappears after laxatives are stopped. Rarely, the condition is associated with cancer of the colon.

## Melasma

See *Chloasma*.

## Melena

Black, tarry feces caused by bleeding, usually in the upper gastrointestinal tract (esophagus, stomach, or duodenum). The blood is blackened by the action of secretions during digestion. Melena is a sign that should never be ignored. It is usually caused by a *peptic ulcer*, but may be an indication of cancer (or other disorders) of the stomach or of the cecum. (An intake of iron, bismuth, or licorice may also color the feces black.)

## Melioidosis

An infectious disease, similar to *glanders*, caused by a bacterium that lives in soil and lakes. Melioidosis does not occur in the US and Europe but has been reported in Asia, Africa, and Australia. It may cause a high fever

M

and symptoms of pneumonia. Given early, antibiotics can cure the illness, but in some cases it is rapidly fatal.

## Melphalan

An *anticancer drug* used mainly in the treatment of *multiple myeloma* (a cancer of the bone marrow). Melphalan is also prescribed to treat certain types of *breast cancer* and ovarian cancer (see *Ovary, cancer of*).

Possible adverse effects include nausea, vomiting, sore throat, and loss of appetite. Melphalan may also cause aplastic anemia, abnormal bleeding, and increased susceptibility to infection.

## Membrane

A layer of tissue, often very thin, that covers a body surface (such as the *meninges*, which cover the surface of the brain); lines a cavity (such as the *peritoneum*, which lines the abdominal cavity); divides a space or organ (such as the tympanic membrane, or eardrum, which separates the *ear* canal from the middle ear); or forms the boundaries of individual *cells*.

## Memory

The ability to remember what has happened in the past. It is a complex process, usually thought of as having three stages—registration, long-term memory, and recall (see box).

Many factors determine how well something is remembered, including its familiarity and how much attention has been paid to it. Techniques advertised for improving memory are generally based on teaching people methods of improving their coding systems by consciously associating new material with what is already known. For example, a person might be taught to visualize a well-known street and then think of each building as representing a new fact.

### MECHANISM OF MEMORY

It is not known where in the brain the memory process takes place. There seems to be no set memory area; stimulating the brain with electrodes can evoke different memories from the same site. However, disturbances of the temporal lobe and limbic lobe typically cause memory disorders. Stimulation of a particular part of the temporal lobe in patients with temporal lobe *epilepsy* may consistently evoke the same memory.

The mechanisms for storing memory also are unknown. Memory may be held within the chemical structure of some substance within brain

### THE STAGES OF MEMORY

**Stage 1**
In the first stage, known as registration, information is perceived and understood. It is then retained in a short-term memory system that seems to be very limited in the amount of material it can store at one time. Unless refreshed by constant repetition, the contents of short-term memory are lost within minutes, to be replaced by other material.

**Stage 2**
If information is important enough, it may be transferred into the long-term memory, where the process of storage involves associations with words or meanings, with the visual imagery evoked by it, or with other experiences, such as smell or sound.

**Stage 3**
The final stage is recall (or retrieval), in which information stored at an unconscious level is brought, at will, into the conscious mind. The reliability of recall depends on how well the material was coded at stage 2.

cells—possibly spare *DNA* that is not being utilized to hold the genetic code. Others stress the role of the brain's electrical circuits in memory storage.

A good memory is usually part of a high *IQ*, although some people have extraordinary "photographic" memories that are unrelated to their other intellectual abilities. Even some severely retarded people have phenomenal memories for specific types of information (the so-called "idiot savant"—learned idiot).

### DISORDERS

Disturbances of memory can result from a problem at any of the three stages. Most disturbances involve an inability to recall past events due to failure at the retention or recall stage (see *Amnesia*). In some cases, the problem occurs at the registration stage (for example, in *mania* because the person's attention is continually distracted, or in *depression* as a result of preoccupation with personal thoughts and feelings). Some people with temporal lobe epilepsy have uncontrollable flashbacks of distant past events.

## Memory, loss of

See *Amnesia*.

## Menarche

The onset of *menstruation*. Menarche usually occurs around age 13, two or three years after the first physical signs of *puberty* start to appear.

## Meniere's disease

A disorder of the inner ear characterized by recurrent *vertigo*, *deafness*, and *tinnitus* (ringing or buzzing in the ear). In 80 to 85 percent of cases, only one ear is affected.

### CAUSES AND INCIDENCE

The disease is caused by an increase in the amount of fluid in the membranous labyrinth (the canals in the inner ear that control balance). This increase damages the labyrinth and sometimes the adjacent cochlea (a spiral organ that receives sound and transmits it to the brain). The cause of the fluid increase is not known in most cases. Meniere's disease is uncommon before age 50.

### SYMPTOMS AND SIGNS

The main symptom is a sudden attack of vertigo, which may be so severe that the person falls to the ground. Vertigo is usually accompanied by nausea, vomiting, nystagmus (jerky eye movement), and, in the affected ear, deafness, tinnitus, and a feeling of pressure or pain. Attacks, which vary considerably in frequency, may last from a few minutes to several hours. However, the deafness and tinnitus tend to persist between the attacks of vertigo.

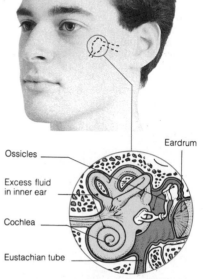

Ossicles

Excess fluid in inner ear

Cochlea

Eustachian tube

Eardrum

**The cause of Meniere's disease**
This condition is caused by excessive fluid in the middle ear, which may become damaged as a result.

## DIAGNOSIS AND TREATMENT

Meniere's disease is usually diagnosed from the results of audiometry (see *Hearing tests*), a *caloric test*, and sometimes other tests.

During an attack, the person should rest in bed. An *antiemetic drug* (such as dimenhydrinate or cyclizine) may be given to relieve nausea and tinnitus.

Hearing tends to deteriorate progressively. If deafness becomes total, the other symptoms of the disease usually disappear.

## Meninges

The three membranes that cover and protect the brain and the spinal cord. The outermost layer, the dura mater, is tough and fibrous; it lines the inside of the skull and forms a loose sheath around the spinal cord. The middle layer, the arachnoid mater, is elastic and weblike. It is separated from the innermost membrane, the pia mater, by the subarachnoid space, which contains *cerebrospinal fluid*. The pia mater is a thin layer that lies directly next to the brain and follows the folds and furrows of its surface.

Inflammation of the meninges, usually from infection, is called *meningitis*. Tumors of the meninges are called *meningiomas*.

---

### ANATOMY OF THE MENINGES
The pia mater lies on the brain, separated from the arachnoid mater by the subarachnoid space. The dura mater lines the inside of the skull.

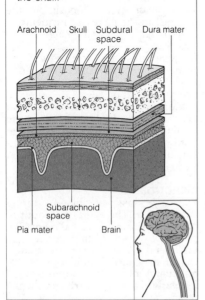

Arachnoid  Skull  Subdural space  Dura mater

Subarachnoid space

Pia mater    Brain

---

## Meningioma

A benign *brain tumor* that develops from the meninges (protective coverings of the brain). The tumor arises from cells in the arachnoid (middle layer of the meninges) and usually becomes attached to the dura mater (outer layer).

Meningiomas are rare, with about one new case diagnosed annually per 100,000 population in the US. They may occur at any age. The tumor expands slowly, sometimes becoming large before it causes symptoms.

### SYMPTOMS

Symptoms can include headache, vomiting, and impaired mental function from raised pressure within the skull; more specific symptoms include speech loss or visual disturbance due to pressure from the meningioma on underlying brain tissue. The tumor may invade the overlying bone, causing thickening and bulging of a region of the skull.

### DIAGNOSIS AND TREATMENT

Meningiomas can be detected by skull X ray, *CT scanning*, and *MRI*. Because they are usually well demarcated from underlying brain tissue, meningiomas can often be completely removed by surgery. Tumors that cannot be removed surgically are treated by *radiation therapy*.

## Meningitis

Inflammation of the *meninges* (the membranes that cover the brain and spinal cord) that usually results from infection by a variety of microorganisms. Viral meningitis is relatively mild; bacterial meningitis is life-threatening and needs prompt treatment.

### CAUSES

The organisms that cause meningitis usually reach the meninges through the bloodstream from an infection elsewhere in the body. Less common means of transmission are through cavities in the skull from an infected ear or sinus, or from the air following a fractured skull.

### INCIDENCE

Viral meningitis is far more common than bacterial meningitis, tending to occur in epidemics in the winter months. It affects between 9,000 and 12,000 people, mostly under the age of 30, in the US each year.

Meningococcal meningitis, the most common form of bacterial meningitis, sometimes occurs in small epidemics; more frequently, it occurs in isolated cases. It probably affects between 2,000 and 5,000 young

people—70 percent under the age of 5—in the US each year. Tuberculous meningitis, which is a less common type of bacterial meningitis, occurs particularly in young children in parts of the world where there is a high incidence of tuberculosis.

### SYMPTOMS

The main symptoms are fever, severe headache, nausea and vomiting, dislike of light, and a stiff neck. In viral meningitis the symptoms are mild and may resemble influenza.

In meningococcal meningitis the main symptoms develop more rapidly, sometimes over a few hours, and are followed by drowsiness and sometimes loss of consciousness. In about half the cases there is also a red, blotchy skin rash.

In tuberculous meningitis, the sufferer may be sick for several weeks before the typical symptoms of meningitis develop.

### DIAGNOSIS AND TREATMENT

Meningitis is diagnosed by *lumbar puncture* and the removal of a small sample of cerebrospinal fluid from the spinal cord for examination.

Viral meningitis requires no treatment. Bacterial meningitis is a medical emergency treated with large doses of intravenous antibiotics.

### OUTLOOK

Viral meningitis is usually not serious, clears up within a week or two, and leaves no aftereffects. Patients with bacterial meningitis who receive prompt treatment usually recover; in some cases, however, some brain damage results.

### PREVENTION

Vaccination may occasionally be valuable in controlling an epidemic caused by certain strains of bacteria. However, giving antibiotics to people who have come into contact with sufferers is generally more effective than vaccination.

Vaccination against meningitis has achieved only limited success because vaccines exist against only some of the organisms responsible and the protection is of limited duration.

## Meningocele

A protrusion of the meninges (protective coverings) of the spinal cord under the skin due to a congenital defect in the spine (see *Spina bifida*). Meningocele is less serious than myelocele, which is protrusion of the spinal cord and of the meninges.

## Meningomyelocele

See *Myelocele*.

M

## Meniscectomy

A surgical procedure in which the whole or part of a *meniscus* (cartilage disk) is removed from a joint. Meniscectomy is almost always performed on the knee.

### WHY IT IS DONE

Meniscectomy is carried out when a meniscus has been badly damaged, usually as a result of injury, causing the knee to lock or give way repeatedly. Removing the damaged part of the meniscus cures these symptoms but may increase the likelihood of premature *osteoarthritis* in the joint. Today, the operation is avoided whenever possible.

### HOW IT IS DONE

*Arthroscopy* (in which a viewing tube is inserted into the joint through a small incision) is performed to confirm that a torn meniscus is the cause of the symptoms and to locate the tear. The torn portion of the meniscus is then removed by means of instruments inserted through the arthroscope. The incision is closed with one stitch, a bandage is applied, and the patient goes home.

Alternatively, the surgeon may need to open up the knee joint through an incision at the side of the patella (kneecap). After the operation, the wound is stitched and an elastic bandage and a plaster splint are applied over the knee.

### RECOVERY PERIOD

Patients can usually go home the day of arthroscopic surgery and are able to walk normally within several days. After an open operation, the patient stays in the hospital for a few days. He or she is allowed to put weight on the affected leg after two or three days; the splint is removed after about a week, but normal activities cannot be resumed for four to six weeks.

After either procedure, patients should do exercises to strengthen the thigh muscles, which help to stabilize the knee.

### OUTLOOK

The procedures are about equally effective in relieving symptoms and restoring the knee to normal function, although the scar after an open operation is larger. In either case, there may be an increased risk of osteoarthritis in later life, although the risk is less than if the damaged meniscus had been left in place.

## Meniscus

A crescent-shaped disk of cartilaginous tissue found in several joints in the body. The *knee* joint has two

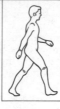

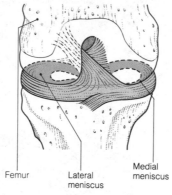

**MENISCI**
The diagram (right) shows the sites of the menisci. The menisci of the knee are shown in detail below.

Femur    Lateral meniscus    Medial meniscus

menisci; the *wrist* joint and *temporomandibular joints* (jaw joints) have one each. The main function of the meniscus, which is held in position by ligaments, is to reduce friction during joint movement.

## Menopause

The cessation of *menstruation*; the term is commonly used to describe the time in a woman's life when physical and psychological changes occur as a result of reduced production of *estrogen hormones* by the ovaries.

Menopause usually occurs between the ages of 45 and 55. The follicles in the ovaries stop producing ova (eggs) and less estrogen is produced. It is this reduction in estrogen that causes the problems associated with the menopause. Other hormonal changes include increased amounts of *gonadotropin hormones* (produced by the pituitary gland) and higher amounts of androgens (male hormones) present in the blood.

### SYMPTOMS AND SIGNS

*Hot flashes* and night sweats occur in about 70 percent of all menopausal women. These symptoms occur with varying frequency and severity. The flashes are usually present for between two and five years, but may continue longer; in 25 percent of women they are so severe that the woman seeks medical help.

Vaginal dryness is the major symptom of 20 percent of menopausal women. Dryness occurs because the vaginal skin thins and its secretions diminish with the fall in estrogen levels. The vagina itself shrinks, loses elasticity, and becomes prone to minor infections; sexual intercourse is often more difficult and painful due to the dryness (see *Vaginitis*). The neck of the bladder and the urethra undergo similar changes, often resulting in the "urethral syndrome," in which the woman feels the need to empty her bladder frequently.

The skin becomes thinner during the menopause and the sebaceous secretions (the skin's natural oils) diminish, resulting in skin dryness. Body and scalp hair becomes dry and brittle and falls out more easily.

Psychological symptoms are often attributed to the menopause, but it is not clear whether these symptoms are caused by the lack of estrogen or are a reaction to the physical symptoms and the sleep disturbance caused by the night sweats. The most common symptoms are poor memory, poor concentration, tearfulness, anxiety, and loss of interest in sex.

Changes in *metabolism* (internal body chemistry) also occur during the menopause, but may not cause symptoms until later. The bones lose calcium more rapidly, especially in the first two to five years of the menopause; over a period of 10 to 15 years, *osteoporosis* (brittle bones) may develop. Other metabolic effects include a rise in blood pressure and an increase in fats in the blood. These changes result in an increase in *atherosclerosis* (fatty deposits in the arteries) and an increased incidence of *coronary heart disease* and *stroke*.

### TREATMENT

If symptoms are severe, *hormone replacement therapy* is recommended to treat the physical and psychological symptoms and also to prevent menopause-related osteoporosis and heart disease. *Beta-blocker drugs* are sometimes given to women for whom hormone replacement therapy is unsuitable (e.g., women who have been treated for breast cancer).

## Menorrhagia

Excessive loss of blood during *menstruation*. The average amount of blood lost during a normal menstrual period is about 2 fluid ounces (60 milliliters). A woman with menorrhagia may lose 3 fluid ounces (90 milliliters) or more. Some women regularly have menorrhagia, while others rarely or never do.

Menorrhagia is usually caused by an imbalance of estrogen and progesterone, the hormones that control menstruation. This imbalance causes an excessive buildup of endometrium (lining of the uterus).

Any disorder that affects the uterus can cause menorrhagia, including *fibroids*, polyps of the uterus, the presence of an *IUD*, or a pelvic infection. In some women with menorrhagia no physical cause can be found.

### TREATMENT
Treatment depends on the severity of the bleeding, the age of the woman, whether or not she wants children in the future, and on any underlying disorder. A *D and C* (dilatation and curettage) may be performed to investigate the cause of menorrhagia. Hormones may be prescribed to reduce the amount of bleeding, especially if the woman is very young. If the condition is severe, a *hysterectomy* (removal of the uterus) may be considered.

## Menotropins
A *gonadotropin hormone* given as a drug to stimulate cell activity in the ovaries and testes. Menotropins is prepared from human menopausal gonadotropin, which is obtained from urine samples of women who have passed the menopause.

### WHY IT IS USED
Menotropins is used together with human chorionic gonadotropin (see *Gonadotropin, human chorionic*) in the treatment of certain types of female and male *infertility*. Menotropins prepares the ovary for ovulation and helps stimulate sperm production.

### POSSIBLE ADVERSE EFFECTS
In women, menotropins may cause multiple pregnancy, abdominal pain, bloating, and weight gain. In men, breast enlargement may occur.

## Menstrual extraction
A procedure in which the endometrium (the lining of the uterus), which is ordinarily sloughed off during *menstruation*, is removed all at one time. The procedure is also known as menstrual regulation. Menstrual extraction is usually performed to terminate a pregnancy.

Menstrual extraction is carried out in the first two weeks after a missed period. The procedure can be performed in a physician's office with or without local anesthetic. A narrow plastic tube is inserted into the uterus and the contents, including any embryo if the woman is pregnant, are suctioned out.

## Menstruation
The periodic cyclical shedding of endometrium (lining of the uterus), accompanied by bleeding, that occurs in a woman who has not become pregnant. Menstruation identifies the fertile years of a woman's life. Menstrual periods usually begin at *puberty* and continue until the *menopause*.

### MECHANISM
Menstruation is the end result of a complicated series of hormonal interactions. At the beginning of the menstrual cycle, *estrogen hormones* cause the endometrium to thicken to prepare the uterus for the possibility of *fertilization*; this is known as the proliferative or follicular phase of the menstrual cycle. *Ovulation* (egg release) usually occurs around midcycle and is accompanied by the increased production of *progesterone hormone*. This hormone induces marked changes in the endometrium, and the cells become swollen and thick with retained fluid. These changes, which occur during the secretory (or luteal) phase of the menstrual cycle, enable a fertilized egg to implant in the endometrium. If pregnancy fails to occur, the production of estrogens and progesterone from the ovaries diminishes. The blood-filled lining of the uterus is not required and both the unfertilized egg and the lining are shed about 14 days after the start of ovulation. Uterine contractions force the menstrual discharge to be expelled through the cervix and into the vagina.

Blood loss varies from cycle to cycle and from woman to woman, averaging about 2 fluid ounces (60 milliliters). The menstrual cycle, which is counted from the first day of bleeding to the last day before the next menstrual period, lasts between 24 and 35 days in 95 percent of women, the average being 28 days. The length of bleeding also varies—usually lasting from one to eight days, with the average length being five days. (See also *Menstruation, disorders of*; *Menstruation, irregular*.)

M

### THE MENSTRUAL CYCLE

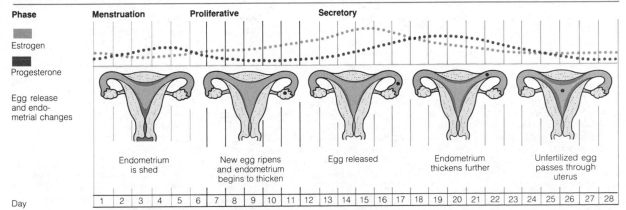

| Phase | Menstruation | Proliferative | | Secretory | |

Estrogen

Progesterone

Egg release and endometrial changes

Endometrium is shed | New egg ripens and endometrium begins to thicken | Egg released | Endometrium thickens further | Unfertilized egg passes through uterus

Day: 1 2 3 4 5 6 7 8 9 10 11 12 13 14 15 16 17 18 19 20 21 22 23 24 25 26 27 28

During menstruation, estrogen and progesterone levels are low, and the unfertilized egg and endometrium are shed. Following menstruation, a pituitary hormone stimulates the ovaries to produce egg follicles. The follicles secrete estrogen, and one eventually releases an egg. The empty follicle also produces progesterone, which, with estrogen, prepares the endometrium to receive the egg. If the egg is unfertilized, follicle hormone levels fall and a new menstrual cycle begins.

## Menstruation, disorders of

An abnormality in the monthly cycle of menstrual bleeding. Regular *menstruation* depends on development of a healthy endometrium (lining of the uterus) and regular cyclical production of *estrogen hormones* and *progesterone hormone*. This delicate balance is easily upset, making abnormal menstruation one of the most common disorders of women. Any change in a woman's periods can indicate a problem in the pelvic area, such as *fibroids*, *endometriosis*, or *pelvic inflammatory disease*.

*Dysmenorrhea* (painful periods) is the most common disorder. In most women the cause is unknown.

*Amenorrhea* (absence of menstruation) is most frequently caused by pregnancy; it may also be caused by a hormonal imbalance, stress, starvation, and *anorexia nervosa*. Polymenorrhea (too frequent menstruation) occurs when the length of the menstrual cycle is reduced to less than 22 days. It is usually due to a hormone imbalance. If the periods occur infrequently or the blood loss is scanty, it is termed oligomenorrhea.

*Menorrhagia* (excessive bleeding) may be caused by a hormone imbalance, the presence of an IUD, fibroids, or *polyps*.

In metrorrhagia, there are extreme variations in the interval between periods, the duration of bleeding, and the amount of blood lost each month (see *Menstruation, irregular*).

## Menstruation, irregular

A variation from the normal pattern of *menstruation*. Menstruation is considered irregular if there are wide variations in the interval between periods, the duration of bleeding, or the amount of blood lost.

### CAUSES

Disturbance of a woman's menstrual pattern can be caused by stress, travel, or changing the method of contraception. Because menstruation depends on a balance of estrogen and progesterone hormones, the cause of irregular menstruation is often a hormone disturbance. For the first few years after menstruation starts, and for the few years before the *menopause*, cycles are often irregular and ovulation does not occur.

A common cause of irregularity is unsuspected pregnancy or early miscarriage. Disorders of the uterus, ovaries, or pelvic cavity (e.g., *endometriosis*) can also lead to irregularity. (See also *Vaginal bleeding*.)

## Mental hospital

A hospital specializing in the treatment of psychiatric illness. Formerly called asylums (or lunatic asylums), many were built in the 19th and early 20th century and were of enormous size. They became infamous as institutionalized backwaters filled with chronic patients who were commonly neglected and abused. Recently, many mental hospitals have been closed as the trend toward care in the community has increased. Still, the debate continues over how much this has contributed to the number of homeless people and how best to protect and treat old, long-stay patients (many of whom are homeless) and new, long-stay patients (such as those suffering from *schizophrenia* or advanced *dementia*).

Today, most admissions to mental hospitals are for acute psychiatric illness. People are admitted to remove them from a stressful or harmful home environment, to provide treatment possible only in the hospital, or to protect them or others from harm. The majority of these admissions are voluntary, but in some cases legal *commitment* is necessary.

## Mental illness

A general term that describes any form of psychiatric disorder. It is common to divide these illnesses into two broad categories, the more severe *psychoses* and the less disturbing *neuroses*. While the former are probably caused by complex biochemical brain disease, the latter seem related to upbringing and personality.

The concept of mental illness is also important, for legal reasons, in determining whether a person can be held responsible for his or her actions. In this respect, there is much uncertainty as to whether *personality disorder*, which is often characterized by antisocial behavior, should be regarded as a form of mental illness.

## Mental retardation

Impaired intellectual function that results in an inability to cope with the normal responsibilities of life.

### CLASSIFICATION AND PREVALENCE

To be classified as mentally retarded, a person must have an IQ below 70 (see *Intelligence tests*) and impairment must be present before the age of 18. Within this group (which comprises about 1 percent of the population) there are various degrees of severity, resulting in different levels of handicap (see table for classification).

### MENTAL RETARDATION

| Severity | IQ |
| --- | --- |
| Mild | 50 to 70 |
| Moderate | 35 to 49 |
| Severe | 20 to 34 |
| Profound | Under 20 |

Mild retardation is the most common form, accounting for 80 percent of the retarded population. The other 20 percent have moderate, severe, or profound retardation.

### CAUSES

The more severe grades of retardation (IQ below 50) usually have a specific physical cause; their incidence is the same in all social classes. About a quarter are due to *Down's syndrome*, another quarter to other inherited or congenital conditions (such as *phenylketonuria* or brain damage due to *hemolytic disease of the newborn*), and about one third result from trauma or infection around birth or early childhood. In about 15 percent of cases the cause is unknown, but the recently discovered *fragile X syndrome* may account for some of them.

By contrast, mild mental retardation usually has no specific cause, is concentrated in the lowest social classes, and seems to run in families. Poverty and *malnutrition* probably contribute to it along with inheritance.

### SYMPTOMS

The mildly retarded usually show no obvious psychological symptoms apart from slowness in carrying out mental tasks, such as arithmetic or problem-solving. Reading is variably impaired and emotions may be expressed in a more childlike manner. However, *hyperactivity*, repetitive involuntary movements, and *autism* are up to four times more common than in the general population.

In more severely retarded people, speech is limited or absent, and epileptic seizures and neurological impairments are common. Fecal and urinary incontinence and self-injury may also occur.

### TREATMENT

There is no specific means of eliminating the intellectual deficit. Special training and behavior modification can enhance the skills and quality of life for retarded people, many of whom are cared for in the community rather than in institutions. Family support and counseling can be crucial in preserving a stable home for the retarded person.

# MENSTRUATION, IRREGULAR

Any variation in the interval between menstrual periods, the duration of bleeding, or the amount of blood lost, or bleeding that occurs in between normal periods, during pregnancy, or after the menopause. An occasional irregular period is generally no cause for concern if it is normal in other respects.

## Absent or reduced bleeding

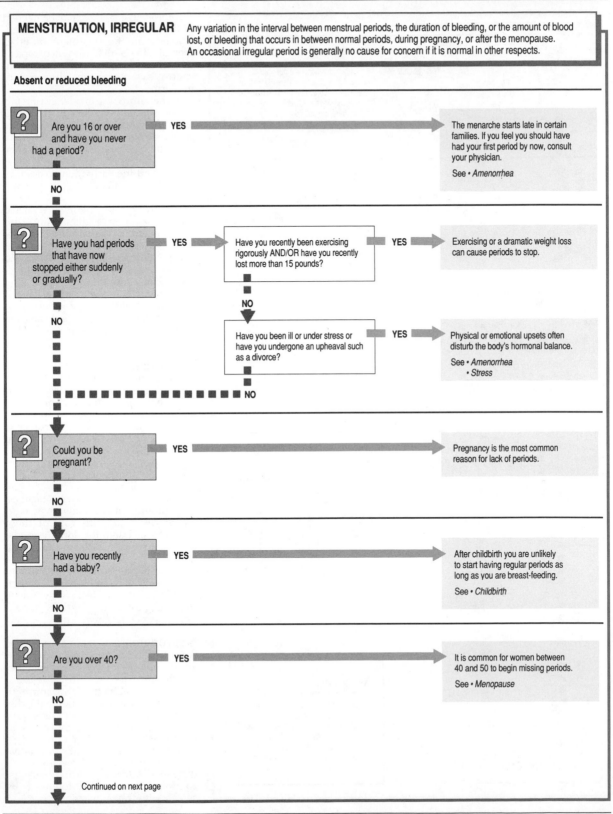

Are you 16 or over and have you never had a period?

**YES** → The menarche starts late in certain families. If you feel you should have had your first period by now, consult your physician.

See • *Amenorrhea*

**NO**

---

Have you had periods that have now stopped either suddenly or gradually?

**YES** → Have you recently been exercising rigorously AND/OR have you recently lost more than 15 pounds?

**YES** → Exercising or a dramatic weight loss can cause periods to stop.

**NO**

Have you been ill or under stress or have you undergone an upheaval such as a divorce?

**YES** → Physical or emotional upsets often disturb the body's hormonal balance.

See • *Amenorrhea*
• *Stress*

**NO**

**NO**

M

---

Could you be pregnant?

**YES** → Pregnancy is the most common reason for lack of periods.

**NO**

---

Have you recently had a baby?

**YES** → After childbirth you are unlikely to start having regular periods as long as you are breast-feeding.

See • *Childbirth*

**NO**

---

Are you over 40?

**YES** → It is common for women between 40 and 50 to begin missing periods.

See • *Menopause*

**NO**

Continued on next page

**Heavier or more frequent than normal bleeding**

**?** Have you had only one heavy period that was also late? — **YES** → An early miscarriage is a possible cause, although a normal period that is late may also be heavier than usual. If you think you have had a miscarriage, consult your physician.

See • *Miscarriage*

**NO** ↓

**?** Have your periods become heavier and do they last longer than they used to? — **YES** → A disorder of the lining of the uterus, such as benign growths or the formation of uterine tissue outside the uterus, is a possible cause. Consult your physician.

See • *Endometriosis*
• *Fibroids*
• *Menorrhagia*

**NO** ↓

**?** Are you taking the birth-control pill OR have you been fitted with an IUD? — **YES** → An IUD can cause heavy menstrual bleeding and both these contraceptive methods may cause spotting between periods. Discuss with your physician.

**NO** ↓

**?** Does bleeding occur after intercourse? — **YES** → ☎
**Consult your physician without delay!**
This may indicate an abnormality of the cells of the cervix.

See • *Cervical erosion*
• *Cervix, cancer of*

**NO** ↓

If you are unable to make a diagnosis from this chart, consult your physician.

**CANCER WATCH**
Any bleeding that occurs between periods can be serious. It may indicate cancer of the cervix or uterus, particularly if you are over 40 and have not had a period for more than six months, or if the bleeding follows intercourse. **Consult your physician without delay!**

---

*Anticonvulsant drugs* may be needed in the treatment of epilepsy and *antipsychotics* in the treatment of other mental illness that may accompany mental retardation; these drugs help control symptoms and thus reduce impairment.

In the future, the incidence of retardation should be reduced by prevention. Preventive measures include *genetic counseling*, the elimination of infections such as *rubella*, reducing the alcohol and drug intake during pregnancy, and the early identification of fetal abnormalities.

**OUTLOOK**

While caring for a mentally retarded relative is often a demanding and time-consuming task, there is evidence that such people, even if severely impaired, can live rewarding and emotionally stable lives. Handicap is caused not by an absolute limit on achievement, but by delay in acquiring skills; as they grow older, the mentally retarded are able to improve in terms of personal and social function.

## Meperidine

A synthetic narcotic *analgesic drug* (painkiller) similar to, but less powerful than, *morphine*. Meperidine, which is used almost exclusively in hospitals, is given as a *premedication* (a drug used to relax and sedate a person before an operation). It is also used to relieve severe pain after a major operation, during childbirth, and, occasionally, in terminal illness.

Since meperidine may cause nausea and vomiting, it is usually given with an *antiemetic drug* to control these symptoms. Used for long periods, meperidine may cause constipation.

**ABUSE**

Meperidine may cause euphoria and is abused for this effect. Taken regularly, it is likely to cause psychological and physical dependence (see *Drug dependence*).

## Meprobamate

An *antianxiety drug* that is used to treat *anxiety* and *stress*. Meprobamate, which also has a muscle-relaxant effect, is combined with aspirin to relieve pain caused by rheumatic disorders (such as *osteoarthritis*) or injury to soft tissues (such as muscles and ligaments).

Since meprobamate has a sedative effect, it may cause drowsiness and dizziness. After long-term use, its discontinuation may be followed by severe withdrawal reactions.

## Mercaptopurine

An *anticancer drug* used to treat certain types of *leukemia* (cancer of white blood cells). Mercaptopurine is also used as a treatment for *Crohn's disease* and for *lymphoma* (cancer of lymph nodes) in children.

Possible adverse effects include nausea, vomiting, mouth ulcers, and appetite loss. Rarely, mercaptopurine may cause liver damage, anemia, and abnormal bleeding.

## Mercury

The only metallic element that is liquid at room temperature. Mercury is used in *thermometers*, *sphygmomanometers* (instruments for measuring blood pressure), and dental *amalgam*. Various compounds of mercury are used in some paints, pesticides, cosmetics, medicines, and in certain industrial processes.

## Mercury poisoning

All forms of mercury are poisonous (except the amalgam in dental fillings), but some forms are absorbed into the body more readily than others and are therefore more dangerous. The liquid metal itself is absorbed very slightly through the intestines, so accidentally swallowing mercury from a broken thermometer is unlikely to lead to poisoning. However, liquid mercury is highly volatile and mercury vapor is readily absorbed into the body via the lungs. Inhalation of mercury vapor—usually as a result of industrial exposure—is the most common cause of poisoning. Mercury compounds (not highly volatile) cause poisoning by absorption through the skin or intestines.

**SYMPTOMS AND SIGNS**
The initial symptoms of mercury poisoning depend on the part of the body affected. Inhalation of mercury vapor may cause shortness of breath from lung damage; mercury compounds that come into contact with the skin may cause severe inflammation. A swallowed mercury compound can cause nausea, vomiting, diarrhea, and abdominal pain.

After mercury has entered the body, it passes into the bloodstream and later accumulates in various organs, principally the brain and kidneys. Mercury deposits in the brain cause a wide range of symptoms, including tiredness, incoordination, excitability, tremors, numbness in the limbs, and, in severe cases, impairment of vision and sometimes *dementia*. Deposits of mercury in the kidneys

may lead to *renal failure*. Without treatment, severe mercury poisoning may be fatal.

**TREATMENT**
Mercury poisoning is treated by giving *chelating agents* (such as penicillamine) to detoxify the mercury and help the body excrete it at a faster rate. In some cases, purification of the blood by hemodialysis (see *Dialysis*) may also be performed, especially if the kidneys have been damaged. Inducing vomiting or pumping out the stomach is helpful only if mercury has been swallowed within the previous few hours.

## Mescaline

 A drug obtained from the Mexican peyote (or peyotl) cactus and classified as a psychedelic or *hallucinogenic drug*. The dried tops of the cactus, known as peyote buttons, have been used historically by Mexican and North American Indians in religious ceremonies. In modern times, psychologists have used mescaline to study the mechanism of *psychosis*, since the drug induces temporary psychotic symptoms.

The effects, which generally last for four to eight hours, are similar to those of *LSD* and *psilocybin*. Effects include illusions, changes in thought and mood, a sense of being in touch with the unknown, intense self-absorption, and an altered sense of time. Although the "trip" is most often pleasant and seemingly insightful, frightening ideas or experiences leading to panic and injury may occur. True psychosis, persisting after the drug has worn off, and addictive craving may occur.

## Mesenteric lymphadenitis

An acute abdominal disorder in which lymph nodes in the mesentery (a membrane anchoring organs to the abdominal wall) become inflamed. Mesenteric lymphadenitis mainly affects children. Its cause is unknown but it may be related to some type of viral infection.

The main symptoms are pain and tenderness in the lower right abdomen, as in appendicitis. There may be mild fever, and sometimes the condition is preceded by a sore throat, chest infection, or swollen neck glands.

The disorder usually clears up rapidly. Analgesics (painkillers) may be given to reduce pain and fever. If the sufferer is no better after six hours or if the symptoms worsen dra-

matically, a *laparotomy* (surgical opening of the abdominal cavity) may be carried out to exclude appendicitis.

## Mesentery

A membrane that attaches various organs to the abdominal wall. The term is used particularly to refer to the membranous fold that encloses the small intestine, attaching it to the back of the abdominal wall. The mesentery contains the arteries, veins, nerves, and lymphatic vessels that supply the large and small intestines.

## Mesothelioma

A tumor of the pleura (lining of the lung and chest cavity). There are two types of mesothelioma—a solitary growth that remains localized in one area of the pleura and a diffuse malignant form. There is an increased incidence of mesothelioma in people exposed to asbestos dust (see *Asbestosis*), especially smokers.

Mesothelioma may cause no symptoms or it may cause cough, chest pain, and breathing difficulty, especially if a *pleural effusion* (collection of fluid around the lung) develops.

A chest X ray may show abnormal shadowing; the diagnosis can be confirmed by examination of a sample of fluid from any effusion or by pleural *biopsy* (removal of a sample of tissue for examination).

Surgical removal of a solitary tumor may result in complete cure. There is no effective treatment for the malignant form, although *radiation therapy* may help alleviate symptoms.

## Mesothelium

A type of *epithelium* (surface cell layer) that lines the body cavities of the *peritoneum* and the *pleura* and makes up the *pericardium* (the saclike covering of the heart).

## Mestranol

An *estrogen drug* used in various *oral contraceptive* preparations.

## Metabolism

A collective term for all the chemical processes that take place in the body. Metabolism is divided into catabolism and anabolism. A catabolic process is a chemical reaction in which a complex substance is broken down into simpler ones, usually with the release of energy. An example is the "burning" of glucose (sugar) in body cells to produce energy and the by-products carbon dioxide and water. An anabolic process is a chemical reaction in which

M

a complex substance is built up from simpler ones, usually with the consumption of energy (which is provided by catabolism). The synthesis of complex *proteins* from *amino acids* is an anabolic process.

### METABOLIC RATE

The basal metabolic rate (BMR) is the energy required to keep the body functioning at rest (that is, to maintain breathing, heart beat, body temperature, and other basic body functions). It is measured in Calories (or joules) per square meter of body surface per hour. The metabolic rate increases in response to factors such as exertion, stress, fear, and illness. It is controlled principally by various endocrine hormones (such as *epinephrine*, *norepinephrine*, *insulin*, *corticosteroid hormones*, and thyroid hormones—see *Thyroid gland*), which influence the rate at which chemical processes are carried out in body cells.

### DISORDERS

The primary types of metabolic disorders include inherited abnormalities in which a specific enzyme (a substance that promotes a metabolic reaction) is lacking or malfunctions in some way (see *Metabolism, inborn errors of*). Other metabolic disorders are endocrine disorders in which there is underproduction or overproduction of a hormone that controls metabolic activity. Examples are *Cushing's syndrome*, *diabetes mellitus*, *insulinoma*, *hyperthyroidism* (overproduction by the thyroid gland), and *hypothyroidism* (underproduction by the thyroid).

## Metabolism, inborn errors of

Inherited defects of body chemistry. These are *genetic disorders* in which the disturbance of body chemistry is caused by a single gene defect.

### TYPES AND INCIDENCE

There are about 180 known inborn errors of metabolism. They vary in severity, from harmless abnormalities to serious diseases that may cause death in a newborn baby or result in severe physical or mental handicap. Examples include *Tay-Sachs disease*, *phenylketonuria*, *galactosemia*, the various *porphyrias*, *Hurler's syndrome* and various other types of *mucopolysaccharidosis*, hereditary fructose intolerance, Lesch-Nyhan syndrome, homocystinuria, glycogen storage diseases, mucolipidoses, and sphingolipidoses.

Individual disorders are rare. Most affect only one child in every 10,000 to 100,000, but the precise incidence is often unknown because sufferers may

have only vague symptoms that are never investigated, or because they die before any characteristic features appear. Collectively, these disorders affect about one child in 1,000.

### CAUSES

All inborn errors of metabolism are caused by abnormal functioning of a specific *enzyme* (protein that stimulates a chemical reaction) caused by a defect of a *gene*. Most defects show an autosomal recessive pattern of inheritance (see *Genetic disorders*).

Individual disorders vary in their effects. In some cases the abnormal enzyme is nonfunctional; in others there is some residual activity.

### SYMPTOMS AND SIGNS

Symptoms are usually present at or soon after birth, although they may not appear until later in childhood. Symptoms may include unexplained illness or failure to thrive in a newborn, developmental delay, floppiness, drowsiness, persistent vomiting, or seizures. Signs may include enlarged body organs, bone deformities, anemia, cataracts, persistent jaundice, unusual body odor, the recurrent development of kidney stones, or a rash brought on by sunlight. The child may be intolerant to specific foods.

Miscarriages, stillbirths, or deaths in early infancy suggest the possibility of an inborn error of metabolism.

### DIAGNOSIS

Investigations include tests to measure the levels of various substances in the affected child's blood, including *liver function tests* and *kidney function tests*. Chemical analysis of a *biopsy* specimen (small piece of tissue removed from the body) may be performed to check the level and function of a specific enzyme.

Early diagnosis can be important in preventing serious complications. Routine tests are done in the newborn for some of the more common disorders, such as phenylketonuria. Additional screening may be performed for disorders that are more common in certain countries or racial groups (for example, Tay-Sachs disease in European Jews).

Certain disorders can now be diagnosed prenatally following *chorionic villus sampling* or *amniocentesis*, allowing for an elective abortion.

### TREATMENT

Some inborn errors of metabolism do not require treatment. Some respond to avoidance of a specific environmental factor to which an affected person is abnormally sensitive. For example,

avoiding exposure to sunlight may help certain types of porphyria, avoiding food containing phenylalanine helps in phenylketonuria.

In some cases, a vitamin supplement can help compensate for defective enzyme function. In others, injections of the defective enzyme are given. Transplanting enzyme-producing cells from a donor has been effective in some cases (such as to treat Hurler's syndrome). Treating inborn errors of metabolism at the gene level is still, however, only theoretical. (See also *Genetic counseling*.)

## Metabolite

Any substance that takes part in a metabolic reaction (a biochemical reaction in the body). In the breakdown of glucose (sugar) to produce energy, the metabolites are glucose, carbon dioxide, and water. The term metabolite is sometimes used to refer only to the products of a metabolic reaction. (See also *Metabolism*.)

## Metacarpal bone

One of five long, cylindrical bones within the body of the hand. The bones run from the base of each digit to the wrist. On the palm of the hand, they are covered by a thick layer of fascia (fibrous connective tissue); on the back of the hand, they can be seen and felt through the skin. The heads of the metacarpal bones form the knuckles, standing out prominently when the hand is clenched. Fracture of the metacarpal bones is fairly common, usually as the result of a fall on the hand or a blow to the knuckles.

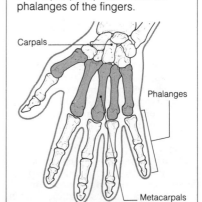

**LOCATION OF METACARPAL BONES**
The five metacarpals lie between the carpal (wrist) bones and the phalanges of the fingers.

Carpals

Phalanges

Metacarpals

## Metaplasia

A change in tissue resulting from the transformation of one type of cell into another. Usually harmless, but occasionally precancerous, metaplasia can affect the lining of various organs, such as the bronchi (airways) and bladder. Metaplasia of the cervix, which occurs in *cervical erosion*, can be detected by a *cervical smear test*.

## Metaproterenol

A *bronchodilator drug* used in the treatment of *asthma*, chronic *bronchitis*, and *emphysema*. Possible adverse effects include anxiety, restlessness, tremor, and palpitations.

## Metastasis

A secondary malignant tumor (one that has spread from a primary *cancer* to affect other parts of the body). A metastasis in the liver may arise as a result of the spread of a cancer in the colon. The term metastasis also applies to the process by which such spread occurs. The degree of malignancy of a tumor depends largely on its ability to invade surrounding normal tissue and on its ability to send metastases to other parts of the body.

Metastases can spread from one part of the body to another through the lymphatic system, in the bloodstream, or across a body cavity (such as that between the inner and outer layer of the peritoneal membrane in the abdomen).

## Metatarsal bone

One of five long, cylindrical bones within the foot. The bones make up the central skeleton of the foot and are held in an arch by surrounding ligaments. Fracture of the metatarsal bones may be caused by a heavy object falling onto the foot, by a twisting

---

**LOCATION OF METATARSAL BONES**

The five metatarsals lie between the tarsal bones (which form the ankle and back of the foot) and the phalanges of the toes.

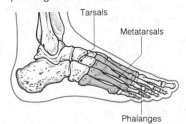

Tarsals

Metatarsals

Phalanges

---

injury in which the foot turns over on its outside edge, or by prolonged walking or running on a hard surface (see *March fracture*).

## Metatarsalgia

Pain in the foot. Causes include a fracture of one of the *metatarsal bones*, *flatfeet*, or a *neuroma* (benign tumor) of one of the nerves in the foot.

## Metatarsophalangeal joint

The joint between each *metatarsal bone* and its adjoining toe bone (see *Phalanges*). The metatarsophalangeal joint at the base of the big toe is commonly affected by *gout* and osteoarthritis (see *Hallux rigidus*). Deformity may result in a bunion (see *Hallux valgus*).

## Methadone

A synthetic narcotic *analgesic drug* (painkiller) that resembles *morphine*. Methadone causes only mild symptoms when it is withdrawn and is therefore used to relieve withdrawal symptoms in people undergoing a supervised heroin or morphine detoxification program.

Possible adverse effects include nausea, vomiting, constipation, dizziness, and dryness of the mouth.

## Methane

A colorless, odorless, highly flammable gas that occurs naturally in the gas from oil wells and in coal mines, where it is an explosion hazard. Methane is also produced by the decomposition of organic matter; it is one of the gases present in intestinal gas (see *Flatus*).

## Methanol

A poisonous type of *alcohol* used as a solvent or paint remover, and as an ingredient in some types of antifreeze. Also known as wood alcohol or methyl alcohol, methanol may cause blindness or death if ingested.

POISONING

Methanol is toxic; poisoning usually occurs as a result of drinking it as a substitute for ordinary alcohol (ethanol, or ethyl alcohol), although its inebriating effect is weaker.

Symptoms of poisoning, which develop 12 to 24 hours after drinking the methanol, include headache, dizziness, nausea, vomiting, and unconsciousness. The symptoms are caused by the breakdown in the liver of methanol into formaldehyde and formic acid. These substances may also damage the retina and optic

nerve, causing blurred vision. If methanol is drunk repeatedly, or if a single large dose is taken, permanent blindness may result.

TREATMENT

If somebody has ingested methanol and is conscious, vomiting should be induced and medical help obtained. Treatment may include pumping the stomach (see *Lavage, gastric*) and inducing vomiting, although this is effective only within about two hours of having drunk the methanol (before it has been absorbed into the bloodstream). In addition, ethanol may be given by injection into the bloodstream because it slows the rate at which the liver breaks down the methanol. An intravenous infusion of sodium bicarbonate may be used to neutralize formic acid in the blood. Occasionally, purification of the blood (by *dialysis*) is also necessary.

## Methimazole

A drug used in the treatment of *hyperthyroidism* (overactivity of the thyroid gland). Methimazole suppresses the production of thyroid hormones by the thyroid gland.

Possible adverse effects include nausea, rash, dizziness, headache, and aching in the joints. Rarely, methimazole may cause increased susceptibility to infection.

## Methocarbamol

A *muscle-relaxant drug* used to relieve stiffness caused by muscle injury and back pain. Methocarbamol is sometimes given to treat symptoms of *tetanus* (lockjaw). During prolonged treatment, methocarbamol may cause drowsiness, dizziness, and, in rare cases, liver damage.

## Methotrexate

An *anticancer drug* used in the treatment of *lymphoma* (cancer of the lymph nodes) and certain forms of *leukemia*. Methotrexate is also used to treat some cancers of the uterus, breast, ovary, lung, bladder, and testis. It is given to treat *rheumatoid arthritis* when other treatments have proved ineffective and is sometimes used to treat severe *psoriasis*.

Methotrexate may cause nausea, vomiting, diarrhea, and mouth ulcers. It may also cause anemia, increased susceptibility to infection, and abnormal bleeding.

## Methoxsalen

A *psoralen drug* used in the treatment of *psoriasis* and *vitiligo* when other

M

treatments have been ineffective. Potential adverse effects are typical of other psoralen drugs.

## Methyclothiazide

A commonly prescribed thiazide *diuretic drug*.

## Methyl alcohol

Another name for *methanol*.

## Methylcellulose

A bulk-forming *laxative drug* commonly used to treat *constipation, diverticular disease,* and *irritable bowel syndrome*. Methylcellulose is also used to increase the firmness of bowel movements in *diarrhea* and to regulate their consistency in people who have had a *colostomy* or *ileostomy*.

In eye-drop form, methylcellulose is given to relieve dryness caused by sun, wind, and other irritants.

**POSSIBLE ADVERSE EFFECTS**
Methylcellulose may cause bloating, flatulence, and abdominal pain, or even bowel obstruction if sufficient amounts of fluids are not taken.

## Methyldopa

An *antihypertensive drug* used in the treatment of *hypertension* (high blood pressure), usually in conjunction with other drugs from this group. Unlike most antihypertensives, methyldopa is safe to use during pregnancy. Adverse effects include drowsiness, depression, and nasal congestion.

## Methylprednisolone

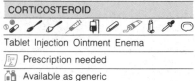

| CORTICOSTEROID |
| --- |
| Tablet Injection Ointment Enema |
| 📋 Prescription needed |
| 🔳 Available as generic |

A *corticosteroid drug* used to replace hormones in *pituitary* or *adrenal gland* disorders that reduce the body's natural corticosteroid production. Methylprednisolone is also used in the treatment of severe *asthma*, skin inflammation, *inflammatory bowel disease*, and types of arthritis, including *rheumatoid arthritis*.

Possible adverse effects are typical of corticosteroid drugs.

## Methysergide

A drug used to prevent *migraine* and cluster *headaches* (recurrent severe headaches). Methysergide is usually given only when other treatments have been ineffective.

Long-term drug treatment with methysergide may cause abnormal tissue growth in the lungs, around the ureters, or around blood vessels (resulting in chest pain, kidney failure, or leg cramps). Other possible adverse effects include dizziness, drowsiness, nausea, and diarrhea.

## Metoclopramide

An *antiemetic drug* used to relieve nausea and vomiting caused by *anticancer drugs, radiation therapy,* or anesthetic drugs (see *Anesthesia, general*).

Metoclopramide is often given with a *premedication* (drug used to relax and sedate a person before an operation) to empty the stomach's contents and thereby reduce the risk of a person inhaling vomit. Metoclopramide is sometimes used to treat *heartburn*.

**HOW IT WORKS**
Metoclopramide reduces nerve activity in the part of the brain that stimulates vomiting. It also increases the speed with which fluid and food pass from the stomach.

**POSSIBLE ADVERSE EFFECTS**
Adverse effects may include rash, dryness of the mouth, agitation, and irritability. Large doses or prolonged use may cause sedation, diarrhea, or uncontrollable movements of the face, mouth, and tongue.

## Metolazone

A *diuretic drug* used in the treatment of *hypertension* (high blood pressure). Metolazone is also given to reduce *edema* (fluid retention) in people with *heart failure* (reduced pumping efficiency of the heart), kidney disorders, *cirrhosis* of the liver, or *premenstrual syndrome*.

Metolazone is also a useful treatment for certain types of kidney stones (see *Calculus, urinary tract*) because it reduces the amount of calcium in the urine.

Possible adverse effects include weakness, lethargy, and dizziness caused by an increase in the amount of potassium excreted in the urine.

## Metoprolol

A cardioselective *beta-blocker drug* used in the treatment of *angina pectoris* (chest pain due to impaired blood supply to heart muscle) and *hypertension* (high blood pressure). Metoprolol is also prescribed to relieve symptoms of *hyperthyroidism* (overactivity of the thyroid gland). It is occasionally given following a *myocardial infarction* (heart attack) to reduce the risk of further damage to the heart.

Possible adverse effects of metoprolol include lethargy, cold hands and feet, nightmares, and rash.

## Metronidazole

An *antibiotic drug* that is particularly effective against infections caused by *anaerobic* bacteria (those that do not depend on oxygen), such as a tooth abscess and *peritonitis*. Metronidazole is also used to treat infections caused by *protozoa,* such as *trichomoniasis, amebiasis,* and *giardiasis*.

Adverse effects include nausea and vomiting, loss of appetite, abdominal pain, and dark-colored urine. Drinking alcohol during treatment often produces severe unpleasant effects such as nausea and vomiting, hot flashes, abdominal pain, palpitations, and headache.

## Mexiletine

An *antiarrhythmic drug* used in the treatment of certain heart rhythm disorders, usually after a *myocardial infarction* (heart attack).

Adverse effects include nausea, vomiting, dizziness, and tremor.

## Miconazole

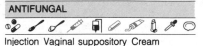

| ANTIFUNGAL |
| --- |
| Injection Vaginal suppository Cream |
| 📋 Prescription needed |
| 🔳 Available as generic |

An *antifungal drug* used to treat *tinea* skin infections, such as ringworm and *athlete's foot,* vaginal *candidiasis* (thrush), and rare fungal infections that affect internal organs, such as the lung.

Miconazole in the form of a cream or vaginal suppository causes a burning sensation and rash in rare cases. Injections of miconazole may cause nausea, vomiting, and fever.

## Micro-

A prefix meaning small, as in microorganisms, tiny living organisms (such as bacteria, viruses, and protozoa), most of which are too small to be seen by the naked eye.

## Microangiopathy

Any disease or disorder of the small blood vessels. Microangiopathy may be a feature of various conditions, including some kidney diseases, such as *glomerulonephritis* (inflammation of the kidneys' filtering units) or *hemolytic-uremic syndrome* (premature destruction of red blood cells accompanied by kidney damage); *eclampsia* (a disorder characterized by seizures in late pregnancy); *septicemia* (blood poisoning); and advanced cancer. When microangiopathy accompanies these conditions, the small blood vessels become distorted, resulting in red blood cells becoming damaged or destroyed. This, in turn, leads to a certain type of anemia called microangiopathic hemolytic anemia (see *Anemia, hemolytic*).

Another cause of microangiopathy is thrombotic thrombocytopenic purpura, a rare, often fatal disease that mainly affects young adults. In this condition, the small blood vessels in many organs throughout the body become blocked and the vessel walls are damaged; hemolytic anemia, fever, and a patchy, purplish rash known as *purpura* develop.

## Microbe

A popular term for a *microorganism*, especially one that causes disease.

## Microbiology

The study of *microorganisms*, particularly pathogenic (disease-causing) ones. Microbiology began in the 17th century with the discovery by the Dutch microscopist Antonj van Leeuwenhoek (1632-1723) of a wide variety of organisms too small to be seen by the naked eye. However, relatively little progress was made until the 19th century when, largely due to the work of scientists such as Louis Pasteur (1822-1895) and Robert Koch (1843-1910), it was recognized that microorganisms cause many infectious diseases and are also responsible for processes such as fermentation and decay. Microbiology continued to progress with the discovery of viruses, the development of vaccines and antibiotics against many diseases, and studies of the chemical processes fundamental to all living cells. Recently, microbiologists have played an important role in the study of genetics by pioneering techniques of *genetic engineering*.

In hospitals, microbiologists help identify the infectious organisms responsible for a patient's illness; they also advise clinicians on the sensitivity of these organisms to drugs.

## Microcephaly

An abnormally small head, usually associated with mental retardation. Microcephaly may occur if the brain is damaged before birth by congenital *rubella* (German measles) or if the mother is exposed to X rays during early pregnancy. It may also be the result of brain damage during birth, or of injury or disease in early infancy. Microcephaly may also occur if the skull bones fuse too early (see *Craniosynostosis*). There is also a rare inherited form of microcephaly in which the forehead slopes backward and the top of the head is pointed.

There is no method of treatment for this condition.

## Microorganism

 Any tiny, single-celled living organism, usually too small to be seen by the naked eye. In medicine, the most important microorganisms are those that are pathogenic (disease-causing), although this group constitutes a relatively small minority of the vast number of microorganisms known to exist.

The principal pathogenic microorganisms are *bacteria*, which cause certain types of pneumonia, typhoid, diphtheria, and some types of food poisoning; *viruses* (usually classified as microorganisms although they are not true cells), which cause numerous infections, including AIDS, the common cold, influenza, and measles; *protozoa*, which are the causative agents of malaria, giardiasis, and amebic dysentery; *fungi*, which cause disorders such as ringworm and thrush; *rickettsiae*, which cause typhus, Rocky Mountain spotted fever, and Q fever; and chlamydiae, which cause various genital, eye, and respiratory infections (see *Chlamydial infections*).

## Microscope

An instrument for producing enlarged images of small objects. There are many types of microscopes, ranging from simple, one-lens instruments (magnifying glasses), to compound microscopes and high-powered electron microscopes.

### HISTORY

The single-lens microscope may date from as early as the 15th century, but the first truly powerful lenses were probably made by Antonj van Leeuwenhoek (1632-1723). His single-lens microscopes were capable of magnifying up to about 300 times. With them, he discovered microorganisms, thereby founding the science of *microbiology* and providing the basis for the development of the germ theory of disease. Probably the greatest of the early microscopists was the Italian Marcello Malpighi (1628-1694), who is generally regarded as the founder of *histology*.

The compound microscope, which has two lens systems, was developed toward the end of the 16th century. However, the single-lens microscope continued to be widely used until the 19th century, when improvements in optical design and glass technology made the compound microscope a practicable instrument.

Light microscopes continued to be refined with the development of the phase-contrast microscope. However, the next major advances were instruments that use electrons in place of light—the transmission electron microscope (TEM), invented in the early 1930s, and the scanning electron microscope (SEM), invented in the middle 1960s.

### LIGHT MICROSCOPES

Compound microscopes are the most widely used instruments. They have two lens systems. The objective and eyepiece are mounted at opposite ends of a tube called the body tube. There is also a stage to hold the specimen, a light source, and an optical condenser (see box, overleaf).

For ordinary light microscopes, the maximum magnification is about 1,500 times. By using a beam of electrons, much higher magnifications are possible.

### ELECTRON MICROSCOPES

TEMs are similar to light microscopes, except that they use a beam of electrons instead of light, and electromagnetic "lenses" instead of glass ones. Furthermore, because electrons are invisible, the image must be formed on a fluorescent screen or photographic film. Modern TEMs can magnify up to about 5 million times, enabling tiny viruses and large molecules (such as DNA) to be seen.

The SEM works in a different way from the TEM (see box). SEMs have a lower maximum magnification (about 100,000 times) than do TEMs. However, unlike TEMs, SEMs produce three-dimensional images. This makes SEMs particularly valuable for studying the surface structures of cells and tissues.

### OTHER MICROSCOPES

Phase-contrast and interference microscopes are types of light microscopes with modified illumination and optical systems that make it possible for unstained transparent specimens to be seen clearly. These microscopes are particularly useful for examining living cells and tissues.

M

# TYPES OF MICROSCOPES

Microscopes are indispensable in medicine. For many purposes, the light microscope, with a magnification of up to 1,500 times, is sufficient. Modern research increasingly requires the much higher magnifications (up to about 5 million times) of a transmission electron microscope or a scanning electron microscope.

## LIGHT MICROSCOPE

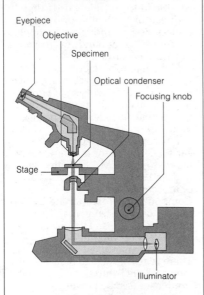

Eyepiece
Objective
Specimen
Optical condenser
Focusing knob
Stage
Illuminator

## TRANSMISSION ELECTRON MICROSCOPE

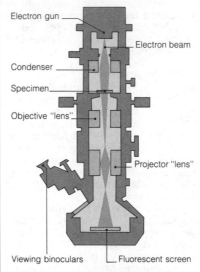

Electron gun
Electron beam
Condenser
Specimen
Objective "lens"
Projector "lens"
Viewing binoculars
Fluorescent screen

## SCANNING ELECTRON MICROSCOPE

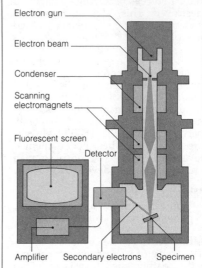

Electron gun
Electron beam
Condenser
Scanning electromagnets
Fluorescent screen
Detector
Amplifier
Secondary electrons
Specimen

Shown is a collection of sperm cells.

Shown here is the sperm's internal structure.

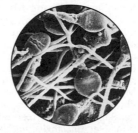

This shows the sperm cells in close detail.

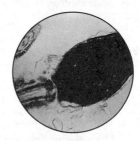

**The compound light microscope**
One lens (the objective) forms a magnified image of the specimen; this image is then magnified further by the eyepiece (viewing) lens. The specimen is held on a stage, beneath which is an optical condenser that concentrates light (usually from a built-in illuminator) onto the specimen. Focusing is carried out by altering the distance between the objective and specimen.

**The transmission electron microscope**
An electron beam (generated by a "gun") is concentrated by an electromagnetic condenser, then passes through the specimen. An electromagnetic objective "lens" then produces a magnified "image" of the specimen; this image is further magnified by an electromagnetic projector "lens," which also focuses the image onto a fluorescent screen, where it can be viewed through special binoculars.

**The scanning electron microscope**
An electron beam (generated by a "gun") is scanned over the surface of the specimen, causing the emission of a beam of secondary electrons, the intensity of which varies according to the surface features of the specimen. A detector converts the secondary electrons into an electric current, which is then amplified and used to control an electron beam that forms an image on a fluorescent screen.

Another instrument, the fluorescence microscope, is used to study the chemical composition of cells. In fluorescence microscopy, a specimen that has been selectively stained with fluorescent dyes is illuminated with ultraviolet light, which makes the stained parts glow.

Operating microscopes are low-powered compound microscopes with several modifications. They do not have a stage, and the illumination system is arranged to shine light down onto the living tissues rather than up through the specimen.

### USES

The microscope is probably the single most important instrument in biological and medical science. Its applications are vast, ranging from the study of molecular structures to *microsurgery*. Microscopes have enabled scientists to examine both the structure and chemical composition of cells (*cytology*) and tissues (histology). They are used to investigate diseased tissues (a specialty called *histopathology*), thereby playing a vital role in diagnosis. In the operating room, microscopes have enabled the development of microsurgery, one application of which is to rejoin individual nerve fibers.

## TECHNIQUES OF MICROSURGERY

Microsurgery started with ophthalmic surgeons, whose demands for more delicate operating instruments led to the adoption of the operating microscope. The results were so favorable that surgeons working in other specialties began to use the technique for intricate operations.

### The operating microscope
This surgeon is performing microsurgery with the aid of an operating microscope. The photograph (below) shows small blood vessels as seen through the microscope.

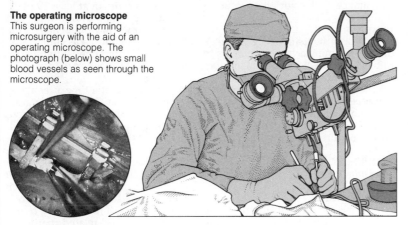

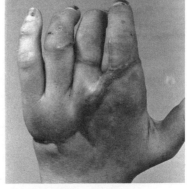

### Replantation microsurgery
A major application of microsurgery is the replantation of severed fingers, toes, hands, feet, or even entire limbs. This is successful only if the severed blood vessels and nerves are accurately rejoined so that regeneration occurs.

## MAIN AREAS OF OPERATION
Microsurgery is most commonly employed in ophthalmic, vascular, neurological, gynecological, urological, and otological surgical procedures, in which delicate structures are involved.

### Ophthalmology
By using microsurgery, even operations on the delicate retina of the eye are now possible.

### Otology
Microsurgery is routinely used for operations on the tiny bones in the middle ear.

### Gynecology
With microsurgery, blockages of the fallopian tubes can often be corrected, restoring fertility.

### Urology
A vasectomy (male sterilization) can sometimes be reversed by using microsurgery to rejoin the cut ends of the vas deferens.

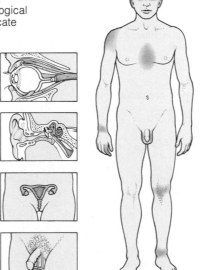

## INSTRUMENTS

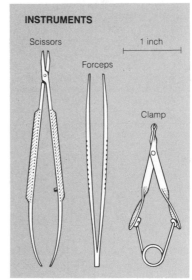

Scissors

Forceps

1 inch

Clamp

Microsurgery is possible only by using extremely delicate operating instruments, such as the fine scissors, forceps, and clamp shown above (their sizes can be judged from the scale bar).

M

## Microsurgery
Delicate surgery in which the surgeon views the operation site through a special binocular *microscope* with pedal-operated magnification, focusing, and movements.

Microsurgery technique is used for surgery involving minute, delicate, or not easily accessible tissues. It has strikingly improved the success rate of some operations and made others possible that were previously impracticable. These operations include removing a diseased cataract from the eye and implanting a new lens (see *Cataract surgery*); transplanting a new cornea to the eye (see *Corneal graft*); replacing a diseased stirrup bone in the middle ear to treat deafness caused by otosclerosis (see *Stapedectomy*); restoring a severed limb by rejoining disconnected blood vessels and nerves; and unblocking and rejoining obstructed fallopian tubes to restore a woman's fertility.

## Micturition
A term for passing *urine*.

## Midbrain
Also known as the mesencephalon, the midbrain is the topmost part of the *brain stem*, situated above the pons.

M

## Middle ear
See *Ear*.

## Middle-ear effusion, persistent
Fluid accumulation in the middle-ear cavity that causes impaired hearing. Persistent middle-ear effusion is most common in children, often accompanied by enlarged *adenoids*; it frequently occurs with viral upper respiratory tract infections, such as colds. Usually both ears are affected.

### CAUSES
The mucus-secreting lining of the middle-ear cavity sometimes becomes overactive, producing large amounts of sticky fluid. If there is blockage of the eustachian tube, which links the middle ear to the back of the nose, the fluid cannot drain away. The fluid subsequently accumulates and inter-

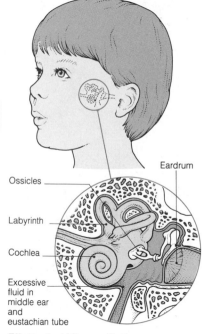

Ossicles

Eardrum

Labyrinth

Cochlea

Excessive
fluid in
middle ear
and
eustachian tube

**Effects of middle-ear effusion**
In this condition, sticky fluid in the middle ear prevents free movement of the eardrum and ossicles, causing deafness.

feres with the movement of the delicate bones in the middle ear.

### SIGNS
The first, and often the only, sign is some degree of deafness. The child may be unaware of it and, unless his or her unresponsiveness is noticed by parents or teachers, the condition may pass undetected.

### DIAGNOSIS
Middle-ear effusion is sometimes first detected through *hearing tests*, which

should be carried out routinely on all children. Once any hearing loss is detected or suspected in a child, a physician uses an *otoscope* (viewing instrument) to examine each eardrum for the characteristic changes in appearance and color that occur in middle-ear effusion.

### TREATMENT
In mild cases the patient is given nose drops containing *decongestant drugs* to unblock the affected eustachian tube, so that the fluid can drain through it.

When the condition is severe, a *myringotomy* (a surgical opening in the eardrum) may be needed to drain the fluid. Removal of the adenoids may also be required (see *Adenoidectomy*).

## Middle-ear infection
See *Otitis media*.

## Mid-life crisis
A popular phrase that describes the feelings of distress that affect some people in early middle age (35 to 45 years) after realizing that they are no longer young. The term is used most often to describe men who strive to recapture their sense of lost youth by having extramarital affairs, suddenly changing jobs, or adopting youthful fashions. Sometimes anxiety or depression, brought on by fears of declining powers and death, can lead to psychiatric illness. Counseling and support are usually effective in helping people come to terms with the changes of age.

## Midwifery
The profession concerned with the assistance of women in pregnancy and childbirth. A midwife provides care and information throughout pregnancy, supervises labor and delivery, and cares for both mother and baby during the period immediately following childbirth.

Certified midwives (called nurse-midwives) have met the graduate training standards of the American College of Nurse-Midwives and are licensed to practice in most states. Unqualified, or lay, midwifery is illegal in most states. The vast majority of qualified midwives practice in hospitals or birthing centers, usually with physician backup in case of complications and emergencies. Others work in private practice, and some midwives deliver in the woman's home.

## Migraine
A severe headache, lasting for two hours to two days, accompanied by

disturbances of vision and/or nausea and vomiting. A sufferer may experience only a single attack; more commonly, he or she has recurrent attacks at varying intervals.

### CAUSES AND INCIDENCE
Migraine occurs in at least 10 percent of the population and is three times more common in women than in men. It may affect children as young as 3; 60 percent of migraine sufferers have their first attack before the age of 20. It is extremely rare for migraine to appear for the first time after age 50.

There is no single cause of migraine. It tends to run in families, although the exact mechanism of inheritance is not understood. A number of factors, singly or in combination, may bring on an attack in a susceptible person. These factors may be stress-related (such as anxiety, anger, worry, excitement, depression, shock, overexertion, changes of routine, and changes of climate), food-related (particularly chocolate, cheese and other dairy products, red wine, fried food, and citrus fruits), or sensory-related (such as bright light or glare, loud noises, and intense or penetrating smells). Menstruation and the birth-control pill may also trigger migraine.

### TYPES
There are two types of migraine: common and classical. In common migraine, the pain of the headache develops slowly, sometimes mounting to a throbbing pain that is made worse by the slightest movement or noise. The pain is often, but not always, on one side of the head only and usually occurs with nausea and sometimes vomiting. Many sufferers, particularly children, recover after they have vomited.

Classical migraine is comparatively rare. The headache is preceded by a slowly expanding area of blindness surrounded by a sparkling edge that increases to involve up to one half of the field of vision of each eye. The blindness clears up after about 20 minutes and is often followed by a severe one-sided headache with nausea, vomiting, and sensitivity to light. Other temporary neurological symptoms, such as weakness in one half of the body, may occur.

### DIAGNOSIS
Special tests are rarely necessary. The physician can usually make a diagnosis from the patient's history and a physical examination. However, if there are accompanying persistent symptoms (such as tingling or weakness of a limb) or if the type of

headache changes or becomes more severe, a full neurological examination may be carried out to exclude the unlikely possibility of a serious condition, such as a brain tumor.

TREATMENT

If migraine attacks occur less frequently than once a month, treatment of the acute attack is all that is required. If the attacks are more frequent, preventive treatment may be necessary. The simplest form of prevention is to avoid known trigger factors; keeping a careful diary can help the sufferer pinpoint them.

The best treatment for an acute migraine attack is with aspirin or acetaminophen plus an *antiemetic drug* (often provided in suppository form). If this combination is not effective, *ergotamine* may also be prescribed. Certain ergotamine preparations may help prevent an attack if taken in the early phases before the headache begins. Most people find that they recover more quickly if they can then sleep in a darkened room.

If migraine attacks occur more than once a month, prophylactic drugs (for example, *beta-blockers* and *calcium channel blockers*) may be prescribed.

## Milia

Tiny, hard, white spots that most commonly occur in clusters on the upper cheeks and around the eyes of young adults. The cause is usually unknown although they may sometimes follow injury or blistering. They are painless and harmless.

## Miliaria

Another name for *prickly heat*.

## Milk

A *nutrient* fluid produced by the mammary gland of any mammal. Human milk differs considerably from cow's milk in the proportions of its ingredients. It contains about the same amount of fat, but twice as much lactose (sugar) and half as much protein.

Virtually all babies can digest milk, but early in childhood some lose the enzyme that breaks lactose down to simpler sugars (see *Lactase deficiency*). Milk allergy occurs in some infants, caused by a *food allergy* or intolerance to the proteins in cow's milk. (See also *Breast-feeding*; *Feeding, infant*.)

## Milk-alkali syndrome

A rare type of *hypercalcemia* (abnormally high level of calcium in the blood) accompanied by *alkalosis* (reduced acidity of the blood) and

*renal failure*. Milk-alkali syndrome is caused by excessive, long-term intake of calcium-containing *antacid drugs* and milk. It is most common in people with the symptoms of a *peptic ulcer* and associated kidney disorders.

The symptoms include weakness, muscle pains, irritability, and apathy. Treatment is to reduce the intake of milk and antacids.

## Milk of magnesia

A magnesium preparation used as an *antacid drug* and a *laxative drug*.

## Milk teeth

See *Primary teeth*.

## Minamata disease

The name given to a severe form of *mercury* poisoning that occurred in the middle 1950s in people who had eaten fish from Minamata Bay, Japan. The fish contained large amounts of mercury as a result of water polluted with industrial mercury waste. By the time the cause of the condition was identified and brought under control, many people had suffered severe nerve damage and some had died.

## Mineralization, dental

The deposition of calcium crystals and other mineral salts in developing teeth. (See *Calcification, dental*.)

## Mineralocorticoid

The term used to describe a corticosteroid hormone (a hormone produced by the *adrenal gland*) that controls the amount of salts, including potassium and sodium, excreted in the urine. Some corticosteroid hormones (e.g., *aldosterone*) have only a mineralocorticoid action; others (such as *hydrocortisone*) also have a glucocorticoid effect (that is, they help regulate the body's use of carbohydrates).

## Mineral oil

A lubricant *laxative drug* obtained from petroleum. Taken orally or given as an enema, mineral oil is used to treat *constipation*. Prolonged use may impair the absorption of vitamins from the intestine into the blood.

## Minerals

Defined in *nutrition* as chemical elements that must be present in the diet for the maintenance of health. At least 13 minerals are essential to health. Important among them are potassium, sodium, calcium, magnesium, and phosphorus. Others, such as iron, zinc, and copper, are

needed in only tiny amounts (see *Trace elements*). A balanced diet usually contains all the minerals the body requires. (See also chart, next page.)

## Mineral supplements

A group of drug preparations containing one or more *minerals*. Mineral supplements, which are available over-the-counter in tablet or liquid form, should be used only when deficiency exists and on the advice of a physician. Most people obtain adequate amounts of minerals from the diet and additional amounts do not have any beneficial effects. Taken in excess, some mineral supplements may have harmful effects.

MEDICAL USES

The most commonly used mineral supplement is iron, which is used to treat iron-deficiency *anemia* and is sometimes needed by a woman who is pregnant or breast-feeding.

Other types of mineral deficiency are rare, with the exception of *magnesium* deficiency, which may occur as a result of alcohol abuse, a kidney disorder, or prolonged treatment with *diuretic drugs*.

Mineral supplements are sometimes needed by people suffering from an intestinal disorder that impairs the absorption of minerals from the diet. (See also individual mineral entries.)

## Minilaparotomy

See *Sterilization, female*.

## Minimal brain dysfunction

A postulated explanation for a variety of behavioral and other problems occurring in young children for which a physical cause might be expected but for which none is found.

Minimal brain dysfunction may be a cause of attentional difficulties, impulsiveness, *hyperactivity*, and some *learning disabilities*.

## Minocycline

A tetracycline *antibiotic drug* used in low doses to treat *acne*. In rare cases, it is used to treat other disorders.

## Minoxidil

A *vasodilator drug* used to treat severe *hypertension* (high blood pressure) when other drugs have been ineffective. Prolonged treatment often stimulates hair growth, especially on the face. Minoxidil in lotion form was approved by the FDA in 1988 as a treatment for male pattern *alopecia* (baldness).

M

## MINERALS AND MAIN FOOD SOURCES

| Mineral | Sources |
|---|---|
| Calcium | Milk, cheese, butter and margarine, green vegetables, legumes, nuts, soybean products, hard water |
| Chromium | Red meat, cheese, butter and margarine, whole-grain cereals and breads, green vegetables |
| Copper | Red meat, poultry, liver, fish, seafood, whole-grain cereals and breads, green vegetables, legumes, nuts, raisins, mushrooms |
| Fluorine | Fish, fluoridated water, tea |
| Iodine | Milk, cheese, butter and margarine, fish, whole-grain cereals and breads, iodized table salt |
| Iron | Red meat, poultry, liver, eggs, fish, whole-grain cereals and breads |
| Magnesium | Milk, fish, whole-grain cereals and breads, green vegetables, legumes, nuts, hard water |
| Phosphorus | Red meat, poultry, liver, milk, cheese, butter and margarine, eggs, fish, whole-grain cereals and breads, green vegetables, root vegetables, legumes, nuts, fruit |
| Potassium | Whole-grain cereals and breads, green vegetables, legumes, fruit |
| Selenium | Red meat, liver, milk, fish, seafood, whole-grain cereals and breads |
| Sodium | Red meat, poultry, liver, milk, cheese, butter and margarine, eggs, fish, whole-grain cereals and breads, green vegetables, root vegetables, legumes, nuts, fruit, table salt, processed foods |
| Zinc | Red meat, fish, seafood, eggs, milk, whole-grain cereals and breads, legumes |

**M**

## Miosis

Constriction (reduction in size) of the pupil of the eye. Miosis may be caused by certain drugs (such as pilocarpine or opium), by a disease affecting the *autonomic nervous system* (such as *Horner's syndrome*), or simply by bright light. A degree of miosis is normal in older people.

## Miscarriage

Loss of the fetus before the 22nd week of pregnancy or before viability (the ability to survive outside the uterus without artificial support). The medical term for miscarriage is spontaneous abortion.

### INCIDENCE

The incidence of miscarriage is difficult to determine, since not all women who miscarry seek medical attention or even realize they are miscarrying. It is estimated that from 10 to 30 percent of all pregnancies end in miscarriage, with the majority occurring in the first 10 weeks.

### CAUSES

A wide range of problems can cause miscarriage. Many miscarriages occur because of abnormalities of the fetus itself, such as *chromosomal abnormalities* or major developmental defects. Severe maternal illness or exposure to toxins may also cause miscarriage. Less common causes of miscarriage include abnormalities such as inadequate progesterone secretion or an *autoimmune disorder* of the pregnant woman.

After the first three months, miscarriage is less common. Of the 3 to 5 percent of pregnancies that miscarry between 12 and 22 weeks, problems include genetic defects, *cervical incompetence* (inability of the cervix to hold the pregnancy), a defect such as a septate (subdivided) uterus, and large uterine fibroid tumors. Severe maternal infection or illness can also trigger a late miscarriage.

### SYMPTOMS AND SIGNS

The symptoms of miscarriage are cramping and/or bleeding. Light bleeding during the early months of pregnancy occurs in up to half of all pregnancies and is often caused by low placental implantation or by *cervical erosion*. Many of these pregnancies continue uneventfully to term.

Heavy bleeding with cramping is generally more serious since it may signal impending miscarriage. Spotting and severe pain can be a symptom of either a threatened miscarriage or *ectopic pregnancy*. A gush of clear or pink fluid caused by rupture of the amniotic sac is an ominous sign.

### DIAGNOSIS AND TREATMENT

In early pregnancy a woman in whom bleeding and cramping develop is often prescribed bed rest to minimize bleeding (although bed rest probably does not influence the outcome). Ultrasound scanning may be recommended to determine that the pregnancy is intrauterine (i.e., not ectopic) and that it appears to be progressing normally. A pelvic examination may be performed to find out if the size of the uterus feels appropriate and to see if the cervix is open or closed.

If a miscarriage is incomplete or inevitable and bleeding is heavy, a *D and C* (scraping out of the uterus) may be required. If the miscarriage seems complete (i.e., all fetal and placental material has been passed), no further treatment may be needed. Missed abortion may require *induction of labor*. Often, women are given antibiotics and other drugs to minimize bleeding. Rh-negative women are given $Rh_o(D)$ immune globulin to prevent future Rh complications (see *Rh incompatibility*).

After the first trimester, any cramping or spotting merits immediate medical attention; at this stage a significant number of possible miscarriages are caused by treatable problems, such as an incompetent cervix, rather than by severe fetal defects.

If there is evidence of an incompetent cervix, the cervix may be stitched shut. Prolonged bed rest may be recommended and uterine relaxants may be administered to women with uterine or cervical abnormalities.

A woman who miscarries three or more times consecutively is called an habitual aborter. Habitual abortion may be caused by genetic or hormonal

## TYPES OF MISCARRIAGE

| | |
|---|---|
| **Threatened abortion** | The fetus remains alive and has not been expelled from the uterus, despite bleeding from the woman's vagina. |
| **Inevitable abortion** | The fetus has died and is being expelled from the uterus. An inevitable abortion may be complete (when all the uterine contents are expelled) or incomplete (when the fetus and/or placenta are not completely expelled). |
| **Missed abortion** | The fetus has died but is retained with the placenta in the uterus. |

abnormalities, chronic infection, autoimmune disease, or uterine abnormalities. Evaluation includes genetic studies for hormonal and infectious problems as well as *hysterosalpingography* (X-ray imaging of the uterus and fallopian tubes).

### OUTLOOK
The majority of women who miscarry can eventually carry a pregnancy to term. Current diagnostic and treatment measures have made the outlook better than ever before. (See also *Abortion*; *Abortion, elective*.)

## Mites and disease

 Mites are small, eight-legged animals, less than one twentieth of an inch (1.2 mm) long, similar to tiny spiders. Many have piercing and blood-sucking mouthparts and may parasitize animals and humans.

Mites can cause problems in a variety of ways. One species, the *scabies* mite, lives solely in human skin, where its burrowing activities cause an intense itch. Another, the house-dust mite, is common in bedding; inhaling dust containing dead mite parts can cause *asthma*.

Other types of mites inhabit grassy areas or affect crops. Chiggers (harvest mites) can be picked up when walking through thick grass. Their bites can produce an itchy rash (see *Chigger bites*). Mites in grain or fruit may cause various types of skin irritation, commonly known as grocers' itch or bakers' itch.

In some parts of the world, certain mites transmit disease, particularly scrub *typhus* and rickettsialpox. Both these diseases are caused by *rickettsiae* (organisms intermediate between bacteria and viruses), which normally infect rodents, but which can be transmitted to humans by mites.

The use of insect repellents (such as dimethyl phthalate) is advisable when walking through mite-infested areas.

## Mitosis
The way in which most cells divide, so that the *chromosomes* (inherited genetic material) within the nucleus of the original cell are exactly duplicated into two daughter cells.

Each person begins as a single cell (a fertilized egg) and, following successive mitotic divisions of this cell, is born as a multicellular being with trillions of cells, most of which contain exactly the same chromosomal material. Mitotic divisions occur in the body thousands of times every second as dead cells are replaced by new ones formed by the division and multiplication of other cells.

Mitosis can be observed in a cell culture under a microscope. The sequence of events as the original cell divides to form two daughter cells is shown below.

A minority of cells (in the ovaries and testes) undergoes a fundamentally different type of division that results in the daughter cells receiving only half of the original cell's chromosomal material. This process, called *meiosis*, occurs in the formation of egg and sperm cells.

M

---

### THE MECHANISM OF MITOSIS

Mitosis is the simplest type of cell division. It provides new body cells to replace those that have died. The new cells each receive an identical copy of the original cell's chromosomes.

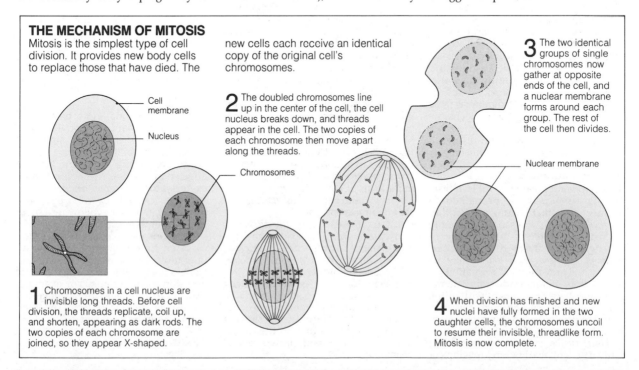

Cell membrane

Nucleus

Chromosomes

**1** Chromosomes in a cell nucleus are invisible long threads. Before cell division, the threads replicate, coil up, and shorten, appearing as dark rods. The two copies of each chromosome are joined, so they appear X-shaped.

**2** The doubled chromosomes line up in the center of the cell, the cell nucleus breaks down, and threads appear in the cell. The two copies of each chromosome then move apart along the threads.

**3** The two identical groups of single chromosomes now gather at opposite ends of the cell, and a nuclear membrane forms around each group. The rest of the cell then divides.

Nuclear membrane

**4** When division has finished and new nuclei have fully formed in the two daughter cells, the chromosomes uncoil to resume their invisible, threadlike form. Mitosis is now complete.

## Mitral insufficiency

Failure of the mitral valve of the heart to close properly, which allows blood to leak back into the left atrium (upper chamber) when pumped out of the left ventricle (lower chamber). Also known as mitral incompetence or mitral regurgitation, the disorder may occur in conjunction with *mitral stenosis* (narrowing of the valve).

In mitral insufficiency, the left side of the heart must work harder to clear the regurgitated blood. Eventually left-sided (and later, right-sided) *heart failure* may develop; generally, however, this is not a life-threatening condition. A buildup of blood from the left side of the heart can result in pulmonary *edema*.

### CAUSES AND INCIDENCE

The most common cause (though much less common than it once was) is damage to the valve as a result of *rheumatic fever*. Other causes include *mitral valve prolapse* (floppy valve syndrome), damage following a *myocardial infarction* (heart attack), and stretching of the valve due to enlargement of the ventricle in left-sided heart failure. Rarely, the disorder may be present from birth or occurs as part of *Marfan's syndrome*.

### SYMPTOMS AND SIGNS

The characteristic symptoms are increasing shortness of breath and fatigue, sometimes accompanied by *palpitations*. Later, as right-sided heart failure develops, the ankles swell.

An occasional complication is *endocarditis* (infection of the valve). Another risk is that a thrombus (blood clot) may form in the left atrium and travel to the brain, resulting in a *stroke*.

### DIAGNOSIS

The physician makes a diagnosis from the patient's history, from a characteristic heart *murmur* heard through a stethoscope, and from the results of chest *X rays*, *ECG*, *echocardiography*, and cardiac *catheterization*.

### TREATMENT AND OUTLOOK

If shortness of breath is troublesome, a *diuretic drug* may be prescribed to reduce fluid in the lungs and other tissues. *Digitalis drugs* may be given to increase the force of the heart's contraction and control rhythm disturbances. *Anticoagulant drugs* may be given to prevent the formation of blood clots. Before undergoing dental or other surgery, a person with mitral valve disease should take *antibiotic drugs* to prevent a blood infection that could cause endocarditis.

*Heart valve surgery* is considered only if severe heart failure develops or if drug treatment fails to prevent the patient's symptoms from becoming severe and disabling.

The outlook for mitral insufficiency is good whether treated by drugs or by valve surgery. Breathlessness and fatigue cannot be relieved by treatment once there has been permanent heart damage.

## Mitral stenosis

Narrowing of the orifice of the mitral valve in the heart. This causes the atrial portion of the left side of the heart to work harder to force blood through the narrowed valve. The consequences are similar to those of *mitral insufficiency* (failure of the valve to close properly), which may accompany stenosis.

### CAUSES AND INCIDENCE

Mitral stenosis is almost always due to scarring of the valve from an earlier attack of *rheumatic fever*, although in about half the cases there is no medical record of the illness. Mitral stenosis is four times more common in women than in men.

### SYMPTOMS AND SIGNS

Symptoms do not usually develop until adulthood, many years after rheumatic fever. The primary symptom is shortness of breath, which at first occurs only on exertion; as the stenosis worsens, breathing difficulty is felt with less exertion and is eventually present when the person is at rest. Other symptoms and signs include *palpitations*, *atrial fibrillation* (rapid, uncoordinated, irregular heart beat), and deeply flushed cheeks. Congestion of the lungs can lead to recurrent chest infections, coughing up of blood, and fatigue.

Possible complications are as for mitral insufficiency.

### DIAGNOSIS

Mitral stenosis is diagnosed from the patient's history, by a physician listening to heart sounds through a stethoscope, and by investigations that may include an *ECG*, chest *X rays*, echocardiography, and cardiac *catheterization*.

### TREATMENT AND OUTLOOK

Drug treatment (with *diuretic drugs* and *digitalis drugs*) is broadly the same as for mitral insufficiency, as are the precautions to help prevent *endocarditis* (infection of the valve).

If symptoms persist despite drug treatment, *heart valve surgery* may be considered to repair or replace the defective valve. The outlook following surgery is good, although the operation may need to be repeated several years later.

## Mitral valve prolapse

A common, slight deformity of the mitral valve, situated in the left side of the heart, that can produce a degree of *mitral insufficiency* (leakage of the valve). Also known as "floppy valve syndrome," the condition affects up to 5 percent of the population and is most common in young to middle-aged women. Mitral valve prolapse causes a characteristic heart *murmur* that may be heard by the physician through a stethoscope during a routine examination.

The cause is not known in most cases, although there is some evidence that the condition is inherited. Occasionally the prolapse results from *rheumatic fever*, *coronary heart disease*, or *cardiomyopathy*.

Usually, there are no symptoms and the condition is of no consequence; treatment is not required. Occasionally, however, it may produce chest pain, *arrhythmia* (disturbance of heart rhythm), or leakage of the valve sufficient to cause *heart failure*. These conditions may require treatment with heart drugs (such as *beta-blockers*, *diuretics*, or *digitalis drugs*) or, rarely, *heart valve surgery*.

## Mittelschmerz

Pain in the lower abdomen that occurs in some women at the time of *ovulation* midway through each menstrual cycle. The pain is usually one-sided and lasts only a few hours; slight spotting (vaginal blood loss) may accompany the pain. Mittelschmerz is usually not severe. However, if it is, *oral contraceptives* may be prescribed to suppress ovulation.

## Mobilization

The process of making a part of the body capable of movement. Mobilization refers to treatment aimed at increasing mobility in a part of the body recovering from injury or affected by disease. Examples include exercises to treat *frozen shoulder* or joint stiffness caused by *arthritis*, and retraining in walking following a *stroke* or lower limb *fracture*.

Surgeons use the term mobilization to refer to the freeing, during an operation, of an organ or structure from surrounding connective tissue and fibrous adhesions. For example, in a *cholecystectomy*, the gallbladder has to be mobilized from the liver before it can be removed.

## Molar

See *Teeth*.

## Molar pregnancy

A pregnancy in which a tumor develops from placental tissue and the embryo fails to develop normally. A molar pregnancy may be benign (*hydatidiform mole*) or malignant, when it is called an invasive mole. *Choriocarcinoma* is an invasive mole that has spread outside the uterus.

A different type of molar pregnancy occurs after a missed abortion (a type of *miscarriage* in which the dead embryo and placenta are not expelled from the uterus). The dead tissue is called a carneous mole.

## Mold

Any of a large group of *fungi* that exist as many-celled, filamentous colonies. Some molds are the source of antibiotics, such as penicillin. Some can cause disease, such as *aspergillosis*.

## Mole

A type of pigmented *nevus*.

## Molecule

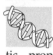

The smallest complete unit of a substance that can exist independently and still retain the characteristic properties of that substance. Almost all molecules consist of two or more atoms that are linked. A molecule of carbon dioxide comprises one carbon atom linked to two oxygen atoms. Certain unusual molecules, called monatomic molecules, consist of only one atom (e.g., molecules of inert gases such as argon and neon).

Molecules vary enormously in size and complexity. At one extreme are the small, simple ones, such as oxygen, consisting of two linked oxygen atoms. At the other extreme are huge, complicated molecules, such as *DNA* (deoxyribonucleic acid), containing thousands of atoms of carbon, hydrogen, oxygen, nitrogen, and phosphorus that are linked to form a double-helix structure shaped like a spiral staircase.

## Molluscum contagiosum

A harmless viral infection characterized by shiny, pearly white papules (tiny lumps) on the skin surface. Each papule is circular, has a tiny central depression, and produces a cheesy fluid if squeezed. A crust forms before healing occurs.

The papules appear in groups, or sometimes alone, on the genitals, the inside of the thighs, the face, or elsewhere. Children or, less commonly, adults may be affected. The infection is easily transmitted by direct skin contact or during intercourse.

Molluscum contagiosum usually clears up in a few months, but may require treatment by a physician.

## Mongolian spot

A blue-black pigmented spot found singly or in groups on the lower back and buttocks at birth. The spot may be mistaken for a bruise, although it is a type of *nevus*. Mongolian spots are common in black or Asian children and are caused by a concentration of melanocytes (pigment-producing cells) deep within the skin. They usually disappear by the age of 3 or 4.

## Mongolism

The outdated name for the disorder now called *Down's syndrome*.

## Moniliasis

See *Candidiasis*.

## Monitor

To maintain a constant watch on a patient's condition so that any change can be detected early and appropriate treatment given. The term also refers to any device used to carry out monitoring, such as the cardiac monitor used in intensive-care units. A cardiac monitor displays the patient's *ECG* (a record of the electrical impulses generated by the heart) on a screen and signals the heart rate both visually and audibly.

## Monoarthritis

Inflammation of a single joint, causing pain and stiffness. Common causes are *osteoarthritis*, *gout*, and infection.

## Monoclonal antibody

See *Antibody, monoclonal*.

## Mononucleosis, infectious

An acute viral infection characterized by a high temperature, sore throat, and swollen lymph glands, particularly in the neck (hence its common name, glandular fever).

### CAUSES AND INCIDENCE

Infectious mononucleosis is caused either by the Epstein-Barr virus or cytomegalovirus, both members of the herpesvirus family. The disease develops only if the virus is encountered for the first time at an age when the response of the body's *immune system* is most vigorous (that is, during adolescence and early adult life). The peak incidence of the illness occurs around ages 15 to 17. Kissing is thought to be a common method of transmitting the virus.

Once in the body, the virus multiplies in the *lymphocytes* (white blood cells that form part of the immune system). Lymphocytes are also called mononuclear cells. When infected with the virus, the lymphocytes change their appearance and are referred to as "atypical."

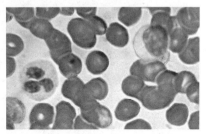

**Blood smear in mononucleosis**
The large cell with one nucleus, surrounded by many red blood cells, is an atypical lymphocyte (it is bigger than normal).

### SYMPTOMS AND SIGNS

The illness usually starts with a fever and headache, followed by swelling of the lymph glands in the neck, armpits, and groin and a severe sore throat due to tonsillitis. The enlarged, inflamed tonsils make swallowing difficult and, in rare cases, may obstruct breathing. Occasionally, mild liver damage may occur, leading to jaundice for a few days. A physician may feel an enlarged spleen in the upper left part of the abdomen.

### DIAGNOSIS

The diagnosis is often obvious from the symptoms and from examination of a blood smear, which shows many atypical lymphocytes in the blood. A test for the infection—the heterophil antibodies test—may also be carried out. This test looks for antibodies (proteins produced by the immune system to counter the virus) that possess the unique ability to cause clumping of red cells taken from sheep's blood. More specific tests are also available when the diagnosis is in doubt.

### TREATMENT AND OUTLOOK

Almost all patients recover after four to six weeks without drugs. If the antibiotic ampicillin is mistakenly given, it may produce a rash and worsening of symptoms. Rest is needed for a month or so to allow the body's immune system to destroy the virus. In rare cases, *corticosteroid drugs* are required to reduce severe inflammation, particularly if breathing is obstructed by swollen tonsils. For two to three

M

months after recovery, patients often feel depressed, lack energy, and feel sleepy during the day. However, the majority of people who have chronic fatigue that they attribute to chronic Epstein-Barr virus disease produce no laboratory results to substantiate this diagnosis.

## Monorchism
The presence of only one testis in a male. Unless a testis has been removed surgically (see *Orchiectomy*), the most likely cause of monorchism is *congenital* absence. The term monorchism should not be used to describe an undescended testis (see *Testis, undescended*).

## Monosodium glutamate
A *food additive* frequently used as a flavor enhancer and seasoning. Until recently, monosodium glutamate (MSG) was suspected to be the cause of *Chinese restaurant syndrome*, in which a sense of pressure in the face, pain in the chest, and a feeling of burning in the head and upper trunk comes on 20 minutes after a meal and lasts for about 45 minutes. Clinical trials have shown that MSG does not produce exactly this symptom pattern, although it may occasionally cause some of these symptoms in sensitive people.

## Monteggia's fracture
Fracture of the ulna (the bone on the inner side of the forearm) just below the elbow, with dislocation of the radius (the bone on the outer side of the forearm) from the elbow joint. Monteggia's fracture can be caused by a fall onto the arm or by a blow to the back of the upper arm.

Treatment usually requires an operation through two incisions on either side of the forearm. First, the radius is replaced in the joint. The fractured bone ends of the ulna are then realigned and fixed with a plate and screws or a long nail. The incisions are sewn up and the limb is immobilized in a plaster cast until healing occurs, which usually takes about 12 weeks.

## Montezuma's revenge
A name given to a type of *gastroenteritis* (especially the resulting diarrhea) that is often contracted by tourists visiting Mexico.

## Moon face
The rounded facial appearance that is a feature of *Cushing's syndrome*.

## MORA
The abbreviation for *mandibular orthopedic repositioning appliance*.

## Morbid anatomy
Also known as pathological anatomy, the study of the structural changes that occur in body tissues as a consequence of disease.

The term morbid anatomy refers especially to those changes that are visible to the naked eye during a postmortem examination (in contrast to changes visible only through a microscope).

## Morbidity
The state or condition of being diseased. The morbidity ratio is the proportion of diseased to healthy people in a community.

In the US, detailed statistics on morbidity are recorded at the *Centers for Disease Control* in Atlanta, Georgia.

## Morbilli
Another name for *measles*.

## Morning-after pill
See *Contraception, postcoital*.

## Morning sickness
See *Vomiting in pregnancy*.

## Moron
An outdated term, derived from the Greek word for dull, for a person with mild *mental retardation* (IQ 50 to 70).

## Morphea
A condition in which one or more well-defined, hard, flat, round or oval patches develop on the skin. Morphea is a nonspreading type of *scleroderma* (a disease in which there is progressive hardening of tissues).

The skin patches of morphea are white or reddish, measuring up to several inches in diameter. They usually occur on the trunk, neck, hands, or feet. Loss of hair or ulceration at the affected site may also occur. The condition most often affects middle-aged women. Although harmless, morphea can be disfiguring. There is no treatment.

## Morphine
The best known narcotic *analgesic* (painkiller), derived from the unripe seed pods of the opium poppy.

## MAJOR CAUSES OF DEATH IN THE US IN A REPRESENTATIVE YEAR

| Cause | Total deaths (per 100,000 population) | Male deaths (per 100,000 men) | Female deaths (per 100,000 women) |
|---|---|---|---|
| Circulatory system diseases | 421.5 | 435.3 | 408.4 |
| Acute myocardial infarction | 122.4 | 145.7 | 100.3 |
| Other ischemic heart disease | 113.8 | 116.0 | 111.7 |
| Hypertension | 13.6 | 12.1 | 15.0 |
| Other forms of heart disease | 79.9 | 81.5 | 78.4 |
| Stroke | 66.5 | 55.3 | 77.1 |
| Atherosclerosis | 11.3 | 8.8 | 13.6 |
| Cancer (all forms) | 189.9 | 209.7 | 170.1 |
| Colon | 19.7 | 19.7 | 19.8 |
| Lung, bronchus, trachea | 49.2 | 70.7 | 28.8 |
| Breast | — | — | 31.6 |
| Prostate | — | 22.0 | — |
| Accidents | 39.5 | 56.2 | 23.8 |
| Traffic accidents | 18.6 | 27.1 | 10.2 |
| Suicide | 12.1 | 19.2 | 5.4 |
| Homicide | 8.5 | 13.4 | 3.9 |
| Pneumonia | 23.3 | 24.2 | 22.4 |
| Bronchitis, emphysema, asthma | 8.7 | 11.3 | 6.3 |
| Other respiratory diseases | 28.1 | 36.7 | 19.9 |
| Diabetes mellitus | 15.5 | 12.9 | 17.9 |
| Other endocrine and metabolic diseases | 4.3 | 4.1 | 4.4 |
| Chronic liver disease and cirrhosis | 11.7 | 15.4 | 8.1 |
| Other digestive system disorders | 14.3 | 13.8 | 14.7 |
| Infections and parasitic diseases | 9.3 | 9.9 | 8.8 |
| Septicemia | 5.7 | 5.6 | 5.8 |

**WHY IT IS USED**

Morphine is given to relieve severe pain caused by *myocardial infarction* (heart attack), major surgery, serious injury, and cancer. It is occasionally used as a *premedication* (a drug used to prepare a person for surgery).

**HOW IT WORKS**

Morphine blocks the transmission of pain signals at specific sites (called opiate receptors) in the brain and spinal cord, thereby preventing the perception of pain.

**POSSIBLE ADVERSE EFFECTS**

Morphine causes drowsiness, dizziness, constipation, nausea, vomiting, and confusion. Short-term use is unlikely to cause *drug dependence*.

**ABUSE**

The euphoric effects of morphine have led to its abuse. Long-term abuse leads to a craving for the drug and *tolerance* (the need for greater amounts to have the same effect). It also causes physical dependence, with flulike symptoms (such as sweating, shaking, and cramping) when the drug is suddenly withdrawn.

## Mortality

The death rate, that is, the number of deaths per 100,000 (or, occasionally, per 1,000 or per 10,000) of the population per year. The total mortality is made up of the individual mortality from different causes (such as accidents, coronary heart disease, and cancer). The study of differences in these proportions between one country and another, or between different periods in the same country, can offer valuable information about the comparative state of health of a population or about disease trends.

Mortality is often calculated for specific groups of the population. For example, *infant mortality* quantifies deaths of live-born infants during the first year of life; perinatal mortality quantifies deaths (including all stillbirths) during the first week (or sometimes month) of life.

Standardized mortality compares the death rate in an occupational or socioeconomic group with the average for the entire population. It is a useful indicator of the relative safety of an occupation, or of whether a specific socioeconomic group is at particular risk. (See also table, left; *Life expectancy*; *Maternal mortality*.)

## Mosaicism

The presence of two (or more) groups of cells containing different chromosomal material within one person.

Usually, each of a person's body cells contains 46 chromosomes. They include the two sex chromosomes, termed XX in females and XY in males (see *Chromosomes*). In a mosaic person, some cells may contain 46 and others 45, 47, or other numbers of chromosomes. The probable cause in most cases is a fault in the process of cell division early in embryonic life. The diagnosis is made by *chromosome analysis* of skin or white blood cells.

Mosaicism can give rise to syndromes associated with *chromosomal abnormalities* (such as *Down's syndrome* and *Turner's syndrome*). A girl with Turner's syndrome mosaicism has some cells with a normal chromosome complement and others missing an X sex chromosome. About 3 percent of children with Down's syndrome have mosaicism. These children carry a mixture of normal cells and others containing an extra number 21 chromosome.

Depending on the proportion of abnormal cells and type of abnormality, people with mosaicism range from looking physically normal to having features typical of a chromosomal abnormality syndrome. People with mosaicism are often less severely affected than those with the abnormality in all their cells.

## Mosquito bites

Mosquitoes are flying insects found throughout the world. The females require blood from humans or animals to produce eggs; they obtain this blood through their bites. The mosquito eggs are laid and hatched in stagnating water, so mosquitoes are most prevalent close to marshes, ponds, reservoirs, and water tanks,

especially after a rainy period. Male mosquitoes do not bite.

Mosquitoes are a nuisance simply because of their bites. However, the main problem with mosquitoes is disease transmission—particularly in the tropics. During a bite, a mosquito may acquire infectious organisms from the blood of an infected person; the organisms multiply within the insect and are transferred to another person during a subsequent bite.

The main disease-transmitting mosquitoes belong to three groups: *ANOPHELES*, *AEDES*, and *CULEX*. They have varying appearances and habits and transmit different diseases (see chart). The only illnesses acquired from mosquito bites in the US are certain types of viral *encephalitis* (inflammation of the brain), such as St. Louis encephalitis, eastern and western equine encephalitis, and California encephalitis. Several thousand cases of these infections occur in the US each year, with features similar to other types of encephalitis. A hundred years ago, malaria was commonly transmitted in parts of the South and middle West.

**TREATMENT**

Mosquito bites should be washed with soap and water, and a soothing cream applied. A physician should be consulted if mosquito bites cause a severe skin reaction.

**PREVENTION**

Protective measures against mosquitoes (to limit the chances of infection) should be taken in the tropics and subtropics and in any area where the insects are rampant. The most effective measures are the wearing of long sleeves and socks at dusk to reduce the amount of exposed skin,

**M**

**DANGEROUS MOSQUITOES**

| Mosquito | Appearance | Habits | Diseases transmitted |
|---|---|---|---|
| *ANOPHELES* species | Head and body in straight line and at an angle to surface | Mainly rural; bite at night | Malaria; filariasis |
| *CULEX* species | Body parallel to surface; head bent down; whining flight; brown color | Urban or rural; bite in evening or at night | Viral encephalitis; filariasis |
| *AEDES* species | Body shape as for *CULEX*, but tropical species are black and white | Urban or rural; bite during day | Dengue; yellow fever; viral encephalitis |

placing mosquito screens over windows, and the use of insect-repellent sprays or slow-burning coils that release a smoke containing insecticide. A mosquito net that surrounds the bed is of value in preventing mosquitoes from biting during sleep.

Attempts to control mosquitoes in the tropics have included direct attack with insecticides, efforts to limit breeding areas, and even the release of vast numbers of sterilized male mosquitoes. However, these efforts have achieved only limited success. (See also *Insect bites; Insects and disease*.)

## Motion sickness

A condition produced in some people by road, sea, or air travel. In its mildest form, motion sickness may be only a feeling of uneasiness and a headache; in severe cases, there may be distress, excessive sweating and salivation, pallor, nausea, and vomiting.

Motion sickness is caused by the effect of any constant pronounced movement on the organ of balance in the inner ear. Other factors also play a part, however. Anxiety based on previous attacks, a stuffy or fume-laden atmosphere, a full stomach, or the sight of food can make the condition worse. So, too, can focusing on nearby objects; sufferers should look at a point on the horizon.

**PREVENTION**

Various *antiemetic drugs* are available to prevent or help control motion sickness. Scopolamine or cyclizine (an *antihistamine drug*) should be taken about an hour before the start of a journey. The longer-acting antihistamines (promethazine or meclizine) need to be taken about a day before the journey.

## Motor

A term used to describe anything that brings about movement, such as a muscle or nerve. The word is usually applied to nerves (including those in the part of the brain called the cerebral cortex) that stimulate muscles to contract and thereby produce movement.

## Motor neuron disease

A group of rare disorders in which the nerves that control muscular activity degenerate within the brain and spinal cord. The result is weakness and *atrophy* (wasting) of the muscles. The cause is unknown.

**INCIDENCE AND TYPES**

The most common motor neuron disease is amyotrophic lateral sclerosis (ALS), often referred to as Lou

Gehrig's disease. About one or two cases of ALS are diagnosed annually per 100,000 people in the US. ALS usually affects people over 50 and is more common in men than women. About 10 percent of ALS cases are familial (run in the family).

Other motor neuron diseases include progressive muscular atrophy and progressive bulbar palsy. While these diseases start with patterns of muscle weakness different from typical ALS, they usually develop into that disease.

Two motor neuron diseases, usually inherited, affect much younger people. In infantile progressive spinal muscular atrophy (Werdnig-Hoffmann paralysis), children are affected at birth or shortly thereafter. The weakness progresses to death in several months to several years with rare exceptions. A more benign form (chronic spinal muscular atrophy) begins any time from childhood through adolescence; it causes a progressive weakness that may never result in serious disability.

**SYMPTOMS**

In ALS, sufferers first note weakness in the hands and arms accompanied by wasting of the muscles. Fasciculations, an involuntary quivering of small areas of the muscle, may also occur. Many sufferers also report cramping or stiffness. Sometimes the weakness starts in the legs but, in every case, all four extremities are soon involved. There is no loss of sensation; bladder function is normal.

The diagnosis is confirmed by *EMG* (measurement of muscle electrical activity) and other tests, such as muscle *biopsy*, blood studies, *myelography*, *CT scanning*, or *MRI*, to rule out other disease.

**TREATMENT AND OUTLOOK**

The weakness usually progresses to involve the muscles of respiration and swallowing, leading to death in two to four years. Exceptions do occur, however, and some people have lived more than 20 years after diagnosis.

There is no means of slowing the nerve degeneration, although physical therapy can sometimes lessen disability. Wheelchairs, walkers, and other aids are available to help patients maintain independence as long as possible.

The final stages may be especially distressing for the patient and family because, although the victim is unable to speak, swallow, or move, awareness and intellect are maintained. Occasionally, life may be prolonged

through the use of feeding tubes and *ventilators*. Care is generally aimed at easing discomfort.

## Motor system disease

See *Motor neuron disease*.

## Mountain sickness

An illness that can affect mountain climbers, hikers, or skiers who have ascended too rapidly to heights above 8,000 feet (2,400 m) or, more commonly, to above 10,000 feet (3,000 m).

**CAUSES**

Mountain sickness is caused by the reduced atmospheric pressure—and thus reduced oxygen—at high altitude, but the exact mechanism by which reduced pressure leads to illness is not fully understood. Broadly, reduced oxygen in the blood, along with other changes in blood chemistry, affects the nervous system, muscles, heart, and lungs.

At altitude there is a higher-than-normal blood flow through the lungs and to the brain; this, combined with an apparent increase in the permeability (leakiness) of blood vessels, can lead to *edema* (waterlogging) of these organs.

Mountain sickness is more likely the younger the person, the faster the ascent, and the higher the altitude.

**PREVENTION**

A person ascending to an altitude above 8,000 feet should do so gradually, stopping for a day or two's rest after each further ascent of 2,000 to 3,000 feet. Ascending higher during the rest day is permissible, provided a return to the lower level is made before night.

**SYMPTOMS AND SIGNS**

In most cases, mountain sickness is mild and short-lived, with symptoms such as headache, nausea, dizziness, and impaired mental processes. No further ascent should be made until the symptoms disappear. Some cases are more severe. Fluid builds up in the lungs, leading to severe breathlessness, cough, and the production of frothy sputum (phlegm). This is called high-altitude pulmonary edema. If fluid builds up around the brain (cerebral edema) the symptoms may include severe headache, seizures, vomiting, unsteadiness, hallucinations, and sometimes coma.

**FIRST AID AND TREATMENT**

In serious cases, the victim must be brought down from the mountain and taken to a hospital as quickly as possible. Any delay can result in brain damage and death. Administering pure oxygen, if available, can help. In the hospital, *diuretic drugs* are often given to help reduce edema.

The conditions of patients with high-altitude pulmonary edema often improve rapidly after descending a few thousand feet. Patients with the cerebral form may take days or weeks in the hospital to recover.

## Mouth

The mouth, where food is broken down for swallowing, forms the first part of the digestive tract (see *Mastication*); it converts vibrations produced by the larynx (voice box) into *speech*; and it is used in breathing.

### STRUCTURE
The roof of the mouth consists of a hard bony *palate* at the front and a soft fleshy palate behind. Most of the floor of the mouth is formed by the *tongue*, which contains specialized cells, sensitive to taste, known as taste buds. Surrounding the palate and tongue are the *teeth*, which are set in the shock-absorbent tissue of the *gums*. Enclosing them all are the cheeks and *lips*, which contain a ring of muscle that helps keep food in the mouth. The inside of the mouth is lined with mucous membrane, which is lubricated with saliva produced by three pairs of *salivary glands*.

### DISORDERS
The most common deformities of the mouth, other than alignment of the teeth (see *Malocclusion*), are *cleft lip and palate* (a split in the upper lip and a gap in the roof of the mouth). They may occur alone or together.

Infections of the mouth are common. They include an abscess around the root of a tooth (see *Abscess, dental*) and oral *candidiasis* (thrush), a fungal infection that produces sore, cream-colored patches on the lining of the mouth. Noninfective conditions that also cause discoloration include *leukoplakia* (marked by thickened white or gray patches) and the more rare *lichen planus* (in which a white network of raised tissue develops).

Extremely common are *mouth ulcers*, painful white or yellow open sores that may develop anywhere on the mucous membrane. *Cysts*, fluid- or semisolid-filled swellings, may also occur on the lining of the cheek or the floor of the mouth.

Any lump, sore, or ulcer in the mouth that persists for more than three or four weeks should be seen by a physician. In rare cases, the abnormality is an early sign of a malignant growth (see *Mouth cancer*).

## ANATOMY OF THE MOUTH
The mouth has a complicated structure, reflecting its various functions. For example, the tongue, lips, teeth, and palate play an essential role in speech production. Together with the salivary glands, the same mouth parts play a role in eating and drinking.

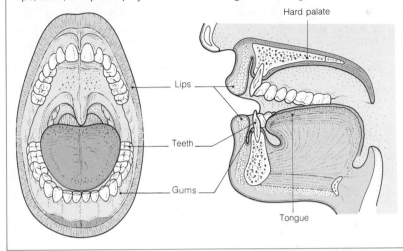

Hard palate

Lips

Teeth

Gums

Tongue

## Mouth cancer
Malignant tumors affecting the oral cavity; most common are *lip cancer* and *tongue cancer*. The floor of the mouth, the salivary glands, the inside of the cheeks, the gums, and the palate are less commonly affected. Most are squamous carcinomas.

### CAUSES AND INCIDENCE
The main cause of oral cancer is smoking. Tobacco smoke and heat irritate the mucous membrane lining the mouth. The risk to pipe and cigar smokers is as great, or greater, than to cigarette smokers. The other chief causes are chewing tobacco, inhaling snuff, and heavy alcohol consumption. Poor oral hygiene and irritation from ill-fitting dentures or jagged teeth are predisposing factors.

Oral cancers represent about 8 percent of all malignancies. Men are twice as commonly affected as women, and most cases occur in men older than 40.

### SYMPTOMS AND SIGNS
Cancer of the lip usually starts with a whitish patch on the lower lip called *leukoplakia*. The lesion is a small ulcer, or a deep, hard-edged fissure, and may be the first sign of a malignant tumor in the mouth. These initial tissue changes may be accompanied by a burning sensation, but are usually painless.

As the tumor grows, it develops into an ulcer that may bleed and that erodes surrounding tissue. If the tongue is affected, it becomes stiff, making chewing, swallowing, and speaking difficult. In its advanced stages, the tumor is usually painful.

### DIAGNOSIS
Any lump, discolored patch, or other tissue change on the lip or in the mouth that does not clear up within a month should be reported to a physician. In some cases, a dentist is the first person to detect such a change. The diagnosis is based on a *biopsy* (removal of a small sample of tissue).

### TREATMENT AND OUTLOOK
Treatment consists of surgical removal of all cancerous tissue, *radiation therapy*, or a combination of both. Extensive surgery may result in facial disfigurement and problems with eating and speaking, which may require reconstructive surgery. Radiation therapy sometimes damages the salivary glands (see *Mouth, dry*).

The rate of spread of oral cancer varies according to the site. Tongue cancer is the most dangerous, spreading rapidly to nearby lymph nodes. When oral cancer in any form is detected and treated early, the outlook is good, resulting in a cure in three quarters of cases. More than half the people with oral cancer survive for more than five years after treatment.

## Mouth, dry
The result of inadequate production of saliva. Dry mouth is usually a temporary condition caused by fear, a salivary gland infection (see *Parotid*

**M**

# MOVEMENT

During life, movement occurs constantly throughout the body. All visible movements are caused by the shortening of muscles, usually for only brief periods at a time. This causes movement of many kinds—of bones, of blood in the vessels, of food in the intestines, of urine from the bladder, of the eye, of facial expression, and of the body as a whole. All movement is either voluntary (willed) or involuntary (automatic).

## SKELETAL MOVEMENT

This always involves moving bones relative to one another. Many muscles are involved. Some act to brace certain bones so that different bones can be moved by other muscles.

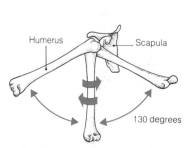

Combined rotation and displacement

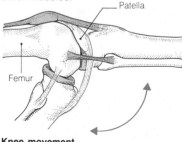

**Knee movement**
A hinge joint, the knee allows movement in one plane only through an arc of about 130 degrees.

### Arm movements
The shoulder—a ball-and-socket joint—allows movement in all directions. Sometimes two or more movements of the arm may be combined.

### Yoga and movement
Yoga (right) teaches a wide range of body movements and postures. It helps to increase joint flexibility, to eliminate tension, and to promote relaxation.

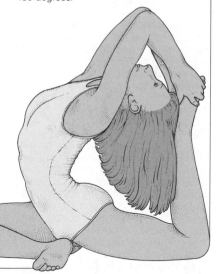

## EYE MOVEMENT

Six muscles work together on the eyeball to give a range of smooth, precise movements.

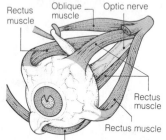

### Eye muscles
The four rectus eye muscles run directly back from the eyeball; the oblique muscles are attached to and pull on the eyeball at an angle.

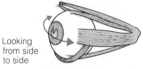

Looking from side to side

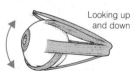

Looking up and down

### Actions of eye muscles
Two rectus muscles control side-to-side eye movements. The other muscles control up-and-down and rotational movements.

## INVOLUNTARY MOVEMENT

Movement of internal organs is not under voluntary control but is regulated by the autonomic nervous system.

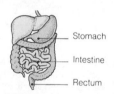

Stomach

Intestine

Rectum

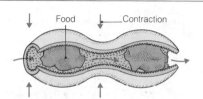

Food   Contraction

### Peristalsis
This is an example of movement caused by involuntary muscle action. Waves of contraction pass along muscles in the intestinal wall, forcing the contents forward and preventing obstruction.

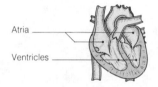

Atria

Ventricles

### Heart beat
The heart differs from other muscles in that it has an impulse-conducting system that ensures contraction in sequence—the atria (upper chambers) first, then the ventricles (lower chambers).

gland), or the action of *anticholinergic drugs*. Permanent dry mouth is rare. It can occur, for unknown reasons, as part of *Sjögren's syndrome* or may result from *radiation therapy* given to treat a tumor of the mouth. In these cases, dry mouth is usually accompanied by difficulty swallowing and speaking, interference with taste, and tooth decay. Dry mouth may be partially relieved by spraying the inside of the mouth with artificial saliva.

## Mouth-to-mouth resuscitation

See *Artificial respiration*.

## Mouth ulcer

An open sore caused by a break in the *mucous membrane* lining the mouth. Mouth ulcers take the form of round or oval, shallow, white, gray, or yellow spots with an inflamed red border. They may occur singly or in clusters anywhere in the mouth.

### TYPES

The most common type of mouth ulcer is a *canker sore*, which occurs on the inside of the cheek and lip and on the tongue. Also common are ulcers caused by the *herpes simplex* virus, which also causes *cold sores*.

Rare types of mouth ulcer include those occurring in *Behçet's syndrome*, *tuberculosis*, *syphilis*, *Vincent's disease*, *leukemia*, *anemia*, and drug allergy.

A mouth ulcer may be the first stage of *mouth cancer*. Any ulcer that fails to heal within three or four weeks, or that recurs, should be seen by a physician. *Blood tests* and/or a *biopsy* (removal of a small sample of tissue for analysis) may be required to determine the cause.

## Mouthwash

A solution for rinsing the mouth. Many mouthwashes make various medicinal claims, but most do no more than leave the mouth feeling fresh and, if used vigorously, remove loose food debris from the teeth (an effect that can be achieved with water). Most antiseptic mouthwashes intended to combat *halitosis* (bad breath) are ineffective because they do not treat the cause of the problem; if used for a prolonged period, they may irritate the mouth.

Some mouthwashes, however, are useful. When the gums are too tender for proper toothbrushing, as in some types of *gingivitis* (inflamed gums), a mouthwash containing hydrogen peroxide can help clean the teeth by its foaming action. Any time routine dental hygiene is not possible (such as

after oral surgery), a mouthwash with chlorhexidine used under the supervision of a dentist acts effectively against the bacteria in dental plaque, the sticky coating on the teeth responsible for decay.

*Fluoride* mouthwashes are helpful in preventing dental caries, probably by strengthening tooth enamel, and possibly also by acting directly against plaque. A mouthwash of warm salt water can help ease painful inflammation caused by tooth disorders, such as impacted wisdom teeth (see *Impaction, dental*) or *dry socket* (infection at the site of a tooth extraction).

## Movement

Bodily movements include skeletal movements and movements of soft tissues and body organs. All movement is brought about by the actions of various types of muscles.

### SKELETAL MOVEMENTS

The simplest skeletal movement consists of a change in the relative position of two bones, brought about by shortening of a muscle attached to the two bones and acting across a *joint*. Simultaneously, other muscles and soft tissues, such as skin, tendons, and ligaments, are stretched.

More complex skeletal movements involve many bones, joints, and muscles, which are arranged to allow an enormous range of possible actions, from turning a screwdriver to turning a somersault. Even in a fairly simple movement, several muscles are active, some contracting to initiate and maintain a movement while others that oppose the movement contract to help prevent sudden, uncontrolled movement.

All voluntary (willed) skeletal movements are initiated in the part of the cerebrum (the main mass of the brain) called the motor cortex. Signals are sent down the spinal cord along nerve fibers, and from there along separate nerve fibers to the appropriate muscles. Control relies on information supplied by sensory nerve receptors, in the muscles and elsewhere, that record the position of the different parts of the body and the amount of contraction in each muscle. This information is integrated in specific areas of the brain (including the cerebellum and basal ganglia) that control coordination, initiation, and cessation of movement. Learning complex sequences (such as piano playing) involves the establishment of unconscious patterns of nerve activity in the cerebellum.

Skeletal movements can also occur as simple *reflexes* in response to certain sensory warning signals. In these instances, the movement is automatic and less controlled, involving far fewer nerve connections.

### OTHER MOVEMENTS

Not all body movements involve the skeleton. Movements of the eyes and tongue are brought about by contractions of muscles attached to soft tissues. Again, they may be voluntary movements (controlled from the motor cortex) or reflexes. Movements of the internal organs are involuntary; they include the *heart beat* and *peristalsis*. (See also *Muscles*.)

### DISORDERS

Disorders of the nervous system, muscles, joints, or bones may impair movement. (See *Nerve injury; Neuropathy; Brain* disorders box; *Spinal cord; Muscles* disorders box.)

## Moxibustion

A form of treatment, often used in conjunction with *acupuncture*, in which a cone (moxa) of wormwood leaves or of certain other plant materials is burned just above the skin to relieve internal pain. The burning material is thought to act as a counterirritant (that is, its irritation of nerve endings in the skin alleviates deep-seated pain in the same area). When used in conjunction with acupuncture, the cone of moxa is placed on a needle over an acupuncture point, and the moxa is lit.

## MRI

Magnetic resonance imaging. MRI is a diagnostic technique that provides high quality cross-sectional images of organs and structures within the body without X rays or other radiation.

### HOW IT WORKS

During the imaging, the patient lies inside a massive, hollow, cylindrical magnet and is exposed to short bursts of a powerful magnetic field. The nuclei (protons) of the body's hydrogen atoms normally point randomly in different directions, but, in a magnetic field, they line up parallel to each other, like rows of tiny magnets. If the hydrogen nuclei are then knocked out of alignment by a strong pulse of radio waves, they produce a detectable radio signal as they fall back into alignment.

Magnetic coils in the machine detect these signals and a computer changes them into an image based on the strength of signal produced by different types of tissue. Tissues that

**M**

contain a lot of hydrogen (such as fat) produce a bright image; those that contain little or no hydrogen (such as bone) appear black.

### WHY IT IS DONE

MRI allows images to be constructed in any plane; it is particularly valuable in studying the brain and spinal cord. This technique reveals tumors vividly, indicating their precise extent, and produces impressive images of the internal structure of the eye and ear.

MRI also produces detailed images of the heart and major blood vessels, provides images of blood flow, and is useful for examining joints and soft tissues, particularly in the knee. The role of MRI in imaging the abdominal organs is becoming established.

Images from MRI are similar in many ways to those produced by *CT scanning*, but MRI generally gives much greater contrast between normal and abnormal tissues.

### HOW IT IS DONE

MRI is usually an outpatient procedure. During the examination the patient must lie still; children may be given a general anesthetic. A scan usually takes about half an hour.

### RISKS

There are no known risks or side effects to MRI. The technique does not use radiation and can therefore be performed repeatedly with no known adverse effects.

However, any person fitted with a pacemaker, hearing aid, or other electrical device should tell his or her physician before undergoing MRI, since the scanner may interfere with these devices.

### OUTLOOK

MRI is a costly test that is not yet widely available; it is still the subject of continuing research. A future application of MRI, known as magnetic resonance spectroscopy, relies on the properties of other chemical elements in the body (such as phosphorus and calcium) and is able to provide information on organ function.

## MS

The abbreviation for *multiple sclerosis*.

## Mucocele

A swollen sac or cavity within the body that is filled with mucus secreted from cells in its inner lining. An example is a mucocele of the appendix, caused by constriction of the opening of the appendix into the intestine. A mucocele of the gallbladder (*hydrops*) may be caused by a gallstone obstructing its outlet.

---

## MAGNETIC RESONANCE IMAGING (MRI)

A valuable diagnostic technique, MRI has been in use since the early 1980s. The patient lies down surrounded by electromagnets and is exposed to short bursts of powerful magnetic fields and radio waves. The bursts stimulate hydrogen atoms in the patient's tissues to emit signals, which are detected and analyzed by computer to create an image of a "slice" of the patient's body.

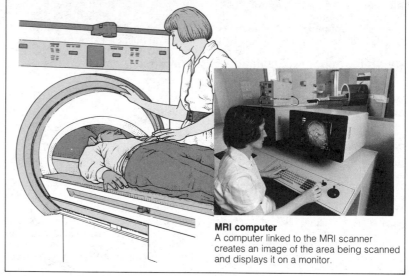

**MRI computer**
A computer linked to the MRI scanner creates an image of the area being scanned and displays it on a monitor.

---

## Mucolytic drugs

Mucolytic drugs (including *acetylcysteine*) make sputum (phlegm) less sticky and easier to cough up.

## Mucopolysaccharidosis

Any of a group of inborn errors of *metabolism*. The best known is *Hurler's syndrome*; others include Hunter's, Sanfillippo's, Morquio's, Maroteaux-Lamy, and Scheie's syndromes. They are rare, collectively affecting about one child in 10,000.

All are *genetic disorders* in which there is an abnormality of a specific *enzyme* in body tissues. The enzyme abnormality affects the way carbohydrates are handled within body cells, leading to an accumulation of unwanted substances called mucopolysaccharides in the tissues.

Depending on the disease, features include abnormalities of the skeleton and/or the central nervous system (brain and spinal cord) with mental retardation and, in some cases, a characteristic facial appearance. There may also be corneal clouding, liver enlargement, and joint stiffness. No specific treatment is available; death often occurs during the childhood or teenage years. However, there are also mild varieties that may allow a reasonably normal life. Some children with Hurler's syndrome have been successfully treated by bone marrow transplantation, which provides a continuing source of the enzyme.

Parents with a seriously affected child should receive *genetic counseling* concerning the risk of any future child being affected.

## Mucosa

Another term for a *mucous membrane*.

## Mucous membrane

The soft, pink, skinlike layer that lines many of the cavities and tubes in the body, including the respiratory tract, alimentary canal, the urinary and genital passages, and eyelids. The mucous membrane secretes a fluid that contains *mucus* to keep such structures moist and well-lubricated. The fluid is produced and released onto the surface of the mucous membrane by millions of specialized cells (goblet cells) within the membrane.

## Mucus

The thick, slimy fluid secreted by *mucous membranes*. Mucus moistens, lubricates, and protects those parts of the body lined by mucous membrane, such as the alimentary and urinary tracts. Mucus prevents stomach acid from damaging the stomach wall and prevents enzymes from digesting the intestine, it eases swallowing and lubricates food as it passes through the alimentary tract, it moistens inhaled air and traps smoke and other foreign particles in the airways (to keep them out of the lungs), and it facilitates sexual intercourse.

## Mucus method of contraception
See *Contraception*.

## Multiple myeloma
A malignant condition of middle to old age, also called myelomatosis. Multiple myeloma is characterized by the uncontrolled proliferation and disordered function of cells called plasma cells in the bone marrow.

Plasma cells are a type of B-*lymphocyte* (class of white blood cell) responsible for making *antibodies*, or *immunoglobulins*, that normally help protect against infection. In multiple myeloma, the proliferating plasma cells produce excessive amounts of a single type of immunoglobulin while the production of other types is impaired, making the patient particularly prone to infection.

Multiple myeloma is rare, with about three new cases annually per 100,000 population.

### SYMPTOMS
As the abnormal plasma cells expand within bone, they cause pain and destruction of bone tissue. If the bones in the spine are affected, they may collapse and compress nerves, causing symptoms such as numbness or paralysis. The level of calcium in the blood may increase markedly as bone is destroyed, as may the level of a breakdown product of the immunoglobulin secreted by the plasma cells. These changes in blood chemistry may damage the kidneys, leading to *renal failure*.

In addition to the increased risk of infection, patients may suffer from *anemia* and a bleeding tendency if healthy bone marrow becomes replaced by malignant plasma cells.

### DIAGNOSIS, TREATMENT, AND OUTLOOK
The disease is diagnosed from the appearance of a *bone marrow biopsy* specimen, the excess of the single type of immunoglobulin in the blood or urine, and the presence of areas of destroyed bone, as shown by X rays.

Treatment includes the use of *anticancer drugs* to reduce the number of abnormal plasma cells, *radiation therapy* to diseased areas of bone, and supportive measures (including blood transfusions to correct anemia, antibiotics to combat infections, and analgesics to relieve pain).

The severity and prognosis of the illness varies, but only about one fifth of patients survive for four years or longer from the time of diagnosis.

## Multiple personality
A rare disorder in which a person has two or more distinct personalities, each of which dominates at different times. The personalities are almost always very different from each other and are often total opposites, as in the story of Dr. Jekyll and Mr. Hyde. They may have no awareness of each other, but are aware of lost periods of time.

Although multiple personality is often called split personality, a phrase also used to describe *schizophrenia*, the two disorders are unrelated. The split in schizophrenia is between thought and feeling.

## Multiple pregnancy
See *Pregnancy, multiple*.

## Multiple sclerosis
A progressive disease of the central nervous system in which scattered patches of myelin (the protective covering of nerve fibers) in the brain and spinal cord are destroyed. This causes symptoms ranging from numbness and tingling to paralysis and incontinence. The severity of multiple sclerosis (MS) varies markedly among sufferers.

### CAUSES
The cause of multiple sclerosis remains unknown. It is thought to be an *autoimmune* disease in which the body's defense system begins to treat the myelin in the central nervous system as foreign, gradually destroying it, with subsequent scarring and damage to some of the underlying nerve fibers.

There seems to be a genetic factor, since relatives of affected people are more likely than others to contract the disease. Environment may also play a part—it is five times more common in temperate zones (such as the US and Europe) than in the tropics. Spending the first 15 years of life in a particular area seems to determine future risk. It is thought that a virus picked up by a susceptible person during this early period of life may be responsible for the disease's later development.

### INCIDENCE
Multiple sclerosis is the most common acquired (not present at birth) disease of the nervous system in young adults. In relatively high-risk temperate areas the incidence is about one in every 1,000 people. More women than men contract the disease.

### SYMPTOMS AND SIGNS
Multiple sclerosis usually starts in early adult life. It may be active briefly and then resume years later. The symptoms vary with which parts of the brain and spinal cord are affected.

Spinal cord damage can cause tingling, numbness, or a feeling of constriction in any part of the body. The extremities may feel heavy and become weak. *Spasticity* (stiffness) sometimes develops. The nerve fibers to the bladder may be involved, causing incontinence.

Damage to the white matter in the brain may lead to fatigue, vertigo, clumsiness, muscle weakness, slurred speech, unsteady gait, blurred or double vision, and numbness, weakness, or pain in the face.

These symptoms may occur singly or in combination and may last from several weeks to several months. In some sufferers, relapses may be precipitated by injury, infection, or physical or emotional stress.

Attacks vary considerably in their severity from person to person. In some, the disease may consist of mild relapses and long symptom-free periods throughout life, with very few permanent effects. Others have a series of flare-ups, leaving them with some disability, but further deterioration ceases. Some become gradually more disabled from the first attack and are bedridden and incontinent in early middle life. A small group suffers gross disability within the first year.

A person disabled with multiple sclerosis may have problems in addition to the paralysis, such as painful muscle spasms, urinary tract infections, constipation, skin ulceration, and changes of mood between euphoria and depression.

### DIAGNOSIS
There is no single diagnostic test for multiple sclerosis; confirmation of the disease is usually by exclusion of all other possible conditions. A neurologist may perform tests to help confirm the diagnosis, including *lumbar puncture* (removal of a sample of fluid from the spinal canal for laboratory analysis), tracing electrical activity in the brain (see *Evoked responses*), *CT scanning*, and *MRI*.

### TREATMENT
The search for a cure is still in progress. Patients are encouraged to

M

adopt as positive an outlook as possible, and to lead as active a life as their disabilities allow. *Corticosteroid drugs* may be prescribed to alleviate the symptoms of an acute episode; other drugs may be given to control specific symptoms, such as incontinence and depression. *Physical therapy* often helps strengthen muscles and various aids can help patients maintain mobility and independence.

## Multivitamin

A group of over-the-counter preparations containing a combination of *vitamins* and used to supplement the intake of vitamins in the diet. (See *Vitamin supplements*.)

## Mumps

An acute viral illness, mainly of childhood. The chief symptom is inflammation and swelling of the parotid (salivary) glands on one or both sides. Serious complications are uncommon. However, in teenage and adult males, mumps can be a highly uncomfortable illness in which one or both testes become inflamed and swollen. One attack of mumps confers lifelong immunity.

**CAUSES AND INCIDENCE**

The mumps virus is spread in airborne droplets. There is an incubation

## FEATURES OF MULTIPLE SCLEROSIS

This disease can affect any area of the white matter of the brain and spinal cord. The plaques of demyelination are areas in which the fatty myelin sheaths of the nerve fibers have been destroyed. Affected fibers cannot conduct nerve impulses, so functions such as movement and sensation may be lost. The patchy distribution of plaques causes very varied effects.

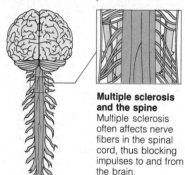

**Multiple sclerosis and the spine**
Multiple sclerosis often affects nerve fibers in the spinal cord, thus blocking impulses to and from the brain.

### Effects of multiple sclerosis
The fiber of the nerve tract is not usually destroyed. But the loss of insulating myelin and its replacement by neuroglia alters normal ion movements, so that the fiber can no longer conduct impulses.

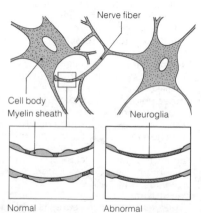

Nerve fiber

Cell body
Myelin sheath

Neuroglia

Normal          Abnormal

### RANGE OF OUTLOOKS IN MULTIPLE SCLEROSIS

Dead
Bedridden
Restricted
Mild
No obvious disease

Dead
Bedridden
Restricted
Mild
No obvious disease

Years   0    5    10    15    20    25    30

**Progress of multiple sclerosis**
Multiple sclerosis is characterized by periods when symptoms are present, alternating with remissions (when symptoms are mild or absent).

5 percent

10 percent

33 percent

Majority

## AFFECTED AREAS

Because the brain and spinal cord control all parts of the body, damage to these parts by multiple sclerosis may affect any function or any organ.

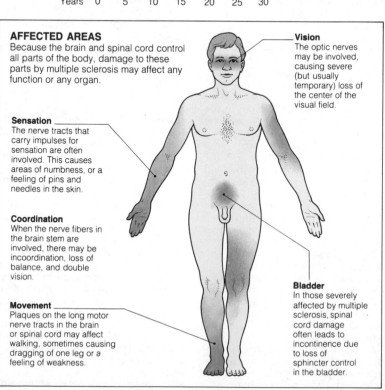

**Vision**
The optic nerves may be involved, causing severe (but usually temporary) loss of the center of the visual field.

**Sensation**
The nerve tracts that carry impulses for sensation are often involved. This causes areas of numbness, or a feeling of pins and needles in the skin.

**Coordination**
When the nerve fibers in the brain stem are involved, there may be incoordination, loss of balance, and double vision.

**Movement**
Plaques on the long motor nerve tracts in the brain or spinal cord may affect walking, sometimes causing dragging of one leg or a feeling of weakness.

**Bladder**
In those severely affected by multiple sclerosis, spinal cord damage often leads to incontinence due to loss of sphincter control in the bladder.

period of two to three weeks between infection and the appearance of symptoms. An affected person may spread the virus to others for about a week before and up to two weeks after symptoms appear. Most infections are acquired at school or from infected family members.

In the US, where many states require proof of mumps vaccination for school entry, the incidence has dropped markedly over the last 20 years, from a peak incidence of more than 185,000 cases in 1967 to a few thousand cases per year currently. In countries where immunization is not given routinely in early childhood, the infection remains common, affecting a large proportion of the population at some time between ages 5 and 10.

**SYMPTOMS AND COMPLICATIONS**

Many infected children have no symptoms or no more than mild sickness and discomfort in the region of the salivary glands (just inside the angle of the jaw). In more serious cases, the child first complains of pain in this region and has difficulty chewing; the glands on one or both sides then become swollen, painful, and tender. Fever, headache, and difficulty swallowing may develop, but the temperature falls after two to three days and the swelling subsides within a week to ten days. When only one side is affected, the second gland often swells as the first is subsiding.

An occasional complication is *meningitis*, which can cause headache, photophobia, drowsiness, fever, and stiff neck. However, these symptoms also resolve without long-term effects in most cases. A less common complication is *pancreatitis*, causing abdominal pain and vomiting.

In males after puberty, *orchitis* (inflammation of the testis) develops in about one quarter of cases. Only one testis is usually affected, becoming swollen, tender, and painful for two to four days. Subsequently, the affected testis shrinks to smaller than normal size. Uncommonly, both testes are affected; extremely rarely this can lead to sterility.

There is no evidence that mumps in pregnancy has any effect on the fetus.

**DIAGNOSIS AND TREATMENT**

Mumps is usually diagnosed from the patient's symptoms; the diagnosis may be confirmed by culturing the virus from saliva or urine or by measuring antibodies to mumps virus in the blood.

There is no specific treatment, but an affected child may be given

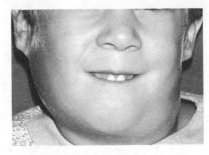

**Appearance of mumps**
The swelling, especially if present on both sides, may give the affected child a somewhat hamsterlike appearance.

*analgesics* (painkillers) and plenty to drink. In moderate to severe cases, the child may need to stay in bed during the first few days of the illness and should not go to school until symptoms have subsided.

For males with severe orchitis, a physician may sometimes prescribe a stronger painkiller, and *corticosteroid drugs* to reduce inflammation.

**IMMUNIZATION**

A safe and effective mumps vaccine is available and routinely given in the US to children in their second year, usually in combination with measles and rubella vaccines. The vaccine should not be given to children under 1, or to anyone with risk factors for vaccination (see *Immunization*).

Males who have already gone through puberty who have never been immunized against mumps or had the infection should avoid contact with any infected person. If symptoms of mumps do develop, passive immunization with antimumps *immunoglobulin* can provide some protection against the development of orchitis.

## Münchausen's syndrome

A form of chronic *factitious disorder* in which the sufferer complains of physical symptoms that are pretended or self-induced. Sufferers are not *malingering*, they simply want to play the patient role. Most afflicted people are repeatedly hospitalized for investigations and treatment.

Pain in the abdomen, bleeding, neurological symptoms (such as dizziness and blackouts), skin rashes, and fever are the usual complaints. Sufferers typically invent dramatic, but often plausible, false histories and, once in the hospital, behave in a disruptive manner. Many show evidence of self-injury or of previous treatment (such as numerous scars or detailed medical knowledge).

It is difficult to determine the causes of the disorder; when challenged, the sufferers deny any allegations of deception or immediately discharge themselves from the hospital. Treatment is aimed at protecting these people from unnecessary operations and treatments.

## Murmur

A sound caused by turbulent blood flow through the heart, as heard by a physician through a *stethoscope*. Murmurs are a separate phenomenon from other types of normal or abnormal *heart sounds*, which are caused mainly by sudden acceleration or deceleration of blood movement.

Heart murmurs are not necessarily a sign of disease, but an unusual sound is regarded as an indication of possible abnormality in the blood flow. Apart from "innocent" murmurs, the most common cause of extra blood turbulence is a disorder of the heart valves, such as stenosis (narrowing) or insufficiency (leakage) with regurgitation. Murmurs can also be caused by some types of congenital heart disease such as *septal defects* (holes in the heart) or *patent ductus arteriosus*, by *pericarditis* (inflammation of the membrane around the heart), or by other, rarer, conditions, such as a *myxoma* in a heart chamber.

By noting the location on the chest wall at which the murmur is best heard and the timing of the murmur in relation to the basic heart sounds, and by considering these factors in conjunction with other signs and symptoms, the physician can usually arrive at a diagnosis, which may be confirmed by *echocardiography*.

## Muscle

A structure composed of bundles of specialized cells capable of contraction and relaxation to create movement, both of the body itself in relation to the environment and of the organs within it. There are three different types of muscle in the body—skeletal, smooth, and cardiac.

**SKELETAL MUSCLE**

The largest part of the musculature consists of skeletal (voluntary) muscles; the body contains more than 600 such muscles.

Skeletal muscles are classified according to the type of action each muscle performs. An extensor muscle opens out a joint, a flexor closes it; an adductor muscle draws a part of the body inward, an abductor moves it outward; a levator raises it, a

M

## THE BODY'S MUSCLES

The most prominent muscles in the body are the skeletal muscles, which account for 40 to 45 percent of body weight. These muscles are called voluntary because they are under conscious control; some important voluntary muscles are indicated on the illustration below. Many internal organs, such as the heart and intestines, also consist partly or entirely of involuntary muscle, which is not under conscious control.

M

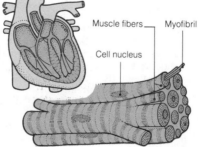

**Trapezius**
Draws shoulder backward and upward

**Deltoid**
Raises arm

**Gluteus maximus**
Extends thigh in walking and climbing

**Biceps femoris**
(hamstring)
Extends thigh or bends knee

**Gastrocnemius**
Bends knee in walking; extends foot in jumping

**Pectoralis major**
Draws arm forward and inward

**Biceps**
Bends arm at elbow

**Serratus anterior**
Draws shoulder blade forward; assists in raising arm and in pushing movements

**Obliquus externus**
Compresses abdominal contents

**Sartorius**
Bends thigh and knee; rotates thigh outward

**Quadriceps**
Bend thigh at the hips; straighten knee

### MUSCLE MOVEMENT
Contraction makes a muscle shorter and draws together the bones to which the muscle is attached.

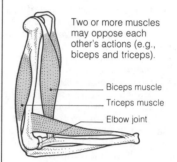

Two or more muscles may oppose each other's actions (e.g., biceps and triceps).

Biceps muscle
Triceps muscle
Elbow joint

Controlled movement at the elbow relies on coordinated relaxation and contraction of the biceps and triceps.

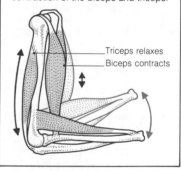

Triceps relaxes
Biceps contracts

### MUSCLE TYPES
Skeletal and cardiac muscles appear striped under the microscope, unlike smooth muscles.

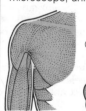
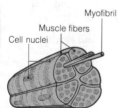

Myofibril
Muscle fibers
Cell nuclei

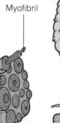

Muscle fibers
Myofibril
Cell nucleus

Separate cells
Cell nucleus

**Skeletal muscle**
Skeletal muscle consists of bundles of fibers (muscle cells), each containing contractile elements (myofibrils).

**Cardiac muscle**
Cardiac muscle contains short, branching cells that interconnect to help spread the signals that cause contraction.

**Smooth muscle**
Smooth muscle consists of more loosely woven, tapering cells. Contraction is slower than in other muscle types.

depressor lowers it; and constrictor or sphincter muscles surround and close body orifices.

Skeletal muscles are composed of groups of muscle fibers in an orderly arrangement.

A small muscle may be made up of only a few bundles of fibers, while the major muscles in the body (such as the gluteus maximus that forms the bulk of the buttock) are made up of hundreds of bundles. A muscle fiber is made up of even smaller longitudinal units called myofibrils, the basic working units of which are microscopic filaments called actin and myosin; these are proteins that control contraction.

Movement of the skeletal muscles is under the voluntary control of the brain. Each muscle fiber is supplied with a nerve ending that receives impulses from the brain. The nerve impulse stimulates the muscle by releasing a *neurotransmitter* called acetylcholine. This starts a chain of chemical and electrical events, involving sodium, potassium, and calcium ions, which results in the filaments of myosin sliding over the actin filaments in much the same way as an extendable ladder moves when it is closed. This movement of myosin over actin filaments causes the muscle to shorten in length.

Each muscle contains a set of specialized nerve fibers that registers the force of contraction; another set in the tendon gauges the stretch. The information received by these fibers is transmitted to the brain and is vital in limiting muscle action.

Skeletal muscle is maintained in partial contraction—called muscle tone. *Spasticity* is one form of abnormally increased muscle tone.

Skeletal muscle activity is affected by changes in chemical composition of the fluid surrounding the muscle cells. A fall in potassium ions causes muscle weakness; a decrease of calcium ions causes muscle spasm.

## DISORDERS OF MUSCLE

The most common muscle disorder is injury, followed by symptoms caused by a lack of blood supply to a muscle (including the heart). In addition, there are a number of other rarer disorders of muscle.

### GENETIC DISORDERS
The *muscular dystrophies* cause progressive weakness and disability. Some types appear at birth, some in infancy, and some develop as late as the fifth or sixth decade.

One type of *cardiomyopathy*, a general term for disease of the heart muscle, is inherited.

### INFECTION
The most important infection of muscle is *gangrene*, which may complicate deep wounds (especially those contaminated by soil). *Tetanus* is acquired in a similar way, causing widespread muscle spasm through the release of a powerful toxin.

Viruses (especially influenza B) may also infect muscles (causing *myalgia*), as may the organism causing *toxoplasmosis*. *Trichinosis* is an infestation of muscle with the worm TRICHINELLA SPIRILIS, which is acquired by eating undercooked meat (usually pork).

### INJURY
Muscle injuries, such as tears and *sprains*, are very common; they cause bleeding into the muscle tissue. Healing leads to formation of a scar in the muscle, which shortens its natural length. Blunt muscle injury may result in *hematoma* formation from bleeding into the muscle. Rarely, bone may form in the hematoma causing *myositis* ossificans.

### TUMORS
Primary muscle tumors may or may not be cancerous. Noncancerous tumors are called *myomas*, those affecting smooth muscle are *leiomyomas*, and those affecting skeletal muscle are rhabdomyomas. Myomas of the uterus (see *Fibroids*) are among the most common of all tumors. Cancerous tumors are called myosarcomas and are very rare; cancers of the skeletal muscle are known as *rhabdomyo-sarcomas*.

Secondary tumors, which spread from a primary site of cancer elsewhere in the body, very rarely involve muscle.

### HORMONAL AND METABOLIC DISORDERS
Muscle contraction depends on the maintenance of proper levels of sodium, potassium, and calcium in and around muscle cells. Any alteration in the concentration of these substances affects muscle function. For example, a severe drop in the level of potassium (hypokalemia) causes profound muscle weakness and may stop the heart. A drop in blood calcium (hypocalcemia) causes increased excitability of muscles and, occasionally, spasms.

Thyroid disease is often associated with muscle disorders, the most common being a swelling of the small muscles that move the eyes, causing a bulging eyeball (see *Exophthalmos*).

*Adrenal failure* causes general muscle weakness.

### IMPAIRED BLOOD SUPPLY
Muscles depend on a good blood supply for normal function. *Cramp* is usually caused by a lack of blood flow, sometimes associated with severe exertion. *Peripheral vascular disease*, which restricts the blood supply,

causes *claudication* (muscle pain on exercise). *Angina pectoris* (chest pain caused by lack of blood supply to heart muscle) occurs in *coronary heart disease*.

The *compartment syndrome* is pain in muscles as a result of swelling that limits the blood supply. It is brought on by injury or exercise, occurring often in athletes with well-developed muscles.

### POISONS AND DRUGS
Several toxic substances can damage muscle. They include alcohol, which can cause damage following a prolonged drinking bout. Other substances that may cause muscle damage include aminocaproic acid, chloroquine, clofibrate, emetine, and vincristine.

### AUTOIMMUNE DISORDERS
*Myasthenia gravis* is a disorder of transmission of nerve impulses to muscles; it usually begins by causing drooping of the eyelids and double vision. Other diseases with an autoimmune basis that may affect muscles are *lupus erythematosus*, *rheumatoid arthritis*, *scleroderma*, *sarcoidosis*, and *dermatomyositis*.

### INVESTIGATION
Muscle disorders are investigated by *EMG* (electromyography), which measures the response of muscles to electrical impulses, and by muscle biopsy.

M

## SMOOTH MUSCLE

This type of muscle is concerned with the movements of internal organs, such as *peristalsis* in the intestine and contractions of the uterus during childbirth. Many other parts of the body, such as the bronchi of the lungs, the bladder, and the walls of the blood vessels, also contain smooth muscle.

Smooth muscle is composed of long, spindle-shaped cells. In most hollow organs, these cells are arranged in bundles organized in an outer longitudinal layer and an inner circular one. However, the mechanism of contraction relies on the same sliding action of actin and myosin as in skeletal muscle.

The nerve supply to smooth muscle comes from the *autonomic nervous system*, which is not under conscious control. Hence, its alternative name—involuntary muscle. Nerves from the autonomic nervous system penetrate into the muscle. There, they divide into many branches from which the neurotransmitter is released to initiate the process that leads to contraction.

In addition to neurotransmitters, smooth muscle responds to a variety of hormones, to the stretch of individual muscle fibers, and to changes in the chemical composition of the fluid surrounding the fibers, such as oxygen levels and acidity.

## CARDIAC MUSCLE

This type of muscle, also called myocardium, is found only in the heart; it has unique properties that enable it to contract rhythmically about 100,000 times a day to propel blood through the circulatory system. The structure of cardiac muscle resembles that of skeletal muscle.

Contraction of cardiac muscle is stimulated by the autonomic nervous system, hormones, and stretching of the muscle fibers.

To act as an efficient pump, the muscles of the heart must contract in an orderly, regular manner. Separate muscle fibers are joined end to end by areas of extensive folds that allow contractions to be transmitted rapidly from one fiber to another. The stimulus for cardiac muscle contraction is initiated in an area of the right atrium (called the sinoatrial node), which stimulates a regular rate of contraction. Specialized conducting cells in cardiac muscle form a network capable of transmitting nerve impulses throughout the cardiac muscle fibers, spreading the contraction through both atria and then both ventricles alternately (see *Heart*).

# Muscle-relaxant drugs

## COMMON DRUGS

*Baclofen Carisoprodol*
*Cyclobenzaprine Dantrolene*
*Diazepam Methocarbamol Orphenadrine*

A group of drugs used to relieve *muscle spasm* and *spasticity*. They are often used in combination with an *analgesic* (painkiller) to relieve muscle stiffness caused by types of *arthritis*, back pain, or a disorder of the nervous system, such as *stroke* or *cerebral palsy*. Muscle-relaxant drugs are occasionally used to relieve muscle rigidity caused by injury.

## HOW THEY WORK

With the exception of *dantrolene*, muscle-relaxant drugs partially block nerve signals from the brain and spinal cord that stimulate different muscles to contract.

Dantrolene acts directly on muscles by interfering with the chemical activity in muscle cells necessary for muscle contraction.

## POSSIBLE ADVERSE EFFECTS

Because muscle-relaxant drugs reduce the strength of muscle contraction, they may cause weakness that is noticed when performing certain activities. Some muscle relaxants affect the brain and spinal cord, causing drowsiness. In rare cases, dantrolene causes liver damage.

# Muscle spasm

Abnormal rigidity of a muscle. Causes include brain damage due to *stroke*, *cerebral palsy*, and severe *head injury*; brain disorders, such as *Parkinson's disease*; and pressure on a nerve from a *disk prolapse*. Other causes include muscle *strain* or injury.

# Muscular dystrophy

An inherited muscle disorder of unknown cause in which there is slow but progressive degeneration of muscle fibers. Different forms are classified according to the age at which the symptoms appear, the rate at which the disease progresses, and the way in which it is inherited. (See box at right for main types.)

## INCIDENCE

All forms of muscular dystrophy are rare. Duchenne muscular dystrophy is the most common type, affecting about one or two in 10,000 boys. It is inherited through a recessive, sex-linked gene (see *Genetic disorders*) so that only males are affected and only females can pass on the disease.

## DIAGNOSIS

Often the diagnosis is suggested to the physician from observing the patient, but tests are needed for confirmation. A blood test may be performed to look for high levels of certain enzymes released from the damaged muscle cells. A test of electrical activity in the

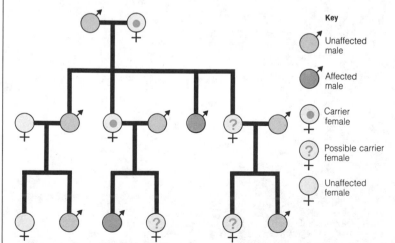

**DUCHENNE MUSCULAR DYSTROPHY: A TYPICAL FAMILY TREE**

**Key**

- Unaffected male
- Affected male
- Carrier female
- Possible carrier female
- Unaffected female

Affected males always inherit the gene for the disorder from their mothers, who are carriers of the gene, although unaffected themselves. About half the sons of carriers are affected; the other sons are neither affected nor carriers. The daughters of carriers have a 50 percent chance of being carriers themselves; complex blood tests provide the only means of knowing whether or not a certain daughter (or granddaughter) is a muscular dystrophy carrier.

muscles (see *EMG*) and muscle *biopsy* may be performed.

### TREATMENT AND OUTLOOK

There is no effective treatment for muscular dystrophy. Affected children should be active for as long as possible to keep the healthy muscles in good condition. The children should not be allowed to become overweight; surgery to the heel cords may assist walking in some cases. The long-term outlook varies.

### PREVENTION

Parents or siblings of an affected child should receive *genetic counseling*. Carriers of sex-linked forms of muscular dystrophy (see box, previous page) can be detected because their blood contains high levels of a particular enzyme.

It is now possible to diagnose some types of muscular dystrophy before birth by *chorionic villus sampling* or *amniocentesis*.

## Musculoskeletal

Relating to muscle and/or bone. The musculoskeletal system is the bony skeleton of the body and the hundreds of muscles that are attached to it.

## Mushroom poisoning

There are many species of poisonous mushrooms and toadstools in the US, but only some of them cause poisoning. Many of the others, although poisonous, have an unpleasant taste and thus are unlikely to be eaten in significant amounts.

### TYPES, SYMPTOMS, AND TREATMENT

Most fatal cases of mushroom poisoning in the US are caused by AMANITA PHALLOIDES (the death cap) and its relatives. This mushroom looks innocuous, bearing a resemblance to the edible field mushroom. However, there are some clear differences. The death cap grows in deciduous woods (mainly beech and oak), has a yellow-olive colored cap, and, most importantly, has white gills on the underside of its cap (not pink-brown as on the edible field mushroom).

The death cap and one or two related species such as AMANITA VIROSA (destroying angel) contain highly poisonous peptides called amanitins, which attack cells in the lining of the small intestine, the liver, and, occasionally, the kidneys. Symptoms such as severe abdominal pain, vomiting, and diarrhea usually develop eight to 14 hours after eating the mushroom. Later, there may be liver enlargement and jaundice; about 10 to 15 percent of victims die of liver failure (this stage of the poisoning resembles acute viral hepatitis). There is no effective antidote. Treatment consists of supportive measures in the hospital. For those who survive the poisoning (after about one week), recovery is usually fairly rapid.

Another species, AMANITA MUSCARIA, or fly agaric, is very similar in shape to the death cap but has a red cap flecked with white. Symptoms of poisoning, which appear within 20 minutes to two hours, may include drowsiness, visual disturbances, delirium, muscle tremors, and nausea and vomiting. Treatment of this type of mushroom poisoning, and of other types in which symptoms develop rapidly, is by gastric lavage (see *Lavage, gastric*) and the administration of activated charcoal. Full recovery usually occurs within 24 hours. Fatal poisoning by fly agaric has never been reported in the US.

"Magic" mushrooms are a species containing the hallucinogenic substance psilocybin. In addition to hallucinations, they may cause high fever in children, which requires medical attention. The effects usually subside within four to six hours; occasionally they persist longer.

## Mutagen

Any physical or chemical agent that, when applied to a group of living cells, increases the rate of *mutation* in those cells. A mutation is a change in the genetic material within a cell, which,

M

### TYPES OF MUSCULAR DYSTROPHY

| | | |
|---|---|---|
| **Duchenne muscular dystrophy** | In this type, the child is slow in learning to sit up and walk, and does so much later than normal. The condition is rarely diagnosed before the age of 3, but progresses rapidly. Affected children tend to walk with a waddle and have difficulty climbing stairs. In getting up from the floor, the child "climbs up his legs," pushing his hands against his ankles, knees, and thighs. Sometimes there | is curvature of the spine. Despite their weakness, the muscles (especially those in the calves) appear bulky; this is because wasted muscle is replaced by fat. By about age 12, affected children are no longer able to walk; few survive their teen years, usually dying from a chest infection or heart failure. Affected boys often have below-average intelligence. |
| **Becker's muscular dystrophy** | This type produces the same symptoms as the Duchenne type, but starts later in childhood and progresses much more | slowly. Patients often reach the age of 50. Both types of dystrophy have sex-linked inheritance. |
| **Myotonic dystrophy** | This form affects muscles of the hands and feet. Infants are floppy and slow to develop. The main feature is that the muscles contract strongly but do not relax easily. Myotonic dystrophy | is associated with cataracts in middle age, baldness, mental retardation, and endocrine problems. The condition has an autosomal dominant pattern of inheritance. |
| **Limb-girdle muscular dystrophy** | This type takes different forms. It starts in late childhood or early adult life, and progression is slow. The muscles of the hips and shoulders are mainly | affected. Other nerve and muscle conditions must be eliminated before this form of dystrophy can be diagnosed confidently. |
| **Facioscapulohumeral muscular dystrophy** | This form usually appears first between the ages of 10 and 40; it affects only the muscles of the upper arms, shoulder girdle, and face. It is inherited in an autosomal | dominant pattern. In this form of muscular dystrophy, progression of the weakness is slow, and severe disablement is rare. |

under certain circumstances, can give rise to a cancer or a hereditary disease.

The most important mutagens are ionizing radiation and some chemicals. The former includes X rays and various types of emission from nuclear explosions, radioactive fallout, and leaks from nuclear reactors, including gamma rays and alpha and beta particles (see *Radiation hazards*). Similar types of radiation are also emitted (at a low intensity) from rocks and from the sky (cosmic rays).

Many chemical *carcinogens* are thought to cause cancers by altering the genetic material within cells, thus acting as mutagens. Chief among them are chemicals in tobacco smoke.

## Mutation

A change in the genetic material within a living cell—that is, in the *DNA*, the main constituent of a cell's *chromosomes* that provides the coded instructions for the cell's activities.

Many mutations are neutral or harmless; some are harmful, giving rise to cancers, birth defects, and hereditary diseases. Very rarely, a mutation may be beneficial.

### CAUSES AND TYPES

A mutation results from a fault in the copying of a cell's DNA to its daughter cells when the cell divides. One of the offspring cells inherits some faulty DNA, and the fault is copied each time the cell divides, creating a population of cells containing the altered DNA.

The change may be a point mutation, affecting only a small part of a section of DNA (called a *gene*). This type may lead to production of defective enzymes or other proteins in the affected cells, thus disrupting their activities. In other cases, entire chromosomes or bits of chromosomes are deleted, added, or rearranged in affected cells, which can produce greater disruptive effects.

The term *mutagen* refers to any physical or chemical agent that makes mutations more likely. The most important mutagens are types of high-energy radiation, and certain chemicals, including some *carcinogens* (cancer-inducing agents).

### EFFECTS

The effects of a harmful mutation depend on whether the affected cell is a "germ" cell in an ovary or testis (capable of giving rise to an egg or sperm) or whether it is one of the other cells in the body (somatic cells).

A mutated somatic cell can, at worst, multiply to form a group of abnormal cells within a particular body region. Often these cells die out, are destroyed by the body's immune system, or have only a minor local effect. Sometimes, however, they may form the basis for a tumor.

A mutation in a germ cell can have a dramatically different effect. It may be passed on, via egg or sperm, to a child, who then carries the mutation in all of his or her cells. This may lead to an obvious birth defect or abnormality in body chemistry. Furthermore, the child may pass on the mutation to some of his or her descendants. *Genetic disorders* (such as *hemophilia* and *achondroplasia*) stem originally from point mutations that have occurred to the germ cell of a parent, grandparent, or more distant ancestor. Some of these mutations occur frequently; about one third of all cases of hemophilia are caused by new mutations. *Chromosomal abnormalities* (such as *Down's syndrome*) generally result from mutations in the formation of a parental egg or sperm.

### PREVENTION

Some mutations are unavoidable, occurring by chance or as the result of natural background radiation from the sky and from radioactivity in rocks. This background radiation causes random mutations in the population.

Minimizing any further risk of a mutation depends on avoiding known mutagens. It is particularly important for people exposed to radiation in the course of their work to have their exposure closely monitored to ensure that it does not exceed safe limits (see *Radiation hazards*). Younger people and those of reproductive age should have their reproductive organs shielded when undergoing X rays or radiation therapy.

Radioactive leaks or explosions from nuclear reactors can cause a rise in mutation rates that affects large populations. This may lead to an increase in the incidence of various cancers and birth defects in succeeding generations.

The chances of a mutation can also be lessened by avoiding exposure to carcinogens (which are a class of mutagen), the most obvious of which are the chemicals in tobacco smoke.

### BENEFICIAL MUTATIONS

Very rarely, a mutation occurs in a germ cell that confers a survival advantage in the face of some environmental stress. People who inherit this mutation tend to survive longer than their peers; some of their children in turn inherit the mutation and pass it on to succeeding generations. Such mutations tend to become more common in a population over many generations as long as the original environmental stress persists.

An example is the mutation that causes sickle cell trait. Carrying this mutation protects against malaria, so it enhances a child's survival chances where malaria is prevalent. The mutation is prevalent in Africa (along with malaria) and affects many people of African origin. A double dose of the mutation (inheriting it from both parents) can lead to *sickle cell anemia*.

## Mutism

Refusal or inability to speak. Mutism may occur as a symptom of severe *manic-depressive illness*, catatonic *schizophrenia*, and a rare form of *conversion disorder*. The term may also be applied to those who have taken a vow of silence for religious reasons.

Elective mutism describes a rare childhood disorder usually starting before age 5. The child understands language and speaks properly, but refuses to speak most of the time, preferring to use nods or gestures. A shy, withdrawn personality and anxiety over leaving home for school are important factors, but mild mental retardation or language problems may be the cause. This condition rarely lasts more than a few months.

Akinetic mutism describes a state of inert passivity that is caused by certain deep-seated tumors of the brain or by *hydrocephalus*. Though conscious and able to follow movements with their eyes, these people are incontinent, require feeding, and respond at most with a whispered "yes" or "no."

Treatment of mutism depends on the underlying cause.

## Myalgia

The medical term for muscle pain. Myalgia is common in viral illnesses (such as influenza) and also occurs in a number of rheumatic disorders, such as *rheumatoid arthritis*, systemic *lupus erythematosus*, and *polymyalgia rheumatica*. Myalgia is the main symptom of *polymyositis* and *dermatomyositis*, disorders that cause inflammation of muscle tissue.

## Myasthenia gravis

A disorder in which the muscles become weak and tire easily. The eyes, face, throat, and limb muscles are most commonly affected. Typically, the sufferer has drooping eyelids, a blank facial expression, and weak, hesitant speech.

## CAUSES AND INCIDENCE

Myasthenia gravis is an *autoimmune disorder* in which, for unknown reasons, the body's *immune system* attacks and gradually destroys the receptors in muscles that are responsible for picking up nerve impulses. As a result, affected muscles fail to respond, or respond only weakly, to nerve impulses.

Myasthenia gravis is a rare disease; two to five new cases per 100,000 people are diagnosed annually. It affects more women than men (in a ratio of 3 to 2). Although it can occur at any age, myasthenia gravis usually appears between the ages of 20 and 30 in women and 50 and 70 in men.

## SYMPTOMS AND SIGNS

The disease may develop suddenly or gradually. It is extremely variable in the way it affects different people and in how it affects the same person from day to day. The affected muscles become worse with use but may recover completely with rest. Symptom-free periods typically alternate with relapses of the condition.

The eye muscles are the most commonly affected, and most sufferers have drooping eyelids and double vision. Weakness is also common in the muscles of the face, throat, larynx (voice box), and neck. This causes difficulty speaking, so that the voice becomes weak, hoarse, nasal, and slurred toward the end of a conversation. Chewing and swallowing become increasingly difficult as a meal progresses, so that the sufferer may choke or regurgitate food through the nose. Sometimes the jaw must be supported to prevent it from hanging.

In some people, the arm and leg muscles are also affected, producing difficulty combing the hair and climbing stairs. In severe cases of myasthenia gravis, respiratory muscles in the chest may be weakened, causing breathing difficulty.

Infection, stress, menstruation, medications, and other factors can exacerbate the condition.

Abnormalities in the thymus gland are present in about three quarters of affected people and, in about 10 to 15 percent of them, a *thymoma* (tumor of the thymus gland) is found.

## DIAGNOSIS

The disease is diagnosed by a physical examination, the patient's history, and various tests. The most commonly used diagnostic test involves the injection of a drug called edrophonium into a vein. Within a minute, power is temporarily restored

to the weak muscles. Electromyography (see *EMG*), which detects muscle weakness by measuring the muscle's electrical activity, and blood tests that reveal the presence of certain antibodies may also be carried out.

In some patients, mainly those over 40, *CT scanning* may be performed to look for a thymoma.

## TREATMENT

In mild cases of myasthenia gravis, regular medication with drugs to facilitate the transmission of nerve impulses to the muscles is often enough to restore the patient's condition to near normal.

In severe myasthenia gravis, thymectomy (removal of the thymus gland) often considerably improves, and sometimes cures, the condition. Otherwise, regular exchanges of the patient's antibody-containing plasma for antibody-free plasma may be carried out; high doses of *corticosteroid drugs*, which block the immune process, may be given.

## OUTLOOK

In mild cases the sufferer is able to live a comparatively normal life. In a minority of patients, progression of the disease cannot be halted and paralysis of the throat and respiratory muscles may lead to death.

## Mycetoma

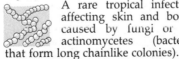 A rare tropical infection affecting skin and bone, caused by fungi or by actinomycetes (bacteria that form long chainlike colonies).

The infection is usually confined to one limb and can be highly disfiguring. It produces a hard swelling covered by the openings of multiple drainage channels, through which pus is discharged. The disease organisms form into visible "grains," which are found in the discharge.

Antibiotic drugs are the main treatment if the disease is caused by actinomycetes. Mycetoma caused by fungal infections may be difficult to treat with drugs; surgical removal of diseased tissue may be necessary.

## Mycology

The study of *fungi* and *fungal infections.*

## Mycoplasma

Any of a group of microorganisms that are the smallest capable of free existence. Mycoplasmas are about the same size as viruses and, like viruses, have no cell wall. However, unlike viruses, mycoplasmas can reproduce outside living cells.

Most types of mycoplasma are harmless to humans, although many cause respiratory diseases in animals such as cattle, sheep, and poultry. One of the species, MYCOPLASMA PNEUMONIAE, causes a special form of *pneumonia* (primary atypical pneumonia) in humans. The pneumonia is treated effectively with antibiotics such as tetracyclines.

## Mycosis

Any disease caused by a fungus. (See *Fungi*; *Fungal infections*.)

## Mycosis fungoides

A type of *lymphoma* (cancerous spread of lymphoid tissue) that primarily affects the skin of the buttocks, back, or shoulders but can also occur in other sites. The cause of this rare disorder is unknown.

The mildest form appears as a red, scaly, nonitching rash; it may spread slowly or remain unaltered for many years. In the more severe forms of the disease, thickened patches of skin and ulcers may develop and lymph glands may enlarge.

## DIAGNOSIS, TREATMENT, AND OUTLOOK

A skin *biopsy* (removal of a small sample of tissue for microscopic examination) is carried out. In mild cases, patients are treated with *PUVA* (*psoralen drugs* plus long-wave ultraviolet light treatment in the A range) or nitrogen mustard applied to the skin. In more severe cases, *anticancer drugs* may be needed.

## Mydriasis

Dilation (widening) of the pupil of the eye. Mydriasis, which occurs naturally in the dark, also occurs if a person is emotionally aroused, after the use of eye drops (such as atropine), and after consumption of alcohol. Adie's syndrome is a benign condition in which one pupil constricts slowly in response to light. The condition may last for years.

## Myectomy

Surgical removal of part or all of a muscle. Myectomy may be performed to alter the power of an eye muscle to correct *strabismus* (squint), or to remove a fibroid in an operation called a *myomectomy*. Myectomy is also part of the treatment of severely injured and infected muscles.

## Myel-

A prefix that denotes a relationship to bone marrow (as in myeloma, a tumor consisting of bone marrow cells) or to

**M**

the spinal cord (as in myelitis, inflammation of the spinal cord). The prefix myelo- is synonymous with myel-.

## Myelin

The fatty material, composed of lipid (a fat) and protein, that forms a protective sheath around some types of nerve fiber. Myelin gives the characteristic appearance to the white matter of the brain, which is composed largely of myelinated nerve fibers.

In addition to having a protective function, myelin acts as an electrical insulator, thereby increasing the efficiency of nerve impulse conduction.

Abnormal breakdown of myelin is called *demyelination*. It occurs in some diseases of the nervous system, notably *multiple sclerosis*.

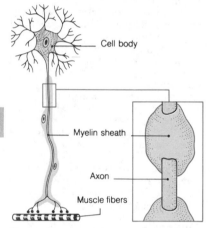

**The myelin nerve sheath**
The axon is the long conducting fiber of a nerve. To transmit impulses, each nerve requires an insulating myelin sheath.

## Myelitis

Inflammation of the spinal cord. Myelitis may be the result of a viral infection—for example, *poliomyelitis* (commonly called polio), *measles*, or *herpes simplex*. The illness starts suddenly with headache, fever, neck stiffness, and pain in the back and limbs, which are followed in some cases by muscle pain and weakness, and eventually paralysis.

Transverse myelitis is a type of myelitis in which there is inflammation of the spinal cord around the middle of the back. It may follow a viral illness but often occurs without obvious cause. Common symptoms are back pain and gradual paralysis of the legs. Many people recover, but some are left with spastic paralysis of the involved limbs.

## Myelocele

A protrusion of the spinal cord and its meninges (protective coverings) under the skin due to a congenital defect in the vertebral column (see *Spina bifida*).

## Myelography

X-ray examination of the spinal cord, nerves, and other tissues within the spinal canal after injection of a substance opaque to X rays.

### WHY IT IS DONE

In the past, myelography was often performed to examine the lower spinal nerves when a disk prolapse was suspected; it was also important in diagnosing tumors of the spinal cord, and in looking for damaged nerves after certain injuries. The procedure is being replaced today by newer imaging techniques, such as *CT scanning* and *MRI*.

### HOW IT IS DONE

The patient lies facedown on the X-ray table. Using local anesthesia, a *lumbar puncture* is performed; X-ray control is used to guide a fine needle into the fluid-filled space that surrounds the spinal cord and spinal nerves. A small sample of fluid is withdrawn for testing, and the radiopaque dye is introduced. By tilting the patient headdown, the dye can be moved up the spinal canal, and X-ray pictures are taken of areas where damage is suspected. The procedure usually takes 15 to 20 minutes. Afterward, the patient must lie down for a few hours with the head slightly raised.

## Myeloma, multiple

See *Multiple myeloma*.

## Myelomeningocele

See *Myelocele*.

## Myelopathy

A term that refers to any disease of the *spinal cord* or of the bone marrow, such as *multiple myeloma* or *leukemia*.

## Myelosclerosis

An increase of fibrous tissue within the bone marrow. It is also known as osteosclerosis or myelofibrosis. Myelosclerosis may occur without any obvious cause (primary myelosclerosis) or may result from some other bone marrow disease (such as *polycythemia* or chronic myeloid *leukemia*). The ability of the bone marrow to produce blood components is impaired. However, this function can be partly taken over by the spleen and the liver.

Primary myelosclerosis is a disease of middle age with a gradual onset. The main symptoms are those of *anemia*, which is caused by impaired red blood cell production by the bone marrow. Enlargement of the spleen, night sweats, itching, loss of appetite, and weight loss are other common symptoms of myelosclerosis. In secondary myelosclerosis, there may be other symptoms connected with the underlying disease.

### TREATMENT

Treatment of primary myelosclerosis is aimed at the relief of symptoms, mainly through blood transfusions. Anticancer drugs are of little or no use. Only half of patients survive for more than three years, and acute leukemia develops in a small number.

In secondary myelosclerosis, treatment is of the underlying cause.

## Myiasis

An infestation of the skin, deeper tissue, or intestines by fly larvae. Myiasis is primarily restricted to the tropical regions of the world.

### TYPES AND SYMPTOMS

In Africa, the tumbu fly lays eggs on clothing left outside to dry; the larvae that hatch from these eggs penetrate the skin to cause boillike swellings. Various other flies may lay eggs in open wounds, on the skin, or in the ears or nose. Sometimes the larvae penetrate deeply into the tissues, causing considerable destruction. Intestinal infestation can occur after eating contaminated food.

### PREVENTION AND TREATMENT

Myiasis can largely be prevented by keeping flies away from food, by covering open wounds, and, in Africa, by thoroughly ironing clothes dried outdoors.

Cutaneous myiasis is treated by placing drops of oil over the swelling caused by the larva. The oil suffocates the larva, which is forced to come to the surface and can be removed with a needle. Infestation in deeper tissues may require surgical treatment. Intestinal myiasis can be adequately treated with a laxative.

## Myo-

A prefix that denotes a relationship to muscle (as in myocarditis, inflammation of the heart muscle).

## Myocardial infarction

Popularly known as a heart attack, sudden death of part of the heart muscle characterized, in most cases,

# FEATURES OF MYOCARDIAL INFARCTION

Myocardial infarction, in which an area of heart muscle is deprived of blood supply and suffers tissue death as a result, is a major cause of death in developed countries. Atherosclerosis of the coronary arteries is the cause in most cases of myocardial infarction.

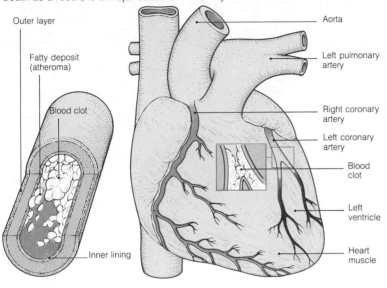

Outer layer

Fatty deposit (atheroma)

Blood clot

Inner lining

Aorta

Left pulmonary artery

Right coronary artery

Left coronary artery

Blood clot

Left ventricle

Heart muscle

### Atherosclerosis

Like all other arteries, the coronary arteries may be affected by atherosclerosis. Patchy plaques of atheroma develop on the inner lining of the arteries, restricting the blood flow and encouraging the formation of blood clots. The clotting results in a sudden stoppage of blood flow to the heart.

## OUTLOOK AFTER AN ATTACK

Myocardial infarction is fatal within 20 days in about one third of cases, and another 3 to 12 percent of patients die between 20 days and one year of the attack. Some further risk persists for several years, but a significant number of patients (about 30 percent) are still alive 10 years after an attack.

### FATALITY RATES

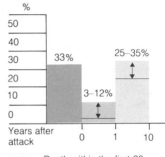

%

50
40
30
20
10
0

33%

3–12%

25–35%

Years after attack

0    1    10

Death within the first 20 days after the attack

Death between 20 days and 1 year after the attack

Death between 1 year and 10 years after the attack

M

### PAIN

Many victims of myocardial infarction have a history of angina pectoris, in which the chest pain is relieved by rest. The pain of infarction usually comes on suddenly, and ranges from a tight ache to intense crushing agony. It lasts for 30 minutes or more, and is not relieved by rest.

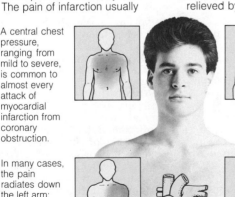

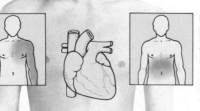

A central chest pressure, ranging from mild to severe, is common to almost every attack of myocardial infarction from coronary obstruction.

In many cases, the pain radiates down the left arm; it may cause a sensation of weakness in the arm muscles.

In some cases, pain radiates up into the jaw and through to the back. Sometimes, it occurs only in these places.

More rarely, pain may be felt in the upper abdomen. If it occurs only here, it may be mistaken for another disorder.

### RISK FACTORS

Uncontrollable factors include a family history of heart disease, old age, and being male.

Habitual cigarette smokers have a substantially increased risk of dying from myocardial infarction.

High blood pressure is a major risk factor, and the risk increases the higher the pressure.

The risk of atherosclerosis and coronary heart disease increases dramatically in those who are more than 30 percent overweight.

A raised blood cholesterol content (for which there may be a genetic tendency) increases the risk. A high-fat diet is also a factor.

Physical inactivity is also a major risk factor.

by severe unremitting chest pain. Each year in the US about 1 million people have a heart attack; attacks are fatal in about one third of cases and are the single most common cause of death in developed countries.

Men are more likely to suffer heart attacks than women, smokers more than nonsmokers, and the children of someone who has died of a heart attack are more likely to die from this cause. Other risk factors include increased age, unhealthy diet, stress, obesity, and disorders such as *hypertension* (high blood pressure), *diabetes mellitus*, and *hyperlipidemia*.

### SYMPTOMS AND COMPLICATIONS

The characteristic symptom is sudden pain in the center of the chest (see box on previous page). The victim may also be short of breath, restless, and apprehensive, have cold clammy skin, feel nauseated or vomit, or lose consciousness.

In mild cases, pain and other symptoms are slight or do not develop at all (in which case the attack is known as a silent infarct). The episode passes unnoticed and may be discovered only by subsequent tests.

Damage to the heart muscle may be so severe that it leads immediately to *heart failure* (reduced pumping efficiency of the heart). *Arrhythmias* (abnormal heart rhythms) are common. Most people who die of a myocardial infarction do so within the first few hours due to a type of arrhythmia called ventricular fibrillation, which seriously interferes with the pumping action. However, if the person can be brought to a hospital, arrhythmias can be controlled with drugs or electrical *defibrillation*.

Possible long-term complications include damage to the mitral valve, leading to *mitral insufficiency*, or the development of a weak area in the wall of the heart or in the muscle dividing the two sides of the heart. Complications may require surgery.

### DIAGNOSIS

The diagnosis is made from the patient's history and from special tests. Those performed immediately include *ECG* and the measurement of certain enzymes released into the blood from damaged heart muscle. Emergency coronary artery *angiography* may be performed if surgery is being considered.

### TREATMENT

If someone is thought to be having a heart attack, a physician or ambulance should be called immediately. Initial treatment may include strong

analgesics (painkillers) and *oxygen therapy*. *Diuretic drugs* may be given to treat heart failure, which can lead to accumulation of fluid in the lungs. Intravenous fluids may need to be given for shock, and *antiarrhythmic drugs* may be given to control arrhythmias. *Beta-blocker drugs* are given in some cases to reduce the risk of further muscle damage.

In many hospitals, patients who arrive within three to six hours of a heart attack are now treated with *thrombolytic drugs* to dissolve any blood clot. Other new methods of treatment include *angioplasty* (widening of narrowed coronary arteries), which may follow the thrombolytic treatment. *Coronary artery bypass* surgery may be considered.

In the past, it was recommended that patients rest in bed for two weeks or more following an attack. Today, patients are encouraged to be out of bed within four or five days.

It is increasingly common for heart attack patients to be supervised in special hospital coronary care units. The nursing and medical staff are trained to recognize and institute early treatment for arrhythmias, and many patients find the environment reassuring. However, some specialists believe coronary care units are actually more stressful and prefer that some patients, particularly the very elderly, be cared for elsewhere in the hospital or at home.

### OUTLOOK

Anyone who has suffered a heart attack has an increased risk of suffering another one in the following few years. The chances of surviving for many years can be improved by attention to risk factors (see table on previous page).

It is important for patients to have their conditions assessed by their physicians at regular intervals for life.

## Myocarditis

Inflammation of the heart muscle. The diagnosis of myocarditis is sometimes made after death when a young person has died unexpectedly during vigorous exercise. In such cases the pathologist finds evidence of inflammation, which is usually assumed to be due to a virus infection sometimes preceded by a sore throat or a cold. Myocarditis is a feature of *rheumatic fever*, which is rare today. It may also, in rare cases, be caused by drugs or radiation therapy.

People with virus infections affecting the lungs often have mild myocar-

ditis, which may be detected only by an *ECG*. Rarely, the inflammation causes a serious disturbance of the heart beat, breathlessness, chest pain, *heart failure* (reduced pumping efficiency), and cardiac arrest leading to death. Acute *pericarditis* (inflammation of the outer lining of the heart) often accompanies myocarditis.

Most cases clear up without treatment, although occasionally *corticosteroid drugs* are prescribed to reduce inflammation. It is generally believed that exercise is dangerous for people with myocarditis; most physicians recommend that exercise be avoided until a patient's electrocardiogram results have returned to normal. Anyone with symptoms of a viral infection (such as a sore throat) should avoid strenuous exercise to reduce the risk of myocarditis developing.

In Central and South America, the most common cause of myocarditis is the parasitic infection *Chagas' disease*. Many years after the initial infection, the parasitic organisms can cause extensive damage to the heart muscle, leading to progressive and often fatal heart failure.

## Myoclonus

Rapid, uncontrollable jerks or spasm of a muscle or muscles that occur at rest or during movement. Myoclonus may be associated with disease of nerves and muscles. It may occur during an epileptic seizure (see *Epilepsy*) or as a symptom of a brain disorder such as *encephalitis* (inflammation of the brain).

Myoclonus also occurs in healthy people, an example being the limb jump that is sometimes experienced just before falling asleep.

## Myofacial pain disorder

See *Temporomandibular joint syndrome*.

## Myoglobin

The oxygen-carrying pigment in muscles. It consists of a combination of iron and protein, and gives muscles their red color. Like *hemoglobin* (the oxygen-carrying pigment in red blood cells), myoglobin takes up and then stores oxygen, which it releases when the muscle tissues are in need of oxygen to contract.

Myoglobinuria is the presence of myoglobin in the urine. Small amounts of myoglobin in the urine may occur when taking prolonged, vigorous exercise. However, severe myoglobinuria is usually caused by the release of myoglobin from a large area of damaged muscle (which can occur in *crush syndrome*, for instance) and may cause *renal failure*.

## Myoma

A noncancerous tumor of muscle. The most common type is a *leiomyoma*, which affects the smooth muscle of the intestine, uterus, and stomach.

## Myomectomy

Surgical removal of a *myoma* (a noncancerous tumor of muscle). The term is commonly applied to the removal of *fibroids* of the uterus.

## Myopathy

A disease of muscle, usually degenerative (see *Muscle* disorders box), but sometimes caused by chemical poisoning, by a drug side effect, or by a chronic disorder of the *immune system*. A myopathy is not caused by disease of the nervous system. An example is *muscular dystrophy*.

## Myopia

An error of *refraction* in which near objects can be seen clearly while those in the distance appear blurred. Commonly known as nearsightedness, myopia is caused by the eye being too long from front to back. As a result,

the corneal lens focuses images of distant objects in front of the retina.

Myopia, which tends to be inherited, usually appears around puberty and increases progressively until the early 20s, when it stabilizes. Myopia that starts in early childhood often progresses into adult life, and may become very severe.

If myopia is detected during a *vision test*, *glasses* or *contact lenses* may be prescribed to reduce the focusing power of the cornea.

## Myositis

Inflammation of muscle tissues that causes pain, tenderness, and weakness. Types of myositis include *pleurodynia* (a viral infection affecting muscles around the rib cage), myositis ossificans (in which the damaged muscle is replaced by bone), *polymyositis* (inflammation of muscles throughout the body), and *dermatomyositis* (inflammation of muscles and the presence of a rash). Polymyositis and dermatomyositis are rare *autoimmune disorders*.

## Myotomy

A procedure that involves cutting into a muscle. An example is pyloromyotomy—cutting into the muscle surrounding the lower end of the stomach to treat *pyloric stenosis* (narrowing of the stomach's exit).

## Myotonia

A rare symptom that describes the inability of a muscle to relax after the need for contraction has passed. Myotonia occurs primarily in two neurological diseases. Myotonia congenita is an inherited condition in which muscle stiffness starts during infancy and usually improves as the person grows older. In myotonic dystrophy, myotonia is combined with muscle weakness. Drugs may help reduce myotonia.

## Myringitis

Inflammation of the eardrum. Myringitis occurs, to some degree, in every case of *otitis media*.

## Myringoplasty

Surgical closure of a perforation (hole) in the eardrum (see *Eardrum, perforated*) by means of a tissue graft. Myringoplasty is done to improve hearing and, sometimes, to stop a recurrent discharge from the ear. The graft material is usually muscle fascia (fibrous lining) taken from the temple or the thigh.

## Myringotomy

A surgical opening made through the eardrum to allow drainage of the middle-ear cavity.

**WHY IT IS DONE**

Myringotomy is usually performed on children to treat persistent *middle-ear effusion*, in which a sticky secretion fills the middle-ear cavity. The fluid causes hearing loss, which may become permanent if the condition is not treated.

Before the advent of antibiotics, myringotomy was performed to treat acute *otitis media* (middle-ear infection) by releasing the pus and thereby relieving pressure on the eardrum.

**HOW IT IS DONE**

Using a general anesthetic, a small incision is made in the eardrum and most of the fluid is removed by suction. At the same time, a small tube may be inserted in the hole to allow any remaining and subsequently produced fluid to drain into the outer ear. In most cases the child can leave the hospital the following day. The tube usually falls out a few months later as the hole in the eardrum closes. If the condition has not cleared up, a second operation may be required to insert another tube.

## Myxedema

A condition in which there is thickening and coarsening of the skin and other body tissues (most noticeable in the face, where the lips become swollen and the nose thickened). Other symptoms usually include weight gain, hair loss, sensitivity to cold, and mental dullness. Myxedema results from *hypothyroidism* and is most common in adults (especially women) over 40. The term myxedema is sometimes used interchangeably with adult hypothyroidism.

## Myxoma

A benign, jellylike tumor composed of soft mucous material and loose fibrous strands. Myxomas usually occur singly, and may grow very large. They usually occur under the skin (typically in the limbs or neck), but may also develop in the abdomen, bladder, or bone. Very rarely, a myxoma may grow inside the heart, which can lead to the formation of thrombi (blood clots) and obstruct blood flow through the heart. In most cases, a myxoma can be successfully removed by surgery. Myxomatosis is a highly infectious viral disease of rabbits in which many myxomas develop throughout the rabbit's body; this disease does not affect humans.

---

**THE CAUSE OF MYOPIA**

Myopia is caused by the combined power of the cornea and lens being too great in relation to the length of the eyeball.

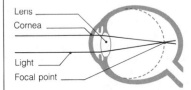

Lens
Cornea
Light
Focal point

**Uncorrected myopia**

With uncorrected myopia, the images of distant objects are focused in front of the retina and appear blurred.

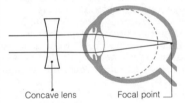

Concave lens    Focal point

**Corrected myopia**

To see distant objects clearly, the power of the eye must be reduced by a concave (negative) lens.

---

M

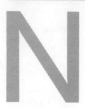

# N

## Nadolol

A *beta-blocker drug* used in the treatment of *hypertension* (high blood pressure), *angina pectoris* (chest pain due to impaired blood supply to heart muscle), certain types of *arrhythmia* (irregularity of the heart beat), and *hyperthyroidism* (overactivity of the thyroid gland).

Possible adverse effects are typical of other beta-blocker drugs.

## Nail

A hard, curved plate on the fingers and toes composed of *keratin* (a tough protein that is also the main constituent of skin and hair). A fingernail takes about six months to grow from base to tip, although there are seasonal growth variations. Toenails take twice as long to grow.

### DISORDERS

The nails are susceptible to damage through injury, usually as a result of crushing or pressure on the nail. Sometimes the nails become abnormally thick and curved—a condition called *onychogryphosis* that mainly affects the big toes of elderly people.

Nails may be damaged by bacterial or fungal infections, especially *tinea* and *candidiasis*. In *paronychia*, the nail folds are infected. The nails may also be affected by skin disease or by more generalized illnesses.

Examples of the effects of skin disease on the nails include pitting of the nails in *alopecia* areata, pitting and *onycholysis* (separation of the nail from its bed) in *psoriasis*, and scarring and onycholysis in *lichen planus*.

Nail abnormalities may be signs of more generalized disease. Brittle, ridged, concave nails are a sign of iron-deficiency *anemia*, onycholysis is seen in *thyrotoxicosis*, and fibrous growths on the nails are a sign of *tuberous sclerosis*. Splinterlike black marks develop beneath the nails (denoting bleeding into the nail bed) in *endocarditis* and *bleeding disorders*.

Abnormalities of nail color may also signify disease. A greenish discoloration may be caused by bacterial infec-

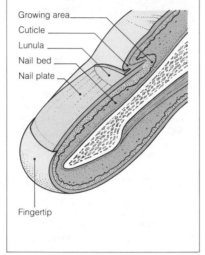

**ANATOMY OF A NAIL**
The nail bed is the area from which the nail grows. At the base of each nail, a half-moon shape, the lunula, is crossed by a flap of skin, the cuticle. The skin that surrounds the nail is the nail fold. The nail is composed of keratin, a tough protein also found in skin and hair.

Growing area
Cuticle
Lunula
Nail bed
Nail plate
Fingertip

tion under the nail, blue nails may be a sign of heart or respiratory disease, and yellow nails that are hard and curved develop in *bronchiectasis* and *lymphedema*. The nails may also be discolored by the color in nail polish and by nicotine staining.

### DIAGNOSIS AND TREATMENT

Nail disorders are usually diagnosed by inspecting the nails and skin, along with a physical examination if necessary. Laboratory examination of nail clippings may be performed.

Treatment of nail disorders is difficult. Creams and lotions seldom penetrate sufficiently; oral medication may take months to be effective.

## Nail-biting

A common activity that does not indicate any underlying medical condition. Many children bite their nails during their first years at school, but most grow out of it. Nail-biting sometimes continues as a nervous habit in adolescents and adults. Persistent nail-biting may make the nails unsightly and cause pain and sometimes bleeding.

Various preparations with an unpleasant taste can be painted on the nails, but many people become accustomed to the taste.

## Nalidixic acid

An *antibiotic drug* used to treat and, occasionally, to prevent *urinary tract infection*. Nalidixic acid is effective against some types of bacteria that are resistant to other antibiotics.

Adverse effects include nausea, vomiting, increased sensitivity to sunlight, blurred vision, drowsiness, and dizziness.

## Naloxone

A drug that blocks the action of *narcotic drugs*. Naloxone reverses breathing difficulty caused by a narcotics overdose. It is also given to newborn babies affected by narcotics used to aid childbirth and to people who have received high doses of a narcotic drug during surgery.

Possible adverse effects include abdominal cramps, diarrhea, nausea, vomiting, and tremors.

## Naltrexone

A drug that blocks the euphoric effects of *narcotic drugs*. Naltrexone is given to addicts who have stopped taking narcotics as part of a supervised detoxification program. It helps prevent the recurrence of *drug dependence*.

Possible adverse effects include nausea, loss of energy, depression, and, in rare cases, liver damage.

## Nandrolone

An anabolic steroid (see *Steroids, anabolic*) sometimes used with *growth hormone* in the treatment of *short stature*. Nandrolone is also used to treat certain types of *anemia*.

Possible adverse effects include swollen ankles, nausea and vomiting, jaundice, and aggressive behavior. In men, nandrolone may cause difficulty passing urine; in women, irregular menstruation and abnormal hair growth may occur.

## Naphazoline

A *decongestant drug* used in the treatment of allergic *rhinitis*, *sinusitis*, or a common *cold*. Naphazoline is also given to clear bloodshot eyes and to relieve minor eye irritation.

Overuse of nasal preparations containing naphazoline may lead to palpitations, headache, drowsiness, restlessness, and "rebound" congestion (worsening of congestion after drug use is stopped).

## Naproxen

A *nonsteroidal anti-inflammatory drug* (NSAID) that is used as an *analgesic* (painkiller) in the treatment of headache, menstrual pain, and injury to soft tissues (such as muscles or ligaments). It is also used to reduce joint pain and stiffness in *arthritis*.

Possible adverse effects are nausea, abdominal pain, and *peptic ulcer*.

## Narcissism

Intense self-love. The term is derived from the Greek myth of Narcissus, who so loved to stare at his own reflection in the water that he fell in and drowned. In *psychoanalytic theory* there is an early stage in childhood development when the ego (self) feels omnipotent. Failure to deal with the frustrations of discovering that this is not so may result in neurosis later.

A narcissistic personality disorder is characterized by an exaggerated sense of self-importance, constant need for attention or praise, inability to cope with criticism or defeat, and poor relationships with other people.

## Narcolepsy

A *sleep* disorder characterized by chronic, excessive daytime sleepiness with recurrent episodes of sleep occurring several times per day. Attacks may last from a few seconds to more than an hour and may be mildly inconvenient or severely disabling, often interfering with work and daily life. *Cataplexy* (sudden loss of muscle tone without loss of consciousness) occurs in about three quarters of cases. Other symptoms may include *sleep paralysis* and vivid hallucinations at the onset of sleep or on awakening.

In narcolepsy, the REM (rapid eye movement) state, which normally occurs only during sleep, intrudes into wakefulness. Narcolepsy is often inherited. Treatment usually involves regular naps, along with *stimulant drugs* to control drowsiness and sleep attacks and *antidepressant drugs* to suppress cataplexy.

## Narcosis

A state of stupor usually caused by a drug (see *Narcotic drugs*) or other chemical. Narcosis resembles sleep, being marked by reduced awareness and by diminished ability to respond to external stimulation. However, unlike a sleeper, a person in narcosis cannot be roused completely.

## Narcotic drugs

| COMMON DRUGS |
| --- |

*Codeine  Meperidine
Morphine  Propoxyphene*

A type of *analgesic* (painkiller) used in the treatment of moderate and severe pain. Abuse of narcotic drugs for their euphoric effects often causes *tolerance* (the need for greater amounts to have the same effects) and physical and psychological *drug dependence*.

## Nasal congestion

Partial blockage of the nasal passage caused by inflammation of the mucous membrane that lines it. Congestion can be caused by an infection of the nasal passage itself (such as a cold), by an infection that has spread from the sinuses (see *Sinusitis*), or by an allergy (see *Rhinitis, allergic*).

A simple, effective, and time-honored method of alleviating nasal congestion is to inhale the steam from a pot of hot water. This loosens the mucus, which enables the sufferer to blow it out through the nose. *Decongestant drugs* in the form of nasal drops and sprays should be used sparingly since extensive use can make congestion worse. Decongestant tablets and syrups are of doubtful value and may cause drowsiness.

Persistent nasal congestion should be investigated by a physician.

## Nasal discharge

The spontaneous emission of fluid from the nose. Nasal discharge is commonly caused by inflammation of the mucous lining and is often accompanied by *nasal congestion*.

In allergic *rhinitis*, the discharge consists of runny, clear mucus. Infection of the nasal passage itself (such as a cold) or infection that has spread from the sinuses (see *Sinusitis*) usually causes a thicker discharge of mucus, often mixed with pus. A newly developed persistent runny discharge may be an early sign of a tumor (see *Nasopharynx, cancer of*).

Bleeding from the nose is usually caused by injury or a foreign body in the nose; it may also be a sign of an underlying bleeding disorder or a tumor (see *Nosebleed*). In rare cases, cerebrospinal fluid may be discharged from the nose as a result of a fracture at the base of the skull.

## Nasal obstruction

Blockage of one or both sides of the nasal passage, which interferes with breathing. The most common cause is inflammation of the mucous membrane that lines the passage (see *Nasal congestion*). Other causes include severe deviation of the *nasal septum*, nasal *polyps*, a *hematoma* (a collection

of clotted blood) usually caused by injury, and, rarely, a malignant tumor. In children, enlargement of the adenoids is the most common cause of nasal obstruction.

## Nasal septum

The central partition inside the nose that divides it into two cavities. The nasal septum consists of cartilage at the front and bone at the rear, both covered by *mucous membrane*.

### DISORDERS

Deviated septum (twisting of the septum to one side) may be present from birth or may be caused by a blow to the nose. It is rarely troublesome, but, if breathing is obstructed, the septum can be straightened by surgery.

Injury can also cause a *hematoma* (a collection of clotted blood) to form between the cartilage of the septum and the wall of one nasal cavity, again sometimes obstructing breathing. The hematoma may become infected, causing an *abscess*, which may require surgical drainage. Occasionally, an abscess develops on a child's septum without prior injury.

Rarely, a hole may be eroded in the septum by *tuberculosis, syphilis, cocaine,* or *Wegner's granulomatosis*.

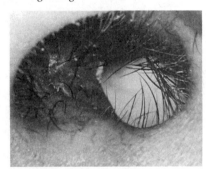
**Destroyed nasal septum**
This photograph of the left nostril was taken with a light shined into the right nostril. There is a hole in the septum.

## Nasogastric tube

A narrow plastic tube that is passed through the nose, down the esophagus, and into the stomach.

### WHY IT IS USED

One of its most common uses is to suck or drain digestive juices from the stomach when the intestine is blocked (as in *pyloric stenosis*) or is not working properly (as may occur after an abdominal operation). The tube is also used to give liquid nourishment to very ill patients who cannot eat (see *Feeding, artificial*), to obtain specimens of stomach secretions for examina-

**N**

tion, and to wash out the stomach after a drug overdose or after swallowing a poison (see *Lavage, gastric*).

### HOW IT IS USED

Inserting the tube is a quick, simple procedure that causes little discomfort and does not require an anesthetic. The tube is lubricated and passed into one nostril; while the patient swallows, it is slid down the throat and into the stomach. To ensure that the tube is in the stomach, a sample of fluid is withdrawn through a syringe and tested on litmus paper for acidity. The stomach contents may then be sucked out through the syringe or through a suction device, or they may be allowed to drain freely into a container. Fluids for lavage or feeding are introduced through a funnel. If the nasogastric tube is to be left in place for some time, the protruding end of the tube is taped to the face.

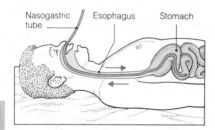

**Using a nasogastric tube**
The tube is passed via a nostril and the esophagus into the stomach. Substances may be delivered into the stomach via the tube, or the stomach contents may be removed through it.

## Nasopharynx

The passage connecting the nasal cavity behind the nose to the top of the throat behind the soft *palate*. Part of the respiratory tract, the nasopharynx forms the upper section of the *pharynx*. During swallowing, the nasopharynx is sealed off (to prevent food from entering it) by the action of the soft palate pressing against the back of the throat.

The nasopharynx contains the openings to the *eustachian tubes* (passages connecting the back of the nose to the middle ear) and, in children, the *adenoids*. The adenoids can enlarge to such an extent that the nasopharynx becomes completely blocked, forcing the child to breathe through his or her mouth.

## Nasopharynx, cancer of

A malignant tumor that originates in the *nasopharynx* (uppermost part of the throat, behind the nose) and usually spreads to the nasal cavity, nasal sinuses, base of the skull, and lymph nodes in the neck. Cancer of the nasopharynx is rare in the West but common in the Far East; it is most common between the ages of 40 and 50 and affects twice as many men as women. One cause is believed to be the *Epstein-Barr virus*.

### SYMPTOMS AND SIGNS

Common first signs are recurrent nosebleeds, a persistently runny nose, and voice change. As the tumor spreads, there may be a bloody discharge from the nose, loss of smell, double vision, deafness, paralysis of one side of the face, and severe facial pain.

### DIAGNOSIS AND TREATMENT

The diagnosis is made from a *biopsy* (removal of a small sample of tissue for analysis). X rays may be taken to determine to what extent the cancer has spread.

Treatment is with *radiation therapy*. The outlook depends on when treatment began; one third of sufferers survive for more than five years.

## Natural childbirth

See *Prepared childbirth*.

## Naturopathy

A form of *alternative medicine* based on the principle that disease is due to the accumulation of waste products and toxins in the body, and that symptoms reflect the body's attempt to rid itself of these substances. Practitioners of naturopathy believe that health is maintained by avoiding anything artificial or unnatural in the diet or in the environment.

## Nausea

The sensation of needing to vomit. Although nausea may occur independently of vomiting, the causes are the same (see *Vomiting*).

## Navel

A popular term for the *umbilicus*, the depression in the abdomen that marks the point at which the umbilical cord was attached to the fetus.

## Nearsightedness

See *Myopia*.

## Nebulizer

A device used to administer a drug in aerosol form through a face mask. Nebulizers are used to administer *bronchodilator drugs*, especially in the emergency treatment of an attack of

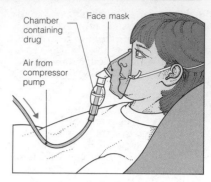

**Using a nebulizer**
An electric or hand-operated pump sends a stream of air or oxygen across a chamber containing the required drug. This stream of air disperses the drug into a fine mist, which is then conveyed to the face mask and inhaled by the user.

*asthma*. A nebulizer is much easier to use than a conventional *inhaler* (pressurized aerosol canister).

## Neck

In addition to supporting the head, the neck is the passageway between the head and brain and the body. It thus contains a number of vital structures. Decapitation kills because it cuts through the *spinal cord* (which carries nerve impulses to and from the brain) and because it severs the *trachea* (windpipe), the *esophagus*, and major blood vessels leading to and from the head. Strangulation kills by compressing major blood vessels and by cutting off the air supply to the lungs.

### DISORDERS

**INJURY** *Torticollis* (wryneck), in which the head is twisted to one side, may result from birth injury to a neck muscle or from skin *contracture* after burns or other injuries.

*Fractures* and *dislocations* of any of the vertebrae in the neck can injure the spinal cord, causing paralysis or even death; *whiplash injuries* can also severely damage the spinal cord.

**DEGENERATION** The joints between vertebrae may be affected by *cervical osteoarthritis*, causing neck pain, stiffness, and sometimes tingling and weakness in the arm and hand. Similar symptoms may be caused by a *disk prolapse*. In *ankylosing spondylitis*, fusion of the vertebrae may result in permanent neck rigidity.

**CONGENITAL DEFECT** *Cervical rib* (a small extra rib in the neck) often causes no symptoms until middle age, when it may result in pain, numbness, and a pins and needles sensation in the forearm and hand.

## ANATOMY OF THE NECK

The neck contains many important structures, including the larynx, the thyroid and parathyroid glands, many lymph nodes, and the carotid arteries. The upper seven vertebrae of the spine are in the neck; a complex system of muscles is connected to these vertebrae, the clavicles, the upper ribs, and the lower jaw. Contraction of these muscles allows the head to turn and the jaw to open and close.

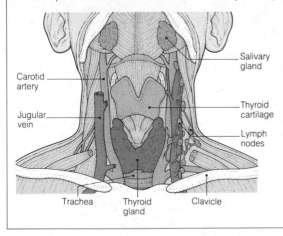

Carotid artery

Jugular vein

Salivary gland

Thyroid cartilage

Lymph nodes

Trachea    Thyroid gland    Clavicle

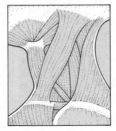

**Muscles of the neck**
Muscles on the back and side of the neck support and move the head.

OTHER DISORDERS Because structures in the neck are so closely packed, any condition that causes swelling (such as inflammation, allergy, bleeding, or tumors) may, if large enough, interfere with breathing or swallowing. Enlargement of the lymph nodes usually results from infection, but may be due to other conditions.

Neck pain of unknown origin is very common. As long as neurological symptoms (such as loss of sensation or muscle power) are absent, it is unlikely to be serious. Most sufferers recover within a few weeks.

### Neck dissection, radical

A surgical procedure for removing cancerous lymph nodes in the neck. The operation is commonly required as part of the treatment of cancer of the tongue, tonsils, or other structures in the mouth and throat.

A flap of skin on the affected side of the neck is raised (using a general anesthetic) to expose the underlying sternomastoid muscle. The muscle is cut through just above the clavicle (collarbone) and lifted up. The entire lymphatic system in the neck (the vessels as well as the nodes) is then removed, along with the internal jugular vein, lower salivary gland, and other surrounding tissue.

### Neck rigidity

Marked stiffness of the neck caused by spasm of the muscles in the neck and spine. Neck rigidity is an important clinical sign of *meningitis* (inflammation of the membranes surrounding the brain and spinal cord). Severe neck rigidity may cause the head to arch backward, especially in babies.

### Necrolysis, toxic epidermal

A severe, blistering rash in which the surface layers of the skin peel off, exposing large areas of red raw skin over the body. The effects of toxic epidermal necrolysis are similar to those of a severe third-degree burn, with the same potentially serious risks of widespread infection and loss of body fluid and salts from the exposed body surface.

In newborn babies, the condition is usually caused by staphylococci (a type of bacteria) and is called the scalded skin syndrome. Treatment is with antibiotic drugs and sometimes intravenous fluid replacement.

In adults, the most common cause of toxic epidermal necrolysis is an adverse reaction to a drug, particularly a barbiturate, sulfonamide, or penicillin. The condition usually clears up when use of the drug is discontinued. Intravenous fluid replacement is sometimes necessary.

### Necrophilia

A rare sexual perversion in which orgasm is achieved by sexual acts, either heterosexual or homosexual, with dead bodies.

### Necropsy

A little-used alternative medical term for an *autopsy* (postmortem examination of a body).

### Necrosis

The death of tissue cells. Necrosis can occur as a result of *ischemia* (inadequate blood supply), which may lead to *gangrene*; infection (such as *tuberculosis*); or damage by extreme heat or cold, noxious chemicals (such as acids), or excessive exposure to X rays or other forms of radiation.

The appearance of dead tissue depends on the cause of the necrosis and, usually, on the type of tissue affected. For example, in necrosis due to tuberculosis, the dead tissue is soft, dry, and cheeselike; fatty tissue beneath the skin that has died as a result of damage or infection develops into tough scar tissue that may form a firm nodule.

### Nematodes

The scientific name for a group of cylindrically shaped worms, some of which can be parasites of humans. (See *Roundworms*.)

### Neologism

The act of making up new words that have a special meaning for the inventor. The term also refers to the invented words themselves. While inventing words is often considered a creative act in novelists and poets, persistent neologism is a sign of *schizophrenia*, in which it occurs with other disordered thoughts.

### Neomycin

An *antibiotic drug* used in the treatment of ear, eye, and skin infections, often in combination with other drugs. Neomycin is given to treat and sometimes prevent some infections of the intestine. It is also used in the treatment of *hyperlipidemia* (high lipid levels in the blood).

Possible adverse effects include rash, itching, diarrhea, nausea and vomiting, hearing loss, dizziness, and ringing in the ears.

### Neonate

A newly born infant (see *Newborn*).

### Neonatologist

A specialist in the care of newborn babies and their special problems. Problems may be short-term (such as those associated with premature or low-weight babies) or lifelong (such as

N

*spina bifida*). The neonatologist cares for the baby for the first four weeks of life. After this time, the child's medical care becomes primarily the responsibility of a *pediatrician*.

## Neonatology

The branch of *pediatrics* concerned with the care of newborn infants and the treatment of their disorders. (See also *Neonatologist*.)

## Neoplasia

A medical term for *tumor* formation, characterized by a progressive, abnormal multiplication of cells. The term neoplasia does not necessarily imply that the new growth is *malignant*; *benign* tumors also develop as a result of neoplasia.

## Neoplasm

A medical term for a *tumor* (any new, abnormal growth). Neoplasms may be *malignant* or *benign*.

## Neostigmine

A drug used in the treatment of *myasthenia gravis* (a rare autoimmune disorder that causes muscle weakness). Neostigmine is also given to treat abnormal retention of urine (see *Urine retention*) and paralytic *ileus* (temporary paralysis of the intestine).

Neostigmine works by increasing the activity of *acetylcholine*, a *neurotransmitter* (chemical released from nerve endings) that stimulates the contraction of muscles.

Possible adverse effects include nausea and vomiting, increased salivation, blurred vision, diarrhea, abdominal cramps, sweating, muscle cramps, twitching, and rash.

## Nephrectomy

Surgical removal of one or both of the *kidneys*.

**WHY IT IS DONE**

One of the most common reasons for nephrectomy is to remove a malignant tumor (see *Kidney cancer*). A kidney may also be removed if it is not functioning normally due to infection or the presence of stones (see *Calculus, urinary tract*), or is causing severe *hypertension* (high blood pressure). Nephrectomy may also be necessary if a kidney is so badly injured that bleeding cannot be stopped.

**HOW IT IS DONE**

Nephrectomy is carried out using general anesthesia. The patient lies on his or her side, bent sharply at the waist over an angled operating table. An incision is made along the lower

edge of the ribs, from the spine at the back to the front of the abdomen to expose the kidney. The *ureter* and renal blood vessels are tied off, and the kidney is removed. The incision is stitched up after insertion of a drainage tube, which is left in position for 24 to 48 hours.

**OUTLOOK**

A person's kidney function becomes virtually normal about six months after removal of a single kidney because the remaining kidney (providing it is healthy) takes over the entire work load. If both kidneys are removed, the patient requires *dialysis* or a *kidney transplant*.

## Nephritis

Inflammation of one or both kidneys. Nephritis may be caused by infection (see *Pyelonephritis*), by abnormal responses of the *immune system* (see *Glomerulonephritis*), and by metabolic disorders, such as gout. (See also *Kidney* disorders box.)

## Nephroblastoma

See *Kidney cancer*.

## Nephrocalcinosis

The deposition of calcium within the substance of one or both kidneys. Nephrocalcinosis is not the same as kidney stones (see *Calculi, urinary tract*), in which calcium particles develop within the drainage channels of the kidney.

Nephrocalcinosis may occur in any condition in which the blood level of calcium is raised. These conditions include *hyperparathyroidism* (overactivity of the parathyroid gland) and *renal tubular acidosis* (in which the kidney produces urine of lower than normal acidity). Nephrocalcinosis may also develop as a result of taking excessive amounts of certain *antacid drugs* or *vitamin D*.

Treatment is of the underlying cause to prevent further calcification.

## Nephrolithotomy

The surgical removal of a *calculus* (stone) from the kidney by cutting through the body of the kidney. Nephrolithotomy can be achieved through an abdominal incision, or through a puncture incision made through the skin in the back and directly into the kidney (percutaneous nephrolithotomy). Instruments allow the stone to be grasped or fragmented and withdrawn.

A more straightforward method of stone removal is *pyelolithotomy*, in

which the stone is removed through a cut at the junction between the kidney and ureter.

An alternative approach to dealing with kidney stones is to pulverize them by means of ultrasonic waves (see *Lithotripsy*). Pulverization may also be achieved with an ultrasonic wand passed through the skin (percutaneous *lithotripsy*).

## Nephrologist

A specialist in the diagnosis and treatment of kidney disease.

## Nephrology

The medical specialty concerned with the normal functioning of the *kidneys*, and with the causes, diagnosis, and treatment of kidney disease.

Methods of investigating the kidneys include kidney *biopsy*, *kidney function tests*, and *kidney imaging* techniques (such as intravenous *pyelography*). Treatment of kidney disorders includes drugs (to control high blood pressure, inflammation, or infection), surgical intervention (for the treatment of stones and tumors), and *dialysis* or, in some cases, a *kidney transplant* (for the treatment of advanced kidney disease).

## Nephron

The microscopic unit of the *kidney* that consists of a glomerulus (filtering funnel) and a tubule. There are about 1 million nephrons in each kidney. The nephrons filter waste products from the blood and modify the amount of salts and water excreted in the urine according to the body's needs.

## Nephropathy

Any disease or damage to the kidneys (see *Kidney* disorders box).

Obstructive nephropathy refers to kidney damage caused by a urinary tract *calculus* (stone), tumor, scar tissue, or pressure from an organ blocking urine flow and creating back pressure within the kidney.

Reflux nephropathy refers to kidney damage caused by backflow of urine from the bladder toward the kidney. It is caused by failure of the valve mechanism at the lower end of each ureter.

Toxic nephropathy refers to damage caused by various poisons or minerals (such as carbon tetrachloride or lead).

## Nephrosclerosis

A process in which normal kidney structures are replaced with scar tissue composed of *collagen*. Nephro-

N

sclerosis usually represents the final healing stage of any of the conditions that cause inflammation within the kidney. Such conditions include *diabetes mellitus*, *glomerulonephritis*, and chronic *pyelonephritis*.

## Nephrosis
See *Nephrotic syndrome*.

## Nephrostomy
The introduction of a small tube into the kidney to drain urine to the abdominal surface, thus bypassing the ureter. Nephrostomy is sometimes performed after an operation (typically, removal of a *calculus*) on the ureter or kidney-ureter junction to allow healing to take place.

## Nephrotic syndrome
A collection of symptoms and signs that results from damage to the glomeruli (filtering units of the *kidney*) causing severe *proteinuria* (loss of protein from the bloodstream into the urine). Loss of large amounts of protein in the urine lowers the protein content of the blood and results in edema (fluid retention).

### CAUSES
Nephrotic syndrome may be caused by *diabetes mellitus*, *glomerulonephritis* (inflammation of the glomeruli), *amyloidosis* (a condition in which amyloid, an abnormal protein, collects in the tissues and organs), severe *hypertension* (high blood pressure), reactions to poisons (including lead, carbon tetrachloride, and poison ivy), and adverse drug reactions.

### SYMPTOMS
Edema causes marked swelling of the legs and face. Fluid may also collect in the chest cavity (producing *pleural effusion*) or within the abdomen (causing *ascites*). Anorexia, lethargy, and diarrhea may also occur.

### TREATMENT
Treatment is of the underlying condition. A low-sodium diet may be recommended, and *diuretic drugs* may be given to reduce edema. If the plasma protein concentration is particularly low, protein may need to be given intravenously.

## Nerve
A bundle of nerve fibers that travels to a common location. Nerve fibers, also called axons, are the filamentous projections of many individual *neurons* (nerve cells).

The most obvious nerves in the body are the peripheral nerves, which extend from the central nervous system (CNS), consisting of the brain and spinal cord, to other parts of the body. Apart from the *optic nerves*, most nerve fiber bundles within the brain and spinal cord are referred to as nerve tracts or nerve pathways rather than simply "nerves."

### STRUCTURE
Including optic nerves, there are 12 pairs of *cranial nerves* (which link directly to the brain) and 31 pairs of *spinal nerves* (which join the spinal cord)—all are peripheral nerves.

In the shoulder and hip regions, the spinal nerves join to form the main nerves to the limbs, such as the median nerve in the arm and the sciatic nerve in the leg. Most nerves divide at numerous points along their length to send branches to all parts of the body, particularly to the sense organs, skin, skeletal muscles, internal organs, and glands.

### FUNCTION
Nerve fibers may have a sensory function, carrying information from a receptor or sense organ at the far end of the nerve toward the CNS, or a motor function, carrying instructions from the CNS to a muscle or a gland. Messages are carried by electrical impulses propagated along the fibers. Some nerves carry only sensory or motor fibers, but most carry both.

Nerve functioning is sensitive to cold, pressure, and to a wide variety of injuries (see *Nerve injury*). The peripheral nerves can be damaged by infection, inflammation, poisoning, nutritional deficiencies, and metabolic disorders (see *Neuropathy*).

## Nerve block
The injection of a local anesthetic into or around a nerve to produce anesthesia (loss of sensation) in a part of the body supplied by that nerve.

### WHY IT IS DONE
A nerve block is performed when it is not possible to inject anesthetic directly into the tissues that are being treated because the area is painfully inflamed or because there is a risk of spreading infection. Nerve block may also be used to anesthetize a large area, or an area not suited for injection because it is deep within the body or is covered with bone.

### HOW IT IS DONE
The local anesthetic is injected at an accessible area into or around the nerve at a point remote from the area to be treated (e.g., the palm of the hand may be anesthetized by injecting points up the arm, thus blocking the ulnar and median nerves).

A nerve may be blocked as it leaves the spinal cord, such as in *epidural anesthesia* (used in childbirth) and in *spinal anesthesia* (used mainly for surgery of the lower abdomen and limbs). In a caudal block, anesthetic is injected into nerves leaving the lowest part of the spinal cord; it produces anesthesia in the buttock and genital areas. A caudal block is occasionally used for childbirth, especially a forceps delivery. A pudendal nerve block involves injection of nerves passing under the pelvis into the floor of the vagina; it is used for forceps delivery. (See also *Anesthesia, local*.)

## Nerve injury
A cut or crush injury to a nerve that severs some or all of its individual conducting fibers. Surgical repair is the only treatment for a severed nerve, and only the peripheral nerves (those outside the brain and spinal cord) are amenable to such repair. (See *Neuropathy* for nerve damage from causes other than injury.)

### CRUSH INJURIES
In a crush injury, individual fibers within a peripheral nerve may be severed while the nerve trunk itself remains intact. The severed fibers degenerate on both sides of the injury, leading to loss of power in the muscles and loss of sensation in the skin area supplied by the nerve. However, if the ends are still aligned, new fibers can regenerate along the channels left by the degenerated fibers. These fibers begin to grow within a few days after an injury and advance at a rate of about 1 inch (2.5 cm) per month.

### COMPLETE SEVERANCE
Total severance of a nerve can result from accidental contact with powered devices (such as rotary saws and propellers), from knife and bullet wounds, or from other penetrating injuries (such as from flying glass).

If the ends of the cut nerve are separated, the fibers try to regenerate but, in the absence of directing channels, they simply bunch up to form a lump of tissue; there is no recovery of function. It is therefore essential in the surgical repair of cut nerves to ensure that the ends are meticulously brought together and stitched into place. This is achieved with *microsurgery* and delicate sutures and needles.

Even with the best surgical repair, recovery is rarely complete. While the fibers with a motor function are regenerating, the paralyzed muscles are kept healthy and free from *contractures* by constant *physical therapy*.

N

Regenerating nerve fibers sometimes pass down the wrong channels; as a result, when function is restored, actions may differ from what was intended (for example, an attempt to move the index finger may move the middle finger as well). Movement skills and the interpretation of sensations may need to be relearned.

**BRAIN AND SPINAL CORD INJURY**

Nerve tracts within the brain and spinal cord are structurally different from the peripheral nerves, and severed fibers there do not regenerate. For example, it is impossible for vision to be restored if the *optic nerves* are cut.

## Nerve, trapped

Compression or stretching of a nerve, causing numbness, tingling, weakness, and sometimes pain in the area supplied by the nerve.

Common examples of a trapped nerve include *carpal tunnel syndrome*, in which symptoms appear in the thumb, index, and middle fingers as a result of pressure on the median nerve as it passes through the wrist; a prolapsed disk (see *Disk prolapse*), in which pressure on the nerve root leading from the spinal cord produces symptoms in the back and legs; and *crutch palsy*, in which the radial nerve is pressed against the humerus (upper arm bone), producing symptoms in the wrist and hand.

A damaged nerve may take some time to heal, causing symptoms to persist. Surgical decompression to relieve pressure on the nerve may be necessary in severe cases.

## Nervous breakdown

A popular term used to describe unusual behavior that is thought to be part of a crisis of severe anxiety or tension or a psychiatric illness. The term has no technical meaning, but is often applied to people suffering from sudden tearfulness, episodes of shouting and screaming, marked social withdrawal, and concerns about the possibility of illness.

## Nervous habit

A nontechnical term for a minor repetitive movement or activity. Sometimes these are involuntary twitches and facial tics, such as in *Gilles de la Tourette's syndrome* and some forms of *dyskinesia*.

Voluntary nervous habits, such as *thumb-sucking* and nose-picking, are common in young children, but usually disappear naturally with time. Also common is *nail-biting*, which

often persists into adult life (20 percent of adults bite their nails). Such habits are thought to be a means of releasing inner tension.

All nervous habits increase during tension or anxiety. They may be severe in some forms of *depression*, an *anxiety disorder*, or drug withdrawal.

## Nervous system

The body's information-gathering, storage, and control system.

The overall function of the nervous system is to gather information about the external environment and the body's internal state, to analyze this information, and to initiate appropriate responses aimed at satisfying certain drives. The most powerful drive is for survival. Many survival responses, which range from running away from danger to shivering in response to cold, are initiated unconsciously and automatically by the nervous system.

Other drives are more complex, revolving around a need to experience positive emotions (pleasure, excitement) and avoid negative ones (pain, anxiety, frustration).

In carrying out its functions, the nervous system has access to many built-in programs, but it can also improve its performance through *learning*, which relies on *memory*.

**STRUCTURE**

The nervous system is organized like a computer system that controls a highly complex machine. The central processing unit for the system is the central nervous system (CNS), comprising the brain and spinal cord, which consists of billions of interconnecting *neurons* (nerve cells).

Input of information to the CNS comes from the sense organs. Output (motor) instructions go to the skeletal muscles, muscles controlling speech, internal organs and glands, and the sweat glands in the skin. The cables along which this information is carried are the *nerves* that fan out from the CNS to the entire body. Each nerve is a bundle of the axons (filamentous projections) of many neurons.

In addition to these anatomical divisions of the nervous system, there are various functional divisions. Two of the most important are the *autonomic nervous system*, which is specifically concerned with the automatic (unconscious) regulation of internal body functioning, and the somatic nervous system, which controls the skeletal muscles responsible for voluntary movement.

**FUNCTION**

The nervous system functions largely through automatic responses to various stimuli (see *Reflex*), although voluntary (willed) actions can also be initiated through the activity of higher, conscious areas of the brain. Certain higher functions (such as visual perception, memory storage, thought, and speech production) are extremely complex and not understood in detail. Overall, however, all nervous activity is based on the transmission of impulses through complex networks of neurons.

**DISORDERS**

Disorders of the nervous system may result from damage to or dysfunction of its component parts (see *Brain* disorders box; *Spinal cord*; *Neuropathy*; *Nerve injury*). Disorders may also be due to impairment of sensory, analytical, or memory functions (see *Vision, disorders of*; *Deafness*; *Numbness*; *Smell, loss of*; *Agnosia*; *Amnesia*) or of motor functions (see *Aphasia*; *Dysarthria*; *Ataxia*).

## Netilmicin

An *antibiotic drug* used in the hospital to treat serious infection, usually when other antibiotic drugs have been ineffective. Netilmicin is often used to enhance the effects of other antibiotics. In rare cases, it causes damage to the inner ear and the kidneys.

## Neuralgia

Pain caused by irritation of, or damage to, a nerve. The pain usually occurs in brief bouts, may be very severe, and can often be felt shooting along the affected nerve.

The neuralgia that often occurs in *migraine* consists of attacks of intense, radiating pain around the eye that can last for up to an hour. Postherpetic neuralgia is a burning pain that may recur at the site of an attack of *herpes zoster* (shingles) for months or even years after the illness.

In glossopharyngeal neuralgia, intense pain is felt at the back of the tongue and in the throat and ear. The structures in this area are served by the glossopharyngeal nerve. The pain may occur spontaneously or be brought on by talking, eating, or swallowing; its cause is generally unknown. The same is true of *trigeminal neuralgia*, a severe paroxysm of pain affecting one side of the face supplied by the trigeminal nerve.

**TREATMENT**

Glossopharyngeal, trigeminal, and postherpetic neuralgia sometimes re-

N

# NERVOUS SYSTEM

The nervous system detects and interprets changes in conditions inside and outside the body and responds to them. The central nervous system analyzes information and initiates responses; the peripheral nervous system gathers information and carries the response signals. Some responses are involuntary; others are dictated by conscious thought. All nervous system activity consists of signals passed through pathways of inter-connected neurons (nerve cells).

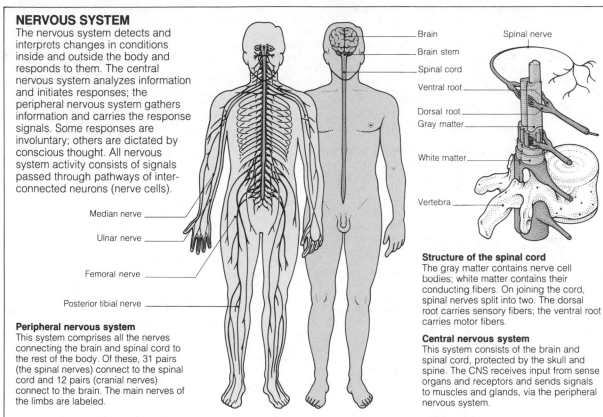

Brain
Brain stem
Spinal cord
Ventral root
Dorsal root
Gray matter
White matter
Vertebra

Spinal nerve

Median nerve
Ulnar nerve
Femoral nerve
Posterior tibial nerve

### Peripheral nervous system
This system comprises all the nerves connecting the brain and spinal cord to the rest of the body. Of these, 31 pairs (the spinal nerves) connect to the spinal cord and 12 pairs (cranial nerves) connect to the brain. The main nerves of the limbs are labeled.

### Structure of the spinal cord
The gray matter contains nerve cell bodies; white matter contains their conducting fibers. On joining the cord, spinal nerves split into two. The dorsal root carries sensory fibers; the ventral root carries motor fibers.

### Central nervous system
This system consists of the brain and spinal cord, protected by the skull and spine. The CNS receives input from sense organs and receptors and sends signals to muscles and glands, via the peripheral nervous system.

N

# HOW IT WORKS

Some possible events in response to a finger touching a hot object are shown. A receptor sends a message, via a sensory fiber, to the spinal cord. This triggers a signal that travels, via a motor fiber, back to a muscle, which contracts to move the finger. This action is called a reflex arc. Other signals pass toward the brain.

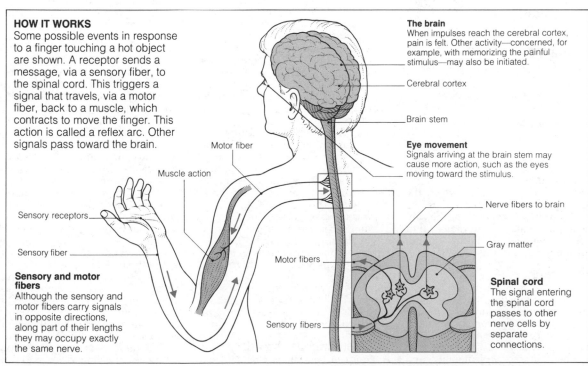

Motor fiber
Muscle action
Sensory receptors
Sensory fiber

Motor fibers
Sensory fibers

### The brain
When impulses reach the cerebral cortex, pain is felt. Other activity—concerned, for example, with memorizing the painful stimulus—may also be initiated.

Cerebral cortex

Brain stem

### Eye movement
Signals arriving at the brain stem may cause more action, such as the eyes moving toward the stimulus.

Nerve fibers to brain

Gray matter

### Spinal cord
The signal entering the spinal cord passes to other nerve cells by separate connections.

### Sensory and motor fibers
Although the sensory and motor fibers carry signals in opposite directions, along part of their lengths they may occupy exactly the same nerve.

spond to carbamazepine. They may also be relieved by analgesics (painkillers) such as acetaminophen.

## Neural tube defect

A developmental failure affecting the spinal cord or brain in the embryo. Very early in fetal development, there is a ridge of neural-like tissue along the back of the embryo. As the fetus develops, this material differentiates into both the spinal cord and body nerves at the lower end and the brain at the upper end. At the same time, the bones that make up the back gradually surround the spinal cord on all sides. If any part of this sequence goes awry, many defects can appear. The worst is total lack of brain (*anencephaly*). Much more common is *spina bifida*, in which the back bones do not form a complete ring to protect the spinal cord. One to two babies per 1,000 born alive in the US have a neural tube defect; many more fetuses are affected but do not survive birth.

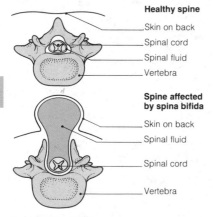

**Healthy spine**
Skin on back
Spinal cord
Spinal fluid
Vertebra

**Spine affected by spina bifida**
Skin on back
Spinal fluid
Spinal cord
Vertebra

**Neural tube defect**
This defect leads to failure of the bony arch to fuse over the back of the spinal cord, thus causing spina bifida.

## Neurapraxia

A type of *nerve injury* in which the outward structure of a nerve appears intact, but in which some of the conducting fibers have been damaged or have degenerated and thus do not transmit signals to muscles.

## Neurasthenia

An outdated term, meaning literally "nervous exhaustion." It was once used to describe a number of mental and physical symptoms, including loss of energy, insomnia, aches and pains (especially in the chest and abdomen), *depression*, irritability, and reduced concentration.

## Neuritis

Literally, inflammation of a nerve. True nerve inflammation may be caused by infection (e.g., by a virus in *herpes zoster* or a bacterium in *leprosy*). The term neuritis is also often applied to nerve damage or disease from causes other than inflammation. Thus, it has become virtually synonymous with *neuropathy*, a term for all disorders of peripheral nerves.

## Neuroblastoma

A tumor of the adrenal glands or sympathetic nervous system (the part of the nervous system responsible for certain automatic body functions, notably the *fight or flight response*). Most neuroblastomas develop in the adrenal glands or in the sympathetic nerves along the back wall of the abdomen. Less commonly, they develop in the sympathetic nerves of the chest or neck, or, very rarely, in the brain.

Neuroblastomas are the most common extracranial (outside the skull) solid tumor of childhood. About 80 percent of cases develop during the first 10 years of life, most commonly in the first four years. The incidence is 8.3 cases per 1 million children.

**SYMPTOMS AND SIGNS**
The symptoms vary according to the site of the tumor and the extent to which it has spread. Common symptoms include weight loss, general aches and pains, paleness, and irritability. There may also be tumors of the abdomen, neck, eyes, or skin. In some cases, the tumor secretes the hormones *epinephrine* and *norepinephrine*, which may cause diarrhea, high blood pressure, and flushing of the skin.

**DIAGNOSIS**
The condition is diagnosed from the symptoms and signs, and from X rays, blood tests, and urine tests. In some cases, it may be necessary to perform a biopsy (removal of a small sample of tissue for examination) of the bone marrow and any accessible tumors.

**TREATMENT AND OUTLOOK**
Treatment consists of surgical removal of the tumor, followed by *radiation therapy* and possibly *anticancer drugs*.

The outlook varies greatly because neuroblastomas range from being relatively harmless to highly malignant. Overall, about one third of those affected survive for at least five years after treatment.

## Neurocutaneous disorders

A group of conditions characterized by abnormalities of the skin as well as

abnormalities of the nerves and/or the central nervous system.

The best known of these disorders is *neurofibromatosis*, in which there are brown patches on the skin and numerous fibrous nodules on the skin and nerves. Another example is *tuberous sclerosis*, characterized by small skin-colored swellings over the cheeks and nose, mental deficiency, and epilepsy.

## Neurodermatitis

An itchy, eczemalike skin condition caused by repeated scratching. (See also *Lichen simplex*.)

## Neuroendocrinology

The study of the interactions between the *nervous system* and the *endocrine system*. These systems control internal body functions and the way in which the body responds to the external environment. However, the two systems do not act separately. Hormones produced by the endocrine system can affect nervous system functions, including behavior (for example, sex hormones affect mood and sexual motivation). Similarly, special nerve cells, called neurosecretory cells (found mainly in the *hypothalamus*), can release hormones in response to stimulation by the nervous system; these hormones can, in turn, affect various endocrine glands. Stress is initially perceived by the nervous system but ultimately causes the release of hormones by the pituitary and adrenal glands.

Neuroendocrinological investigations range from recording the electrical activity of neurosecretory cells to experiments showing the relationship between hormones and behavior.

## Neurofibromatosis

An uncommon inherited disorder, also called von Recklinghausen's disease. Neurofibromatosis is characterized by numerous soft, fibrous swellings (called neurofibromas) that grow from nerves in the skin and sometimes elsewhere in the body. In addition, there are *café au lait spots* (pale, coffee-colored patches) on the skin of the trunk and pelvis.

**SYMPTOMS AND SIGNS**
In most cases, neurofibromatosis affects only the skin. However, the swellings and spots may be unsightly. If neurofibromas occur in the central nervous system, they can cause *epilepsy* and other complications, sometimes affecting vision and hearing. Rarely, bone deformities occur.

### TREATMENT

Surgical removal of neurofibromas is necessary only if they are causing complications. Anyone who has the disorder, and parents of an affected child, should seek *genetic counseling*.

## Neurologist

A specialist in the diagnosis and treatment of diseases and disorders of the nervous system. Neurologists conduct examinations of the patient's nerves, reflexes, motor and sensory functions, and muscles to determine the cause and extent of a problem.

## Neurology

The study of the nervous system and its disorders, particularly their diagnosis and treatment (the specialty of *neuropathology* is concerned with the causes and effects of neurological conditions). In addition to a detailed knowledge of the structure and function of the brain, spinal cord, and nerves, neurologists must understand the many conditions that can affect them. To aid in the diagnosis of such conditions, extensive use is made of modern imaging techniques (such as *CT scanning* and *MRI*). Because the nervous system is profusely supplied with blood vessels that may be involved in a neurological disorder, *angiography* (an X-ray imaging technique to show blood vessels) is often used in diagnosis.

In the past, relatively few disorders of the nervous system could be treated effectively. Today, however, with better understanding of the biochemical and structural bases of neurological disorders, new treatments are being developed, including the surgical removal of tumors, repair of damaged nerves (see *Neurosurgery*), transplantation of adrenal tissue in *Parkinson's disease*, and drug treatment of some forms of *dementia*.

## Neuroma

A benign tumor of nerve tissue that may affect any nerve in the body. In most cases, the cause is unknown; rarely, a neuroma develops as a result of damage to a nerve.

The symptoms vary according to the nerve involved. In general, there is intermittent pain in parts of the body supplied by the nerve. The same areas may also become numb and weak if the neuroma develops in a confined space and presses on the nerve.

If the symptoms are troublesome, the tumor may be surgically removed. (See also *Acoustic neuroma*.)

## Neuron

A nerve cell. There are billions of neurons in the nervous system; they act in various combinations to do everything from writing a symphony to scratching a fleabite. The neurons are analogous to the wires in a complex electrical machine.

There are three main types of neuron—interneurons, motoneurons, and sensory neurons (see illustrated box, overleaf).

### FUNCTION

The function of a neuron is to signal, or "fire" (that is, to transmit an electrical impulse along its axon), under certain specific conditions. The electrical impulse causes the release of a neurotransmitter from the axon terminals, which in turn may cause a muscle cell to contract, cause an endocrine gland to release a hormone, or affect the next neuron in a circuit.

Different stimuli excite different types of neurons to fire. Sensory neurons may be excited by physical stimuli, such as light of a certain wavelength, pressure, or cold. The activity of most neurons is controlled by the effects of neurotransmitters released from adjacent neurons.

The ability of a neuron to fire depends on a small difference in electric potential between the inside and outside of the cell. Under the direct influence of an excitatory neurotransmitter, a sudden change occurs in this potential at one point on the cell's membrane. The change, called an "action potential," then flows along the membrane (and thus along the axon of the cell) at speeds up to several hundred miles per hour. A neuron may be able to fire in this way several times every second.

There are also neurotransmitters that stabilize neuronal membranes, preventing an action potential. Thus, the firing pattern of a neuron depends on the balance of excitatory and inhibitory influences acting on it.

### LIFE SPAN

If the cell body of a neuron is damaged or degenerates, the cell dies and is never replaced. A baby starts life with the maximum number of neurons; their number decreases continuously thereafter. We seem to be born with an excess number of neurons, so problems arise only when disease, injury, or persistent alcohol abuse affects the central nervous system, dramatically increasing the rate of neuron loss.

If a peripheral nerve is damaged, its individual fibers can regenerate (see *Nerve injury*; *Neuropathy*).

## Neuropathic joint

A joint damaged by a series of injuries, which pass unnoticed because of neuropathy (loss of sensation) affecting that joint. Neuropathic joints develop in a number of conditions, including *diabetes mellitus* and untreated *syphilis*.

When sensation to pain is lost, abnormal stress and strain on a joint do not stimulate the protective reflex spasm of the surrounding muscles; this allows exaggerated movement that can damage the joint. Severe recurrent damage to a joint may lead to *osteoarthritis*, swelling, and deformity; there is minimal pain because of the lack of sensation.

### DIAGNOSIS AND TREATMENT

Severe joint degeneration and deformity are visible on X rays. A brace or caliper splint may be necessary to restrict abnormal joint movement. Occasionally, an arthrodesis (joint fusion) is performed. The nerve damage is irreversible.

## Neuropathology

The study of diseases and disorders of the nervous system. Neuropathologists are concerned principally with the causes and effects of neurological conditions rather than with their diagnosis and treatment (usually handled by a *neurologist* or *neurosurgeon*).

## N

## Neuropathy

Disease, inflammation, or damage to the peripheral nerves, which connect the central nervous system, or CNS (brain and spinal cord), to the sense organs, muscles, glands, and internal organs. Symptoms caused by neuropathies include numbness, tingling, pain, or muscle weakness, depending on the nerves affected.

### TYPES

Most nerve cell axons (the conducting fibers that make up nerves) are insulated within a sheath of a fatty substance called *myelin*, but some are unmyelinated. Most neuropathies arise from damage or irritation either to the axons or to their myelin sheaths. An axon may suffer thinning, complete loss of, or patchy loss of its myelin sheath. This may cause a slowing or a complete block to the passage of electrical signals.

Various types of neuropathy are described according to the site and distribution of damage. For example, a distal neuropathy starts with damage at the far end of a nerve (farthest from the brain or spinal cord). A symmetrical neuropathy

## STRUCTURE OF A NEURON

A neuron (nerve cell) consists of a cell body and several branching projections called dendrites. Every neuron has a filamentous projection called an axon (nerve fiber). Axons vary in length from a fraction of an inch to several feet. An axon branches at its end to form terminals, via which signals are transmitted to target cells, such as the dendrites of other neurons, muscle cells, or glands. Bundles of the axons of many neurons are known as nerves or, within the brain or spinal cord, as nerve tracts or pathways.

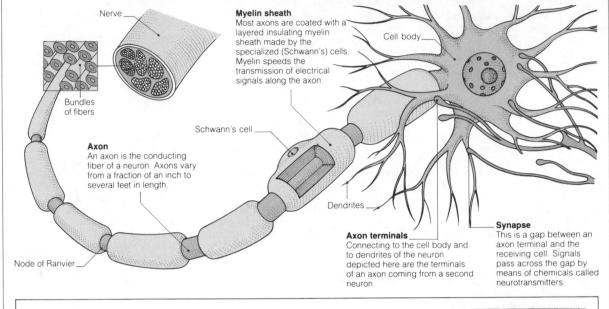

Nerve

Bundles of fibers

**Myelin sheath**
Most axons are coated with a layered insulating myelin sheath made by the specialized (Schwann's) cells. Myelin speeds the transmission of electrical signals along the axon.

Cell body

Schwann's cell

**Axon**
An axon is the conducting fiber of a neuron. Axons vary from a fraction of an inch to several feet in length.

Node of Ranvier

Dendrites

**Axon terminals**
Connecting to the cell body and to dendrites of the neuron depicted here are the terminals of an axon coming from a second neuron.

**Synapse**
This is a gap between an axon terminal and the receiving cell. Signals pass across the gap by means of chemicals called neurotransmitters.

**N**

### BASIC TYPES OF NEURON

Sensory neurons carry signals from sense receptors along their axons into the CNS. Motoneurons carry signals from the CNS to muscles or glands; the axon terminals form a motor end-plate. Interneurons form all the complex interconnecting electrical circuitry within the CNS itself. For each sensory neuron in the body, there are about 10 motoneurons and 99 interneurons.

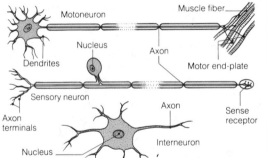

Motoneuron

Muscle fiber

Nucleus

Dendrites

Axon

Motor end-plate

Sensory neuron

Axon terminals

Axon

Sense receptor

Nucleus

Interneuron

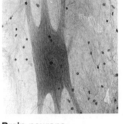

**Brain neurons**
Electron micrograph of interneurons in the brain.

affects nerves at the same places on each side of the body. Some neuropathies are described according to their underlying cause (e.g., diabetic neuropathy and alcoholic neuropathy).

The term neuritis is now used virtually interchangeably with neuropathy. Polyneuropathy (or polyneuritis) literally means damage to several nerves; mononeuropathy (or mononeuritis) indicates damage to a single nerve. *Neuralgia* describes pain caused by irritation or inflammation of a particular nerve.

### CAUSES

In some cases of neuropathy there is no obvious or detectable cause. Among the many specific causes are *diabetes mellitus*, dietary deficiencies (particularly of B vitamins), persistent excessive alcohol consumption, and metabolic upsets such as *uremia*. Other causes include *leprosy*, *lead poisoning*, or poisoning by drugs.

Nerves may become acutely inflamed. This often occurs after a viral infection (for example, in *Guillain-Barré syndrome*). Neuropathies may result from autoimmune disorders such as *rheumatoid arthritis*, systemic *lupus erythematosus*, or *periarteritis nodosa*. In these disorders, there is often damage to the blood vessels supplying the nerves. Neuropathies may occur secondarily to malignant tumors such as *lung cancer*, or with *lymphomas* and *leukemias*. Finally, there is a group of inherited neuropathies, the most common being *peroneal muscular atrophy*.

### SYMPTOMS

The symptoms of neuropathy depend on whether it affects mainly sensory nerve fibers or motor nerve fibers. Damage to sensory nerve fibers may cause numbness and tingling, sensations of cold, or pain, often starting in the hands and feet and spreading toward the body center. Damage to motor fibers may cause muscle weakness and muscle wasting.

Damage to nerves of the autonomic nervous system may lead to blurred vision, impaired or absent sweating, episodes of faintness associated with falls in blood pressure, and disturbance of gastric, intestinal, bladder, and sexual functioning, including incontinence and impotence. Some neuropathies are linked with particular symptoms (for example, very painful neuropathies may arise in diabetes mellitus and in *alcohol dependence*).

**DIAGNOSIS**
To determine the extent of damage, studies of nerve conduction are performed, along with *EMG* tests, which record the electrical activity in muscles. To determine the cause of neuropathy, *blood tests*, X rays, nerve or muscle *biopsy* (removal of tissue for analysis), and various other tests may be required.

**TREATMENT**
When possible, treatment is aimed at the underlying cause. For example, in diabetes mellitus, scrupulous attention to the control of the blood sugar level affords the best chances for recovery. Other people may need to stop drinking alcohol, or, if a nutritional deficiency has been diagnosed, may be given injections of vitamins such as thiamine (vitamin $B_1$).

If treatment is successful and the cell bodies of the damaged nerve cells have not been destroyed, a full recovery from the neuropathy is possible.

## Neuropsychiatry
The branch of medicine that deals with the relationship between psychiatric symptoms and distinct neurological disorders. These conditions are usually forms of brain disease, such as *temporal lobe epilepsy*, tumors, or infections. Research and brain imaging are revealing evidence that subtle forms of brain damage underlie certain psychotic illnesses.

## Neurosis
A term commonly used to describe a range of relatively mild psychiatric disorders in which the sufferer remains in touch with reality.

Neurotic symptoms are distressing to the afflicted person, who is aware of a change from his or her usual psychological state. By contrast, people suffering from psychotic illnesses do not recognize that they are sick (see *Psychosis*). Neurotic symptoms generally do not lead to distinctly abnormal behavior, although they can severely limit work or social activities. They tend to fluctuate in intensity,

often in response to social or personal stresses. No physical abnormality has been shown to underlie them.

The major neurotic disorders are *depression* (the mild form); *anxiety disorders*, including *phobias* and *obsessive-compulsive behavior*; *somatization disorder*; and *dissociative disorders*. *Psychosexual disorders* have recently been included in this category.

## Neurosurgeon
A surgeon who operates on the brain, spinal cord, or other parts of the nervous system (see *Neurosurgery*).

## Neurosurgery
The specialty concerned with the surgical treatment of disorders of the nervous system. Many generalized nervous system disorders do not respond to surgical treatment, but neurosurgery can deal with most conditions in which a localized structural change interferes with nerve function.

Conditions treated by neurosurgery include tumors of the brain, spinal cord, or meninges (membranes that surround the brain and spinal cord), certain abnormalities of the blood vessels that supply the brain, such as an *aneurysm* (a bulge in a weak point of an artery), bleeding inside the skull (see *Extradural hemorrhage*; *Intracerebral hemorrhage*; *Subdural hemorrhage*), *brain abscess*, some birth defects (such as *hydrocephalus* and *spina bifida*), certain types of *epilepsy*, and nerve damage caused by illness or accidents. Neurosurgeons are also concerned with the surgical relief of otherwise untreatable pain.

## Neurosyphilis
Infection of the brain or spinal cord that occurs in untreated *syphilis* many years after the initial infection.

Damage to the spinal cord due to neurosyphilis may cause tabes dorsalis, characterized by poor coordination of leg movements when walking, urinary incontinence, and intermittent pains in the abdomen and limbs. Damage to the brain may cause *dementia*, muscle weakness, and, in rare cases, extensive neurologic damage (when it is called general paralysis of the insane).

## Neurotoxin
A chemical that damages nervous tissue. The principal effects of neurotoxic nerve damage are numbness, weakness, or paralysis of the part of the body supplied by the affected nerve. Neurotoxins are pres-

ent in the venom of certain snakes (see *Snakebites*), and are released by some types of bacteria (such as those that cause *tetanus* and *diphtheria*). Some chemical poisons, such as arsenic and lead, are also neurotoxic.

## Neurotransmitter
Although nerve impulses are electrical, the transmission of these impulses from one neuron (nerve cell) to another, or to a muscle cell, is achieved chemically rather than electrically. The chemical that transmits the message is a neurotransmitter. Scores of different chemicals fulfill this function in different parts of the nervous system (see box, overleaf).

Many neurotransmitters are similar to, or identical to, substances used by our bodies as hormones. These neurotransmitters also act as messenger molecules, but are released into the bloodstream to act on their target cells at a distance.

**TYPES**
One of the most important neurotransmitters is *acetylcholine*. It is released by neurons connected to skeletal muscles (causing them to contract) and by neurons that control the sweat glands and the heart beat. It also transmits messages between neurons in the brain and spinal cord.

Interference with the action of acetylcholine on skeletal muscles is the cause of the disease *myasthenia gravis*; depletion of the nerve cells that release acetylcholine in the brain may be a cause of *Alzheimer's disease*.

Another transmitter, *norepinephrine*, is important in nerve pathways controlling heart beat, blood flow, and response to stress. In addition to being produced in the body by neurons, norepinephrine is made by the *adrenal glands*. Dopamine plays an important role in parts of the brain that control movement, and malfunction of the neurons that respond to dopamine is thought to be important in causing *Parkinson's disease*. *Serotonin* is one of the primary neurotransmitters in parts of the brain concerned with conscious processes.

Over the last 20 years, a whole new family of transmitters, called the neuropeptides, has been discovered. Neuropeptides are small proteins; they are larger molecules than the previously known neurotransmitters, which are all very small molecules. The best studied of these neuropeptides are the *endorphins*, which are used by the brain to control sensitivity to pain.

N

## Nevus

A skin blemish that can be flat, raised slightly above the skin's surface, or on a stalk; a nevus can be colored or not colored, and with or without hair growth. Some nevi are present at birth, others develop at any age.

### TYPES

There are two main types of nevus: melanocytic (pigmented) nevi, caused by abnormality or overactivity of skin cells producing the pigment *melanin*, and vascular nevi, caused by an abnormal collection of blood vessels.

The most common type of pigmented nevi are *freckles*, which are small, flat, light to dark brown areas found on any part of the body that is exposed to the sun. A *lentigo* is a pale to brown spot very similar to a freckle. *Café au lait spots* are another type of light brown pigmented nevus.

A mole (a brown to dark brown spot that is not usually present at birth) is another common type of nevus. As a child grows, moles may spread, forming an average number of 15 to 20 per person by adulthood. In rare cases these moles become cancerous (see *Melanoma, malignant*).

Unusual types of moles include hairy, pigmented nevi found on the shoulders of some young men, halo nevi (in which the skin surrounding the nevus lightens in color to give a characteristic "halo" appearance), and juvenile melanomas (see *Melanoma, juvenile*), which are red-brown nevi that occur in childhood.

Some nevi have a bluish coloration; these so-called blue nevi are often found on the backs of the hands of young girls. Most black and Asian infants are born with one or more blue-black spots on their lower backs (see *Mongolian spot*).

Another type of nevus is a vascular nevus (*hemangioma*), caused by an abnormal collection of blood vessels; a port-wine mark is an example.

### TREATMENT

Most nevi are harmless and do not require treatment. However, if a nevus suddenly appears, grows, bleeds, or changes color, medical advice should be sought without delay to exclude the possibility of cancer. (See also *Spider nevus*.)

## Newborn

An infant at birth and during the first few weeks of life.

### INITIAL EXAMINATION

Immediately after birth, the newborn baby is briefly checked by the nurse, midwife, or physician in attendance.

---

## HOW NEUROTRANSMITTERS WORK

When an electrical impulse travels down a nerve cell axon, it causes the release of a chemical neurotransmitter at the axon terminals. The chemical is not the same in every case; acetylcholine, norepinephrine, dopamine, and serotonin are all important examples.

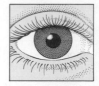 

**Example of neurotransmitter activity**
Neurotransmitters enable the pupil to change size in different light conditions.

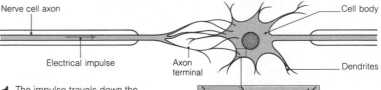

Nerve cell axon — Cell body

Electrical impulse — Axon terminal — Dendrites

**1** The impulse travels down the neuronal axon (above), from the cell body toward the axon terminals; neurotransmitter is released from tiny swellings, called synaptic knobs, at the axon terminals.

**2** The neurotransmitter crosses the gap, or synapse, to the surface membrane of the target cell (right), where it binds to a protein called a receptor.

**3** If sufficient target cell receptors are activated by neurotransmitter binding, an impulse is initiated and passes in turn down the target cell's axon (below right).

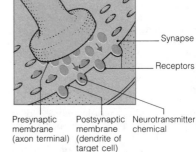

Synapse

Receptors

Presynaptic membrane (axon terminal)   Postsynaptic membrane (dendrite of target cell)   Neurotransmitter chemical

Electrical impulse to target

---

This examination includes checking the heart rate with a *stethoscope* and establishing that breathing is normal. The *Apgar score* and other tests are performed to check the baby's health. The baby's sex is noted and a check made for any obvious *birth defect*.

### NURSING PROCEDURE

The baby is labeled with his or her name and date of birth; the birth weight, length, and head circumference are recorded. Usually a handprint or footprint is recorded along with the mother's fingerprint or thumbprint for identification.

At birth, the baby is usually covered with vernix, a greasy, white substance that protects it in the uterus. It is wiped off and the baby is wrapped in a blanket and given to the mother to hold and to feed, or placed in a warm crib. If very small or sick, the baby is kept in an *incubator* and treated in a neonatal intensive-care unit or other intensive-care unit.

The frequency of the baby's urine and *meconium* (the newborn stool) is recorded. During the second week of life, two special blood tests are performed. The *Guthrie test* is performed on all babies to check for *phenylketonuria*. The other test done at this time checks for *hypothyroidism*.

### MEDICAL EXAMINATION

Within 24 hours of birth, the baby is usually given a complete medical examination by his or her physician. This examination assesses the baby's general health and identifies any birth defects (such as cleft palate). The skull, eyes, face, abdomen, heart, spine, hips, genitals, and limbs are checked, and the baby's posture, movements, behavior, cry, reflexes, and responsiveness are noted (see *Reflexes, primitive*).

### ABNORMALITIES IN THE NEWBORN

The newborn baby may have a swollen or misshapen head due to pressure during labor. Less commonly, there may be more notable evidence of *birth injury*, such as *cephalhematoma* (swelling of the scalp caused by bruising around the skull). Most problems caused by the pressure of delivery resolve themselves within a few days.

*Jaundice* is extremely common in the newborn, especially if the baby is breast-fed. Usually appearing on the second or third day, the jaundice generally disappears over the next few days. In most cases, jaundice in the newborn is harmless. However, it may be serious if it appears during the first 24 hours or occurs in a very premature infant.

Some newborn girls have slight vaginal bleeding or discharge, and babies of either sex may have enlargement of the breasts. These harmless conditions are caused by maternal sex hormones that reached the fetus through the placenta. Any extra hormones soon leave the baby's body.

The umbilical cord, which may be painted with a dye to prevent infection, usually dries and drops off within a week or so of birth. Serious infections of the cord stump can occur.

Minor, harmless abnormalities of the newborn include *milia* (tiny, white spots on the face), *hemangioma*, *mongolian spot*, and *urticaria* of the newborn (a blotchy, red rash that occurs around the second day). See also *Prematurity*; *Postmaturity*.

## Niacin
See *Vitamin B*.

## Nickel
A metallic element that is present in the body in minute amounts. Its exact role is poorly understood. Nickel is thought to activate certain *enzymes* (substances that promote biochemical reactions). It also may play a part in stabilizing chromosomal material in the nuclei of cells.

Disease due to a deficiency of nickel is unknown. However, excessive exposure to it—which occurs most commonly in industrial workers—may cause *dermatitis* (inflammation of the skin) or, rarely, *lung cancer*.

## Niclosamide
An *antihelmintic drug* used in the treatment of *worm infestation*. Niclosamide acts on tapeworms in the intestine, causing them to loosen their grip and be passed out of the body in the feces.

Adverse effects are uncommon and are typical of those produced by other antihelmintic drugs.

## Nicotine

A drug in tobacco that acts as a stimulant and is responsible for dependence on tobacco. The drug has no medical use, but certain of its derivatives are used as pesticides.

After inhalation, the nicotine in tobacco smoke passes rapidly into the bloodstream. Nicotine in chewing tobacco is absorbed more slowly through the lining of the mouth. Once in the bloodstream, the drug acts on the nervous system until it is eventually broken down by the liver and excreted in the urine.

**EFFECTS**
Nicotine acts primarily on the *autonomic nervous system*, which controls involuntary body activities such as the heart rate. The effects of the drug vary from one person to another, and also depend on dosage and past usage. In someone unused to smoking, even a small amount of nicotine may slow the heart rate and cause nausea and vomiting. However, in habitual smokers, the drug increases the heart rate, narrows the blood vessels (the combined effect of which is to raise blood pressure), and stimulates the central nervous system, thereby reducing fatigue, increasing alertness, and improving concentration.

Regular tobacco smoking results in tolerance to nicotine, so that a higher intake is needed to bring about the same effect. However, this process is much less notable with tobacco than with other addictive drugs.

**NICOTINE AND DISEASE**
Although it is the tar in tobacco smoke that damages lung tissue and causes lung cancer, tobacco smoking is also clearly associated with *coronary heart disease*, *peripheral vascular disease*, and other cardiovascular disorders. It is uncertain whether these disorders are caused by the nicotine or by the carbon monoxide content of the smoke.

Excessively large amounts of nicotine can cause poisoning, which may result in vomiting, seizures, and, very occasionally, death.

**WITHDRAWAL**
Because most smokers are physically dependent on nicotine, stopping smoking often causes withdrawal symptoms, such as drowsiness, headaches, fatigue, and difficulty concentrating. To reduce these symptoms in a person who is trying to stop smoking, a physician may prescribe nicotine chewing gum, which has a less harmful effect on the circulatory system. (See also *Tobacco smoking*.)

## Nicotinic acid
See *Vitamin B*.

## Nifedipine
A *calcium channel blocker* used mainly to prevent and treat *angina pectoris*. It is also often used to treat *hypertension* (high blood pressure) and disorders affecting the circulation, such as *Raynaud's disease*.

Possible adverse effects are *edema* (fluid retention), flushing, headache, and dizziness.

## Night blindness
The inability to see well in dim light. Many people with night blindness show no discernible eye disease. In other people, the condition may be an inherited functional defect of the retina or an early sign of *retinitis pigmentosa*. Night blindness is sometimes caused by vitamin A deficiency.

## Nightmare
An unpleasant vivid dream, often accompanied by a sense of suffocation. Nightmares occur during REM (rapid eye movement) *sleep*, in the middle and later parts of the night, and are often clearly remembered if the dreamer awakens completely.

Nightmares are very common, especially in children aged 8 to 10. They are particularly likely to occur when the child's breathing is slightly difficult because of a cold or illness, or when there is anxiety over separation from parents or home. In adults, nightmares may be a side effect of certain drugs, including *beta-blocker drugs* and *benzodiazepine drugs*. Traumatic events (such as accidents, torture, or prolonged imprisonment) seem to be particularly associated with disturbing and repeated nightmares. However, there is no specific relationship to psychiatric illness.

Nightmares should not be confused with hypnagogic *hallucinations*, which occur while falling asleep, or with *night terror*, which occurs in NREM (nonrapid eye movement) sleep and is not remembered the next day.

## Night terror
A disorder, occurring mainly in children, consisting of abrupt arousals from sleep in a terrified state. Night terror (also called sleep terror) usually starts between the ages of 4 and 7, and gradually disappears in early adolescence. Episodes occur during NREM (nonrapid eye movement) *sleep*, usually half an hour to three and a half hours after falling asleep.

N

Sufferers awaken screaming in a semiconscious state and remain frightened for some minutes. They do not recognize familiar faces or surroundings, and usually cannot be comforted. Physical signs of agitation, such as sweating or an increased heart rate, are also common. Gradually, the sufferer falls back to sleep and has no memory of the event the next day.

Though distressing to parents, night terror in children has no serious significance. In adults, it is likely to be associated with an *anxiety disorder*.

## NIH

The abbreviation for the National Institutes of Health. The institutes are a part of the Department of Health and Human Services and comprise a research hospital, a computerized medical library, and 11 of the largest and best-financed research organizations in the world. One of them concentrates on cancer; the others have broader charters—the National Institute of Allergy and Infectious Diseases, for example, and the National Heart, Lung, and Blood Institute. The major focus of medical and dental research in the US, the NIH finance additional research programs in universities, hospitals, and other nongovernment institutions.

## Nipple

The small prominence at the tip of each breast. Each of a woman's nipples contains tiny openings through which milk can pass. The nipple and the surrounding areola are darker than the surrounding skin, darkening more and increasing in size during pregnancy. Muscle in the nipple allows it to become erect.

### DISORDERS

Structural defects of the nipple are rare. One or both nipples may be absent, or there may be additional nipples along a line extending from the armpit to the groin.

An inverted nipple is usually an abnormality of development. It can be corrected by drawing out the nipple between finger and thumb daily for several weeks. Inversion of a previously normal nipple in an adult is much more significant and may be due to *breast cancer*.

Cracked nipples are common during the last months of pregnancy and during breast-feeding. Daily washing, drying, and moisturizing of the nipple can help prevent it. In addition to causing discomfort, cracks may lead to infective *mastitis*.

---

### LOCATION OF THE NIPPLE

The protrusion at the tip of the breast, surrounded by the areola. Milk ducts emerge at the nipple.

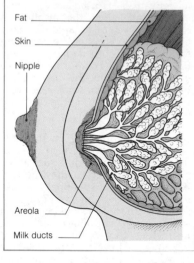

Fat
Skin
Nipple
Areola
Milk ducts

---

Papilloma of the nipple is a benign swelling attached to the skin by a stalk. *Paget's disease of the nipple* appears initially as persistent eczema of the nipple. It is caused by a slowly growing cancer arising in a milk duct, and surgical treatment is required.

Discharge from the nipple occurs for a variety of reasons. A clear, straw-colored discharge may develop in early pregnancy. A milky discharge may occur after the period of breast-feeding is over. *Galactorrhea* (discharge of milk in someone who is not pregnant or breast-feeding) may be caused by a hormone imbalance; rarely, it may be due to a galactocele (a cyst under the areola). A discharge containing pus indicates a breast *abscess*. A bloodstained discharge may be due to mammary dysplasia (abnormal tissue), chronic mastitis, or cancer.

## Nit

The egg of a louse. Both head lice and pubic lice produce eggs, which they glue to the base of hairs growing from their host's head or pubes. The nits are tiny—about one fiftieth of an inch (0.5 mm) in diameter—and yellow (newly laid) or white (hatched). They hatch within eight days, and the empty eggshells are carried outward as the hair grows.

Louse infestations are often diagnosed from the presence of nits. The distance from the base of hairs to the furthest nits provides a rough approximation of the duration of the infestation. (See *Lice*; *Pubic lice*.)

## Nitrate drugs

### COMMON DRUGS

*Isosorbide dinitrate Nitroglycerin*

A group of *vasodilator drugs* used in the treatment of *angina pectoris* (chest pain due to impaired blood supply to heart muscle) and severe *heart failure* (reduced pumping efficiency).

Possible adverse effects of nitrate drugs include headache, flushing, and dizziness. *Tolerance* (the need for greater amounts of the drug to have the same effect) may develop when the drug is used regularly.

## Nitrites

Salts of nitrous acid (a nitrogen-containing acid). Some of these chemicals, notably sodium nitrite, are added to certain foods in small quantities (mainly meat products such as sausages) because they act as preservatives and destroy bacteria that cause *food poisoning*. In large amounts, nitrites can cause dizziness, nausea, and vomiting.

Within the intestine, nitrites are converted to substances called nitrosamines. In laboratory tests, nitrosamines have been shown to cause cancer in animals. However, there is no conclusive proof that they have the same effect in humans or that eating food containing nitrites is harmful to health.

## Nitrofurantoin

An *antibacterial drug* used in the treatment of *urinary tract infection*.

Nitrofurantoin should be taken with food to reduce the risk of irritating the stomach, which can prompt abdominal pain and nausea. More serious adverse effects, such as breathing difficulty, numbness, and jaundice, are rare.

## Nitrogen

A colorless, odorless gas that makes up 78 percent of the Earth's atmosphere. Atmospheric nitrogen has no biological action, although, in scuba diving, bubbles of nitrogen gas may form in body fluids if a diver ascends to the surface too rapidly, causing the condition commonly called the "bends" (see *Decompression sickness*).

Although nitrogen gas cannot be utilized by the body, compounds of nitrogen are essential to life. Probably

N

the most important of such compounds are *amino acids*, the building blocks of *proteins*, which represent the fundamental structural substances of all cells and tissues. Because humans cannot make amino acids, they must be obtained from the diet in the form of animal and plant proteins. The proteins are then broken down into their constituent amino acids so that they can be absorbed and reconstituted into the specific proteins needed by the body. These processes of protein breakdown and reconstitution produce a variety of nitrogen-containing waste products, primarily *urea*, which is excreted from the body in the urine. (See also *Nitrate drugs; Nitrites*.)

## Nitroglycerin

A *vasodilator drug* used to treat and prevent symptoms of *angina pectoris* (chest pain due to an inadequate blood supply to the heart). Nitroglycerin may cause headache, flushing, and dizziness; adverse effects are usually relieved by a reduction in the dose.

## Nitrous oxide

A colorless gas (sometimes called laughing gas) with a sweet taste that is used with oxygen to provide *analgesia* (pain relief) and light anesthesia (see *Anesthesia, general*) during dental procedures, childbirth, and minor surgery. For major surgery requiring deeper anesthesia, nitrous oxide and oxygen need to be combined with other drugs.

The advantages of the combination of nitrous oxide and oxygen over other agents are their rapid action and nonflammability. Possible adverse effects include nausea and vomiting during the recovery period.

## NMR

Abbreviation for nuclear magnetic resonance. The preferred term for this technique is magnetic resonance imaging (see *MRI*).

## Nocardiosis

An infection caused by a funguslike bacterium. The infection usually starts in the lung and spreads via the bloodstream to the brain and tissues under the skin. The causative organism is present in the soil in all parts of the world and is acquired by inhalation. Nocardiosis is rare except in people with *immunodeficiency disorders* or those already suffering from other serious disease.

The infection causes a pneumonia-like illness, with fever and cough. It fails to settle under normal, short-term, antibiotic treatment, and signs of progressive lung damage occur. Brain abscesses may follow. The condition is diagnosed by microscopic examination of sputum (phlegm). Treatment, which may have to be continued for 12 to 18 months, is with *sulfonamide drugs*, sometimes in conjunction with other antibiotics (such as trimethoprim).

## Nocturia

The disturbance of a person's sleep at night by the need to pass urine. In most people, a moderately full bladder does not usually disturb sleep, although light sleepers are more likely to wake to empty their bladders. Drinking alcohol in the evening stimulates urine production and may result in nocturia.

A common cause of nocturia is enlargement of the prostate gland (see *Prostate, enlarged*), which obstructs the normal outflow of urine and causes the bladder to be full at night.

Another common cause is *heart failure* (reduced pumping efficiency of the heart) leading to the retention of excess fluid, which is absorbed into the bloodstream and carried to the kidneys at night to make more urine.

Also common is *cystitis* (inflammation of the bladder), in which irritation of the bladder wall increases its sensitivity so that smaller volumes of urine trigger a desire to pass urine.

Rarer causes of nocturia include *diabetes mellitus* (in which greater volumes of urine are produced both day and night) and chronic *renal failure* (in which the kidney loses its ability to produce a reduced quantity of more concentrated urine at night).

## Nocturnal emission

Ejaculation that occurs during sleep, commonly called a "wet dream." Nocturnal emission is normal in male adolescents and is a common cause of unnecessary anxiety. Nocturnal emissions may also occur in adult males whose sexual activity is limited.

## Node

A small, rounded mass of tissue that may be normal or abnormal. The term most commonly refers to a *lymph node*, which is a normal structure in the lymphatic system. Abnormal nodes are often called *nodules*.

## Nodule

A small lump of tissue, usually more than one quarter of an inch (6 mm) in diameter. A nodule may protrude from the skin's surface or it may form deep under the skin. Nodules may be either hard or soft.

## Noise

Sound that is disordered, unwanted, or that interferes with hearing.

*Hearing* may be damaged by exposure to intensely loud noise for a short period (such as an explosion at close range) or by prolonged exposure to lower levels of noise (such as might occur in a machine room or foundry). Any noise above 90 decibels may cause damage; the louder the noise, the shorter the time required for damage to occur (see chart).

### HOW NOISE DAMAGES HEARING

Exposure to a sudden very loud noise, usually above 130 decibels, can cause immediate and permanent damage. Normally, muscles in the middle ear respond to loud noise by altering the stiffness of the chain of bones that pass vibrations to the inner ear, thus reducing their efficiency. But when the noise occurs without warning, these protective reflexes have no time to respond. The full force of the vibrations is carried to the inner ear, causing severe damage to delicate hair cells in the cochlea. Occasionally, loud noises can rupture the eardrum.

**COMPARATIVE NOISE LEVELS**

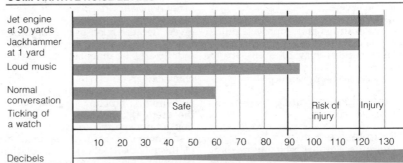

| | | | |
|---|---|---|---|
| Jet engine at 30 yards | | | |
| Jackhammer at 1 yard | | | |
| Loud music | | | |
| Normal conversation | Safe | Risk of injury | Injury |
| Ticking of a watch | | | |

10  20  30  40  50  60  70  80  90  100  110  120  130

Decibels

More commonly, damage from loud noise occurs over a period of time, with gradual destruction of the hair cells of the cochlea and permanent hearing loss.

### SYMPTOMS OF NOISE DAMAGE
Sound at 90 decibels or above usually causes pain, which is a warning that hearing may be damaged unless the source of the noise is removed. Prolonged *tinnitus* (ringing or buzzing in the ears) that occurs after a noise has ceased is an indication that some damage has probably occurred.

Prolonged exposure to loud noise leads initially to a loss of ability to hear certain high tones. Later, deafness extends to all high frequencies and the perception of speech becomes impaired. Eventually, lower tones are also affected.

### PREVENTION OF NOISE DAMAGE
Regulations governing maximum noise levels apply to places of work and to some other potential hazards, such as noise from low-flying aircraft. People who cannot avoid exposure to loud noise (for example, workers using pneumatic drills) should wear earplugs. People who are persistently exposed to loud noise should have their hearing monitored regularly.

## N Noma
Also known as cancrum oris, death of tissue in the lips and cheeks caused by bacterial infection. Noma is most often seen in (and largely confined to) young, severely malnourished children in developing countries. It may complicate other diseases, especially *measles*, and sometimes occurs during the last stages of *leukemia*.

### SYMPTOMS
The first symptom is inflammation of the gums and the inner surface of the cheeks. Without treatment, this leads to severe ulceration (with a foul-smelling discharge) and eventual destruction of the bones around the mouth and loss of teeth. Healing occurs naturally after a time, but scarring may be severe.

### TREATMENT
Penicillin drugs and improved nutrition halt the progress of the disease. Plastic surgery may be necessary to reconstruct damaged bones or to improve facial appearance.

## Nonaccidental injury
See *Child abuse*.

## Noninvasive
A term used to describe any medical procedure that does not involve penetration of the skin or entry into the body through any of the natural openings; examples include *CT scanning* and *echocardiography*. The term noninvasive is sometimes applied to benign tumors that do not spread throughout body tissues.

## Nonspecific urethritis
Also called nongonococcal urethritis, inflammation of the urethra due to a cause or causes other than *gonorrhea*. Worldwide, nonspecific urethritis is the most common type of *sexually transmitted disease*.

### CAUSES
The name nonspecific urethritis was given to the disorder at a time when few laboratory tests were available for the detection of microorganisms. Today, about 40 percent of cases are known to be caused by CHLAMYDIA TRACHOMATIS (see *Chlamydial infections*); others are caused by HERPESVIRUS HOMINIS (the virus that causes *herpes simplex*) or TRICHOMONAS VAGINALIS infections. In about 50 percent of cases, however, the cause remains unknown.

### SYMPTOMS
Nonspecific urethritis has an incubation period of about two to three weeks. In men, the infection usually causes a clear or pus-containing urethral discharge often accompanied by pain or discomfort on passing urine. Sometimes these symptoms are very mild or even absent. Women with nonspecific urethritis may have no symptoms; some have a vaginal discharge, mild discomfort on passing urine, or pain in the pelvic region.

### DIAGNOSIS AND TREATMENT
Laboratory tests are performed to find the organism responsible for the infection. Because a woman may have no symptoms, a diagnosis often rests on the fact that she has a male partner with nonspecific urethritis.

Treatment is difficult because in many cases the cause cannot be determined. The cure rate is roughly 85 percent. *Antibiotic drugs*, including oxytetracycline and erythromycin, are given. Because relapses are common, follow-up visits are necessary for three months after treatment to examine the urine and any discharge.

### COMPLICATIONS
In men, *cystitis*, *epididymitis*, *prostatitis*, and urethral stricture (narrowing of the urethra) can occur as complications of nonspecific urethritis.

In women, *salpingitis* (inflammation of the fallopian tubes), cysts of the Bartholin's glands, and *cervicitis* may occur. *Ophthalmia* neonatorum, a type of conjunctivitis, sometimes develops in babies born to women with chlamydial cervicitis.

*Reiter's syndrome* (in which there is arthritis and conjunctivitis as well as urethritis) develops in about 5 percent of people with nonspecific urethritis.

## Nonsteroidal anti-inflammatory drugs

| COMMON DRUGS |
| --- |
| Diflunisal Fenoprofen Ibuprofen Indomethacin Meclofenamate Naproxen Phenylbutazone Piroxicam Sulindac Tolmetin |

> **WARNING**
> Report abdominal pain or indigestion to your physician.

A group of drugs that has an *analgesic* (painkilling) action and also reduces inflammation in joints and soft tissues, such as muscles and ligaments. The name nonsteroidal anti-inflammatory drugs is commonly abbreviated NSAIDs.

### WHY THEY ARE USED
NSAIDs are widely used to relieve symptoms caused by types of arthritis, such as *rheumatoid arthritis*, *osteoarthritis*, and *gout*. They do not cure or halt the progress of disease but improve mobility of the affected joint by relieving pain and stiffness.

NSAIDs are also used in the treatment of back pain, menstrual pain, headaches, pain after minor surgery, and soft tissue injuries.

### HOW THEY WORK
NSAIDs reduce pain and inflammation by blocking the production of prostaglandins (chemicals that cause inflammation and trigger transmission of pain signals to the brain).

### POSSIBLE ADVERSE EFFECTS
Nausea, indigestion, diarrhea, and *peptic ulcer* may occur.

## Norepinephrine
A hormone secreted by certain nerve endings (principally those of the *sympathetic nervous system*) and by the medulla (center) of the *adrenal glands*. Norepinephrine's primary function is to help maintain a constant blood pressure by stimulating certain blood vessels to constrict when the blood pressure falls below normal. For this reason, an injection of the hormone may be given in the emergency treatment of *shock* or severe bleeding. (See also *Epinephrine*.)

## Norethindrone

A *progesterone drug* that is used with an *estrogen drug* in several *oral contraceptive* preparations and in *hormone replacement therapy*.

On its own, norethindrone is sometimes used to treat women who are suffering from *endometriosis*, *amenorrhea* (absent periods), or irregular menstrual bleeding (see *Menstruation, disorders of*).

## Norgestrel

A synthetic *progesterone drug* used in some *oral contraceptive* preparations.

## Nortriptyline

An *antidepressant drug* that also has a sedative effect. Nortriptyline is useful in the treatment of *depression* that may follow a *stroke*.

## Nose

The uppermost part of the respiratory tract and the organ of *smell*.

### STRUCTURE

The nose is an air passage connecting the nostrils at its front to the *nasopharynx* (the upper part of the throat) at the rear. The *nasal septum*, made of cartilage at the front and bone at the rear, divides the passage.

Two small bones, the nasal bones, project from the front of the cranium and form the top of the bridge of the nose; the remainder of the bridge is cartilage. The roof of the nasal passage is formed by bones at the base of the skull, the walls by the maxilla (upper *jaw*), and the floor by the hard *palate*. Projecting from each wall are three conchae (thin, downward-curling plates of bone). The entire nasal passage is lined with *mucous membrane*, which bears tiny hairs that considerably increase the surface area.

The bones surrounding the nose contain air-filled, mucous membrane-lined cavities known as paranasal *sinuses*, which open into the nasal passage. In each wall of the nose is the opening to a nasolacrimal duct, which drains away the tears that bathe the front of the eyeball.

Projecting into the roof of the nasal passage through tiny openings are the hairlike nerve endings of the *olfactory nerves*, which are responsible for the sense of smell.

### FUNCTION

One of the main functions of the nose is to filter, warm, and moisten inhaled air before it passes into the rest of the respiratory tract. Just inside the nostrils small hairs trap large dust particles and even larger foreign bodies

## ANATOMY OF THE NOSE

The nose is involved in breathing and also in the sense of smell; it is a hollow passage connecting the nostrils and the top of the throat. The upper part of the nose transmits sensations of smell.

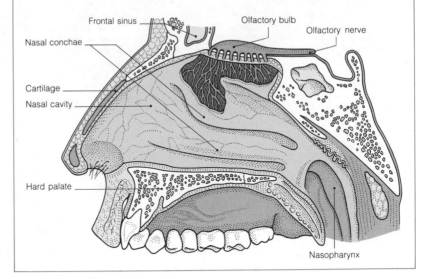

Frontal sinus — Olfactory bulb — Olfactory nerve — Nasal conchae — Cartilage — Nasal cavity — Hard palate — Nasopharynx

and induce sneezing to remove them. Smaller dust particles are filtered from the air by the hairs of the conchae. All air entering the nose passes over the blood vessels and mucus-secreting cells on the surface of the conchae. The mucus on the conchae flows inward, carrying harmful microorganisms and other foreign bodies back toward the nasopharynx so that they can be swallowed and destroyed by the gastric acid in the stomach.

The nose detects smells by means of the olfactory nerve endings, which, when stimulated by inhaled vapors, transmit this information to the olfactory bulb in the brain.

The nose also is a resonator, giving each voice its characteristic tone. (See also *Nose* disorders box, overleaf.)

## Nosebleed

Loss of blood from the mucous membrane that lines the nose, most

---

### FIRST AID: NOSEBLEED

**WARNING**
If a nosebleed starts after a heavy blow to the head, it could indicate a fractured skull. Take the victim to the hospital immediately.

**1** Have the victim sit, ensuring he or she leans forward slightly with the mouth held open so that blood or clots do not obstruct the airway.

**2** Pinch the lower part of the nostrils for about 15 minutes. The victim should breathe through the mouth.

**3** The nostrils should be released slowly and the victim should avoid touching or blowing the nose. If the bleeding has not stopped after 20 minutes, seek medical attention.

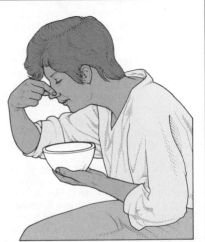

## DISORDERS OF THE NOSE

The nose is susceptible to a wide range of disorders. Infections and allergic conditions, leading to stuffiness or sneezing and sometimes some loss of smell, are common. Because of its prominent position, the nose is also particularly prone to injury.

### CONGENITAL DEFECTS

In choanal atresia, one or both nasal cavities fail to develop fully. If both sides are affected, the baby cannot breathe properly. An abnormality affecting one side may not cause any problems until later in life.

*Syphilis* that is transmitted to a fetus during pregnancy may lead to a failure of full development of the nasal bones, with flattening of the bridge of the nose.

### INFECTION

The common *cold*, a virus infection, causes inflammation of the lining of the nasal passages and excessive production of mucus, leading to nasal congestion. Small *boils* (infected hair follicles) are common just within the nostril, where they may cause severe pain. Backward spread of infection from the nose can rarely cause *cavernous sinus thrombosis*, a serious condition that, without antibiotics, may be fatal.

### TUMORS

*Hemangiomas* (benign tumors of blood vessels) commonly affect the nasal cavity in babies. Many disappear spontaneously before puberty.

*Basal cell carcinoma* and *squamous cell carcinoma* (skin cancers) may occur in and around the nostril. The nose may also be invaded by cancers originating in the surrounding sinuses.

### INJURY

Fracture of the nasal bones (see *Nose, broken*) is a common sports injury that can lead to deformity; it may require corrective surgery. *Nosebleeds* are also common, particularly in children; they may be caused by fragile blood vessels, infection of the lining of the nose, or a blow to the nose.

### DRUGS

Repeated sniffing of cocaine interferes with the blood supply to the mucous membrane lining the nose and can cause perforation of the nasal septum. Persistent inhalation of snuff can lead to nasopharyngeal cancer.

### ALLERGIES

Allergic rhinitis (hay fever) is one of the most common allergies. Common causative allergens include pollens, animal dander, house mites, and fungal spores. (See *Rhinitis, allergic*.)

### OBSTRUCTION

A nasal *polyp* (a projection of swollen mucous membrane) may block a nostril, causing a sensation of congestion.

Young children frequently insert foreign bodies, such as beads, peas, or pebbles, into their nostrils. They often become stuck, causing obstruction and a discharge.

### INVESTIGATION

To inspect the inside of the nose, the physician uses a speculum to open up the nostrils. If a fracture is suspected, *X rays* are taken. For suspected cancer, nasal endoscopy and a *biopsy* are done.

often from inside one nostril only. Nosebleeds are most common in childhood, when they are usually insignificant and easily stopped. They are infrequent in healthy young adults, but become more common and more serious in old age.

### CAUSES

The most common causes of a nosebleed are a blow to the nose, fragile blood vessels, or dislodging crusts that form in the mucous membrane as a result of a cold or other infection. Rarely, recurrent nosebleeds are a sign of an underlying disorder, such as *hypertension* (high blood pressure), a *bleeding disorder*, or a tumor of the nose or sinuses.

### TREATMENT

Most nosebleeds can be controlled by simple first-aid measures (see box on previous page).

If first-aid treatment fails to stop bleeding within 20 minutes, a physician should be consulted. He or she may pack the affected nostril firmly with gauze (to apply constant pressure to the wound) or may cauterize the wound. In rare cases, surgery may be needed to stop the bleeding.

## Nose, broken

Fracture of the nasal bones, sometimes with dislocation of the adjacent cartilage. A blow from the side may knock the bones or cartilage out of position or cause displacement of the *nasal septum*. A frontal blow tends to splay the nasal bones out-

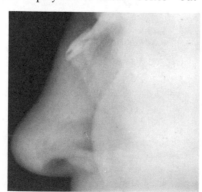

**X ray showing broken nose**
The nasal bones under the bridge of the nose and part of the ethmoid bone, which forms the top part of the nasal septum (partition between the two sides of the nose), have been broken.

ward, depressing the bridge. Usually, the fracture is accompanied by severe swelling of overlying soft tissue, which can mask a minor fracture (revealed only when X rays are taken).

A fractured nose is painful and remains tender for about three weeks after the injury.

### TREATMENT

Resetting is usually carried out either before the swelling has started or when it has subsided, about 10 days after the injury. Occasionally, the displaced bridge can be manipulated into position using a local anesthetic, but usually a general anesthetic is needed. A plaster splint is sometimes required during healing.

## Nose reshaping

See *Rhinoplasty*.

## Nuclear energy

Also known as atomic energy, the energy released (principally in the form of heat, light, and "hard" *radiation* such as gamma rays) as a result of changes in the nuclei of atoms. Nuclear energy is released in certain natural processes, such as the spontaneous decay of naturally occurring radioactive substances (uranium ores, for example), and the nuclear reactions that power the sun and other stars. It is also released in man-made devices such as nuclear reactors and nuclear weapons.

## Nuclear magnetic resonance
See *MRI*.

## Nuclear medicine
Techniques that use radioactive substances to detect or treat disease.

The most important application of nuclear medicine is in diagnosis. Radioactive materials (which are injected or swallowed) are taken up by body tissues or organs in different concentrations, and an instrument called a gamma camera is used to detect and map the distribution of radiation within the body. The technique requires only a small amount of radiation, and produces images that reflect bodily functions—not simply anatomy. (See *Radionuclide scanning*.)

In techniques for treatment, higher doses of radiation are used. Diseased tissues are destroyed by exposing them to an external radioactive source or by inserting a radioactive substance into a body tissue or cavity. (See *Radiation therapy; Interstitial radiation therapy; Intracavitary therapy*.)

## Nucleic acids
Substances found in all living matter that have a fundamental role in the propagation of life. Nucleic acids provide the inherited, coded instructions (or "blueprint") for an organism's development; they also provide some of the apparatus by which these instructions are carried out.

There are two types of nucleic acid, called deoxyribonucleic acid (DNA) and ribonucleic acid (RNA). In all plant and animal cells (including humans), it is the DNA that permanently holds the coded instructions; RNA helps transport, translate, and implement the instructions. The DNA is the main constituent of *chromosomes*, which are carried in the nucleus (central unit) of the cell.

### STRUCTURE
DNA and RNA are similar in their structure. Both have long, chainlike molecules. The main difference is that DNA usually consists of two intertwined chains, whereas RNA is generally single stranded.

The basic structure of DNA (shown at right) has been likened to a very long rope ladder, the chains of the DNA forming the two sides of the ladder with interlinking structures between the chains forming the rungs. The ladder is not straight, however, but twisted into a helical (spiral) shape, which gives it great stability. This shape is called a double helix.

If the two DNA chains are separated, it is found that each has a "backbone" (the side of the ladder) consisting of a string of sugar and phosphate chemical groups. Attached to each sugar in this string is a chemical called a base. The base can be any of four types, called adenine, thymine, guanine, and cytosine (or A,T,G, and C), and each forms half of one "rung" of the DNA ladder. The four bases can occur in any sequence along the chain (a sequence might be, for example, GTCGTATTTAGTCC). The sequence itself, which may be many millions of individual bases long, provides the code for the activities of the cell, just as the sequence of letters on this page provides a message to the reader (see *Genetic code*).

Because the two bases that form each rung of the ladder conform to certain pairings (A always pairing with T, and G with C), the sequence of bases on one chain always determines exactly the sequence on the second chain. This is of fundamental importance for the copying of DNA molecules when a cell divides.

RNA is like a single strand of DNA, except that the nucleotide base thymine in DNA is replaced by another base, uracil, in RNA, and the sugar and phosphate chain in RNA is slightly different chemically.

### FUNCTION
DNA controls a cell's activities by specifying and regulating the synthesis of enzymes and other proteins in the cell, with different *genes* (sections of DNA) regulating the production of different proteins. For a particular protein to be made, an appropriate section of DNA acts as a template for an RNA chain. This "messenger" RNA then passes out of the nucleus into the cell cytoplasm, where it is decoded to form proteins (see *Genetic code; Protein synthesis*).

When a cell divides, identical copies of its DNA must go to each of the two daughter cells. The structure of DNA makes this process possible. Starting at one end of the molecule, the two chains separate, or "unzip." As they do so, two more chains are formed side by side to the original chains (these new chains are formed by the linking of free, unlinked, nucleotides that are present in cells). Because only certain base pairings are possible, the new double chains are identical to the original DNA molecule.

Thus, when a cell divides, it provides an exact copy of its DNA to its daughter cells. Each of a person's cells carries the same DNA replica that was present in the fertilized ovum. The DNA message is thus passed from one generation to another.

N

---

## DNA STRUCTURE
A DNA molecule consists of two intertwined strands, the margins of which are chains of sugar and phosphate groups. The chains are linked by pairs of substances called bases, of which there are four types—adenine, guanine, thymine, and cytosine. An adenine on one chain is always paired with thymine on the second; similarly, cytosine is always paired with guanine. The sequence of bases in one chain thus exactly determines the sequence in the other chain.

**Nucleotides**
Each base, along with the sugar and phosphate groups to which it is attached, forms a unit called a nucleotide.

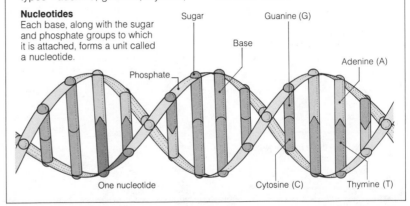

Sugar
Base
Phosphate
Guanine (G)
Adenine (A)
One nucleotide
Cytosine (C)
Thymine (T)

## NUMBNESS AND TINGLING   Loss of feeling and/or a pins and needles sensation in any part of the body

**?** Did you notice the numbness AND/OR tingling after sitting in one position for a long time or after waking from a deep sleep?

**YES** → Pressure on a nerve, which stretches it, or temporarily cuts off its blood supply, is often the cause of these sensations. Feeling should return to normal in a few minutes.

NO ↓

**?** Are only your hands affected?

**YES** → Have you noticed any stiffness in your neck?

**YES** → These symptoms suggest a disorder of the nerves and bones of the neck, especially if you are over 50.

See • *Cervical osteoarthritis*

NO ↓

Are the symptoms worse at night AND/OR do you have pains that shoot up the hand from your wrist?

**YES** → This suggests a disorder of the nerves that pass through the wrist.

See • *Carpal tunnel syndrome*

NO

NO ↓

**?** Does the numbness AND/OR tingling affect only one side of your body?

**YES** → Have you also noticed one or more of the following symptoms?
• blurred vision
• confusion
• difficulty speaking
• loss of movement in your arms or legs
• dizziness

**YES** → ☎ **EMERGENCY!**
**GET MEDICAL HELP NOW!**
Your symptoms may be caused by a disruption of the blood supply to the brain.

See • *Stroke*
      • *Transient ischemic attack*

NO

NO ↓

**?** Do your fingers or toes get numb and turn blue in cold weather, and then become red and painful as feeling returns?

**YES** → You may have a disorder that affects the small blood vessels in the extremities.

See • *Raynaud's disease*

NO ↓

If you are unable to make a diagnosis from this chart, consult your physician.

**N**

# Nucleus

The central core, structure, or focal point of an object.

The nucleus of a living cell is a roughly spherical unit at the center of the cell. It contains the *chromosomes* (composed mainly of *nucleic acid*) responsible for directing the cell's activities, and is surrounded by a membrane. There are small pores in the membrane through which various substances can pass between the nucleus and the cytoplasm (the rest of the cell).

The nucleus of an atom, composed of protons and neutrons, accounts for nearly all the mass of an atom but only a tiny proportion of its volume. Nuclear energy is produced through changes in the mass and structure of atomic nuclei.

A nerve nucleus is a group of neurons (nerve cells) within the brain and spinal cord that work together to perform a particular function.

# Numbness

Loss of sensation in part of the body caused by interference to the passage of impulses along sensory nerves.

### CAUSES

Numbness can occur naturally and harmlessly (such as when blood supply to a nerve in the leg is cut off temporarily by sitting cross-legged), it can be induced artificially (e.g., by a dentist anesthetizing a nerve before filling a tooth), or it may be the result of a disorder or damage to the nervous system or its blood supply.

*Multiple sclerosis* can cause loss of sensation in any part of the body through damage to nerve pathways in the central nervous system (CNS). In *neuropathy*, it is the peripheral nerves (outside the CNS) that are damaged. In a *stroke*, pressure on, or reduced blood supply to, nerve pathways in the brain often causes loss of feeling on one side of the body.

Severe cold, as in frostbite, causes numbness by a direct action on the nerves. Numbness may also be a feature of various psychological disorders, such as *anxiety*, *panic attack*, or a hysterical *conversion disorder*.

### DIAGNOSIS AND TREATMENT

Examination by a physician usually reveals an area of sensory loss or impairment that corresponds to the skin distribution of a single peripheral nerve, several nerves, or a sensory area in the CNS. The distribution of the affected area may suggest the site and mechanism of nerve damage. Treatment can then be prescribed.

# Nurse

A person trained in *nursing care*. Registered nurses (RNs) are registered and licensed by a state to care for the sick and to promote health. They work in hospitals, nursing homes, physicians' offices, clinics, workplaces, schools, and patients' homes.

Some RNs concentrate on a particular field, engaging in the full-time practice of *anesthesia*, *psychiatry*, *pediatrics*, or *surgery*. Specific types of RN also exist. Nurse-midwives have special training in prenatal and postnatal care, labor, and delivery (see *Midwifery*). Nurse practitioners or nurse clinicians are trained to provide health services (such as preventive care, monitoring of chronic conditions, physical examinations, and health counseling) under the supervision of a physician.

Other types of nurses include licensed practical nurses (LPNs), who are trained to provide basic care for patients under the supervision of physicians and RNs. Nurses' aides assist nurses in hospitals, nursing homes, and clinics.

# Nursing

See *Breast-feeding*.

# Nursing care

The process by which a patient is helped by a *nurse* to recover from an illness or injury, or to regain as much independence as possible. The nurse is more concerned with the patient's overall reaction to the disorder than with the disorder itself, and is devoted to the control of physical pain, the relief of mental suffering, and, when possible, the avoidance of complications. In terminal cases, the nurse's responsibility is to help the patient meet death with as little distress and as much dignity as possible.

Working closely with physicians and other health care professionals, the nurse exercises continuous surveillance over the patient. This involves the measurement and recording of many bodily functions. The patient's pulse rate, respiratory rate, temperature, weight, and urine output are recorded daily—or more frequently in acute illness. The nurse may also monitor blood pressure and the ECG in an intensive-care unit, and may record the output of fluids and the intake of fluids and food.

In patients recovering from surgery, the nurse monitors the level of consciousness, ensures that there is no obstruction to breathing, maintains the correct rate of flow of any intravenous infusion, and records vital functions, such as pulse rate.

Prevention is another important aspect of nursing care. The nurse moves unconscious or immobile patients every few hours to prevent the development of bedsores; washing out the mouth, cleaning the teeth, and removing urine and feces guards against infection.

The nurse is also responsible for administering drugs.

From the patient's perspective, the most important quality the nurse can offer may be understanding care, which involves listening with patience to anxieties and fears, and providing emotional support and comfort.

# Nursing home

A residential facility for the care of elderly people or, in some cases, for people who have serious illnesses or disabilities.

The rapid increase in the number of elderly people in the US (more than 11 percent of the population is now over 65) has resulted in an increased need for provision of long-term care. There are currently some 19,000 nursing homes in the US caring for more than 1.4 million people, including 20 percent of the people over 85.

Nursing homes as they exist today are partly a result of the Social Security Act of 1935, which refused benefits to people who were in public residential institutions. Consequently, many of the people concerned moved to private facilities.

### TYPES OF NURSING HOME

There are three basic types of nursing home. Residential care facilities (RCFs) provide accommodation and food; staff members monitor the basic health of the residents. RCFs are appropriate for elderly people who are fairly independent and able, but who want someone to take over responsibility for basic housekeeping chores.

Intermediate care facilities (ICFs) provide food and lodging and regular custodial care for people who are too ill or frail to look after themselves. Recreational activities may be provided, and some ICFs have rehabilitation programs.

Skilled nursing facilities (SNFs) are overseen by physicians and provide 24-hour nursing. These facilities are for people who require intensive medical and rehabilitation care.

Most care in nursing homes is long-term, but short-term homes are available for people who are primarily

N

nursed at home. This allows caregivers (usually family members) some respite from their responsibility.

**CARE IN NURSING HOMES**

Approximately 50 percent of nursing home residents are demented, and most suffer from a number of medical conditions related to *aging*. In addition, because of changes in the Medicare system, patients tend to be discharged from hospitals to nursing homes at earlier stages in their convalescence. These factors place great demands on the medical care provided by nursing homes.

The ideal nursing home is well equipped with registered nurses as well as nurses' aides, has regular visits from a physician, provides access to advanced medical care facilities, and is closely linked, both organizationally and geographically, to community hospitals. It is also important for a nursing home to have a pleasant atmosphere, to treat its patients in a caring and sensitive manner, and to respect their rights to privacy. (See also *Geriatric medicine*.)

## Nutrient

A substance that provides nourishment. Essential nutrients are those necessary for body function that are not synthesized in the body. They include proteins, carbohydrates, fats, vitamins, and minerals.

## Nutrition

The science and study of the foodstuffs people eat and drink and the ways they are digested and assimilated. Both physicians and the public have shown growing interest in the relationship between diet and health. Until about 30 years ago the primary concern of nutritionists was dietary deficiencies; their recommendations concentrated on the minimum amounts of nutrients required for health. In Western societies the focus is now on the dangers of too much fat or sugar in the diet, and the effects of food additives, colorings, and preservatives on health.

**ELEMENTS OF GOOD NUTRITION**

Basic elements of the diet are proteins, carbohydrates, fats, fiber, vitamins, minerals, and water (see also entries on individual nutrients). A balanced diet contains adequate, not excessive, amounts of each (see box).

**EATING A BALANCED DIET**

People require different amounts of nutrients and energy. A precise assessment of each person's requirements would be ideal, but a general

## ESSENTIAL NUTRIENTS

| | | |
|---|---|---|
| **Proteins** | The main structural component of tissue and organs. We need proteins for growth and repair of cells.<br>Each protein contains hundreds and sometimes thousands of units called amino acids in specific combinations. In the body there are 20 amino acids; 12 of these are manufactured by the body itself and | the remaining eight are obtained from a balanced diet.<br>A vegetarian diet containing eggs, milk, and cheese provides sufficient amounts of all essential amino acids. A vegan diet, which also excludes dairy products, needs careful planning to prevent protein deficiency (see *Vegetarianism*). |
| **Carbohydrates** | The two carbohydrate food groups, sugars and starches, are the main energy sources required for metabolism (chemical processes that take place within cells).<br>Carbohydrates should make up at | least half of our diet. Unrefined (unprocessed) carbohydrates found in cereals and fruit are usually richer in fiber and nutrients than refined carbohydrates, such as sugar and white flour. |
| **Fats** | Fats provide energy for metabolism and are a structural component of cells. Most people in developed countries eat too much fat; fats should constitute no more than 30 percent of total calorie intake.<br>There are three kinds of dietary fats—saturated fats (found mostly in meat and dairy products), monosaturated fats (found in olive oil and avocados), and polyunsaturated fats (found in fish and vegetable oils). Saturated fats | tend to increase the amounts of unwanted types of cholesterol in the blood whereas polyunsaturated fats and monosaturated fats have the opposite effect.<br>Studies have indicated that a high level of low-density lipoprotein cholesterol in the blood is associated with coronary heart disease. Our bodies produce enough cholesterol for our needs; any excess is primarily due to eating too much saturated fat. |
| **Fiber** | This is the indigestible structural material in plants. Although fiber passes through the intestine unchanged, it is an essential part of a healthy diet. A low fiber diet may lead to constipation, diverticular disease, and other disorders.<br>High fiber diets (including plenty | of fruit, raw vegetables, grains, and cereals) provide bulk without excess calories. Low fiber diets tend to be high in refined carbohydrates and fats, and thus are more likely to encourage obesity, heart disease, and other unwanted effects. |
| **Water** | Our bodies are composed of about 60 percent water. Water constitutes a high proportion of many foods and is essential to maintain metabolism | (chemical processes within cells) and normal bowel function. It also determines the volume of blood in our circulation. |
| **Vitamins** | Regulators of metabolism. Vitamins ensure the healthy functioning of the brain, nerves, muscles, skin, and bones. Although vitamins do not supply energy, some enable energy to be released from the food.<br>A healthy, balanced diet contains enough vitamins for most people's needs and supplements are not | usually necessary. Indeed, some vitamins, especially A, D, E, and K, are dangerous if taken in excess. Water-soluble vitamins (B and C) are stored in the body less well than fat-soluble vitamins, but even on a very restricted diet vitamin deficiency is rare until several months have elapsed. |
| **Minerals** | A balanced diet provides enough minerals for most people. Calcium is necessary for the maintenance of healthy bones and teeth. Other minerals, such as zinc and magnesium, are needed in minute amounts to control cell metabolism. | The only mineral commonly required as a supplement is iron, which is used to prevent anemia in women who experience heavy periods.<br>Sodium chloride (table salt) is needed to maintain fluid balance. Excess may cause *hypertension*. |

N

guide can be useful as well. The figures for the recommended daily allowances (RDAs) are based on average requirements to cover the needs of the majority; the variables are usually body size, age, sex, and lifestyle (active or sedentary).

## Nutritional disorders

Nutritional disorders may be caused by a deficiency or an excess of one or more nutrients or by a toxin or poisonous element in the diet.

### NUTRIENT DEFICIENCY

A diet deficient in carbohydrate is almost inevitably deficient in protein too (protein-calorie malnutrition). This deficiency is most often seen in people in Africa and Asia as a result of poverty and famine (see *Kwashiorkor*; *Marasmus*).

Inadequate intake of protein and calories may also occur in people who restrict their diet in an attempt to lose weight (see *Anorexia nervosa*); it can also occur because of mistaken beliefs about diet and health (see *Food fad*) or because of loss of interest in food associated with *alcohol dependence* and *drug dependence*.

In Western societies, deficiency of nutrients is usually associated with a disorder of the digestive system, such as *celiac sprue*, *Crohn's disease*, or pernicious anemia (see *Anemia, megaloblastic*).

### NUTRIENT EXCESS

*Obesity* and dental *caries* are two of the most common disorders in the US; both are due to excessive intake of nutrients. Obesity is caused by an excess of refined carbohydrates and fat. Dental caries develop mainly in people who eat large amounts of refined carbohydrates.

### TOXIC EFFECTS

A nutritional disorder may arise from the presence of toxic substances in the food. These may be naturally occurring substances, such as the *aflatoxin* fungus found on peanuts (which can cause *liver cancer*) or the *ergot* fungus found on rye (which can cause ergotism). Industrial pesticides, fertilizers, pollutants, and other chemicals may also contaminate food.

## Nymphomania

A *psychosexual disorder* in which a woman is dominated by an insatiable appetite for sexual activity with numerous different male partners. Nymphomaniacs are often distressed by their own behavior and by their inability to see men as anything other than objects for sexual conquest. Nymphomania is generally thought to be an expression of some deep psychological disorder.

A similar behavior in men is called satyriasis or Don Juanism. It is said to be caused by intense narcissism and the need to control feelings of inferiority through sexual success.

## Nystagmus

A condition in which there is involuntary movement of the eyes; the movement is usually horizontal, but can be vertical or rotary. In almost all types, both eyes move together.

### CAUSES AND TYPES

In the most common type, called jerky nystagmus, the eyes repeatedly move slowly in one direction and then rapidly in the other, giving a jerking effect. The disorder is almost always congenital and is usually unassociated with any abnormality of the eyes; the cause is unknown. Jerky nystagmus is permanent and, because steady gaze is impossible, there is almost always a moderate to severe defect of visual acuity. Nystagmus also occurs in *albinism* and as a result of any very severe defect of vision, such as congenital *cataract*, retinal disease, or *optic atrophy*, present at birth.

Persistent nystagmus appearing later in life indicates the presence of a disorder of the nervous system (such as *multiple sclerosis* or a brain tumor) or a disorder of the balancing mechanism in the inner ear. Nystagmus may also occur as a normal effect of a person's attempts to follow a sequence of objects rapidly passing the eyes. This phenomenon is known as "optokinetic nystagmus."

*Electronystagmography*, a method of recording eye movements, may be performed to identify different types of nystagmus.

## Nystatin

### ANTIFUNGAL

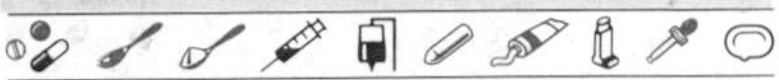

Tablet Liquid Powder Vaginal suppository Cream Ointment Eye drops

Prescription needed

Available as generic

An *antifungal drug* used in the treatment of *candidiasis* (thrush). Nystatin may be safely used during pregnancy. High doses taken by mouth may cause diarrhea, nausea, vomiting, and abdominal pain.

---

## THE FOUR FOOD GROUPS AND RECOMMENDED DAILY SERVINGS

| Food group | | Typical servings | |
| --- | --- | --- | --- |
| Milk group<br><br>Servings required per day: 2 | 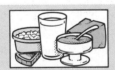 | Milk<br>Yogurt, plain<br>Hard cheese<br>Cheese spread<br>Cottage cheese | 8 ounces (1 cup)<br>1 cup<br>1¼ ounces<br>2 ounces<br>2 cups |
| 'Meat' group<br><br>Servings required per day: 2 | 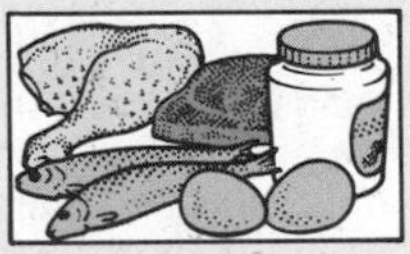 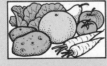 | Meat, lean<br>Poultry<br>Fish<br>Eggs<br>Peanut butter | 2 to 3 ounces (cooked)<br>2 to 3 ounces<br>2 to 3 ounces<br>2 to 3<br>4 tablespoons |
| Fruit and vegetable group<br><br>Servings required per day: 4 | 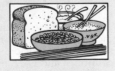 | Vegetables<br>Fruits<br>Grapefruit<br>Potato<br>Lettuce | ½ cup<br>½ cup<br>½ medium<br>1 medium<br>1 wedge |
| Bread and cereal group<br><br>Servings required per day: 4 | | Bread<br>Cooked cereal<br>Pasta<br>Rice<br>Dry cereal | 1 slice<br>½ to ¾ cup<br>½ to ¾ cup<br>½ to ¾ cup<br>1 ounce |

Essential nutrients are found in differing amounts in foods, so a varied diet is needed to ensure you get all you need. An easy way to plan a balanced diet is to use the above chart to select foods from each of the four basic food groups. Note that the meat group contains other protein-rich foods, such as eggs and peanut butter, as well as meat.

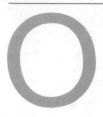

## Obesity

A condition in which there is too much body fat. Being obese is not the same as being overweight. A person is usually not considered obese unless he or she weighs 20 percent or more over the maximum desirable weight for his or her height (see *Weight*).

### INCIDENCE

It is estimated that about 25 percent of the US population carries too much fat. About 5 to 10 percent of children are overweight or obese. Between 13 and 23 percent of all adolescents (especially girls) are obese; 80 percent of obese teenagers are likely to grow into obese adults.

### CAUSES

The reasons why some people become obese are unclear. Although obesity occurs when the net energy intake exceeds the net energy expenditure (that is, when more calories are taken in than are being used by the body), obese people do not always eat considerably more than thin people.

A person's energy requirements are determined partly by his or her basal metabolic rate (the amount of energy needed to maintain vital body functions at rest—see *Metabolism*) and partly by his or her level of physical activity. Obese people may have a very low basal metabolic rate, or they may need fewer calories because they are less physically active.

It is thought that genetic factors play a part in the development of obesity; children of obese parents are 10 times more likely to be obese than children with parents of normal weight. Some hormonal disorders are accompanied by obesity, but the overwhelming majority of obese people do not suffer from such disorders.

### COMPLICATIONS

Obesity increases a person's chance of becoming seriously ill. *Hypertension* (high blood pressure) and *stroke* are twice as likely to occur in obese people than in lean people. *Coronary heart disease* is more common, particularly in obese men under the age of 40. Adult-onset *diabetes mellitus* is five times more common among obese people, the risk increasing with the degree and duration of obesity. Increasing degrees of extra weight in men are associated with an increased risk of cancer of the colon, rectum, and prostate. With increasing weight, women show a progressive increase in risk of cancer of the breast, uterus, and cervix. *Osteoarthritis* may be agravated by obesity. Extra weight on the hips, knees, and back places undue strain on these joints. Weight loss does not reverse the disease but does help relieve stress and pain.

### TREATMENT

The first line of treatment for obesity is a weight-loss diet (see *Nutrition; Weight reduction*). An obese person should follow a diet that provides 500 to 1,000 calories less than his or her energy requirements. The energy deficit is met by using some of the excess stored fat, which is reflected by an average weight loss of 1 to 2 pounds a week. Regular exercise (especially *aerobics*) increases weight loss by burning extra calories and by increasing the metabolic rate.

Fad diets may cause a dramatic weight loss within a short period of time, but, in almost all cases, the weight is quickly regained when normal eating habits are resumed. The use of drugs as appetite suppressants was once popular, but is usually no longer recommended by physicians.

Various radical procedures are available for severely obese people who have failed to lose weight, but because of the possible adverse effects they are attempted only if the person's health is in danger.

Wiring the jaw to prevent the mouth from opening more than about half an inch makes it impossible to chew. Reduced calorie meals in liquid form are taken through a straw. The jaw is usually wired for up to a year and the patient is kept under constant medical supervision. Weight is often regained once the wiring is undone.

An operation in which part of the stomach is stapled together reduces its size and has the effect of making the person feel full after eating a small amount of food.

Intestinal bypass operations were popular in the 1970s but are now uncommon due to the frequency and variety of adverse effects. A large part of the small intestine is bypassed by cutting the jejunum and joining it to the ileum, thus reducing the length of the digestive tract and allowing less food to be absorbed.

### OUTLOOK

Some people who have been seriously obese for much of their lives can lose weight without regaining it. As when trying to give up smoking or alcohol, the essential element in weight reduction is psychological motivation.

## Obsessive-compulsive behavior

A neurosis in which sufferers are constantly troubled by persistent ideas (obsessions) that make them carry out repetitive, ritualized acts (compulsions). Obsessive-compulsive disorder usually starts in adolescence and runs a fluctuating course.

### CAUSES AND INCIDENCE

The condition is partly inherited, but environmental factors also play a part. Personality traits of orderliness and cleanliness are said to be related, as is a tendency for other neurotic symptoms. Certain forms of brain damage (especially *encephalitis*) can result in obsessional symptoms.

Obsessive-compulsive disorder is rare, although minor obsessional symptoms probably occur in about one sixth of the population.

### SYMPTOMS

People with this disorder usually suffer from both obsessions and compulsions, often accompanied by *depression* and *anxiety*.

Obsessions are recurrent thoughts or feelings that come into the mind seemingly involuntarily. Sufferers regard these thoughts as senseless and sometimes unpleasant, but are unable to ignore or resist them. Thoughts of violence, fears of being infected by germs or dirt, and constant doubts (e.g., whether or not the front door is shut) are the most common obsessions. One form is obsessional rumination, in which a person broods constantly over a word, phrase, or an unanswerable problem.

Compulsions are repetitive, apparently purposeful acts that are carried out in a ritualized fashion. They are performed for the purpose of warding off fears or relieving anxiety and are thus the physical form of an obsessional state. Sufferers do not usually derive any pleasure from performing the activities, but feel increasingly anxious if they try to resist the compulsion. Handwashing, counting, and checking are the most common compulsions.

Compulsive acts may have to be performed so many times in a particular way that they seriously disrupt work and social life. It may take some sufferers two or three hours just to get up and wash in the morning. In addition, the constant use of soap may irritate the skin.

**TREATMENT**
Traditionally, obsessive-compulsive symptoms have been treated by *psychoanalysis*. Today, treatment may also consist of *behavior therapy*. It is often combined with *antidepressant drugs* (especially clomipramine) or *antianxiety drugs*.

**OUTLOOK**
At least two thirds of all people who have obsessive-compulsive disorder respond well to therapy. Symptoms may recur under stress but can usually be controlled. In severe cases, the affected person may become housebound and severely handicapped by indecision. In less than 3 percent of cases, sufferers go on to have psychotic symptoms (see *Psychosis*).

## Obstetrician
A physician who specializes in the care of a woman during pregnancy, labor, delivery, and the period immediately afterward. Prenatal care may include periodic examinations of the woman and her developing baby with recommendations for changes in activity or diet. The obstetrician delivers the baby, performing a cesarean section if necessary. In many cases, the obstetrician is also the woman's *gynecologist*.

## Obstetrics
The branch of medicine concerned with *pregnancy*, *childbirth*, and *postnatal care*. In conjunction with *gynecology*, obstetrics also involves the study of the structure and function of the female reproductive system (see *Reproductive system, female*).

## Obstructive airways disease
See *Lung disease, chronic obstructive*.

## Occiput
The lower back part of the head, where it merges with the neck.

## Occlusion
Blockage of any passage, canal, opening, or vessel in the body. Occlusion may be the result of disease (as in *pulmonary embolism*) or may be induced for medical reasons (see *Embolism, therapeutic*). The term is also used to refer to the covering of the better-seeing eye during treatment of *amblyopia*. In dentistry, occlusion is the relationship between the upper and lower teeth when the jaw is shut.

## Occult
A term meaning hidden or obscure. Occult blood in a sample of feces is invisible to the naked eye but can be detected by chemical tests.

## Occult blood, fecal
The presence in the feces of blood that cannot be seen by the naked eye but can be detected by chemical tests. It may be a sign of various disorders of the gastrointestinal tract, including *esophagitis*; *gastritis* (inflammation of the stomach lining); *stomach cancer*; intestinal cancer (see *Intestine, cancer of*); rectal cancer (see *Rectum, cancer of*); *diverticular disease*; *polyps* in the colon; *ulcerative colitis*; or the use of medications that irritate the stomach or intestine, such as aspirin. Bleeding gums or *hemorrhoids* may also cause occult blood in the feces, although in most cases of hemorrhoids the blood is visible.

**DETECTION**
Screening for colorectal cancer is done by testing the stools of asymptomatic people for occult blood.

A thin film of feces is smeared on a chemically coated paper and a drop or two of oxidizing agent is placed on it. If blood is present, the feces-covered paper turns blue. (See also *Feces, abnormal*; *Rectal bleeding*.)

## Occupational disease and injury
Illnesses, disorders, or injuries that occur as a result of work practices or exposure to chemical or physical agents or factors (e.g., dusts, poisons, or radiation) in the workplace. The efforts of specialists in this field mean that serious occupational diseases are much less common than they once were. Overall, however, occupational diseases make up an important and fairly common group of conditions (see table, overleaf).

**TYPES**
Some of the main types of occupational diseases are described below.

**DUST DISEASES** *Pneumoconiosis* refers to *fibrosis* of the lung caused by inhaled inorganic and organic dusts. It includes various diseases associated with mining (including coal and quartz mining), china clay processing, metal grinding, and foundry work. *Asbestosis* is a similar hazard for workers in the asbestos, mining, milling, and product manufacturing industries, and in shipbuilders.

Allergic *alveolitis* is a lung condition caused by inhalation of organic dusts (often containing fungal spores). It is

often occupationally related and includes such conditions as *farmers' lung* in agricultural workers.

**CHEMICAL POISONING** A vast number of industrial chemicals can cause damage to the lungs if inhaled, or to the liver, kidneys, bone marrow, or other organs if they reach the bloodstream via the lungs or skin.

Exposure to the fumes of cadmium (in the welding and electroplating industries) or beryllium (in high-technology industries) can damage the lungs. Lead and arsenic compounds (in metal processing and other industries) and benzene (in various industries where solvents are used) can damage the bone marrow, leading to *anemia* and other blood abnormalities. Carbon tetrachloride and vinyl chloride (in chemicals and plastics manufacture) are causes of liver disease. Many of these compounds can also cause kidney damage.

**OCCUPATIONAL SKIN DISEASE** Contact *dermatitis* (skin inflammation) can occur as a result of an allergy or of direct irritation by chemicals contacting the skin at work. Many substances may be responsible, from wet cement to processing chemicals used in the rubber goods industry. Other skin problems may also be occupationally related (e.g., severe itching caused by glass fiber or *squamous cell carcinoma* through exposure to tar).

**RADIATION HAZARDS** People with outdoor occupations in sunny climates are at increased risk of skin disease (such as *basal cell carcinoma*).

Workers in the nuclear energy industry and in some health care professions should use precautions to reduce the risk of developing a disease caused by ionizing radiation (see *Radiation hazards*).

**INFECTIOUS DISEASES** Rare infectious diseases are more common in certain occupations. They include *brucellosis* and *Q fever* (acquired from livestock) among farmworkers, *psittacosis* (from birds) in pet store owners, and *leptospirosis* (from rats) in sewer workers, miners, ditchdiggers, and fishermen. Viral *hepatitis* and *AIDS* are hazards for people who work with blood and blood products.

**MISCELLANEOUS** Disorders caused by repetitive actions, or overuse of parts of the body, range from writers' cramp to *carpal tunnel syndrome* and *singers' nodes*. *Raynaud's phenomenon* is associated with the handling of vibrating tools; *deafness* may be caused by exposure to noise and *cataracts* by exposure to intense heat.

O

## SAFETY AT WORK

A major method of preventing occupational disease and injury is the use of suitable protective clothing. This may include an air-filter mask in the presence of dust or fumes; earplugs where there is a noise hazard; eye shields to protect against radiation, chemicals, or metal dust; gloves for handling machinery; protective headgear and reinforced footwear where there is a risk of falling objects.

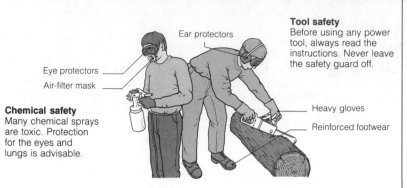

**Tool safety**
Before using any power tool, always read the instructions. Never leave the safety guard off.

Ear protectors

Eye protectors
Air-filter mask

**Chemical safety**
Many chemical sprays are toxic. Protection for the eyes and lungs is advisable.

Heavy gloves
Reinforced footwear

## OCCUPATIONAL INJURIES OR DISEASES

| Injuries or diseases | Approximate no. of cases in US annually | Deaths | Examples |
|---|---|---|---|
| Disabling injuries at work caused by falls | 250,000 | Many thousands | All types of fractures, wounds, crush and penetrating injuries, sprains, burns, electrical injuries |
| All other disabling injuries at work | 1,650,000 | | |
| Skin conditions | 40,000 | Few | Contact allergic or irritant dermatitis, some squamous cell carcinomas |
| Disorders associated with repeated trauma or overuse injury | 26,000 | Very few | Bursitis, tenosynovitis, tennis elbow, singers' nodes |
| Respiratory diseases caused by inhaled dusts or toxic agents | 10,000 | Several thousand | Pneumoconiosis, asbestosis, byssinosis, berylliosis, farmers' lung |
| Disorders caused by effects of physical phenomena | 9,000 | Few | Cancers, blood disorders (radiation), hearing loss (noise), cataract (heat), Raynaud's phenomenon (vibration) |
| Other types of poisoning | 3,000 | Several hundred | Diseases of the liver, kidneys, bone marrow, heart, nervous system, bladder |
| Other occupational diseases | 18,000 | Few | Brucellosis (slaughterhouse workers), decompression sickness (divers), viral hepatitis (health-care workers) |

O

### DIAGNOSIS AND PREVENTION

Sometimes the link between a disease and occupation may be obvious; sometimes it may become apparent only when a patient with mysterious symptoms mentions his or her occupation to the physician. Part of every medical history is a question regarding the patient's occupation. Even when an occupational disease is suspected, it may require extensive investigation at the workplace to determine the exact cause.

In more serious cases, the patient must quit his or her occupation, but then can make a claim for workers' compensation. In all cases, measures to prevent a recurrence are needed.

## Occupational medicine

A branch of medicine concerned with the effects of a person's job on his or her health, with preventing *occupational disease and injury*, and with promoting general health in workers.

Occupational medicine has a long history. As early as the middle ages, it was recognized that miners were at risk of lung diseases caused by dust, and attempts were made to improve their working conditions by increasing ventilation. The scope of occupational medicine widened during the industrial revolution as research revealed the hazards of working with metals (such as lead and mercury) and minerals (such as phosphorus).

The occupational physician uses epidemiological (see *Epidemiology*) techniques to analyze patterns of absenteeism, injury, illness, and causes of death in working populations, and investigates and monitors the health of a particular work force. Health risks can be reduced in two ways: by primary prevention—the reduction of exposure to harmful substances and work practices by attention to dust control, safe work stations, and the disposal of wastes—and by secondary prevention, which involves regular screening of workers for early evidence of occupational disorders, such as dust diseases or damage to the liver from chemicals.

Today, the occupational physician is increasingly concerned with psychological stress at work, with the investigation of the hazards (known and unknown) of new technologies, and with promoting healthy personal habits in workers.

## Occupational mortality
Death caused by disease contracted at the workplace or by injuries related to a person's work.

The death rate from work-related injuries in the US has been decreasing steadily for 50 years—from about 40 deaths annually per 100,000 working population in the 1930s to about 10 deaths per 100,000 in the middle 1980s. This last figure still represents approximately 10,000 injury-related deaths in the US each year.

In addition, there are several thousand deaths annually in the US attributable to occupational disease—principally to *pneumoconiosis* (dust disease of the lungs)—and to lung disease or cancers caused by exposure to asbestos.

While the precise number is unknown, it is estimated that one person in 200 in the US dies as a direct result of his or her occupation.

## Occupational therapy
Treatment aimed at enabling people disabled by physical illness or a serious accident to relearn muscular control and coordination, to cope with everyday tasks (such as dressing), and, when possible, to resume some form of employment. Treatment, carried out by specially trained therapists, usually starts in the hospital and may be continued at an outpatient clinic or in the person's home.

## Ocular
Relating to or affecting the eye and its structures. The term is also used to refer to the eyepiece of an optical device, such as a microscope.

## Oculogyric crisis
A state of fixed gaze, lasting for minutes or hours, in which the eyes are turned in a particular direction (usually upward). The fixed-eye position is sometimes associated with spasm of the muscles of the tongue, mouth, and neck.

The crisis may occur in people with *parkinsonism* or those who have had *encephalitis*, or it may be induced by drugs (such as *reserpine* or the *phenothiazine* derivatives). It is often precipitated by emotional stress.

## Oculomotor nerve
The third *cranial nerve*. The oculomotor nerve stimulates only motor functions. This nerve controls all the muscles that move the eye, except for two—the superior oblique muscle (which rotates the eyeball downward and outward and is controlled by the *trochlear nerve*) and the lateral rectus muscle (which moves the eye outward and is controlled by the *abducent nerve*). The oculomotor nerve also supplies the muscle that constricts the pupil, the ciliary muscle (which focuses the eye), and the muscle that raises the upper eyelid.

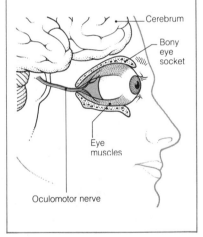

**LOCATION OF THE OCULOMOTOR NERVE**
The oculomotor nerve originates high in the brain stem and passes forward through a slit in the bony eye socket to reach the muscles that move the eye and eyelids.

Cerebrum
Bony eye socket
Eye muscles
Oculomotor nerve

The oculomotor nerve may be damaged as a result of a basal skull fracture or a disorder that distorts the brain, such as a tumor. Depending on the severity of damage, the following symptoms may occur: *ptosis* (drooping of the upper eyelid), *strabismus* (squint), dilation of the pupil, inability to focus the eye, double vision, and slight protrusion of the eyeball.

## Oedipus complex
A term used in *psychoanalytic theory* to describe the unconscious sexual attachment of a child for the parent of the opposite sex and the consequent jealousy of, and desire to eliminate, the same-sexed parent. The name is derived from the Greek myth in which, unknowingly, Oedipus kills his father Laius and marries his mother Jocasta.

Sigmund Freud believed that the Oedipus complex (sometimes called the Electra complex in females) was present in all young children and that normal psychological development depended on the child coming to identify with the parent of the same sex and, later, making sexual attachments with members of the opposite sex outside the family.

## Oils
See *Fats and oils*.

## Ointment
A greasy, semisolid preparation that is applied to the skin. Ointments are used to apply drugs to an area of skin or to act as a protective agent. Most ointments contain petrolatum or wax and have an *emollient* (soothing, moisturizing) effect.

## Olecranon
The bony projection at the upper end of the ulna (the inner bone of the forearm) that forms the point of the *elbow*. The olecranon is commonly known as the "funny bone"; a blow to the nerve that passes across it produces a tingling sensation that passes down the forearm to the fourth and fifth fingertips.

O

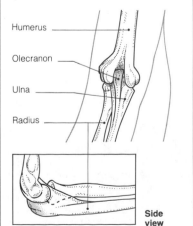

**LOCATION OF THE OLECRANON**
This is the curved projection at the upper end of the ulna. It acts to prevent elbow overextension.

Humerus
Olecranon
Ulna
Radius
Side view

## Olfactory nerve
The first *cranial nerve*, which conveys *smell* sensations (as nerve impulses)

from the *nose* to the brain. Each of the two olfactory nerves detects smells with hairlike receptors (nerve endings specialized in detecting stimuli) in the mucous membrane lining the roof of the nasal cavity. Nerve fibers pass from the receptors through tiny holes in the roof of the nasal cavity and come together to form two structures called the olfactory bulbs. From the bulbs, nerve fibers travel to the olfactory center in the brain.

**LOCATION OF OLFACTORY NERVE**

Each olfactory bulb lies on top of a thin bony plate in the roof of the nose and connects to the brain via an olfactory nerve. Nerve twigs pass through the bony plate to enter the nasal lining.

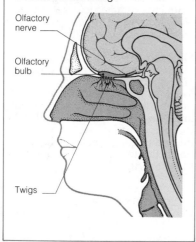

Olfactory nerve

Olfactory bulb

Twigs

Damage to the olfactory nerves, which is usually caused by head injury, may result in loss or impairment of the sense of smell.

## Oligo-

A prefix meaning few, little, or scanty, as in oligospermia (too few sperm in the semen). The prefix olig- is synonymous with oligo-.

## Oligodendroglioma

A rare, slow-growing type of primary *brain tumor* that mainly affects young or middle-aged adults. Several hundred cases of oligodendroglioma occur in the US each year. Symptoms, diagnosis, and treatment are as for other types of brain tumor. Surgical removal of the tumor can, in some cases, lead to a complete cure. About one third of patients survive for five years or more.

## Oligohydramnios

A rare condition in which there is an abnormally small amount of *amniotic fluid* surrounding the fetus in the uterus during pregnancy.

**CAUSES**

Amniotic fluid is normally produced by the placenta, swallowed by the fetus, and excreted as fetal urine. Oligohydramnios may occur if the placenta is not functioning properly, as in severe *preeclampsia* or *eclampsia*. Oligohydramnios may also occur if there is an abnormality of the fetal urinary tract or if a pregnancy continues beyond 41 weeks' gestation.

**TREATMENT AND OUTLOOK**

In some cases, the underlying disorder can be treated, but sometimes it cannot (particularly if the fetus is abnormal). If oligohydramnios occurs early in pregnancy, it usually results in *miscarriage*. If it occurs later in pregnancy, the pressure of the uterus on the fetus may cause deformity, such as *clubfoot*. If it occurs in an overdue pregnancy, induction of labor or cesarean section may be beneficial.

## Oligospermia

 A deficiency in the number of sperm per unit volume of seminal fluid; there are normally more than 20 million sperm per milliliter of semen. Oligospermia may be temporary or permanent. It is a major cause of *infertility*, especially when present with certain other disorders of the sperm.

**CAUSES**

Oligospermia may be caused by a number of different disorders, including *orchitis* (inflammation of a testis), failure of a testis to descend into the scrotum (see *Testis, undescended*), and, infrequently, a *varicocele* (varicose vein of the testis). Stress, cigarette smoking, alcohol abuse, and some drugs may cause temporary oligospermia.

**DIAGNOSIS AND TREATMENT**

A sperm count is performed as part of *semen analysis*. Treatment is of the underlying cause. *Gonadotropin hormones* may be prescribed for a short period when the cause is unknown. (See also *Azoospermia*.)

## Oliguria

The production of a smaller-than-normal quantity of urine in relation to the volume of fluid taken in. Oliguria may be due simply to excessive sweating (without adequate fluid replacement) in a hot climate. In other cases oliguria may be a sign of failure of normal kidney function (see *Renal failure*).

## Olive oil

 An oil obtained from the fruit of the olive tree *OLEA EUROPAEA*. Warm olive oil is sometimes used to soften *earwax* before the ears are syringed. Olive oil is also used for its *emollient* (soothing, moisturizing) effect in the treatment of *cradle cap*.

## -oma

A suffix that denotes a tumor, as in lipoma, a benign tumor of fatty tissue.

## Omentum

An apronlike double fold of fatty membrane that hangs down in front of the intestines. The omentum contains blood vessels, nerves, lymph vessels, and lymph nodes. In addition to acting as a fat store, the omentum may limit the spread of infection within the abdominal cavity by adhering to the affected area.

## Omphalocele

An alternative name for *exomphalos*.

## Onchocerciasis

 A tropical disease that is caused by infestation with the worm *ONCHOCERCA VOLVULUS*. The disease, which is a type of *filariasis*, affects more than 20 million people in portions of Central and South America and Africa. Many sufferers are blinded by the condition.

**CAUSES AND SYMPTOMS**

The disease is transmitted from person to person by small, fiercely biting, black *SIMULIUM* flies. These flies breed in, and always remain near, fast-running turbulent streams (hence the disease's alternative name, "river blindness").

The transmission of the disease and life cycle of the worm are shown opposite. Blindness may result as an allergic reaction to dead microfilariae (tiny worms) near the eyes.

**TREATMENT AND PREVENTION**

The microfilariae are quickly killed by the drug diethylcarbamazine. This drug must be used with great care, however, because of the severe reactions caused by the dead worms.

Travelers to areas where the disease is prevalent should take measures to discourage the insects from biting (see *Insect bites*).

## Oncogenes

Genes, found in all cells, that are responsible for cells becoming malignant (cancerous). Out of the complete

O

human gene complement of 50,000 genes, fewer than 100 are probably oncogenes; about half of them have been identified.

Cancer cells differ from healthy ones in various ways. Their growth is unrestrained, and they infiltrate and destroy normal tissues (see *Cancer*). These differences are induced by mutations (alterations) in certain key genes—the oncogenes—that cause them to be "switched on." Switching on of a cell's oncogenes may increase its rate of multiplication, alter its responsiveness to hormonal growth factors, or increase its invasiveness.

Oncogenes may be switched on by the various environmental factors that are known to cause cancer, such as ultraviolet light, radioactivity, tobacco smoke, alcohol, asbestos particles, carcinogenic chemicals, and certain viruses. To transform a cell from normal to malignant seems to require the switching on of between two and four oncogenes. Thus, cancer of the cervix may develop in a woman who smokes and whose cervix has been infected with papillomavirus (a potentially cancer-causing virus), whereas either of these factors by itself might not be sufficient to cause cancer.

## Oncologist

A specialist in the diagnosis and treatment of *cancer*. Many oncologists specialize in a particular type of cancer, such as leukemia. The oncologist conducts tests to determine the location, type, and extent of the cancer. He or she administers or supervises treatment, which may involve several other specialists and take a number of forms, such as *radiation therapy*, *anticancer drugs*, surgery, or a combination of these.

## Oncology

The study of the causes, development, characteristics, and treatment of *tumors*, particularly malignant (cancerous) ones. Because there are many different types of tumors, which can derive from virtually any tissue in the body, oncology encompasses a wide range of experimental techniques and investigative approaches. These include surveying the frequency and distribution of tumors, testing new treatments, investigating the biochemical processes involved in tumor formation, and studying abnormal genes associated with tumors.

## Onlay, dental

A tooth restoration of gold made outside the mouth and fixed onto the biting surface and over one or more cusps of a tooth. An onlay may be used to strengthen an extensively restored tooth. It is also sometimes needed to build up teeth in cases of *malocclusion* in which the biting surfaces of certain upper and lower teeth fail to meet when the jaw is closed.

## Onychogryphosis

Abnormal thickening, hardening, and curving of the nails, which occurs

### Onychogryphosis
This extraordinary thickening and overgrowth, resembling the claws of the mythological griffin, may affect toenails or fingernails.

mainly in elderly people. Its cause is unknown, but onychogryphosis is associated with fungal infection or poor circulation.

## Onycholysis

Separation of the nail from its bed, beginning at the tip. It occurs in many skin conditions, including *psoriasis* and fungal infections.

## Onychosis

A general term for disease, deformity, or wasting of the *nails*. Onychosis caused by fungal infection is called onychomycosis.

## Oophorectomy

Removal of one or both ovaries.

**WHY IT IS DONE**
Oophorectomy is performed to treat *ovarian cysts* or ovarian cancer (see *Ovary, cancer of*). In women under 40, the surgeon attempts to preserve ovarian function by performing only a partial oophorectomy.

Both ovaries may be removed during a *hysterectomy* if disease has spread from the uterus to the ovaries. Removing both ovaries can also reduce the risk of ovarian cancer in women past the menopause.

**HOW IT IS DONE**
Oophorectomy is performed using general anesthesia and usually takes less than one hour. The ovaries are removed through an incision in the lower abdominal wall.

**RECOVERY PERIOD**
There is some pain and tenderness around the operation site. Most activities can be resumed within about a month of surgery, and sexual intercourse after about six weeks.

**OUTLOOK**
There are usually no adverse effects when one ovary or part of an ovary is

---

**THE CYCLE OF ONCHOCERCIASIS**
The infestation is spread by a fly that ingests microfilariae (tiny worms) from an infested person; the worms grow into larvae and are deposited in the skin of a new host when the fly bites.

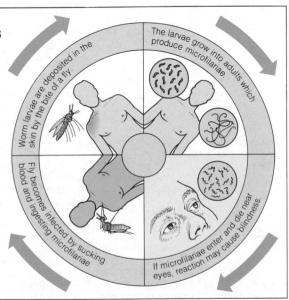

Worm larvae are deposited in the skin by the bite of a fly.

The larvae grow into adults which produce microfilariae.

Fly becomes infected by sucking blood and ingesting microfilariae.

If microfilariae enter and die near eyes, reaction may cause blindness.

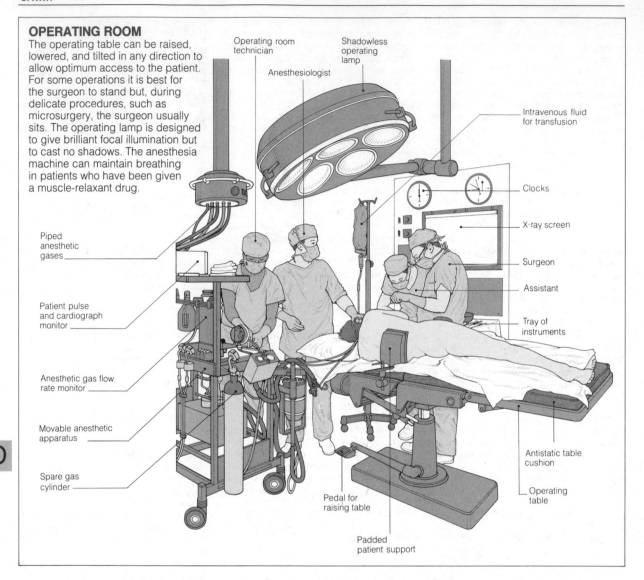

## OPERATING ROOM

The operating table can be raised, lowered, and tilted in any direction to allow optimum access to the patient. For some operations it is best for the surgeon to stand but, during delicate procedures, such as microsurgery, the surgeon usually sits. The operating lamp is designed to give brilliant focal illumination but to cast no shadows. The anesthesia machine can maintain breathing in patients who have been given a muscle-relaxant drug.

Operating room technician

Anesthesiologist

Shadowless operating lamp

Intravenous fluid for transfusion

Clocks

X-ray screen

Surgeon

Assistant

Tray of instruments

Piped anesthetic gases

Patient pulse and cardiograph monitor

Anesthetic gas flow rate monitor

Movable anesthetic apparatus

Spare gas cylinder

Pedal for raising table

Padded patient support

Antistatic table cushion

Operating table

---

removed because ovulation and hormone production continue. If both ovaries are removed, *hormone replacement therapy* may be necessary.

## -opathy

A suffix that denotes a disease or disorder (often a noninflammatory one), as in neuropathy, any disorder of the peripheral nerves. The suffix -pathy is synonymous with -opathy.

## Open heart surgery

Any operation on the heart in which the heart beat is temporarily stopped and its function taken over by a mechanical pump. The early heart surgeons carried out closed operations, inserting their fingers and

specially designed knives into the heart (to open the channel of a narrowed valve) while the organ continued to beat. Such operations had only limited scope.

With the development of reliable *heart-lung machines* in the 1950s, the picture changed. Once the pump was connected, the surgeon could open the heart, repair defects, and even reconstruct the main chambers. During the operation, the heart is kept cool through techniques of surgical *hypothermia*, which help prevent damage to the heart muscle from lack of oxygen.

The main applications of open heart surgery have been the correction of congenital heart defects (see *Heart*

*disease, congenital*), surgery for heart valve insufficiency or narrowed heart valves (see *Heart valve surgery*), and *coronary artery bypass* surgery.

## Operable

A term applied to any condition that is suitable for surgical treatment, such as an accessible benign tumor that requires removal because it is causing symptoms. (See also *Inoperable*.)

## Operating room

A hospital room in which surgical procedures are performed. The room is designed to reduce the risk of bacteria infecting open surgical wounds. A ventilation system provides a constant supply of clean, filtered air, the walls and floors are easily washable and are cleaned at least once daily, and there are annexes with foot- or elbow-operated faucets where surgeons, assistants, and nurses use sterile brushes and bactericidal soaps to scrub their hands and forearms before putting on sterile gowns, masks, and gloves. Often built into the walls are light boxes for viewing images obtained by *X ray*, *CT scanning*, or *MRI*.

**EQUIPMENT**

During an operation using general anesthesia, the anesthesia machine stands at the head of the operating table (see *Anesthesia, general*) connected by tubes to oxygen and various anesthetic gases.

The surgeon's sterile instruments, covered with sterile towels before use, are arranged on stainless steel wheeled tables. There is also a *diathermy* machine, which controls bleeding. If required, other equipment, such as a *heart-lung machine* (which can take over the function of the patient's heart and lungs), is brought into the operating room.

## Operation

Any surgical procedure, usually carried out with instruments but sometimes using only the hands (as in the

### COMMON SURGICAL OPERATIONS

| Operation | No. performed in US per year |
|---|---|
| Inguinal hernia repair | 585,000 |
| Cholecystectomy (gallbladder removal) | 490,000 |
| Releasing of peritoneal adhesions | 300,000 |
| Appendectomy (removal of appendix) | 285,000 |
| Biopsy or local removal of breast abnormality | 235,000 |
| Debridement of wound, burn, or infection | 220,000 |
| Partial colectomy (excision of large intestine) | 170,000 |
| Hemorrhoidectomy | 130,000 |
| Free skin graft | 120,000 |
| Mastectomy (breast removal) | 115,000 |

manipulation of a simple fracture). Operations range from procedures performed quickly using a local anesthetic (such as draining a skin abscess) to surgery using general anesthesia lasting several hours (such as a heart or liver transplant).

## Ophthalmia

A word once used to describe any inflammatory eye disorder; its use is now restricted to the following two specific disorders.

Ophthalmia neonatorum (literally "eye inflammation of the newborn") is a discharge of pus from the eyes of an infant that starts within 21 days of birth. In many cases the cause is an infection (such as *gonorrhea* or a *chlamydial infection*) acquired during birth. It is treated with antibiotics.

Sympathetic ophthalmia is a rare condition that occurs at least 10 days after a penetrating eye injury. If the injured eye is not removed within this time, severe *uveitis* (inflammation of the iris and choroid) that threatens blindness in the uninjured eye may develop. *Corticosteroid drugs* are used to treat the inflammation.

## Ophthalmologist

A physician who specializes in care of the *eyes*. Ophthalmologists conduct examinations to determine the quality of *vision* and the need for corrective *glasses* or *contact lenses*. Ophthalmologists also check for the presence of any disorders, such as *glaucoma* or *cataracts*. Ophthalmologists may prescribe glasses and contact lenses, medication, or surgery, as necessary.

## Ophthalmology

The study of the *eye*, and the diagnosis and treatment of disorders that affect it. Ophthalmology includes not only the assessment of *vision* and the prescription of *glasses* or *contact lenses* to correct defects, but also the surgery required to treat eye disorders such as *cataracts*, *glaucoma*, *retinal detachment*, and obstruction of tear ducts.

Ophthalmologists frequently work closely with other physicians because many disorders of the retina at the back of the eye are signs of nonoptical disorders, such as *hypertension* (high blood pressure), *atherosclerosis* (narrowing of arteries due to the deposition of fatty material inside them), or *diabetes mellitus*. Careful analysis of a person's field of vision (see *Eye, examination of*) can reveal defects that indicate neurological damage, such as that caused by a brain tumor.

## Ophthalmoplegia

Partial or total paralysis of the muscles that move the eyes. Ophthalmoplegia may be caused by disease of the muscles themselves (as in *Graves' disease*) or by one of the conditions affecting the brain or the nerves supplying the eye muscles (including *stroke*, *encephalitis*, *brain tumor*, and *multiple sclerosis*).

## Ophthalmoscope

An instrument used to examine the inside of the eye. The ophthalmoscope, by means of a deflecting prism or a perforated angled mirror, allows illumination and viewing of the entire area of the retina, the head of the optic nerve, the retinal arteries and veins, and the vitreous humor.

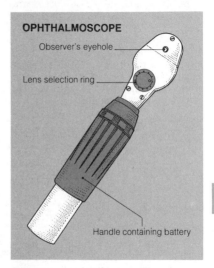

**OPHTHALMOSCOPE**

Observer's eyehole

Lens selection ring

Handle containing battery

## Opiate

Any drug derived from, or chemically similar to, *opium*. The term opiate is also used to refer to certain *receptors* (specific sites on the surface of cells) with which opiate drugs combine to initiate their effects.

## Opium

A milky substance obtained from the unripe seed pods of the poppy *PAPAVER SOMNIFERUM*. Used as a drug for thousands of years, opium has an analgesic (painkilling) effect and may also cause sleepiness and euphoria. Opium and its derivatives, which include *codeine* and *morphine*, are among the drugs collectively known as *narcotic drugs*.

## Opportunistic infection

Infection caused by organisms that do not usually produce disease in healthy people; or widespread infection by organisms that normally produce only mild, local, infection.

Many of the causative organisms are normally present on or in the human body and cause disease only when the host's *immune system* is impaired. Impairment of natural defenses may be due to treatment with anticancer and immunosuppressant drugs, to radiation therapy, or to diseases such as leukemia. Opportunistic infections also affect premature or malnourished infants and people with *immunodeficiency disorders*.

Opportunistic infections, especially *pneumocystis pneumonia*, are the cause of death in most *AIDS* patients. Many fungal infections (such as *cryptococcosis* and *candidiasis*) and some viral infections (such as *cytomegalovirus* and the virus that causes *herpes simplex*) are opportunistic infections.

Opportunistic infections are often unavoidable because the underlying defects in the host's defenses cannot easily be rectified. However, treatment with appropriate antimicrobial drugs may be lifesaving.

## Optic atrophy
A shrinkage or wasting of the *optic nerve* fibers, which results in some or near total loss of vision. Optic atrophy is caused by disease or injury to the optic nerve and may occur without prior signs of nerve disease, such as inflammation or swelling.

## Optic disk edema
Swelling of the head of the *optic nerve*, visible when the eye is examined with an ophthalmoscope. Optic disk edema usually indicates a dangerous rise in the pressure of *cerebrospinal fluid* within the skull, but may also arise from conditions affecting the nerve itself, including damage from restriction of blood supply. Optic disk edema may be followed by *optic atrophy*. (See also *Papilledema*.)

## Optician
A person who fits, supplies, and adjusts *glasses* or *contact lenses*. Because their training is limited, opticians may not examine or test eyes or prescribe glasses or drugs.

## Optic nerve
The second *cranial nerve*. The nerve of *vision*, the optic nerve consists of a collection of about 1 million nerve fibers that transmit impulses from the *retina* (the layer of light receptors at the back of the eye) to the brain.

## THE FUNCTION OF THE OPTIC NERVE

Each optic nerve is a bundle of long fibers originating from nerve cells in the retina and passing to the back of the brain. Because of the arrangement of the nerve fibers, disease or injury at any point causes a unique pattern of visual loss. Charting the pattern of visual loss allows accurate location of damage to the nerve.

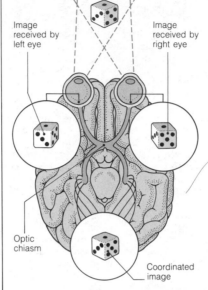

Image received by left eye

Image received by right eye

Optic chiasm

Coordinated image

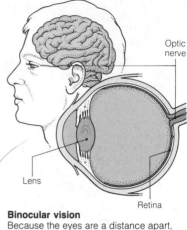

Optic nerve

Lens

Retina

**Binocular vision**
Because the eyes are a distance apart, they form slightly different images of a nearby object. The fusion of these two images into one provides the illusion of solidity. This is called stereopsis.

The two optic nerves converge at the optic junction behind the eyes, where fibers from the inner halves of the retinas cross over. As a result of this crossing over, nerve fibers from the right halves of both retinas pass to the right side of the occipital lobes at the back of the brain. The nerve fibers from the left halves of the retinas go to the left side of the brain.

Disorders of the optic nerve include *optic neuritis* (inflammation of the optic nerve) and *optic disk edema*, caused by external pressure from disease within the orbit or a brain tumor.

## Optic neuritis
Inflammation of the optic nerve that often causes sudden loss of part of the field of vision. Optic neuritis is usually accompanied by pain on moving the eyes and tenderness when the eyes are touched. In some cases, however, there may be little or no pain.

The cause of optic neuritis often remains uncertain, but most cases are thought to be due to *demyelination* (destruction of the myelin sheaths) of the optic nerve fibers, which occurs in *multiple sclerosis*. The condition may also result from inflammation or infection of tissues around the optic nerve.

Optic neuritis causes loss of vision, usually in the central part of the visual field. Vision usually improves substantially within six weeks, but each attack causes damage to a proportion of the optic nerve fibers; recurrent attacks usually lead to permanent loss of visual acuity.

Treatment with *corticosteroid drugs* may aid the return of vision but seems to have little effect on the long-term outcome of the inflammatory process. (See also *Optic atrophy*.)

## Optometrist
A specialist trained to examine the *eyes* and to prescribe, supply, and adjust *glasses* or *contact lenses*. Because they are not physicians, optometrists may not prescribe drugs or perform surgery. An optometrist refers patients requiring these types of treatment to an *ophthalmologist*.

## Optometry
The practice of assessing *vision* and establishing whether *glasses* or, for certain people, *contact lenses* are needed to correct any visual defect. (See also *Optometrist*.)

## Oral
Concerning the mouth.

# Oral contraceptives

## COMMON DRUGS

**Estrogens**
*Conjugated estrogens Diethylstilbestrol Ethinyl estradiol*

**Progesterones**
*Norethindrone Norgestrel*

> **WARNING**
> If you vomit or have diarrhea while taking an oral contraceptive, follow the advice for missing a pill. If you have missed two consecutive periods, you should have a pregnancy test.

A group of oral drug preparations containing a *progesterone drug*, often combined with an *estrogen drug*, taken by women to prevent pregnancy. All types of oral contraceptives—combined pills, phased pills, and minipills—are commonly known as the pill.

### HOW THEY ARE TAKEN

All types of oral contraceptives need to be taken on a monthly cycle for as long as a woman wishes to avoid pregnancy. The first course of pills is started on the first day of a period or on the fifth day after bleeding starts. Additional contraceptive precautions are usually needed for the duration of the first course of combined pills or phased pills or if the minipill is commenced on day 5.

Each course of pills is usually taken as described (right). Some brands of phased pills contain seven additional inactive pills, which may contain an iron supplement, so that the habit of taking a pill each day is not broken. It is possible to take a combined or phased pill continuously and thus avoid bleeding, but most physicians do not recommend this.

In some women, the use of oral contraceptives may cause menstruation to cease.

### MISSING A PILL

For maximum contraceptive effect, each type of pill should be taken at approximately the same time each day. This is particularly important with the minipill, which should be taken within three hours of the chosen time each day.

A forgotten combined or phased pill should be taken as soon as remembered even if it means taking two pills the next day. Pills for the rest of the course should be taken at the correct time. A different form of contraception should be used for seven days after missing the pill.

If between three and 12 hours have elapsed from the time a minipill was due to be taken, the pill should be taken and additional contraceptive precautions used for 48 hours. If more than 12 hours have elapsed, the minipill should be taken and additional contraceptive precautions used for as long as your physician advises. (For more information, see the illustration below.)

### EFFECTIVENESS

Used correctly, oral contraceptives have a failure rate of less than one

## HOW ORAL CONTRACEPTIVES WORK

The combined and phased pills increase the levels of estrogen and progesterone in the body, which interferes with the production by the pituitary gland of two *gonadotropin hormones* called follicle-stimulating hormone (FSH) and luteinizing hormone (LH). This action in turn prevents ovulation.

The minipill works mainly by making the mucus that lines the inside of the cervix (neck of the uterus) so thick that it is impenetrable to sperm.

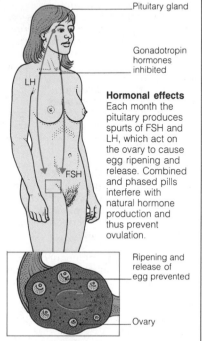

**Hormonal effects**
Each month the pituitary produces spurts of FSH and LH, which act on the ovary to cause egg ripening and release. Combined and phased pills interfere with natural hormone production and thus prevent ovulation.

Ripening and release of egg prevented — Ovary

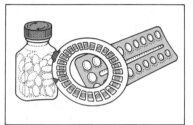

**Pill packaging**
Most oral contraceptives come in packs that clearly indicate the day on which each pill should be taken.

**Effects on eggs**
FSH normally brings about egg ripening and LH the egg's release from the ovary; combined and phased pills prevent this.

**Combined pill**
This pill contains an estrogen and a progesterone drug in fixed doses. A course usually consists of one pill per day for 21 days, followed by seven tablet-free days, during which bleeding may occur. A new course is then started, whether or not bleeding has occurred.

**Phased pill—a typical program**
These pills contain both an estrogen and a progesterone drug, but are divided into two or three groups or phases. The dose of the progesterone drug, and sometimes of estrogen as well, changes from phase to phase. A course lasts for 21 days followed by seven tablet-free days.

**Minipill—progesterone only**
These pills contain a progesterone drug only in a fixed dose. The pills are taken continuously, one every day with no tablet-free days. Bleeding usually occurs during the last few days of each cycle. The minipill has a slightly higher failure rate than the combined and phased pills.

pregnancy per 100 woman-years (i.e., the number of pregnancies among 100 women using the method for one year). Allowing for incorrect use or other factors, the actual failure rates may be as high as between two and three pregnancies per 100 woman-years for the combined or phased pill, and between two and a half to four pregnancies for the minipill.

Certain other drugs (such as *barbiturate drugs*, *anticonvulsant drugs*, *griseofulvin*, and some *antibiotic drugs*) may impair the effectiveness of oral contraceptives. A woman should always inform her gynecologist if she is taking other medication.

### ADVANTAGES AND DISADVANTAGES
In addition to providing excellent protection against pregnancy, the main advantage of oral contraceptives is that they do not interfere with the spontaneity of sex.

Estrogen-containing pills seem to protect against cancer of the uterus and ovaries, *ovarian cysts*, *endometriosis*, and iron-deficiency *anemia*. They also tend to make periods regular, lighter, and relatively free of menstrual pain.

The main disadvantages of oral contraceptives are that they are medically unsuitable for some women and that they may produce adverse effects.

### CONTRAINDICATIONS
Estrogen-containing pills increase the risk of certain disorders and are therefore not usually prescribed if a woman suffers from *hypertension* (high blood pressure), *hyperlipidemia* (high levels of fat in the blood), *liver* disease, *migraine*, *otosclerosis* (an ear disorder), or if she has previously had a *thrombosis* (abnormal blood clot).

The chances of a thrombosis occurring are increased in women who smoke or who are over the age of 35. An estrogen-containing pill is usually not given during the first few months after childbirth or in the four weeks before a major operation because of the increased risk of thrombosis. *Obesity* and *diabetes mellitus* also make a woman more susceptible to thrombosis.

Oral contraceptives are not usually prescribed to women with heart or circulatory disorders, a family history of certain disorders, or unexplained vaginal bleeding.

Combined or phased pills interfere with milk production and should not be taken during breast-feeding. The minipill is usually considered unsuitable for a woman who has had an ectopic pregnancy.

### POSSIBLE ADVERSE EFFECTS
Estrogen-containing pills may cause nausea and vomiting, weight gain, depression, breast swelling, reduced sex drive, increased appetite, cramps in the legs and abdomen, headaches, and dizziness. A more serious adverse effect of these pills is the risk of a thrombosis causing a *stroke*, *embolism*, or *myocardial infarction* (heart attack). Estrogen-containing pills may also aggravate heart disease or cause hypertension, *gallstones*, *jaundice*, and, very rarely, *liver cancer*.

Medical evidence suggests that cancer of the cervix is more common in women taking estrogen-containing pills. This risk may be outweighed by the reduced risk of other cancers of the reproductive system.

All forms of oral contraception can cause bleeding between periods, but this is especially true of the minipill. Other possible adverse effects of the minipill are irregular periods, ectopic pregnancy, and ovarian cysts.

There is no evidence that use of an oral contraceptive reduces a woman's fertility permanently (although menstruation may be irregular or absent for some months after stopping the pill). Likewise, there is no evidence that a fetus can be harmed if conceived while the woman is taking the pill or has recently stopped doing so.

Adverse effects usually disappear within a few months. If they persist, it may be necessary to change to a different type of pill or to an alternative method of contraception. Because adverse effects are more likely to occur with high doses of estrogen, low-estrogen preparations are prescribed whenever possible. The minipill may be used by women who suffer adverse effects even with low estrogen doses or who should not take estrogen drugs for other medical reasons.

Women taking oral contraceptives should receive checkups, including blood pressure and weight checks and *cervical smear tests*. (See also *Contraception*; *Contraception, hormonal methods*.)

## Oral hygiene
Measures that keep the mouth and teeth clean and healthy. Good oral hygiene reduces the incidence of tooth decay (see *Caries, dental*), prevents *gingivitis* and other *gum* disorders, and helps prevent *halitosis* (bad breath). Oral hygiene is broadly divided into personal and professional care.

### PERSONAL CARE
The most important aspect of personal oral hygiene is daily removal of dental

*plaque* (a sticky, bacteria-containing substance) by thorough *toothbrushing* and use of dental floss (see *Floss, dental*). Use of a fluoride mouth rinse or an oral irrigator (a device that produces a forceful water stream) may also be helpful, but these are aids that cannot remove plaque or replace brushing and flossing. *Disclosing agents* can help make tooth cleaning more efficient by showing the location of plaque. Dentures must always be kept scrupulously clean by brushing every surface and soaking them in a cleansing solution.

### PROFESSIONAL CARE
A *dentist* or hygienist (see *Hygienist, dental*) removes stubborn plaque and *calculus* (a hard mineral deposit that forms on the teeth above and below the gums) by *scaling* and polishing. These procedures are usually carried out during a routine checkup; in cases of *periodontal disease*, they may need to be performed more often.

## Oral surgeon
A surgeon who specializes in operations on the teeth, jaws, and other parts of the mouth and face (see *Oral surgery*). The qualifications required include a degree in general dentistry and specialization through a four-year training program in oral and maxillofacial (pertaining to the upper jaw and face) surgery. Many oral surgeons also have medical degrees, although it is not required.

## Oral surgery
Surgery to treat disease, deformity, or injury of the mouth, face, and jaws.

Among the dental procedures carried out by oral surgeons are the extraction of severely impacted wisdom teeth (see *Impaction, dental*) and *alveolectomy* (removal of part of the jaw that holds the teeth) to improve the fitting of dentures.

More complicated oral surgery includes *orthognathic surgery* to correct deformities of the jaw that result in an abnormal relationship between the upper and lower teeth; repairing a broken jaw; plastic surgery to correct *cleft lip and palate*; and the removal of certain types of benign tumors from tissues within the mouth.

## Orbit
The socket in the skull that contains the eyeball, protective pads of fat, and various blood vessels, muscles, and nerves. An opening in the back of the orbit allows the *optic nerve* to pass from the eyeball into the brain.

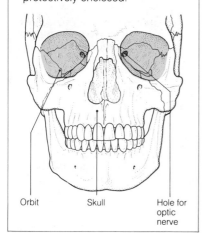
## DISORDERS

**INJURY** A blow of great force, as in a car crash or a sports injury, may fracture the orbit; the eyeball itself often escapes damage because it is squeezed backward by protective muscles during reflex blinking. Many such fractures heal without treatment, but some result in facial deformity that requires corrective surgery. An operation also may be needed to reinforce the floor of the orbit if a fracture causes downward displacement of the eye.

**INFECTION** Rarely, bacteria infect the fatty tissue lining the orbit, causing orbital *cellulitis.* Usually the infection originates in a nearby sinus, but sometimes it spreads in the blood from a facial infection. The affected eye protrudes, is extremely painful and red, and there is severe swelling of the lids and conjunctiva (the membrane lining the inside of the lids and front of the eye).

Orbital cellulitis is a serious disorder. The pressure on the eye may damage it and there is a slight risk that the infection may spread inward to the meninges (the membranes covering the brain) and the brain itself, causing *meningitis.* Prompt treatment with high doses of antibiotics usually clears up the condition.

## Orchiectomy

The surgical removal of a single testis or of both the testes.

**WHY IT IS DONE**

Orchiectomy may be performed to deal with a testicular cancer (see *Testis,*

*cancer of*) or *gangrene,* or to reduce production of the hormone testosterone as part of the treatment of cancer of the prostate gland (see *Prostate, cancer of*). Because the prostate gland depends on male sex hormones for its normal growth, orchiectomy is often effective in reducing the growth of a prostatic cancer. It is especially effective in controlling the symptoms of secondary tumors in the bones.

**HOW IT IS DONE**

The scrotum is cut open (using spinal and local anesthesia), the blood vessels and nerves leading to the scrotum are cut free, the testis is cut away from surrounding tissue and removed, and the skin is stitched.

After the operation, *analgesics* (painkillers) may be needed and an *ice pack* may be applied to the surgical area for the first 24 hours to prevent excessive swelling.

**OUTLOOK**

Complete healing can be expected without complications. Removal of one testis does not affect sex drive, potency, or the ability to have children. The patient is advised to wear an athletic supporter and to avoid vigorous exercise for a month or so after the operation.

## Orchiopexy

An operation in which an undescended testis (see *Testis, undescended*) is brought down into the scrotum. It is usually performed before a boy is 5 to avoid the risk of the condition causing infertility or even cancer of the testis (see *Testis, cancer of*).

An incision is made in the groin (using a general anesthetic) and the testis is gently maneuvered down the inguinal canal leading from the abdomen to the scrotum. The base of the testis is then usually attached to the scrotum with a few stitches to prevent it from retracting.

Pain and swelling are relieved with *analgesics* (painkillers) and an *ice pack.* Healing usually takes place without any complications.

## Orchitis

Inflammation of a testis. Orchitis may be caused by infection with the virus that causes *mumps.*

Orchitis develops in about one quarter of males who contract mumps after puberty. It is characterized by swelling and severe pain in the affected testis and a high fever. In *epididymo-orchitis* (which has different causes), the tube that carries sperm from the testis is also inflamed.

Treatment is with *analgesics* (painkillers) and *ice packs* to reduce swelling and pain; antibiotics are usually given. The condition usually begins to subside after three to seven days. Occasionally, orchitis is followed by shrinking of the testis.

## Organ

A collection of various *tissues* integrated into a distinct structural unit that performs specific functions. For example, the brain consists of nerve tissue and supporting tissue (called neuroglia) organized to receive, process, and send out information.

## Organ donation

The agreement of a person (or his or her relatives) to the surgical removal of one or more organs for use in *transplant surgery.* Most organs used as transplants are removed immediately after death, but a kidney is also commonly taken from living *donors.*

The donation of kidneys by living donors is usually confined to relatives of the transplant patient. This occurs for medical reasons (because a relative is more likely to have the same or a similar tissue type as the patient) and for ethical reasons (because physicians discourage the sale of living organs). The risks of donation are carefully explained and the kidney is removed only after the donor gives clear voluntary consent.

The range of organs removed after death is much greater, including the heart, lungs, liver, pancreas, and kidneys. Most organs can be transplanted successfully only if removed immediately after death; the best results often require surgical removal of organs before the donor's heart has stopped beating. In practice this means that most donations of major organs are made from patients who die in an intensive-care unit and are certified as "brain dead" while still having the heart and lung function maintained by a machine (see *Death*).

People who want to donate some or all of their organs after death should make their intentions clear to their relatives and sign a donor card. In most Western countries the demand for donated organs is far greater than the supply. Some countries have introduced laws that allow physicians to remove organs after death unless the patient has specifically forbidden it. In practice, physicians are reluctant to carry out such legislation and the supply of donor organs continues to depend on voluntary donations. (See

O

also *Corneal graft; Heart valve surgery; Heart transplant; Heart-lung transplant; Kidney transplant; Liver transplant.*)

## Organic

Related to a body organ; having organs or an organized structure; or related to organisms or to substances from them. In chemistry, the term refers to any of the group of compounds that contain carbon, with the exception of carbon oxides (such as carbon dioxide) and sulfides and metal carbonates (such as calcium carbonate). The term also signifies the presence of disease, in contrast to a *functional disorder* or psychosomatic complaint. (See also *Inorganic.*)

## Organic brain syndrome

See *Brain syndrome, organic.*

## Organism

A general term for any individual animal or plant. Medically, the most important are humans and disease-causing *microorganisms*, such as *bacteria, fungi, protozoa,* and *viruses.*

## Orgasm

Intense sensations resulting from the series of muscular contractions that occur at the peak of sexual excitement. Orgasm is usually followed by physical relaxation and often drowsiness.

In men, contractions of the muscles of the inner pelvis massage seminal fluid from the prostatic area into the urethra, from which it is forcefully propelled from the urethral orifice (see *Ejaculation*). Following orgasm, the penis becomes soft again and there is a refractory period during which there is no physical response to further sexual stimulation.

Orgasm in women is associated with irregular contractions of the voluntary muscles of the walls of the vagina and, in some women, of the uterus, followed by relief of congestion in the pelvic area. Orgasm usually lasts about three to 10 seconds, but can last up to a minute in some women. There is no refractory phase; some women experience multiple orgasms if stimulation is continued.

Both men and women may have problems with orgasm (see *Ejaculation, disorders of; Orgasm, lack of*).

## Orgasm, lack of

The inability to achieve orgasm. Lack of orgasm is the most common sexual problem in women. Between 30 and 50 percent experience difficulties at some time in their lives. The once-used term "frigidity" to describe lack of orgasm is outmoded and considered perjorative by many women. Lack of orgasm is rarer in men (see *Ejaculation, disorders of*).

Some women (10 to 15 percent) are not able to achieve orgasm under any circumstances. Others experience orgasm only occasionally or under special circumstances.

**CAUSES**

Lack of orgasm is usually caused by sexual inhibition, inexperience, lack of knowledge, or psychological factors (such as anxiety or early sexual trauma). In some cases it may be due to alcohol dependence, certain drugs, or pain during intercourse (see *Intercourse, painful*).

Inability to achieve orgasm under any circumstances may stem from poor sex education or lack of familiarity with the body's sexual responses. Psychological attitudes also contribute. Some women are ashamed of their bodies, are inhibited about the sex act, have deep-seated guilt feelings about sexual pleasure, fear pregnancy, feel uncertain about intimacy, or fear "letting go" or losing momentary control during an orgasm. They therefore cannot relax during sex. Additionally, some women have difficulties with physical arousal and never reach or get past the excitement stage (see *Sexual desire, inhibited*) due to not receiving or not allowing sufficient foreplay.

A woman may be able to achieve orgasm through masturbation but fail to achieve orgasm with her partner. This may occur with a new partner who is unfamiliar with the woman's sexual responses. In other cases, a woman may be able to achieve orgasm through stimulation by a partner, but not through intercourse. This is sometimes attributable to the longer time a woman needs to attain coital climax (about 13 minutes for a woman compared to less than three minutes for the average man). Lack of experience or knowledge, impatience, or premature ejaculation of the partner are factors. Problems in a long-term relationship may be due to underlying feelings of hostility, boredom, or distrust. Performance anxiety caused by the pressure to have an orgasm may also be an inhibiting factor, which in time sets up a cycle of failure.

**TREATMENT**

Any physical problems should be treated. Otherwise, women may be helped to achieve orgasm or to increase the frequency of orgasms through *sex therapy* or *marital counseling. Psychotherapy* may be helpful for women in whom the problem is related to deep-seated feelings of guilt or insecurity.

## Ornithosis

A disease of birds that is caused by the microorganism *CHLAMYDIA PSITTACI.* It can be transmitted to humans, causing *psittacosis,* a feverish illness accompanied by pneumonia.

## Orphan drugs

Drugs that have been developed to treat rare conditions but are not manufactured because the potential sales are small while the cost of carrying out the necessary safety tests is high. Reluctance to market an orphan drug may increase if the drug is out of patent (i.e., available for other companies to market) or cannot be patented because it is a known substance. However, changes in the law have made it profitable to provide certain orphan drugs.

An example of an orphan drug is tetrahydroaminoacridine (THA). Although clinical trials suggest THA may improve orientation and memory in people who have *Alzheimer's disease,* it has not been manufactured because the patent has expired.

## Orphenadrine

A *muscle-relaxant drug* used to relieve painful muscle spasm caused by injury to soft tissues (such as muscles and ligaments). Orphenadrine is also given to reduce muscle rigidity in *Parkinson's disease.*

Possible adverse effects include dryness of the mouth and blurred vision.

## Ortho-

A prefix meaning normal, correct, or straight, as in orthopedics (from the Greek for "straight child"), which originally concerned the correction of skeletal deformities in children. Today it includes all bone or joint problems in any age group.

## Orthodontic appliances

Devices, commonly known as braces, worn to correct *malocclusion* (poorly positioned teeth). Braces are most commonly fitted during childhood and adolescence when the teeth and jaws are still developing.

**WHY THEY ARE USED**

Braces are usually worn to correct overcrowded teeth that splay outward, tilt inward, or rotate (see *Overcrowding, dental*). Braces are fre-

O

quently used on *buck teeth* (projecting upper front teeth) and may also be used to reposition upper and lower premolars and molars (back teeth) when a faulty relationship between the upper and lower jaws prevents the teeth from meeting properly and interferes with chewing. Sometimes braces are required when permanent teeth fail to develop; in such cases, it may be necessary to move teeth to create room for artificial teeth.

### TYPES

**FIXED APPLIANCES** These braces, which cannot be removed by the wearer, exert a continuous pressure and can move teeth in any direction. They are usually fitted to all the upper and/or lower teeth and are used when many teeth need repositioning.

The tooth-moving part of a fixed appliance is the arch wire, an adjustable, high-tensile steel wire, threaded through a bracket on each tooth.

To allow extra force to be applied to specific teeth, some brackets may be fitted with small hooks to which headgear (straps that fit around the back and over the top of the head) can be attached when the wearer is at rest.

Fixed appliances are kept in the mouth until the teeth have moved into the correct position, which may take a year or more. Thereafter, a fixed or removable retainer plate may need to be worn for anywhere from six months to five years to hold the teeth in their correct place until tooth and jaw growth stop in late adolescence.

Fixed appliances give more precise control over tooth movement than removable braces, but they are more expensive and take longer to fit and adjust. They also trap *plaque* (the sticky coating that forms on teeth and causes decay) and make cleaning of the teeth more difficult.

Lingual braces ("invisible" braces) also can be used by some people in the inner arch (the tongue side) of teeth. These braces pull rather than push teeth into place.

**REMOVABLE APPLIANCES** These braces are used when only one or several teeth need correcting. They consist of a plastic plate that covers the roof of the mouth (or, much less commonly, the floor of the mouth) with attachments that anchor over the back teeth. Force is applied by means of springs, wire bows, screws, or rubber bands fitted to the plate, sometimes combined with the use of headgear.

Occasionally, removable appliances are used in younger children before facial growth has stopped. They con-

## HOW ORTHODONTIC APPLIANCES WORK

The tooth sockets are remarkably responsive to sustained pressure against the teeth. Orthodontic appliances, which may be fixed or removable, provide such pressure. Even gentle pressure applied in a particular direction will move teeth. As they move, bone is remodeled so that the new position is stable.

### FIXED APPLIANCES

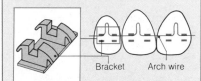

Bracket    Arch wire

**Appearance of brackets and wires**
Brackets are fixed appliances cemented to the outer surface of the teeth; they have slots into which arch wires can be fitted.

By careful design of the arrangement of wires and springs, force can be exerted in any direction to move a tooth into the desired position.

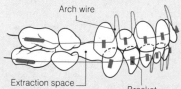

Arch wire

Extraction space

Bracket

**1** Teeth are removed to create space and an appliance made to correct the alignment of the remaining teeth and to close gaps between them.

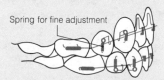

Spring for fine adjustment

**2** Once the teeth in the upper and lower jaws are aligned, the appliance is adjusted to tip or rotate the teeth to give a good appearance and bite.

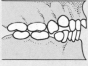

**Overcrowding**
This is frequently associated with malocclusion (poor alignment between upper and lower teeth). Teeth may have to be extracted to make room for those to be straightened.

### REMOVABLE APPLIANCES

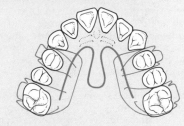

These are easier to keep clean than fixed appliances and are less obtrusive, but they may interfere with speech; their efficiency relies on patients using them as directed. This type exerts pressure to push the teeth at the sides outward.

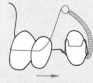

**Bow device**
This simple wire spring acts by exerting force to straighten the tooth. Many bow devices are more complicated.

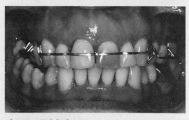

**A removable bow**
One of the many forms of orthodontic wire appliance, this bow device exerts pressure on the teeth at the sides, which straightens and moves them outward.

sist of interconnected upper and lower plates that force the jaw into a position of slight tension against the pull of the surrounding muscles, translating this force to move the teeth.

Potential disadvantages of removable appliances are that their bulk may interfere with speech and that wearers may remove them so often that they become ineffective.

## Orthodontics

A branch of dentistry concerned with the prevention and treatment of *malocclusion* (irregularities of the position of teeth or an abnormal relationship between the upper and lower teeth). In most cases, the orthodontist performs orthodontic procedures on children and adolescents while the teeth are still developing and are relatively maneuverable. However, adults are also able to benefit from orthodontic treatment.

Diagnosis of the exact type of malocclusion involved may require making models of the teeth (see *Impression, dental*) to see clearly how they come together when clenched, taking X rays of the head to relate the position of the teeth to that of the facial bones, and taking X rays of the jaws to study their structure and relationship.

Orthodontic treatment consists of moving poorly positioned teeth by means of gentle pressure exerted by *orthodontic appliances* (braces). To achieve this, the orthodontist may first need to extract certain teeth, often the first molars, to provide growing room for the teeth being moved.

## Orthodontist

A dentist who specializes in preventing or correcting crooked, crowded, or irregularly spaced teeth and abnormal relationships between the upper and lower teeth (see *Malocclusion*). To achieve this, the orthodontist makes use of various *orthodontic appliances*.

## Orthognathic surgery

An operation to correct deformity of the jaw and the severe *malocclusion* (abnormal relationship between the upper and lower teeth) that is invariably associated with it.

### HOW IT IS DONE

The operation, which usually requires a stay in the hospital, is carried out using a general anesthetic.

A jaw that projects too far can be shortened by removing a block of bone from each side and maneuvering the front of the jaw backward. A jaw that is too short can be remedied by dividing the bone on each side, sliding the front of the jaw forward, and inserting bone grafts (taken from elsewhere in the body) into the gaps.

After repositioning, the bones often require splinting (see *Splinting, dental*) until healing occurs.

## Orthopedics

The branch of surgery concerned with disorders of bones and joints and the muscles, tendons, and ligaments associated with them. Orthopedists perform many tasks, including setting broken bones and putting on casts; treating joint conditions, such as dislocations, slipped disks, arthritis, and back problems; treating bone tumors and birth defects of the skeleton; and surgically repairing or replacing hip, knee, or finger joints.

## Orthopedist

A physician who specializes in problems affecting bones, joints, and related structures (see *Orthopedics*).

## Orthopnea

Breathing difficulty brought on by lying flat. Orthopnea is a symptom of *heart failure* (reduced pumping efficiency) and is caused by *edema* (fluid collection) in the lungs. It also occurs with *asthma* and chronic obstructive lung disease (chronic *bronchitis* with or without *emphysema*).

## Orthoptics

A technique used to measure and evaluate *strabismus* (misalignment of the eyes). Orthoptics sometimes includes eye exercises, which may or may not help the strabismus.

## Os

An anatomical term for a bone, as in os coxae, the hip bone. The plural of os is ossa, as in ossa cranii, the skull bones. The term os also refers to an opening in the body, usually the cervical os (entrance to the uterus).

## Osgood-Schlatter disease

Painful enlargement of the tibial tuberosity, the bony prominence of the tibia (shin) just below the knee. Osgood-Schlatter disease occurs in children (usually boys) aged 10 to 14.

The condition is caused by excessive, repetitive pulling of the quadriceps muscle (at the front of the thigh) on the patellar tendon, which is attached to the tibial tuberosity. There is usually pain above and below the knee, which is worse during strenuous activity, and the tibial tuberosity is tender when touched.

Osgood-Schlatter disease usually clears up completely without treatment; if pain is severe, the knee may be immobilized in a plaster cast.

## Osmosis

The passage of a solvent (such as water) through a semipermeable membrane (one that acts like a sieve) from a less concentrated (weaker) solution to a more concentrated (stronger) one. Osmosis occurs whenever solutions of different strengths are separated by a semipermeable membrane and continues until the two solutions are of equal strength unless the movement of solvent is opposed by applying pressure to the stronger solution. The pressure needed to stop the movement completely is called the osmotic pressure.

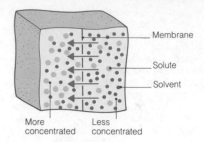

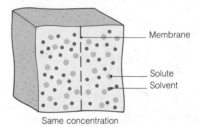

**Osmosis**
If two solutions, consisting of different concentrations of a solute (e.g., salt) in a solvent (e.g., water), are separated by a semipermeable membrane, solvent moves from the weaker to stronger solution until the two solutions attain equal concentration.

Semipermeable membranes are widespread in the body—they surround all cells. These membranes allow water, salts, simple sugars (such as glucose), and amino acids (but not proteins) to pass through. Consequently, osmosis plays an important part in regulating the distribution of water and other substances.

## Ossicle

A small bone, particularly the malleus (hammer), incus (anvil), and stapes (stirrup)—the three tiny bones in the middle *ear* that conduct sound from the eardrum to the inner ear.

## Ossification

The process by which *bone* is formed, renewed, and repaired. Ossification begins in the embryo and continues throughout life. There are three main types of ossification: bone growth, during which new bone is formed mainly from *cartilage* at the *epiphyses* (bone ends); bone renewal, which occurs as part of the normal regeneration process; and bone repair, which fuses broken bones after a fracture.

## Osteitis

Inflammation of bone. The most common cause is infection (see *Osteomyelitis*). Other causes are *Paget's disease* and *hyperparathyroidism*.

## Osteo-

A prefix that denotes a relationship to bone, as in *osteoporosis*, a condition in which the bones become thin and weak. The prefix oste- is synonymous with osteo-.

## Osteoarthritis

A joint disease aggravated by mechanical stress. Osteoarthritis is characterized by degeneration of the cartilage that lines joints or by *osteophyte* (bony outgrowth) formation, which leads to pain, stiffness, and occasionally loss of function of the affected joint.

### INCIDENCE

Osteoarthritis occurs in almost all people over age 60, although not all have symptoms. Various factors lead to the development of osteoarthritis earlier in life, including an injury to a joint or a congenital joint deformity. Osteoarthritis may occur with *rheumatoid arthritis*. Severe osteoarthritis affects three times as many women as men.

### SYMPTOMS

Osteoarthritis causes pain, swelling, creaking, and stiffness of one or more joints. Pain and stiffness may interfere with activities (such as walking and dressing) and may disrupt sleep.

Weakness and shrinkage (*atrophy*) of surrounding muscles may occur if pain prevents the joint from being used regularly. The affected joints become enlarged and distorted by osteophytes, which account for the gnarled appearance of hands affected by osteoarthritis.

### DIAGNOSIS AND TREATMENT

A diagnosis is generally made on the basis of a person having a history of joint pain with use and on physical findings of joint tenderness, swelling, and pain on motion. An X ray can confirm cartilage loss and osteophyte formation and assess the extent of the degenerative process. As yet there is no cure for osteoarthritis; symptoms may be relieved by *analgesics* (painkillers) and *nonsteroidal anti-inflammatory drugs*, which reduce joint inflammation. Sometimes a painful joint can be eased by injection of a *corticosteroid drug*.

*Physical therapy*, including exercises and heat treatment, can often relieve symptoms. If the condition is severe, various aids can make coping at home easier (see *Disability*).

Surgical treatment for severe osteoarthritis includes *arthroplasty* (joint replacement surgery) and *arthrodesis* (immobilization of a joint).

## OSTEOARTHRITIS

This differs from rheumatoid arthritis and has a better outlook. It results from excessive wear on joints, sometimes due to obesity or to slight deformity or misalignment of bones in a joint. Inflammation from disease, such as gout, may also proceed to osteoarthritis. Weight-bearing joints, such as those in the neck, the lower back, and the knees and hips, are the most commonly affected by this type of arthritis.

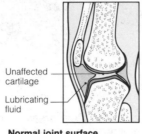

**Normal joint surface**
The healthy joint is lined with smooth cartilage and lubricated by synovial fluid.

Unaffected cartilage

Lubricating fluid

**Osteoarthritic joint**
In osteoarthritis (below), the cartilage becomes rough and flaky and small pieces break off to form loose bodies.

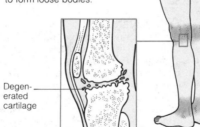

Degenerated cartilage

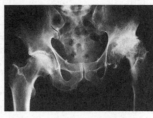

**X-ray signs of osteoarthritis**
This X ray shows narrowing of the joint space with osteophyte production and an increase in density of the bone ends.

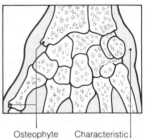

Osteophyte

Characteristic swelling

**Osteophytes**
These are outgrowths of new bone that tend to occur at the margins of the joint surfaces in osteoarthritis.

O

---

### TREATMENT AND SELF-HELP MEASURES

An important self-help measure is to shed excess weight to reduce wear and tear on joints. Measures to increase muscle power help to stabilize the affected joint and reduce symptoms.

**Swimming**
Regular exercise, to strengthen muscles and maintain joint mobility, can be valuable. Swimming in a heated pool increases muscle power without putting undue strain on joints.

**Other treatment**
Drugs such as aspirin or indomethacin are useful; sometimes corticosteroid injections are advised. There is little evidence that special diets or herbal treatments are effective.

---

## Osteochondritis dissecans

Degeneration of a bone just under a joint surface, causing fragments of bone and cartilage to become separated from surrounding bone.

Osteochondritis dissecans frequently affects the knee and usually starts in adolescence. The exact cause is unknown but the disorder is thought to be caused by damage to a small blood vessel beneath the joint surface, which may be initiated by injury. The separated fragment sometimes reattaches but usually forms a *loose body* within the joint. Symptoms include aching discomfort and intermittent swelling of the affected joint. The presence of a loose body may cause locking of a joint in one position.

*X rays* show damage to the joint and reveal the presence of any loose bodies. If a fragment has not completely separated, the joint may be immobilized in a cast to allow reattachment. Loose bodies of the knee are removed during *arthroscopy*.

The cavity left in the bone by a detached fragment disrupts the smoothness of the joint surface, increasing the likelihood of developing *osteoarthritis* in later life.

## Osteochondritis juvenilis

Inflammation of an *epiphysis* (growing area of bone) in children and adolescents. The exact cause is unknown, but the condition is thought to be due to disrupted blood supply to the bone.

There are several distinct types of osteochondritis juvenilis, each involving different bones in the body. *Perthes' disease* affects the epiphysis of the head of the femur (thigh bone), while Scheuermann's disease affects epiphyses of several adjoining vertebrae. Other types affect certain bones in the foot and wrist.

### SYMPTOMS AND SIGNS

Osteochondritis juvenilis causes localized pain and tenderness and, if the epiphysis forms part of a joint, restricted movement. Inflammation leads to softening of the bone, which may result in deformity because of surrounding pressure. X rays of the affected area show a patchy appearance and flattening of the bone.

### TREATMENT AND OUTLOOK

Immobilization by use of a brace or plaster cast may be used to relieve pain and reduce the risk of deformity. In some cases of Perthes' disease, an operation is required to relieve the pressure on the diseased bone to prevent more deformity.

The bone usually regenerates within three years and rehardens. In many cases, however, deformity is permanent and increases the likelihood of the development of *osteoarthritis* in later life.

## Osteochondroma

A benign bone tumor made up of a stalk of bone capped with cartilage. It grows from the side of a bone, usually at the end of a long bone in the region of the knee or shoulder. The osteochondroma develops in late childhood and early adolescence and stops growing when the skeleton is fully developed.

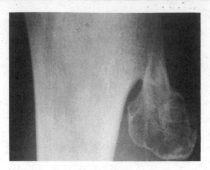

**X ray of osteochondroma**
The X ray shows a typical osteochondroma protruding from the bone. The tumor has a bony stalk and a cap made of cartilage.

The tumor, which appears as a hard round swelling near a joint, causes problems only if it interferes with the movement of tendons or the surrounding joint. In such cases, surgical removal may be necessary. A large osteochondroma can interfere with skeletal growth, causing deformity.

## Osteochondrosis

See *Osteochondritis juvenilis*.

## Osteodystrophy

Any generalized defect of the bones caused by a metabolic disorder (an abnormality of the body chemistry). Examples include *rickets*, a childhood condition in which the bones fail to harden properly due to a deficiency of vitamin D; *osteomalacia*, the equivalent condition in adults; *osteoporosis* (wasting away of bone) when it is caused not by aging but by the hormonal disorder *Cushing's syndrome* or by an excessive intake of *corticosteroid drugs*; and bone cysts and reduction of bone mass, which occasionally occur in chronic *renal failure* or *hyperparathyroidism* due to a disturbance in calcium metabolism in the body.

An osteodystrophy is usually reversible if the underlying cause can be treated effectively.

## Osteogenesis imperfecta

Abnormally brittle bones from birth caused by a familial (inherited) congenital defective development of the *connective tissue* that forms the basic material of bone.

### SYMPTOMS AND SIGNS

Severely affected infants, born with multiple fractures and a soft skull, usually do not survive. Those less severely affected have many fractures, often brought about by minimal force, during infancy and childhood. A physician examining such children

may sometimes find it difficult to determine whether the cause is osteogenesis imperfecta or *child abuse*. Very mild cases may not be detected until adolescence or later.

A common accompanying sign of the disorder is abnormal thinness of the sclera (whites of the eyes), making them appear blue. In addition, sufferers of osteogenesis imperfecta may be deaf due to *otosclerosis*.

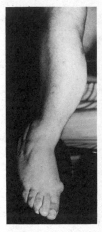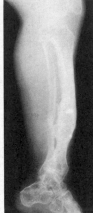

**Osteogenesis imperfecta**
Affected children may suffer recurrent fractures of the limbs that lead to deformity and shortening, and to abnormal growth. At right is an X ray of the leg of a sufferer.

### TREATMENT AND OUTLOOK

Fractures are generally treated in the usual way (by immobilization); otherwise, there is no specific treatment for the condition. The fractures usually heal quickly but often cause severe shortening and deformity of limbs, resulting in stunted, abnormal growth. Skull fractures may cause brain damage or death.

## Osteogenic sarcoma

See *Osteosarcoma*.

## Osteoid osteoma

An abnormal area of bone that causes deep pain, which is usually worse at night. An osteoid osteoma is extremely small—about 0.2 inch (0.5 cm)—and can be definitely diagnosed only by X ray. It most commonly affects a long bone of the arm or leg.

Pain can usually be relieved by *aspirin*. The condition is cured by removing the affected area of bone. (See also *Osteochondroma; Osteoma*.)

## Osteoma

A benign bone tumor. It is hard, usually small, and may occur on any bone. An osteoma is usually harmless, but surgical removal may be necessary if the tumor causes symptoms by pressing on surrounding structures.

## Osteomalacia

Softening, weakening, and demineralization of the bones in adults due to *vitamin D* deficiency (in children, the condition is called *rickets*).

The development of healthy bone requires an adequate intake of calcium and phosphorus from the diet, but these minerals cannot be absorbed by the body without a sufficient amount of vitamin D. A deficiency of this vitamin, which is obtained from certain foods and from the action of sunlight on the skin, results in softening and weakening of the bones, which then become vulnerable to distortion and fractures.

### CAUSES

Osteomalacia is usually caused by any of the following, alone or in combination: an insufficient amount of vitamin D in the diet (due to a lack of milk, butter, eggs, or fish liver oils), insufficient exposure to sunlight, or inadequate absorption of vitamin D from the intestine (see *Malabsorption*), which may be caused by a disorder such as *celiac sprue* or by intestinal surgery. Rare causes include *renal failure*, *acidosis* (increased acidity of body fluids), and certain metabolic disorders that are inherited.

Osteomalacia is rare in developed countries. Most commonly affected are people with an inadequate diet, people who rarely or never go outdoors, and dark-skinned immigrants living in a country that has much less sunlight than their countries of origin.

### SYMPTOMS AND SIGNS

Osteomalacia causes pain in the bones (particularly those in the neck, legs, hips, and ribs), muscle weakness, and, if the blood level of calcium is very low, *tetany* (muscle spasms) in the hands, feet, and throat. If the bones become greatly weakened, they may break after a minor injury.

### DIAGNOSIS AND TREATMENT

Osteomalacia is diagnosed from the symptoms and signs, along with blood tests, urine tests, and bone X rays. In some cases, a bone *biopsy* (removal of a small sample of bone for examination) is performed.

Treatment consists of a diet that is rich in vitamin D and regular supplements of the vitamin. Supplements are usually taken as tablets; if tablets cannot be absorbed by the intestine, injections may be necessary. In some cases of osteomalacia due to malabsorption, calcium supplements may also be taken.

## Osteomyelitis

Infection of bone and bone marrow, usually by bacteria. It can affect any bone in the body, is more common in children, and most often affects the long bones of the arms and legs and the vertebrae. In adults, it usually affects the pelvis and the vertebrae. In developed countries, adequate nutrition and a generally high resistance to infection have made the disease, which may be acute or chronic, much rarer than it once was.

### ACUTE OSTEOMYELITIS

The infecting microorganism (generally the bacterium *STAPHYLOCOCCUS AUREUS*) enters the bloodstream via a skin wound or an infection (usually in the nose or throat) and is carried to the bone in the blood. The infected bone and marrow become inflamed and pus forms, causing fever, severe pain and tenderness in the infected bone, and inflammation and swelling of the skin over the affected area.

The diagnosis may be confirmed by blood *culture*, bone scanning, and bone *X rays*. Treatment is with high doses of *antibiotic drugs* over several weeks or months. With prompt antibiotic treatment, acute osteomyelitis usually clears up completely. If the condition fails to respond to antibiotics, an operation is performed to expose the bone, to clean out the areas of infected and dead bone, and to drain the pus.

### CHRONIC OSTEOMYELITIS

This form may develop when an attack of acute osteomyelitis is neglected or fails to respond to treatment. It may also occur after a compound *fracture* or, occasionally, as a result of *tuberculosis* spreading from another part of the body.

Chronic osteomyelitis causes constant pain in the affected bone. Complications include persistent deformity and, in children, arrest of growth in the affected bone. In the later stages of the disease (which may have been recurring for many years) *amyloidosis* (harmful deposits of a starchy substance in vital organs) may develop.

Chronic osteomyelitis requires surgical removal of all affected bone, sometimes followed by a *bone graft* to replace the removed bone; antibiotics are also prescribed. If the cause is tuberculosis, antituberculous drugs are prescribed for at least one year after surgery.

## Osteopathic medicine

A system of diagnosis and treatment that recognizes the role of the musculoskeletal system (bones, muscles, tendons, tissues, nerves, and spinal column) in the healthy functioning of the human body.

Osteopathic medicine was founded on the Missouri frontier in 1874 by Andrew Taylor Still, MD. It is based on the concept of the human body as a unified organism, with the musculoskeletal system as central to the patient's well-being.

The Doctor of Osteopathy (DO) is a fully licensed physician with additional training in osteopathic palpatory diagnosis and manipulative therapy. The DO prescribes drugs and is qualified to practice all branches of medicine and surgery.

Osteopathic physicians emphasize that all body systems operate in unison, and that disturbances in one system can alter the functions of other systems in the body.

The osteopathic physician uses manipulation techniques, as well as traditional diagnostic and therapeutic procedures, to diagnose and treat dysfunction. Manipulation includes thrusting techniques and rhythmic stretching and pressure to restore motion to the joints.

## Osteopetrosis

A rare, inherited disorder in which bones harden and become more dense. The growth of healthy bone is a balance between the activity of its two constituent cells, bone-forming osteoblasts and bone-reabsorbing osteoclasts. In osteopetrosis, there is a deficiency of osteoclasts, which results in the disruption of normal bone structure.

The mildest form of osteopetrosis may not cause any symptoms. More severe forms can result in greater susceptibility to fractures, stunted growth, deformity, and anemia. Pressure on nerves may cause blindness, deafness, and facial paralysis.

Bone marrow transplants have been attempted on an investigational basis. The transplant supplies the recipient with cells from which healthy osteoclasts might develop.

## Osteophyte

A localized outgrowth of bone that forms at the boundary of a joint. Osteophytes are a characteristic of *osteoarthritis* and are partly responsible for the deformity and restricted movement of affected joints.

O

## OSTEOPOROSIS

In osteoporosis, the density of bones decreases, and their brittleness increases, although there is no change in size or composition. Women past the menopause are the most commonly affected because their ovaries no longer produce estrogen, which helps to maintain bone mass. The risk of the condition is greater in a woman who undergoes the menopause early, or whose mother had osteoporosis.

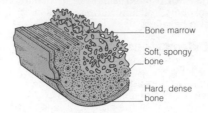

**Normal bone cross section**
Bone consists of fibers of collagen (a protein), which give elasticity, and calcium, which gives hardness.

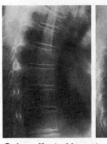

**Osteoporotic bone**
Thinning is mainly due to loss of collagen, which takes calcium with it. Both hard and spongy bone tissue are affected.

**Bone loss with age**
The graph at right shows how the percentage of bone lost increases in both sexes from age 30 onward, with the losses particularly marked in women after the menopause. By age 75, about half of all women have sustained at least one fracture due to osteoporosis, a much higher proportion than in men.

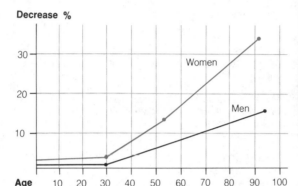

**Decrease %**

Women

Men

Age  10  20  30  40  50  60  70  80  90  100

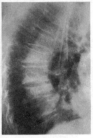

**Spine affected by osteoporosis**
The X rays show progressive thinning of the vertebrae, giving a characteristic "codfish" appearance to the spine.

## Osteoporosis

Loss of protein matrix tissue from bone, causing it to become brittle and easily fractured.

Many physicians do not discriminate between osteoporosis and *osteomalacia*, diagnosing any decreased density of bone (thinning) as osteoporosis. In fact, decreased density may be caused by osteomalacia or by osteomalacia with osteoporosis.

Osteoporosis is a natural part of aging. By age 70, the density of the skeleton has diminished by about one third. However, for hormonal reasons, the condition is much more common in women than in men. Also, for reasons that are unknown, osteoporosis is more common in whites than in blacks.

### CAUSES

Bone naturally becomes thinner as a person ages, but women are especially vulnerable to osteoporosis after the *menopause* because their ovaries no longer produce *estrogen hormone*, which helps maintain bone mass.

Other causes of the disorder include removal of the ovaries; a diet deficient in calcium, which is essential for bone health; certain hormonal disorders, such as *Cushing's syndrome*, or prolonged treatment with *corticosteroid drugs*; and prolonged immobility.

Osteoporosis is more common in smokers and drinkers and, for unknown reasons, is associated with chronic obstructive lung disorders, such as *bronchitis* and *emphysema*.

### SYMPTOMS AND SIGNS

In many cases, osteoporosis produces no obvious symptoms; the first sign is often a fracture after a fall that would not cause a fracture in a young adult. Typical sites for such fractures are just above the wrist and the top of the femur (thigh bone). Another type of fracture that occurs in osteoporosis is a spontaneous fracture of one or several vertebrae, which causes the bones to be compressed, leading to a progressive loss of height or to pain due to compression of a spinal nerve.

### DIAGNOSIS

The condition is diagnosed from the symptoms and from bone X rays. In some cases, blood tests and a bone *biopsy* (removal of a sample of bone for examination) may also be necessary to exclude osteomalacia.

### TREATMENT AND PREVENTION

Lost bone tissue cannot easily be replaced, but more bone loss can be minimized by preventive measures. For example, both men and women should ensure that their *calcium* intake is adequate. The richest dietary sources of this mineral are milk and milk products, green leafy vegetables, citrus fruits, sardines, and shellfish. Calcium tablets may be needed.

Exercise also helps to build bones, but anything less than three brisk three-mile walks a week (or the equivalent) is unlikely to be of much benefit in preventing osteoporosis.

*Hormone replacement therapy* to compensate for reduced estrogen production after the menopause has been shown to prevent osteoporosis in women; in the US, it has halved the rate of fractures caused by osteoporosis in menopausal women.

## Osteosarcoma

A malignant bone tumor that occurs primarily in adolescent and elderly people. It spreads rapidly to the lungs and, less commonly, to other areas.

In young people, osteosarcoma develops for no known reason; in elderly people, it is a late, rare complication of *Paget's disease*.

### SYMPTOMS AND DIAGNOSIS

The most common site of the tumor in young people is in a long bone of the leg or arm, or around the knee, hip, or shoulder. The first symptom is usually a painful visible swelling of the affected bone (if it is near the surface) or a deep-seated pain (if the affected bone cannot be felt through the skin).

O

As a complication of Paget's disease, an osteosarcoma may develop in several bones; its pain may be indistinguishable from that caused by the original disease.

Diagnosis is usually based on *X rays* of the bone. Other imaging techniques (e.g., *MRI*) may also be used.

**TREATMENT AND OUTLOOK**

Although *radiation therapy* is sometimes used to treat the tumor, the bone is usually surgically removed. In most cases, this means *amputation* of a limb; in some cases, a prosthesis can be fitted immediately after the amputation (see *Limb, artificial*). The tumor can also be treated by removal and bone graft or bone transplant.

Treatment with *anticancer drugs* is usually given for several months after the operation to destroy any cancer cells that may have spread to other parts of the body. With this additional treatment, the outlook is good; about half of all patients whose disease is discovered early are cured.

## Osteosclerosis

Increased bone density, usually detected on *X-ray* film as an area of extreme whiteness.

Localized osteosclerosis may be caused by a severe injury that compresses the bone; by *osteoarthritis*, in which bone around affected joints thickens; by chronic *osteomyelitis*, in which healthy bone next to the infected area thickens and becomes more dense; or by an *osteoma* (benign bone tumor), which consists of a hard, dense, usually harmless outgrowth of normal bone tissue.

Osteosclerosis occurs throughout the body in *osteopetrosis*, an inherited bone disorder.

## Osteotomy

An operation in which a bone is cut to change its alignment or to shorten or lengthen it.

**WHY IT IS DONE**

Osteotomy is performed on a deformity of the big toe that has caused a bunion (see *Hallux valgus*). It is also performed to straighten a long bone that has healed crookedly after a *fracture* or to shorten the uninjured leg after a fractured leg has shortened during healing (see *Leg, shortening of*).

Osteotomy may be used to correct the deformity caused by congenital dislocation of the hip (see *Hip, congenital dislocation of*) that has not been detected until after about age 10. It is also used to correct *coxa vara* (hip deformity usually caused by injury).

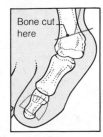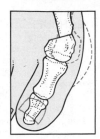

Bone cut here

**Example of an osteotomy**
This procedure is performed to correct a hallux valgus (outward protrusion of the joint at the base of the toe), usually because it has caused a bunion. Part of the top of the first metatarsal bone is removed.

**HOW IT IS DONE**

Using general anesthesia, bones are straightened by cutting through them and repositioning the ends; sometimes a wedge of bone is inserted or removed to achieve the correct alignment. Bones can be lengthened by making an oblique cut and displacing the two parts slightly before rejoining them. Bones can be shortened by cutting out a section of bone and rejoining the two parts.

After the operation, bones that were corrected during surgery are held in position by a metal plate or nail or by a plaster cast or splint.

## Ostomy

The term used to describe a surgical opening or junction of two hollow organs (e.g., *colostomy* and *ileostomy*).

## Ot-

A prefix that denotes a relationship to the ear, as in otitis, inflammation of the ear. The prefix oto- is also used to denote the ear.

## Otalgia

The medical term for *earache*.

## OTC

The abbreviation for over-the-counter. OTC refers to drug preparations that may be purchased from a drugstore without a prescription from a physician.

## Otitis externa

Also called swimmers' ear, inflammation of the outer-ear canal that is caused by infection.

**CAUSES**

Generalized infection, affecting the whole canal and sometimes also the pinna (the external ear), may be caused by bacteria or by fungi, which produce a persistent inflammation known as otomycosis. Bacterial infection may also cause a localized infection in the form of a *boil*. In some cases, the outer-ear canal becomes inflamed as part of a generalized skin disorder, such as atopic *eczema* or seborrheic *dermatitis*.

Malignant otitis externa is an uncommon and occasionally fatal form of the disorder caused by the bacterium *PSEUDOMONAS AERUGINOSA*. It usually affects elderly diabetics, whose resistance to infection is reduced, and spreads rapidly into surrounding bones and soft tissue.

**SYMPTOMS AND SIGNS**

Otitis externa usually causes redness and swelling of the skin of the ear canal, a discharge from the ear, and sometimes an area of eczema around the opening of the ear. The ear may itch only in the early stages, but can become painful. Occasionally, pus blocks the ear, causing deafness.

**DIAGNOSIS AND TREATMENT**

The physician examines the ear with an *otoscope* (a viewing instrument) and may take a sample of any pus for laboratory analysis.

Often the only treatment required is a thorough cleaning and drying of the ear by the physician, sometimes using a suction apparatus. Antibiotic, antifungal, or anti-inflammatory drugs are often necessary. Oral antibiotics are used for the treatment of severe bacterial infections. If the ear canal is very swollen, a wick should be placed in the canal to allow drops to enter. The sufferer should avoid getting the ear canal wet until the infection has cleared up.

## Otitis media

Inflammation of the middle ear (the cavity between the eardrum and the inner ear).

**CAUSES**

The inflammation occurs as the result of an upper respiratory tract infection (such as a cold) extending up the eustachian tube, the passage that connects the back of the nose to the middle ear. The tube may become blocked by the inflammation or sometimes by enlarged *adenoids*, which are often associated with infections of the nose and throat. As a result, fluid produced by the inflammation—along with pus in bacterial infections—is not drained off through the tube but accumulates in the middle ear.

The chronic phase of otitis media (otitis media with effusion) follows an upper respiratory infection that has produced acute otitis media.

O

## INCIDENCE

Children are particularly susceptible to otitis media, probably because of the shortness of their eustachian tubes. About one in six children suffers from the acute form in the first year of life and about one in 10 in each of the next six years. Some children have recurrent attacks. Chronic otitis media is much less common because, in most cases, attacks of acute middle-ear infection clear with treatment.

## SYMPTOMS AND SIGNS

Acute otitis media is marked by sudden, severe earache, a feeling of fullness in the ear, deafness, tinnitus (ringing or buzzing in the ear), and fever. Sometimes the eardrum bursts, relieving the pain and resulting in a discharge of pus. In this case, healing usually occurs in several days.

In chronic otitis media, pus constantly exudes from a perforation in the eardrum and there is some degree of deafness. Complications of the condition include *otitis externa* (inflammation of the outer ear); damage to the bones in the middle ear, causing more deafness (sometimes total) in the affected ear; or a *cholesteatoma* (a matted ball of sometimes infected skin debris). In rare cases, infection spreads inward from an infected ear, causing *mastoiditis* or a *brain abscess*.

## DIAGNOSIS

The diagnosis is usually made from examining the ears with an *otoscope* (a viewing instrument). A swab may be taken of any discharge so that the organism responsible for the infection can be cultured and identified.

## TREATMENT

Acute otitis media is treated by giving antibiotic drugs and analgesics (painkillers). Usually, the condition clears up completely with treatment, but in some cases there is continual production of sticky fluid in the middle ear, a condition known as persistent *middle-ear effusion*.

Chronic otitis media is treated by sucking out pus and infected debris from the ear as necessary. Antibiotic ear drops may be given if this does not adequately control the condition.

## Otolaryngologist, head and neck surgeon

A specialist in the medical and surgical treatment of disorders of the head and neck, excluding the brain, eyes, spinal cord, and spinal column. The term "head and neck surgery" refers to surgical procedures on certain tumors of the sinuses, throat, and neck, and to facial plastic surgery.

---

### EAR INFECTIONS

Inflammation of the middle ear (otitis media) or ear canal (otitis externa) usually results from infection and may cause an earache. Otitis media is more common in children and may be acute (with sudden onset of pain) or chronic (continuing painlessly over a long period).

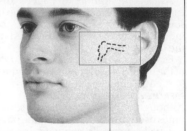

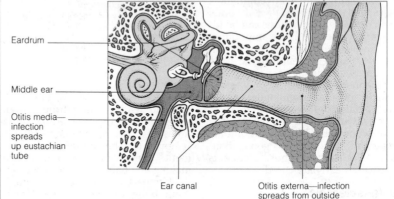

Eardrum

Middle ear

Otitis media—infection spreads up eustachian tube

Ear canal

Otitis externa—infection spreads from outside

**Otitis media**
This usually occurs through spread of infection from the back of the nose to the middle ear via the eustachian tube.

**Otitis externa**
The ear canal is susceptible to infection if it is moist (after swimming) or damaged by attempts to remove earwax.

---

Much of an otolaryngologist's time is spent treating common conditions, such as *sinus* infections, acute *otitis media* (middle-ear infection), persistent *middle-ear effusion*, *tonsillitis*, and minor hearing loss. The otolaryngologist is often faced with complex and difficult problems, such as *otosclerosis*, *Meniere's disease*, airway problems in children, uncontrollable bleeding from the nose, and cancer of the larynx and sinuses.

## Otoplasty

Cosmetic or reconstructive surgery on the outer ear. Otoplasty is usually performed to flatten protruding ears. It may also be done to construct or repair a missing or badly damaged ear.

### PROTRUDING EARS

The operation, as described at right, is usually done as an outpatient procedure using local anesthesia. After the operation, the ear is dressed until the wound has healed 10 to 14 days later, when the stitches are removed. The scar is hidden in the crease between the ear and scalp.

### LACK OF AN OUTER EAR

Some children are born with part or all of the outer ear missing. These children may also lack an external ear passage; in some cases there is also underdevelopment of the same side of the face.

Treatment involves transferring a piece of rib cartilage, which is sculpted to resemble the normal ear, to a pocket of skin in the position that the ear will be placed. The procedure usually involves three operations. Hearing in the reconstructed ear may be abnormal but, if the child has a normal range of hearing in the other ear, no attempt is made to improve hearing in the reconstructed ear.

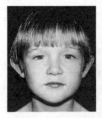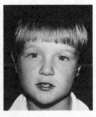

**Otoplasty for protruding ears**
A strip of skin is removed from behind each ear. The underlying cartilage is remolded and the two edges of the wound stitched together, thus pulling the ear closer to the head. The appearances before and after are shown.

## Otorhinolaryngology

The full title for the surgical specialty concerned with diseases of the ear, nose, and throat (see *Otolaryngologist, head and neck surgeon*).

## Otorrhea

The medical name for a discharge from the ear (see *Ear, discharge from*).

## Otosclerosis

A disorder of the middle ear that causes progressive deafness. Otosclerosis is often inherited.

**CAUSES AND INCIDENCE**
Otosclerosis occurs when, for unknown reasons, an overgrowth of bone immobilizes the stapes (the innermost bone of the middle ear). This prevents sound vibrations from being passed to the inner ear, resulting in conductive *deafness*. In most cases of otosclerosis, both ears are ultimately affected.

About one person in 200 is affected by the disease, which usually starts in early adulthood. It is more common in women than in men and often develops during pregnancy.

**SYMPTOMS AND SIGNS**
Sound is heard as muffled but is more distinguishable when there is background noise. Affected people tend to talk quietly. Hearing loss progresses slowly over a period of 10 to 15 years and is often accompanied by *tinnitus* (noises in the ear) and sometimes by *vertigo* (dizziness). Some sensorineural deafness (caused by damage spreading to the inner ear) may eventually occur, making high tones difficult to hear and resulting in the sufferer speaking loudly.

**DIAGNOSIS AND TREATMENT**
The diagnosis is based on abnormal results of *hearing tests*. A *hearing aid* is an excellent treatment for otosclerosis; the deafness can be cured only by *stapedectomy*, an operation in which the stapes is replaced with an artificial substitute. Stapedectomy is usually performed on only one ear at a time because there is a risk that total deafness may result in the operated ear.

## Otoscope

An instrument for examining the ear. An otoscope includes magnifying lenses, a light, and a speculum (a funnel-shaped tip that is inserted into the ear canal). The instrument allows easy inspection of the outer-ear canal and the eardrum. With an otoscope it is also possible to detect certain diseases of the middle ear through the semitransparent eardrum.

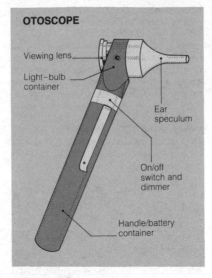

**OTOSCOPE**

Viewing lens

Light–bulb container

Ear speculum

On/off switch and dimmer

Handle/battery container

## Ototoxicity

Having a poisonous effect on the ear. High doses of certain drugs (especially aminoglycoside *antibiotic drugs*) can damage the cochlea and the semicircular canals in the inner ear, impairing hearing and balance.

## Outpatient treatment

Medical care given to a person on a day basis in a clinic or other facility.

## Ovarian cyst

An abnormal, fluid-filled swelling in an ovary. Ovarian cysts are common and are benign in about 95 percent of cases. Many ovarian cysts disappear without treatment.

**TYPES**
The most common type of ovarian cyst is a follicular cyst, in which the egg-producing follicle of the *ovary* enlarges and fills with fluid. Cysts may also occur in the corpus luteum, a yellow mass of tissue that forms from the follicle after *ovulation*.

Other types of ovarian cysts include *dermoid cysts* and malignant cysts (see *Ovary, cancer of*).

**SYMPTOMS AND SIGNS**
Ovarian cysts often cause no symptoms, but some cause abdominal discomfort, pain during intercourse, or menstrual irregularities including *amenorrhea* (lack of menstruation), *menorrhagia* (heavy periods), or *dysmenorrhea* (painful periods). Severe abdominal pain, nausea, and fever, which necessitate surgery, may develop if twisting of a cyst occurs.

**DIAGNOSIS AND TREATMENT**
A cyst may be discovered during a routine *pelvic examination. Ultrasound*

*scanning* or a *laparoscopy* (examination of the abdominal cavity through a viewing tube) may be necessary to confirm the diagnosis and to determine the size and position of the cyst.

Simple cysts (thin-walled and filled with fluid) often go away on their own, but complex cysts (such as dermoid cysts) do not. They often require surgical removal. In many cases, only the cyst needs to be removed, but if a cyst is large it is sometimes necessary for the surgeon to remove the entire ovary (see *Oophorectomy*).

## Ovary

One of a pair of almond-shaped glands situated on either side of the *uterus* immediately below the opening of the *fallopian tube*. Each ovary is about 1.25 inch (30 mm) long and 0.75 inch (20 mm) wide and contains numerous cavities called follicles in which egg cells (see *Ovum*) develop. In addition to producing ova, the ovaries also produce the female sex hormones estrogen and progesterone.

**DISORDERS**
Absence or failure of normal development of the ovaries is a rare disorder usually caused by a chromosomal abnormality (see *Turner's syndrome*).

Oophoritis (inflammation of the ovary) may be caused by the *mumps* virus or by other infections such as *gonorrhea* or *pelvic inflammatory disease*.

*Ovarian cysts* may develop at any age; about 95 percent of them are benign. *Polycystic ovary* syndrome, in

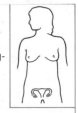

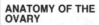

**ANATOMY OF THE OVARY**
Each ovary consists of glandular cells and egg-producing follicles. After ovulation, each follicle forms a corpus luteum.

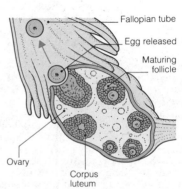

Fallopian tube

Egg released

Maturing follicle

Ovary

Corpus luteum

which multiple ovarian cysts form, is an uncommon disorder thought to be due to the body's inappropriate hormonal stimulation of the ovaries. The cysts may produce male sex hormones, leading to *amenorrhea*, *infertility*, and *hirsutism*.

Cancer of the ovary (see *Ovary, cancer of*) occurs mainly in women over 50 and usually causes few symptoms (if any) in the early stages, although it can cause symptoms similar to those of an ovarian cyst.

Ovarian failure, in which the ovaries cease to function, causes premature *menopause* in about 5 percent of all women.

## Ovary, cancer of

Malignant growth of the *ovary*. Ovarian cancer is the fourth leading cause of cancer death in women. Cancer of the ovary can occur at any age but is most common after 50. It is three times more common in women who have never had children and less common in women who have taken oral birth-control pills.

The growth may be primary (arising in the ovary) or may be a secondary growth that has spread to the ovary from some other part of the body, often the breast.

### SYMPTOMS AND SIGNS

In most cases ovarian cancer causes no symptoms until it is widespread. The first symptom is usually vague abdominal discomfort and swelling. There may be digestive disturbances, such as nausea and vomiting, abnormal vaginal bleeding, and ascites (excess fluid in the abdominal cavity). A physical examination may reveal a swelling in the pelvis.

### DIAGNOSIS AND TREATMENT

A *laparoscopy* (examination of the abdominal cavity through a viewing tube) or *laparotomy* (opening of the abdomen wall) may be necessary to confirm the diagnosis. Treatment is surgery to remove the cancer or as much of the malignant tissue as possible. This usually involves *salpingo-oophorectomy* (removal of the ovaries and fallopian tubes) and *hysterectomy* (removal of the uterus). Surgery is usually followed by *radiation therapy* and *anticancer drugs*.

### OUTLOOK

If the growth is confined to one or both ovaries, 60 to 70 percent of patients survive at least five years. If the growth is more widespread, only about 10 to 20 percent of patients survive five years. New drug combinations may improve this survival rate.

## Overbite

Overlapping of the lower front teeth by the upper front teeth. A slight degree of overbite is normal because the upper jaw is larger than the lower one. In *malocclusion*, overbite may be greater than normal or may be reversed (with the lower teeth projecting in front of the upper ones).

## Overcrowding, dental

Excessive crowding of the teeth so that they are unable to assume their normal positions in the jaw.

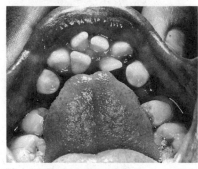

**Severe case of overcrowding**
The front teeth are crowded together because the two molars, just behind them, have grown too far forward.

### CAUSES

Overcrowding frequently occurs through heredity when the teeth are relatively too large or there are too many for a person's jaw. The condition also can occur or worsen with the premature loss of primary molar teeth. This can cause the permanent teeth growing beneath them to move out of position and leave insufficient space for the developing permanent teeth further forward in the mouth.

### PROBLEMS

Overcrowded teeth may lead to *malocclusion* (incorrect relationship between the upper and lower teeth) and may prevent certain teeth from erupting through the gum (see *Impaction, dental*). There is an increased risk of dental decay in crowded teeth because they are more difficult to clean. Overcrowding can also increase the risk of *periodontal disease* because of more difficult cleaning and more unusual stress being placed on supporting tissues.

### TREATMENT

An orthodontist decides whether one or more teeth should be extracted to allow room for others to grow. Often the remaining teeth require fitting with an *orthodontic appliance* to move them into their correct positions.

## Overuse injury

A term for any injury that has been caused by repetitive movement of part of the body. A common example is *epicondylitis*, painful inflammation of one of the epicondyles (bony prominences) at the elbow, caused by the pull of the attached forearm muscles during gardening, painting, or playing certain sports (see *Golfers' elbow*; *Tennis elbow*).

Overuse injuries of the finger and wrist joints may affect assembly line workers and typists. Musicians are also prone to a variety of problems; the thumb may be affected in players of woodwind instruments and the neck may be affected in violinists.

Symptoms, which usually disappear with rest, include pain and stiffness in the affected joints and muscles. It is sometimes possible to avoid a recurrence by altering technique during the activity.

## Overweight

See *Obesity*.

## Ovulation

The development and release of an *ovum* (egg) from a follicle within the *ovary*. Ovulation occurs midway through the menstrual cycle and is regulated by hormones. During the first half of the cycle, the follicle-stimulating hormone (FSH) causes several ova to mature in the ovary. At mid-cycle, the luteinizing hormone causes one ripe ovum to be released. The follicle then forms a small mass of yellow tissue called the corpus luteum, which secretes the hormone *progesterone* during the second half of the menstrual cycle.

After its release, the ovum travels along the fallopian tube and, unless *fertilization* occurs, is shed during *menstruation*. Regular menstruation usually means that a woman ovulates, but this is not always the case, especially around *puberty* and approaching the *menopause*.

Some forms of contraception (see *Contraception, periodic abstinence*) are based on predicting when ovulation occurs each month and avoiding sexual intercourse at that time. Signs of ovulation include a rise in body temperature and changes in the amount and consistency of cervical mucus; there may also be mild abdominal pain (see *Mittelschmerz*).

If a woman does not ovulate, she cannot conceive. Investigation of female *infertility* includes tests to determine whether ovulation occurs.

## Ovum

 The egg cell (female cell) of reproduction. Each ovum measures about 0.04 inch (0.1 mm) in diameter. There are about 1 million immature ova present in each ovary at birth; only about 200 per ovary ever mature to be released at *ovulation* during a woman's fertile years. If *fertilization* occurs, the ovum develops into an *embryo*.

## Oxacillin

A *penicillin*-type *antibiotic drug*. Oxacillin is especially useful in the treatment of *staphylococcal infections* resistant to other antibiotic drugs.

## Oxandrolone

An anabolic steroid (see *Steroids, anabolic*) used after a major illness or injury to help increase weight. It is also sometimes used in the treatment of *hyperlipidemia*.

Oxandrolone may cause swollen ankles and, in women, irregular periods. Rare adverse effects include nausea, vomiting, jaundice, and, in men, difficulty passing urine.

## Oxazepam

A *benzodiazepine drug* used in the treatment of *anxiety* and *insomnia*. Like other benzodiazepines, oxazepam may cause dependence if taken regularly for more than two weeks (see *Drug dependence*).

## Oxtriphylline

A *bronchodilator drug* related to *theophylline*, used in the treatment of *asthma* and *bronchitis*. Oxtriphylline may cause adverse effects, such as nausea, vomiting, and headache.

## Oxycodone

A narcotic *analgesic* (painkiller) derived from *morphine*. It is used in the treatment of severe pain.

## Oxygen

A colorless, odorless gas that makes up 21 percent of Earth's atmosphere. Oxygen is essential for almost all forms of life, including humans, because it is necessary for the metabolic "burning" of foods to produce energy—a process known as *aerobic* metabolism.

To reach the body cells, where aerobic metabolism takes place, oxygen in the air is absorbed through the lungs and into the blood, where it binds to the *hemoglobin* in red blood cells. In this form, the oxygen is distributed throughout the body, being released from the hemoglobin and taken up by cells in areas where the oxygen level is low.

Oxygen is used therapeutically to treat conditions such as severe *bronchitis* or *hypoxia* (an inadequate supply of oxygen to body tissues). In some cases, high pressure oxygen (see *Hyperbaric oxygen treatment*) is used to treat the bends (*decompression sickness*) or poisoning from *carbon monoxide*. (See also *Ozone*.)

## Oxygen therapy

Supplying a person with oxygen-enriched air to relieve severe *hypoxia* (inadequate oxygen in the tissues).

In hospitals, oxygen is usually piped to a terminal at the patient's bedside and is administered as necessary through a face mask or nasal cannulas (tubes inserted into the nostrils). The concentration of oxygen is varied according to the patient's needs.

People at home can be supplied with oxygen in cylinders for use during acute attacks of hypoxia (which occur in severe *asthma*). People with persistent hypoxia due to severe, chronic *bronchitis* or *emphysema* may benefit from long-term oxygen therapy. These patients may be supplied with a machine called an oxygen concentrator, which separates oxygen from the air and remixes it in a higher-than-normal concentration. Oxygen-rich air is then piped to different rooms for prolonged inhalation.

People receiving oxygen therapy should not smoke, since smoking not only presents a fire risk but also reduces the oxygen-carrying capacity of the blood and aggravates the underlying condition for which the oxygen is being given. (See also *Hyperbaric oxygen treatment*.)

## Oxymetazoline

A *decongestant drug* used in the treatment of allergic *rhinitis* (hay fever), *sinusitis*, and the common *cold*. Oxymetazoline has a longer-lasting effect than other decongestants; it needs to be taken only twice a day.

Oxymetazoline may irritate the nose. Prolonged use causes rebound congestion (increased congestion when the drug is withdrawn).

## Oxytetracycline

A type of *antibiotic drug* known as a *tetracycline drug*. Oxytetracycline is used to treat *chlamydial infections* such as *nonspecific urethritis*, *psittacosis*, and *trachoma*. It is also used to treat a variety of other infections, including bronchitis, pneumonia caused by *mycoplasma*, *syphilis*, *brucellosis*, *Rocky Mountain spotted fever*, and *cholera*. Oxytetracycline may be used to treat severe *acne*.

**POSSIBLE ADVERSE EFFECTS**
Oxytetracycline occasionally causes nausea, vomiting, diarrhea, rash, or increased sensitivity of the skin to sunlight. It may also discolor developing teeth and is therefore not prescribed for children under 12 or during pregnancy.

## Oxytocin

A hormone produced by the *pituitary gland* that causes contractions of the uterus during labor and stimulates the flow of milk in nursing women.

**USE AS A DRUG**
Synthetic oxytocin is commonly used to induce childbirth (see *Induction of labor*). It is sometimes used to help expel the placenta (afterbirth) after delivery or to empty the uterus after an incomplete *miscarriage* or a fetal death. Oxytocin is sometimes given as a nasal spray to stimulate milk flow.

**POSSIBLE ADVERSE EFFECTS**
Contractions may be stronger and more painful than usual, increasing the need for stronger *analgesic drugs* (painkillers). Rare adverse effects include nausea, vomiting, palpitations, seizures, and coma.

## Ozena

A severe and rare form of *rhinitis* (inflammation of the mucous membrane in the nose) in which the membrane atrophies (wastes away) and a thick nasal discharge dries to form crusts. It often causes severe *halitosis* (bad breath).

## Ozone

A rare form of oxygen, ozone is a poisonous, faintly blue gas that is produced by the action of electrical discharges (such as lightning) on oxygen molecules.

Ozone occurs naturally in the upper atmosphere (about 15 to 20 miles above the Earth's surface), where it screens the Earth from most of the sun's harmful ultraviolet radiation.

However, there are claims that the ozone layer is being depleted by various environmental chemicals (notably the chlorofluorocarbons in aerosols). The result is that stronger and more potent forms of ultraviolet radiation are reaching the Earth's surface. Increased ultraviolet levels could lead to an increase in the incidence of skin cancer and cataracts.

O

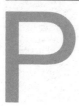

# PABA

The abbreviation for *para-aminobenzoic acid*, a sunscreen ingredient.

# Pacemaker

A device that supplies electrical impulses to the heart to maintain the heart beat at a regular rate. A pacemaker consists of a small electronic device and power source connected to the heart via an electrical wire.

In a healthy heart, the beat is maintained by a nucleus of specialized muscle called the sinoatrial node; it sends out regular electrical impulses that pass through the heart muscle and trigger heart contractions. An artificial pacemaker is implanted when a person's sinoatrial node is not functioning properly, or when there is some impairment to the passage of the normal electrical impulses (see *Heart block*; *Sick sinus syndrome*). Each year, tens of thousands of Americans have a pacemaker implanted.

Two main types of pacemaker—fixed rate and demand—are shown in the box below. More advanced types can increase the heart rate during exercise. Dual-chamber devices utilize one electrode in the atrium and another in the ventricular wall.

### IMPLANTATION

Implantation is carried out using local anesthetic. Patients can expect complete healing without complications and should return to normal work and activity as soon as possible. Vigorous exercise should be avoided for two weeks after the operation.

Modern microelectronic circuits require little power and lithium batteries have a long life. Unless the demand on the battery is excessive, a pacemaker usually runs satisfactorily for several years. Battery replacement requires a minor operation.

### PRECAUTIONS

Modern pacemakers are relatively insensitive to interference but may be affected by powerful electromagnetic pulses. Anyone with a pacemaker should avoid powerful radio or radar transmitters and should not pass through security screens at airports. Precautions may also be required with some physical therapy or surgical *diathermy* machines.

# Paget's disease

A common disorder of middle-aged and elderly people in which the normal process of bone formation is disrupted, causing the affected bones to weaken, thicken, and become deformed. Also known as osteitis deformans, Paget's disease usually involves only limited areas of the skeleton. The bones usually affected are the pelvis, skull, collarbone, vertebrae, and long bones of the leg.

### CAUSE AND INCIDENCE

The normal maintenance of healthy bones by the body involves a balance between the actions of cells that break down bone tissue and those that rebuild it. In Paget's disease, this balance is disturbed. The disease varies in frequency from one part of the country to another, suggesting an infective cause, which is thought to be

---

## PACEMAKERS

A pacemaker may be external (worn on a belt) or internal (implanted in the chest), like those shown below.

External pacing is used only as a temporary measure. There are two main methods of implantation.

### TYPES OF PACEMAKERS
The two main types are shown. In some cases, an external programmer can adjust the rate.

**Transvenous implantation**
An insulated wire is inserted into a major vein in the neck and guided down into the heart until the electrode at its far end is secured within the part of the heart muscle to be stimulated. The free end is connected to the pacemaker, which is fitted into a pocket created under the skin of the abdomen or below the collarbone.

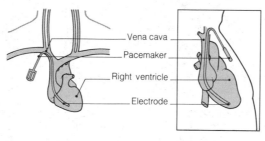

Vena cava
Pacemaker
Right ventricle
Electrode

**Side view**
The pacemaker is usually well hidden by overlying tissue

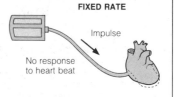

**FIXED RATE**

Impulse

No response to heart beat

**Fixed-rate pacemaker**
This type discharges impulses at a steady rate, irrespective of the heart's activity.

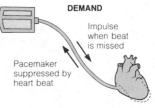

**DEMAND**

Impulse when beat is missed

Pacemaker suppressed by heart beat

**Epicardial implantation**
The electrode is attached to the outer surface of the part of the heart muscle to be stimulated and the pacemaker is fitted into a pocket constructed underneath the skin of the abdomen.

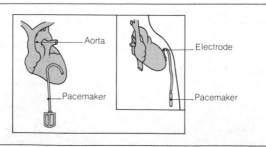

Aorta
Electrode
Pacemaker
Pacemaker

**Demand pacemaker**
This type discharges impulses only when the heart rate slows or a beat is missed. A normal heart rate and beat suppresses the pacemaker.

viral. Overall, Paget's disease affects about 3 percent of the population over the age of 40, the incidence increasing with age. The disorder has a tendency to run in families and affects more men than women.

### SYMPTOMS AND SIGNS

Paget's disease often causes no symptoms and is usually discovered from an X ray taken for some other reason. The most common symptoms are bone pain and deformity, especially bowing of the legs. Affected bones are prone to fracture.

Changes in the skull may lead to leontiasis (distortion of the facial bones that produces a lionlike appearance) and to inner-ear damage, sometimes resulting in deafness, tinnitus (ringing in the ear), vertigo, or headaches. Enlarged vertebrae may press on the spinal cord, causing pain and sometimes paralysis of the legs. If the pelvis is affected, it can result in severe arthritis of the hips. Occasionally, *bone cancer* may develop, and, in rare cases, when many bones are involved, increased blood flow through the affected bones may cause *heart failure*.

### DIAGNOSIS

X rays reveal areas of porous, thickened bone. *Blood tests* that show an elevated level of the enzyme alkaline phosphatase (which is associated with bone cell formation) give an indication of the extent and activity of the disease.

### TREATMENT AND OUTLOOK

Most people with the disorder do not require treatment, and many others simply need to take *analgesic drugs* (painkillers). In severe cases, the hormone *calcitonin* may be prescribed. It relieves pain, reduces alkaline phosphatase levels, and promotes normal bone formation. Other drugs that have the same effect (including disodium etidronate and plicamycin) may also be used. Surgery may be required to correct deformities or treat secondary arthritis.

## Paget's disease of the nipple

A rare *breast cancer* in which the tumor starts in the milk ducts of the nipple. Paget's disease of the nipple looks similar to *eczema*, causes the nipple to itch and burn, and may feature a sore on the nipple that will not heal. Usually only one nipple is affected. If left untreated, the tumor may gradually spread into the breast. Eczema of the nipple should be reported to a physician and a *biopsy* of the underlying breast taken.

## Pain

A localized sensation that can range from mild discomfort to an unbearable and excruciating experience. Pain is the result of stimulation of special sensory nerve endings following injury or caused by disease.

### THE MECHANISM OF PAIN

The basic mechanism of pain is shown in the illustrated box on the next page. The skin contains many specialized nerve endings (nociceptors). Stimulation of these receptors leads to transmission of pain messages to the brain. Nociceptors have different sensitivities, some responding only to severe stimulation, such as cutting, pricking, or heating the skin to a high temperature; others respond to warning stimuli, such as firm pressure, stretching, or temperatures not high enough to burn. Pain receptors are present in structures other than the skin, including blood vessels and tendons. Most internal organs have few, if any, nociceptors. The large intestine, for example, can be cut without causing any pain. It does, however, have nociceptors that respond to stretching, which, in severe cases, may cause pain.

### PSYCHOLOGICAL ASPECTS OF PAIN

Pain is usually associated with distress and anxiety, and sometimes with fear. People vary tremendously in their pain thresholds (the level at which the pain is felt and the person feels compelled to act). The cause and circumstances of the pain may also affect the way it is perceived by the sufferer. The pain of cancer, because of fear of the disease, may seem much greater and cause more suffering than similar pain resulting from persistent indigestion. Unexplained pain is often worse because of the anxiety it can cause; once a diagnosis is made and reassurance given, the pain may be perceived as less severe.

The experience of pain may be reduced by arousal (e.g., an injury sustained during competitive sport or on the battlefield may go unnoticed in the heat of the moment); strong emotion can also block pain. Some people believe that mental preparation for pain (e.g., in childbirth or in experiments to test pain) can greatly reduce the response.

A person's response to pain is greatly modified by past experience; the outcome of previous episodes of pain may affect the way the individual copes with subsequent pain. Factors such as insomnia, anxiety, and depression, which often accompany incapacitating illness, lower pain tolerance. Treatment for these symptoms is given along with treatment for the pain to allow the minimum dose for pain relief.

Cultural differences exist in the expression of pain. In some parts of the world self-inflicted torture and the ability to withstand great pain are a mark of a person's strength and character. However, the pain of even mild torture inflicted by captors may be perceived as much worse than a similar degree of pain that occurs under different circumstances.

### TYPES OF PAIN

Many adjectives are used to describe different types of pain. Common descriptive terms include throbbing, penetrating, gnawing, aching, burning, and gripping. The extent to which a patient is accurately able to describe his or her pain to the physician is highly variable, even though it can be a vital clue to the diagnosis.

Attempts have been made to categorize pain according to intensity, ranging from a minor cut or sore throat at the lower end to childbirth and renal or biliary colic at the upper.

If the pain comes from an internal organ it is often difficult for the sufferer to pinpoint its origin with any precision. For example, in the early stages of appendicitis, pain may be felt in the region above the navel. In the later stages, when infection has caused inflammation of the peritoneum (lining of the abdominal cavity), the pain becomes localized above the right groin.

Pain may be felt at a point some distance from the disorder. This is called *referred pain* (see illustrated box overleaf). A person who has lost a limb may experience pain that seems to come from the amputated limb (see *Phantom limb*). Sometimes the person can localize the pain (e.g., to a toe, despite having had a mid-thigh amputation). See also *Endorphins; Enkephalins*.

## Painful arc syndrome

A condition in which pain occurs when the arm is lifted between 45 degrees and 160 degrees away from the side of the body. Movement either side of this range is pain-free. Painful arc syndrome is usually caused by inflammation of tendons or bursae (see *Bursa*) around the shoulder joint. The pain is caused by the inflamed tendon or bursa being squeezed between the upper parts of the shoulder blade and the *humerus*.

P

# PAIN

Pain mechanisms exist to provide a useful warning of possible injury or to caution against repeating an action that has led to injury. Certain diseases, such as arthritis and extensive cancer, may set off these same mechanisms, causing chronic pain that has no apparent function.

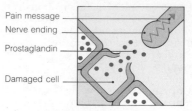

Pain message
Nerve ending
Prostaglandin
Damaged cell

### Initiation of pain signals
The signals are set off by stimulation of special nerve endings—by pressure, heat, or release of chemicals, including prostaglandins, by damaged cells.

### Reflex action
The nerve pathways that warn of noxious stimuli (through the sensation of pain) may also initiate automatic, reflex actions that help prevent harm.

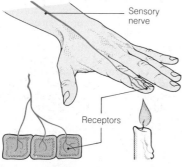

Sensory nerve

Receptors

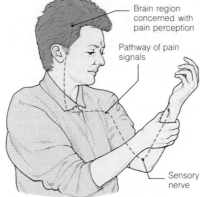

Brain region concerned with pain perception

Pathway of pain signals

Sensory nerve

### Perception of pain
When an injury occurs, signals pass along nerve pathways concerned with pain, first to the spinal cord and then to the thalamus in the brain; there the pain is perceived.

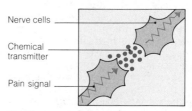

Nerve cells

Chemical transmitter

Pain signal

### Signal transmission to brain
Within the brain and spinal cord, pain signals pass between nerve cells by means of chemicals that cross the gaps between the cells.

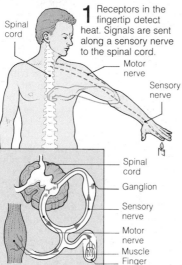

Spinal cord

**1** Receptors in the fingertip detect heat. Signals are sent along a sensory nerve to the spinal cord.

Motor nerve

Sensory nerve

Spinal cord

Ganglion

Sensory nerve

Motor nerve

Muscle

Finger

**2** The signals arriving in the spinal cord pass instantaneously to a motor nerve that connects to a muscle in the arm. The signals received via the motor nerve cause the muscle in the arm to contract, moving the arm away from the source of danger (the flame).

### REFERRED PAIN
A referred pain is one felt in a site other than an injured or diseased part. Sensory nerves from certain body areas converge before they enter the brain, causing confusion about the source of pain signals.

#### Tooth to ear region
A toothache may be felt in the ear, because the same sensory nerve supplies both parts.

#### Diaphragm to right shoulder
Inflammation of the diaphragm, often due to pneumonia, may be felt as a pain in the right shoulder.

#### Heart to left arm
Angina, a pain caused by reduced blood supply to the heart muscle, is often felt in the left shoulder or arm.

#### Knee to hip
Disorders affecting the knee, such as arthritis, may be felt as pain in the hip.

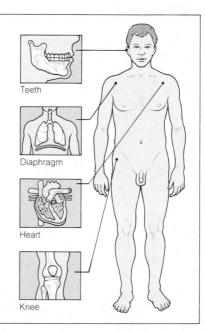

Teeth

Diaphragm

Heart

Knee

P

## Painkillers
See *Analgesic drugs*.

## Pain relief
The treatment of *pain*, usually with *analgesic drugs*. Methods of treatment depend on the severity, duration, location, and cause of the pain.

### DRUG TREATMENT
Mild analgesics, available over-the-counter, are usually effective in the treatment of mild pain, such as headache, toothache, or dysmenorrhea (menstrual pain). *Acetaminophen* and *aspirin* are the most widely used drugs in this group.

Mild or moderate pain, such as that caused by arthritis or sports injuries, is often treated with a *nonsteroidal anti-inflammatory drug* (NSAID).

Severe pain, such as that caused by serious injury or kidney stones, may require treatment with a *narcotic* analgesic. Narcotic analgesics are also used to prevent pain after surgery. Long-term use of narcotic analgesics may be necessary to prevent or relieve pain in cancer.

**NONDRUG TREATMENT**
*Massage, ice packs,* or *poultices* may be used for the relief of localized pain caused by muscle spasm, inflammation, or injury.

Chronic or recurrent pain that has not responded to drug treatment may be relieved by *acupuncture* or *hypnosis*.

Surgical procedures to relieve pain may be performed if all other treatments have failed. These procedures may involve destruction of nerves that transmit pain (as is done in a *cordotomy*). Alternatively, nerve fibers in the thalamus (the part of the brain that responds to pain) may be cut to prevent perception of pain.

## Palate

The roof of the mouth. The palate separates the mouth from the nasal cavity. Covered with *mucous membrane*, it consists, in the front, of the hard palate, whose substructure is a plate of bone forming part of the *maxilla* (upper jaw). At the rear is the soft palate, a flap of muscle and fibrous tissue that projects into the *pharynx* (throat). During swallowing, the soft palate presses against the rear wall of the pharynx, preventing food from being regurgitated into the nose.

About one in 500 babies is born with a gap along the midline of the palate (see *Cleft lip and palate*).

## Palliative treatment

Therapy that relieves the symptoms of a disorder but does not cure it. Treatment for the symptoms of widespread cancer is considered palliative.

## Pallor

Abnormally pale skin, particularly of the face. Pallor may be a symptom of disease, but more often has an innocent explanation. Possible causes include a deficiency of the skin pigment *melanin*, constriction of the small blood vessels in the skin, or *anemia*.

Melanin deficiency may result from lack of exposure to the sun, occurring in people (such as nightworkers or miners) who spend very little time in daylight. A deficiency of melanin can also be hereditary when it is associated with *albinism*.

Constriction of small blood vessels in the skin may occur in response to shock, severe pain, injury, heavy blood loss, fainting, or extreme cold. Cutting off the blood flow to the skin

---

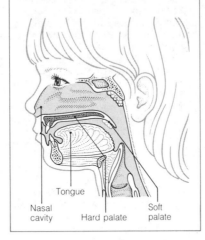

**LOCATION OF THE PALATE**
The palate forms the floor of the nasal cavity and roof of the mouth, providing a surface against which the tongue can push during chewing and swallowing.

Tongue
Nasal cavity
Hard palate
Soft palate

---

ensures that the brain and other vital organs are adequately supplied and that body heat is conserved. In anemia, pallor results from lack of *hemoglobin* pigment in blood vessels in the skin.

Certain kidney disorders, such as *pyelonephritis* and *renal failure*, produce a sallow appearance akin to pallor, as does *hypothyroidism*. Rare conditions that give rise to pallor include *scurvy* and lead poisoning.

## Palpitation

Awareness of the heart beat.

**CAUSES**
A palpitation is usually felt after strenuous exercise, in tense situations, or after a severe scare, when the heart is beating harder and/or faster than normal. When experienced at rest or in a calm mood, palpitation is usually due to *ectopic heart beats* (premature beats followed by a prolonged pause) and is felt as a fluttering or thumping in the chest, sometimes with a brief but alarming sense that the heart has stopped beating. Ectopic beats do not normally indicate heart disease; they are often caused by heavy smoking, alcohol, or a large intake of caffeine.

An *arrhythmia* (irregularity of the heart beat) may cause palpitation. An example of an arrhythmia is atrial *tachycardia*, a condition in which the heart suddenly starts to beat very rapidly; the affected person may feel

---

faint and breathless. The pulse may be as high as 200 beats per minute but remains regular. In *atrial fibrillation*, the atria (upper chambers of the heart) beat in a disorganized manner and the impulses passed to the ventricles (lower pumping chambers) are very irregular. *Hyperthyroidism* (overactive thyroid gland) may cause palpitation by speeding up the heart beat.

**DIAGNOSIS AND TREATMENT**
If palpitation lasts for several hours or recurs over several days, or if it causes chest pain, breathlessness, or dizziness, a physician should be consulted as soon as possible, as there may be a serious underlying disorder. Recurrent palpitations can be investigated by means of a *Holter monitor* and *thyroid function tests*. Treatment depends on the underlying cause.

## Palsy

A term applied to certain forms of *paralysis*. Examples are *cerebral palsy*, Bell's palsy (paralysis of one side of the face), and Erb's palsy (paralysis of the upper arm and shoulder on one side of the body).

## Panacea

A remedy for all diseases; a cure-all. No such remedy is known, despite claims to the contrary made by numerous quacks through the ages.

## Pancreas

An elongated, tapered gland that lies across the back of the abdomen, behind the stomach. Its right-hand end (called the head) is the broadest part and lies in the loop of the duodenum. Tapering from the head, the main part of the gland (the body) extends left and slightly upward; the left-hand, narrower end (the tail) terminates near the spleen.

**STRUCTURE**
Most of the pancreas consists of exocrine tissue, embedded in which are "nests" of endocrine cells (the islets of Langerhans). The exocrine cells secrete digestive enzymes into a network of ducts that meet to form the main pancreatic duct. This duct joins the common bile duct (which carries bile from the gallbladder) to form a small chamber, called the ampulla of Vater, that opens into the duodenum. The islets of Langerhans are surrounded by many blood vessels into which they secrete hormones.

**FUNCTION**
The pancreas has two functions: digestive and hormonal. The exocrine tissue secretes various digestive

P

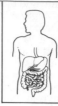

## LOCATION OF THE PANCREAS

This organ lies under the stomach, except for its head, which lies within the curve of the duodenum.

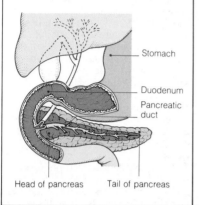

Stomach

Duodenum

Pancreatic duct

Head of pancreas    Tail of pancreas

enzymes that break down carbohydrates, fats, proteins, and nucleic acids (see *Digestive system*). Most of these enzymes are secreted in inactive form and are activated in the duodenum by other enzymes. Also secreted by the exocrine tissue is bicarbonate, which neutralizes stomach acid entering the duodenum. The endocrine cells in the islets of Langerhans secrete the hormones *insulin* and *glucagon*, which regulate the level of glucose in the blood. (See also *Pancreas* disorders box.)

## Pancreas, cancer of

A malignant tumor of the exocrine tissue of the *pancreas* (the main tissue in the gland). The cause of the condition is unknown, although it has been linked to heavy smoking and to certain dietary factors, such as a high intake of fats or alcohol.

The incidence of pancreatic cancer in the US has increased threefold during the past 50 years, to about 11 per 100,000 people. Today, it is the fourth most common cancer in men, and the sixth most common in women. Approximately 80 percent of cases occur in people older than 50.

### SYMPTOMS AND DIAGNOSIS

The most common symptom is pain in the upper abdomen, which often spreads to the back. Other common symptoms are appetite and weight loss, and jaundice. There may also be indigestion, nausea, vomiting, diarrhea, and tiredness. In most cases, the symptoms do not appear until the cancer is well advanced, often not until it has spread to other parts of the body (typically to the liver or lungs).

Diagnosis of pancreatic cancer usually requires *ultrasound scanning* or *CT scanning* of the upper abdomen, or endoscopic examination of the ducts of the pancreas (see *ERCP*). In some cases, the condition is detected during exploratory surgery on the abdomen (see *Laparotomy, exploratory*).

### TREATMENT AND OUTLOOK

If the condition is detected in its early stages, surgical removal of the malig-

---

**P**

## DISORDERS OF THE PANCREAS

Serious disruption of pancreatic function occurs only when the secretory tissue of the gland has been damaged or destroyed in advanced disease. The most common pancreatic disorder is *diabetes mellitus*, in which the insulin-producing cells in the gland are destroyed.

### CONGENITAL AND GENETIC DISORDERS

About 85 percent of people with the genetic disorder *cystic fibrosis* produce totally inadequate quantities of pancreatic digestive enzymes, which results in *malabsorption* of fats and proteins. This, in turn, may produce steatorrhea (excess fat in the feces) and muscle wasting.

Genetic factors are thought to play some part in diabetes mellitus, although they are not the primary cause of the disease.

Chronic *pancreatitis* (inflammation of the pancreas) may, in rare cases, be hereditary; chronic pancreatitis often causes diabetes.

### INFECTION

Acute pancreatitis may result from certain viral infections, especially infection with the *mumps* virus. Other viruses, such as coxsackievirus and echoviruses, may

also cause pancreatitis. In some cases, coxsackievirus infection may contribute to the development of diabetes.

### TUMOR

Pancreatic cancer is one of the most common cancers in the US (see *Pancreas, cancer of*). It is difficult to diagnose and often has spread extensively by the time it is detected.

### TRAUMA

Injury to the pancreas—which may result from a powerful blow to the abdomen, for example—may cause acute pancreatitis. The mechanism by which this happens is not fully established, but it is believed that pancreatic enzymes (most of which are inactive until they reach the intestine) are released within the tissue of the gland and then activated, with the result that they digest the pancreas.

### POISONS AND DRUGS

Excessive alcohol intake is a common cause of pancreatitis. It can also be caused by various drugs, such as sulfa drugs, estrogens (including estrogen-containing contraceptive pills), and thiazide *diuretic drugs; corticosteroid drugs* may also cause pancreatitis.

### AUTOIMMUNE DISORDERS

The cause of the damage to the pancreas in diabetes mellitus remains controversial. However, there is increasing evidence that, possibly in response to a viral infection, the body's immune system produces *antibodies* (proteins with a role in the defense against infection) that inappropriately attack and destroy the pancreatic cells.

### OTHER DISORDERS

Other than alcohol overuse, the condition most commonly associated with pancreatitis is *gallstones*. They occasionally block the exit of the pancreatic duct into the duodenum, which leads to inflammation of the pancreas.

### INVESTIGATION

Diagnosis of pancreatic disorders may involve *ultrasound scanning* of the abdomen, tests to measure levels of pancreatic enzymes in the blood or duodenum, and endoscopic examination of the gland (see *ERCP*).

---

nant tissue (see *Pancreatectomy*) along with *radiation therapy* and *anticancer drugs* may cure it. However, in most cases the cancer is not diagnosed until it is well advanced, and little can be done apart from relieving the pain with *analgesics* (painkillers), alleviating any other symptoms, and bypassing the growth if it is causing obstruction of the bile duct or bowel. In such cases, the outlook is poor; death occurs in about 90 percent of the cases within a year of diagnosis.

## Pancreatectomy
Removal of all or part of the pancreas. Pancreatectomy may be performed to treat *pancreatitis* (inflammation of the pancreas), localized pancreatic cancer (see *Pancreas, cancer of*), or carcinoma of the ampulla of Vater (the small chamber formed by the union of the common bile duct and pancreatic duct that opens into the duodenum). Rarely, it is done to treat some endocrine tumors, such as *insulinomas* (*insulin*-producing tumors).

Removal of all or part of the gland depends on the disorder involved and/or on how much of the pancreas is affected. Obstruction of the pancreatic duct may require removal of only the tail of the gland (the narrower end, nearest the spleen) and the linking of the duct with a small piece of small intestine. Disease of the head of the pancreas (the broader end, situated in the loop of the duodenum) may necessitate removal of both the pancreatic head and duodenal loop (Whipple's operation).

### COMPLICATIONS
Because the pancreas produces insulin and a variety of digestive enzymes, removal of the entire gland results in *diabetes mellitus* (which requires insulin therapy) and *malabsorption* (which requires oral supplements of pancreatic enzymes). Such treatment may also be necessary after a partial pancreatectomy, depending on how much function remains.

## Pancreatin
A drug obtained from the pancreas of pigs and used to supplement a deficiency of pancreatic *enzymes* (proteins that stimulate digestion of nutrients).

## Pancreatitis
Inflammation of the pancreas. In acute pancreatitis, the gland usually returns to normal after a single attack (although sometimes attacks recur). In chronic pancreatitis, there is permanent damage to the structure and to

the function of the pancreas due to persistent inflammation, which causes fibrosis (the formation of fibrous scar tissue) in the gland.

### CAUSES
The principal causes of acute pancreatitis are *gallstones* and alcohol abuse. Less commonly, pancreatitis results from a viral infection (such as *mumps*), injury (such as through surgery on the biliary tract or a blow to the abdomen), or certain drugs (such as *tetracycline*).

The most common cause of chronic pancreatitis is alcohol abuse. It may also result from *hemochromatosis* (excess iron in the body) or, rarely, it may be hereditary. In some cases, severe acute pancreatitis causes it.

### SYMPTOMS AND DIAGNOSIS
Acute pancreatitis produces a sudden attack of severe upper abdominal pain, often accompanied by nausea and vomiting. The pain may spread to the back and is made worse by movement; sitting up may relieve it. An attack, which usually lasts for about 48 hours, is accompanied by the release of pancreatic enzymes into the blood; measurement of these enzymes is an important diagnostic test. *Ultrasound scanning* or *CT scanning* of the abdomen may also be performed.

Chronic pancreatitis usually produces the same symptoms as the acute form, although the pain may last from hours to several days, and attacks become more frequent as the condition progresses. However, in some cases there may be no pain and the principal signs may be *malabsorption* (due to a deficiency of pancreatic enzymes) or *diabetes mellitus* (due to insufficient *insulin* production by the pancreas). Measuring pancreatic enzyme levels in the blood is of little value in diagnosing chronic pancreatitis, although measuring the output of such enzymes into the duodenum may be useful. Abdominal X rays or scans are the principal diagnostic methods, along with endoscopic examination of the ducts of the gland (see *ERCP*) to visualize the extent of tissue damage.

### COMPLICATIONS
If acute pancreatitis causes severe damage to the gland, hypotension (low blood pressure), failure of the heart, kidneys, and respiratory system, and *ascites* (accumulation of fluid in the abdomen) may occur. In some cases, cysts or abscesses may develop in the damaged gland.

Ascites and cysts may also develop as a result of chronic pancreatitis.

Other possible complications include obstruction of the common bile duct (which drains the gallbladder and joins the pancreatic duct), permanent diabetes mellitus, and blood clots in the splenic vein (which drains the spleen and pancreatic veins).

### TREATMENT
There is no specific remedy for acute pancreatitis. Treatment consists of giving fluids and salts by intravenous infusion to replace those lost through vomiting; pain is relieved by giving narcotic analgesics. Nothing is given by mouth, because anything in the digestive tract stimulates pancreatic activity and makes the symptoms worse. A recurrence of the condition may be prevented by treating the underlying cause, when possible. Occasionally, surgery is necessary to remove the pancreas (see *Pancreatectomy*) or any gallstones that are blocking the drainage of pancreatic juice.

Chronic pancreatitis is treated by providing pain relief, controlling blood sugar levels by giving insulin, and giving preparations of pancreatic enzymes to correct the underproduction that the condition causes. In some cases, a pancreatectomy may be necessary to relieve pain.

## Pancreatography
Imaging of the pancreas or its ducts. The methods usually used include *CT scanning*, *ultrasound scanning*, *X rays* (with a radiopaque dye) during exploratory surgery of the pancreas, and endoscopic retrograde cholangiopancreatography (see *ERCP*), an X-ray procedure in which a radiopaque dye is introduced into the ducts of the pancreas through an *endoscope* (flexible viewing tube).

## Pancrelipase
A preparation of *enzymes* (proteins that stimulate chemical reactions) obtained from the pancreas of pigs.

Pancrelipase is given by mouth to supplement a deficiency of pancreatic enzymes and thus prevent *malabsorption* of fats, carbohydrates, and proteins. Deficiency may be caused by *pancreatectomy* or by disorders that affect the pancreas, such as chronic *pancreatitis*, cancer of the pancreas, and *cystic fibrosis*.

## Pandemic
A medical term applied to a disease that occurs over a large geographical area (sometimes the whole world) and affects a high proportion of the population; a widespread *epidemic*.

# Panic attack

A brief period of acute *anxiety*, often dominated by an intense fear of dying or losing one's reason. Panic attacks occur unpredictably at first, but tend to become associated with certain places, such as a crowded supermarket or a cramped elevator.

The symptoms begin suddenly and usually include a sense of breathing difficulty, chest pains, palpitations, feeling light-headed and dizzy, sweating, trembling, and faintness. *Hyperventilation* (fast, shallow breathing) often accompanies and worsens the symptoms, leading to a *pins and needles sensation*, and to feelings of *depersonalization* and *derealization*.

Most often, these symptoms are the result of underlying emotional conflicts (such as a fear of being trapped or fear of loss of dependency). Psychoanalytically, the person is often unconsciously feeling threatened by the loss of his or her relationship with the mother. Anxiety about heights may represent the fear of losing emotional support. Fear of being closed in may symbolize fear of being trapped or overwhelmed.

Although unpleasant and frightening, panic attacks last for only a few minutes, cause no physical harm, and are rarely associated with serious physical illness. The symptoms of hyperventilation may be relieved by covering the mouth and nose with a small paper bag and breathing into the bag for a few minutes.

In general, panic attacks are a symptom of *panic disorder*, *agoraphobia* (if they lead to avoidance of certain situations), or other *phobias*. Less often they are part of a *somatization disorder* or *schizophrenia*.

# Panic disorder

A common form of *anxiety disorder* dominated by repeated *panic attacks* that are not caused by other illnesses or brought on by intense exercise or truly dangerous situations. A panic disorder runs a fluctuating course, tending to become worse during periods of stress. Underlying emotional anxieties cause panic reactions.

Psychotherapy is an effective treatment. Medication is often effective in treating the symptoms.

# Papaverine

A *vasodilator drug* sometimes used in the treatment of patients with *peripheral vascular disease* (reduced blood supply to the legs and sometimes the arms) and in those with *transient ischemic attacks* and *impotence* of unknown cause.

Possible adverse effects of papaverine include flushing, nausea, loss of appetite, and drowsiness.

# Papilla

Any small, nipple-shaped projection from the surface of a tissue, such as the mammary papilla (the nipple of the breast) and the lingual papillae (the numerous projections from the surface of the tongue, some of which contain taste buds).

# Papilledema

*Optic disk edema* (swelling of the head of the optic nerve) caused by a rise in pressure within the brain. Papilledema, which is visible through an *ophthalmoscope*, may be a sign of a *brain tumor*.

# Papilloma

A usually nonmalignant tumor, often resembling a wart, that arises from *epithelium* (the cell layer that forms the skin and mucous membranes, and that lines most of the hollow organs of the body). Although papillomas may develop from epithelium anywhere in the body, they are most common on the skin, tongue, or larynx (voice box), and in the urinary tract, digestive tract, or breasts.

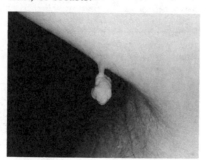

**Skin papilloma**
This harmless type of growth is common in elderly people. It can easily be snipped off at skin level and the base cauterized.

# Pap smear

See *Cervical smear test*.

# Papule

A small, solid, slightly raised area of skin. Papules are usually less than half an inch (1 cm) in diameter and may be rounded or flat, with a smooth or warty texture. Papules may be the color of surrounding skin or pigmented. Many skin conditions, including *acne* and *lichen planus*, start as papules.

# Par-/para-

Prefixes with several meanings: beside or beyond, as in the parathyroid glands (which are situated behind the thyroid at its sides); closely related to or closely resembling, as in paratyphoid fever (a disease that is similar to typhoid); faulty or abnormal, as in paresthesia (abnormal sensation); or associated with an accessory capacity, as in paramedical workers (personnel who supplement the work of physicians).

# Para-aminobenzoic acid

The active ingredient in many *sunscreen* preparations, commonly abbreviated to PABA.

# Paracentesis

A procedure in which a body cavity is punctured with a needle from the outside. Paracentesis is most often performed to remove fluid for analysis to aid diagnosis of conditions causing *ascites*, in which fluid collects in the abdominal cavity. It may also be performed to relieve pressure due to excess fluid or to instill drugs. Abdominal or thoracic paracentesis is most common, but other sites include the pericardium and the scrotum.

The procedure is usually carried out using local anesthesia; it is quick and relatively painless.

# Paraffinoma

A tumorlike swelling under the skin caused by prolonged exposure to paraffin. Paraffinomas may occur in the lungs due to inhalation of paraffin, usually in someone who uses liquid paraffin as a laxative. They were once an uncommon side effect of augmentation *mammoplasty* (enlargement of the breast) when paraffin wax was used in this operation.

# Paraldehyde

An unpleasant-smelling hypnotic sedative that has been used in the treatment of alcohol withdrawal. Paraldehyde is administered as an enema or by injection. This drug dissolves plastic, so a glass syringe must be used to inject it.

# Paralysis

Complete or partial loss of controlled movement caused by the inability to contract one or more muscles. Weakness, rather than complete loss of movement, is often referred to as *paresis*. Paralysis may be temporary or permanent, and can affect a range of muscles—from a small facial muscle to many of the major muscles in the body. Loss of feeling in the affected parts may accompany the inability to move them.

**TYPES**

Paralysis of one half of the body is called *hemiplegia*; paralysis of all four limbs and the trunk is called *quadriplegia*. *Paraplegia* is paralysis of both legs and sometimes part of the trunk. *Palsy* is an outdated general term for paralysis; it is still used in the names of certain disorders (such as *cerebral palsy*).

Paralysis may be flaccid, which gives the limbs a floppy appearance, or spastic, in which case the affected parts of the body are rigid.

**CAUSES**

Muscles that control movement of the body are stimulated to contract by impulses originating in the motor cortex of the brain; they travel via the spinal cord and peripheral nerves to reach the muscle. Paralysis may be caused by any form of injury or disorder anywhere along this nerve pathway, or by a muscle disorder.

**BRAIN DISORDERS** A very common cause of paralysis is a *stroke*, in which damage to part of the brain is caused by bleeding from or blood clotting in a blood vessel that supplies that area of the brain. Because motor fibers cross in the brain stem, paralysis occurs on the side opposite to the site of the brain damage.

Hemiplegia can be caused by any brain disorder in which the portion of the brain that controls movement is damaged—by a *brain tumor, brain abscess, brain hemorrhage, cerebral palsy,* or *encephalitis* (brain infection).

Some forms of paralysis are caused by damage to those parts of the nervous system concerned with the fine control of movement (such as the *cerebellum* and *basal ganglia*). *Parkinson's disease* is caused by lack of dopamine in the basal ganglia.

**SPINAL CORD DISORDERS** Paralysis can be caused by damage to the spinal cord from a fractured spine caused by a motor vehicle accident. Pressure on the spinal cord may cause paralysis in *disk prolapse* or *cervical osteoarthritis*. Muscles supplied by nerves below the damaged area are affected.

Diseases affecting nerves in the spinal cord (e.g., *multiple sclerosis, poliomyelitis, myelitis, Friedreich's ataxia, meningitis,* and *motor neuron disease*) may also cause paralysis.

**PERIPHERAL NERVE DISORDERS** A range of disorders (known as *neuropathies*) affects the peripheral nerves and causes paralysis of varying degrees. A neuropathy may be caused by a variety of conditions, including *diabetes mellitus*, vitamin deficiency, liver disease, cancer, and the toxic effects of some drugs or metals (such as lead); it may also occur as an inherited disorder.

A type of neuropathy that often causes paralysis of the shoulder, arm, or hand is injury to the *brachial plexus* (a collection of nerves that serves the arm and hand).

**MUSCLE DISORDERS** *Muscular dystrophy* causes progressive muscular weakness and may lead to paralysis. Temporary paralysis sometimes occurs in *myasthenia gravis*.

**TREATMENT**

The underlying cause is treated if possible. *Physical therapy* is used to prevent joints from becoming locked into useless positions, which is important in both temporary and permanent paralysis. When the paralysis is temporary (such as in a mild stroke), physical therapy is used to retrain and strengthen the muscles and joints so that some degree of mobility is possible after recovery.

For paralyzed people confined to bed or a wheelchair, nursing care is essential to avoid complications (such as bedsores, deep vein thrombosis, urinary tract infections, constipation, and limb deformities) of prolonged *immobility*. In addition, various aids are available to help the totally or partially paralyzed person.

## Paralysis, periodic

A rare, inherited condition that affects young people. Periodic paralysis is characterized by episodes of weakness and paralysis of limb muscles that may last from a few minutes to two days, occurring every six weeks or so. The attacks often begin during the night and wake the sufferer.

The exact cause of periodic paralysis is unknown, although, in many cases, there is a drop in the level of potassium (which is essential for normal muscle function) in the blood. A meal that is rich in carbohydrates often triggers an attack.

The frequency of attacks can be lessened by reducing the intake of carbohydrates and by taking *acetazolamide* or other potassium-sparing, weak *diuretic drugs*. An episode can sometimes be curtailed by taking potassium or by gentle exercise at the first sign of muscle weakness. The condition often disappears without treatment by the age of 30.

## Paramedic

A person trained to provide emergency resuscitation after an accident or when someone has collapsed from a myocardial infarction (heart attack) or other medical condition. Paramedics work from ambulances and in the emergency room.

The term is also used as an abbreviation for paramedical, to describe any health care worker other than a physician, nurse, dentist, or podiatrist. Examples of paramedical staff include physical therapists, X-ray technologists, and laboratory technicians.

## Paranoia

A condition whose central feature is the *delusion* (a false idea not amenable to reasoned argument) that people or events are in some way specially related to oneself. The term is also used popularly to describe a person's feelings of persecution.

A person suffering from paranoia gradually builds up an elaborate set of beliefs based on the interpretation of chance remarks or events. Typical themes include persecution, jealousy (see *Jealousy, morbid*), love, and grandeur (belief in one's own superior position and powers).

**TYPES AND CAUSES**

Psychoanalytically, paranoia stems from deep, underlying insecurity. Chronic paranoia may result from brain damage, amphetamine or alcohol abuse, *schizophrenia*, or *manic-depressive illness*. The condition is especially likely to develop in people with paranoid *personality disorder*—suspicious, oversensitive people who seem emotionally cold and take offense easily.

Acute paranoia, lasting for less than six months, may occur in people who have experienced radical changes in their environment, such as immigrants, refugees, people entering military service, or people leaving home for the first time.

In shared paranoia (folie à deux), delusion develops as a result of a close relationship with someone who already has a delusion.

**SYMPTOMS**

Feelings and activities often seem relatively normal in that they are appropriate for the beliefs held. There are usually no other symptoms of mental illness apart from occasional *hallucinations*. However, anger, suspiciousness, and social isolation mark an increasing change in the person toward difficult and eccentric behavior. Paranoid individuals rarely

P

see themselves as ill and usually receive treatment only when brought by friends or relatives.

**TREATMENT AND OUTCOME**

When acute illness is treated early with *antipsychotic drugs*, the outlook is good. In chronic disorders, delusions are usually firmly entrenched, although antipsychotic drugs may make them less prominent. However, long-term control through medication is difficult in someone with poor insight into his or her illness.

## Paraparesis

Partial *paralysis* or weakness of both legs and sometimes part of the trunk.

## Paraphilia

See *Deviation, sexual.*

## Paraphimosis

Constriction of the penis behind the glans (head) by an extremely tight foreskin that has been retracted (pulled back), causing swelling and pain. Paraphimosis often occurs as a complication of *phimosis* (an abnormally tight foreskin).

Often the foreskin can be returned to its normal position manually. The swelling in the glans may be reduced by first applying an ice pack and then squeezing the glans. If manual return proves impossible, an operation to cut the foreskin (using a general anesthetic) or an injection may be necessary. *Circumcision* (surgical removal of the foreskin) is usually required to prevent recurrence.

## Paraplegia

Weakness or *paralysis* of both legs, and sometimes part of the trunk; it is often accompanied by loss of sensation and by loss of urinary control.

Paraplegia is a result of nerve damage in the brain or spinal cord. It is usually caused by a motor vehicle or sports accident, a fall, or gunshot wounds. Twice as many men as women are victims, and the incidence is highest between the ages of 19 and 35 years.

## Parapsychology

The branch of psychology dealing with experiences and events that cannot be accounted for by scientific understanding. Such paranormal phenomena include telepathy (communicating thoughts from one person's mind to another), telekinesis (the movement of objects simply by thinking), clairvoyance (the ability to "see" events at a distance without

using one's eyes), and precognition (being able to see into the future). These are all forms of extrasensory perception (ESP).

The basis of most paranormal experiences can probably be explained by various brain disorders (see *Brain disorders box*) and mental disturbances. Thought broadcasting (in which individuals have the impression that their thoughts can be heard by others) is a common symptom of *schizophrenia*.

Other apparently paranormal experiences are a result of coincidence or self-deception, while some, such as psychic surgery (removal of objects from the body apparently without an incision), are no more than sleight-of-hand trickery.

## Paraquat

A poisonous defoliant weedkiller that, if swallowed, causes respiratory failure, acute or progressive lung damage, and kidney failure, which

may be fatal. The main symptom of paraquat poisoning is difficulty breathing. It may be severe, depending on the amount swallowed.

If paraquat poisoning is known or suspected, medical help should be obtained immediately. First-aid treatment consists of having the victim eat charcoal or fuller's earth (a clay-containing earthy substance), which inactivate paraquat.

In some cases, medical treatment may include hemodialysis (removal of toxic substances from the blood, see *Dialysis*) and other measures to remove the chemical from the body.

If paraquat has been splashed into the eyes or onto the skin, it should be washed away immediately with plenty of water.

Marijuana is sometimes contaminated with paraquat. Smoking it can cause any or all of the following: stinging eyes, a burning sensation in the mouth and throat, vomiting, and mouth ulcers.

---

### PARASITES

|  |  |  |  |  |
|---|---|---|---|---|
| **Head louse** | **Bedbug** | **Cat flea** | **Tapeworm** | **Hookworm** |

**ECTOPARASITES** (present in skin or on body surface)

| Common examples | Activities | How acquired |
|---|---|---|
| Head lice<br>Ticks<br>Bedbugs<br>Cat fleas<br>Aquatic leeches | Suck host's blood. | Through contact with other people (lice, scabies mites, warts), animals (ringworm fungi, ticks), vegetation (ticks, mites), water (aquatic leeches), or locker-room floors (some fungi). Bedbugs live in bedroom walls or mattresses and visit their host at night. Cat and dog fleas may visit humans when the pet is absent. |
| Scabies mites | Burrow in skin. | |
| Ringworm fungi | Multiply in skin. | |
| Wart viruses | | |

**ENDOPARASITES** (live within body)

| | | |
|---|---|---|
| Tapeworms<br>Flukes<br>Roundworms<br>Pinworms<br>Hookworms | Adults live in human gut, blood vessels, bile ducts, or elsewhere and produce eggs that are passed out of body. | By eating infected meat, swallowing eggs on food, contaminating fingers with fecal material, or contact with infected water. |
| Various disease-causing protozoa, fungi, bacteria, and viruses | Organisms multiply locally or spread throughout the body, causing disease. | By inhalation, water- or food-borne transmission, sexual transmission, or blood-borne infection, among other mechanisms. |

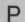

## Parasite

Any organism living in or on any other living creature and deriving advantage from doing so, while causing disadvantage to the host. The parasite satisfies its nutritional requirements from the host's blood or tissues or from the host's diet, which allows the parasite to reproduce and multiply.

Parasites may remain permanently with their host or may spend only part of their life cycles in association. Some cause few symptoms, others cause disease and even death of the host.

Animal parasites of humans include various *protozoa* (single-celled animals), *worms*, *flukes*, *leeches*, *lice*, *ticks*, and *mites*. *Viruses* and disease-causing *fungi* and *bacteria* are also essentially parasites. Some types of bacteria actually benefit their hosts (by helping to control the populations of more harmful organisms), so they are not strictly parasites.

## Parasitology

The scientific study of organisms that treat others as their living environment (see *Parasite*), especially the study of their life cycles and reproductive behavior, the ways in which they cause disease, and their susceptibility to drug treatment and other methods used to halt their multiplication. Although viruses and many types of bacteria and fungi are parasites, their study is conducted under the general title of *microbiology*.

Medical parasitology is concerned primarily with animal parasites of humans, especially the protozoa, worms, flukes, and arthropod parasites (insects and related animals) such as lice and the scabies mite.

## Parasuicide

See *Suicide, attempted*.

## Parasympathetic nervous system

One of the two divisions of the *autonomic nervous system*. In conjunction with the other division (the sympathetic nervous system), the parasympathetic system controls the involuntary activities of the organs, glands, blood vessels, and other tissues in the body.

## Parathion

An agricultural organophosphate insecticide that is highly poisonous to both humans and animals. Poisoning may occur by absorption through the skin, inhalation, or swallowing and is most common in agricultural workers.

Symptoms of poisoning include nausea, vomiting, abdominal cramps, involuntary defecation and urination, excessive salivation and sweating, blurred vision, headache, confusion, and muscle twitching. If poisoning is severe, there may also be difficulty breathing, palpitations, seizures, and unconsciousness. Without treatment, parathion poisoning may be fatal.

If parathion has been swallowed, treatment consists of inducing vomiting or washing out the stomach (see *Lavage, gastric*). If poisoning occurred through skin absorption, clothing is removed and contaminated areas of skin are thoroughly washed. To counteract the effects of the poison, injections of atropine and pralidoxime may be given. It may also be necessary to support breathing by giving oxygen and/or artificial ventilation. With rapid treatment, many people survive doses of parathion much greater than the usual fatal dose.

## Parathyroidectomy

The surgical removal of abnormal parathyroid tissue. Parathyroidectomy may be performed to treat *hyperparathyroidism* (excess secretion of parathyroid hormone) when it is caused by an *adenoma* (a small, benign tumor) of a parathyroid gland or, less commonly, by overgrowth of all of the glands or by parathyroid cancer.

In the case of an adenoma, usually only one of the glands is involved and requires removal. If all glands are enlarged and overactive, all but a whole gland or a half of a gland may require excision (cutting out). Removal of all parathyroid tissue leads to a dangerously low level of calcium in the blood and the condition of *tetany* (painful, cramplike spasms).

The operation is performed using general anesthesia. An incision is made in the neck, just beneath the Adam's apple. A section of suspected abnormal tissue is taken and examined to decide how much should be removed. It is then cut out, and the incision sewn up.

The average hospital stay for the operation is less than a week. Patients can expect complete healing without complications, although some people need treatment for *hypoparathyroidism*.

## Parathyroid glands

Two pairs of oval, pea-sized glands, located adjacent to the two lobes of the thyroid gland in the neck. Occasionally, only one or (rarely) an extra gland is present in the neck or chest.

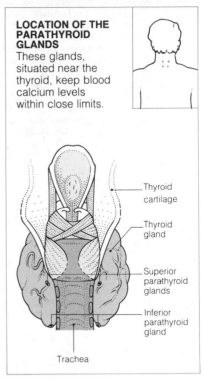

**LOCATION OF THE PARATHYROID GLANDS**
These glands, situated near the thyroid, keep blood calcium levels within close limits.

Thyroid cartilage

Thyroid gland

Superior parathyroid glands

Inferior parathyroid gland

Trachea

**FUNCTION**
The glands produce parathyroid hormone, which helps control the level of calcium in the blood. This requires constant regulation, since even small variations from normal can impair muscle and nerve function.

If the blood's calcium level drops, the parathyroid glands respond by increasing their output of hormone. This causes the bones to release more calcium into the blood, the intestines to absorb more from food, and the kidneys to conserve calcium. These actions quickly restore the blood calcium level. If the blood level of calcium rises too high, the glands reduce their output of hormone, reversing the above processes.

In rare cases, the glands may become overactive (see *Hyperparathyroidism*), causing thinning of the bones (*osteoporosis*) and *calculi* in the urinary tract. In other cases, the glands become underactive (see *Hypoparathyroidism*), resulting in painful spasms or seizures.

## Parathyroid tumor

A growth within one of the parathyroid glands. A parathyroid tumor may result in excess secretion of parathyroid hormone into the bloodstream, leading to the symptoms of *hyperparathyroidism*.

**P**

Most parathyroid tumors are benign *adenomas*. Cancers of the parathyroid are very rare (with an incidence of less than one per 100,000 population per year) and are not highly malignant, although occasionally they may spread to other organs in the body.

When a tumor is causing hyperparathyroidism, it is surgically removed (see *Parathyroidectomy*). If the tumor is an adenoma, surgery usually gives a complete cure. Occasionally the tumor may recur or, after surgery, the patient may need treatment for *hypoparathyroidism*.

In people who have parathyroid cancer, surgery allows long-term survival without recurrence, provided the entire tumor can be completely removed before it has spread.

## Paratyphoid fever

An illness identical in most respects to *typhoid fever*, except that it is caused by a slightly different bacterium, SALMONELLA PARATYPHI, and is usually less severe. The causative organism is spread in a similar way to the typhoid bacterium, but long-term carriers of infection are less common.

## Parenchyma

The functional tissue of an organ, as distinct from accessory structures such as the framework (*stroma*) and the fibrous outer layer (capsule) that holds the organ together.

## Parenteral

A term applied to the administration of drugs or other substances by any route other than via the gastrointestinal tract (e.g., by injection into a blood vessel or muscle or by suppository into the vagina).

## Parenteral nutrition

See *Feeding, artificial*.

## Paresis

Partial *paralysis* or weakness of one or several muscles.

## Paresthesia

Altered sensation in the skin that causes *numbness* or tingling (see *Pins and needles sensation*).

## Parietal

A medical term that refers to the wall of a body cavity or organ, as in the parietal peritoneum (the membrane that lines the walls of the abdomen and pelvis and the underside of the diaphragm), or to the parietal bones (the two joined bones that form much of the top, sides, and upper back part of the skull), as in the parietal lobes of the brain (the parts of the cerebral hemispheres that are covered by the parietal bones).

## Parkinsonism

A neurologic disorder characterized by a masklike face, rigidity, and slowness of movements. The most common type, which is of unknown cause, is *Parkinson's disease*.

Known causes of parkinsonism include *antipsychotic drugs*, the rare *encephalitis lethargica* infection, *carbon monoxide* poisoning, *cerebrovascular disease*, and the use of certain *designer drugs* of abuse.

## Parkinson's disease

A brain disorder that causes muscle tremor, stiffness, and weakness. The characteristic signs are trembling, a rigid posture, slow movements, and a shuffling, unbalanced walk.

---

## CAUSE OF PARKINSON'S DISEASE

This disorder results from damage, of unknown origin, to the basal ganglia (nerve cell clusters in the brain). The difference between the healthy state and Parkinson's disease is shown below.

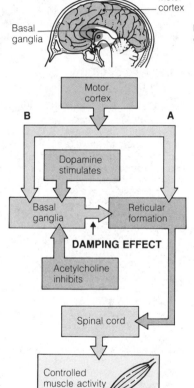

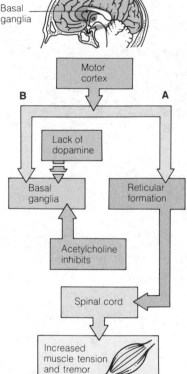

**Healthy state**
During movement, signals pass from the brain's cortex, via reticular formation and spinal cord (pathway A), to muscles, which contract. Other signals pass, by pathway B, to the basal ganglia; these damp the signals in pathway A, reducing muscle tone so that movement is not jerky. Dopamine, a nerve transmitter made in the basal ganglia, is needed for this damping effect. Another transmitter, acetylcholine, inhibits the damping effect.

**Parkinson's disease**
In Parkinson's disease, degeneration of parts of the basal ganglia causes a lack of dopamine within this part of the brain. The basal ganglia are thus prevented from modifying the nerve pathways that control muscle contraction. As a result, the muscles are overly tense, causing tremor, joint rigidity, and slow movement. Most drug treatments increase the level of dopamine in the brain or oppose the action of acetylcholine.

P

### CAUSES AND INCIDENCE

Parkinson's disease is caused by degeneration of or damage to nerve cells within the *basal ganglia* in the brain. The way this affects muscle tension and movement is shown in the illustrated box at left.

About one person in 200 (mostly elderly) is affected by the disease, with 50,000 new cases a year in the US. Men are more likely to be affected than women. The incidence of Parkinson's disease is lower among smokers.

### SYMPTOMS AND SIGNS

The disease usually begins as a slight tremor of one hand, arm, or leg. In the early stages, the tremor is worse when the hand or limb is at rest; when it is used, the shaking virtually stops.

Later, the disease affects both sides of the body and causes stiffness and weakness, as well as trembling, of the muscles. Symptoms include a stiff, shuffling, overbalancing walk that may break into uncontrollable, tiny, running steps; a constant trembling of the hands, more marked at rest and sometimes accompanied by shaking of the head; a permanent rigid stoop; and an unblinking, fixed expression. Eating, washing, dressing, and other everyday activities gradually become very difficult to manage.

The intellect is unaffected until late in the disease, although speech may become slow and hesitant; handwriting usually becomes very small. Depression is common.

### TREATMENT

Although there is no cure for Parkinson's disease, much can be done for sufferers to improve their morale and mobility through exercise, special aids in the home, and encouragement. Organizations exist to provide help and advice for sufferers and their families. This is often all that is needed in the early stages of the disease.

Later, treatment is with drugs, which minimize symptoms but cannot halt the degeneration of brain cells. Such treatment is often complex because several different types of drugs may need to be administered in various combinations.

*Levodopa*, which the body converts into dopamine, is usually the most effective drug and is often the first drug tried. The beneficial effects of levodopa often suddenly wear off, when another drug may be given; levodopa usually can be successfully reintroduced some weeks later.

Drugs used in conjunction with or as substitutes for levodopa include bromocriptine and amantadine. Other drugs that provide effective relief for specific symptoms, such as tremor, include *anticholinergic drugs*.

Occasionally, an operation on the brain may be performed to reduce the tremor and rigidity. This operation is reserved for relatively young, active sufferers who are otherwise in good health and who are in the early stages of the illness.

### OUTLOOK

Untreated, the disease progresses over 10 to 15 years to severe weakness and incapacity. However, with modern drug treatment, a person suffering from Parkinson's disease can obtain considerable relief from the illness and a much improved quality of life. About one third of patients do eventually show signs of *dementia*.

Experimentation with transplantation of dopamine-secreting adrenal tissue is now taking place.

## Paronychia

An infection of the skin fold at the base of the nail. Paronychia is usually caused by CANDIDA ALBICANS (a yeast), although in some cases bacteria are responsible.

The condition is most common in women—particularly those who have poor circulation and whose work involves frequent hand washing. Paronychia is also likely to develop in people with skin disease that affects the nail fold.

Treatment is with *antifungal drugs* or *antibiotic drugs*. It is important to keep the hands as dry as possible (by wearing rubber gloves for wet work and by drying the hands thoroughly each time they are washed). If an abscess forms, it may be drained surgically.

## Parotid glands

The largest of the three pairs of *salivary glands* (the other two are the sublingual glands and submandibular glands). The parotid glands lie, one on each side, above the angle of the jaw, below and in front of the ear. The parotid glands continuously secrete saliva, which passes along the duct of the gland and into the mouth through an opening in the inner cheek, level with the second upper molar tooth. The output of saliva is increased substantially by thinking about or seeing food.

### DISORDERS

Certain conditions, including *dehydration* and *Sjögren's syndrome*, may cause reduced secretion of saliva by the gland, resulting in a dry mouth (see *Mouth, dry*).

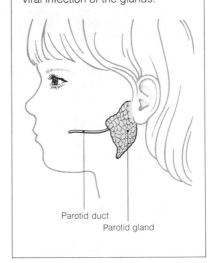

**LOCATION OF THE PAROTID GLANDS**
The glands are situated deep in the angle of the jaw and secrete saliva into the mouth. Mumps is a viral infection of the glands.

Parotid duct
Parotid gland

Parotitis, inflammation of the gland, is usually due to infection with the mumps virus but may also be caused by a bacterial infection due to poor oral hygiene, by dehydration, or by severe illness. In some cases, an *abscess* forms in the inflamed gland.

*Calculi* (stones) may block the duct of the parotid gland, causing a painful swelling of the gland. Painless enlargement may be caused by *sarcoidosis, tuberculosis,* a *lymphoma,* or a benign tumor. Rarely, carcinoma (a type of malignant tumor) of the gland causes a hard, painful growth.

## Paroxysm

A sudden attack, worsening, or recurrence of symptoms or of a disease; a *spasm* or *seizure*.

## Parturition

The process of giving birth (see *Childbirth*).

## Passive-aggressive personality disorder

Failure to keep up with tasks at home or at work as a result of passive resistance to demands for improved performance rather than of active refusal to cooperate. People with the disorder may delay or "forget" to perform tasks, or be deliberately inefficient. Their resulting ineffectiveness and unreliability prevents promotion at work and interferes with social func-

P

tioning. Depression often compounds the problem. Hidden aggression is thought to be the cause of passive-aggressive personality disorder.

## Pasteurization

The process of heating foods, usually milk and milk products, to destroy or retard the development of pathogenic (disease-causing) microorganisms and thus protect against putrefaction and fermentation.

The process is named for its inventor, the French scientist Louis Pasteur (1822-1895).

Pasteurization consists of heating food to a moderate temperature for a specific period, then cooling it rapidly. For example, milk is heated to between 145°F and 150°F (63°C and 66°C) for 30 minutes, then its temperature is raised to 161°F (72°C) for 15 seconds, and finally it is quickly cooled. This process does not sterilize the milk, but it does destroy most types of pathogenic microorganisms. Pasteurization has been an important factor in dramatically decreasing the incidence of milk-borne diseases, such as tuberculosis.

## Patella

The medical name for the kneecap, the triangular bone at the front of the knee joint. The patella is held in position by the *quadriceps muscle* (at the front of the thigh), the lower end of which surrounds the patella and is attached to the upper part of the tibia (shin) by the patellar tendon. The patella protects the knee.

### DISORDERS

Dislocation of the patella is usually due to a congenital abnormality, such as underdevelopment of the lower end of the femur (thigh bone) or excessive laxity of ligaments that support the knee. Fracture is usually caused by a direct blow.

Inflammation and roughening of the undersurface of the patella, resulting in knee pain that worsens when bending the knee or climbing stairs, is caused by *chondromalacia patellae* in adolescents and by retropatellar inflammation in adults.

## Patent

In medicine, a term meaning open or unobstructed, as in *patent ductus arteriosus*, a condition in which the ductus arteriosus (a blood vessel that enables blood to bypass the lungs in the fetus) remains open after birth. The term patent is also applied to nonprescription medications.

## Patent ductus arteriosus

A type of heart defect present at birth.

### CAUSES AND INCIDENCE

The ductus arteriosus is a channel between the pulmonary artery and the aorta (two large vessels emerging from the heart) through which, in the fetus, blood pumped by the right side of the heart is able to bypass the lungs (see *Fetal circulation*).

The duct usually closes at or shortly after birth so blood will go to the lungs. However, in some babies born prematurely or with breathing difficulties, this closure fails to happen. Some of the blood pumped by the left side of the heart and intended for the body is misdirected via the duct to the lungs. As a result, the heart must work harder to pump sufficient blood to the body.

Patent ductus arteriosus accounts for about 8 percent of all heart defects present from birth (see *Heart disease, congenital*), affecting about 60 babies per 100,000.

### SYMPTOMS AND SIGNS

Usually, the defect is not severe enough to cause symptoms. Occasionally, however, when a large amount of blood is misdirected, strain is placed on the heart; as a result, the baby fails to gain weight, becomes short of breath on exertion, and has frequent chest infections. Eventually, *heart failure* (reduced pumping efficiency) may develop. Bacterial *endocarditis* (inflammation of the lining of the heart) is a common complication of patent ductus arteriosus.

### DIAGNOSIS AND TREATMENT

The diagnosis is made by a physician listening to the heart with a stethoscope (the defect produces a characteristic *murmur*), from *chest X rays*, and from an *ECG* (electrocardiogram) and *echocardiography*.

The drug indomethacin often causes the duct to close in premature babies. If this treatment fails, the channel is closed surgically. The operation is straightforward, carries little risk, and enables the child to thrive normally.

## Paternity testing

The use of blood tests to help decide whether a particular man is or is not the father of a particular child. Tests are carried out on blood samples taken from the child, from the man who is suspected to be the father, and, if available, from the child's mother.

### WHY IT IS DONE

The investigation may be requested, or ordered by a court, in any of various legal situations in which the paternity of a child is disputed.

### HOW IT IS DONE

The blood tests are performed by a special investigator, who examines the samples for the presence of various genetically determined substances. These substances may include proteins found on the surface of red blood cells that determine *blood groups*, other proteins in the blood plasma, *histocompatibility antigens*, and short lengths of *DNA*, the genetic material itself. Comparison of these genetic markers in the different blood samples can provide useful information. For example, if a particular marker is present in the child but not in the mother, it must be determined by a gene present in the real father. If the man claimed to be the father does not display this marker in his blood, he can be excluded from paternity.

Techniques have advanced to the stage where it is now possible, through extensive tests, to exclude a wrongly named father in nearly 100 percent of cases. Until recently, it was never possible to prove beyond reasonable doubt that a man was the father of a particular child; the new technique of DNA fingerprinting (see illustrated box opposite) changes this situation almost beyond doubt. Using this technique, an investigator may be able to state that the similarities between a man's and a child's DNA could have occurred by chance with a probability of just one in 30 billion—which would amount to positive proof of paternity.

## Patho-

A prefix denoting a relationship to disease, as in pathogen, a disease-causing agent.

## Pathogen

Any agent, particularly a *microorganism*, that causes disease.

## Pathogenesis

The processes by which a disease (or disorder) originates and develops. Pathogenesis applies particularly to the cellular and physiological events involved in these processes.

## Pathognomonic

A medical term applied to a symptom or sign that is itself characteristic of a specific disease or disorder, and is therefore sufficient to establish a diagnosis. Koplik's spots (small red spots with white centers) on the lining of the mouth are pathognomonic of measles.

## PATERNITY TESTING USING DNA FINGERPRINTS

A new method of paternity testing, DNA fingerprinting, is replacing older techniques because it gives a decisive result in more cases.

Blood samples are taken from the mother, child, and suspected father, and some DNA (hereditary material) from each is specially processed.

### PATERNITY ESTABLISHED

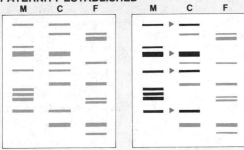

M   C   F     M   C   F     M   C   F

**1** Each person's DNA has a unique banding pattern, or "fingerprint," detectable by X rays after the processing.

**2** A child's DNA bands come from the biological parents. First the bands from the mother are identified.

**3** The other bands are compared with the suspected father's bands. Here they match, proving paternity.

### PATERNITY DISPROVED

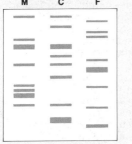
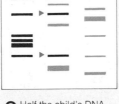

M   C   F     M   C   F     M   C   F

**1** The mother's, child's, and suspected father's DNA have different banding patterns.

**2** Half the child's DNA bands can be seen to have come from the mother, as before.

**3** The other bands are not shared by the suspected father, meaning he is not the biological father.

**Key**   **M** = Mother   **C** = Child   **F** = Father

## Pathological
Relating to disease or to *pathology* (the study of disease).

## Pathologist
A physician who conducts the laboratory studies of tissues and cells that help other physicians reach accurate diagnoses and who supervises other laboratory personnel in the testing and microscopic examination of blood and other body fluids. Pathologists also conduct *autopsies*. (See also *Pathology*.)

## Pathology
The study of disease, its causes, mechanisms, and effects on the body.

Various factors can cause pathological changes in tissues and cells. These factors include pathogens (disease-causing microorganisms), poisonous chemicals, radiation, *inflammation*, degeneration (see *Degenerative disorders*), the accumulation of abnormal substances (see *Infiltrate*), metabolic defects (see *Metabolism, inborn errors of*), *nutritional disorders*, and *carcinogens* (agents that cause *cancer*).

The study of the pathological changes that occur in cells is known as cytopathology (a branch of *cytology*); histopathology (a branch of *histology*) is concerned with changes in tissues. Both rely on examining cell or tissue samples under the *microscope*.

It was the growth of postmortem pathology in the 18th and 19th centuries that formed the basis of modern scientific medicine. Study of the body after death enabled a patient's symptoms to be linked with observable changes in the internal organs. It also made it possible for physicians to assess the accuracy of their diagnoses and the effects of their treatment.

## Pathology, cellular
Also called cytopathology, the branch of *cytology* concerned with the effects of disease on cells.

## Pathophysiology
The study of the effects of disease on body functions (e.g., how bronchitis impairs lung function).

## -pathy
A suffix that denotes a disease or disorder, as in myopathy, any disorder of the muscles. The suffix -opathy is synonymous with -pathy.

## Peak flow meter
A piece of equipment that measures the maximum speed at which air can flow out of the lungs. Because narrowed airways slow the rate at which air can be forced from the lungs, a peak flow meter is useful in assessing the severity of *bronchospasm* (narrowing of the airways in the lungs).

The most common use of a peak flow meter is to monitor patients with *asthma* and to assess their response to treatment with *bronchodilator drugs*. It is also useful to confirm whether people who suffer from intermittent coughing or breathing difficulty without wheezing have asthma.

People with asthma are encouraged to measure their peak flow every day as a means of monitoring their health, just as diabetics measure their blood sugar level. A diary of readings is kept to record the difference in airflow when symptoms are present and during other times in the day.

The peak flow is measured by taking a deep breath in and then breathing out with maximum effort through the mouthpiece of the meter.

## Peau d'orange
A condition in which the skin resembles orange peel. The skin remains a normal color but develops a dimpled appearance due to retention of fluid in the nearby lymph vessels. Causes of blockage of the lymph vessels include *breast cancer* in the region of the nipple and *elephantiasis*.

P

## Pectoral

A medical term that means relating to the chest, as in the major and minor pectoral muscles.

The pectoralis major is a large, fan-shaped muscle that covers much of the upper part of the front of the chest; it arises from the sternum (breastbone) and cartilages of the second to sixth ribs, and converges on the humerus (upper arm bone) just below the shoulder. Its main function is to move the arm across the body.

The pectoralis minor is a smaller, triangular muscle that underlies the pectoralis major; it arises from the third to fifth ribs, and converges on the scapula (shoulder blade), which it moves down and forward.

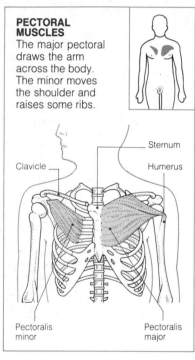

**PECTORAL MUSCLES**
The major pectoral draws the arm across the body. The minor moves the shoulder and raises some ribs.

Sternum
Humerus
Clavicle
Pectoralis minor
Pectoralis major

## Pediatrician

A specialist in the care of children from infancy through adolescence (usually to age 18, occasionally into the early 20s). Pediatricians advise on the care of the child and conduct periodic "well baby" examinations to assess general health and detect any problems. They also give vaccinations and treat childhood disorders. (See also *Neonatologist*.)

## Pediatrics

The branch of medicine concerned with the growth and development of children, and the diagnosis, treat-ment, and prevention of childhood diseases. Special aspects of pediatrics include the care of newborn infants and disabled children.

## Pedicle

A stemlike structure by which some tumors are attached to tissue and through which they receive their blood supply. Also called pedicles are the two bars of bone that extend backward from the body of each vertebra and form the sides of the bony arch that surrounds the spinal cord.

## Pediculosis

Any type of louse infestation. (See *Lice*; *Pubic lice*.)

## Pedophilia

An illegal sexual perversion in which sexual activity with a prepubertal child is the preferred recurrent means of reaching orgasm. Pedophiles are almost exclusively male (heterosexual, bisexual, or homosexual) and are rarely diagnosed as suffering from psychosis. However, they often show personality problems and little concern for the effect of their behavior on the minor.

Pedophiles fantasize about sex with a child, and fondle the child more commonly than they have intercourse. Actual research is rudimentary. However, the prevalence of child prostitution and of child sexual abuse within families seems much higher than previously thought. Nearly 10 percent of women in some studies report some form of sexual interference in childhood or early adolescence. (See also *Child abuse*; *Incest*.)

## Peduncle

A stalklike connecting structure. The term usually refers to bands of nerve fibers that connect different parts of the brain, or to the ropelike connection of a polyp to the surface of the organ to which it is attached.

## Peer review

Various processes by which physicians review the work, including clinical decisions and scientific writings, of other physicians.

## Pellagra

A nutritional disorder caused by a deficiency of niacin (see *vitamin B complex*), resulting in dermatitis, diarrhea, and dementia. Pellagra occurs primarily in poor rural communities in parts of India and southern Africa where people subsist on corn.

**CAUSES**
Although the niacin content of corn is no lower than that of some other cereals, much of the vitamin occurs in an unabsorbable form unless it is first treated with an alkali such as lime water. (People living in communities in Mexico who prepare the cereal in this way before making tortillas do not suffer from the disease.)

Corn is also low in tryptophan, an amino acid that is converted into niacin in the body. Certain disorders, such as *carcinoid syndrome* (which increases the breakdown of tryptophan) and *inflammatory bowel disease* (which reduces its absorption from the intestine) may also cause pellagra.

**SYMPTOMS**
The first symptoms are weakness, weight loss, lethargy, depression, irritability, and itching and inflammation of skin exposed to sunlight. In acute attacks, weeping (leaking) blisters may develop on the affected skin; the tongue becomes bright red, swollen, and painful. In chronic cases, the exposed skin darkens, thickens, and becomes rough and dry. Diarrhea is a common symptom, and severe mental disturbance, including confusion and memory loss, may develop.

**DIAGNOSIS AND TREATMENT**
Pellagra is diagnosed from the patient's physical condition and dietary history. Daily intake of a regulated amount of niacin and a varied diet rich in protein and calories usually are enough to bring about a complete cure.

## Pelvic examination

Examination of a woman's external and internal genitalia, performed as part of a complete physical examination or to investigate the cause of abdominal pain or symptoms. A pelvic examination is sometimes performed by the primary care physician, who may refer the woman to a *gynecologist* for more tests.

A pelvic examination should be a part of a physical examination; it may also be performed as part of contraceptive counseling. Women with symptoms such as abdominal pain, vaginal bleeding or discharge, urinary incontinence, or infertility require a pelvic examination to establish the cause of the symptoms. During childbirth, a pelvic examination is performed to help assess the position and descent of the baby.

The main aspects of a pelvic examination are shown in the illustrated box opposite.

## PROCEDURE FOR PELVIC EXAMINATION

The examination is usually performed with the woman lying on her back with knees bent. If it is carried out because of uterine prolapse or incontinence, she may be asked to lie on her side. The physician usually begins by inspecting the external genitals for ulceration or swelling and then does an internal examination.

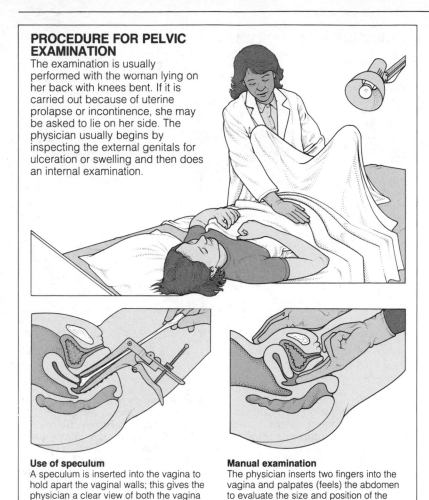

**Use of speculum**
A speculum is inserted into the vagina to hold apart the vaginal walls; this gives the physician a clear view of both the vagina and cervix. A *cervical smear test* may also be performed at this time.

**Manual examination**
The physician inserts two fingers into the vagina and palpates (feels) the abdomen to evaluate the size and position of the uterus and ovaries, and to detect any abnormal pelvic swelling or tenderness.

## Pelvic floor exercises

A program of exercises to strengthen the muscles and tighten the ligaments at the base of the abdomen. These muscles and ligaments, which form the pelvic floor, support the uterus, vagina, bladder, urethra, and rectum. Stretching or slackening of the pelvic floor is common during childbirth and is also a part of the aging process.

Performing pelvic floor exercises, especially during pregnancy and following childbirth, tones these structures and may help to prevent prolapse of the uterus (see *Uterus, prolapse of*) and urinary stress incontinence (see *Incontinence, urinary*).

Pelvic floor exercises also can sometimes help women who are having difficulty achieving orgasm.

One exercise, carried out during urination, involves stopping and starting the flow of urine several times by contracting and then relaxing the muscles around the vagina, each time for a count of six. Another exercise involves placing two fingers inside the vagina and contracting the muscles around the fingers. The exercises should be done two or three times a day for at least a month.

## Pelvic infection

An infection in the female reproductive system. Severe or recurrent pelvic infection is referred to as *pelvic inflammatory disease* (PID). The infection can result in damage to the fallopian tubes and can cause female infertility.

Occasionally, nongynecologic conditions affecting surrounding organs, such as *appendicitis* and *inflammatory bowel disease*, can cause damage to the female genital tract.

## Pelvic inflammatory disease

Infection of the internal female reproductive organs. Pelvic inflammatory disease (PID) is one of the most common causes of pelvic pain in women. The infection may not have any obvious cause, but often occurs after a sexually transmitted disease, such as *gonorrhea* or a *chlamydial infection*. PID may also occur after miscarriage, abortion, or childbirth. *IUD* users have a higher incidence of PID, as do young, sexually active women.

**SYMPTOMS AND SIGNS**
Abdominal pain and tenderness, fever, and an unpleasant-smelling vaginal discharge are the most common symptoms of PID. The pain often occurs immediately after menstruation and may be worse during intercourse. There may also be malaise, vomiting, or backache.

**DIAGNOSIS AND TREATMENT**
The physician performs a *pelvic examination* and takes samples of any discharge for analysis. A *laparoscopy* may be done to detect any abscess or abnormal growth.

*Antibiotic drugs* are prescribed to clear up the infection, and *analgesics* may be given. If the woman has an IUD, it may need to be removed.

**OUTLOOK**
Some women have repeated attacks of PID with or without reinfection. PID may cause *infertility* or an increased risk of *ectopic pregnancy*, primarily due to scarring in the fallopian tubes that prevents the egg from traveling down the tube into the uterus.

## Pelvic pain

See *Abdominal pain*.

## Pelvimetry

Assessment of the shape and dimensions of a woman's pelvis. Pelvimetry is usually carried out about the 37th week of pregnancy to determine whether the woman is likely to have difficulty delivering her baby.

A rough indication of the size of the pelvic outlet can be obtained during an internal examination by the gynecologist checking the distance between the ischial tuberosities (the prominent bones in the lower pelvis). Radiological pelvimetry (assessing the dimensions by X ray) allows more precise measurement and may be carried out in unusual circumstances. However, the risk of subsequent development of leukemia or solid tumors in children exposed to this procedure mandates great care in balancing the benefit with the risk of the procedure.

P

# Pelvis

The ring of bones in the lower trunk, bounded by the coccyx and the hip bones. The pelvis protects abdominal organs such as the bladder, rectum, and, in women, the uterus.

## STRUCTURE

The pelvis consists of two innominate bones (hipbones), which are joined by rigid sacroiliac joints to the sacrum (the triangular spinal bone below the lumbar vertebrae) at the back; the hipbones curve forward to join at the pubic symphysis at the front. Attached to the pelvis are the muscles of the abdominal wall, the buttocks, the lower back, and the insides and backs of the thighs.

Each innominate bone consists of three fused bones: the ilium, ischium, and pubis. The ilium, the largest and uppermost, consists of a wide, flattened plate with a long curved ridge (called the iliac crest) along its upper border. The ischium is the bone that bears much of the body weight when sitting. The pubis is the smallest pelvic bone; from the ischium it extends forward and round to the pubic symphysis, where it is joined to the other pubis bone by tough fibrous tissue. All three bones meet in the acetabulum, the cup-shaped cavity that forms the socket of the hip joint.

The pelvis varies considerably between men and women. In women, the pelvis is generally shallow and broad, and the pubic symphysis joint is less rigid than a man's. These differences facilitate childbirth. In men, the pelvis is usually larger and built more heavily to bear a greater body weight.

## DISORDERS

Fractures of the pelvis may be caused by a direct blow, or by a force transmitted through the femur (thigh bone). Considerable force is required to cause such a fracture, and it is usually the result of a motor vehicle accident; motorcycle riders are particularly at risk. The fracture itself often heals without problems, but it is frequently accompanied by damage to internal organs within the pelvis, especially the bladder, which may require immediate surgical treatment.

Osteitis pubis (inflammation of the pubic symphysis) is usually caused by repeated stress on the pelvis. It is most common in soccer players as a result of continually kicking a ball. The symptoms include pain in the groin and tenderness over the front of the pelvis. In most cases, the condition clears up with rest.

## STRUCTURE OF THE PELVIS

The pelvis is a basin-shaped bony structure at the base of the trunk. It consists of the sacrum and coccyx at the back and, at the sides, the two hipbones, which curve around to meet at the front. The pelvis supports the upper half of the body and protects the lower abdominal organs. The female pelvis is shallower and wider.

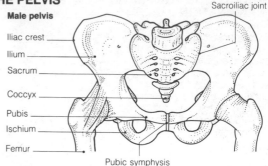

**Male pelvis**

Sacroiliac joint
Iliac crest
Ilium
Sacrum
Coccyx
Pubis
Ischium
Femur
Pubic symphysis

**Female pelvis**

# Pemoline

A central nervous system *stimulant drug* used in the treatment of *narcolepsy* (a rare condition characterized by paroxysms of sleep) and *hyperactivity* in children. Pemoline may cause insomnia, loss of appetite, and, in rare cases, drowsiness, depression, and hallucinations.

# Pemphigoid

An uncommon, chronic skin disease in which large, soft blisters form on the skin. The blisters in pemphigoid are intensely itchy, unlike those in *pemphigus*, a similar, but more serious, disorder. Pemphigoid, which is considered to be an *autoimmune disorder* (one in which the body reacts against its own tissues), primarily affects elderly people.

The diagnosis is confirmed by a skin *biopsy* (removal of a small sample of tissue for analysis). Treatment is usually a long-term course of *corticosteroid drugs* or, in some cases, *immunosuppressant drugs*.

# Pemphigus

An uncommon, serious skin disease in which blisters appear on the skin and on mucous membranes in the mouth and sometimes elsewhere. Pemphigus primarily affects people between the ages of 40 and 60.

## SYMPTOMS AND SIGNS

The blisters usually begin in the mouth (and sometimes the nose), then appear on the skin. They rupture easily, forming raw, often painful areas that may become infected and that later crust over. Apparently unaffected skin may also blister after gentle pressure. When the blisters occur over a great area of the body, the resultant severe skin loss can lead to secondary bacterial infection and, sometimes, death.

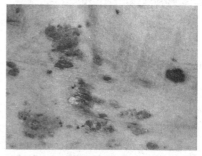

**Pemphigus on back**
The typical appearance is of numerous large, raw areas of skin where the fragile blisters have broken down.

## DIAGNOSIS AND TREATMENT

A diagnosis of pemphigus is confirmed by a skin *biopsy* (removal of a small sample of tissue for analysis).

The usual treatment is with *corticosteroid drugs* given over long periods to keep the disease under control. In addition, other *immunosuppressant drugs* may help. *Antibiotic drugs* may need to be taken for skin and secondary infections.

## Penicillamine

An *antirheumatic drug* sometimes used to treat *rheumatoid arthritis* when symptoms are severe and not relieved by *nonsteroidal anti-inflammatory drugs* (NSAIDs).

Penicillamine is also a *chelating agent* used in the treatment of copper, mercury, lead, or arsenic poisoning. It is used to treat *Wilson's disease* (a rare brain and liver disorder caused by copper deposits in these tissues) and primary *biliary cirrhosis* (a liver disorder). Penicillamine has also been given to people with cystinuria (excessive excretion of cystine in the urine) to prevent stones from forming in the urinary tract.

**POSSIBLE ADVERSE EFFECTS**
Penicillamine frequently causes allergic rashes, itching, nausea, vomiting, abdominal pain, and loss of taste. Infrequently, it causes blood disorders or impaired kidney function.

## Penicillin drugs

| COMMON DRUGS |
| --- |
| *Amoxicillin Ampicillin Penicillin G Penicillin* |

The first group of *antibiotic drugs* to be discovered, natural penicillins are derived from the mold PENICILLIUM. Also made synthetically, penicillins are used in the treatment of many infections, including *tonsillitis, pharyngitis, bronchitis,* and *pneumonia.*

Penicillins are also given to prevent the recurrence of *rheumatic fever* and to treat bacterial *endocarditis, syphilis, gonorrhea,* and *Vincent's disease.*

**POSSIBLE ADVERSE EFFECTS**
The most common adverse effect is an allergic reaction that causes a rash. Any person who has an allergic reaction to one type of penicillin should not be given any other type of penicillin or its derivatives without great caution. Other adverse effects include vomiting and diarrhea.

## Penile implant

A prosthesis inserted into the penis to help a man suffering from *impotence* to achieve intercourse. Penile implants are usually used for men who are permanently impotent.

---

## INFLATABLE PENILE IMPLANT

There are various types of penile implants for the treatment of impotence. The type below gives full control over erection. It is implanted surgically, entirely within the body.

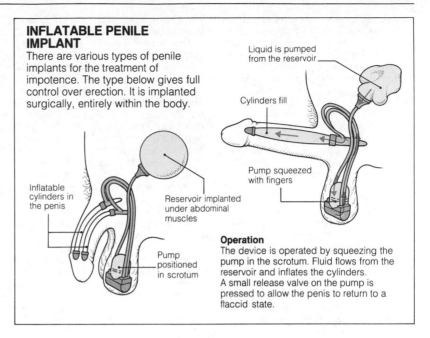

Inflatable cylinders in the penis

Reservoir implanted under abdominal muscles

Pump positioned in scrotum

Liquid is pumped from the reservoir

Cylinders fill

Pump squeezed with fingers

**Operation**
The device is operated by squeezing the pump in the scrotum. Fluid flows from the reservoir and inflates the cylinders. A small release valve on the pump is pressed to allow the penis to return to a flaccid state.

---

One treatment involves inserting a silicone splint between the loose skin of the upper surface of the penis and the underlying tissue. The penis can be inserted into the vagina, but does not become erect or increase in size.

Alternatively, an inflatable prosthesis may be implanted in the penis. This type makes the penis larger and firmer for intercourse and is operated by squeezing a small bulb placed in the scrotum.

## Penile warts

See *Warts, genital.*

## Penis

The male sex organ through which urine and semen pass. The penis consists mainly of three cylindrical bodies of erectile tissue (spongy tissue full of tiny blood vessels) that run the length of the organ. Two of these bodies, the corpora cavernosa, lie side by side in the upper part of the penis. The third, the corpus spongiosum, lies centrally beneath them, expanding at its end to form the tip of the penis, the glans.

Through the center of the corpus spongiosum runs the *urethra,* a narrow tube that carries urine and semen out of the body through an opening at the tip of the glans. Surrounding the erectile tissue is a sheath of fibrous connective tissue enclosed by skin. Over the glans, the skin forms a loose fold known as the *foreskin,* which is sometimes removed soon after birth (see *Circumcision*).

---

**DISORDERS**
The most common congenital abnormality is *hypospadias,* in which the urethra opens on the undersurface of the penis anywhere from the base of the glans to the root. *Pseudohermaphroditism,* which is also congenital,

---

## ANATOMY OF THE PENIS

The corpora cavernosa and spongiosum are the erectile tissues of the penis. A network of nerves controls the blood flow into them.

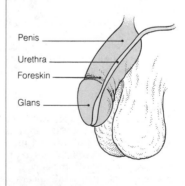

Penis

Urethra

Foreskin

Glans

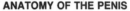

**Cross section of penis**

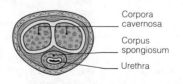

Corpora cavernosa

Corpus spongiosum

Urethra

causes the penis to be very small; it is usually complicated by hypospadias.

*Balanitis* (inflammation of the glans and foreskin) is usually caused by *candidiasis*, although other organisms, including those that cause *gonorrhea* and *syphilis*, may cause inflammation. Balanitis may lead to *phimosis* (abnormally tight foreskin) or *paraphimosis*, in which the foreskin retracts at erection but is too tight to move over the glans.

Penile warts (see *Warts, genital*) are caused by a sexually transmitted virus. Cancer of the penis is rare and is more common in uncircumcised men (see *Penis, cancer of*).

*Impotence* (failure to attain or maintain an erection) is usually psychological in origin. However, it may be caused by nerve damage associated with *diabetes mellitus*, *alcohol dependence*, *atherosclerosis*, or spinal cord injury. The causes of *priapism*, in which an erection is painful and prolonged, and of *Peyronie's disease*, in which the erect penis bends to one side, are unknown.

## Penis, cancer of

A rare form of malignant tumor that is more common in uncircumcised men whose personal hygiene is poor. Both virus infection and smoking have been shown to be additional factors.

The tumor usually starts on the glans (head) of the penis or on the foreskin as a dry, painless, wartlike lump or a painful ulcer, and develops into a cauliflowerlike mass. The growth usually spreads slowly, but a highly malignant tumor can spread to the lymphatic glands in the groin within a few months; the glands swell and the skin over them may ulcerate.

Any growth or sore area on the penis that persists for more than two or three weeks should be reported to a physician. A *biopsy* (removal of a sample of tissue for analysis) will show whether the condition is due to cancer or to some other cause, such as warts (see *Warts, genital*) or *syphilis*.

Because it spreads slowly, cancer of the penis can usually be treated successfully by *radiation therapy* if it is reported early. Otherwise, surgical removal of part or all of the penis may be necessary.

## Pentazocine

A narcotic *analgesic drug* (painkiller) used as a *premedication* (drug used to prepare a person for an operation). Pentazocine is also given to relieve pain caused by *cancer*, during *childbirth*, and, occasionally, after a *myocardial infarction* (heart attack).

Possible adverse effects are typical of other narcotic analgesics. Such effects include depression of respiration and the cough reflex and an ability to induce addiction.

## Pentobarbital

A *barbiturate drug* sometimes used to treat *insomnia*. Pentobarbital is also used as a *premedication* (drug used to prepare a person for an operation). Possible adverse effects are typical of other barbiturate drugs.

## Pentoxifylline

A drug related to *caffeine* that is promoted for the relief of *claudication* (leg pain during exercise) in *peripheral vascular disease*.

Possible adverse effects include dizziness, headache, nausea, flushing, and, in rare cases, chest pain and palpitations.

## Peppermint oil

An oil obtained from the peppermint plant MENTHA PIPERITA. It is used as a flavoring in some drug preparations. Peppermint oil may cause *heartburn*.

## Peptic ulcer

A raw area that occurs in the gastrointestinal tract, where it is bathed by acid gastric juice. A peptic ulcer may occur in the esophagus, stomach, or duodenum. Rarely, it occurs in the jejunum (as it does in *Zollinger-Ellison syndrome*) or ileum (as in *Meckel's diverticulum*). Usually about 0.33 inch to 1 inch (10 to 25 mm) across, and about 0.01 inch deep, an ulcer may occur singly or in several places. The typical symptom is a gnawing pain in the abdomen when the stomach is empty.

**CAUSES AND INCIDENCE**
The lining of the stomach and duodenum is constantly at risk of erosion from acid produced by the stomach wall. The lower esophagus is at risk only when reflux of acid juice from the stomach occurs. Ulcers in the jejunum occur only with massive outpouring of gastric acid, while ulcers in a Meckel's diverticulum occur when misplaced gastric lining grows there. Some of the main factors that may be involved in causing peptic ulcer are shown in the illustrated box opposite. In some people, there is a strong family history of peptic ulceration. Psychological stress may play a part in making an existing ulcer worse.

In the US, a duodenal ulcer develops in about one in 10 people at some time in their lives; a gastric ulcer develops in about one in 30. The incidence of gastric ulcers is about equal in men and women, but more males than females suffer from duodenal ulcers. Middle age is the most likely time for either type of ulcer to develop, although the peak age for duodenal ulcers to develop is somewhat earlier than the peak age for gastric ulcers.

**SYMPTOMS**
Many people found to have a peptic ulcer have no symptoms, but a greater number complain of a burning or gnawing pain in the abdomen, which sometimes wakes them at night. The pain of a duodenal ulcer is often relieved by eating, but usually recurs a few hours later.

Other symptoms accompanying both types of ulcer include loss of appetite (though sometimes a duodenal ulcer increases appetite), belching, feeling bloated, weight loss, nausea, and vomiting (which usually relieves the pain).

**COMPLICATIONS**
In some cases, complications develop, usually bleeding from the ulcer, which, if considerable, results in vomiting blood and passing black feces; this is a medical emergency. Chronic blood loss may cause iron-deficiency *anemia*.

Rarely, an ulcer may penetrate (make a hole in) the back wall of the digestive tract and extend to the pancreas, usually causing pain that spreads through to the sufferer's back. If the affected area is on the front wall of the duodenum, the leaking digestive juices may cause *peritonitis* (inflammation of the abdominal lining), producing sudden, severe pain and requiring emergency hospital admission.

Chronic ulcers can cause extensive scarring of the stomach or duodenum, narrowing the outlet of the stomach into the duodenum (a condition called *pyloric stenosis*) and obstructing the passage of food. This may cause vomiting and rapid weight loss.

A small number of gastric ulcers are malignant and should be removed as soon as they are diagnosed.

**DIAGNOSIS**
The condition can be diagnosed with certainty only after a *barium X-ray examination* or *endoscopy* (inspection through a viewing tube) of the stomach and duodenum.

P

## SITES AND CAUSES OF PEPTIC ULCER

A peptic ulcer develops in about one in eight Americans at some time in their lives. Some of the mechanisms involved in causing ulcers are shown below. Most ulcers respond to self-help measures or to drug treatment, but occasionally surgery is necessary.

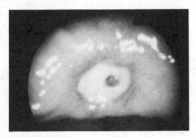

**Gastric ulcer**
This photograph of an ulcer in the wall of the stomach was taken via a viewing tube passed down the esophagus.

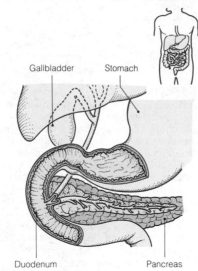

Gallbladder    Stomach

Duodenum    Pancreas

**Site of ulcers**
Peptic ulcers are most common in the first part of the duodenum or lower half of the stomach, but esophageal ulcers also occur.

### ULCER CARE

**Self-help methods**

Avoid smoking, the most important step in self-help.

Avoid drinking alcohol, coffee, and tea.

Avoid using aspirin and nonsteroidal anti-inflammatory drugs.

Eat several small meals a day, at regular intervals, rather than two or three large ones.

**Drug treatment**

Antacids neutralize acid in the stomach.

$H_2$-blockers, such as ranitidine, cimetidine, and famotidine, reduce acid secretion by blocking nerve receptors on acid-producing cells.

Drugs such as sucralfate work by forming a protective coat over the ulcer crater.

---

### HOW AN ULCER IS FORMED

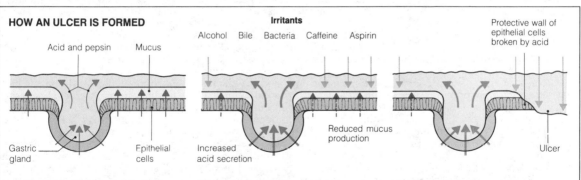

Acid and pepsin    Mucus

Gastric gland    Epithelial cells

**1** Gastric glands in the lining of the stomach secrete acid and the enzyme pepsin, which help break down food. The acid and pepsin would quickly eat away the stomach and duodenum if other cells in the lining did not secrete a protective mucus.

**Irritants**
Alcohol    Bile    Bacteria    Caffeine    Aspirin

Increased acid secretion

Reduced mucus production

**2** Peptic ulcers may be caused by one or more of the following: increased acid secretion; reduced mucus production; or factors that irritate the lining, such as alcohol. Drugs of the aspirin group act as irritants and reduce mucus production.

Protective wall of epithelial cells broken by acid

Ulcer

**3** If damaging influences overcome the protective factors in the stomach or duodenal lining, the mucous layer and mucus-secreting cells are eroded and an ulcer forms. Stress is probably not a prime cause of ulcers but may aggravate an existing ulcer.

---

**TREATMENT AND OUTLOOK**

*Antacid drugs* neutralize excess acidity and assist in the healing of ulcers. They ultimately relieve pain if taken regularly, and, along with the other self-help measures listed above, may be enough to heal the ulcer. If not, and if symptoms persist, professional treatment is necessary. It usually consists of *ulcer-healing drugs* (such as cimetidine, ranitidine, or famotidine), which reduce acid production, or sucralfate, which may form a protective covering on the ulcer.

In more than two thirds of cases, the drugs promote healing within six to eight weeks of the start of treatment. In the remaining one third, long-term drug treatment is usually required; very rarely, if the ulcer fails to respond to medication, surgery is necessary. Usually the surgery is a *vagotomy* (cutting the fibers of the vagus nerve that control digestive acid production).

Occasionally, a partial *gastrectomy* (surgical removal of a portion of the stomach) is performed to treat the ulcer and reduce acid production.

Substantial bleeding from an ulcer sometimes requires a *blood transfusion* to be performed.

Perforation, obstruction, or penetration into the pancreas usually necessitate surgery to correct the problem. In some cases of perforation, however, passing a suction tube into the stomach via the nose to drain off digestive juices may be treatment enough. This procedure sometimes allows the perforation to heal of its own accord in the absence of irritation from acidic juices.

P

## Peptide

A fragment of protein consisting of two or more *amino acids*. Peptides are formed by the linking of amino acids by chemical bonds (peptide bonds) between the amino and carboxyl groups of adjacent acids. Larger peptides, consisting of many linked amino acids, are known as polypeptides; still longer chains of amino acids, made up of linked polypeptides, are called *proteins*.

Peptides are widely distributed in the body's endocrine and nervous systems. Many hormones are peptides, including some *gastrointestinal hormones* and several pituitary hormones, such as *oxytocin*, *ADH* (antidiuretic hormone), and *ACTH* (adrenocorticotropic hormone). In the nervous system, peptides are found in nerve cells throughout the brain and the spinal cord; examples include *endorphins* and substances involved in the control of the pituitary gland.

## Perception

The interpretation of a sensation. People receive information about the environment through the five senses—*taste*, *smell*, *hearing*, *vision*, and *touch*—but the way in which this information is interpreted depends on other factors.

First, the information must be organized into a pattern. Objects must be distinguished from their background and recognized as moving or stationary. The object then requires identification (e.g., as a chair or a friend), a process that relies on memory. The final interpretation depends on an individual's attitudes, expectations, and current mood. Valued objects often appear larger, and hungry people are more likely to notice food sooner than those who have just eaten.

False perceptions, which occur in the absence of sensory stimuli, are *hallucinations*. They are a symptom of psychotic illness (see *Psychosis*).

## Percussion

A diagnostic technique for examining the chest or abdomen by tapping it with the fingers and listening to the resonance of the sound produced. In this way, the condition of internal organs can be deduced. For example, a fluid-filled lung produces a dull note when tapped, as opposed to the hollow sound yielded by air filling one side of the chest in *pneumothorax*. (See also *Examination, physical*.)

## Percutaneous

A medical term meaning performed through the skin. Percutaneous procedures include the injection of drugs into veins, muscles, or other body tissues, and biopsies in which tissue or fluid is removed with a needle.

## Perforation

A hole made in an organ or tissue by a disease or injury. Among the more common types of perforation due to a disorder are a hole in the wall of the stomach or duodenum (the first part of the small intestine) caused by a *peptic ulcer*, and a rupture of the eardrum, usually caused by middle-ear infection (see *Eardrum, perforated*).

Perforating *wounds* (which penetrate through outer layers of tissue to an internal organ or cavity) usually require exploratory surgery to check for and remove any foreign material; they are then repaired.

## Peri-

A prefix meaning around, as in pericardium, the membranous sac that surrounds the heart.

## Periarteritis nodosa

An uncommon disease of small and medium-sized arteries, also called polyarteritis nodosa. Areas of arterial wall become inflamed, weakened, and liable to the formation of *aneurysms* (ballooned out segments). Many different groups of blood vessels may be involved, including the coronary arteries that supply blood to the heart muscle, or the arteries of the kidneys, intestine, skeletal muscles, and nervous system. The seriousness of the condition depends on which organs are affected and how severely they are affected.

### CAUSES AND INCIDENCE

The disease seems to be the result of a disturbance of the *immune system* (body's defenses against infection), triggered in some cases by exposure to the *hepatitis B* virus. It may develop at any age but is most common in adults. More men than women are affected.

### SYMPTOMS AND COMPLICATIONS

In the early stages the patient has a fever and aching muscles and joints. There is general malaise, loss of appetite and weight, and, if blood vessels supplying nerves are affected, nerve pain. Damage to blood vessels leads to obstruction of the blood supply, causing *hypertension* (raised blood pressure), muscle weakness, ulceration of the skin, and *gangrene* (tissue death). If the coronary arteries

are affected, *myocardial infarction* (heart attack) may occur. Because blood vessels supplying the intestines are frequently affected, a high proportion of patients suffer abdominal pain, nausea, vomiting, and diarrhea, and pass blood in the feces.

### DIAGNOSIS

The condition is diagnosed by examination of the blood vessels in a *biopsy* specimen taken from an affected organ. Inflammation is seen under the microscope. *Angiography* (X rays of blood vessels injected with radiopaque dye) may show areas of narrowing, irregularity of the walls, and/or aneurysms.

### TREATMENT AND OUTLOOK

*Corticosteroid drugs* in large doses, supplemented, if necessary, by *immunosuppressant drugs*, are effective in improving an otherwise unfavorable outlook. Without treatment, few victims of the condition survive for five years; death often occurs from a heart attack, *renal failure*, severe bleeding into the intestine, or from complications of hypertension. With modern drug treatment, however, about 50 percent of patients survive for five years or more.

## Pericarditis

Inflammation of the *pericardium* (the membrane that encloses the heart), leading, in many cases, to chest pain and fever. In addition to inflammation, there may be an effusion (increased amount of fluid) in the pericardial space, which separates the two smooth layers of the pericardium. This excess fluid may compress the heart, restricting its action.

Long-standing inflammation can cause constrictive pericarditis, in which the pericardium becomes scarred, thickens, and contracts, interfering with the heart's action.

### CAUSES

There are many causes of pericarditis. They include certain bacterial, viral, and fungal infections; *myocardial infarction* (heart attack); cancer spreading from a nearby tumor in the lung or breast or by way of the blood from a remote site; and injury to the pericardium from a penetrating wound or after open heart surgery. Pericarditis sometimes accompanies *rheumatoid arthritis*, systemic *lupus erythematosus*, and *renal failure*. It can also occur for no known reason.

### SYMPTOMS AND SIGNS

The characteristic symptom of pericarditis is pain behind the breastbone, sometimes spreading to the neck and shoulders. The pain often becomes more severe if the person takes a deep breath, changes posture, or even swallows; sitting up and leaning forward sometimes relieves it. Fever is another common symptom.

When pericarditis is due to infection, pus may accumulate in the pericardial space. When, rarely, the cause is a tumor, blood may collect there. If heart action is impeded, heart output and blood pressure fall—a condition known as cardiac tamponade. This results in breathing difficulty and in swollen neck veins. The main symptom of constrictive pericarditis is *edema* (an accumulation of fluid in the tissues) of the legs and abdomen, causing them to swell.

**DIAGNOSIS**

The condition is diagnosed by the findings of the physician during a physical examination, including listening to the heart with a stethoscope, and from the result of an *ECG* (electrocardiogram) and chest *X rays*. *Echocardiography* may be used to confirm that enlargement of the heart shown on X rays is due to effusion.

**TREATMENT**

Treatment is aimed at the underlying cause whenever possible. *Analgesics* (painkillers) or *anti-inflammatory drugs* may be given to relieve pain. If effusion is seriously affecting heart action, the excess fluid is drawn off through a needle inserted through the chest wall into the pericardial space.

Severe constrictive pericarditis may require surgical removal of the thickened pericardium.

## Pericardium

The membranous bag that completely envelops the heart and the roots of the major blood vessels that emerge from the heart. The pericardium has two layers. The outer layer is tough, inelastic, and fibrous and is attached to the diaphragm below. It is attached to the sternum (breastbone) in front by fibrous bands. The inner layer is separated into two sheets. Of these, the innermost is firmly attached to the heart and the outer is attached to the fibrous layer. The space between the smooth, inner surfaces of these sheets is called the pericardial space; it contains a small quantity of fluid that lubricates the movements of the heart.

## Perimetry

A visual field test to determine the extent of peripheral vision. Perimetry, which is not usually done as a routine procedure, may be performed to pro-

vide vital information in certain neurological disorders, such as a brain tumor. (See *Eye, examination of.*)

## Perinatal

Relating to the period just before or just after birth. Perinatal is often defined more precisely as the period from the 28th week of pregnancy to the end of the first week after birth. Perinatal mortality is a statistical expression of the number of stillbirths and infant deaths occurring during the first week after birth.

## Perinatologist

An obstetrician who specializes in caring for mother and baby during late pregnancy and after birth.

## Perinatology

A branch of *obstetrics* and *pediatrics* concerned with the study and care of mother and baby during the late stages of pregnancy and early days after birth.

## Perineum

There are two definitions. Internally, the perineum is bounded by the pelvic floor (the muscles that form the supportive base of the pelvis) and the surrounding bony structures. The perineum is pierced by the genitourinary and digestive organs. Externally, the perineum is represented by the area between the thighs that lies behind the genital organs and in front of the anus.

## Periodic fever

An inherited condition causing recurrent bouts of fever. (See *Familial Mediterranean fever.*)

## Period, menstrual

See *Menstruation.*

## Periodontal disease

Any disorder of the periodontium (the tissues surrounding and supporting the teeth). The most common type is chronic *gingivitis* (inflammation of the *gums*), which, if untreated, leads to *periodontitis* (inflammation of the periodontal membranes around the base of the teeth and erosion of the bone holding the teeth).

## Periodontics

The branch of dentistry concerned with the study and treatment of diseases that affect the periodontium (the structures that surround and support the teeth). Of particular concern are *gingivitis* (inflammation of the

*gums*) and *periodontitis* (inflammation of the periodontium).

A periodontist makes considerable use of X rays in diagnosis (to detect erosion of the bones in which the teeth are embedded) and is concerned with *preventive dentistry*. Treatment includes *scaling*, curettage (see *Curettage, dental*), *gingivectomy*, and root planing (removal of the *calculus* from the root surface).

## Periodontitis

Inflammation of the periodontium (the tissues that support the teeth). There are two types. Periapical periodontitis is a complication of neglected dental *caries* and affects the area around a root tip. Chronic periodontitis is a complication of untreated *gingivitis* (inflammation of the gums). It affects the whole of the periodontium and is the major cause of tooth loss in adults.

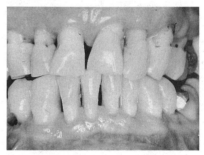

**Periodontal disease**
The gums are inflamed and have receded. Many of the teeth are eroded at their bases; the tooth sockets may also be in decay.

**CAUSES**

If dental caries is untreated, enamel and the dentin beneath eventually are destroyed, allowing bacteria to enter the tooth pulp. From there, bacteria spread to the root tip and into the surrounding tissues, sometimes leading to the formation of a dental *abscess*, *granuloma*, or dental *cyst*.

If gingivitis, which is usually the result of poor *oral hygiene*, is neglected, inflamed gum tissue at the base of the teeth becomes damaged and pockets form between the gums and the teeth. Dental *plaque* (a sticky deposit of mucus, food particles, and bacteria) and calculus (a hard, mineralized coating that forms from plaque and saliva) then collect in these pockets. The bacteria in the plaque and calculus attack the periodontal tissues, causing them to become inflamed and detached from the teeth. The bacteria also eventually erode the bones surrounding

P

the teeth. In time, the teeth become loose in their sockets and fall out.

### SYMPTOMS AND SIGNS

In periapical periodontitis, there may be localized toothache, especially when biting. An abscess may cause some bone and ligament destruction, thus causing the tooth to become loose; a large dental cyst may cause visible swelling of the jaw.

In chronic periodontitis, the signs of gingivitis are present (red, soft, shiny, tender gums that bleed easily) along with an unpleasant taste and bad breath. The deepening pockets in the gums gradually expose the sensitive dentin of the roots of the teeth, causing aching when hot, cold, or sweet food or liquids are consumed.

Occasionally, there is a discharge of pus from the gums or a gumboil (an abscess in the gum); in late stages of chronic periodontitis, there may be bone loss and loosening of teeth.

### DIAGNOSIS AND TREATMENT

In periapical periodontitis, the dentist usually finds a deep cavity beneath a filling, and X rays may show bone destruction around the root tip.

The condition is treated either by draining pus through the root canal and then cleaning and filling the tooth or, if the tooth cannot be salvaged, by dental *extraction*. A minor operation may be required to remove dental cysts or large granulomas. Root canal treatment may also be necessary.

The dentist assesses the extent of chronic periodontal disease by measuring the depth of the gum pockets and by taking X rays to determine the extent of bone loss. If the disease has not reached an advanced stage, regular, scrupulous cleaning of the teeth can, by preventing further plaque and calculus formation, halt destruction of the tissues surrounding the teeth. The dentist removes the plaque and calculus by *scaling* and, in some cases, root planing.

*Gingivectomy* (surgical trimming of the gums using a local anesthetic) may be required to reduce the size of the gum pockets; curettage (see *Curettage, dental*) may be carried out to remove the diseased lining from the pocket so that healthy underlying tissue will reattach itself to the tooth.

Loose teeth can sometimes be anchored to firmer ones by splinting (see *Splinting, dental*); if they are very loose, they may require extraction and replacement with dentures.

## Period pain

See *Dysmenorrhea*.

## Periosteum

The tissue that coats all the bones in the body except the surfaces inside joints. Periosteum contains small blood vessels that supply nutrients to the underlying bone, and nerves that respond to pain caused by injury or disease. New bone is produced by the periosteum in the initial stages of healing after a *fracture*.

## Periostitis

Inflammation of the *periosteum* (connective tissue covering bone). The usual cause is a blow that presses directly onto bone. Rarely, periostitis is caused by infection, such as syphilis. Symptoms include pain, tenderness, and swelling over the affected area of bone.

## Peripheral nervous system

All the nerves that fan out from the central nervous system (brain and spinal cord) to the muscles, skin, internal organs, and glands (see *Nerve*; *Cranial nerves*; *Spinal nerves*).

Diseases and disorders affecting the peripheral nerves are grouped under the heading *Neuropathy*.

## Peripheral vascular disease

Narrowing of blood vessels in the legs, and sometimes in the arms, restricting blood flow and causing pain in the affected area. In severe cases, *gangrene* (death of tissue supplied by the vessels) may develop, requiring amputation of the limb.

### TYPES AND CAUSES

In most cases, peripheral vascular disease is caused by *atherosclerosis*, in which fatty plaques form on the inner walls of arteries. Factors that contribute to the risk of atherosclerosis, such as *hypertension* and inadequately controlled *diabetes mellitus*, are associated with peripheral vascular disease. However, the greatest risk factor is cigarette smoking; more than 90 percent of patients are, or were, moderate to heavy smokers.

Diseases affecting the peripheral arteries that are not caused by atherosclerosis include *Buerger's disease* (which mainly affects smokers) and *Raynaud's disease*; deep vein *thrombosis* and *varicose veins* are diseases of the peripheral veins.

### SYMPTOMS AND COMPLICATIONS

When narrowing of the arteries develops gradually because of atherosclerosis, the first symptom is usually an aching, tired feeling in the leg muscles when walking. It occurs most often in the calf, but may be felt anywhere in the leg. Typically, the pain is relieved by resting the leg for a few minutes, but recurs after roughly the same amount of walking as before. This symptom is called intermittent *claudication*. Prolonged use of the arms may produce a similar symptom.

As the disease worsens, the amount of activity possible before symptoms develop decreases, until eventually pain is present at rest. This pain may be severe and continuous, disturbing sleep; to relieve it, the sufferer may dangle the limb over the edge of the bed. At this stage, an affected leg is dangerously short of blood supply; the foot and lower leg are cold and often numb, the skin is dry and scaly, and *leg ulcers* tend to develop after minor injury. In the final stage there is gangrene, which usually starts in the toes and then spreads upward.

Sometimes, sudden arterial blockage occurs. It may be caused by a clot developing rapidly on top of a plaque of atherosclerosis, by a dissecting *aneurysm* (splitting of an arterial wall), or by an *embolism* arising from a clot formed in the heart and carried to obstruct a peripheral artery. Blockage causes sudden severe pain in the affected limb, which becomes cold and either pale or blue. There is no pulse in the limb, and movement and sensation in it are lost.

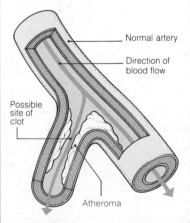

**HOW PERIPHERAL VASCULAR DISEASE DEVELOPS**

The disease usually starts with the formation of fatty plaque on artery walls. Smokers are among those at highest risk.

Normal artery

Direction of blood flow

Possible site of clot

Atheroma

**Clot formation**
Clots may form on top of the plaque, restricting blood flow to tissues. This may cause pain and tissue death.

P

## DIAGNOSIS
The diagnosis is based on comparing blood pressure readings taken at the ankle, calf, upper thigh, and arm and use of *Doppler* ultrasound blood velocity detection or *plethysmography*, which traces the pulse pattern.

## TREATMENT
By far the most important part of treatment is for the sufferer to stop smoking. Exercise is also extremely important; an affected person should walk for up to an hour each day, stopping whenever claudication occurs and resuming when it stops.

Regular inspection of the feet and scrupulous care of them (ideally by a *podiatrist*) are essential to prevent infection, which can lead to gangrene. Feet should be washed and stockings changed daily. Shoes should fit well to avoid pressure on the feet, and toenails should be cut straight across.

Surgery on the diseased blood vessels is sometimes required (*arterial reconstructive surgery* to bypass them, *endarterectomy* to remove the obstructing fatty deposits on their linings, and balloon *angioplasty* to widen them).

In severe cases in which gangrene has developed, *amputation* is necessary, usually to just below the knee to leave a suitable stump for fitting an artificial limb.

# Peristalsis
Wavelike movement as a result of contraction and relaxation of the muscles in the walls of the digestive tract and of the ureters. Peristalsis is responsible for the movement of food and waste products through the digestive system and for transporting urine from the kidneys to the bladder.

Peristalsis occurs in the esophagus during swallowing so that food can be moved toward the stomach even when the body is upside down. Stomach peristalsis helps to mix food with gastric juices and moves the partially digested food into the duodenum. In the small intestine, peristalsis changes to a slow back-and-forth churning motion that allows more time for absorption of nutrients.

In the large intestine, peristaltic contractions occur only once every 30 minutes. Two or three times a day, usually following a meal, a strong, sustained wave of peristalsis passes over the colon. This forces the contents into the rectum and prompts the urge to defecate.

# Peritoneal dialysis
See *Dialysis*.

# Peritoneum
The two-layered membrane that lines the wall of the abdominal cavity and covers the abdominal organs; it contains blood vessels, lymph vessels, and nerves. The peritoneum has a large surface area equal to that of the entire skin surface.

The most important functions of the peritoneum are to support the abdominal organs, to produce a lubricating fluid that allows the organs to glide smoothly over each other and the abdominal wall, and to protect against infection. In addition, the peritoneum is able to absorb fluid; it is a natural filtering system made use of in peritoneal *dialysis*.

The peritoneum may become inflamed as a complication of an abdominal disorder (see *Peritonitis*).

# Peritonitis
Inflammation of the peritoneum (the membrane that lines the wall of the abdomen and covers the abdominal organs). It is a serious, usually *acute*, and painful condition, almost always due to bacterial infection caused by another abdominal disorder.

## CAUSES
The most common cause of peritonitis is *perforation* of the stomach or intestine, which allows bacteria and digestive juices to escape from the digestive tract into the abdominal cavity. The perforation is usually the result of a *peptic ulcer*, *appendicitis*, or *diverticular disease*. Less commonly, intestinal contents may leak into the abdominal cavity after surgery on the intestine. Peritonitis may also be associated with acute *salpingitis*, *cholecystitis*, or *septicemia*.

## SYMPTOMS AND SIGNS
Peritonitis is usually marked by severe abdominal pain, either localized (in one place) or generalized (covering a larger area). Occasionally, however, pain may be mild or absent. After a few hours, the muscles in the abdominal wall go into spasm, making the abdomen feel hard, and *peristalsis* (wavelike contractions of the intestinal muscles) stops (see *Ileus, paralytic*). Other symptoms include fever, bloating, nausea, and vomiting. Dehydration and shock may occur.

## DIAGNOSIS AND TREATMENT
The condition, diagnosed from a physical examination, requires immediate admission to the hospital.

Prompt surgery may be needed to deal with any underlying cause—for example, removal of a perforated appendix (see *Appendectomy*) or repair of a perforated peptic ulcer. When the cause is unknown, an exploratory operation called a *laparotomy* may be performed. *Antibiotic drugs* are often given, sometimes requiring a delay in surgery. Dehydration is treated by an *intravenous infusion* of fluid.

## OUTLOOK
In most cases, the patient makes a full recovery following treatment.

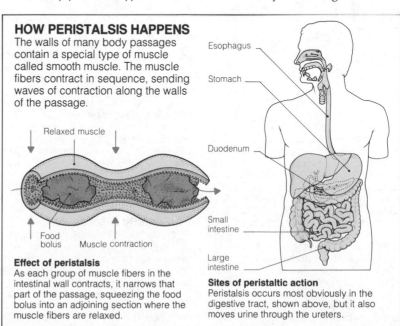

## HOW PERISTALSIS HAPPENS
The walls of many body passages contain a special type of muscle called smooth muscle. The muscle fibers contract in sequence, sending waves of contraction along the walls of the passage.

Esophagus

Stomach

Relaxed muscle

Duodenum

Food bolus    Muscle contraction

Small intestine

Large intestine

**Effect of peristalsis**
As each group of muscle fibers in the intestinal wall contracts, it narrows that part of the passage, squeezing the food bolus into an adjoining section where the muscle fibers are relaxed.

**Sites of peristaltic action**
Peristalsis occurs most obviously in the digestive tract, shown above, but it also moves urine through the ureters.

P

Occasionally, however, an abscess develops within the abdomen, requiring more surgery. Intestinal obstruction, resulting from the formation of *adhesions* (fibrous bands of scar tissue between loops of the intestine), may occur later.

## Peritonsillar abscess
See *Quinsy*.

## Permanent teeth
The second *teeth*, which usually start to replace the primary teeth at about age 6. There are 32 permanent teeth, 16 in each jaw. Each set of 16 consists of four incisors (biting teeth) at the front, flanked by two canines (tearing teeth), with four premolars and six molars (grinding teeth) at the back of the mouth. (See also *Eruption of teeth*.)

## Pernicious anemia
A type of anemia caused by failure to absorb vitamin $B_{12}$, which is essential for normal red blood cell production in the bone marrow. A deficiency leads to the production of abnormal, large, red cells. The vitamin is also essential for normal nerve cell metabolism. (See *Anemia, megaloblastic*.)

## Pernio
An itchy, purple-red swelling, usually on a toe or finger, caused by excessive constriction of small blood vessels below the surface of the skin in cold weather conditions.

Pernios are most common in the young and the elderly, and women are more susceptible than men. Pernios generally heal without treatment; talcum powder may partially relieve itching. Those susceptible to pernios can help prevent them by keeping feet and hands warm in cold weather.

## Peroneal muscular atrophy
A rare, inherited disorder characterized by wasting of the muscles, first in the feet and thighs and then in the hands and forearms. The condition, also known as Charcot-Marie-Tooth disease, is a result of degeneration of some of the peripheral nerves. It can affect both sexes, but is more common in boys, and usually appears in late childhood or adolescence.
### SYMPTOMS AND SIGNS
Wasting of the muscles stops abruptly halfway up the arms and legs, giving them the appearance of inverted bottles; sensation may be lost in the affected areas. Muscle weakness in the legs causes a characteristic high-stepping walk and clawing of the toes.

### TREATMENT AND OUTLOOK
No treatment is available but the condition tends to progress so slowly that the sufferer rarely becomes completely incapacitated; sometimes the deterioration stops for no apparent reason. Life expectancy for an affected person is normal.

## Perphenazine
A *phenothiazine*-type *antipsychotic drug* used to relieve symptoms in certain psychiatric disorders, especially in *schizophrenia* and *mania*. Perphenazine is also often used as an *antiemetic drug* to relieve nausea and vomiting caused by anesthesia, *radiation therapy*, chemotherapy, and certain drugs.

Possible adverse effects include abnormal movements of the face and limbs, drowsiness, blurred vision, stuffy nose, and headache. Long-term use may cause *parkinsonism*.

## Personality
The sum of a person's traits, habits, and experiences. There is much disagreement as to precisely what personality is, what defines it, and how it can be assessed. However, three different aspects are usually considered to be important in any definition: temperament, intelligence, and emotion and motivation.

The notion of temperament originates from the four ancient humors, which divided people into choleric, melancholic, sanguine, and phlegmatic types. It reflects differences in the nature and speed of an individual's responses. For example, some people are easily angered, while others are placid and react slowly. Intelligence defines a person's capabilities in comparison with a theoretical norm, while emotion and motivation describe feelings, attachments to others, moral standards, and aspirations.

The development of personality seems to depend on the interaction of two basic factors: heredity (the qualities a person is born with) and environment (a person's life experiences that affect his or her ways of thinking and behaving).

## Personality disorders
A group of conditions characterized by a general failure to learn from experience or adapt appropriately to changes, resulting in personal distress and impairment of social functioning.

Personality disorders are not forms of illness, but ways of behaving that may become especially obvious during periods of stress. They are usually first recognizable in adolescence and continue throughout life, often leading to *depression* or *anxiety*. Some people realize that they have personality problems; others fail to see their personalities as in any way unusual or difficult, blaming circumstances, bad luck, or other people for their constant failures in life.
### TYPES
Specific types of personality disorders are divided into three groups; there is often overlap among types, particularly within each group. The first group is characterized primarily by eccentric behavior. Paranoid people show unwarranted suspiciousness and mistrust of others, schizoid people are cold emotionally and have difficulty forming social relationships, and schizotypal personalities show oddities of behavior similar to those of *schizophrenia*, but less severe.

In the second group, behavior tends to be dramatic and emotions intensely expressed. Histrionic individuals are very excitable and constantly crave stimulation, narcissists have an exaggerated sense of their own importance (see *Narcissism*), and those with *antisocial personality disorder* consistently fail to conform to social standards.

General anxiety and fear characterize people in the third group. Included are people with *avoidant personality disorder*, who are extremely sensitive to criticism; dependent personalities, who lack self-confidence and cannot function independently (see *Dependence*); compulsive people, who are perfectionists, rigid in their habits, and emotionally cold (see *Obsessive-compulsive behavior*); and passive-aggressive types, who resist demands from others to improve their performances at work and at home (see *Passive-aggressive personality disorder*).
### TREATMENT AND OUTLOOK
The usual forms of treatment are counseling and individual *psychotherapy*. Because such people are often uncooperative, it may be difficult to attain even simple goals, such as avoiding the complications of drug abuse or hospitalization, or maintaining personal relationships and jobs. Drug therapy is used only for treating additional illnesses.

In *psychoanalysis*, a therapeutic, helping relationship may be established between sufferer and therapist. Ideally, this forms a foundation for gradual changes in personality as the sufferer begins to understand the causes that motivate his or her maladaptive behavior.

P

## Personality tests

Questionnaires designed to define various *personality* traits or types. Personality tests are used to assist in psychiatric diagnosis, in research, and to assess the suitability of candidates or employees for positions in colleges or industry. The validity and reliability of the tests are uncertain.

The Minnesota Multiphasic Personality Inventory (MMPI) has more than 500 questions, some relating to psychiatric symptoms (such as *depression* or *paranoia*) and others relating to underlying personality traits (such as *intelligence*). Another personality test is said to measure "extroversion-introversion" (how outgoing or reserved a person is) and "neuroticism" (predisposition to developing neurotic illness). Closely related to this test is a third questionnaire, in which a person is rated on pairs of factors, such as tense versus relaxed, or timid versus adventurous.

## Perspiration

The production and excretion of sweat from the *sweat glands*. Perspiration is another name for sweat.

## Perthes' disease

Inflammation of an epiphysis (growing area) of the head of the *femur*. A type of *osteochondritis juvenilis*, Perthes' disease is thought to be due to disrupted blood supply to the bone.

The condition most commonly occurs in children aged 5 to 10, and usually affects one hip. Symptoms include pain in the thigh and groin and a limp on the affected side. Movement of the hip is restricted and painful. X rays may show fragmentation and, at a later stage, shrinking of the head of the femur.

Treatment may consist of rest for a few weeks until the pain subsides, followed by splinting of the hip to reduce pressure on the femur, or an *osteotomy* operation to change the angle of the head of the femur so that it fits more securely into the pelvis.

Perthes' disease usually clears up by itself within three years, but may leave the hip permanently deformed. Severe deformity may increase the likelihood of *osteoarthritis* later in life.

## Pertussis

A distressing infectious disease, also called whooping cough, that mainly affects infants and young children. Paroxysms of coughing, often ending in a characteristic "whoop" as breath is drawn in, are the main symptoms of the illness, which may last for weeks and can have some serious complications. Before the introduction of a vaccine against pertussis in the 1950s, this disease killed more children every year in the US than all other infectious diseases combined.

---

### DEATH RATE FROM PERTUSSIS IN US

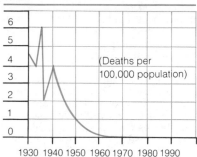
(Deaths per 100,000 population)

1930 1940 1950 1960 1970 1980 1990

**The decline of pertussis**
Pertussis caused thousands of deaths annually in the 1930s and 1940s. Now there are just a handful of deaths each year.

#### CAUSES AND INCIDENCE

Pertussis is caused by a bacterium, *BORDETELLA PERTUSSIS*, that is spread from an infected person to others in coughed-out airborne droplets. The disease leads to inflammation of the entire respiratory tract. The illness occurs worldwide. Infants are susceptible from birth, and the illness is most dangerous in infants. Adults are occasionally affected.

In developed countries such as the US, most infants are vaccinated in the first year of life. However, the vaccine is not completely effective in preventing the illness, and not all children are suitable for vaccination, so epidemics of the illness still occur. Probably about 20,000 to 30,000 cases occur annually in the US, although not all of them are reported.

Experience has shown that, if the percentage of children vaccinated drops significantly (as occurred in the UK in the 1970s), the number affected in epidemics climbs severalfold. Because the illness is potentially serious, it is important that as many infants as possible who are suitable for vaccination be vaccinated. The risks of vaccination are far less than the dangers of having pertussis.

#### PREVENTION

Pertussis vaccine is usually given in combination with diphtheria and tetanus vaccines to children at 2, 4, and 6 months of age in the US; a "booster" dose is given at age 5.

An infant often becomes mildly feverish or fretful for a day or two after an injection, but this is no cause for concern. Giving the child a dose of acetaminophen before the vaccination helps reduce the side effects.

Very rarely (in about one in 100,000 cases), a baby may have a severe reaction, with high-pitched screaming or seizures and, in about one in 300,000 cases, may suffer permanent brain damage. To lessen these already very small risks, the vaccine is not given to an infant who has a history of seizures, who has a feverish illness, or who has suffered a previous reaction to the pertussis vaccine.

Infants should be kept away from anyone with pertussis.

#### SYMPTOMS AND COMPLICATIONS

After an incubation period of one to three weeks, the illness starts with a mild cough, sneezing, nasal discharge, fever, and sore eyes; this is the period when the child is most infectious. After a few days, the cough becomes more persistent and severe. Whooping occurs in most but not all cases. Sometimes the cough induces vomiting. In infants, there is a risk of temporary *apnea* (cessation of breathing) after a coughing spasm.

The illness continues for up to 10 weeks and can be exhausting for the whole family, especially if the child's coughing continues at night. Complications include the development of *pneumonia*; the mechanical effects of the coughing may cause nosebleeds and bleeding from blood vessels on the surface of the eyes. Recurrent vomiting can cause dehydration and malnourishment.

#### DIAGNOSIS AND TREATMENT

Pertussis is diagnosed by identifying the causative bacterium in a culture grown from a nasal swab in the early stages of the illness.

Antibiotics are not particularly helpful once the severe coughing stage of the illness has begun. However, if the illness is recognized early, erythromycin is often given; it reduces the child's infectivity to others and may shorten the length of the illness.

A child with pertussis should be kept warm, given small, frequent meals and plenty to drink, and protected from stimuli that can cause coughing (such as drafts or smoke). An infant or child who becomes blue or keeps vomiting after coughing needs to be admitted to the hospital.

## Perversion

See *Deviation, sexual*.

P

## Pes cavus
See *Clawfoot*.

## Pessary
One of a variety of devices placed in the vagina. Some types of pessaries are used to correct the position of the uterus (see *Uterus, prolapse of*).

## Pesticides
Poisonous chemicals used to eradicate pests of any kind. The most frequently used types are insecticides, herbicides (weedkillers), and fungicides. Most cases of pesticide poisoning occur in children who have swallowed a garden herbicide or insecticide, such as *paraquat* or a chlorate pesticide (see *Chlorate poisoning*). However, poisoning also occurs in agricultural workers, usually by inhalation or absorption through the skin—as in *parathion* poisoning.

In addition, indirect exposure to pesticides can occur through eating food in which the chemicals have accumulated as a result of repeated crop spraying. Some authorities believe the result of eating such foods may be insidious long-term damage to health. For this reason, and because of environmental dangers, pesticide manufacturers in the US must reveal the results of their toxicity studies before the Environment Protection Agency will approve a new product. (See also *DDT*; *Defoliant poisoning*.)

## Petechiae
Red or purple, flat, pinhead spots that occur in the skin or mucous membrane. Petechiae are caused by a localized hemorrhage from small blood vessels. They occur in *purpura* (a group of bleeding disorders) and sometimes in bacterial *endocarditis*.

## Petit mal
A type of seizure that occurs in *epilepsy*. Petit mal attacks occur in children and adolescents but rarely persist into adult life. They are characterized by a momentary loss of awareness; an observer may think that the sufferer is daydreaming. Petit mal attacks may occur hundreds of times a day and sometimes last as long as half a minute each.

## Petroleum jelly
A greasy substance obtained from petroleum, also known as petrolatum and yellow soft paraffin. Petroleum jelly is commonly used as an *ointment* base, as a protective dressing, and as an *emollient* to soothe the skin.

## PET scanning
Positron emission tomography, a diagnostic technique based on the detection of positrons (positively charged particles) that are emitted by labeled substances introduced into the body. PET scanning produces three-dimensional images that reflect the metabolic and chemical activity of tissues being studied.

### HOW IT WORKS
Substances that take part in biochemical processes in the body are labeled with radioisotopes (radioactive forms of elements, such as carbon 11, nitrogen 13, or oxygen 15). These substances are injected into the blood and are taken up in greater concentrations by areas of tissue that are more metabolically active. In the tissue, the substances emit positrons, which, in turn, release photons. It is the detection of these photons that actually forms the basis of PET scanning.

By surrounding the patient with an array of detectors linked to a computer, the origin of the photons can be computed and a picture built of the distribution of the radioisotope within body tissues.

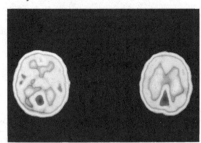

**PET scan images of brain sections**
Features within the brain appear as light or dark areas according to their uptake of radioactively labeled glucose.

### WHY IT IS DONE
PET scanning is particularly valuable for investigating the brain. It is used for detecting tumors (which are more or less metabolically active than surrounding brain tissue), for locating the origin of epileptic activity within the brain, and for examining brain function in various mental illnesses.

### OUTLOOK
PET scanning equipment is expensive to buy and operate; it is available in only a few centers where there is also a cyclotron, which makes the necessary isotopes. However, because PET scanning can provide valuable information not obtainable by other techniques, it seems likely that its use will become more widespread in the future.

## Peutz-Jeghers syndrome
An inherited condition in which numerous polyps occur in the small intestine and small, flat, brown spots appear on the lips and in the mouth. The syndrome usually produces no symptoms but occasionally the polyps cause abdominal pain, bleed, or lead to *intussusception* (in which the intestine telescopes in on itself and causes obstruction).

Tests may include *barium X-ray examination* of the small and large intestines and *colonoscopy* (inspection through a viewing tube). Bleeding polyps may be removed.

## Peyote
A cactus plant found in northern Mexico and the southwestern US, the dried blossoms of which are prepared as an *hallucinogenic drug*. The active ingredient is *mescaline*, which produces visual hallucinations and altered consciousness lasting for several hours.

## Peyronie's disease
A disorder of the *penis* in which part of the sheath of fibrous connective tissue within the penis thickens. Peyronie's disease causes the penis to bend at an angle during erection, usually to one side, often making intercourse difficult and painful. The disorder usually affects men over 40 and the cause is unknown.

The thickened area can usually be felt as a firm nodule when the penis is flaccid. Eventually, some of the erectile tissue (spongy tissue in the penis responsible for erection) may also thicken, interfering with erection.

In some cases, Peyronie's disease improves without treatment. Local injections of *corticosteroid drugs* sometimes improve the condition. If it persists, the thickened area may be removed surgically and replaced with a graft of normal tissue. The drawback to this operation is that it sometimes results in more scarring, making the problem worse.

## pH
A measure of the acidity or alkalinity of a solution. The pH scale ranges from 0 to 14, with 7 denoting neutrality; the smaller the pH value below 7, the more strongly acidic a solution is; the larger the value above 7, the more strongly alkaline it is.

The pH of body fluids must be maintained very near 7.4 (close to neutrality) for the body's metabolic reactions to proceed properly (see

*Acid-base balance*). If the pH falls below about 7.3, a condition called *acidosis* results; if it rises above about 7.5, *alkalosis* results.

## Phagocyte

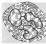A cell capable of surrounding, engulfing, and digesting microorganisms (such as bacteria and viruses), foreign particles that have entered the body (such as dust inhaled into the lungs), and cellular debris.

Phagocytes form part of the body's *immune system* (natural defenses against infection) and are found in the blood, spleen, and lymph nodes, in the alveoli (small air sacs) within the lungs, and elsewhere.

Some types of white *blood cells*, especially granulocytes and some monocytes, are phagocytes. They are "free" phagocytes, able to wander through the tissues and engulf organisms and debris.

## Phalanges

The small bones that make up the skeleton of the fingers, thumb, and toes. Each finger has three phalanges, the thumb and big toe have two, and the other toes have three.

## Phallus

Any object that is considered to symbolize the penis.

## Phantom limb

The perception that a limb is present after *amputation*. Impulses from the nerves in the remaining stump are interpreted by the brain as if they were coming from the original limb.

## Pharmaceutical

Any medicinal drug. The term is also used to describe the manufacture and sale of drugs.

## Pharmacist

A person who is professionally concerned with the preparation and dispensing of drugs.

## Pharmacokinetics

The term used to describe how the body deals with a drug, including how the drug is absorbed into the bloodstream, distributed to different tissues, broken down, and excreted from the body.

## Pharmacologist

A specialist in the composition of drugs and their effects on the body. A pharmacologist also undertakes research to help develop new drugs and find new ways to use existing drugs. Although most drugs come in prepackaged forms and dosages, the clinical *pharmacist* is often called upon in a hospital to develop special preparations for special needs, and to advise on dosage, methods of administration, and side effects.

## Pharmacology

The branch of science concerned with the discovery and development of drugs; with their chemical structure and the ways in which they act in the body; with their uses in the prevention or treatment of disease; and with their side effects and toxicity. Pharmacological chemists are also concerned with devising methods of synthesizing naturally occurring drugs, producing completely new synthetic drugs, finding new combinations of drugs, and modifying existing drugs to extend or improve their effectiveness.

## Pharmacopeia

Any book that lists and describes almost all drugs used in medicine, especially an official national publication, such as the United States Pharmacopeia (USP).

Used as a standard book of reference by physicians and pharmacists, a pharmacopeia describes sources, preparations, doses, and tests that can be used to identify individual drugs and to determine their purity. Pharmacopeias may also contain additional information, such as how a drug works, and possible adverse effects.

## Pharmacy

The practice of preparing drugs and making up prescriptions, or a place where this activity is carried out.

## Pharyngitis

Acute inflammation of the pharynx (the part of the throat between the tonsils and the larynx), the chief symptom of which is a *sore throat*.

### CAUSES

Pharyngitis is most often caused by a viral infection; sometimes it is due to infection by bacteria, such as streptococci, mycoplasma, or chlamydial infection. A common symptom of a cold (see *Cold, common*) or *influenza*, pharyngitis may also be an early feature of mononucleosis (see *Mononucleosis, infectious*) or *scarlet fever*. *Diphtheria* is a rare, but serious, cause of pharyngitis.

Pharyngitis may also be caused by swallowing substances that scald, corrode, or scratch the lining of the throat. The condition can be aggravated by smoking or excess consumption of alcohol.

### SYMPTOMS AND SIGNS

In addition to a sore throat, there may be discomfort when swallowing, slight fever, earache, and tender, swollen lymph nodes in the neck. In severe cases, the fever may be high and the soft palate and throat may swell so much that breathing and swallowing become difficult. One potential complication is edema (an accumulation of fluid in the tissues) of the larynx (voice box), which is a life-threatening condition.

### TREATMENT

Other than gargling with warm salt water, avoiding lying flat, and taking *analgesics* (painkillers), no treatment is usually required; pharyngitis most often clears up on its own. Antiseptic lozenges and sprays may aggravate the condition and should therefore not be used.

Particularly severe and/or prolonged sore throats should be reported to a physician, who may take a throat culture and prescribe *antibiotic drugs*. Severe edema of the larynx may require *intubation* (establishment of an air passage by placing a tube through the larynx into the trachea) or *tracheostomy* (creating an opening in the trachea to insert a breathing tube).

## Pharyngoesophageal diverticulum

An abnormal blind-ending sac that bulges back and down from the back of the throat or top of the esophagus. (See *Esophageal diverticulum*.)

## Pharynx

The passage that connects the back of the mouth and the nose to the esophagus. This muscular tube, lined with *mucous membrane*, forms part of the respiratory and the digestive tract. The uppermost part, the *nasopharynx* (an air passage), connects the nasal cavity to the region behind the soft *palate* of the mouth. The middle section, the oropharynx (a passage for both air and food), runs from the nasopharynx to below the tongue. The lowest portion, the laryngopharynx (a passage for food only), lies behind and to each side of the larynx and merges with the esophagus.

### DISORDERS

Acute *pharyngitis* (inflammation of the pharynx), which causes sore throat, is

**P**

the most common disorder affecting the pharynx. A foreign body, such as a fish bone, may become lodged in the pharynx, causing pain and *choking*.

*Pharyngoesophageal diverticulum* (also called Zenker's diverticulum) is a rare disorder in which a small sac develops in the rear wall of the laryngopharynx.

Malignant tumors of the nasopharynx (see *Nasopharynx, cancer of*), though common in the Far East, are rare in the West, as are cancer of the oropharynx and laryngopharynx (see *Pharynx, cancer of*). The latter two are found in association with smoking and heavy drinking.

### LOCATION OF THE PHARYNX

The pharynx, or throat, plays an essential part in breathing and eating and can change shape to help form vowel sounds in speech. It has a mucous membrane lining.

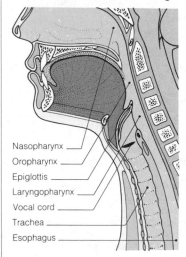

Nasopharynx
Oropharynx
Epiglottis
Laryngopharynx
Vocal cord
Trachea
Esophagus

## Pharynx, cancer of

A malignant tumor of the *pharynx* (the passage that connects the back of the nose with the esophagus). It usually develops in the squamous (flattened, scalelike) cells of the *mucous membrane* that lines the passage. Tumors of the nasopharynx, the uppermost part of the passage, have different causes and symptoms than those occurring elsewhere in the pharynx (see *Nasopharynx, cancer of*).

#### CAUSES AND INCIDENCE

In the West, almost all pharyngeal cancer is related to smoking (of pipes and cigars as well as cigarettes) and drinking alcohol, with the highest incidence in those who both smoke and drink.

In the US, the incidence of the disease is about six cases per 100,000 population per year. The incidence rises with age, and the disorder is more common in men.

#### SYMPTOMS AND SIGNS

Malignant tumors of the oropharynx (the middle section of the pharynx, running from behind the soft palate to below the tongue) usually cause difficulty swallowing, often with a sore throat and earache. In addition, blood-stained sputum (phlegm) may be coughed up. Sometimes the disease causes no more than the feeling of a lump in the throat or a visible enlarged lymph node in the neck.

Cancer of the laryngopharynx (the lowest part of the pharynx), which lies behind the larynx and merges with the esophagus, initially causes an uncomfortable sensation of incomplete swallowing. As the tumor spreads, symptoms include a muffled voice, hoarseness, and increased difficulty swallowing. A sensation of incomplete swallowing may have a different, harmless cause, but it should always be reported to a physician.

#### DIAGNOSIS

*Biopsy* (removal of a small sample of tissue for analysis) of suspicious pharyngeal lesions is mandatory and is often done in the operating room in conjunction with *laryngoscopy*, *bronchoscopy*, and *esophagoscopy* (inspection through a viewing tube of the larynx, lungs, and esophagus).

#### TREATMENT AND OUTLOOK

The growth may be removed surgically or treated with *radiation therapy*; anticancer drugs may be given. The outlook varies considerably according to the site and type of tumor, its degree of malignancy, the stage of the disease at the time of treatment, and the age of the patient.

## Phenazopyridine

An *analgesic drug* (painkiller) used to relieve pain in the urinary tract (caused, for example, by *cystitis* or the insertion of a *catheter*). When pain is due to an infection, phenazopyridine is given with an *antibiotic drug*.

Phenazopyridine may cause abdominal discomfort, orange or red discoloration of the urine, and, rarely, headache and dizziness. Diabetics may find that the drug causes false readings of urine sugar test results.

## Phenelzine

A monoamine oxidase inhibitor *antidepressant drug*. Like other drugs of this type, phenelzine may cause a

dangerous increase in blood pressure if taken with certain drugs, foods, or drinks. For this reason, it is usually given only when other antidepressant drugs are ineffective.

Phenelzine may cause dizziness, and, rarely, jaundice and rash. Headache, unexplained sweating, nausea, and vomiting may indicate a dangerous rise in blood pressure.

## Phenobarbital

A *barbiturate drug* used mainly as an *anticonvulsant drug*. Although phenobarbital has to some extent been replaced by newer anticonvulsant drugs, it is widely used with *phenytoin* to treat *epilepsy* in children.

Phenobarbital is occasionally used as a daytime sedative and is combined with *antispasmodic drugs* for the treatment of *irritable bowel syndrome*.

Possible adverse effects include drowsiness, clumsiness, dizziness, excitement, and confusion.

## Phenothiazine drugs

### COMMON DRUGS

*Chlorpromazine Fluphenazine Perphenazine Thioridazine Trifluoperazine*

A group of drugs derived from the chemical phenothiazine. These drugs are widely used to treat psychotic illness (see *Antipsychotic drugs*) and are also commonly used as *antiemetic drugs* and antihistamine drugs.

## Phentermine

An *appetite suppressant* promoted for the treatment of *obesity*. Phentermine may cause dryness of the mouth, palpitations, and *insomnia*.

## Phenylbutazone

A *nonsteroidal anti-inflammatory drug* (NSAID) used to relieve the symptoms of certain types of arthritis, such as *ankylosing spondylitis* and *rheumatoid arthritis*. Because of the risk of adverse effects, phenylbutazone is not commonly given; it is usually prescribed only when other similar drugs have proved ineffective.

Phenylbutazone is sometimes given illegally to lame horses to improve their performance.

#### POSSIBLE ADVERSE EFFECTS

Phenylbutazone may cause nausea, fluid retention, rash, and *peptic ulcer*. It may also increase the risk of *blood disorders*, such as agranulocytosis (lack of white blood cells). Regular blood tests are therefore carried out if treatment lasts for longer than two weeks.

P

## Phenylephrine

| DECONGESTANT |
| --- |

Eye drops  Nose drops  Nasal spray
Nasal jelly

Nasal preparations available
over-the-counter

Available as generic

A *decongestant drug* commonly used in the treatment of seasonal allergic *rhinitis* (hay fever) and the common *cold*. Phenylephrine is also used to relieve pain in *conjunctivitis* and to dilate the pupils during examination of or surgery on the eyes.

Combined with a local anesthetic (see *Anesthesia, local*), phenylephrine slows down the anesthetic's spread into surrounding tissues (by narrowing blood vessels) and thereby prolongs its effect.

### POSSIBLE ADVERSE EFFECTS

Eye drops may irritate the eyes. High doses or prolonged use of nasal preparations may lead to worse congestion and may cause headache, blurred vision, and raised blood pressure.

## Phenylketonuria

An inherited disorder in which the enzyme that converts phenylalanine (an amino acid) into tyrosine (another amino acid) is defective. Unless phenylalanine is excluded from the diet, it builds up in the body and causes severe mental retardation.

### INCIDENCE AND DIAGNOSIS

About one baby in 16,000 has phenylketonuria (PKU). All newborn babies are routinely given the *Guthrie test* (sometimes called a PKU test), in which a sample of blood is taken from the baby's heel so that the level of phenylalanine can be checked. If the level of phenylalanine is high, more sensitive tests are carried out during the first few weeks of life.

### SYMPTOMS AND SIGNS

Newborn babies show few signs of abnormality, but, early in infancy, neurologic disturbances, including *epilepsy*, become evident. Affected children have an unpleasant, musty, mousy smell due to the excretion in the sweat and urine of a breakdown product of phenylalanine. Ninety percent of those affected have blond hair and blue eyes. Some skeletal changes are associated with phenylketonuria, such as a small head, short stature, and flat feet. About one third to half the patients have eczema.

### TREATMENT

The only treatment is to restrict the intake of phenylalanine, which is a natural constituent of most protein-containing foods. Babies must be given special milk substitutes. After weaning, they are given a very low-protein, mainly vegetarian, diet. Some physicians believe that a strict low-protein diet should be followed throughout life. Other physicians maintain that a normal diet can be introduced at the age of 10 to 12 years; the special diet must be followed during pregnancy.

## Phenylpropanolamine

| DECONGESTANT |
| --- |

Tablet Capsule Liquid Lozenge

Available over-the-counter

Available as generic

A *decongestant drug* commonly used in the treatment of seasonal allergic *rhinitis* (hay fever), *sinusitis*, and the common *cold*. Phenylpropanolamine is also given to relieve stress incontinence (see *Incontinence, urinary*) and is sometimes promoted as an *appetite suppressant* in the treatment of *obesity*.

Prolonged use of phenylpropanolamine as a decongestant may cause a worsening of the condition. High doses may cause anxiety, nausea, and a rise in blood pressure.

## Phenytoin

An *anticonvulsant drug* commonly used in the long-term treatment of *epilepsy*. Phenytoin is used occasionally to treat *migraine* and infrequently to control certain types of *arrhythmia* (irregular heart beat).

Prolonged use may cause slurred speech, dizziness, confusion, and overgrowth of the gums.

## Pheochromocytoma

A rare, nonmalignant tumor of cells secreting the hormones epinephrine and norepinephrine, which regulate heart rate and blood pressure. The tumor increases production of these hormones, causing intermittent or sustained hypertension (high blood pressure). Pheochromocytomas may be single or multiple, and usually develop in the medulla (core) of one or both adrenal glands. Sometimes they occur in similar tissue in the brain and elsewhere. The tumors may develop at any age but are most common in young to middle-aged adults.

### SYMPTOMS AND SIGNS

Most patients have hypertension, but, for much of the time, there are usually no other signs or symptoms. However, pressure on the area of the tumor, emotional upset, a change in posture, or taking *beta-blocker drugs* can cause a surge of hormones from the tumor, bringing on a sudden rise in blood pressure, rapid pulse, palpitations, headache, nausea, vomiting, clammy skin, and sometimes a feeling of impending death.

### DIAGNOSIS AND TREATMENT

Diagnosis involves blood and urine tests to check for excessive epinephrine and norepinephrine and their metabolites. *CT scanning* and investigational *radioisotope scanning* may be used to locate tumors.

Treatment consists of surgical removal of the tumors. Before surgery, drugs are usually given to control the patient's blood pressure. The outlook after treatment is very good in almost all cases. In some patients, hypertension recurs and requires treatment with drugs.

## Pheromone

An odorous chemical, released by an animal, that affects the behavior or development of other individuals of the same species. Many animals secrete pheromones to attract mates or mark their territory. However, although humans also give off distinctive body odors, whether or not these are true pheromones, able to alter the behavior of other humans, remains open to debate.

## Phimosis

Tightness of the foreskin, preventing it from being drawn back over the underlying glans (head) of the penis.

In uncircumcised males, some degree of phimosis is normal until the age of 6 months. In some boys it persists for several years after, sometimes making urination difficult and causing the foreskin to balloon out. Phimosis prevents proper cleaning of the glans, leading to *balanitis* (infection of the glans and foreskin). There may also be an increased risk of cancer (see *Penis, cancer of*). Phimosis makes erection painful and *paraphimosis* may occur as a complication. The condition is treated by *circumcision*.

## Phlebitis

Inflammation of a vein, often accompanied by clot formation. The preferred medical name for this condition is *thrombophlebitis*.

P

## Phlebography

The obtaining and interpretation of X-ray images of veins after they have been injected with a radiopaque substance. (See *Venography*.)

## Phlebotomy

Puncture of a vein for the purpose of letting blood. (See *Venesection*.)

## Phlegm

See *Sputum*.

## Phobia

A persistent, irrational fear of, and desire to avoid, a particular object or situation. Many people have minor phobias, experiencing some anxiety when unable to avoid contact with spiders, for example. However, these phobias do not impair the ability to cope with day-to-day life. It is only when a fear causes significant distress and interferes with normal social functioning that it is considered a psychiatric disorder.

### TYPES

Simple phobias, also known as specific phobias, are the most common. They may involve fear of particular animals (most often dogs, snakes, spiders, or mice) or of particular situations, such as enclosed spaces (*claustrophobia*), heights, or air travel. Animal phobias usually start in childhood, but other forms may develop at any time. Treatment is not usually required, unless the feared object is so common that it is not easily avoided (e.g., fear of elevators in a person who lives in a large city).

*Agoraphobia* (fear of open spaces or entering public places) is a more serious type of phobia, often causing severe impairment and disruption of family life. It is the most common phobia for which treatment is sought. The disorder usually starts in the late teens or early 20s.

Social phobia, which is relatively rare, is fear of being exposed to the scrutiny of others. Examples include fear of eating, speaking, or performing in public, using public toilets, or writing in the presence of others. The disorder usually begins in late childhood or early adolescence.

### CAUSES

According to some theories, simple phobias are a form of learned response (see *Conditioning*). People with such phobias often have been brought up by someone with a similar fear or have had an early frightening experience that has become associated with the feared object or situation. According to other theories, the phobia has a symbolic meaning (e.g., a fear of snakes may result from repressed sexual feelings).

*Separation anxiety* in childhood, an introverted or dependent personality, and an unstable or conflict-ridden background may predispose a person to the development of agoraphobia.

### SYMPTOMS

Exposure to the feared object or situation causes intense *anxiety* and sometimes a *panic attack*. Phobic individuals may also suffer from *depression* and generalized anxiety and may indulge in minor obsessional rituals (see *Obsessive-compulsive behavior*). People with agoraphobia or social phobia may attempt to relieve their anxiety with alcohol, barbiturates, or antianxiety drugs, and may become psychologically dependent on them, thus compounding the problems.

### TREATMENT

The most effective treatment is *psychotherapy*, sometimes combined with *antidepressant drugs*. People with social phobia may benefit from training in social skills.

## Phocomelia

A type of *limb defect* in which the feet and/or the hands are joined to the trunk by short, stubby stumps resembling seal fins. The condition is rare and was seen in people whose mothers took the drug *thalidomide* early in pregnancy.

## Phosphates

Salts containing a combination of phosphorus, oxygen, and another element such as *sodium* or *calcium*. Phosphates are an essential part of the diet and are present in cereals, dairy products, eggs, and meat.

### FUNCTION

About 85 percent of the body's phosphate is combined with calcium to form the structure of bone and teeth. The remainder is deposited in small amounts in most of the body's tissues and plays a part in maintaining the acid-alkaline balance of the blood, urine, saliva, and other body fluids. Adenosine triphosphate (see *ATP*) is a phosphate compound that provides energy for chemical reactions in cells.

### DISORDERS

In most people, the kidneys maintain a constant level of phosphates in the body by regulating the amount excreted in the urine. A slight deficiency of phosphates in the diet is compensated for by a reduction in the amount lost in the urine.

Hypophosphatemia (an abnormally low level of phosphates in the blood) may occur in some forms of kidney disease, *hyperparathyroidism*, long-term treatment with *diuretic drugs*, *malabsorption* (inadequate absorption of incompletely digested foods from the intestine), or prolonged starvation. Hypophosphatemia causes bone pain, weakness, seizures, and, in severe cases, coma and death.

Accidental poisoning with a phosphate-containing fertilizer may cause hyperphosphatemia (excessive levels of phosphates in the blood). Although this condition does not usually cause symptoms, it sometimes leads to the formation of calcium deposits in tissues.

### DRUG THERAPY

Phosphates may be taken by mouth as tablet preparations or milk to treat hypophosphatemia. Phosphates are also used to treat *hypercalcemia*. Diarrhea is a possible side effect of phosphate drugs.

## Phosphorus poisoning

There are two forms of phosphorus—yellow and red. Yellow phosphorus is readily absorbed by the body and is highly poisonous. Red phosphorus cannot be absorbed and is nontoxic.

Yellow phosphorus is used in matches, fireworks, some insecticides, and certain rodent poisons. Most cases of poisoning occur in industrial workers who accidentally ingest the chemical or inhale its vapor. Acute poisoning, due to absorption of comparatively large amounts of phosphorus over a short period, causes damage to the liver, kidneys, central nervous system, and other organs. Symptoms of acute poisoning include burning abdominal pain, an odor of garlic on the breath, nausea, vomiting, bloody diarrhea, jaundice, and symptoms of kidney failure (see *Renal failure*) and *liver failure*. In severe cases, or untreated milder ones, delirium, seizures, unconsciousness, and death may occur within about 48 hours of poisoning.

Chronic poisoning, caused by taking in small amounts of phosphorus over a relatively long period, may cause gradual destruction of the jaw bones (phossy jaw), *cirrhosis* of the liver, and kidney damage.

Treatment of acute poisoning consists of washing out the stomach (see *Lavage, gastric*) with copper sulfate, along with injections of calcium and treatment for any resultant liver or kidney failure.

P

## Photocoagulation

The destructive heating of tissue by intense light focused to a fine point, as with *laser treatment*. Photocoagulation is used to treat disorders of the retina, especially diabetic retinopathy.

## Photophobia

An abnormal sensitivity or intolerance to light. Photophobia causes pain and occurs with some eye disorders, such as corneal abrasion and ulceration, acute *keratitis* (inflammation of the cornea), acute *uveitis* (inflammation of the iris and the ciliary body), and congenital *glaucoma*.

Photophobia is commonly, and inaccurately, used to describe any discomfort caused by bright light.

## Photosensitivity

Abnormal reaction to sunlight. Photosensitivity usually takes the form of a skin rash that occurs as a reaction to the effects of light on the skin. It often occurs because a substance has been ingested or topically applied to the skin. Examples of such substances, called photosensitizers, are certain drugs, dyes, chemicals used in perfumes and soaps, and plants such as buttercups, parsnips, and mustard.

Photosensitivity is also a feature of certain disorders that affect internal organs as well as the skin, such as systemic *lupus erythematosus* and *porphyria*; exposure to light may worsen the disease.

### TREATMENT

Known photosensitizers should be avoided when possible. If the reaction occurs independently of photosensitizers, a susceptible person should avoid exposure to sunlight, especially between 10 AM and 4 PM (when the light is at its most intense), and should use a *sunscreen*.

## Phototherapy

Treatment with light. Phototherapy may involve the use of sunlight, nonvisible ultraviolet light, visible blue light, or *lasers*.

Moderate exposure to sunlight is the most basic form of phototherapy. It is helpful in treating about 75 percent of people with *psoriasis* and probably accounts for its lower incidence in sunny climates.

A newer form of phototherapy is *PUVA*, which combines the use of long-wave ultraviolet light with a *psoralen drug* (such as methoxsalen), which sensitizes the skin to light. PUVA is particularly effective in treating psoriasis and is also used in treating some other skin diseases, such as *vitiligo* and *mycosis fungoides*. Shortwave ultraviolet light, sometimes combined with application of coal tar, may also be used to treat psoriasis. Several treatments are given; the exposure time is gradually increased according to the reaction of the patient's skin to the therapy.

Visible blue light is used in treating *jaundice* in the newborn (caused by accumulation of the bile pigment bilirubin as a result of an insufficiently developed liver). The light is thought to cause the chemical breakdown of bilirubin, allowing it to be excreted in urine. With eyes shielded, the infant is completely exposed to the light for 12 hours or more; he or she may need additional fluids to compensate for water loss.

## Phrenic nerve

The principal nerve supplying the *diaphragm*. It carries all the motor impulses to, and some of the sensory impulses from, the diaphragm, and plays an important part in controlling breathing. Each of the two phrenic nerves arises from the third, fourth, and fifth cervical nerves in the neck, and passes down through the chest to one side of the diaphragm. Injury to, or surgical cutting of, one of the nerves results in paralysis of the corresponding half of the diaphragm.

The phrenic nerve may be deliberately crushed by a surgeon to produce temporary paralysis of the diaphragm after an operation to repair a *hiatal hernia*, or, very rarely, as a treatment for intractable *hiccup*. Crushing the nerve was once commonly performed as a part of the treatment for lung disorders such as *tuberculosis* and *bronchiectasis*.

## Physical examination

See *Examination, physical*.

## Physical medicine and rehabilitation

A medical specialty that concentrates on patients recovering from or overcoming disabilities or impairments caused by injury (especially of the joints and muscles), illness, or neurological conditions such as paralytic strokes. The physician specializing in rehabilitation examines and tests the patient, establishes a rehabilitation program, and supervises a team of therapists who help the patient carry out the program.

## Physical therapy

Treatment of disorders or injuries with physical methods or agents, such as exercise, *massage*, *heat treatment* (including *ultrasound treatment* and short-wave *diathermy*), cold (see *Ice packs*), water (see *Hydrotherapy*), light (see *Phototherapy*), and electrical currents (see illustrated box overleaf).

Exercises may be passive, in which the physical therapist moves parts of the patient's body, or active, in which the patient is taught to contract and to relax certain muscle groups or to perform specific movements.

Physical therapy is used to prevent or reduce joint stiffness and to restore muscle strength in the treatment of arthritis or after a fracture has healed. It is also used to reduce pain, inflammation, and muscle spasm, and to retrain joints and muscles after stroke or nerve injury.

## Physician

A person licensed to practice medicine and surgery in all branches of medicine. The term commonly refers to a doctor of medicine (MD) or a doctor of osteopathy (DO). However, the term is popularly used by other practitioners of the healing arts whose licenses to practice may be more limited (e.g., doctors of podiatric medicine). See also *Licensure*.

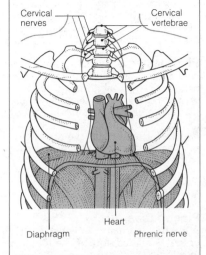

**LOCATION OF PHRENIC NERVES**
There are two phrenic nerves, one on each side of the body. Each follows a tortuous course from its origin in the neck, through the chest, to the diaphragm.

Cervical nerves

Cervical vertebrae

Heart

Diaphragm

Phrenic nerve

P

## TECHNIQUES OF PHYSICAL THERAPY

Physical therapy may be given after a stroke, nerve damage, or a fracture, or for muscle pain or arthritis. In addition to the techniques shown, heat and electrical treatments are often used.

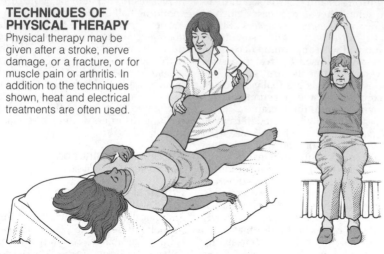

**Passive exercise**
The therapist moves the affected part. This preserves joint mobility and is valuable after nerve injuries and in the treatment of patients with polio.

**Active exercise**
This may help restore function to weak muscles. Stroke patients may benefit, for example, by exercises in which the stronger arm supports the weaker.

### THERAPEUTIC MASSAGE

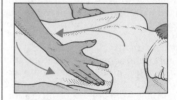
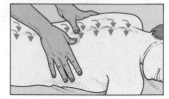

**Massage**
Massage is given mainly to relieve muscle pain and spasm. Long, sweeping strokes can be alternated with "circling" techniques.

## Physiology

The study of the functioning of the body, that is, the physical and chemical processes of its cells, tissues, organs, and systems, including their various interactions. Along with *anatomy* (the study of body structure), physiology constitutes the foundation of all medical science.

Strictly, physiology is concerned with normal functioning, but the boundary between normality and abnormality is not always distinct. Thus a specialty has developed called pathophysiology, which is concerned with the functional changes associated with diseases and disorders. There are also other physiological specialties, such as renal physiology (the study of kidney function), neurophysiology (the study of the functioning of the nervous system), and endocrine physiology (the study of the functions of endocrine glands and their hormone secretions).

## Physiotherapy

See *Physical therapy*.

## Physostigmine

A drug used as eye drops in the treatment of *glaucoma* (raised pressure in the eyeball), often with *pilocarpine*.

## Phytonadione

A *hemostatic drug* used to treat certain *bleeding disorders*. A synthetic preparation of *vitamin K*, phytonadione is used to treat bleeding caused by certain *anticoagulant drugs*, malnutrition, or the inadequate absorption or production of vitamin K in the intestine.

Phytonadione is also used to prevent bleeding in newborns because it carries less risk of anemia and jaundice than other hemostatic drugs.

Possible adverse effects include dizziness, flushing, and, rarely, an unpleasant taste in the mouth.

## Pica

A craving to eat substances (such as dirt, coal, chalk, or wood) that are not food. Pica sometimes occurs during pregnancy and may be a feature of various nutritional or iron deficiency disorders. It may also occur in severe psychiatric disorders.

## Pickwickian syndrome

An unusual disorder characterized by extreme *obesity*, abnormally shallow breathing, excessive sleepiness, and *sleep apnea*. It is named for the fat boy Joe in Charles Dickens' "Pickwick Papers." The cause of the disorder is unclear; symptoms usually improve with weight loss.

## PID

See *Pelvic inflammatory disease*.

## Pigeon toes

A minor abnormality in which the leg or foot is rotated, forcing the foot and toes to point inward.

## Pigmentation

Coloration of the skin, hair, and iris of the eyes by the *melanin* (a yellow, brown, or black pigment) produced by special cells called melanocytes. The greater the amount of melanin, the darker the coloration. The amount of melanin produced is determined by heredity and by exposure to sunlight. Blood pigments can also color skin (such as in a bruise).

### ABNORMALITIES OF PIGMENTATION

**LIGHTENED SKIN** Patches of pale skin occur in various skin disorders. In *psoriasis*, *pityriasis alba*, and *tinea versicolor*, skin scales flake off, resulting in loss of melanin. In *vitiligo*, areas of skin stop producing melanin.

The rare, inherited disorder *albinism* is caused by generalized melanin deficiency, resulting in pale skin and white hair. In *phenylketonuria*, another

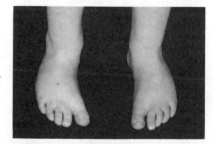

**Appearance of pigeon toes**
This is a common condition in toddlers. In almost all cases it corrects itself by age 7. Severe cases may require surgery.

genetic condition, sufferers have a reduced melanin level, making them paler-skinned and fairer-haired than other members of the family.

DARKENED SKIN Patches of dark skin mingled with lighter areas may follow an episode of *eczema* or psoriasis, or may occur in tinea versicolor. In *chloasma*, hormonal changes cause dark areas to develop on the face; this may occur in women taking oral contraceptives, or during pregnancy or the menopause. Dark facial patches may also be caused by some perfumes and cosmetics, particularly when they contain chemicals that cause *photosensitivity*. All such patches of discoloration usually fade with time.

Permanent areas of pronounced deep pigmentation are usually due to an abnormality in the melanocytes, as is the case with moles and freckles (see *Nevus*). *Acanthosis nigricans*, which may be inherited or acquired, is characterized by dark patches of velvetlike, thickened skin, primarily in body creases.

Darkening of the skin, unrelated to sun exposure, may occur in certain hormonal disorders, such as *Addison's disease* and *Cushing's syndrome*.

OTHER SKIN DISCOLORATION Some abnormal skin pigmentation is caused by an excessive blood level of other pigments. An excess of the bile pigment bilirubin in *jaundice* turns the skin yellow and too much iron in *hemochromatosis* turns the skin bronze. Discoloration may also be caused by an abnormal collection of blood vessels, such as the one that produces a port-wine stain (see *Hemangioma*).

## Piles
A common name for *hemorrhoids*.

## Pill, birth-control
See *Oral contraceptives*.

## Pilocarpine
A drug obtained from the plant *PILOCARPUS*, used for *glaucoma* (raised pressure in the eyeball). Because pilocarpine causes the pupils to constrict, it is also used to reverse dilation (widening) of the pupils (which may be caused by drugs given during surgery or examination of the eyes).

Pilocarpine often causes blurred vision. Other possible effects include headache and irritation of the eyes.

## Pilonidal sinus
A pit in the skin, often containing hairs, in the upper part of the cleft between the buttocks. It is usually harmless, but it can become infected, resulting in recurrent painful abscesses that discharge pus. The condition is probably due to hair fragments burrowing inward. Pilonidal sinus is most common in young, hairy, white males, but is frequently found in others.

Treatment of an infected sinus is by surgically removing a wide area around the infection; the wound is usually left open to allow slow healing from below. Recurrence of infection is common, and plastic surgery is occasionally required.

## Pimozide
A drug used in the treatment of *Gilles de la Tourette's syndrome* (a rare neurological disorder). Pimozide may cause sedation, dry mouth, constipation, and blurred vision.

## Pimple
The common name for a small *pustule* or *papule*. Pimples are usually found on the face, neck, or back, particularly in adolescents suffering from *acne*.

## Pindolol
A *beta-blocker drug* used in the treatment of *angina pectoris* (chest pain due to inadequate blood supply to heart muscle), *arrhythmias* (irregularities of the heart beat), and *hypertension* (high blood pressure). Pindolol is currently under investigation as a treatment for control of *glaucoma* (raised pressure in the eyeball).

Pindolol is less likely than some beta-blockers to cause *bradycardia* (abnormally slow heart beat). Otherwise, possible adverse effects are typical of other beta-blockers.

## Pineal gland
A tiny, cone-shaped body within the brain, whose sole function appears to be the secretion of the hormone melatonin. The amount of hormone secreted varies over a 24-hour cycle, being greatest at night. Control over this secretion is possibly exerted through nerve pathways from the retina in the eye; a high light level seems to inhibit secretion. The exact function of melatonin is not understood, but it may help to synchronize circadian (24-hour) or other *biorhythms*.

The pineal gland is situated deep within the brain, just below the back part of the corpus callosum (the band of nerve fibers that connects the two halves of the cerebrum). In rare cases, it is the site of a tumor.

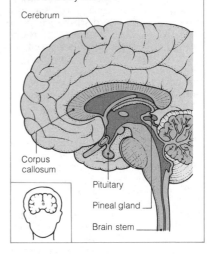

**LOCATION OF THE PINEAL GLAND**
Long considered a mystery, this gland is now thought to act as a sort of body clock.

Cerebrum
Corpus callosum
Pituitary
Pineal gland
Brain stem

## Pinguecula
A small, benign, yellowish spot on the *conjunctiva* over the exposed areas of the white of the eye. Pingueculas are common in the elderly and are caused by ultraviolet radiation in sunlight. Occasionally, a pinguecula enlarges and may threaten to extend onto the cornea to cause a *pterygium*. In such cases the pinguecula may be removed.

## Pinkeye
A common name for *conjunctivitis*.

## Pink puffer
A term sometimes used by physicians to describe one of the two main categories of patients with the lung disease *emphysema*. The other category is the *blue bloater*.

Pink puffers are able to maintain adequate oxygen in their bloodstream—and thus remain "pink" despite serious lung damage—through an increase in their breathing rate. However, this causes almost constant shortness of breath. (Treatment is described under *Emphysema*.)

## Pinna
The fleshy part of the outer *ear*, formed of a flap of cartilage and skin. It is also known as the auricle. The pinna appears to have little practical value; its loss barely affects hearing.

Cosmetic problems affecting the pinna, such as *cauliflower ear*, can usually be corrected by plastic surgery (see *Otoplasty*).

P

## Pins and needles sensation

Medically called paresthesia, a tingling or prickly feeling in an area of skin. It is usually associated with *numbness* (loss of sensation) and occasionally with a burning sensation. Temporary pins and needles sensation is caused by a disturbance in the conduction of impulses through nerves that carry sensation from the skin to the brain (e.g., after sleeping with an arm bent awkwardly under the body). Persistent pins and needles sensation may be caused by *neuropathy* (a group of nerve disorders).

## Pinta

A skin infection occurring in some remote villages in tropical America. The organism responsible, *TREPONEMA CARATEUM*, is closely related to the bacterium that causes syphilis. It is uncertain how the disease is transmitted. A large spot, surrounded by smaller ones, appears on the face, neck, buttocks, hands, or feet, and, one to 12 months later, is followed by red skin patches that turn blue, then brown, and finally white. A course of penicillin or tetracycline clears up the infection, but the skin may be left permanently disfigured.

## Pinworm infestation

 A common infestation with a small parasitic worm, *ENTEROBIUS VERMICULARIS*, that lives in the intestines. This species is also sometimes called threadworm.

**CAUSES, INCIDENCE, AND SYMPTOMS**
The pinworm primarily affects children; it is the most common worm parasite of children in temperate areas. Possibly one fifth of all children in the US are affected at any time.

The female adult pinworms are white and about a third of an inch (10 mm) long. They lay eggs in the skin around the anus, and their movements cause tickling or itching in the anal region, often at night, which may cause the child to scratch. Eggs are transferred directly via the fingers to the mouth to cause reinfestation, or are carried on toys or blankets to other children. Swallowed eggs hatch in the intestine and the worms reach maturity after two to six weeks.

**DIAGNOSIS AND TREATMENT**
Pinworm infestation is easily diagnosed by a physician seeing the worm eggs under a microscope (after the worm eggs have been picked up from the patient's anal area with some sticky tape).

Ointments may be used to relieve the anal itching and the physician may prescribe an *antihelmintic drug*. Treatment of all members of the family is advisable.

Preventive and self-help measures include the wearing of pajamas to discourage scratching, keeping fingernails short, and washing the hands scrupulously before meals. Sheets and nightwear should be changed frequently, washed at high temperature, and ironed.

## Piperazine

An *antihelmintic drug* used in the treatment of intestinal *worm infestations*. Rare adverse effects include nausea, vomiting, and diarrhea.

## Piroxicam

A *nonsteroidal anti-inflammatory drug* (NSAID) used to relieve the symptoms of types of arthritis, such as *osteoarthritis, rheumatoid arthritis,* and *gout*. Piroxicam is also used to relieve pain in *bursitis, tendinitis,* and after minor surgery. Piroxicam may cause nausea, indigestion, abdominal pain, *peptic ulcer,* and swollen ankles.

## Pituitary gland

Sometimes referred to as the master gland, the pituitary is the most important of the endocrine glands (glands that release hormones directly into the bloodstream). The pituitary regulates and controls the activities of other endocrine glands and many body processes (see *Endocrine system*).

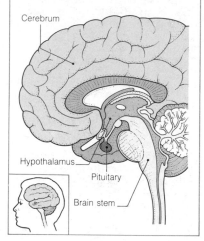

**LOCATION OF PITUITARY GLAND**
This master gland is itself controlled by the hypothalamus, located immediately above it.

Cerebrum

Hypothalamus

Pituitary

Brain stem

**STRUCTURE**
The pituitary is a pea-sized structure that hangs from the base of the brain, just below the optic nerves, and lies in a cavity in the skull. It is attached by a short stalk of nerve fibers to the *hypothalamus,* a region of the brain that controls the function of the pituitary by nervous stimulation and by hormone-releasing factors. The pituitary consists of three parts—the anterior lobe, the intermediate lobe, and the posterior lobe.

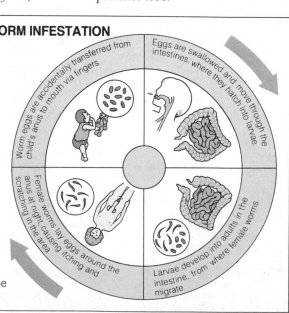

**CYCLE OF PINWORM INFESTATION**
This is probably the most common worm infestation of humans. The adult worms live in the large intestine, from where the females migrate to lay eggs around the anal region. Eggs may be transferred to the mouth (via fingers, sheets, or toys), are swallowed, and hatch to start a new infestation. Occasionally, in a girl, an adult worm migrates into the vagina or bladder, leading to a discharge or to cystitis.

Worm eggs are accidentally transferred from child's anus to mouth via fingers.

Eggs are swallowed and move through the intestines, where they hatch into larvae.

Larvae develop into adults in the intestine, from where female worms migrate.

Female worms lay eggs around the anus at night, causing itching and scratching in the area.

P

## HORMONES SECRETED BY THE PITUITARY GLAND

**Growth hormone**
stimulates cell division and protein synthesis in tissues such as bone and cartilage, leading to growth.

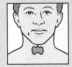

**Thyroid-stimulating hormone (TSH)**
stimulates the thyroid gland to secrete various hormones vital to body metabolism.

**Adrenocorticotropic hormone (ACTH)**
stimulates the adrenal glands to secrete hormones, with multiple effects on metabolism.

**Prolactin**
stimulates female breast development, and, in response to sucking of the infant, milk production.

**Luteinizing and follicle-stimulating hormones (LH and FSH)**
help control the function of male and female sex organs.

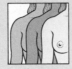

**Melanocyte-stimulating hormone (MSH)**
controls skin darkening by stimulating pigment cells.

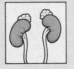

**Antidiuretic hormone (ADH)**
acts on the kidneys to decrease water loss in the urine and thus reduces urine volume.

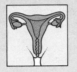

**Oxytocin**
stimulates contraction of the uterus during childbirth and milk release from the breasts.

### FUNCTION
The different lobes of the pituitary produce a range of hormones.

The anterior pituitary produces six hormones: *growth hormone*, which stimulates growth; prolactin, which stimulates the production of milk after giving birth (see *Breast-feeding*); *ACTH* (adrenocorticotropic hormone), which stimulates hormone production by the adrenal glands; TSH (thyroid-stimulating hormone), which stimulates hormone production by the *thyroid gland*; and the *gonadotropins* FSH (follicle-stimulating hormone) and LH (luteinizing hormone), which stimulate the *gonads*.

The intermediate part of the pituitary secretes one hormone, melanocyte-stimulating hormone (MSH), which controls darkening of the skin.

The posterior pituitary produces two hormones—*ADH* (antidiuretic hormone), which increases reabsorption of water into the blood by the kidneys and therefore decreases urine production; and *oxytocin*, which stimulates contractions of the uterus during labor and the ejection of milk during breast-feeding.

## Pituitary tumors
Growths that arise in the pituitary gland. Pituitary tumors are rare, comprising about 10 percent of primary *brain tumors*. Most are benign (noncancerous). However, because the pituitary is situated in a bony hollow at the base of the skull, enlargement of the tumor is upward, where it tends to press on the optic nerves, causing visual field defects.

### CAUSES AND TYPES
The causes of pituitary tumors are unknown. The most common type is called an endocrine inactive tumor. As it grows, it leads to destruction of some of the hormone-secreting cells in the gland, which causes hypopituita-

## DISORDERS OF THE PITUITARY GLAND
Any abnormality of the pituitary gland usually means that it produces either too much or too little of one or more hormones, and this causes changes elsewhere in the body. Locally, serious effects may be caused by enlargement of the gland; for example, it may press on the nearby optic nerves and cause visual defects.

### CONGENITAL AND GENETIC DISORDERS
Deficiency of *growth hormone* may be a genetic disorder, or it may be due to congenital absence or undergrowth of the pituitary, or to damage to the gland sustained during birth. Whatever the cause, deficiency of growth hormone leads to *short stature*.

Congenital growth hormone deficiency may also be associated with deficiency of other pituitary hormones, notably *ACTH* (adrenocorticotropic hormone), *gonadotropin hormones*, and thyroid-stimulating hormone (TSH).

### TUMORS
*Pituitary tumors* are usually benign but may cause either excess production of pituitary hormones (hyperpituitarism) or reduced production (hypopituitarism), depending on the type of cell involved.

### INJURY
Birth injury or a later head injury may cause loss of pituitary function.

### IMPAIRED BLOOD SUPPLY
Rarely, the pituitary may suffer deprivation of its blood supply as a result of pressure on its blood vessels from a growing tumor. This may cause a sudden loss of pituitary function, which may be fatal, or a more gradual loss, which produces signs of general underactivity of the gland. A similar deprivation of blood supply may occur as a complication of massive blood loss associated with childbirth (Sheehan's syndrome). This may lead to failure of milk production, and a range of secondary effects due to the resultant underactivity of other endocrine glands.

Impaired blood supply may also occur from *vasculitis*, or from pressure on the gland from an *aneurysm* of a nearby artery.

### RADIATION
Radiation therapy for a pituitary tumor may cause general underactivity of the gland.

### INVESTIGATION
Techniques used to investigate pituitary disorders include analysis of the levels of pituitary hormones in the blood or urine, and of hormones from other endocrine glands under pituitary control; *X rays, CT scanning*, or *MRI* of the pituitary; and *angiography*, to show displacement of blood vessels by a pituitary tumor. A visual field test (see *Vision tests*) may be done.

P

rism (reduced hormone production). This often leads to a failure of sexual function, with cessation of menstrual periods in women and reduced sperm production in men.

Other types of tumors cause the gland to produce too much of a certain hormone. For example, a tumor of the anterior pituitary can cause excess growth hormone production, leading to *gigantism* or *acromegaly*. Too much thyroid-stimulating hormone (TSH) can lead to *hyperthyroidism* and excess adrenocorticotropic hormone (ACTH) can cause *Cushing's syndrome*. Finally, an increased production of prolactin can cause *galactorrhea* (abnormal milk production), absence of menstrual periods, and infertility in women. In men, increased production can cause impotence, infertility, feminization, and galactorrhea.

Tumors that affect the posterior pituitary may disrupt production of antidiuretic hormone (ADH) and lead to *diabetes insipidus*.

### DIAGNOSIS AND TREATMENT

The diagnosis is made from measurements of the levels of different hormones in the blood and urine, from *CT scanning* or *MRI* of the brain, and from visual field testing (see *Vision tests*).

Treatment may be by surgical excision of the tumor, *radiation therapy*, or replacement of missing hormones, or a combination of these techniques. The drug bromocriptine is sometimes used for hormone-secreting tumors because it suppresses production of some of the hormones.

## Pityriasis alba

A common skin condition of children and adolescents in which irregular, fine, scaly, pale patches appear on the face, usually the cheeks. The condition is caused by mild *eczema* and is often more pronounced after exposure to sun because the patches tan poorly. The condition usually clears up with emollients.

## Pityriasis rosea

A common mild skin disorder in which flat, scaly-edged, round or oval, dark pink or copper-colored spots appear over the trunk and upper arms, usually in a "T-shirt" distribution. The rash is preceded about a week beforehand by a single, larger, round spot (called a herald patch) of the same type on the trunk. The condition, which is not contagious, mainly affects children and young adults. Its cause is unknown.

The rash, which lasts for about six to eight weeks, can occasionally cause itching but is otherwise symptomless. Although the rash usually clears up without treatment, a physician should be consulted to rule out other conditions that cause similar rashes.

Calamine lotion alleviates mild itching; more severe itching can be relieved by *antihistamine drugs*.

## PKU test

See *Guthrie test*.

## Placebo

A chemically inert substance given in the place of a *drug*. Some physicians may prescribe a placebo if a person's symptoms, such as fatigue, are not caused by an illness that requires drug treatment. The benefit gained from taking a placebo occurs because the person taking it believes it will have a positive effect.

Since the effectiveness of any drug may be due in part to this "placebo effect," which is based on a person's expectations of the drug, many new drugs are tested against a placebo preparation. The placebo is made to look and taste identical to the active preparation; volunteers are not told which preparation they are taking.

A comparison of the results enables a more accurate assessment of the drug's efficacy.

## Placenta

The organ that develops in the uterus during pregnancy and links the blood supplies of the mother and baby.

### STRUCTURE

The placenta develops from the chorion (the outermost layer of cells that develops from the fertilized egg). It is firmly attached to the lining of the woman's uterus and is connected to the baby by the umbilical cord. By the end of pregnancy it is about 8 inches (20 cm) wide and 1 inch (2.5 cm) thick. Shortly after the baby is born, the placenta is expelled (thus its common name, "afterbirth").

### FUNCTION

The placenta acts as an organ of respiration and excretion for the fetus. It transfers oxygen from the mother's circulation into the fetus's circulation, and removes waste products from the fetus's blood into the mother's blood for excretion by her lungs and kidneys. The placenta also conveys nutrients from mother to baby.

The placenta produces three hormones—estrogen, progesterone, and human chorionic gonadotropin

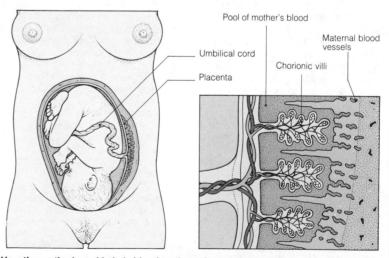

### FUNCTION OF THE PLACENTA

The mother's and baby's blood do not completely mix in the placenta, but are brought sufficiently close so that exchange of nutrients and oxygen (from mother to baby) and waste products (from baby to mother) can occur between the two blood circulations.

Pool of mother's blood

Umbilical cord

Maternal blood vessels

Chorionic villi

Placenta

**How the mother's and baby's blood are brought together**
The baby's blood flows via the umbilical cord to the placenta, where it enters numerous tiny blood vessels arranged in "fingers" (chorionic villi). These are surrounded by a pool of maternal blood brought to the placenta by a major artery.

(HCG; see *Gonadotropin, human chorionic*). High levels of HCG appear in the woman's urine during pregnancy and detection of them in the urine forms the basis of *pregnancy tests*. The hormones enter the mother's blood to help her body adapt to the conditions of pregnancy; they also prepare the breasts for lactation (see *Breastfeeding*).

## Placenta previa

Implantation of the placenta in the lower part of the uterus, near or over the cervix. Placenta previa occurs in approximately one in 200 pregnancies; it is less common in first pregnancies.

The condition varies in severity, depending on how much of the placenta is situated close to the cervix. In some cases, mild placenta previa is detected by *ultrasound scanning* but has no adverse effect on the pregnancy. More severe placenta previa often causes sudden painless vaginal bleeding in late pregnancy, when placental tissue separates from the uterus.

If the bleeding is minor and the pregnancy still has several weeks to run, bed rest may be all that is necessary. If the bleeding stops, the woman may be allowed to get up but she will probably be advised to remain resting in bed until the baby is born because of the risk of sudden severe hemorrhage. The baby is usually delivered by cesarean section at the 38th week.

If the bleeding is heavy or if the pregnancy is near term, an immediate delivery is carried out.

## Plague

A serious infectious disease that mainly affects rodents but is transmissible to humans by the bites of rodent fleas. Plague has been a scourge to people since early history. One of the largest pandemics (worldwide epidemics) was the "black death" of the 14th century, which killed 25 million people in Europe alone. Today, human plague occurs sporadically in various parts of the world (including the US), but can be treated with antibiotics.

CAUSES, TYPES, AND INCIDENCE
The bacterium responsible for the disease, YERSINIA PESTIS, circulates among rodents and their fleas in many parts of the world. The great pandemics of the past were caused by spread of plague from wild rodents to rats in cities and then to humans (via rat fleas) when the rats died. Today, human disease is usually the result of

## SPREAD OF PLAGUE

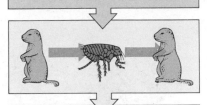

**1** Plague bacteria circulate mainly among wild rodents, such as prairie dogs, ground squirrels, and chipmunks, in the US. They are spread from rodent to rodent by rodent fleas.

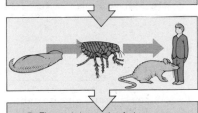

**2** Sometimes so many wild rodents die that the fleas transfer to and infest new wild hosts, such as rats, or even humans who enter plague-affected areas.

**3** The real danger is of plague spreading to, and killing, large numbers of urban rats; rat fleas might then transfer from dead rats to humans en masse, causing an epidemic.

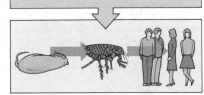

being bitten by fleas of wild rodents. A bite from an infected flea leads to bubonic plague, a form of the disease characterized by swollen lymph glands (called "buboes"). Pneumonic plague, which affects the lungs, can occur as a complication of bubonic plague; it is also spread from person to person in infected droplets expelled during coughing.

In recent years, outbreaks of plague have been confined mainly to parts of Africa, South America, and Southeast Asia. In the US, plague is present in rodents such as ground squirrels, prairie dogs, and marmots in parts of Arizona, New Mexico, California, Colorado, and Nevada. Some 10 to 50 cases of human plague occur in these areas of the US each year, mainly in the spring or summer.

PREVENTION
There is a constant risk of plague spreading to urban rat populations, and the main measures to prevent this are rat control and surveillance of the disease in wild rodents. Hikers in areas where plague is present should not touch rodents or any carcass.

A vaccine against plague is available for people in high-risk occupations, such as agricultural workers within plague areas and workers conducting research on the plague organism.

SYMPTOMS AND SIGNS
Bubonic plague usually starts two to five days after infection with fever, shivering, and severe headache. Soon the buboes appear. They are smooth, oval, reddened, intensely painful swellings usually in the groin, less commonly in the armpits, neck, or elsewhere. There may be bleeding into the skin around the buboes, resulting in dark patches. The victim may have seizures and, in about half the cases, will die if not treated. Occasionally, *septicemia* (blood poisoning) is an early complication and may cause death before buboes appear.

In pneumonic plague, there is severe coughing that produces a bloody, frothy sputum (phlegm) and labored breathing. Death is almost inevitable unless the disease is diagnosed and treated early.

DIAGNOSIS AND TREATMENT
A sample of fluid taken from a bubo, or of sputum in the case of suspected pneumonic plague, is cultured to confirm the presence of plague bacteria and establish the diagnosis.

Prompt treatment with the antibiotics streptomycin, chloramphenicol, or tetracycline reduces the risk of death to less than 5 percent.

All contacts of anyone with pneumonic plague are watched closely and their temperatures checked regularly for a week. Antibiotics are given as a preventive measure and at the first suspicion of illness.

## Plantar wart

A hard, horny, rough-surfaced area on the sole of the foot caused by a virus called a papillomavirus. Plantar warts (verrucae plantaris) may occur singly or in mosaiclike clusters.

Infection is usually acquired from contaminated floors in swimming pools and communal showers. Because of pressure from the weight of the body, the wart is flattened and forced into the skin of the sole, sometimes causing discomfort or pain when standing or walking.

**P**

## TREATMENT

Many plantar warts disappear without treatment, but some persist for years or may recur. To relieve discomfort, a foam pad may be worn in the shoe. Plantar warts can be removed by *cryosurgery*, *electrodesiccation*, *curettage*, *laser treatment*, or applying salicylic acid plasters.

## Plants, poisonous

Several species of plants are poisonous to eat or can cause a severe allergic reaction if their leaves brush against the skin.

### SKIN CONTACT

In the US, poison ivy, poison oak, and poison sumac can cause severe skin reactions. They grow as vines or bushes, and the leaves have three leaflets (poison ivy, poison oak) or a row of paired leaflets (poison sumac). Itching, burning, and blistering develop at the site of skin contact. In some people, these skin reactions can be extremely severe.

First-aid treatment includes thorough washing of the affected area, sponging with alcohol, and application of calamine lotion. Washing any clothing that may have come in contact with the plant is also advised. In the case of a severe reaction, it is wise to consult a physician, who may prescribe *corticosteroid drugs* to be taken by mouth or injection.

### INTERNAL POISONING

Plants that are poisonous to eat include foxglove, aconite, hemlock, laburnum seeds, and many types of berry, including the berries of deadly nightshade (which are black) and holly (red). Young children are the most commonly affected as a result of eating colorful berries. Symptoms of poisoning vary according to the plant but may include abdominal pain, vomiting, excitement, flushing, breathing difficulties, delirium, and coma. Medical help should be sought at once. The usual treatment is gastric *lavage* and measures to relieve symptoms as they arise.

Fatal poisoning is rare. Children should be taught not to sample berries or any type of wild plant.

Paradoxically, many poisonous plants are a source of useful drugs (e.g., *atropine* from deadly nightshade and *digitalis drugs* from foxglove). See also *Mushroom poisoning*.

## Plaque

The term given to an area of *atherosclerosis* (a disease that affects the inner lining of arteries). The

## POISONOUS PLANTS

There are hundreds of different poisonous plants—including many common houseplants and flowers—in addition to those shown. Therefore, it is best to eat only plants known to be harmless.

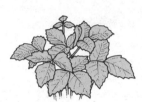

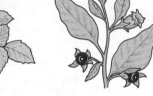

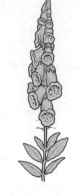

**Poison ivy**
Poison ivy occurs throughout the US, growing as a bush or vine; each leaf consists of three shiny leaflets. On skin contact, an oily substance on the surface of the plant causes irritation, which can be severe.

**Nightshade**
Sometimes called belladonna, the nightshade is about 3 feet high, with shiny black berries. Eating any part can lead to symptoms such as rash, blurred vision, swallowing difficulty, confusion, and coma.

**Foxglove**
This plant has purplish pink flowers; it is a source of the heart drug digitalis. Eating the plant irritates the mouth and causes abdominal pain, diarrhea, and disturbance to the heart beat.

atheromatous plaques give no indication of their presence until they become so large that they reduce blood flow in a vessel or until some disturbance of the plaque surface develops, causing *thrombosis* (clotting of blood) at the site. When this occurs in a small or medium-sized vessel, blockage is likely (see *Peripheral vascular disease*). Plaques in the coronary arteries (which supply blood to the heart muscle) are the cause of *coronary heart disease*.

## Plaque, dental

A rough sticky coating on the teeth that consists of saliva, bacteria, and food debris. It is the chief cause of tooth decay (see *Caries, dental*) and *gingivitis*; if allowed to accumulate, plaque forms the basis of a hard deposit (see *Calculus, dental*).

Plaque begins to form on teeth within a few hours of cleaning and is responsible for the furry feeling of unbrushed teeth. Salivary mucus, consisting mainly of proteins, forms on the teeth. Bacteria that live in the mouth then multiply within this mucus, building up a layer of plaque. Some of these microorganisms, notably *STREPTOCOCCUS MUTANS*, break down the sugar in the remains of carbohydrate food that stick to the mucus, adding to the plaque and creating an acid that erodes enamel.

Plaque should be thoroughly removed at least once a day by *toothbrushing* and use of dental floss (see *Floss, dental*). It can be made more visible by the use of harmless dyes known as *disclosing agents*.

## Plasma

The fluid part of blood that remains if the blood cells are removed. It is a solution containing many important nutrients, salts, proteins, and other chemicals (see *Blood*).

## Plasmapheresis

A procedure, also called plasma exchange, for removing or reducing the concentration of unwanted substances in the blood. Blood is withdrawn from the patient in the same way as for *blood donation*, and the plasma portion of the blood is removed by special machines called cell separators. The blood cells are then mixed with a plasma substitute and returned to the circulation in the same way as for *blood transfusion*. The procedure usually takes approximately two hours.

The main use of plasmapheresis is to remove damaging antibodies or antibody-antigen particles (immune complexes) from the circulation in some *autoimmune disorders*, such as *myasthenia gravis*, *Goodpasture's syndrome*, kidney disease associated with systemic *lupus erythematosus*, and thrombotic *thrombocytopenia*.

## Plasma proteins

All the proteins present in blood plasma (see *Blood*). They include *albumin*, fibrinogen, and other substances important to *blood clotting* and *immunoglobulins* (proteins with a role in the *immune system*).

Apart from their specific roles, the plasma proteins help maintain blood volume by preventing loss of water from the blood into the tissues. The proteins keep the water in the blood by a phenomenon called osmotic pressure (see *Osmosis*).

## Plasminogen activator

See *Tissue plasminogen activator*.

## Plaster of Paris

A white powder composed of a calcium compound that reacts chemically with water, giving off heat and producing a paste that can be molded and shaped before it sets. Plaster of Paris is used for constructing *casts* to immobilize parts of the body and for making dental models (see *Impression, dental*).

## Plastic surgeon

A surgeon who uses special techniques to repair visible defects of skin and underlying tissue present from birth or caused by burns, injuries, certain types of operation, aging, or disease (see *Plastic surgery*). Plastic surgeons also perform operations to improve the appearance of healthy people (see *Cosmetic surgery*).

## Plastic surgery

Any operation carried out to repair or reconstruct skin and underlying tissue that has been damaged or lost by injury or disease, has been malformed since birth, or has changed with aging. Every attempt is made to maintain function of the affected part of the body and to create as natural an appearance as possible.

Operations performed mainly to improve appearance in a healthy person are known as *cosmetic surgery*.

WHY IT IS DONE

Plastic surgery is usually performed to treat damage caused by severe burns or injuries, cancer, certain types of operation, such as *mastectomy* (breast removal), or the effects of aging. Among the more common congenital conditions that may require correction by plastic surgery are *cleft lip and palate*, *hypospadias*, and imperforate anus (see *Anus, imperforate*).

HOW IT IS DONE

A variety of techniques is used to provide skin cover for damaged areas, including *skin grafts*, *skin and muscle flaps*, *Z-plasty*, and tissue expansion (in which skin is stretched by inserting a silicone balloon beneath the surface and gradually increasing its size). These techniques may be combined with a *bone graft* or *implants* to provide underlying support.

The scope of plastic surgery has been much broadened over the past 10 years by the use of microsurgical techniques (see *Microsurgery*) to join blood vessels, thus allowing the transfer of blocks of skin and muscle from one part of the body to another.

## -plasty

A suffix meaning shaping by surgery; performing plastic surgery on. *Rhinoplasty* is plastic surgery on the nose; *mammoplasty* is reshaping or reconstruction of the breasts.

## Platelet

The smallest type of blood particle, also called a thrombocyte (see *Blood cells*). Platelets play a major role in *blood clotting*. A deficiency of platelets (*thrombocytopenia*) can cause *bleeding disorders* or *purpura*.

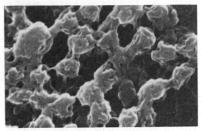

**Electron micrograph of platelets**
Normal and activated (spiky) platelets can be seen. Activated platelets clump to seal defects in blood vessel walls after injury.

## Platyhelminth

 A flat, or ribbon-shaped, parasitic worm. Flukes, *tapeworms*, and schistosomes are types that cause disease in humans. (See *Liver fluke*; *Schistosomiasis*.)

## Play therapy

A method used in the *psychoanalysis* of young children. Play therapy is based on the principle that all play in children has some symbolic significance.

The child is allowed to choose from the toys, drawing materials, and games in the therapist's room. Watching the child at play helps the therapist diagnose the source of the child's problems; the child can then be helped to "act out" particular thoughts and feelings that are causing anxiety. An improvement in the child's state may be indicated by changes in play, such as drawing smiling faces.

## Plethora

A florid, bright-red, flushed complexion. It may be caused by dilation of blood vessels near the skin surface, or, more rarely, by *polycythemia* (excessive numbers of red blood cells).

## Plethysmography

A method of estimating the blood flow in vessels by measuring changes in the size of a body part. Plethysmography

---

## DEVELOPMENT OF PLAQUE

Plaque starts with a deposit of salivary mucus on the teeth. The mucus is colonized by various types of bacteria. initially, the predominant bacteria are spherical cocci. After a day or two, long filamentous colonies of bacteria spread over the surface of the teeth.

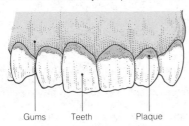

**Areas of plaque buildup**
Plaque develops predominantly at the margin of teeth and gums. If the gums are inflamed or otherwise unhealthy, the plaque tends to develop more rapidly.

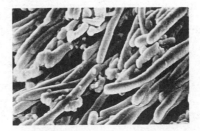

**Mature plaque**
This picture, taken with a scanning electron microscope, shows a mass of filamentous bacterial colonies in plaque, magnified about 2,000 times.

is used on the penis to establish whether a patient with *impotence* gets an erection during sleep. It is occasionally used in the investigation of deep vein *thrombosis* to detect an obstruction of the blood flow back toward the heart.

## Pleura

A thin membrane with two layers, one lining the outside of the lungs and the other the inside of the chest cavity. Fluid between the two layers provides lubrication and thus allows smooth, uniform expansion and contraction of the lungs during breathing.

### DISORDERS

*Pleurisy* (inflammation of the pleura) is usually caused by a lung infection, such as *pneumonia* or *tuberculosis*, and may lead to *pleural effusion* (excessive fluid between the layers of the pleura). *Pneumothorax* (air in the pleural cavity) may occur spontaneously or be caused by a penetrating injury.

## Pleural effusion

An accumulation of fluid between the layers of the *pleura* (the membrane lining the lungs and chest cavity). Pleural effusion may be caused by *pneumonia*, *heart failure*, *cancer*, *pulmonary embolism*, or *mesothelioma* (pleural tumor). The effusion may affect one or both sides of the chest.

Pleural effusion causes compression of the underlying lung, leading to breathing difficulty. Diagnosis is confirmed by *chest X ray*. To determine the cause of the effusion, some of the fluid may be aspirated (removed with a needle and syringe) and examined. A *biopsy* (removal of a tissue sample for microscopic analysis) of the pleura may also be necessary.

Treatment is of the underlying cause. The fluid may require draining with a needle or tube to help breathing. In some cases, depending on the cause, *tetracycline* or *anticancer drugs* are injected into the pleural space to prevent a recurrence.

## Pleurisy

Inflammation of the *pleura* (the membrane lining the lungs and chest cavity). Pleurisy is usually caused by a lung infection, such as *pneumonia* or *pleurodynia* (a viral infection). Rarer causes include *pulmonary embolism*, *lung cancer*, and *rheumatoid arthritis*.

Pleurisy causes a sharp chest pain that sometimes travels to the tip of the shoulder on the involved side. The pain, which is worse when breathing in, arises because the two inflamed membranes rub across each other. Treatment is of the underlying cause, along with *analgesics* (painkillers).

## Pleurodynia

Pain in the chest due to an infectious disease. Sometimes called Bornholm disease, pleurodynia is caused by coxsackievirus B and often occurs in epidemics; it usually affects children but can occur at any age.

Symptoms include sudden severe pain in the lower chest or upper abdomen, with fever, sore throat, headache, and malaise. The disease usually settles in three or four days without treatment, but sometimes recurs several times over a period of weeks. Occasionally, pleurodynia is complicated by *orchitis* (inflammation of the testis), *pericarditis* (inflammation of the lining of the heart), or *meningitis* (inflammation of the lining of the brain and spinal cord).

## Plexus

A network of interwoven nerves or blood vessels, such as the *brachial plexus* (a network of nerves in the neck and upper arm) and the choroid plexus (in the brain).

## Plication

A surgical procedure in which tucks are taken in the walls of a hollow organ and then stitched to decrease the organ's size. One type of plication is fundoplication, used to treat *hiatal hernia*. In this operation, the fundus (upper part) of the stomach is folded up around the lower end of the esophagus to create an inkwell-like valve to prevent reflux of gastric acid from the stomach into the esophagus.

## Plummer-Vinson syndrome

Difficulty swallowing caused by the formation of webs of tissue across the upper esophagus, and usually occurring with severe iron-deficiency *anemia*. The condition primarily affects middle-aged women.

The diagnosis is made by a barium swallow (see *Barium X-ray examinations*) and by inspection of the esophagus with an *endoscope* (flexible viewing instrument). Treatment of the anemia usually relieves symptoms; swallowing is relieved when the web is broken, which often occurs at the time of endoscopy.

## Plutonium

A radioactive metallic element that occurs naturally only in infinitesimal amounts in uranium ores; it is produced artificially in breeder reactors by the bombardment of uranium with neutrons. Plutonium is used as a fuel in nuclear reactors and as an explosive in nuclear weapons, such as the atomic bomb that was dropped on Nagasaki in 1945. The element is highly toxic if it enters the body because of its high rate of *radiation* emission (in the form of alpha particles) and its specific absorption in bone marrow.

## PMS

See *Premenstrual syndrome*.

## Pneumaturia

The presence of gas in the urine. Pneumaturia usually indicates that a *fistula* (an abnormal connection) has developed between the bladder and the intestine. It is an unusual complication of a number of disorders, including *Crohn's disease*, *cancer*, or *diverticular disease*.

## Pneumo-

A prefix meaning related to the lungs, to air, or to the breath. Pneumonia is a disease in which there is inflammation and the accumulation of cells and fluid in the lungs; pneumothorax is air in the pleural space in the chest.

## Pneumoconiosis

Any of a group of lung diseases caused by the inhalation of certain mineral dusts. These dusts originate from nonfibrous materials, so they do not include asbestos (see *Asbestosis*).

Only dust particles smaller than about one five thousandth of an inch across—small enough to reach the smallest air passages and alveoli (air sacs) in the lungs—are likely to cause harm. The dust particles cannot be destroyed within or removed from the lungs, so they accumulate and eventually cause thickening and scarring. The lungs become less efficient in supplying oxygen to the blood.

### TYPES, CAUSES, AND INCIDENCE

The main types of pneumoconiosis are coal workers' pneumoconiosis (caused by coal dust) and silicosis, caused by dust containing silica (a constituent of sand and many types of rock, and the sole constituent of quartz). Silicosis is a hazard for workers in occupations such as quartz mining, stone cutting, blasting, and tunnel construction.

The risk of having either disease develop is directly related to the amount of dust inhaled over the years. Both diseases primarily affect workers

P

over 50, although acute cases of silicosis can occur with 10 months' exposure to a high level of dust.

Other, far less common, types of pneumoconiosis are caused by dusts containing beryllium (used in various high-technology industries), kaolin (from china-clay processing), shale, or hematite (from mining iron ore).

Overall, about 1,700 new cases of pneumoconiosis, causing about 1,000 premature deaths, are diagnosed each year in the US. The incidence is falling due to better preventive measures (e.g., by enforcing maximum permitted dust levels in industry and by use of protective clothing).

**SYMPTOMS AND COMPLICATIONS**

Pneumoconiosis is often detected by a *chest X ray* before it causes any symptoms; if exposure to the dust is stopped at this point, further progression of the disease is sometimes prevented. In other cases, the main symptom is shortness of breath, which gradually gets worse.

In severe cases, *cor pulmonale* (a type of failure of the right side of the heart caused by the lung damage) may develop. There is also a variant of the disease called progressive massive fibrosis, in which damage continues relentlessly (mainly affecting the upper parts of the lungs) even though exposure to dust has stopped.

Complications include the development of *emphysema* and an increased risk of *tuberculosis* in people who have silicosis. One type of pneumoconiosis—caused by hematite—is associated with an increased risk of lung cancer.

**DIAGNOSIS, TREATMENT, AND OUTLOOK**

The diagnosis depends on *pulmonary function tests*, a chest X ray, and a history of exposure to dusts.

There is no treatment for pneumoconiosis aside from treating complications such as lung infections and cor pulmonale. Further exposure to dust must be avoided.

Anyone in whom pneumoconiosis develops at an early age or in whom progressive massive fibrosis develops at any age is at increased risk of a premature death. In the US, compensation can be claimed by anyone in whom pneumoconiosis develops.

## Pneumocystis pneumonia

 An infection of the lungs that is caused by the microorganism *PNEUMO-CYSTIS CARINII*, a type of protozoan (single-celled) parasite. Pneumocystis pneumonia is an *oppor-tunistic infection* that is dangerous only to people with impaired immunity (resistance) to infection—such as people who are suffering from *AIDS* or *leukemia*. Pneumocystis pneumonia is a major cause of death in people who have AIDS.

Symptoms include fever, dry cough, and shortness of breath. They may last from a few weeks to a few months. Diagnosis is by examination of the sputum (phlegm) or a lung *biopsy*. High doses of antibiotics may help eradicate the infection, although it can recur.

## Pneumonectomy

An operation to remove an entire lung. Pneumonectomy is sometimes performed to treat *lung cancer*. It once was used to treat *tuberculosis*, *bronchiectasis*, and lung infection, but these conditions are usually treated today by drugs or removal of only part of the lung (see *Lobectomy, lung*).

Before a pneumonectomy is performed, *pulmonary function tests* are carried out to make sure that the remaining lung is healthy enough to cope with the increased demands that will be placed on it.

**HOW IT IS DONE**

Using general anesthesia, a curved incision is made (starting under the armpit and extending across the back) following the line of the lower edge of the shoulder blade. The muscles are cut through and the ribs gently spread apart to expose the lung. Sometimes a rib is removed for better exposure. The arteries, veins, and bronchi (air passages) leading to the lung are tied off and divided, and the lung is removed. A drain is usually inserted into the pleural space (see *Pleura*) and the incision is then stitched.

**RECOVERY PERIOD**

The drain is usually removed the day after the operation, and the stitches are taken out after about 10 days, when the patient can usually leave the hospital. Many patients require *ventilator* support for hours to days after the operation. At home, normal activities should be resumed slowly; most people are able to return to work after about two months.

## Pneumonia

Inflammation of the lungs due to infection. Pneumonia is the sixth most common cause of death in the US, primarily because it is a common complication of any serious illness. It is more common in males, during infancy and old age, and in those who have reduced immunity to infection (such as alcoholics).

There are two main types of pneumonia: lobar pneumonia and bronchopneumonia. In lobar pneumonia one lobe of one lung initially is affected. In bronchopneumonia, inflammation starts in the bronchi and bronchioles (airways) and then spreads to affect patches of tissue in one or both lungs.

**CAUSES**

Most cases of pneumonia are caused by viruses or bacteria. Causes of viral pneumonia include adenovirus, respiratory syncytial virus, or a coxsackievirus. The most common bacterial pneumonia is caused by *STREPTOCOCCUS PNEUMONIAE*. Other causes of bacterial pneumonia include *HEMOPHILUS INFLUENZAE, LEGIONELLA PNEUMOPHILIA* (see *Legionnaires' disease*), and *STAPHYLOCOCCUS AUREUS*. Pneumonia may also be caused by a *mycoplasma* (an organism that is intermediate between a bacterium and a virus) or by a *chlamydial infection*; *Q fever* is a type of pneumonia caused by a *rickettsia*.

Rarely, pneumonia may be due to a different type of organism, such as fungi, yeasts, or protozoa. These types usually occur only in people with *immunodeficiency disorders* (e.g., pneumocystis pneumonia, caused by a protozoon, commonly occurs in people with *AIDS*).

**SYMPTOMS AND SIGNS**

Symptoms and signs typically include fever, chills, shortness of breath, and a cough that produces yellow-green sputum and occasionally blood. Chest pain that is worse when breathing in may occur because of *pleurisy* (inflammation of the membrane lining the lungs and chest cavity).

Potential complications include *pleural effusion* (fluid around the lung), *empyema* (pus in the pleural cavity), and, rarely, an *abscess* in the lung.

**DIAGNOSIS**

The physician gives the patient a physical examination, listening to chest sounds through a stethoscope. The diagnosis may be confirmed by a *chest X ray* and by examination of sputum and, occasionally, of blood for microorganisms.

**TREATMENT**

Patients with mild pneumonia can usually be treated at home, but hospitalization is necessary in severe cases. The drugs prescribed depend on the causative microorganism; they may include *antibiotic drugs* or *antifungal drugs*. Aspirin or acetaminophen

**P**

may be given to reduce fever. In severe cases, *oxygen therapy* and artificial *ventilation* may be required.

OUTLOOK
The majority of sufferers recover completely within two weeks. However, some elderly or debilitated people fail to respond to treatment; progressively more lung tissue is affected and death occurs as a result of respiratory failure.

## Pneumonitis
Inflammation of the lungs that causes coughing, breathing difficulty, and sometimes wheezing. Pneumonitis may be due to a wide range of causes, including infection, allergic reaction caused by inhalation of dust containing animal or plant material (see *Alveolitis*), exposure to radiation (see *Radiation hazards*), and inhalation of

vomit. It may also occur as a rare side effect of some drugs, such as acebutolol and azathioprine.

## Pneumothorax
A condition in which air enters the pleural cavity (the space between the two layers of pleura lining the lungs and the chest wall) from the lungs or from the outside.

---

## PNEUMONIA
Pneumonia is not a single disease, but the name for several types of lung inflammation caused by infectious organisms. In some cases, accidental inhalation of vomit or a liquid starts the infection. The symptoms, treatment, and outcome vary greatly, depending on the cause and on the general health of the patient.

### Lobar pneumonia
In this type, which is rare in most developed countries today, the inflammation is usually confined to just one lobe of one lung—often a lower lobe.

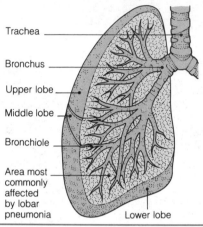

Trachea
Bronchus
Upper lobe
Middle lobe
Bronchiole
Area most commonly affected by lobar pneumonia
Lower lobe

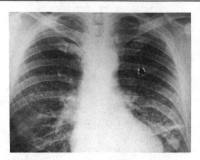

**Chest X ray in bronchopneumonia**
The X ray clearly shows bronchopneumonia. The blotchy, white areas within the darker areas correspond to patches of inflamed lung.

---

### TYPES, CAUSES, AND TREATMENT OF PNEUMONIA

| Types | Causes | Symptoms | Drug treatments | Other treatments |
|---|---|---|---|---|
| **Pneumonias always or usually caused by bacteria** | | | | |
| Lobar pneumonia | *Streptococcus pneumoniae* | Cough, painful breathing, high temperature, rust-colored sputum | Penicillin | Machine ventilation of the lungs to help breathing may be required in some cases. Respiratory therapy to clear sputum out of the lungs may also be needed. |
| Bronchopneumonia | *Hemophilus influenzae* or other organisms | Cough, often a fever, green or yellow sputum | Antibiotics | |
| Aspiration pneumonia | Various organisms. Occurs following inhalation of sputum, vomit, liquids, and so on. | Fever, cough | Antibiotics | |
| Legionnaires' disease | *Legionella pneumophila* | Fever, cough, chest pain, headache, aches and pains | Erythromycin | |
| **Pneumonias not caused by bacteria** | | | | |
| Viral pneumonia | Chickenpox virus, influenza virus, and adenovirus | Cough, fever, not much sputum | Antibiotics (if lungs become infected by bacteria) | Machine ventilation of the lungs to help breathing may be required in severe cases. |
| Psittacosis | *Chlamydia psittaci*, a bacterialike organism caught from birds | Cough, raised temperature, not much sputum | Tetracycline or erythromycin | |
| Q fever | *Coxiella burnetti*, a rickettsia | Cough, raised temperature, not much sputum | Tetracycline or erythromycin | |
| Mycoplasmal pneumonia | *Mycoplasma pneumoniae*, a bacterialike organism | Cough, raised temperature, not much sputum | Tetracycline or erythromycin | |

P

## CAUSES

Spontaneous pneumothorax, which usually occurs for no apparent reason, is six times more common in men than women. Most often, it occurs in thin young adults who have no underlying lung disease; in many cases, it is thought to be due to rupture of a congenital blister (*bleb*) at the top of the lung. There is a 30 percent chance of a recurrence of spontaneous pneumothorax, usually on the same side. Pneumothorax may also be a complication of lung disease (particularly *asthma* or *emphysema*) or it may follow a penetrating injury (e.g., rib fracture).

A pneumothorax may be caused accidentally when a catheter is inserted into a vein in the neck for artificial *feeding*.

## SYMPTOMS

A pneumothorax may cause chest pain or shortness of breath. The degree of breathlessness is proportional to the size of the pneumothorax and any underlying lung disease may be severe. If there is continual leakage of air, the pneumothorax may become progressively bigger and produce a tension pneumothorax, which may occasionally be life-threatening because of compression of the heart.

## DIAGNOSIS AND TREATMENT

A chest X ray confirms the diagnosis and may also show any underlying lung disease.

A small pneumothorax in a healthy adult usually disappears within a few days without treatment. A larger pneumothorax, or a small one in the presence of underlying lung disease, requires treatment. Treatment usually involves removing the air from the pleural cavity through a suction tube inserted through the chest wall; the tube often needs to stay in place for several days. A small pneumothorax can be treated by drawing out the air through a needle and syringe. If the lung fails to expand, or if the pneumothorax recurs, surgery may be required to seal the pleural cavity.

## Pocket, gingival

See *Periodontitis*.

## Podiatrist

A specialist in diagnosing, treating, and preventing diseases and malfunctions of the foot (see *Podiatry*). A podiatrist earns a Doctor of Podiatric Medicine (DPM) degree after completion of college and four years of podiatric medical education (some podiatrists take additional years of residency training).

Podiatrists are licensed to prescribe medications and perform surgery. While most surgery can be performed in the podiatrist's office or in an ambulatory care facility, podiatrists may also use hospital facilities. Podiatrists often work closely with physicians to assure that comprehensive care is provided to the patient.

## Podiatry

The branch of medicine that deals with the examination, diagnosis, treatment, and prevention of diseases and malfunctions of the foot and its related structures. Podiatric medicine is concerned with many different types of foot problems, including walking disorders in children, ankle injuries among adolescents, fractures among athletes and joggers, *bunions* and *hammer toes* among men and women of all ages, and care of foot ulcers, toenails, and infections among people who have diabetes.

## Podophyllin

A drug used in the treatment of genital warts (see *Warts, genital*). It may damage normal skin if not applied carefully. Overuse may in rare cases cause serious adverse effects, such as kidney damage and reduced production of white blood cells.

## Poison

A substance that, in relatively small amounts, disrupts the structure and/or function of cells. Although *toxin* is often used interchangeably with poison, toxin refers strictly and specifically to poisonous proteins produced by pathogenic (disease-causing) bacteria, some animals, and certain plants. (See also *Drug poisoning*; *Poisoning*.)

## Poisoning

Poisons enter the body by various routes. They may be swallowed, inhaled, absorbed through the skin, or injected under the skin (as with an *insect sting* or *snakebite*). They may also originate within the body itself.

For example, bacteria can produce poisonous *endotoxins*, *enterotoxins*, or *exotoxins*. Various disorders, such as *renal failure*, *liver failure*, and certain metabolic disorders (see *Metabolism*), may cause poisonous substances to be produced or to accumulate within the body.

Poisoning may be acute or chronic. In acute poisoning, a large amount of poison enters, or is produced in, the body over a short time (as may occur in *food poisoning*). Chronic poisoning results from the gradual accumulation of a poison.

P

---

**FIRST AID: POISONING**

> **DO NOT**
> ■ make the victim vomit if he or she has swallowed corrosives

**1** If the victim is conscious, quickly ask what he or she has swallowed.

**2** Call an ambulance and say what the victim has taken.

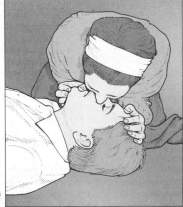

**4** If the victim is not breathing, *artificial respiration* is necessary. Use the mouth-to-nose method to avoid contact with the poison.

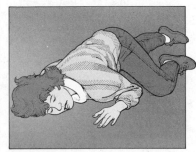

**3** If the victim is unconscious but breathing, place him or her in the *recovery position*.

**5** If you are certain the victim has swallowed only tablets or berries, it may help to induce vomiting by placing your fingers at the back of the throat.

Accidental poisoning is one of the most common types of accident in the home. It occurs primarily in young children, although adults sometimes accidentally poison themselves, often by mistaking the dosage of a prescribed drug (see *Drug poisoning*) or, less commonly, by unthinkingly taking very high doses of certain vitamin or mineral supplements. Exposure to poisonous substances in industry is another important cause of unintentional poisoning in adults, as is *drug abuse*.

Poisoning may be a deliberate attempt to commit *suicide*. However, most such attempts are unsuccessful or are not intended to prove fatal. Taking a drug overdose (often in combination with alcohol, which increases the toxicity of many drugs) is a common method of suicidal poisoning. (See also *Poisoning* first-aid box and articles on individual poisons.)

## Poison ivy
See *Plants, poisonous*.

## Polio
An abbreviation of *poliomyelitis*.

## Poliomyelitis
An infectious disease once known as infantile paralysis but now usually called polio. Poliomyelitis is caused by a virus, which usually provokes no more than a mild illness. However, in more serious cases it attacks the central nervous system (brain and spinal cord). This may lead to extensive paralysis (including paralysis of the muscles involved in breathing) or may be fatal.

Since the development of effective vaccines in the 1950s, polio has virtually been eliminated from the US and Europe; cases still occur in people who have not been fully vaccinated. Polio also remains a serious risk for anyone not vaccinated and traveling in southern Europe, Africa, or Asia.

### INCIDENCE OF PARALYTIC POLIO (US)

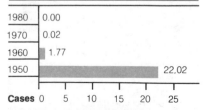

| | |
|---|---|
| 1980 | 0.00 |
| 1970 | 0.02 |
| 1960 | 1.77 |
| 1950 | 22.02 |

Cases 0 5 10 15 20 25

**New cases per 100,000 population**
The incidence has dropped dramatically since the 1950s. In 1986, there were just three reported cases in the entire US.

### CAUSES AND INCIDENCE
There are three closely related polioviruses. Infected people pass large numbers of virus particles in their feces, from where they may be spread indirectly, or directly via fingers, to food to infect others. Airborne transmission also occurs.

In countries where standards of hygiene and sanitation are low, most children become infected and immunity to polio develops early in life, when the infection rarely causes serious illness. In countries with better standards of hygiene, children do not become immune in this manner; if they are not vaccinated, disastrous epidemics occur. Immunization is thus of vital importance.

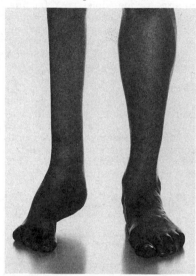

**Wasted limb of polio patient**
Muscle bulk is severely reduced in the paralyzed (right) leg. Muscle function can sometimes be helped by physical therapy.

### PREVENTION
Vaccination is given during infancy, usually in doses at 2, 4, and 18 months of age in the US, with an optional extra dose at 6 months and a booster dose at 5 years (see *Immunization*). The vaccine contains all three types of poliovirus, and immunity develops against each in turn. There are two alternative types of vaccine: IPV (inactivated polio vaccine), which contains dead viruses and is given by injection, and OPV (oral poliovirus vaccine), which contains live but harmless strains of virus and is given by mouth. OPV is the vaccine of choice in the US, except for children who have an *immunodeficiency disorder*, which lowers resistance to infection.

There is an extremely small risk (about one in 5 million doses) of the live vaccine causing polio in the vaccinated person or in a close contact.
### SYMPTOMS AND SIGNS
Minor forms of polio are by far the most common. About 85 percent of children infected with the virus have no symptoms at all. In the rest, after an incubation period of three to five days, there is a short illness with slight fever, sore throat, headache, and vomiting. This lasts for a few days, after which the majority of children recover completely.

In some children, however, after a short period of apparent health there is a major illness with symptoms of *meningitis* (inflammation of the coverings of the brain and spinal cord). The symptoms are fever, severe headache, stiffness of the neck and back, and aching in the muscles, sometimes with widespread twitching. In some cases the condition progresses, often in the course of a few hours, to extensive paralysis of muscles. The legs and lower trunk are the most frequently paralyzed. If infection spreads to the brain stem (lowest part of the brain), the result may be difficulty (or inability) swallowing and breathing.
### DIAGNOSIS
To make a firm diagnosis, the causative virus must be isolated from a sample of cerebrospinal fluid, taken by *lumbar puncture*, or from a throat swab or sample of feces. Muscle paralysis combined with an acute feverish illness is so characteristic of severe polio that it usually enables an immediate diagnosis to be made.
### TREATMENT
There is no effective drug treatment for polio. Nonparalytic patients do not usually need treatment except for bed rest and *analgesics*. When muscles are paralyzed, *physical therapy* is essential to prevent muscle damage while the virus is active. Later, during convalescence, it is needed to help retain muscle function.

When the lower part of the body is paralyzed, the bladder does not function properly and may need catheterization (see *Catheterization, urinary*). Respiratory paralysis requires *tracheostomy* (making an opening in the windpipe to insert a breathing tube) and artificial *ventilation*.
### OUTLOOK
Recovery from nonparalytic polio is complete. Of those who become paralyzed, more than half eventually make a full recovery, more than a quarter suffer only minor permanent

P

muscle weakness, less than a quarter are left with severe disability, and less than one in 10 dies (mainly adults and those in whom the brain stem has been severely affected). Years after extensive paralysis with some recovery, there is a "postpolio" deterioration with new weakness and pain of some of the recovered muscles.

## Pollution
Contamination of the environment by poisons, microorganisms, or radioactive substances.

Serious public concern about pollution developed in the 1950s with the growing realization that *pesticides* were destroying wildlife and poisoning the food chain, and that atmospheric nuclear tests were disseminating radioactive fallout over a wide area (see *Radiation*). This concern was strengthened by incidents of industrial pollution, such as the release of mercury waste into Minamata Bay, Japan (see *Minamata disease*); the release into the atmosphere of the poisonous chemical dioxin by a factory explosion in Italy (see *Defoliant poisoning*); damage to seabirds and beaches from oil tanker spillages; and, more recently, acid rain and radioactive fallout from the nuclear reactor explosion at Chernobyl in the Soviet Union.

Probably the most serious pollutant in its long-term effects is *carbon dioxide*, vast amounts of which are discharged into the atmosphere by the burning of fossil fuels. The continual increase in the atmospheric carbon dioxide level is producing what is called the "greenhouse effect," which is increasing the average global temperature. If the level continues to increase, many experts believe it could cause catastrophic climatic changes within the next 50 years.

Perhaps as serious is the gradual destruction of the *ozone* layer (which blocks harmful ultraviolet radiation from the sun) as a result of the extensive use of aerosols. Other important pollutants include lead (see *Lead poisoning*), cadmium (see *Cadmium poisoning*), *DDT*, and agricultural pesticides, such as *parathion*.

## Poly-
A prefix that means many, much, or excessive, as in polymyositis (inflammation of many muscles) and polyuria (excessive urination).

## Polyarteritis nodosa
Another name for *periarteritis nodosa*.

## Polycystic disease of the kidney
See *Kidney, polycystic*.

## Polycystic ovary
A condition, also known as Stein-Leventhal syndrome, characterized by oligomenorrhea (scanty menstruation) or *amenorrhea* (absence of menstruation), *infertility*, *hirsutism* (excessive hairiness), and *obesity*. Often, but not always, the ovaries contain multiple cysts.

In most women with polycystic ovaries, menarche (the onset of menstruation) occurs at the normal age. After a year or two of regular menstruation, the periods become highly irregular, and then cease. Hirsutism, which often becomes evident around menarche, occurs in about 50 percent of cases, as does obesity.
### CAUSE
The condition is due to an imbalance between the pituitary *gonadotropin hormones* luteinizing hormone (LH) and follicle-stimulating hormone (FSH); there is excessive stimulation of the ovaries by LH and a relative deficiency of FSH. This results in lack of *ovulation* and in increased *testosterone* production by the ovaries.
### DIAGNOSIS
Tests to determine the level of hormones in the blood are needed to confirm the diagnosis. *Ultrasound scanning* of the ovaries and/or *laparoscopy* may be helpful.
### TREATMENT
Methods include drug treatment with clomiphene, progestins, luteinizing hormone-releasing hormone, or oral contraceptives. In rare cases, surgical removal of a wedge of ovarian tissue is performed. The method of treatment used depends on the severity of the symptoms and on whether the woman wishes to become pregnant. Spontaneous ovulation is not unusual in women with polycystic ovary.
### OUTLOOK
Since women with polycystic ovary often have high estrogen levels and irregular menstrual periods, they are at increased risk of heavy periods at menopause and, subsequently, are at increased risk of endometrial (uterine) cancer. Treatment with progesterone may be recommended to restore hormonal balance and decrease the risk of this cancer.

## Polycythemia
A condition characterized by an unusually large number of red cells in the blood due to increased production of red cells by the bone marrow. This condition usually results from some other disorder or is a natural response to *hypoxia* (reduced oxygen in the blood and tissues). In such cases, it is called secondary polycythemia. Rarely, it occurs for no apparent reason and is called polycythemia vera or primary polycythemia.
### SECONDARY POLYCYTHEMIA
Polycythemia occurs naturally in people living at (or visiting) high altitudes due to the reduced air pressure and level of oxygen. It can also result from any disorder that impairs the supply of oxygen to the blood (e.g., chronic *bronchitis*). In these cases, the low blood oxygen stimulates production of the hormone erythropoietin by the kidneys, which in turn stimulates the bone marrow to produce more red cells. The result is an increase in the oxygen-carrying efficiency of the blood, which compensates for the reduced oxygen supply. Descending to sea level, or effective treatment of an underlying disorder, soon returns the blood to normal.

Polycythemia can also be secondary to *liver cancer* or certain kidney disorders that cause excess production of erythropoietin. Treatment of the underlying disorder quickly returns the blood to normal.
### POLYCYTHEMIA VERA
This rare disorder of the bone marrow develops primarily in people over 40. The estimated incidence is about five new cases per million people annually in the US.

The large number of red cells results in an increased volume and thickening of the blood, which may cause headaches, blurred vision, and *hypertension* (high blood pressure). There may also be a flushed skin, dizziness, night sweats, and widespread itching, particularly after a hot bath. Often, the sufferer's spleen is enlarged. In addition, there may be abnormalities in the platelets in blood, causing a tendency to bleed or to form blood clots. Other complications include *stroke* and, at a late stage, other types of bone marrow disease, such as *myelosclerosis* or myelogenous leukemia (see *Leukemia, chronic myeloid*).

The diagnosis is made from a physical examination and *blood tests* and by ruling out any other causes of polycythemia. Treatment of polycythemia vera consists of regular *venesection* (removal of blood through a vein), sometimes in combination with *anticancer drugs* or with radioactive phosphorus taken by

807

mouth to control the overproduction of red cells in the marrow.

Treatment enables most patients to survive for 10 to 15 years. Death usually occurs from a stroke or other complications of the disease.

## Polydactyly

A *birth defect* in which there is an excessive number of fingers or toes. The extra digits may be fully formed and look like the other fingers or toes or they may be fleshy stumps.

Polydactyly affects about 50 babies in every 100,000. It often runs in otherwise normal families, but may also occur as part of the *Laurence-Moon-Biedl syndrome*.

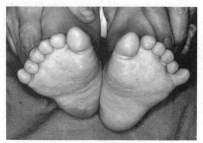

**Polydactyly affecting the feet**
The extra toes can cause problems with footwear and are usually removed surgically during childhood.

## Polydipsia

A medical term for persistent excessive thirst. Polydipsia is an important symptom in people with *diabetes mellitus* and *diabetes insipidus* (see *Thirst, excessive*).

## Polyhydramnios

See *Hydramnios*.

## Polymyalgia rheumatica

An uncommon disease of elderly people that is marked by pain and stiffness in the muscles of the hips, thighs, shoulders, and neck.

### CAUSES AND INCIDENCE

The cause of polymyalgia rheumatica is unknown, but it may be associated with *temporal arteritis*, *rheumatoid arthritis*, systemic *lupus erythematosus*, and, sometimes, cancer.

The disorder affects twice as many women as men and is unusual before the age of 50.

### SYMPTOMS

The pain and stiffness, which may develop gradually or suddenly, make movement difficult. Morning stiffness is notable and often makes getting out of bed a problem. Weight loss and depression may also occur.

### DIAGNOSIS AND TREATMENT

The diagnosis, which is often difficult to confirm, is based on a physical examination, the patient's history, and blood tests (including an *ESR*). If temporal arteritis is suspected, a *biopsy* (removal of a small sample of tissue for analysis) may be performed on an artery in the temple.

Small doses of *corticosteroid drugs* (higher doses when temporal arteritis is present) usually bring about a notable improvement in the disorder within a few days. The dosage is gradually reduced and use of the drug may be discontinued within two years.

## Polymyositis

A rare disease in which the muscles become inflamed and weak. Polymyositis shares the features of *dermatomyositis*, but there is no rash.

## Polymyxins

A group of *antibiotic drugs* derived from the bacterium BACILLUS POLYMYXA. Polymyxins, which include *colistin* and polymyxin B, are commonly given in drop or ointment form to treat eye, ear, and skin infections. Polymyxins are very infrequently given by injection to treat severe infections but in this form may cause nerve or kidney damage. Taken orally, colistin is associated with pseudomembranous enterocolitis (a severe, sometimes life-threatening diarrhea caused by some antibiotics).

## Polyp

A growth that projects, usually on a stalk, from the lining of the nose, the cervix, the intestine, the larynx, or any other *mucous membrane*.

Polyps may need to be removed surgically if they are responsible for symptoms. Some polyps are liable to develop into cancer.

## Polypeptide

A compound that consists of many *amino acids* linked by *peptide* bonds.

## Polypharmacy

The practice of prescribing several different drugs to one person at the same time. Polypharmacy increases the risk of drug interactions (effects that differ from those occurring when a drug is taken alone) and, thus, the risk of adverse effects.

## Polyposis, familial

A rare, inherited disorder, also known as polyposis coli, in which numerous (often a thousand or more) polyps are present in the colon and rectum. The probability of one or more polyps becoming cancerous is extremely high. Without preventive treatment, the development of cancer of the colon (see *Intestine, cancer of*) by age 40 is almost a certainty.

### SYMPTOMS AND DIAGNOSIS

The polyps are not present at birth but usually appear by the age of 10 and may cause bleeding and diarrhea. However, there are often no symptoms until cancer has developed; it is therefore extremely important that a diagnosis be made as early as possible. The polyps are detected by air contrast *barium X-ray examination* and *colonoscopy* (investigation of the colon with a viewing tube).

### PREVENTION AND TREATMENT

Since there is a 50 percent chance that the children of an affected parent will inherit the disease, close medical surveillance is necessary from the age of about 10. This screening, by the diagnostic methods mentioned, is performed every two years until the age of about 40, after which time it is unlikely that polyps will appear.

Because there is such a high risk of cancer, preventive treatment is usually carried out. This often takes the form of total *colectomy* (removal of the entire colon) and the creation of an artificial opening of the ileum (the lower part of the small intestine) through the abdominal wall (see *Ileostomy*). Alternatively, the end of the ileum is joined to the rectum so that a normal passage for bowel movements exists. However, the rectum must be examined regularly to detect polyps, which must be treated immediately before there is a chance for cancerous changes to occur.

## Polyuria

See *Urination, excessive*.

## Pompholyx

An acute form of *eczema* in which itchy blisters form over the palms and/or soles. The condition, often called dyshydrotic eczema, often develops for no apparent reason but is sometimes due to an allergic response to a substance in contact with the skin. It rarely is associated with *ringworm*.

Treatment is with an astringent, which causes the skin to shrink and dry, or with a *corticosteroid drug*.

## Pons

The middle part of the *brain stem*, situated between the midbrain (above) and the medulla oblongata (below).

P

## Pore

A tiny opening. The term usually describes an opening in the skin that releases sweat or sebum (an oily substance secreted by sebaceous glands). Most of the pores from which sebum arises are also hair follicles.

## Porphyria

Any of a group of uncommon inherited disorders caused by the accumulation in the body of substances called porphyrins. Victims often have a rash or skin blistering brought on by sunlight and may have abdominal pain and nervous system disturbances from certain drugs.

### CAUSES, TYPES, AND INCIDENCE

The porphyrins are chemicals with a complex structure and are precursor substances formed in the body during the manufacture of heme—a component of *hemoglobin* (the oxygen-carrying pigment in blood) and of various other important body substances.

The porphyrias result from blocks in the chemical processes by which heme is formed, resulting in accumulation of porphyrins. The blocks are the results of deficiencies of various enzymes in the body; these deficiencies are inherited, usually in an autosomal dominant pattern (see *Genetic disorders*).

Six types of porphyria are recognized—acute intermittent porphyria, variegate porphyria, and porphyria cutanea tarda (the more common types); and hereditary coproporphyria, protoporphyria, and congenital erythropoietic porphyria (all very rare). The prevalence of each varies throughout the world. The combined prevalence in the US is unknown, but is probably about one affected person per 10,000 to 50,000 population.

### SYMPTOMS

Features are as follows.

**ACUTE INTERMITTENT PORPHYRIA** This type usually first appears in early adulthood with attacks of abdominal pain, which may mimic appendicitis. Limb cramps, muscle weakness, and psychiatric disturbances are common. There are no skin symptoms, but the patient's urine turns red when left to stand. A large number of drugs are known to precipitate attacks, including barbiturates, phenytoin, birth-control pills, and tetracyclines.

**VARIEGATE PORPHYRIA** This type is similar in many respects to acute intermittent porphyria, but with blistering of sun-exposed skin. Attacks may be brought on by the same drugs that precipitate acute intermittent porphyria.

**HEREDITARY COPROPORPHYRIA** This type of porphyria is similar to acute intermittent porphyria, with additional skin symptoms in some sufferers.

**PORPHYRIA CUTANEA TARDA** This type also causes blistering on sun-exposed skin, but no abdominal or nervous system disturbance. Wounds are characteristically slow to heal. The urine is sometimes pink or brown. Many cases are precipitated by liver disease, including alcoholic liver disease.

**PROTOPORPHYRIA** This type usually causes mild skin symptoms after exposure to sunlight.

**CONGENITAL ERYTHROPOIETIC PORPHYRIA** This type is extremely rare; it is characterized by red discoloration of urine and teeth, excessive hair growth, severe skin blistering and ulceration, and hemolytic *anemia*. Death may occur in childhood.

### DIAGNOSIS AND TREATMENT

The porphyrias are diagnosed by finding abnormal levels of porphyrins in the urine. More specific tests are available for some types.

Treatment is difficult. Avoiding exposure to sunlight and/or to precipitating drugs is the most important measure. Attacks of acute intermittent porphyria, variegate porphyria, and hereditary coproporphyria can sometimes be helped by administration of glucose or a drug called panhematin, which is chemically related to heme. Porphyria cutanea tarda can be helped by *venesection* (removal of blood through a vein).

## Portal hypertension

Increased blood pressure in the portal vein, a large blood vessel that carries blood from the stomach, intestine, and spleen to the liver. The pressure in the veins of the upper stomach and lower esophagus is raised, causing them to widen (a condition known as *esophageal varices*) and sometimes to rupture. In addition, fluid is forced from the overloaded portal vein, resulting in *ascites*, an accumulation of fluid in the abdomen.

### CAUSES

The most common cause of portal hypertension is the liver disease *cirrhosis*; the scarring and regenerative tissue that form in the organ obstruct the portal vein. Another cause is *thrombosis* (blood clotting) in the vein. This may occur shortly after birth or later in life, when it is usually the result of narrowing of the vein by cirrhosis, compression by enlarged lymph nodes, or inflammation resulting from an infection. Portal hypertension may also be caused by narrowing of the vein from birth.

Rarely, the disorder is due to an abnormal connection between the

P

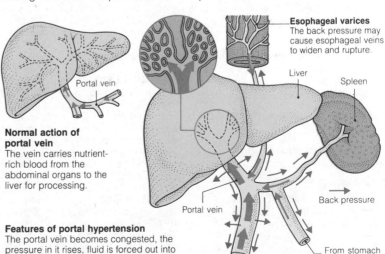

**PORTAL HYPERTENSION**

The most common cause of this condition is liver cirrhosis or some other obstruction to blood flow through the liver. The portal vein becomes congested with blood, and back pressure develops through the system of veins that join the portal vein.

**Esophageal varices**
The back pressure may cause esophageal veins to widen and rupture.

Liver

Spleen

**Normal action of portal vein**
The vein carries nutrient-rich blood from the abdominal organs to the liver for processing.

Portal vein

Back pressure

**Features of portal hypertension**
The portal vein becomes congested, the pressure in it rises, fluid is forced out into the abdomen, and veins that supply the portal vein are widened and may rupture.

From stomach

From intestines

portal vein and an artery (*arteriovenous fistula*), usually as the result of injury. It can also be caused by increased blood flow from the spleen if disease has caused this organ to enlarge.

**SYMPTOMS AND SIGNS**

If the veins in the esophagus and stomach rupture, it causes massive recurrent vomiting of blood and the passing of black feces. Ascites results in abdominal swelling and discomfort and sometimes difficulty breathing.

**DIAGNOSIS**

Portal hypertension is usually diagnosed from the patient's symptoms and signs. The cause can be determined by examining the liver and surrounding blood vessels by means of *ultrasound scanning* and arteriography (see *Angiography*).

**TREATMENT**

Bleeding from ruptured blood vessels is stopped by sclerotherapy, which consists of injection of a solution into or around the veins. This induces inflammation, subsequent scarring, and consequent thickening of the vessels' walls so that the veins are blocked off. Ascites is controlled by dietary sodium chloride (salt) restriction and *diuretic drugs*, which increase urine production.

In some cases, an operation known as a *shunt* may be carried out to divert blood from the portal vein to some other blood vessel, thus relieving the high pressure.

However, studies fail to show any substantial improvement in survival time using sclerotherapy or a shunt for esophageal varices.

The outlook depends on how successfully the underlying cause of the condition can be treated.

## Port-wine stain

A large, purple-red birthmark that is level with the skin's surface. A port-wine stain is a permanent and often unsightly type of *hemangioma*.

## Positron emission tomography

See *PET scanning*.

## Postcoital contraception

See *Contraception, postcoital*.

## Posterior

Relating to the back of the body. In human anatomy, the term is synonymous with *dorsal*.

## Postmaturity

A condition in which a pregnancy persists for longer than 42 weeks; the average length of a normal pregnancy

is 40 weeks from the first day of the last menstrual period (see *Gestation*). Postmaturity may be due to a family tendency to prolonged pregnancy, or it may be an indication that the head is bigger than the mother's pelvis and that the baby is unable to descend properly (see *Engagement*). Many obstetricians attempt to avoid postmaturity by *induction of labor* as the pregnancy nears 42 weeks' gestation.

**COMPLICATIONS**

Because the postmature baby is larger than average and the bones of the baby's skull harder and able to mold less readily, postmaturity is associated with a prolonged labor and an increased risk of a traumatic delivery. The major risk of postmaturity is fetal death and consequent stillbirth; the risk of this occurring doubles by the 43rd week of pregnancy and triples by the 44th week when compared to the normal 40 week pregnancy. This increase in fetal death is in part a consequence of diminished placental efficiency, resulting in the fetus being starved of nutrients and oxygen.

## Postmortem examination

Another term for an *autopsy*.

## Postmyocardial infarction syndrome

Another name for *Dressler's syndrome*.

## Postnasal drip

A watery or sticky discharge from the back of the nose into the *nasopharynx* (the uppermost part of the throat, behind the nose). As the fluid trickles down the throat, it may cause a cough, hoarseness, or a foreign body sensation. The condition is usually caused by *rhinitis* (inflammation of the mucous membrane in the nose); treatment is of the underlying cause.

## Postnatal care

Care of the mother after *childbirth* until about six weeks after delivery.

After delivery the mother's temperature, pulse, and blood pressure are monitored, especially after a *cesarean section* or if there have been any complications, such as *preeclampsia* or kidney disease.

The length of stay in the hospital depends on whether or not there have been any complications; typically, in the US, women stay one to three days after delivery. During the hospital stay, a daily check is made for any signs of *puerperal sepsis* (infection of the genital tract after childbirth), including inspection of the *lochia*

(vaginal discharge after childbirth). If the woman had an *episiotomy* or tears around the vagina, the wounds are checked daily.

The woman is encouraged to walk as soon as possible after delivery to reduce the risk of *thrombosis* (abnormal blood clots). If necessary, help is given with infant feeding techniques (see *Bottle-feeding; Breast-feeding*). There may also be instruction on various abdominal and *pelvic floor exercises*, which can help restore muscle tone.

A final postnatal checkup usually takes place about six weeks after delivery. The obstetrician checks the woman's blood pressure and weight, examines the uterus and bladder to make sure they are in the correct position, and ensures that any wounds are healing properly. Advice on contraception may also be given.

## Postnatal depression

See *Postpartum depression*.

## Postpartum depression

Depression in a woman after childbirth. It is probably caused by a combination of sudden hormonal changes and a variety of psychological and environmental factors. Psychological stress is the major component. Postpartum depression ranges from an extremely common and short-lived attack of mild depression ("baby blues") to a depressive psychosis in which the woman is severely depressed and requires admission to the hospital to prevent harm to herself or her baby.

**MILD DEPRESSION**

Probably more than two thirds of mothers have the "blues," usually starting about four to five days after childbirth. The woman feels miserable, discouraged, irritable, sometimes mentally confused, and may cry easily. Apart from hormonal changes, psychological factors may play a role, including a sense of anticlimax after the birth or an overwhelming sense of responsibility for the baby's care. With reassurance and support from family and friends, the depression usually passes in two or three days.

**MORE SEVERE DEPRESSION**

In about 10 to 15 percent of women the depression is more marked and persists for weeks. There may be a constant feeling of tiredness, difficulty sleeping, loss of appetite, and restlessness. This type of postpartum depression seems more likely to develop if the woman has a strained relationship with her partner, no support from her family, financial or other worries, or a *personality disorder*. At particular risk are women who suffered from depression or anxiety during the pregnancy, first-time mothers, and single-parent mothers. The condition usually clears up of its own accord or responds to treatment with *antidepressant drugs*.

DEPRESSIVE PSYCHOSIS
This severe form of postpartum depression occurs in about one in 1,000 pregnancies and usually starts two to three weeks after childbirth. Since psychosis tends to run in families, its appearance after childbirth probably results from the triggering of latent emotional conflicts by the stress of the birth. Depressive psychosis is marked by severe mental confusion, feelings of worthlessness, threats of suicide or of harm to the baby, and sometimes *delusions*. The woman's moods may change rapidly.

Treatment requires sensitive counseling and *family therapy*. Antidepressant drug therapy may be necessary.

## Postpartum hemorrhage
Excessive blood loss after *childbirth*. Postpartum hemorrhage occurs in about 2 percent of all births. It is more common after a long labor, after a multiple birth, or if the woman required general anesthesia. Before the development of *blood transfusion*, postpartum hemorrhage was a common cause of maternal death.

CAUSES
Most cases of postpartum hemorrhage occur immediately after delivery and are due to excessive bleeding from the site where the placenta was attached to the uterus. Such bleeding may be caused by failure of the uterus to contract efficiently after delivery or by the retention of placental tissue within the uterus.

Postpartum hemorrhage immediately after delivery may also be caused by tears anywhere along the birth canal. Tearing is more likely to occur during a *forceps delivery* or breech delivery. In some cases, postpartum hemorrhage occurs because the mother has a *bleeding disorder*.

Occasionally, postpartum hemorrhage occurs with pain and fever between five and 10 days after delivery. In these cases, the cause of the hemorrhage is usually infection of a retained fragment of placenta.

TREATMENT
A blood transfusion may be given to replace lost blood and emergency treatment may be needed for shock. Other treatment depends on the cause of the hemorrhage. Any retained placental tissue may need to be removed using a general anesthetic, an injection of *ergonovine* may be given to stimulate uterine contractions, and any lacerations in the vagina or on the cervix are sutured. *Antibiotic drugs* are used to treat infection.

## Post-traumatic stress disorder
A specific form of *anxiety* that comes on after a stressful or frightening event. Common causes include natural disasters (such as earthquakes), violence, rape, torture, and serious physical injury. The condition may also result from military combat, when it is sometimes known as battle fatigue or shell shock.

The symptoms include recurring memories or dreams of the event, a sense of personal isolation, and disturbed sleep and concentration. There may be a deadening of feelings, or irritability and painful feelings of guilt, sometimes building to form a true depressive illness (see *Depression*). Symptoms may begin immediately after the trauma or may develop many months later. The symptoms are made worse by any reminder of the traumatic experience.

Most people recover given time, emotional support, and counseling. However, prolonged physical deprivation (such as that experienced in a concentration camp) may scar people psychologically for life.

## Postural drainage
A technique that assists a person whose lungs are clogged with sputum (phlegm) or other secretions to drain them. The person lies in such a way that the secretions drain by gravity into the trachea (windpipe), from

P

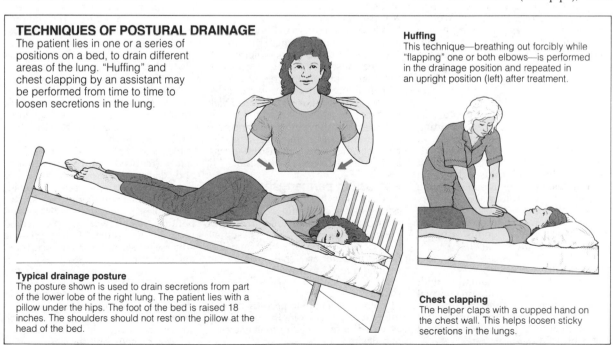

### TECHNIQUES OF POSTURAL DRAINAGE
The patient lies in one or a series of positions on a bed, to drain different areas of the lung. "Huffing" and chest clapping by an assistant may be performed from time to time to loosen secretions in the lung.

**Huffing**
This technique—breathing out forcibly while "flapping" one or both elbows—is performed in the drainage position and repeated in an upright position (left) after treatment.

**Typical drainage posture**
The posture shown is used to drain secretions from part of the lower lobe of the right lung. The patient lies with a pillow under the hips. The foot of the bed is raised 18 inches. The shoulders should not rest on the pillow at the head of the bed.

**Chest clapping**
The helper claps with a cupped hand on the chest wall. This helps loosen sticky secretions in the lungs.

where they are coughed up. Postural drainage is used to treat disorders in which stagnant secretions have become infected (as in acute chest infections in those suffering from chronic *bronchitis*) or are at risk of becoming infected (as in *bronchiectasis* or *cystic fibrosis*).

Postural drainage is sometimes done in association with chest clapping (in which another person gently strikes the chest), theoretically to loosen sticky secretions.

### HOW IT IS DONE

The affected person lies on a bed and each lobe of the lung is drained in turn by the adoption of a different position (see illustration). The different postures are achieved by the person lying supine, prone, or on his or her side; by raising the foot of the bed by varying amounts; and by the use of pillows to elevate different parts of the body. At the same time, the secretions are loosened by the person "huffing" (breathing out forcibly) and raising and lowering the elbows, and by the helper clapping with a cupped hand on the chest wall. A mechanical *vibrator* may be used.

## Postural hypotension

See *Hypotension*.

## Posture

The relative position of different parts of the body at rest or during movement. Good posture consists of efficiently balancing the body weight around the body's center of gravity in the lower spine and pelvis. It is dependent on the shape of the *spine* and on balanced contraction of *muscles* around the spine and in each limb. Maintaining good posture helps prevent neck pain and *back pain*.

Many people have bad posture as the result of habit, such as sitting slumped in a chair or standing with the shoulders and back hunched. Obesity increases the likelihood of bad posture because it increases the strain on muscles. Poor posture may also be caused by neurological disorders (such as *Parkinson's disease*), by muscle disorders (such as *muscular dystrophy*), or by disorders of the joints or bones (such as *ankylosing spondylitis*).

## Potassium

A mineral that; in combination with *sodium* and calcium, maintains normal heart rhythm, regulates the body's water balance, and is responsible for the conduction of nerve impulses and the contraction of muscles.

The body of an average-sized person contains about 5 ounces (140 g) of potassium. Blood levels of the mineral are controlled by the kidneys, which eliminate any excess in the urine. Almost all foods contain potassium, so dietary deficiency is rare. Particularly rich sources include lean meat, whole grains, green leafy vegetables, beans, and many fruits (especially bananas and oranges).

### POTASSIUM DEFICIENCY

A low level of potassium in the blood (called hypokalemia) usually occurs as a result of *gastroenteritis* or some other digestive tract disorder that causes loss of potassium-rich gastrointestinal fluids through diarrhea and/or vomiting. Children are especially vulnerable to this type of potassium loss.

Other potential causes of hypokalemia include prolonged treatment with *diuretic drugs* or *corticosteroid drugs*; overuse of *laxative drugs*; *diabetes mellitus*; *Cushing's syndrome* (overproduction of steroid hormones by the adrenal cortex); *aldosteronism* (overproduction of the hormone aldosterone by the adrenal cortex); certain kidney diseases; excessive intake of sugar, coffee, or alcohol; and extremely profuse sweating.

The effects of mild hypokalemia include fatigue, drowsiness, dizziness, and muscle weakness. In more severe cases, there may be abnormalities of heart rhythm and paralysis of the muscles.

### POTASSIUM EXCESS

Much less common than hypokalemia is an excess of potassium in the blood, a condition called hyperkalemia. It may be caused by taking more than the daily potassium requirement, usually in the form of supplements to correct hypokalemia; by severe *renal failure*; or by *Addison's disease*.

The effects of hyperkalemia include numbness and tingling, muscle paralysis, heart rhythm disturbances, and, in severe cases, *heart failure*.

## Potassium permanganate

A drug that has an *antiseptic* and *astringent* effect, useful in the treatment of *dermatitis* (skin inflammation). Potassium permanganate is sometimes applied to a dressing, may be placed in water as a soak, or may be applied directly to the skin.

## Potency

The ability of a man to perform sexual intercourse; the strength of a drug assessed from its ability to cause certain desired effects.

## Pott's fracture

A combined fracture and dislocation of the *ankle* caused by excessive or violent twisting. In a Pott's fracture, the fibula (the outer of the two bones of the lower leg) is broken just above the ankle, and the tibia (shin) also breaks or the ligaments tear, resulting in dislocation.

Treatment consists of manipulating the bones back into position using a general anesthetic, followed by immobilization of the foot, ankle, and lower leg in a cast for eight to 10 weeks. Screws may be inserted to hold the bone fragments in place.

Severe fracture-dislocations may result in stiffness of the ankle; they increase the likelihood of *osteoarthritis* in later life.

## Poultice

A warm pack consisting of a soft, moist substance (such as *kaolin*) spread between layers of soft fabric. Poultices were once widely used for reducing local pain or inflammation and improving local circulation.

## Pox

Any of various infectious diseases characterized by blistery skin eruptions (e.g., chickenpox). Pox is an outdated term for *syphilis* and still survives as slang.

## Praziquantel

An *antihelmintic drug* used to treat *tapeworm* and *fluke* infestations. Adverse effects include dizziness, drowsiness, and abdominal pain.

## Prazosin

A *vasodilator drug* used as an *antihypertensive drug* in the treatment of *hypertension* (high blood pressure). Prazosin is usually given with a *diuretic drug* and sometimes with other antihypertensive drugs.

Prazosin is also used to treat *heart failure* (reduced pumping efficiency) and *Raynaud's phenomenon* (a circulatory disorder characterized by cold, painful hands and feet).

Prazosin may cause dizziness and fainting by lowering the blood pressure too much. Other possible adverse effects are nausea, headache, and dry mouth.

## Precancerous

A term applied to any condition in which cancer has a tendency to develop. There are three types of such conditions. In the first, there are no tumors present but the condition is

P

known to carry an increased risk of cancer. Examples include *ulcerative colitis* (which carries an increased risk of malignant tumors of the colon or rectum) and *Down's syndrome* (which carries an increased risk of leukemia).

In the second type, there are benign tumors that tend to become malignant themselves or are associated with the development of malignant tumors elsewhere in the body. Examples of this type include *neurofibromatosis* (von Recklinghausen's disease), in which there are large numbers of tumors on the nerves, any of which may become malignant; and *tuberous sclerosis*, in which cancer may develop in the brain, the back of the eye, and various endocrine glands.

The third type comprises disorders that have chronic, sometimes inflammatory or irregular features from the beginning, but which do not always become fully malignant. Disorders within this group include cervical dysplasia (see *Cervix, cancer of*); *leukoplakia* of the mouth (see *Mouth cancer*); and papillomas of the bladder (see *Bladder tumors*).

## Predisposing factors

Factors that lead to increased susceptibility to a disease. Predisposing factors that make a person more likely to have coronary heart disease are a family history of the disease, tobacco smoking, high blood pressure, high *lipid* levels in the blood, being overweight, lack of regular exercise, and mental stress.

## Prednisolone

A *corticosteroid drug* used to reduce inflammation and improve symptoms in a variety of disorders, including *eczema, psoriasis, conjunctivitis, iritis, ulcerative colitis, rheumatoid arthritis,* and *asthma*.

Prednisolone is also used in the treatment of blood disorders, such as *thrombocytopenia* and *leukemia*.

High doses or prolonged treatment may cause adverse effects typical of other corticosteroids, including facial rounding, *acne, hypertension, osteoporosis, peptic ulcer,* and *diabetes mellitus*.

## Prednisone

| CORTICOSTEROID |
| --- |
| Tablet Liquid |
| Prescription needed |
| Available as generic |

A *corticosteroid drug* used to reduce inflammation and improve symptoms in a variety of disorders, including *rheumatoid arthritis* and *ulcerative colitis*. Prednisone is also used in the treatment of severe *asthma*.

Other disorders that are occasionally treated with prednisone include *Addison's disease* and blood disorders, such as *leukemia*. Prednisone is also used to prevent organ rejection after *transplant surgery*.

Large doses taken over a prolonged period may cause adverse effects typical of other corticosteroid drugs.

## Preeclampsia

A serious condition in which *hypertension* (high blood pressure), *edema* (fluid retention), and *proteinuria* (protein in the urine) develop in a woman in the second half of pregnancy. Additional symptoms include headache, nausea and vomiting, abdominal pain, and visual disturbances.

Preeclampsia affects about 7 percent of pregnancies. It is more common in first pregnancies and in women under 25 or over 35; it is also more common if *diabetes mellitus*, hypertension, or kidney disease already exists. Untreated preeclampsia may lead to *eclampsia*, which is characterized by seizures; eclampsia may cause maternal or fetal death.

**TREATMENT**
For mild cases of preeclampsia, the woman is confined to bed, and *antihypertensive drugs* may be used to reduce blood pressure. If the woman is close to term or if eclampsia is imminent, emergency *induction of labor* and delivery may be necessary.

## Pregnancy

The period from conception to birth. Pregnancy begins with conception, the *fertilization* of an ovum (egg) by a sperm and the subsequent implantation of the egg. The fertilized egg develops into the *placenta* and *embryo*, and later into the *fetus*. Most fertilized eggs implant into the uterus. However, occasionally, an egg implants into an abnormal site, such as a fallopian tube, resulting in an *ectopic pregnancy*. (See boxes overleaf on the stages and features of pregnancy and on the effects of hormones during pregnancy.)

**WEIGHT GAIN DURING PREGNANCY**
The average increase in pregnancy is 28 pounds (12.7 kg)—70 percent of it occurring during the last 20 weeks. At term, the typical fetus weighs 7.5 pounds (3.4 kg) and the placenta and fluid together weigh another 3 pounds (1.4 kg). The remaining weight is largely due to water retention and increased fat stores. Within six weeks of delivery, most women return to their pre-pregnancy weight.

**STAYING WELL**
Provided the pregnancy is desired and the woman takes care of herself and has adequate *prenatal care*, there is no reason why she should not overcome some of the early symptoms and feel healthy during pregnancy.

A balanced and nutritious diet is important. Appetite will increase, but pregnant women should avoid filling up on high-calorie snacks, such as potato chips, that are low in nutritional value. It is better to eat frequent, smaller meals. Many physicians prescribe *folic acid* and *iron* supplements during pregnancy.

*Tobacco smoking* and *alcohol* should be avoided throughout pregnancy, and no other drug should be taken except under medical supervision (see *Pregnancy, drugs in*).

Exercise can be continued during pregnancy but overexertion and potentially dangerous sports are generally best avoided.

Sex can continue throughout pregnancy (unless there is bleeding or if the waters break). Adopting different positions may make intercourse more comfortable. Libido may decrease during early and late pregnancy, but many women enjoy sex throughout pregnancy.

**PROBLEMS DURING PREGNANCY**
In addition to the expected features of pregnancy, such as nausea and tiredness, some women experience other minor problems. The symptoms may be troublesome but generally disappear after delivery.

During pregnancy, food passes through the intestine more slowly, which enables more nutrients to be absorbed for the fetus, but which also tends to cause *constipation*. *Hemorrhoids* are fairly common during late pregnancy, as is *heartburn* due to *acid reflux*. The gums may become spongy and bleed easily. *Pica* (a craving to eat substances other than foods, such as clay or coal) is fairly common.

Swollen ankles are common during the second half of pregnancy, especially during the evening. *Varicose veins* may appear in the later months in susceptible women. Leg cramps, backache, and breathlessness are also common during late pregnancy. Pigmentation tends to increase and may cause *chloasma* (mask of pregnancy).

P

*Elective abortion up to 12 wks* (handwritten)

## STAGES AND FEATURES OF PREGNANCY

Pregnancy typically lasts 40 weeks, counted from the first day of the pregnant woman's last menstrual period, and is conventionally divided into three trimesters, each lasting three months. For the first eight weeks following conception, the developing baby is called an embryo; thereafter, it is known as a fetus. It is during the early part of pregnancy (first trimester) that the growing baby is most vulnerable to damage.

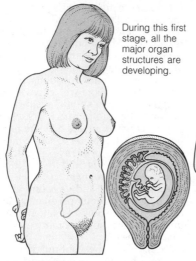

During this first stage, all the major organ structures are developing.

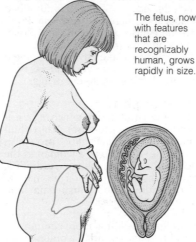

The fetus, now with features that are recognizably human, grows rapidly in size.

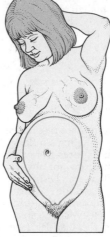

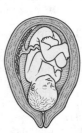

The fetal organs mature in preparation for birth and life outside the uterus.

**First trimester (0 to 12 weeks)**
The first sign of pregnancy is usually the absence of a menstrual period, though some women have breakthrough bleeding. The breasts start to swell and may become tender as the mammary glands develop to prepare for *breast-feeding*. The nipples start to enlarge and the veins over the surface of the breasts become more prominent. A supportive bra should be worn.

Nausea and vomiting are common, are often worse in the morning, and usually persist for six to eight weeks (see *Vomiting in pregnancy*). Urine is passed more frequently and there is often a creamy white discharge from the vagina. Many women feel unusually tired during the early weeks. Some notice a metallic taste in the mouth or a craving for certain foods. Weight begins to increase.

**Second trimester (13 to 28 weeks)**
From 16 weeks, the enlarging uterus is easily felt and the woman begins to look noticeably pregnant. The nipples enlarge and darken, and skin pigmentation may deepen. Some women may feel warm and flushed. Appetite tends to increase and weight rises rapidly. Facial features tend to become heavier. By 22 weeks (usually between the 18th and 20th weeks), most pregnant women have felt the baby moving around (sometimes called "quickening").

During the second trimester, nausea and frequency of urination diminish, and the woman may feel generally better and more energetic than during the early weeks. The heart rate increases, as does the volume of blood pumped by the heart, to allow the fetus to develop properly. These changes put an extra strain on the heart of women who have preexisting heart disease.

**Third trimester (29 to 40 weeks)**
In some women, stretch marks develop on the abdomen, breasts, and thighs. A dark line may appear running from the umbilicus to the pubic hair. *Colostrum* can be expressed from the nipples.

Minor problems are common. Many women become hot and sweat easily, as body temperature rises slightly. More rest may be needed at this stage, though many women find it difficult to find a comfortable position. *Braxton Hicks'* contractions may get stronger.

The baby's head engages (drops down low into the pelvis) around the 36th week in a first pregnancy, but not until a few weeks later in subsequent pregnancies. This "lightening" may relieve pressure on the upper abdomen and on breathing, but increases pressure on the bladder and may result in more vaginal discharge.

---

*Urinary tract infections* are more common during pregnancy, and stress incontinence (see *Incontinence, urinary*) may occur, especially during the later weeks. Vaginal *candidiasis* (thrush) is also more common when a woman is pregnant.

Women may find that their moods are more changeable, which may be the result of hormonal effects on the brain. In addition, women often feel more lethargic than usual, and may experience bouts of depression, may be easily annoyed or angered, and may be prone to bouts of crying.

For complications of pregnancy, see *Antepartum hemorrhage*; *Diabetic pregnancy*; *Hydramnios*; *Miscarriage*; *Preeclampsia*; *Prematurity*; *Rh incompatibility*; *Vomiting in pregnancy*. (See also *Childbirth*; *Fetal heart monitoring*; *Pregnancy, multiple*.)

## Pregnancy, drugs in

Drugs taken during pregnancy may pass from the mother through the placenta to the developing baby. Although only several drugs have been proved to cause harm to a developing baby, no drug should be considered completely safe, especially during early pregnancy. For this reason, a pregnant woman should not take any drug (including over-the-counter drugs) without first consulting her physician.

Drug treatment during pregnancy is usually prescribed only if the potential benefits of treatment outweigh any risk to the baby. Treatment for long-term conditions, such as *epilepsy* or *diabetes mellitus*, is continued during pregnancy but drug therapy may require modification (sometimes even before the woman conceives if pregnancy is planned).

Problems in a developing baby may also be caused if a pregnant woman drinks alcohol (see *Alcohol* in pregnancy box) or smokes tobacco (see *Tobacco smoking* in pregnancy box).

P

## EFFECTS OF HORMONES DURING PREGNANCY

A pregnant woman undergoes many changes that enable her to maintain the pregnancy, nourish the baby, and prepare for breast-feeding.

These adaptations are brought about by increased levels of the female sex hormones *estrogen* and *progesterone*, and by the action of two other

hormones, human chorionic gonadotropin (HCG) and human placental lactogen (HPL), produced only by the placenta.

### EFFECTS OF HORMONES DURING PREGNANCY

| Progesterone | Decreases excitability of smooth muscle, so helps prevent uterine contractions and premature labor. Induces constipation and esophageal acid reflux as a result of its effects on smooth muscle. Increases body temperature. Affects mood. Increases breathing rate. | Estrogens | Are important for the development of the reproductive system and breasts. Stimulate growth of the uterine muscle to enable the powerful contractions of labor. Increase vaginal secretions. Increase size of nipples and help the development of milk glands in breasts. Increase protein production, which is essential for healthy growth of woman and fetus. Alter collagen and other substances to allow body tissues to soften and stretch in preparation for labor. Relax ligaments and joints. May cause sciatica and backache, and contribute to formation of varicose veins as a result of effects on body tissue. |
| --- | --- | --- | --- |
| Human placental lactogen (HPL) | Increases energy production necessary for fetal development. Causes enlargement of breasts and development of milk glands. Induces temporary diabetes mellitus (gestational diabetes) in susceptible women as a result of its effects on metabolism. | | |
| Human chorionic gonadotropin (HCG) | Increases energy production necessary for fetal development. Induces gestational diabetes in susceptible women. | Melanocyte-stimulating hormone (MSH) | Stimulates pigmentation (in combination with estrogens), particularly of the nipples. May also produce chloasma (darkening of facial skin). |

*Drug abuse* during pregnancy can cause serious problems. The babies of women who use *heroin* during pregnancy tend to have a low birth weight and have a higher death rate than normal during the first few weeks after birth. They may suffer withdrawal symptoms, such as feeding and sleeping difficulties, trembling, and seizures. Babies born to women who are intravenous drug abusers have a high risk of being infected with HIV, the *AIDS* virus.

### RISKS

Drugs taken during the first three months of pregnancy may interfere with the normal formation of the baby's organs, causing *birth defects*.

Drugs taken later in pregnancy may slow the rate at which the baby grows, causing a low birth weight. Or they may damage specific fetal tissue, such as developing teeth, which may be damaged by *tetracycline drugs*.

Drugs taken toward the end of pregnancy or during labor and delivery may cause problems for the newborn baby. Narcotic analgesics, for example, may cause breathing difficulty. (See also *Childbirth* pain relief box.)

## Pregnancy, false

An uncommon psychological disorder, medically known as pseudocyesis, in which a woman has the physical signs of pregnancy, including morning sickness, amenorrhea (lack of periods), breast enlargement, and abdominal swelling. Although the results of *pregnancy tests* prove negative and the fetal heart cannot be heard during examination, the woman believes she is pregnant.

Many women with pseudocyesis are childless or approaching the menopause and have an intense desire to have children.

Treatment of pseudocyesis may involve counseling or *psychotherapy*. (See also *Conversion disorder*.)

## Pregnancy, multiple

The presence of more than one fetus in the uterus. Multiple pregnancy can occur if two or more ova (eggs) are released from the ovary and fertilized at the same time. It can also result if a single fertilized ovum divides at an early stage of development. Today, most pregnancies in which there are three or more babies result from the use of *fertility drugs*.

### INCIDENCE

Twins occur in about one in 90 pregnancies, triplets in about one in 8,000 pregnancies, and quadruplets in about one in 73,000 pregnancies.

Multiple pregnancies are more common than average in women who are successfully treated with fertility drugs or if multiple fertilized ova are implanted during *in vitro fertilization*.

### DIAGNOSIS AND TREATMENT

During the woman's prenatal examination, the physician may be able to feel more than one fetus, and may find that the abdomen is larger than expected for the duration of gestation. The physician may also be able to hear more than one fetal heartbeat when listening through a stethoscope. *Ultrasound scanning* may confirm the diagnosis.

The woman is advised to rest during pregnancy and to increase her protein intake. Iron and folic acid tablets are usually recommended.

**COMPLICATIONS**

Hypertension (high blood pressure), *hydramnios*, *postpartum hemorrhage*, and *malpresentation* occur more frequently in a multiple pregnancy. *Prematurity* is a common complication, and the weight of each baby is usually less than that of a single baby. Cesarean section is necessary more often than in single pregnancies.

## Pregnancy tests

Tests on urine or blood performed to determine whether or not a woman is pregnant; some can be performed at home. Pregnancy tests check for the presence of human chorionic gonadotropin (HCG; see *Gonadotropin, human chorionic*), which is produced by the placenta.

**HOW IT IS DONE**

Urine tests are used most often. Most can detect pregnancy about two weeks after a missed period, although some of the newer tests can detect pregnancy within five days. The test is usually done on an early morning midstream urine specimen (because HCG is most concentrated at this

### MULTIPLE PREGNANCY

About one pregnancy in 89 is multiple (e.g., twins or triplets). The rate is highest among women in their 30s. Problems arise more often in multiple pregnancies than in single pregnancies. For example, twins are much more likely than single babies to be born prematurely.

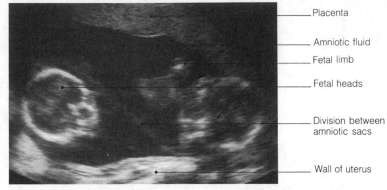

**Ultrasound scan revealing twins**
*Ultrasound scanning* of the woman's uterus can reveal twins within the first several weeks of pregnancy. Here, two fetal heads, a limb belonging to the fetus on the right, and the membrane dividing the two amniotic sacs are visible.

time). Urine tests are about 97 percent accurate if the result is positive and about 80 percent accurate if the result is negative. If the result is negative and there is no menstrual period within about a week, the pregnancy test should be repeated.

Blood tests are normally used only when a very early diagnosis of pregnancy is needed. Blood tests measure

### PREGNANCY TEST KIT

Just one of the many types of pregnancy test kit is shown. No kit is 100 percent accurate. Whether a test indicates pregnancy or gives a negative result despite a missed period, it is wise to consult a physician for confirmation.

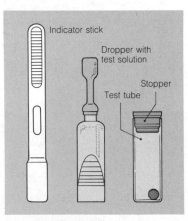

**Components of test kit**
The kit has three main parts—a dropper tube containing a test solution, a test tube with stopper, and an indicator stick.

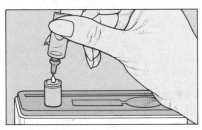

1 The end of the dropper tube is squeezed gently to introduce the test solution into the test tube, which is held upright in a stand provided.

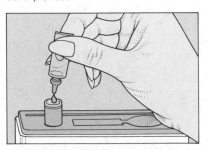

3 Five drops of urine are added to the solution in the test tube. The stopper is put in the test tube, the contents shaken, and the stopper removed.

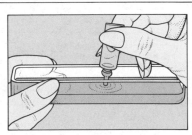

2 The lid of the test kit is used to collect a urine sample early in the morning. Some urine is drawn up into the dropper tube by squeezing and releasing.

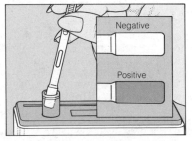

4 The indicator stick is placed in the test tube. The result can be read after 30 minutes. If the end of the stick changes color, it signifies a pregnancy.

the level of HCG in the blood by a laboratory technique called *immunoassay*. It produces a result within nine to 12 days of conception but is more expensive to perform.

## Premature ejaculation

See *Ejaculation, disorders of.*

## Prematurity

Birth of a baby before 37 weeks' *gestation*. A premature labor carries little risk for the mother, but the premature infant may be insufficiently developed to cope with independent life and needs special care.

Prematurity was once a major cause of infant mortality, but improved medical techniques have dramatically increased survival rates of premature infants in developed countries. Approximately 10 percent of babies in the US are born prematurely.

### CAUSES

Some 40 percent of all premature deliveries occur for no known reason. The remainder are due to conditions affecting the mother or fetus.

*Preeclampsia* is the most common maternal cause of premature labor. Other maternal causes include *hypertension* (high blood pressure), longstanding kidney disease, *diabetes mellitus*, and heart disease. Women who have any of these conditions carry an increased tendency to go into labor prematurely. However, more commonly, the pregnancy is curtailed early by *cesarean section* or *induction of labor* by the obstetrician to avoid further risk to mother and baby.

Similarly, *antepartum hemorrhage*, which may result if the *placenta* separates from the uterus before the baby is born, may result in premature labor due to the irritant effect of blood within the uterus. It sometimes makes induction of labor necessary. Other common causes of premature labor are intrauterine infection or premature rupture of membranes.

The most common fetal cause of prematurity is multiple pregnancy (see *Pregnancy, multiple*), which accounts for approximately 15 percent of all premature births. Multiple pregnancy may cause problems in the mother that make cesarean section or induction of labor necessary, or it may cause excessive stretching of the uterus, which stimulates contractions and leads to premature labor. A similar mechanism may occur with *hydramnios* (excessive amniotic fluid) or if the woman's uterine cavity is smaller than normal.

### PREVENTION

If labor begins prematurely and there is no underlying cause, the obstetrician may attempt to stop labor by administering a drug (such as ritodrine) that inhibits contractions of the uterus.

### THE PREMATURE INFANT

The premature infant is not only smaller than a full-term baby but has a characteristic physical appearance—the infant lacks subcutaneous fat, is covered with downy hair called lanugo, and has a very thin, gelatinous skin.

The baby's internal organs are also immature and incompletely developed, making it necessary for the baby to be monitored in a special hospital environment until he or she has developed sufficiently to sustain independent life.

The major complication for a premature infant is *respiratory distress syndrome*, which results from lung immaturity. Other organs, particularly the liver, may also be immature, leading to increased risk of brain hemorrhage, *jaundice*, and *hypoglycemia* (low blood sugar). A premature baby has a limited ability to suck and to maintain body temperature. Additionally, the immune system is poorly developed and the baby is more prone to infection.

### TREATMENT

Premature infants are usually nursed in a special baby unit that provides intensive care. The baby is placed in an *incubator*, which provides warmth and allows easy observation. Other special care may include artificial *ventilation* to assist breathing, artificial feeding through a stomach tube or into a

## PREMATURITY

A premature baby may need to be nursed in an incubator where the temperature and humidity are carefully controlled and the baby can be closely observed. If breathing difficulties develop, they may be treated by artificial ventilation. Very small babies cannot suck so they must be fed intravenously or via a tube passed into the stomach. If jaundice develops, it may be treated by *phototherapy* (light therapy), which breaks up the bilirubin that causes the yellow discoloration of the skin.

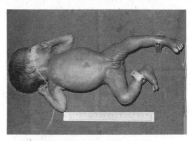

**Premature infant**
This baby girl was born several weeks prematurely. She is being fed via a flexible tube that passes via the nose and esophagus into the stomach.

P

### FEATURES AND COMPLICATIONS OF PREMATURITY

| Physical features | Complications |
| --- | --- |
| Low birth weight (often less than 5.5 pounds) | Increased risk of birth injury |
| Small size | Respiratory distress syndrome |
| Relatively large head and hands | Recurrent bouts of breathing arrest |
| Thin, smooth, shiny skin | Jaundice |
| Veins visible under the skin | Infection |
| Little fat under the skin | Poor temperature control |
| Wizened, wrinkled features | Anemia |
| Soft, flexible ear cartilage | Hypoglycemia (low blood sugar level) |
| Short toenails | and other disturbances of body |
| Downy (lanugo) hair | chemicals |
| Reduced vernix (greasy substance that covers newborn) | Rickets |
| Protuberant abdomen | Increased bleeding tendency |
| Enlarged clitoris (girls) | Brain hemorrhage |
| Small scrotum (boys) | Necrotizing enterocolitis (severe |
| Feeble, whining cry | intestinal inflammation) |
| Irregular breathing | |
| Poor sucking and swallowing ability | |
| Tendency to regurgitate | |

vein, and treatment with *antibiotic drugs* and iron and vitamin supplements. The baby is usually kept in the hospital until he or she reaches a weight of at least 5 pounds (2.25 kg).

### OUTLOOK

The survival chances of a premature baby increase with the length of the pregnancy. With modern techniques, some infants now survive even if they are born as early as 23 weeks' gestation and while weighing less than 2 pounds (1 kg), but this remains exceptional. Of babies born at 28 weeks' gestation, approximately 80 percent survive. Most premature babies catch up with full-term babies before the end of their first year.

## Premedication

The term applied to drugs given one to two hours before an operation to prepare a person for surgery. Premedication usually contains a narcotic *analgesic* (painkiller) to help relieve pain and anxiety and to reduce the dose of anesthesia needed to produce unconsciousness (see *Anesthesia, general*). An *anticholinergic drug* is also sometimes included because it reduces secretions in the airways.

## Premenstrual syndrome

The combination of various physical and emotional symptoms that occurs in women the week or two before *menstruation*. Premenstrual syndrome (PMS) begins at or after *ovulation* and continues until the onset of menstruation. PMS affects more than 90 percent of fertile women at some time in their lives and in some women is so severe that work and social relationships are seriously disrupted.

### CAUSES

Many theories exist for the cause of PMS. Hormonal changes that occur throughout the menstrual cycle clearly influence PMS, but an imbalance between estrogen and progesterone levels has not been consistently found. Similarly, deficiencies of vitamins E and $B_6$ (pyridoxine), magnesium, or prostaglandins have been suggested but not confirmed.

### SYMPTOMS AND SIGNS

The most frequent emotional symptoms of PMS are irritability, tension, depression, and fatigue. Physical symptoms include breast tenderness, fluid retention, headache, backache, and lower abdominal pain.

### TREATMENT

No single method of treatment has proved completely successful. Treatments that may relieve specific symptoms include relaxation techniques to relieve anxiety and tension; *diuretic drugs* to relieve fluid retention; and dietary changes during the latter half of the menstrual cycle (such as avoidance of salt, caffeine, and chocolate). Taking vitamin $B_6$ or evening primrose oil may help some women with breast symptoms, irritability, and depression. *Oral contraceptives*, by eliminating the normal menstrual cycle, can be effective. Progesterone supplements are widely used but do not help all women.

## Premolar

One of eight permanent grinding *teeth*, two on either side in each jaw, located between the canines and molars. (See also *Permanent teeth; Eruption of teeth*.)

## Prenatal care

Care of a pregnant woman and her unborn baby throughout pregnancy with the aim of making sure both are healthy at delivery. Such care involves regular tests on the woman and the fetus to detect disease, defects, or potential hazards, and advising the woman on general aspects of pregnancy, such as diet and exercise.

### FIRST VISIT

A woman should see her obstetrician as soon as she believes she is pregnant. At this time, he or she will take down the medical history of the woman and her family. The physician then examines the woman to confirm that she is actually pregnant and to check her general health. A vaginal examination is carried out to check that the reproductive organs and pelvis are normal and will not present any problems at delivery and to confirm the estimated date of the pregnancy, calculated from the first day of the woman's last period.

The first of a series of screening tests to detect any abnormalities in the woman or baby may be carried out at this visit—see the prenatal screening procedures chart. Some of these tests, such as *ultrasound scanning*, to detect any gross abnormality, usually need to be carried out only once; others, such as *blood tests* to detect *anemia* or *diabetes mellitus* in the woman, may be performed periodically throughout the pregnancy.

At this first visit, too, the woman is given advice about diet and the need not to drink any alcohol and not to smoke, since smoking can stunt the baby's growth and alcohol can result in *fetal alcohol syndrome*.

### SUBSEQUENT VISITS

If there are no problems, the woman visits the physician every month until the 28th week, then every two weeks until the 36th week, and then weekly until the delivery date, which on average is the 40th week from the mother's last menses (menstrual period). If the pregnancy is a high-risk one—for example, if the woman is over 35 years old or is suffering from *hypertension* or diabetes—or if problems develop, visits will be more frequent and, in some cases, the woman may need to be admitted to the hospital for closer observation.

At each visit, as well as undergoing the tests detailed in the chart, the woman is weighed, her blood pressure is taken, and the size of the uterus is estimated to confirm that the baby is growing well.

After the 32nd week, the position of the baby in the uterus (whether it is head-down as it should be) is determined, and the degree of engagement (how far the baby's head has descended into the woman's pelvis) is regularly recorded. The woman is also asked about the baby's movements; frequent pronounced movements indicate an active, healthy baby.

### PREPARATION FOR CHILDBIRTH CLASSES

Childbirth preparation classes (see *Prepared childbirth*) are given in hospitals, physicians' offices, community meeting places, or private homes. Such classes aim to provide information on all aspects of pregnancy, labor, and delivery, including advice on exercise, diet, and sexual activity. The woman learns what happens during labor and the different types of pain relief available during it, and may learn breathing exercises to help her cope with labor and delivery.

## Prepared childbirth

A program of classes for pregnant women and their partners that encourages active involvement in the process of childbirth. Prepared childbirth, also known as natural childbirth or psychoprophylaxis, involves learning relaxation techniques to cope with labor pains so that the use of anesthesia or analgesia (medications for *pain* relief) can be minimized. An important feature of the prepared childbirth method is the involvement of a partner, usually the baby's father, who learns relaxation techniques and breathing exercises along with the expectant mother. The partner provides encouragement, support, and comfort during labor.

## PRENATAL SCREENING PROCEDURES

| When performed | Procedure | Reason for procedure |
| --- | --- | --- |
| First visit | Blood tests | To check the woman's *blood group* and, sometimes, to check for presence of *hepatitis B* virus which might be transmitted to the baby. |
| | Cervical smear test (Pap smear) | To test for an early cancer of the cervix (if a test has not been performed recently). |
| First visit and throughout the pregnancy | Blood tests | To check for *anemia* in the woman and, in women with Rh-negative blood groups, to look for the presence of Rhesus antibodies. |
| | Urine test | To check for *proteinuria*, which could indicate a *urinary tract infection* or *preeclampsia*. |
| | Blood and urine test | To check for *diabetes mellitus*. |
| | Blood pressure check | To screen for *hypertension*, which interferes with blood supply to the placenta and is a sign of preeclampsia. |
| First visit and after any infection | Blood tests | To screen for *rubella*, which can cause defects in the baby, and for *syphilis* and HIV (the *AIDS* virus), which can also be passed on. |
| First 12 weeks | Chorionic villus sampling | May be performed if there is a risk of certain genetic (inherited) disorders being passed on. |
| 16 to 18 weeks | Ultrasound scanning | Is carried out to date the pregnancy accurately and to detect any abnormalities present in the fetus. |
| | Amniocentesis | Carried out on older women and those who have children with *spina bifida* or *Down's syndrome* to detect possible abnormalities in the fetus. |
| | Blood test | In some cases, the amount of *alpha-fetoprotein* in the blood is tested to determine whether the baby has spina bifida. |
| | Fetoscopy and fetal blood sampling | In some cases, these are carried out if there is doubt about the normality of the baby. |
| High-risk or overdue pregnancies | Blood and urine tests | May be administered to assess placental function and well-being of the fetus. |
| | Electronic fetal monitoring | To check on the fetal heart beat. |
| | Ultrasound scanning | Extra scans may be recommended to assess fetal growth and development, the location of the placenta, and the amount of amniotic fluid. |

There are a number of prepared childbirth organizations. In the US, prepared childbirth is often associated with the Lamaze method, which began in the 1940s.

**METHODS**

Prepared childbirth classes are taught by midwives or other qualified childbirth educators. The weekly classes usually begin during the last three months of pregnancy. Most classes are small, containing from six to 10 couples. Information is provided about female anatomy, the physiology of pregnancy, fetal development, labor, delivery, and the postnatal period. Other topics (such as nutrition, breast-feeding, and parenting skills) are also covered.

The primary purpose of the classes is to teach relaxation techniques, often using breathing exercises to help expectant women cope with the pain of uterine contractions and labor. For example, a woman may be taught to concentrate on her breathing pattern, inhaling slowly and deeply initially, then increasing the rate and reducing the depth as the pain of contractions increases. At the end of each contraction, the woman breathes out slowly and relaxes completely. Relaxation techniques help the mother to be aware of muscle tension and to relax during labor.

**OUTCOME**

Of women who use psychoprophylactic preparation for childbirth, about 45 percent require no analgesia during labor; another 45 percent request some analgesia. The remaining 10 percent of women who have attended classes require epidural anesthesia or some other method of pain relief.

## Prepuce
See *Foreskin*.

## Presbycusis
The progressive loss of hearing that occurs with age. Presbycusis is a form of sensorineural *deafness* (degeneration of the hair cells and nerve fibers in the inner ear), which makes sounds less clear and tones, especially higher tones, less audible.

**SYMPTOMS AND CAUSES**

People with presbycusis often have difficulty understanding speech and are usually unable to hear well in the presence of background noise. The severity and progression of the condition vary considerably from person to person (some people who are 80 have far better hearing than others who are only 60).

P

The natural process of presbycusis may be exacerbated by exposure to high *noise* levels, diminished blood supply to the inner ear due to an arterial disease such as *atherosclerosis*, and toxic damage to the inner ear by certain drugs (such as aminoglycoside; see *Antibiotic drugs*).

**TREATMENT**
*Hearing aids* can help most people, except for those with a poor ability to discriminate among speech sounds (and who thus have difficulty understanding what is being said). A person speaking to someone with presbycusis should remember to speak loudly, slowly, and clearly. (If the person with presbycusis is wearing a hearing aid, there is no need to speak in a loud voice.)

## Presbyopia
The progressive loss of the power of *accommodation* for near vision. The focusing power of the eyes weakens with age until, around 65, little or no focusing power remains. Presbyopia is usually noticed around the age of 45 when the eyes cannot accommodate within normal reading distance. Large print can still be seen, but small print may be impossible to focus on; newspapers may need to be read at arm's length.

Simple, convex lens reading *glasses* are used to correct presbyopia. They may need to be changed four to five times over the course of about 20 years, until eventually all the focusing is being done by the glasses.

## Prescription
An instruction written by a physician that directs the *pharmacist* to dispense a particular drug in a specific dose. A prescription also details how often the drug must be taken, how much is to be dispensed, and any other relevant facts. Drugs that require a prescription (prescription medicines) are available only on the authorization of a physician because they are dangerous, powerful, habit-forming, or used to treat a disease that needs to be monitored by a physician.

All prescriptions must bear the name and address of the patient and the physician's signature. The pharmacist keeps a record of all prescriptions dispensed.

## Preservative
A substance that prevents foods and drugs from spoiling. Preservatives include sulfur dioxide and nitrates. (See also *Food additives*.)

## Pressure points
Places on the body where arteries lie near the surface and where pressure can be applied to limit severe arterial *bleeding*. Applying pressure at these points will not stop venous bleeding.

Arterial bleeding can be identified because blood from arteries is bright red and is pumped in regular spurts as the heart beats. To stop bleeding, pressure is applied by hand to compress the appropriate artery against the underlying bone. (See illustrated box, below.)

## Pressure sores
Another common name for *bedsores* (decubitus ulcers).

## Prevalence
The total number of cases of a disease in existence at any one time in a defined population. Prevalence is usually expressed as the number of cases per 100,000 people. Prevalence is one of the two chief measures of how common a disease is; the other is *incidence*. (See also box on next page.)

## Preventive dentistry
An aspect of dentistry concerned with the prevention of tooth decay and gum disease rather than their treatment. Preventive dentistry consists of encouraging the practice of good *oral hygiene* and a reduced intake of sugary foods, *fluoride* treatment to strengthen tooth enamel, and *scaling* to remove any accumulated dental *plaque* and *calculus* from the teeth. (See also *Public health dentistry*.)

## Preventive medicine
The branch of medicine that deals with the prevention of disease by public health measures, such as the provision of pure water supplies; by health education aimed at discouraging smoking and the overuse of alcohol, promoting exercise, and giving advice about a prudent diet; by specific preventive treatments, such as immunization against infectious diseases; and by screening programs to detect diseases such as glaucoma, tuberculosis, and cancer of the cervix before they cause symptoms.

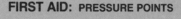

**FIRST AID: PRESSURE POINTS**

**Mechanism of indirect pressure**
If direct pressure on a wound fails to control bleeding, apply indirect pressure by compressing a major artery at a point between the wound and the heart where the artery can be pressed against a bone. In the example at right, the brachial pressure point is used, pressing the artery against the bone of the upper arm, between the armpit and the elbow.

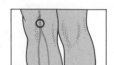

**THE MAJOR PRESSURE POINTS**

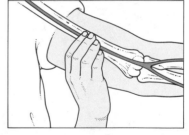

**Temporal**
At the side of the head in front of the ear (for control of scalp bleeding)

**Brachial**
Middle part of upper arm (for control of arm bleeding)

**Radial**
Lower part of arm (for control of bleeding in hand and forearm)

**Femoral**
Center of the fold in the groin (for control of upper leg bleeding)

**Carotid**
At the side of the neck, below the jaw (for control of head and neck bleeding)

**Subclavian**
Between the collarbone and first rib (for control of bleeding in armpit, shoulder, and upper chest)

**Popliteal**
The back of the knee joint (for control of lower leg bleeding)

Most of the increase in the world's population during the 19th century was due to improvements in public health, particularly improvements in the overall standard of nutrition, and the provision of pure water supplies and proper sanitation. Today, these measures remain the priorities of preventive medicine in developing countries, and, along with a program of immunization in childhood, have been targeted as major objectives by the World Health Organization.

However, in developed countries, the primary objective is to persuade the adult population to adopt a healthier life-style. In the US, most premature deaths in adults (that is, deaths before the age of 65) are preventable, being due to accidents and/or linked to such factors as an unhealthy diet, smoking, and excessive drinking. Adoption of a healthier life-style, the wider use of screening for cancers, and measures to reduce accidents could lead to substantial improvements in the nation's health.

## Priapism

Persistent, painful erection of the penis without sexual arousal. Priapism is a dangerous condition that requires emergency treatment.
### CAUSES
Priapism occurs because blood fails to drain from the spongy tissue of the penis, keeping the penis erect. Possible causes include damage to nerves that control the supply of blood to the penis; a blood disease (such as *leukemia* or *sickle cell anemia*) that causes partial clotting of blood in the penis; and, rarely, blockage of the normal outflow of blood from the penis as a result of an infection (such as *prostatitis* or *urethritis*).
### TREATMENT
Urgent treatment is needed because of the risk of permanent damage to the penis. Treatment may involve *spinal anesthesia* (injection of local anesthetic into the spinal canal) or withdrawal of blood from the penis through a wide-bore needle.

## Prickly heat

An irritating skin rash that is associated with profuse sweating. The medical name for prickly heat, miliaria rubra, literally means "red millet seeds." This term describes the numerous tiny, red, itchy spots that cover the mildly inflamed, affected areas of skin. Prickly heat is accompanied by aggravating, prickling sensations. The irritation tends to affect

sites on the body where sweat collects, particularly the waist, upper trunk, armpits, and insides of the elbows.

A milder type (miliaria crystallina) sometimes precedes true prickly heat and produces clear, shiny, fluid-filled blisters that tend to dry up quickly without treatment.
### CAUSES
The mechanism by which prickly heat is caused is not fully understood, but unevaporated sweat is known to be an important factor. The skin becomes unhealthy and waterlogged. Sweat ducts become blocked with debris and eventually leak sweat into the skin. Sleep is often possible only in cool surroundings, and lack of sleep combined with the intense irritation of the rash can make the sufferer irritable.
### TREATMENT AND PREVENTION
Frequent cool showers and sponging the affected areas relieve the itching, although ordinary soap should not be used on affected areas. Application of calamine lotion and dusting powder can further relieve the discomfort.

Clothing should be clean, starch-free, and loose fitting to help sweat evaporation. The chances of developing prickly heat are much reduced by slow acclimation to hot weather. If the sweating has occurred because of fever, *antipyretic drugs* (such as aspirin or acetaminophen) may be helpful.

## Primaquine

A drug used in the treatment of *malaria*. Primaquine is often given after prophylactic treatment with *chloroquine*. It is not effective in the prevention of a malaria attack but kills the parasites in the liver. Primaquine is also used to treat *Chagas' disease*.

Adverse effects include nausea, vomiting, and abdominal pain. In people with *G6PD deficiency*, primaquine may cause hemolytic *anemia*.

## Primary

A term applied to a disease that has originated within the organ or tissue affected, and is not derived from any other cause or source. Primary liver

P

### PREVALENCE OF VARIOUS CHRONIC CONDITIONS IN THE US

(Number of people with the condition per 100,000 population)

| Prevalence | Categorization | Examples |
|---|---|---|
| More than 25,000 | Extremely common | Myopia (nearsightedness) |
| 5,000 to 25,000 | Very common | Male-pattern baldness, partial or total deafness, hypertension (high blood pressure), osteoarthritis |
| 1,000 to 5,000 | Common | Alcohol dependence, asthma, chronic bronchitis, coronary heart disease, all types of diabetes mellitus, psoriasis, schizophrenia |
| 200 to 1,000 | Fairly common | Blindness, epilepsy, rheumatoid arthritis, symptomatic gallstones |
| 50 to 200 | Uncommon | Ankylosing spondylitis, celiac sprue, Down's syndrome, megaloblastic anemia, multiple sclerosis, Parkinson's disease, ulcerative colitis |
| 5 to 50 | Rare | Autism, cystic fibrosis, Crohn's disease, gout, myasthenia gravis, sarcoidosis, sickle cell anemia, systemic lupus erythematosus |
| 0.5 to 5 | Very rare | Achondroplasia, albinism, galactosemia, polycythemia vera, periarteritis nodosa |
| Less than 0.5 | Extremely rare | Alkaptonuria, congenital erythropoietic porphyria |

cancer, for example, is the result of some cancer-producing change in liver cells. Secondary liver cancer results from the spread of cancer cells from another part of the body to the liver.

The term primary is also applied to the first of several diseases to affect a tissue or organ in turn. For example, when a viral infection of the lungs is succeeded by a bacterial infection, the viral infection is called primary and the bacterial infection is termed secondary. Primary also occasionally is used to mean "of unknown cause."

## Primary teeth

The first teeth (also known as deciduous, or milk, teeth), which usually start to appear at the age of 6 months and are gradually replaced by the permanent teeth from about the age of 6 years.

There are 20 primary teeth, 10 in each jaw. Each set of 10 consists of four incisors (biting teeth) at the front, flanked by two canines (tearing teeth), with four molars (grinding teeth) at the back. (See also *Teeth; Eruption of teeth; Teething*.)

## Primidone

An *anticonvulsant drug* used in the treatment of *epilepsy* and, occasionally, *tremor*. Primidone is usually prescribed with another anticonvulsant. Adverse effects include drowsiness, clumsiness, and dizziness.

## Probenecid

A drug used in the long-term treatment of *gout* that reduces the level of uric acid in the body by increasing the amount excreted in the urine.

Probenecid also slows the excretion of *antibiotic drugs* (such as *penicillin drugs* and *cephalosporin drugs*) from the kidneys and is therefore occasionally prescribed with these drugs to boost their levels and thus their effects.

Probenecid may cause nausea and vomiting. It also increases the risk of kidney stones in some people.

## Probucol

A *lipid-lowering drug*. Probucol is often prescribed with other lipid-lowering drugs to boost their effect. Treatment is usually monitored by blood tests.

Possible adverse effects include diarrhea, flatulence, abdominal pain, and, rarely, dizziness.

## Procainamide

An *antiarrhythmic drug* used in the treatment of certain types of *tachycar-*

*dia* (abnormally rapid heart beat) or certain ventricular *arrhythmias*.

Procainamide may cause nausea, vomiting, loss of appetite, and, rarely, confusion. Prolonged treatment may induce *lupus erythematosus*, causing fever, joint pain, swelling, and rash.

## Procaine

A local anesthetic (see *Anesthesia, local*) used before surgical or dental treatment and, sometimes, during childbirth. Procaine has largely been replaced by drugs that are quicker to take effect or are longer-acting.

Occasionally, procaine causes an allergic reaction, with a rash or swelling of the face, lips, mouth, or throat. Rare adverse effects include anxiety, drowsiness, or ringing in the ears.

## Procarbazine

An *anticancer drug* particularly useful in the treatment of *lymphomas*. Procarbazine is also used to treat brain tumors and certain cancers of the skin, lungs, and bone marrow.

In addition to typical anticancer drug adverse effects, procarbazine may cause a sudden rise in blood pressure if taken with certain foods or drinks (e.g., cheese and red wine).

## Prochlorperazine

A *phenothiazine*-type *antipsychotic drug*. Prochlorperazine is used to relieve the symptoms of certain psychiatric disorders, including *schizophrenia* and *mania*. In smaller doses, it is also used as an *antiemetic drug* to relieve nausea and vomiting.

Prochlorperazine may cause involuntary movements of the face and limbs, lethargy, dry mouth, blurred vision, and dizziness.

## Procidentia

A medical term for severe prolapse (displacement of an organ from its normal position in the body), usually of the uterus.

## Proctalgia fugax

A severe cramping pain in the rectum unconnected with any disease. It may be due to muscle spasm, sometimes associated with stress or anxiety. The pain, which may occur at any time, is of short duration and subsides of its own accord.

## Proctitis

Inflammation of the rectum, causing soreness, bleeding, and sometimes a discharge of mucus and pus. Proctitis commonly occurs with inflammation

of the colon as a feature of *ulcerative colitis*, *Crohn's disease*, or *dysentery*. In cases where inflammation is confined to the rectum, the cause is often unknown. However, especially in male homosexuals, it is sometimes due to *gonorrhea* or another sexually transmitted disease. Rare causes include *tuberculosis, amebiasis, bilharziasis*, injury, certain drugs, allergy, or radiation injury.

### DIAGNOSIS AND TREATMENT

The diagnosis is made by *proctoscopy* (inspection of the rectum with a viewing tube). A *biopsy* (removal of a small sample of tissue for laboratory analysis) is sometimes required to determine the precise cause of the rectal inflammation.

Successful treatment of any underlying cause usually clears the problem. *Corticosteroid drugs*, in the form of suppositories or enemas, may relieve symptoms, especially in cases of ulcerative colitis or Crohn's disease.

## Proctoscopy

Examination of the anal canal and rectum by means of a proctoscope (a rigid viewing tube) inserted through the anus. A short, flexible sigmoidoscope (see *Sigmoidoscopy*) is sometimes used and is more comfortable for the person being examined.

## Procyclidine

An *anticholinergic drug* used in the treatment of *Parkinson's disease*. Procyclidine reduces excessive salivation and muscle rigidity and may also improve tremor. Possible adverse effects include dry mouth, blurred vision, and urinary symptoms.

## Prodrome

An early warning symptom of illness. A *migraine* headache attack may be preceded by paresthesia (pins and needles sensation) of an extremity or by an aura composed of visual symptoms—both are prodromes. Awareness of this prodromal period enables a migraine headache sufferer to use certain preventive medications that are far less effective once the headache is established.

## Progeria

Premature old age. There are two distinct forms of the condition, both of which are extremely rare.

In Hutchinson-Gilford syndrome, aging starts around the age of 4, and by 10 or 12 the affected child has all the external features of old age, including gray hair, baldness, and loss of fat, resulting in thin limbs and sagging skin on the trunk and face. There are also internal degenerative changes, such as widespread *atherosclerosis* (fatty deposits lining the artery walls). Death usually occurs at puberty.

Werner's syndrome, or adult progeria, starts in early adult life and follows the same rapid progression as the juvenile form.

The cause of progeria is unknown, although cells taken from affected people show only a few generations of cell division before they stop reproducing, instead of the 50 or so generations that occur in cells taken from healthy young people.

## Progesterone drugs

**COMMON DRUGS**

*Hydroxyprogesterone Medroxyprogesterone Megestrol Norethindrone Norethisterone Norgestrel*

A group of drugs similar to *progesterone hormone*, including natural progesterone and synthetic progesterone derivatives.

**WHY THEY ARE USED**

Progesterone drugs are used in birth-control pills, either on their own (in the mini pill) or with *estrogen drugs* (in combined and phased pills). They work by making the cervical mucus impenetrable to sperm, altering the lining of the uterus so that it prevents the implantation of a fertilized egg, and reducing the production of *gonadotropin hormones*, which may prevent eggs from ripening in the ovary (see *Oral contraceptives*).

Progesterone drugs are also prescribed, sometimes with estrogens, to treat menstrual problems (see *Menstruation, disorders of*).

In *hormone replacement therapy*, a progesterone drug is used in combination with an estrogen drug to reduce the risk of cancer of the uterus (see *Uterus, cancer of*) that occurs if estrogens alone are taken over a long period. The progesterone induces the monthly shedding of the uterine lining.

Progesterone drugs are used also to treat *premenstrual syndrome, endometriosis* (a disorder in which fragments of the lining of the uterus occur elsewhere in the pelvic cavity), and *hypogonadism* (underdevelopment of the ovaries). Progesterone drugs are sometimes effective as *anticancer drugs* in the treatment of certain types of cancers (such as uterine endometrial cancer) that are sensitive to progesterone hormones.

**POSSIBLE ADVERSE EFFECTS**

Adverse effects include weight gain, *edema*, appetite loss, headache, dizziness, rash, irregular periods, breast tenderness, and *ovarian cysts*.

## Progesterone hormone

A female sex hormone essential for the healthy functioning of the female reproductive system. Progesterone is produced in the ovaries during the second half of the menstrual cycle (see *Menstruation*) and by the placenta during *pregnancy*. Small amounts of progesterone are also produced in the adrenal glands and testes.

Following *ovulation*, increased production of progesterone causes the endometrium (lining of the uterus) to thicken in preparation for the implantation of a fertilized egg. If fertilization does not take place, the production of progesterone and also of *estrogen hormones* falls, resulting in shedding of the uterine lining and unfertilized egg in the monthly period.

During pregnancy, progesterone is essential for normal functioning of the placenta and thus for the healthy development of the baby. Progesterone also passes into the developing baby's circulation, where it is converted in the adrenal glands to corticosteroid hormones. At the end of pregnancy, a fall in the level of progesterone helps initiate labor.

Other effects of progesterone produce changes in the cervix and vagina during the menstrual cycle, increased deposition of fat, and increased *sebum* production by glands in the skin.

## Progestin

Another name for a *progesterone hormone* or a synthetic *progesterone drug*.

## Prognathism

Abnormal protrusion of the lower jaw or both jaws. If the condition interferes with biting and chewing (see *Malocclusion*) or is disfiguring, *orthognathic surgery* may be performed.

## Prognosis

A medical assessment of the probable course and outcome of a disease. It is based on the recorded history of the disease (e.g., 90 percent of people with small cell carcinoma of the lung die within five years of the condition developing), the physician's own experience of treating the disease, and the patient's general condition and age. However, every prognosis is no more than an informed guess, and any patient may prove it wrong.

## Progressive muscular atrophy

A type of *motor neuron disease* in which the muscles of the hands, arms, and legs become weak and wasted and twitch involuntarily. This is a progressively debilitating condition that eventually spreads to other muscles in the body.

## Prolactinoma

A benign tumor of the pituitary gland that causes overproduction of the hormone prolactin. In a woman, prolactinoma may result in *galactorrhea* (breast secretion at any time other than a few days before childbirth or during breast-feeding), *amenorrhea* (absence of periods), or *infertility*. In a man, a prolactinoma may cause *impotence* and *gynecomastia* (breast enlargement). In either sex, it may cause headaches, *diabetes insipidus*, and, if it presses on the optic nerves, gradual loss of the outer field of vision.

The condition is diagnosed from blood tests to measure prolactin levels, and from *CT scanning* or *MRI* of the brain. Treatment may consist of removal of the tumor, *radiation therapy*, or the drug bromocriptine, which inhibits prolactin secretion.

## Prolapse

Displacement of part or all of an organ or tissue from its normal position. Common structures that prolapse include the uterus (see *Uterus, prolapse of*) and the disk between two vertebrae (see *Disk prolapse*).

## Promazine

A *phenothiazine*-type *antipsychotic drug* sometimes used as a sedative. Promazine also acts as an *antiemetic drug* and is used to relieve nausea and vomiting after anesthesia.

Possible adverse effects include abnormal movements of the face and limbs, drowsiness, lethargy, dry mouth, constipation, and blurred vision. Long-term treatment may be associated with *parkinsonism*.

## Promethazine

An *antihistamine drug* used to relieve itching in a variety of skin conditions, including *urticaria* (hives) and *eczema*. Promethazine is also used as an *antiemetic drug* to relieve nausea and vomiting caused by *motion sickness* and *Meniere's disease*.

Promethazine has a sedative effect and is therefore sometimes used as a *premedication* (drug used to prepare a person for surgery) and as a short-term sleeping drug for children. Occasionally, promethazine is given to produce sedation during *childbirth*.

Adverse effects of promethazine may include dry mouth, blurred vision, and drowsiness.

## Pronation
The act of turning the body to a prone (facedown) position, or the hand to a palm backward position. The opposite movements are called *supination*.

## Propantheline
An *antispasmodic drug* used in the treatment of *irritable bowel syndrome* and certain types of urinary *incontinence*. Propantheline is rarely used today in the treatment of certain forms of *peptic ulcer*.

Possible adverse effects include dry mouth, blurred vision, and abnormal retention of urine.

## Prophylactic
A drug, procedure, or piece of equipment used to prevent disease; the term prophylactic is popularly used to refer to a *condom*.

## Propoxyphene
A weak narcotic *analgesic* (painkiller) sometimes combined with other analgesics, such as *aspirin* or *acetaminophen*, to boost their effects.

Propoxyphene may cause drowsiness, dizziness, nausea, and vomiting. Used long-term, it may produce dependence (see *Drug dependence*).

## Propranolol
A *beta-blocker drug* used to treat *hypertension* (high blood pressure), *angina pectoris* (chest pain due to inadequate blood supply to the heart muscle), and cardiac *arrhythmias* (irregularities of the heart beat). It is also used to reduce the risk of further damage to the heart after *myocardial infarction*.

Propranolol is used to relieve symptoms of *hyperthyroidism* (overactivity of the thyroid gland) or of *anxiety* (e.g., stage fright), and to prevent attacks of *migraine*.

Possible adverse effects are typical of other beta-blocker drugs.

## Proprietary
A drug patented for production by one company. The patent protects the drug's name, ingredients, and process of manufacture.

## Proprioception
The body's internal system for collecting information about its position relative to the outside world and the

state of contraction of its muscles. This is achieved by means of sensory nerve endings within the muscles, tendons, joints, and sensory hair cells in the balance organ of the inner ear. These structures are called proprioceptors (literally "position sensors").

Information from the proprioceptors passes to the spinal cord and brain and is used to make adjustments in the state of contraction of muscles so that posture and balance are maintained. During movement, there is a continuous feedback of information to the brain from the proprioceptors and from the eyes. This helps ensure that actions are smooth and coordinated.

## Proptosis
A term for protrusion of the eyeball (see *Exophthalmos*).

## Propylthiouracil
A drug used to treat *hyperthyroidism* (overactivity of the thyroid gland) or to control symptoms before *thyroidectomy* (removal of the thyroid gland).

Possible adverse effects include itching, headache, rash, and joint pain. Propylthiouracil may reduce the production of white blood cells by the bone marrow and thus increase the risk of infection.

## Prostaglandin
One of a group of *fatty acids* that is made naturally in the body and that acts in a similar way to *hormones*. Prostaglandins are divided into broad groups according to their chemical structure. They were first discovered in semen but are now known to occur in many different body tissues, including the uterus, brain, and kidneys. Some prostaglandins are prepared synthetically for use as drugs (see *Prostaglandin drugs*).

**EFFECTS**
Prostaglandins produce a wide range of effects on the body, including causing pain and inflammation in damaged tissue, protecting the lining of the stomach and duodenum against ulceration, and stimulating contractions during labor (see box).

Certain drugs counteract the effects of prostaglandins on the body. *Nonsteroidal anti-inflammatory drugs* (NSAIDs), *aspirin*, and *corticosteroid drugs* relieve pain and inflammation by reducing prostaglandin production in tissues. Taken long-term, however, NSAIDs and aspirin may increase the risk of a *peptic ulcer*, in part by reducing production of prostaglandins that protect the stomach lining.

## Prostaglandin drugs
Synthetically produced *prostaglandins* that have a variety of therapeutic uses.

Dinoprostone is an $E_2$ prostaglandin used to stimulate contractions of the uterus for *induction of labor* at full term, after a fetal death, or to induce a late abortion (see *Abortion, elective*).

Carboprost and dinoprost are $F_2$ prostaglandins that resemble dinoprostone by inducing contractions of the uterus.

*Alprostadil* is an $E_1$ prostaglandin used (temporarily) to treat newborn infants awaiting surgery for certain types of congenital heart disease. Alprostadil is also being investigated for use in the treatment of people with *Raynaud's disease*.

Other prostaglandin drugs are under investigation for use in a variety of disorders, including *peptic ulcer*.

## Prostate, cancer of
A malignant growth arising in the outer zone of the *prostate gland*. Cancer of the prostate is the second most common cancer in men. It sometimes develops in middle age but most often occurs in the elderly. While its precise cause is unknown, the hormone *testosterone* appears to be involved.

### EFFECTS OF SOME PROSTAGLANDINS

| Type | Effect |
|---|---|
| $PGA_1$ | Lowers blood pressure<br>Protects against peptic ulcer |
| $PGD_2$ | Causes inflammation |
| $PGE_1$ | Stimulates contractions of the uterus<br>Lowers blood pressure<br>Protects against peptic ulcer<br>Reduces stickiness of platelets in blood |
| $PGE_2$ | Causes inflammation<br>Widens airways<br>Increases stickiness of platelets in blood<br>Stimulates contractions of the uterus |
| $PGF_2$ | Stimulates contractions of the uterus<br>Narrows airways |
| $PGG_2$ | Causes inflammation |
| $PGI_2$ | Reduces stickiness of platelets in blood |

## SYMPTOMS AND SIGNS

Symptoms are caused by enlargement of the prostate (see *Prostate, enlarged*) and include difficulty starting urination, poor flow of urine, and increased frequency of urination. Eventually the flow of urine may cease completely either because the urethra is completely blocked or because the cancer has spread to the bladder and ureters. In advanced cases, pain may be caused by involvement of nerves within the pelvis or by spread of cancer to bones anywhere in the body.

## DIAGNOSIS

Cancer of the prostate is usually diagnosed at a physical examination in which the physician feels the prostate through the rectum; a diseased gland feels hard and knobby. The diagnosis may be confirmed by *ultrasound scanning*, *pyelography*, and prostatic biopsy (removal of a sample for analysis). Blood tests and a bone scan may be performed to assess the extent to which a cancer has spread.

## TREATMENT

Treatment may be by *prostatectomy* (surgical removal of the prostate) or *radiation therapy*; if the disease has spread to other parts of the body, patients may be helped by reducing the level of testosterone. This may be done by *orchiectomy* (surgical removal of the testes), by giving *estrogen drugs*, or by giving drugs that resemble *luteinizing hormone-releasing hormone*.

## OUTLOOK

When the growth is discovered at an early stage, the outlook is very good. However, if the cancer has spread outside the prostate gland and does not respond to hormone treatment, the prognosis is poor. The cancer is so advanced in a majority of people discovered to have cancer of the prostate that radical surgery offers little hope for cure.

## Prostatectomy

An operation to remove part or all of the *prostate gland*. Prostatectomy is usually performed when enlargement of the gland is causing obstruction to the flow of urine (see *Prostate, enlarged*). The operation may also be performed to treat cancer of the prostate (see *Prostate, cancer of*) and, in some cases, *prostatitis*.

## HOW IT IS DONE

The most common method is transurethral prostatectomy, which is performed by means of *cystoscopy*. If the prostate gland is very enlarged, retropubic prostatectomy may be performed (see box, overleaf).

## RECOVERY PERIOD

After removal of the catheter and drainage tube, the patient can begin to pass urine as the bladder fills in the normal way. Initially, urination may be frequent and sometimes painful; occasionally, there is mild incontinence for a few weeks. Patients are encouraged to drink large amounts of fluid to help wash out remaining blood in the urine.

Rarely, bleeding after the operation is severe, and blood transfusions are required. Blood clots that may form within the bladder can be washed out through the catheter.

The hospital stay is about three to five days for transurethral prostatectomy and about eight to 10 days for the retropubic operation. After several weeks, patients may resume all activities, including intercourse.

## OUTLOOK

The operation may affect potency or sexual sensation in a small percentage of men. The majority of men are sterile after prostatectomy because semen is expelled backward into the bladder instead of being ejaculated. Seminal fluid in the bladder is not harmful and is excreted in the urine.

## Prostate, enlarged

Often called benign prostatic hypertrophy, an increase in size of the inner zone of the *prostate gland*, usually affecting men over 50. The cause is unknown.

## SYMPTOMS AND SIGNS

Symptoms usually develop gradually as the enlarging prostate compresses and distorts the urethra. The flow of urine is obstructed, and there is difficulty starting urination and a weak stream.

Initially the bladder muscle becomes overdeveloped to force urine through the obstructed urethra. Eventually the bladder is unable to expel all the urine (see *Urine retention*) and becomes distended, causing abdominal swelling.

There may be *incontinence* due to overflow of small quantities of urine, and the bladder may become overactive, resulting in frequency of urination (see *Urination, frequent*). This is a sign of bladder muscle failure and usually means surgery is required.

Severe abdominal pain and the ability to pass only a few drops of urine indicates acute urinary retention and requires immediate treatment.

## DIAGNOSIS

Enlargement of the prostate can be detected during a *rectal examination* (in which the physician inserts a gloved finger into the rectum). The physician also feels the abdomen for signs of bladder distention.

A sample of urine may be tested for infection and a blood test performed to provide a measurement of kidney function. *Ultrasound scanning*, *pyelography*, and a recording of the strength of urine flow may be performed to give additional information about the severity of the obstruction and any effects elsewhere in the urinary system, especially the kidneys.

## TREATMENT

Mild symptoms of prostatic enlargement do not require treatment. If symptoms are more severe, the usual treatment is *prostatectomy* (removal of the prostate). Retention of urine is treated initially by urinary *catheterization* and then by prostatectomy. If surgery is considered too dangerous because of age or ill health, a catheter is sometimes kept in place permanently to drain urine.

## Prostate gland

A solid, chestnut-shaped organ surrounding the first part of the urethra in the male. The prostate gland is situated immediately under the bladder and in front of the rectum.

P

---

**LOCATION OF PROSTATE GLAND**
Located under the bladder and in front of the rectum, the prostate gland secretes substances into the semen as the fluid passes through ducts leading from the seminal vesicles into the urethra.

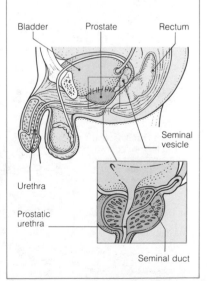

Bladder  Prostate  Rectum

Seminal vesicle

Urethra

Prostatic urethra

Seminal duct

The prostate gland produces secretions that form part of the seminal fluid during ejaculation. The ejaculatory ducts from the seminal vesicles pass through the prostate gland to enter the urethra.

The prostate gland weighs only a few grams at birth. Enlargement starts at puberty from the effect of *androgen hormones* and stops at around the age of 20, when it reaches its adult weight of about 20 grams. In most men, the prostate begins to enlarge further after the age of 50.

The prostate gland consists of two main zones: an inner zone (which produces secretions responsible for keeping the lining of the urethra moist) and an outer zone (which produces seminal secretions).

**DISORDERS**

Prostatic problems very rarely occur before the age of 30. *Prostatitis* (inflammation of the prostate) is usually caused by bacterial infection and may be sexually transmitted. It usually affects men in their 30s and 40s, but can occur later in life.

Enlargement of the prostate (see *Prostate, enlarged*) usually affects men over 50 and may interfere with urination by compressing the urethra.

Cancer of the prostate (see *Prostate, cancer of*) is common in old age and may cause symptoms similar to those that occur with enlargement of the prostate gland.

**Prostatism**

Symptoms resulting from enlargement of the prostate gland (see *Prostate, enlarged*).

---

## PROSTATECTOMY—REMOVAL OF THE PROSTATE GLAND

Of the two possible methods of removal shown, the transurethral method is the most commonly used.

It avoids the disadvantages of an abdominal incision and usually permits a shorter stay in the hospital.

The retropubic method may be necessary if the prostate is very enlarged or if a cancer is suspected.

### TRANSURETHRAL PROSTATECTOMY

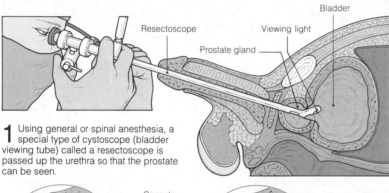

1 Using general or spinal anesthesia, a special type of cystoscope (bladder viewing tube) called a resectoscope is passed up the urethra so that the prostate can be seen.

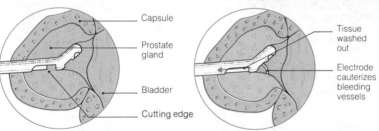

2 A heated wire loop, or sometimes a cutting edge, is inserted through the resectoscope and used to cut away as much of the prostatic tissue as possible.

3 The pieces of tissue are washed out through the resectoscope and any bleeding vessels are cauterized by means of an electrode passed up the tube.

4 The resectoscope is then withdrawn and a catheter passed via the urethra into the bladder. The catheter is left in place for several days to drain urine from the bladder and allow blood to be washed out.

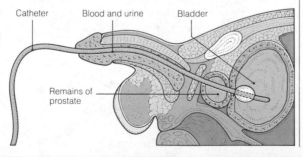

### RETROPUBIC PROSTATECTOMY

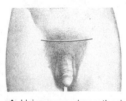

**Site of incision**

1 Using general anesthesia, an incision is made in the abdomen to expose the bladder and prostate. The surgeon cuts open the capsule containing the gland.

2 The surgeon then removes the prostatic tissue by hand. Bleeding vessels are cauterized and a catheter passed up the urethra to drain urine from the bladder.

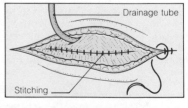

3 A tube is inserted into the empty capsule to drain fluid and blood; the abdomen is sewn up. The tube and catheter are left in for about a week.

## Prostatitis

Inflammation of the *prostate gland*, usually affecting men between the ages of 30 and 50. Prostatitis is often caused by a bacterial infection that has spread from the urethra. The infection may or may not be sexually transmitted. Presence of a urinary catheter increases the risk of prostatitis.

### SYMPTOMS AND SIGNS

Prostatitis causes pain when passing urine and increased frequency of urination; it sometimes causes fever and a discharge from the penis. There may be pain in the lower abdomen, around the rectum, and in the lower back, and blood in the urine.

### DIAGNOSIS AND TREATMENT

The physician examines the prostate by inserting a gloved finger into the rectum; the gland will be tender and enlarged. To investigate the cause of infection, tests are carried out on a urine sample and on urethral secretions obtained after massaging the prostate gland.

Treatment is with *antibiotic drugs*, although the condition may be slow to clear up and tends to recur. If an abscess develops, surgical drainage may be necessary.

## Prosthesis

An artificial replacement for a missing or diseased part of the body. Examples of a prosthesis used to restore normal function include a false leg or arm fitted after amputation (see *Limb, artificial*) or an artificial heart valve used to replace a valve damaged by disease (see *Heart valve surgery*).

Prostheses are also used for cosmetic reasons. Examples include a breast prosthesis fitted after *mastectomy* (removal of a breast) and a glass eye inserted following removal of a diseased eye (see *Eye, artificial*).

## Prosthodontics

The branch of dentistry concerned with the replacement of missing teeth and their supporting structures. Prosthodontics includes three basic kinds of replacement—partial or complete *dentures* (which are easily removed for cleaning), semipermanent appliances such as overdentures (fittings that are attached over existing teeth), and permanent restorations such as crowns and bridges (see *Crown, dental*; *Bridge, dental*).

## Proteins

Large molecules that consist of hundreds or thousands of *amino acids* linked (by peptide bonds) to form long chains, which are often folded in various ways. In addition to amino acids, proteins may contain constituents such as sugars and lipids.

There are two main types of proteins: fibrous and globular. Fibrous proteins are insoluble and form the structural basis of many body tissues, such as hair, skin, muscles, tendons, and cartilage. Globular proteins are soluble and include all *enzymes* (substances that promote biochemical reactions in the body); many *hormones*, such as growth hormone and prolactin; and various proteins in the blood, including *hemoglobin* and *antibodies*. In addition, the *chromosomes* in cell nuclei are formed of proteins linked with *nucleic acids*; proteins linked with lipids constitute a major part of cell membranes (see *Cell*).

### PROTEINS AND DIET

Proteins are needed in the diet primarily to supply the body with amino acids. Ingested proteins are broken down in the *digestive system* to amino acids, which are then absorbed and rebuilt into new body proteins (see *Protein synthesis*). In general, animal proteins have a higher nutritional value than do plant proteins, because they have more essential amino acids. (See also *Nutrition*.)

## Protein synthesis

The formation of *protein* molecules inside cells through the linking of much smaller substances called amino acids. Because proteins provide many of the structural components and the *enzymes* that promote biochemical reactions in the body, their manufacture—in the correct numbers and order—is essential to all aspects of development and growth.

Different cells manufacture a different range of proteins. The instructions for their manufacture are held by the hereditary material—the *genes*, which consist of *DNA* (deoxyribonucleic acid)—within the nucleus of the cell. Protein synthesis starts with a gene (a particular length of DNA) acting as a template for the manufacture of a strand of a substance called messenger RNA. Like DNA, RNA is a *nucleic acid* and consists of a string of building blocks called nucleotide bases. There are four different types of nucleotide bases; their sequence in the strand of messenger RNA provides the coded instructions (the *genetic code*) for making a certain protein.

The strand of messenger RNA passes out of the cell nucleus, where it is then decoded (see diagram, next page) to cause a polypeptide chain (string of amino acids) to be produced. Several polypeptide chains may be manufactured and combine to form one protein molecule.

The rate of protein synthesis is regulated through adjustments in the amount of the relevant messenger RNA formed within the cell nucleus. Highly complex mechanisms exist for "blocking" or "unblocking" messenger RNA copying from DNA; this ensures that the cell makes the right type of proteins, in the right quantities, and at the right time.

## Proteinuria

The passage of increased amounts of protein in the urine. Proteinuria may result from damage to the glomeruli (filtering units in the *kidney*), allowing proteins to leak from the blood into the urine (see *Glomerulonephritis*). The condition may also result from damage to the kidney tubules, preventing the normal reabsorption of protein from the urine. Increased protein in the urine may also occur because of a generalized disorder (such as *myeloma*) that causes an increase in the blood protein level.

Proteinuria rarely causes any symptoms, although the urine may appear frothy. The condition is usually discovered during a routine *urine test* or during investigation of an underlying disorder.

## Protoplasm

An obsolescent term for the entire contents of a cell, including the cytoplasm and organelles such as the nucleus. Today, the word protoplasm has largely been replaced by specific terms for the individual cell components (see *Cell*).

## Protozoa

The simplest, most primitive type of animal; each protozoon consists of a single cell. All types of protozoa are of microscopic size, but bigger than bacteria. The more advanced types are capable of excretion, respiration, and engulfing food particles; they move around through jellylike movements or the use of whiplike or hairlike attachments called flagella. Some protozoa are parasites of larger animals during various stages of the life cycle.

About 30 different types of protozoa are troublesome parasites of humans. Included among them are the organisms that cause *amebiasis* and

P

## STEPS IN PROTEIN SYNTHESIS

Proteins consist of one or more subunits called polypeptides. These are formed, within cells, from building blocks called amino acids, which are provided to each cell as raw materials. The instructions for making polypeptides are encoded in the DNA within the cell nucleus.

**1** To make a specific protein or polypeptide, the relevant section of DNA (or *gene*) in a cell nucleus is used as a template to make a strand of a substance called messenger RNA. Like DNA, this consists of a string of substances called nucleotide bases.

**2** The messenger RNA passes out of the cell nucleus into the cytoplasm, where it is latched onto by several decoding particles called ribosomes. Starting at one end, the ribosomes travel along the RNA strand.

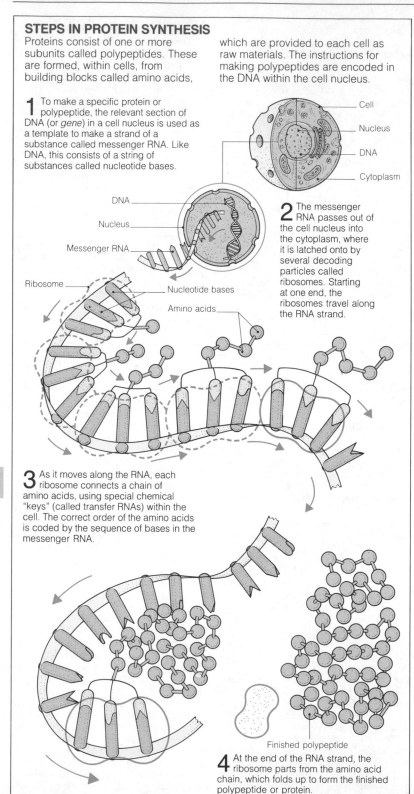

Cell
Nucleus
DNA
Cytoplasm

DNA
Nucleus
Messenger RNA
Ribosome
Nucleotide bases
Amino acids

**3** As it moves along the RNA, each ribosome connects a chain of amino acids, using special chemical "keys" (called transfer RNAs) within the cell. The correct order of the amino acids is coded by the sequence of bases in the messenger RNA.

Finished polypeptide

**4** At the end of the RNA strand, the ribosome parts from the amino acid chain, which folds up to form the finished polypeptide or protein.

*giardiasis* (intestinal infections that cause diarrhea); the sexually transmitted infection *trichomoniasis*; and the insect-borne tropical diseases *malaria, sleeping sickness,* and *leishmaniasis*. *Toxoplasmosis* (a disease acquired from cats) is also caused by a protozoon.

## Protriptyline

An *antidepressant drug*. Protriptyline is especially useful in treating narcolepsy and when *depression* is accompanied by lethargy and tiredness, because it is less likely than other antidepressants to cause drowsiness.

## Proximal

Describing a part of the body that is nearer to a central point of reference, such as the trunk of the body. The hip joint is proximal to the knee; the knuckle is proximal to the fingernail. The opposite of proximal is *distal*.

## Prurigo

A nonspecific term for an itchy rash.

## Pruritus

The medical term for *itching*. Types include pruritus ani (itching of the skin around the anus) and pruritus vulvae (itching of the external genital area in women).

## Pseud-/pseudo-

Prefixes that mean false, as in pseudocyesis (a false pregnancy).

## Pseudarthrosis

A false joint. The term is used to describe an operation in which the ends of two opposing bones in a joint are removed and a piece of tissue (usually muscle) is fixed between the resulting gap to act as a cushion.

The procedure is used to restore mobility and reduce pain when a hip *arthroplasty* (joint replacement operation) has failed. It results in shortening of the affected leg and instability of the joint. A walking aid is usually required after the operation.

Pseudarthrosis also describes a rare condition in children in which congenital abnormality of the bone of the lower half of the tibia (shin) leads to spontaneous fracture without injury. Treatment of this condition consists of inserting a nail through the bone ends and applying a *bone graft*. If the bone ends fail to unite, amputation of the leg, followed by fitting of an artificial limb, may be necessary.

## Pseudocyesis

See *Pregnancy, false*.

P

## Pseudodementia

A form of severe *depression* in elderly people that mimics *dementia*. Features of both illnesses include intellectual impairment and loss of memory. Nearly one in 10 of those initially thought to be suffering from dementia may turn out to have a depressive illness. Unlike dementia, depression is treatable; many people respond well to *antidepressant drugs*.

## Pseudoephedrine

A *decongestant drug* used to relieve *nasal congestion*. Pseudoephedrine is an ingredient of a variety of cough and cold remedies.

High doses may cause anxiety, nausea, dizziness, and, occasionally, hypertension (high blood pressure), headache, and palpitations.

## Pseudoepidemic

An outbreak of an illness in a community or in an institution (such as a school) that has no detectable physical cause but is thought to be due to a form of *hysteria*. Typically, the symptoms are vague and mild—headache and a general feeling of sickness—and are induced by group suggestibility combined with anxiety provoked by contact with somebody who has the symptoms. *Sick building syndrome* is an example of a condition that may be a pseudoepidemic.

## Pseudogout

A form of *arthritis* that results from the deposition of calcium pyrophosphate crystals in a joint. The underlying cause of pseudogout is unknown; in rare cases, it is a complication of *diabetes mellitus, hyperparathyroidism,* and *hemochromatosis.*

Symptoms include intermittent attacks of arthritis similar to *gout*. Pseudogout can be distinguished from gout only by examining a sample of the joint fluid under a microscope to identify the crystals, which are different from the urate crystals found in gout.

Treatment is with *nonsteroidal anti-inflammatory drugs.*

## Pseudohermaphroditism

A congenital abnormality in which the external genitalia resemble those of the opposite sex. Thus, a female pseudohermaphrodite may have an enlarged clitoris resembling a penis and enlarged labia resembling a scrotum. Conversely, a male may have a very small penis and a divided scrotum resembling labia.

Pseudohermaphroditism is usually caused by an endocrine disorder, such as *adrenal hyperplasia.*

The condition differs from true *hermaphroditism*; in pseudohermaphroditism, the person has only ovarian or testicular tissue and not both.

## Psilocybin

A *hallucinogenic drug* similar to *LSD*.

## Psittacosis

A rare illness resembling *influenza* that is caused by a microorganism, CHLAMYDIA PSITTACI, and is spread to humans from birds such as parrots, pigeons, or poultry.

The infection is contracted by inhaling dust contaminated by the droppings of infected birds. Most cases occur among poultry farmers, pigeon owners, and pet store owners, although anyone who acquires a pet parrot is at slight risk. A hundred or so cases are reported in the US each year, though there are probably many more undiagnosed cases.

### SYMPTOMS, DIAGNOSIS, AND TREATMENT

The illness in birds is occasionally serious or even fatal, but often causes no more than lethargy.

Human illness is extremely variable in its features, the most common symptoms being fever, severe headache, and cough. They develop a week or more after exposure to infected birds. Other symptoms include muscle pains, sore throat, nosebleed, lethargy, and depression. In some severe cases, there is also breathing difficulty.

The cause of the condition is often suspected from the patient's occupation; it is diagnosed by the finding of *antibodies* (proteins with a defense role) specific to the causative organism in the patient's blood. Treatment with tetracycline antibiotics is usually effective. Without treatment, the illness may continue for several weeks or months before subsiding; it may occasionally be fatal if unrecognized and not treated.

## Psoas muscle

A muscle that bends the hip upward toward the chest. The psoas muscle is composed of two parts (psoas major and psoas minor) that originate from the lower spine.

The lower end of psoas minor is attached to the margin of the pelvis; the lower end of psoas major is joined to the prominence just below the neck of the femur (thigh bone).

### LOCATION OF PSOAS MUSCLE

The muscle has two parts—major and minor. The psoas major acts to flex the hip (bend it upward toward the trunk) and rotates the thigh inward. The psoas minor acts to bend the spine down toward the pelvis.

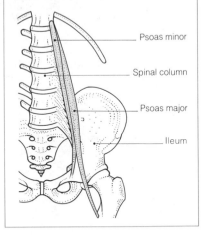

- Psoas minor
- Spinal column
- Psoas major
- Ileum

A rare disorder of the psoas muscle is an *abscess* (collection of pus), which develops as a complication of *osteomyelitis* (bone infection) of the spine, usually caused by *tuberculosis*.

## Psoralen drugs

### COMMON DRUGS

*Methoxsalen Trioxsalen*

> **WARNING**
> During psoralen treatment, always protect eyes and lips from the sun and avoid overexposure to ultraviolet light.

Drugs containing chemicals called psoralens, which occur in certain plants (such as buttercups) and are present in some perfumes. When absorbed into the skin, psoralens react with *ultraviolet light* to cause darkening or inflammation of the skin. Psoralen drugs may be taken by mouth or applied to the skin.

### WHY THEY ARE USED

Psoralen drugs may be used to treat *psoriasis* and *vitiligo* (a disorder in which patches of skin lose color).

### HOW THEY WORK

Used in *phototherapy* in conjunction with ultraviolet light, psoralen drugs stimulate the production of skin pigment and, in psoriasis, slow the rate at which skin cells grow and multiply.

P

### POSSIBLE ADVERSE EFFECTS

Overexposure to ultraviolet light during psoralen treatment or too high a dose of a psoralen drug may cause redness and blistering of the skin. Psoralens in perfumes may cause a rash when the skin is exposed to ultraviolet light (see *Photosensitivity*). The use of psoralens in suntanning preparations is prohibited in the US because these chemicals can cause *sunburn*.

## Psoriasis

A common skin disease characterized by thickened patches of inflamed, red skin, often covered by silvery scales. Although psoriasis does not usually cause itching, the affected area may be so extensive that great physical discomfort and social embarrassment may result.

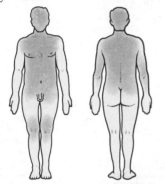

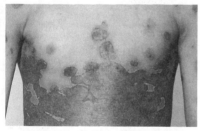

**Distribution and appearance of psoriasis**
The knees, elbows, scalp, trunk, and back are common sites for psoriasis. The usual appearance is of patches of thickened skin covered by dry, silvery, adherent scales.

### CAUSES AND INCIDENCE

The exact cause of psoriasis is not known but it tends to run in families. Psoriasis occurs in about 2 percent of people in the US and Europe and is probably less common in blacks and Asians. It affects men and women equally. Psoriasis usually appears between ages 10 and 30, but infants occasionally suffer from the condition and it may also sometimes develop in old age.

The underlying abnormality in psoriasis is that new skin cells are produced about 10 times faster than normal, but the rate at which old cells are shed remains unchanged. As a result, the live cells accumulate and form the characteristic thickened patches covered with dead, flaking skin.

Psoriasis tends to recur in attacks of varying severity; attacks may be triggered by a number of factors, such as emotional stress, skin damage, and physical illness.

The skin eruption is sometimes accompanied by a painful swelling and stiffness of the joints that can be highly disabling (see *Arthritis*).

### TYPES

The disease has different forms that may need different treatment.

**DISCOID OR "PLAQUE" PSORIASIS** In this type, the most common form, patches appear on the trunk and limbs, particularly the elbows and knees, and on the scalp. In addition, the nails may become pitted, thickened, or separated from their beds.

**GUTTATE PSORIASIS** This form occurs most frequently in children. It consists of numerous small patches that develop rapidly over a wide area of skin, often after a sore throat.

**PUSTULAR PSORIASIS** This form is characterized by small pustules, all over the body or confined to the palms, soles, and other isolated locations.

### TREATMENT

Mild psoriasis may be helped by moderate exposure to sunlight or an ultraviolet lamp (see *Phototherapy*) and use of an emollient (soothing cream). Moderate attacks are usually treated with an ointment containing coal tar or anthralin. Other methods of treating psoriasis include *corticosteroid drugs*, *PUVA* (a type of phototherapy), and some types of *anticancer drugs*, such as methotrexate.

The arthritis is treated with *non-steroidal anti-inflammatory drugs*, *antirheumatic drugs*, or methotrexate.

### OUTLOOK

For most people, psoriasis is a long-term condition with no permanent cure, although individual attacks can be completely relieved with appropriate treatment.

## Psych-

A prefix meaning mental processes or activities, as in psychiatry.

## Psyche

A term meaning mind (as opposed to body) that was derived from the ancient Greek for soul or spirit. The most influential description is provided by Freud's *psychoanalytic theory*, which treats the psyche as an organ of the body that is divided into the conscious and unconscious. Each has its own set of functions.

## Psychedelic drugs

Drugs (many illicit) that may produce hallucinations, also known as *hallucinogenic drugs*.

## Psychiatrist

A physician who specializes in the treatment of mental, emotional, or behavioral problems. A psychiatrist conducts physical examinations, performs laboratory tests, and traces the patient's personal and family history to seek the cause of the problem. Treatment may include medication with counseling or *psychotherapy* (individually or in groups), *psychoanalysis*, or *behavior therapy*.

## Psychiatry

The branch of medicine concerned with the study, prevention, and treatment of mental illness and emotional and behavioral problems. Psychiatry is differentiated from *psychology*, which is principally concerned with the normal mental processes and behavior of people.

Psychiatry is broad in scope; it approaches the understanding and treatment of mental problems from psychological, social, and physical aspects. Some psychiatrists assert that major mental illness is due to genetic and biochemical factors, while psychoanalytically oriented psychiatrists believe that environmental experiences are still the major cause of mental illness. Laboratory investigations and drug treatments have played an increasingly important role in modern psychiatry.

Within psychiatry there are a number of subspecialties, including child and adolescent psychiatry, social psychiatry (focusing on social factors as a cause of mental illness), community psychiatry (addressing care of the mentally ill outside psychiatric hospitals), forensic psychiatry (dealing with legal issues, such as rape), and neuropsychiatry (relating to brain disorders with mental symptoms).

## Psychoanalysis

A treatment for mental illness based on *psychoanalytic theory*. The system was developed by Sigmund Freud at the beginning of the 20th century as a result of treating, under hypnosis, patients who were supposedly suffering from hysteria. He believed that mental disorders were a result of the failure of normal emotional development during childhood. By encouraging the patient to reenact these years and verbalize any problems (past or present), Freud believed that the cause of any internal strife would be uncovered and resolved, and the illness would be cured.

**WHY IT IS DONE**
Psychoanalysis can help *neurosis* and *personality disorders*. A modified psychoanalytic approach has also been used to treat *psychosis* (when medication is often an important adjunct). Psychoanalysis aims to help the patient understand his or her emotional development and to help the person make appropriate adjustments in particular situations.

**HOW IT IS DONE**
The treatment involves interviews between a trained analyst and the patient, each lasting perhaps an hour, repeated up to six times a week and continuing for an indefinite period, usually for several years. Traditionally, the patient lies on a couch with the analyst behind and out of sight, although some therapists prefer to face the patient, who sits in a chair. In dealing with psychotic patients, the psychoanalyst refrains from having the patient lie down on a couch because, in some cases, the structure and reality of face-to-face contact with the psychiatrist is an extremely important element.

The patient is encouraged to talk as freely as possible about his or her life history and any problems that may have occurred in the past or are currently causing concern. This stream of talk is one of free association, with one word or idea leading to another without conscious control so that any repressed material has the opportunity to surface. The analyst interprets these associations in the light of psychoanalytic theory, paying particular attention to areas of resistance that may contain clues to the person's problem. This leads to different trains of thought, more experiences relived, and sometimes exposure of reasons for symptoms.

Psychoanalysis relies on a number of other key processes. A very close relationship develops with the analyst, who eventually comes to be associated in the patient's mind with important people in his or her history (e.g., mother, father, or sister). This experience is called *transference*.

Interpretation of the patient's dreams is another important aspect of the treatment. It is believed that material normally repressed comes to the surface while the patient dreams, usually in the form of symbolic representations (see *Dream analysis*).

The patient is often reluctant to accept the analyst's interpretations and may introduce *defense mechanisms* (such as denial) to cope with the unfolding explanation of his or her behavior. This reaction is a defense against the anxiety that is stimulated as these repressed conflicts break through into consciousness. Understanding the self-destructive patterns of living is an essential aspect of psychoanalytic treatment.

## Psychoanalyst

A person who treats people with certain mental illnesses using the methods of *psychoanalysis*.

The psychoanalyst is usually a doctor of medicine. Following a residency in psychiatry, the psychiatrist is accepted to an accredited institute for psychoanalysis. Finally, the psychiatrist undergoes his or her own psychoanalysis at the institute to resolve as much as possible his or her own emotional problems.

## Psychoanalytic theory

A system of ideas developed by Sigmund Freud early in this century that explains the development of personality and behavior in terms of unconscious wishes and conflicts.

Psychoanalytic theory has undergone considerable distillation by psychoanalysts over the years. However, its basic concepts and the use of *psychoanalysis* (therapy based on the concepts of psychoanalytic theory) have dominated psychiatry in the US for half a century.

**KEY FEATURES OF FREUDIAN THEORY**
Freud placed great emphasis on the importance of sexuality (in its broadest sense) in psychological development. His theory postulates that, during the first 18 months, an infant passes through three phases—oral, anal, and genital—each representing the area of the body that the child devotes attention to at a particular age. After these phases, the child is able to direct attention to people outside himself or herself. Sexual attraction to the parent of the opposite sex develops with consequent desire to eliminate the other parent, who prevents fulfilment of the desire—the *Oedipus complex*.

By the age of 5 or 6, sexual feelings become latent, but reemerge at puberty. At this time, psychological and emotional problems may occur if the individual has not developed normally through the successive stages and has become fixed at a primitive level (see *Fixation*). Problems may also occur if the Oedipus complex has not been successfully dealt with.

Less specifically sexual aspects of psychological development are seen as depending on the interaction among the three parts that make up the personality—the id, ego, and superego. The id is the basic component that guides the individual unconsciously and instinctively toward pleasure; the ego mediates, by conscious reasoning, between internal desires and the reality of the outside world; the superego is also a controlling force but is unconscious, being derived from moral and social standards indoctrinated by parents and other authorities.

It is thought that mental illness results if conflict between the three aspects of personality cannot be satisfactorily resolved. Freud believed that under normal circumstances tension is dealt with by (among other *defense mechanisms*) repression (in which painful ideas or unacceptable thoughts are kept out of consciousness) and sublimation (in which emotional drives that cannot openly be expressed are channeled into an acceptable activity, such as sports). These normally healthy unconscious processes can become harmful if they occur inappropriately or in excess.

Psychoanalysis has, however, progressed since Freud. In general, modern psychoanalysis is based on the observation that emotional problems for the most part are the result of troubled childhood experiences in the family. The pre-Oedipal problems that are caused by difficulties in the early mother-child relationship are probably even more important than later Oedipal conflicts. Such conflicts can form the basis of later neurotic or psychotic disturbances.

It is necessary for the child to separate from the mother to become an individual and comprehend reality. A healthy mother and father help the child to become an individual. Conflict-ridden parents distort reality and program patterns of disturbed self-destructive behavior. Psychoanalysis in practice attempts to bring to light these unconscious conflicts with the parent (which have led to distortions

P

of reality). The aim is to free the individual from the past and help him or her become a real person in the present. The relationship and interaction between physician and patient is an essential part of this process.

## Psychodrama
An adjunct to *psychotherapy* in which the patient acts out certain roles or incidents. They may relate to people closely involved with the patient or may concern situations that he or she finds particularly stressful. The aims of psychodrama are to bring out hidden concerns and to allow a person's disturbing feelings to be expressed. Psychodrama is often carried out with a partner or in a group of patients; music, dance, and pantomime may also be used.

## Psychogenic
A symptom or disorder that originates from psychological or emotional problems and is not produced or caused by any physical illness.

## Psychologist
A nonmedical specialist in the diagnosis and treatment of mental and emotional problems. Because psychologists are not physicians, they cannot prescribe drugs. Their role with patients generally involves testing, *counseling*, or *psychotherapy*.

## Psychology
The scientific study of mental processes. Psychology deals with all internal aspects of the mind, such as *memory*, feelings, *thought*, and *perception*, as well as external manifestations, such as *speech* and behavior. It also addresses *intelligence*, *learning*, and the development of *personality*. Methods employed in psychology include direct experiments, observations, surveys, study of personal histories, and special tests (such as *intelligence tests* and *personality tests*).

Within psychology, a number of different approaches are used. Neuropsychology attempts to relate human behavior to brain and body functions. Behavioral psychology studies the way people react to events and learn to adapt accordingly. Cognitive psychology concentrates on thought processes; it is based on the theory that what a person thinks about his or her behavior is of equal importance to the behavior itself. Psychoanalytic psychology stresses the role of the unconscious and childhood experiences (see *Psychoanalytic theory*).

There are many specialized areas within the science. Educational psychologists study learning and intelligence, clinical psychologists work with emotional and behavioral problems, social and industrial psychologists consider the effects of work and the environment on behavior, and experimental psychologists concentrate on research into new ways of understanding mental events. The emergence of developmental psychology as a specialist area is due to the work of the Swiss psychologist Jean Piaget, who noted that there are certain stages in a child's intellectual development—from simple motor skills to logical and abstract thought.

## Psychometry
The measurement of psychological functions. Psychometry includes statistical assessment of intelligence and personality (see *Intelligence tests*; *Personality tests*) as well as numerous methods of testing specific aptitudes, such as memory, logic, concentration, and speed of response. The design of such measurements has become increasingly sophisticated, but the validity of many tests (that is, whether they measure what they are supposed to measure) is less certain.

## Psychoneurosis
A term now used interchangeably with *neurosis*. Neurosis originally referred to any disorder of the nerves; psychoneurosis specifically described nervous disorders associated with psychological symptoms.

## Psychopathology
The study of abnormal mental processes. There are two main approaches in psychopathology—the descriptive and the psychoanalytic.

Descriptive psychopathology aims to record, as objectively as possible, the symptoms that make up a diagnosis of psychiatric illness. It is particularly concerned with *thought disorders* (such as *delusion*), with mood disturbances, and with the various forms of *hallucination*. The ability to recognize such symptoms when interviewing patients is an important part of the psychiatrist's job.

The psychoanalytic approach is concerned with the unconscious feelings and motives of the individual; they are studied by *psychoanalysis*.

## Psychopathy
An outdated term for *antisocial personality disorder*.

## Psychopharmacology
The study of drugs that affect mental states. Since the early 1950s, more effective medications for a wide range of mental illness have been developed. Particular advances have occurred in the treatment of psychotic illnesses, with the development of *antipsychotic drugs* and *antidepressant drugs*. *Antianxiety drugs* have proved to be extremely effective in relieving symptoms in neurotic illness, but the dangers of dependence have been recognized recently.

## Psychosexual disorders
A range of conditions related to sexual function. Psychosexual disorders are assumed to stem from psychological problems, although some (e.g., *impotence*) may also be caused by physical injury or illness. Psychosexual disorders include *transsexualism* (a sense that one's anatomical sex is inappropriate), *psychosexual dysfunction* (interference with the normal process of sexual response), and sexual deviations (sexual behavior in which intercourse between adults is not the final aim; see *Deviation, sexual*).

## Psychosexual dysfunction
A disorder in which there is interference with the normal process of sexual response in the absence of any known organic cause. Psychosexual dysfunctions are very common in both men and women. They usually start in early adult life, often disappearing spontaneously with experience and increased confidence.

The main dysfunctions affecting men are lack of sexual desire (see *Sexual desire, inhibited*), *impotence*, and premature ejaculation (see *Ejaculation, disorders of*); those affecting women are lack of sexual desire, painful intercourse (see *Intercourse, painful*), *vaginismus*, and lack of orgasm (see *Orgasm, lack of*).

Most psychosexual problems start in early adult life. Some are associated with certain personality traits, including anxiety and obsessiveness. Unpleasant early experiences, such as sexual interference in childhood or problems with the first sexual encounters, are especially likely to inhibit later sexual performance. Unrealistic ideas about normal sexual behavior or a strict upbringing may also increase the likelihood of sexual problems. Many different kinds of feelings and conflicts (basically nonsexual) can be expressed sexually or interfere with normal sexual expression.

Psychosexual dysfunctions are common and not usually evidence of serious illness. About 80 percent of people respond well to *sex therapy*, which is usually brief behavioral therapy with the couple. Sex therapy is also done with an individual or a group of solo men and solo women. Instructors offer sex education and instructions for home practice of helpful techniques in relaxation and sensual pleasuring.

## Psychosis
A severe mental disorder in which the individual loses contact with reality. It contrasts with *neurosis*, which describes the milder group of mental illnesses. Neurotic individuals generally know they are ill, but psychotic illness so disturbs the ability to think, perceive, and judge clearly that sufferers often do not realize they are sick. Psychosis is what people commonly think of as "madness."

### TYPES
Three main forms of psychosis are generally recognized, although the symptoms overlap and there is considerable debate as to whether each is truly a separate category. They are *schizophrenia, manic-depressive illness*, and organic brain syndrome (see *Brain syndrome, organic*).

Paranoid illness (see *Paranoia*) is sometimes regarded as a fourth form of psychosis, but many psychiatrists see it as a distinctive disorder.

### SYMPTOMS
The main feature of psychotic symptoms is that they may lead the person to view life in a distorted way. Symptoms include *delusions, hallucinations, thought disorders*, loss of *affect* (emotion), *mania*, and *depression*.

### CAUSES
Some physicians believe that psychotic symptoms are due to disordered brain function. Psychoanalytically oriented physicians tend to believe that psychotic behavior is a result of deep disturbances in the mother-child relationship and overwhelming emotional trauma.

Research is centered on the role of *neurotransmitters* (chemicals released by nerve endings), such as dopamine, and on the importance of the limbic system and frontal lobes of the brain. As yet no specific physical abnormality that might be isolated by a blood test or X ray has been clearly related to psychosis. However, a new form of brain imaging, *PET scanning*, may begin to reveal hints as to the causes of these disorders.

### TREATMENT AND OUTLOOK
*Antipsychotic drugs* are usually very effective in controlling symptoms, usually as an adjunct to *psychotherapy*. Treatment may need to be long-term, but many sufferers are able to lead normal working lives. The relationship of patient to therapist (see *Transference*) is extremely important because in many cases it is through this relationship that the patient reestablishes contact with reality.

## Psychosomatic
A term used to describe physical disorders that seem to have been caused, or worsened, by psychological factors. Just as a physical reaction (such as crying) may be due to emotion, so it is presumed that worries or unpleasant events can cause physical illness.

For a disorder to be labeled psychosomatic, the psychological factor and physical effect must be closely connected in time and repeatedly related. This is because many chronic illnesses constantly vary in severity, regardless of a person's psychological state, and because there is a tendency to assume that an event was stressful just because a person has become ill.

Common examples of conditions that may fit the psychosomatic label are headache, breathlessness, nausea, *asthma, irritable bowel syndrome, peptic ulcer*, and certain types of *eczema*. (See also *Somatization disorder*.)

## Psychosurgery
Any operation on the brain carried out as a treatment for mental symptoms. Psychosurgery is performed only as a last resort to treat severe mental illnesses that have not responded to other forms of treatment.

### TYPES
Prefrontal *lobotomy* was once the most widely used form of psychosurgery, but it often resulted in harmful side effects and has now largely been replaced by other, safer operations.

The most commonly performed operations today are forms of *stereotaxic surgery*. In these operations, a small hole is drilled in the skull above one temple. A scalpel or diathermy probe is inserted and, under X-ray control, guided to specific areas of the brain, where small cuts are made in nerve fibers. Stereotaxic procedures are most often carried out to provide relief of severe *depression* or *anxiety* or to treat disabling *obsessive-compulsive behavior*.

Performed less often are the more complex, "open" operations, in which a complete portion of the skull is cut through and lifted up to expose the brain so that specific areas can be removed. Parts of the temporal lobe are cut out to treat *temporal lobe epilepsy*. In rare cases, complete lobes are removed in an attempt to treat violent or aggressive behavior.

### OUTLOOK
Psychosurgery has produced good results in some people, enabling those who would otherwise be chronically disabled to lead more useful lives. However, the operations often have inconsistent and unpredictable results, and can produce adverse changes in personality and intellect. They remain a controversial form of treatment for psychiatric illness.

## Psychotherapist
Any person who uses *psychotherapy* as a formal method of treatment. Treatment varies according to the approach used (e.g., if it is based on *Freudian theory* or *Jungian theory*). Many psychotherapists have no medical background, but certain personal characteristics are deemed especially important, notably empathy (the ability to understand what a patient is feeling), genuineness (the therapist appears to mean what he or she says), and warmth. The psychotherapist also requires sufficient maturity and experience to be able to cope with the demanding task of dealing with the mental and emotional problems of his or her patients.

## Psychotherapy
The treatment of mental and emotional problems by psychological methods. In psychotherapy, the patient talks to a therapist about symptoms and problems and establishes a therapeutic relationship with the therapist.

### WHY IT IS DONE
Psychotherapy is used to help people suffering from *neurosis* or *personality disorders*, as well as individuals with specific personal problems. The aim is to help patients learn about themselves, develop new insights into past and present relationships, and change fixed patterns of behavior.

### HOW IT IS DONE
*Counseling* is the simplest form of psychotherapy, consisting of advice and psychological support. At the opposite end of the spectrum is *psychoanalysis*, which attempts to explore the deep unconscious feelings and early childhood experiences of the individual.

Dynamic psychotherapy is based on psychoanalytic principles. The therapist tries to understand and interpret the patient's unconscious messages (without the benefit of formal psychoanalysis) so that the individual can develop a better understanding of his or her underlying feelings and cope with them more effectively.

A course of treatment may be brief, consisting of two or three sessions, or it may extend over many years, depending on the problems involved. It may vary in intensity from a simple, supportive approach during a difficult period to an in-depth analysis aimed at reconstructing the personality.

Psychotherapy may involve one person, a couple (see *Marital counseling*), a family (see *Family therapy*), or a group (see *Group therapy*).

## Psychotropic drugs
Drugs that have an effect on the mind. They include *hallucinogenic drugs, sedative drugs, sleeping drugs, tranquilizer drugs*, and *antipsychotic drugs*.

## Psyllium
A bulk-forming *laxative drug* used in the treatment of *constipation, diverticular disease*, and *irritable bowel syndrome*. Psyllium is also given to increase the firmness of bowel movements in a person with an *ileostomy*.

Adverse effects include bloating, excess gas, and abdominal pain.

## Pterygium
A wing-shaped thickening of the *conjunctiva* that extends across the margin of the cornea toward the center. Pterygium is caused by prolonged exposure to bright sunlight and is common in tropical areas. Unless vision is notably affected, no treatment is usually necessary. If the pterygium is surgically removed, it may be followed by a recurrence that is larger than the original.

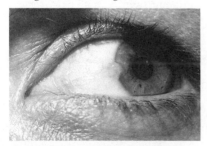

**Appearance of pterygium**
The conjunctiva (outer lining of the eyeball) has extended onto the cornea (transparent front part of the eye).

## Ptomaine poisoning
An obsolescent general term for any form of *food poisoning* caused by bacteria or bacterial poisons.

## Ptosis
A drooping of the upper eyelid. Ptosis may be congenital or may occur as a result of disease (e.g., *myasthenia gravis*) or injury. It is usually due to a weakness of the levator muscle of the lid or to interference with the nerve supply to the muscle.

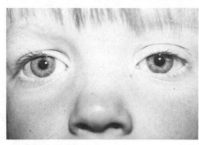

**Ptosis in a child**
This condition, present from birth, should be corrected surgically to prevent any disturbance of visual development.

Severe congenital ptosis, in which the drooping lid covers the pupil, should be surgically corrected to avoid the development of *amblyopia* (failure of visual development).

Acquired ptosis without obvious cause may be a sign of neurologic disease, such as a brain tumor or an aneurysm, and should be investigated by a physician.

## Ptyalism
Excessive salivation caused by irritation of the inside of the mouth by ill-fitting dentures, digestive tract disorders (such as *esophagitis* or a *peptic ulcer*), or, rarely, damage to the nervous system (e.g., by *mercury poisoning* or infection with *rabies*).

## Puberty
The period when secondary sexual characteristics develop and the sexual organs mature, allowing reproduction to become possible. Puberty is the term used for the physical changes that underlie the emotional changes of *adolescence*. It usually occurs between the ages of 10 and 15 in both sexes; it is initiated by the *pituitary gland* producing hormones (known as *gonadotropins*) that stimulate the *ovaries* to increase secretion of *estrogen hormones* and the *testes* to increase secretion of *testosterone*. It is not known what triggers this action by the pituitary gland.

Puberty is accompanied by a significant growth spurt and increase in weight. Body weight may double during this period, due primarily to muscle growth in boys and increased fat in girls.

### PUBERTY IN GIRLS
The first sign of puberty in girls is usually breast budding, which occurs around the age of 11; in about one third of girls, pubic hair appears first. The rate of growth of the breasts may be unequal but any difference usually disappears by the time full maturity is reached. The first menstrual period usually does not occur for a year or more, by which time pubic and underarm hair are in the fully developed adult pattern.

Other secondary sexual characteristics, such as the wider pelvis and the female distribution of fat, develop progressively during this period. Puberty is considered to be complete when menstrual periods occur at regular, predictable intervals.

The age at which menstruation starts has been decreasing for the past century, probably because of a general improvement in nutrition and living standards, but has now become stable. Girls who are overweight tend to start menstruating earlier than the average; those who are malnourished start later. Strenuous sports or other hard physical activity (such as ballet) and debilitating disease can also delay the onset of periods.

### PUBERTY IN BOYS
In boys, puberty is heralded by a sudden increase in the rate of growth of the testes and scrotum, followed by the appearance of pubic and facial hair. The penis begins to grow around the age of 13 and reaches its adult size about two years later. However, there is a wide range of variation so that, at the age of 14, some boys may be sexually mature while others still have immature genitals.

The body's increased secretion of testosterone stimulates sperm production and causes the prostate gland and seminal vesicles to mature. It leads to the development of the typical male distribution of hair on the face, chest, and abdomen. The larynx enlarges and the vocal cords become longer and thicker, causing the pitch of the voice to drop.

### ABNORMAL PUBERTY
Extremely rarely there are instances in which the normal events of puberty occur at a very young age, sometimes within the first five years of life; the youngest mother on record gave birth

P

to a healthy baby at the age of 5 years 8 months. This precocious puberty can occur in either sex. In boys it is often caused by a brain tumor; in girls the cause is usually not known.

## Pubes

The pubic hair or the area of the body covered by this hair.

## Pubic lice

 Small, wingless insects that live in the pubic hair and feed on blood. Also called crabs (because of their crablike claws, which they use to grasp hair), they are usually spread by sexual contact. Their scientific name is *PHTHIRUS PUBIS*.

Each louse has a flattened body, up to one twelfth of an inch (2 mm) across, and can be seen with the naked eye. The females lay minute, pale eggs (called nits) on the hair, where they hatch about eight days later. Pubic lice do not transmit infection.

### SYMPTOMS AND SIGNS

Both lice and eggs can be seen on close inspection. On hairy men the lice may also be found in hair around the anus, on the legs, and on the trunk, and occasionally even in facial hair. The bites sometimes cause itching. Pubic lice can infest children, usually by transmission from parents. In children, the lice may attach to the eyelids.

### TREATMENT

An insecticide lotion containing malathion or carbaryl kills the lice and eggs soon after application. An infested person's sexual partner should also be treated; clothes and bedding should be washed in water hotter than 140°F (60°C) before use.

## Public health

A branch of medicine that developed in the 19th century as physicians became aware of the importance to health of the provision of pure water supplies and safe systems for the disposal of sewage. The medical pioneers in this field instigated the construction of reservoirs and of water and sewage systems. Later, they turned their attention to working conditions in factories and mines, and to improvements in the care of women during pregnancy and of infants in the first few years of life, with programs to improve nutrition and provide immunization against infectious diseases.

Today, the functions of the public health physician are so extensive that they are divided among many different agencies, ranging from the Centers for Disease Control and its reporting laboratories to the Food and Drug Administration.

## Public health dentistry

The aspect of dentistry, sometimes also known as community dentistry, that deals with the dental health of the population at large rather than of the individual. It includes studying the distribution and prevalence of dental disorders, particularly tooth decay (see *Caries, dental*); making sure that enough dentists are trained to cope with demand for treatment; providing information on the need for *oral hygiene*; monitoring *fluoridation* of water supplies to reduce the incidence of tooth decay; and providing special dental facilities for people who have disabilities.

## Pudenda

See *Genitalia*.

## Pudendal block

A type of *nerve block* used during childbirth to provide pain relief for a *forceps delivery*. A local anesthetic (see *Anesthesia, local*) is injected into either side of the floor of the vagina near the pudendal nerve, which passes under the bony prominences on each side of the lower pelvis. The lower part of the vagina becomes insensitive to pain within about five minutes.

## Puerperal sepsis

Infection that originates in the genital tract within 10 days after childbirth, miscarriage, or abortion. Puerperal sepsis is rare, occurring in between 1 and 3 percent of pregnancies. Infection usually starts in the vagina and spreads to the uterus.

---

## CHANGES OF PUBERTY

There is considerable variation in the age of onset of puberty, but girls, on average, undergo puberty earlier than boys. The entire process takes about three to four years to complete. In addition to the sex-specific changes, height and weight both increase rapidly.

10 to 12          15 to 16          12 to 14          15 to 18

**Girls**
Puberty most often starts between the ages of 10 and 12 in girls. Major changes include growth of breasts and pubic hair, widening of the hips, enlargement of the uterus, and the onset of menstruation.

**Boys**
The main changes are enlargement of the sex organs, widening of the shoulders, deepening of the voice, and the growth of facial and pubic hair. The onset is usually between the ages of 12 and 14.

P

### CAUSES

Infection may be caused by bacteria that normally inhabit the vagina but usually cause harm only if the woman's resistance is low or if placental tissue has been retained in the genital tract. Puerperal sepsis may also be caused by bacteria entering the genital tract from other parts of the body or from outside.

### SYMPTOMS AND TREATMENT

The main symptoms are fever, offensive-smelling *lochia* (vaginal discharge after childbirth), headache, chills, and pain in the lower abdomen. If infection spreads to the fallopian tubes (see *Salpingitis*), the tubes may become blocked and cause *infertility*. Further spread of infection may lead to *peritonitis* and *septicemia*, which may be fatal.

Treatment includes *antibiotic drugs* and removal of any remaining placental remnants.

## Puerperium

The period of time following *childbirth* during which the woman's uterus and genitals return to their state before the pregnancy.

## Pulmonary

Pertaining to the lungs. For example, the pulmonary artery is the blood vessel that carries blood from the heart to the lungs.

## Pulmonary embolism

Obstruction of the pulmonary artery or one of its branches in the lung by an *embolus*, usually a blood clot that originated in a vein in the leg or pelvis as a complication of deep vein thrombosis (see *Thrombosis, deep vein*). If the embolus is large enough to block the main pulmonary artery leading from the heart to the lungs, or if there are many clots, the condition is life-threatening. Pulmonary embolism affects about twice as many women as men; recent surgery, pregnancy, and immobility increase the risk. Pulmonary embolism is responsible for 50,000 deaths in the US each year.

### SYMPTOMS

Symptoms depend partly on the size of the embolus. A massive embolus that blocks the main pulmonary artery can cause sudden death. Smaller emboli may cause severe shortness of breath, a rapid pulse, dizziness due to low blood pressure, sharp chest pain that is worse when breathing, and coughing up blood. Small pulmonary emboli may produce no symptoms, but, if recurrent, may eventually lead

---

# PULMONARY EMBOLISM

This condition results when one or more emboli (fragments of material) break off from a blood clot in a vein and are carried, via the heart, to the lungs. The effects depend on the size and numbers of emboli and on the general health of the person's lungs and heart.

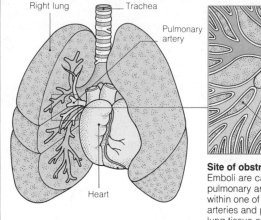

Right lung — Trachea — Pulmonary artery — Heart

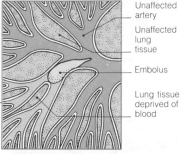

Unaffected artery — Unaffected lung tissue — Embolus — Lung tissue deprived of blood

**Site of obstruction**
Emboli are carried into the lungs by the pulmonary artery. Most of them lodge within one of the larger or medium-sized arteries and partially deprive a section of lung tissue of blood.

---

to *pulmonary hypertension* (increased pressure of blood flow in the lungs).

### DIAGNOSIS

Investigation of the lung may include a *chest X ray*, *radionuclide scanning*, and pulmonary *angiography*. An *ECG* may show changes in the electrical activity of the heart, and *venography* helps determine the source of the embolus.

### TREATMENT

Treatment depends on the size and severity of the embolus. A small embolus gradually dissolves but there is a risk of more emboli developing. *Anticoagulant drugs* (such as heparin and warfarin) are usually given to reduce the clotting ability of the blood and to reduce the chance of more clots occurring. *Thrombolytic drugs* may hasten the process of clot dissolution. If the embolus is very large, an emergency operation may be necessary to remove it.

## Pulmonary fibrosis

Scarring and thickening of lung tissue, usually as a result of previous lung inflammation, such as *pneumonia* or *tuberculosis*. Pulmonary fibrosis may occur throughout both lungs (see *Interstitial pulmonary fibrosis*) or may affect only part of one lung.

Shortness of breath is a common symptom. Diagnosis is confirmed by chest X ray. Treatment depends on the underlying cause, but the fibrosis may be irreversible.

---

## Pulmonary function tests

A group of procedures used to evaluate the function of the lungs and confirm the presence of some lung disorders. Pulmonary function tests are also performed before any major operation on the lungs, such as *lobectomy* (removal of a lobe of the lung), to ensure that the person will not be disabled by the reduction in his or her lung capacity.

*Spirometry* and measurement of lung volume are performed to detect any restriction of normal lung expansion or to detect obstruction of air flow. A *peak flow meter* is used to assess the degree of *bronchospasm* (narrowing of the airways), while a test of *blood gases* (measurement of the concentration of oxygen and carbon dioxide in the blood) demonstrates the efficiency of gas exchange in the lungs.

Another test of lung function (diffusing capacity) shows the efficiency of the lungs in absorbing gas into the blood. This is done by measuring the volume of carbon monoxide breathed out after a known volume of the gas has been inhaled.

## Pulmonary hypertension

A disorder in which the blood pressure in the arteries supplying the lungs is abnormally high. Pulmonary hypertension develops in response to an increased resistance to blood flow through the lungs. To maintain an

P

adequate blood flow, the right side of the heart, which pumps blood to the lungs, must contract more vigorously than was necessary before. This causes an enlargement of the heart's muscle wall. Eventually, right-sided *heart failure* may develop.

**CAUSES**
Several conditions can lead to increased resistance to blood flow through the lungs. The most important is an inadequate supply of oxygen to the lungs' small air sacs (e.g., due to chronic *bronchitis* or *emphysema*). The oxygen lack causes the small branches of the arteries in the lungs to constrict and to thicken their muscular walls, thus causing a permanent increase in resistance. Other causes are *pulmonary embolism* (in which a blood clot blocks off one or several arteries in the lungs) and *interstitial pulmonary fibrosis* (thickening and scarring of lung tissue, which can have many causes).

Primary pulmonary hypertension is the term used to describe cases in which the cause of the increased lung resistance is not known.

**SYMPTOMS AND SIGNS**
As long as the enlargement and strengthening of the right side of the heart is sufficient to maintain a normal blood circulation, there is little indication of trouble. But, with the onset of *heart failure* as the right side of the heart falters in its work load, symptoms develop. Symptoms include enlargement of veins in the neck, enlargement of the liver, and generalized *edema* (swelling due to fluid collection in tissues).

**TREATMENT**
Treatment is directed at the underlying disorder (if known) and to the relief of the effects of right-sided heart failure. *Diuretic drugs* may be valuable in relieving edema and *oxygen therapy* is sometimes useful.

## Pulmonary insufficiency
A defect of the pulmonary valve at the exit of the ventricle (lower, pumping chamber) on the right side of the heart. The valve fails to close properly after each contraction of the ventricle, allowing blood pumped out of the chamber to leak back again.

Pulmonary insufficiency is a rare type of heart valve defect. When it does occur, it is usually the result of *rheumatic fever*, *endocarditis*, or severe *pulmonary hypertension* (raised pressure in the pulmonary artery). It may cause a heart *murmur* that is audible through a stethoscope.

Usually the condition is of little significance. When accompanied by pulmonary hypertension, the eventual result may be right-sided *heart failure*. In such cases, the condition is usually approached by treating the pulmonary hypertension rather than by attempting to repair or replace the defective valve.

## Pulmonary stenosis
A heart condition in which the outflow of blood from the ventricle (lower, pumping chamber) on the right side of the heart is obstructed. With pulmonary stenosis, the heart muscle must work much harder to pump blood to the lungs.

The obstruction may be caused by narrowing of the pulmonary valve at the exit of the chamber, by narrowing of the pulmonary artery (large blood vessel beyond the valve) that carries blood to the lungs, or by narrowing within the upper part of the ventricle itself.

**CAUSES AND INCIDENCE**
Pulmonary stenosis is nearly always congenital (present from birth). About one baby in 8,000 is born with the defect alone or as part of a more complex set of heart defects, called the *tetralogy of Fallot*. Very rarely, pulmonary stenosis develops later in life, usually in a person who has had *rheumatic fever*.

**SYMPTOMS**
In severe cases, a newborn baby's heart begins to enlarge as soon as breathing is established. If the blood supply to the lungs is inadequate, the baby becomes breathless, and damming of blood behind the valve may lead to liver and abdominal swellings. The baby may also not nurse. This is an emergency that can often be helped by surgery.

In less severe cases (which are more common), symptoms may not appear until the child gets older and becomes more active. The main symptom is breathlessness. Marks resembling *pernios* may appear on the cheeks, hands, and feet as a result of the slower blood circulation. In mild cases there are no symptoms, and the condition is detected only when a physician hears a heart *murmur* through a stethoscope.

When pulmonary stenosis exists with other heart defects, such as a *septal defect* (hole in the heart), some deoxygenated blood bypasses the lungs and goes back into the general circulation, leading to *cyanosis* (blue-purple skin coloration).

Pulmonary stenosis that occurs in later life may lead to the symptoms of *heart failure*.

**DIAGNOSIS**
A *chest X ray* may show enlargement of the heart. *ECG* (measurement of the electrical activity of the heart), *echocardiography*, and Doppler *ultrasound* techniques (imaging of the heart using sound waves) can help diagnose the severity of the narrowing.

---

## PULMONARY HYPERTENSION
In this condition, there is increased resistance to blood flow through the lungs (red arrows), usually due to lung disease. The result is a rise in pressure in the pulmonary artery, the right side of the heart (gray lines and arrows), and in the veins that bring blood to the heart.

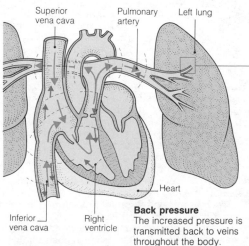

Superior vena cava
Pulmonary artery
Left lung
Heart
Inferior vena cava
Right ventricle

**Back pressure**
The increased pressure is transmitted back to veins throughout the body.

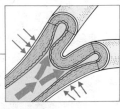

**Causes**
The most common cause of increased resistance to blood flow through the lungs is constriction of the small arteries in the lungs and thickening of their muscular walls. This thickening usually results from a lung disease such as chronic bronchitis or emphysema.

P

## TREATMENT

In some cases a *balloon catheter* is used to relieve the narrowing without the need to open the chest. Alternatively, *heart valve surgery* or other types of *open heart surgery* are often successful in correcting or improving it.

## Pulp, dental

The soft tissue in the middle of each tooth. It receives a rich supply of blood vessels and contains nerves that respond to heat, cold, pressure, and pain. (See also *Teeth*.)

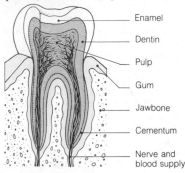

Enamel
Dentin
Pulp
Gum
Jawbone
Cementum
Nerve and blood supply

**Location of the dental pulp**
The pulp forms the soft core at the center of a tooth. If tooth decay reaches as far as the pulp, the latter degenerates rapidly and must be removed to save the tooth.

## Pulpectomy

The complete removal of the pulp of a tooth (the soft tissue inside the tooth that contains blood vessels and nerves). The procedure is part of *root-canal treatment*.

## Pulpotomy

Removal of part of the pulp of a tooth (the soft tissue inside the tooth that contains blood vessels and nerves) when it has become inflamed, usually as a result of bacterial infection. The infection is most commonly the result of extensive dental *caries* (tooth decay) or a dental *fracture* that exposes the pulp. Successful pulpotomy prevents further degeneration of the pulp.

Using a local anesthetic, the dentist removes the damaged pulp and covers the wound with a dressing that encourages it to heal. The gap in the overlying dentin and enamel is then sealed with a restoration such as amalgam (see *Filling, dental*). If the treatment is unsuccessful, *root-canal treatment* may be required.

## Pulse

The rhythmic expansion and contraction of an artery as blood is forced through it, pumped by the heart.

The pulse is usually checked during the course of a *physical examination* because it can give clues to the patient's state of health or illness. It is detected by pressing one or more fingers or thumb against the skin over an artery, usually at the wrist, although it can also easily be felt in the neck or the groin. The pulse may be visible at the temple or in the neck.

The pulse can be described in terms of its rate (number of expansions per minute), rhythm, strength, and whether the blood vessel is hard or soft. The rate is easily determined by counting the beats in a set period (minimum 15 to 20 seconds) and multiplying to give the beats per minute. The pulse rate usually corresponds to the *heart rate*, which varies according to the person's state of relaxation or physical activity.

Abnormally high or low rates, or abnormal rhythms, may be a sign of a heart disorder (see *Arrhythmia*). When the heart is beating very fast, some of its beats may be too weak to be detectable in the pulse, making the pulse rate slower than the heart rate.

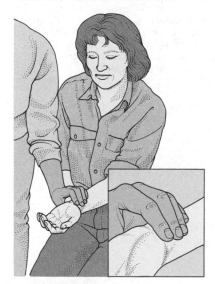

**Taking the pulse**
Two fingertips are pressed against the wrist just below the base of the thumb to feel the pulse in the radial artery.

If the pulse feels weak, it may be a sign of *heart failure*, *shock*, or an obstruction to the blood circulation. A weak or absent pulse in one or both legs is a sign of *peripheral vascular disease*. The vessel wall should feel soft when the pulse is felt. If the vessel wall feels hard, it may be a sign of *arteriosclerosis*.

## Pump, infusion

A machine for the administration of a continuous, controlled amount of a drug or other fluid through a needle that may be inserted into a vein or under the skin.

An infusion pump consists of a small battery-powered pump that controls the flow of fluid from a syringe into the needle. The pump, which is strapped to the patient, is preprogrammed to deliver fluid at a constant rate.

Infusion pumps are frequently used in administering morphine and other drugs to patients suffering from cancer. They are also used to give insulin to patients who have diabetes mellitus (see *Pump, insulin*; see also *Intravenous infusion*).

## Pump, insulin

A type of infusion pump (see *Pump, infusion*) used to administer a continuous dose of insulin in some patients with *diabetes mellitus*.

The needle of the insulin pump is inserted under the skin, usually in the upper arm or the abdominal wall. The rate of flow is adjusted so that the level of blood glucose (sugar) is constantly controlled.

## Punchdrunk

A condition characterized by slurred speech, impaired concentration, and slowed thought processes. It develops as a result of brain damage caused by several episodes of brief loss of consciousness as a result of a head injury. The name punchdrunk comes from the high incidence of the condition in boxers.

## Pupil

The circular opening in the center of the *iris*. In bright conditions, the pupil constricts (narrows) to reduce the amount of light admitted to the *eye*; in dim light, it dilates (widens) to allow more light to reach the retina. Constriction and dilation are controlled by muscles in the iris.

Several drugs affect the size of the pupil. For example, *atropine* eye drops dilate the pupil and *pilocarpine* eye drops constrict it.

### DISORDERS

The pupil may be congenitally small, irregular in shape, or displaced to one side; there may also be a coloboma (a missing segment or fissure in the iris). Adie's pupil is a condition in which the affected pupil is larger than the other, with poor constriction in response to light and slow dilation in

P

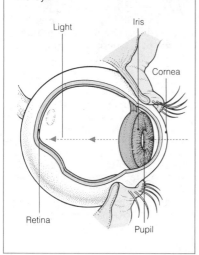

**LOCATION OF THE PUPIL**
The pupil can be widened or narrowed by muscles in the iris to adjust the amount of light entering the eye.

the dark. The Argyll Robertson pupil, usually caused by *syphilis*, is small and irregular; it does not constrict in response to light but does so when an effort at *accommodation* is made.

Injury to the iris frequently affects the pupil, producing either permanent dilation of the pupil or distortion of its shape.

## Purpura

Any of a group of disorders characterized by purplish or reddish-brown areas or spots of discoloration, visible through the skin, and caused by bleeding within underlying tissues. Purpura also refers to the discolored areas themselves, which can range from the size of a pinhead to an inch or so in diameter. The smaller bleeding points are sometimes called *petechiae*; larger, darker areas of discoloration are called bruises or ecchymoses.

### TYPES AND CAUSES

There are many different types and causes of purpura.

Common purpura, also called senile purpura, is the most frequent of all bleeding disorders, affecting primarily middle-aged or elderly women. Large discolored areas appear on the thighs or the back of the hands and forearms. They are caused by thinning of the tissues supporting blood vessels beneath the skin, which as a result rupture easily. Bleeding may also be visible under the membrane that lines the mouth.

*Schönlein-Henoch purpura* (also called anaphylactoid purpura) is caused by inflammation of blood vessels beneath the skin, sometimes as a result of an allergic reaction. Similar changes may occur in patches within the gastrointestinal tract.

Purpura can also occur as a result of a lack of platelets in the blood—a condition called *thrombocytopenia*. Platelets are the small blood cells that play a crucial role in clotting. A lack of platelets may occur as a result of a disease of the bone marrow (such as *leukemia* or aplastic *anemia*), as a side effect of certain drugs or excessive radiation, or for no apparent reason.

Other types of purpura include that seen in *scurvy* due to vitamin C deficiency and forms of the condition caused by damage to blood vessels by certain infections, *autoimmune disorders*, *septicemia* (blood poisoning), or blood chemical disturbances such as uremia (see *Renal failure*).

### DIAGNOSIS AND TREATMENT

Purpura is investigated by a physician studying the signs and symptoms and by a full examination and testing of the blood, including *blood-clotting tests*. The state of the blood platelets is of primary interest. It is essential for the physician to determine exactly the type and cause of the purpura, because treatment depends on the exact type.

Common purpura may be helped by estrogen replacement therapy or by *corticosteroid drugs*, but these often do little to help in Schönlein-Henoch purpura. In this form, *immunosuppressant drugs* can help; in severe cases, *plasmapheresis* (removal of blood, replacement of plasma, and retransfusion) has been effective. Platelet deficiency is treated according to the cause. In some cases, transfusions of platelets must be given. Autoimmune thrombocytopenia (sometimes called

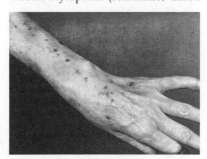

**Appearance of senile purpura**
This common condition of middle to old age is caused by thinning of the tissues that support blood vessels beneath the skin.

idiopathic thrombocytopenic purpura) is usually treated with corticosteroid drugs or *splenectomy*.

## Purulent

A term that means containing, producing, or consisting of *pus*.

## Pus

A pale yellow or green, creamy fluid found at the site of bacterial infection. Pus is composed of millions of dead white blood cells, partly digested tissue, dead and living bacteria, as well as minute quantities of other substances. A collection of pus in a solid tissue is called an *abscess*.

The main pus-forming organisms include streptococci, pneumococci, and *ESCHERICHIA COLI*. Many bacteria produce a distinctive type of pus (*PSEUDOMONAS AERUGINOSA* produces pus with a bluish tinge).

## Pustule

A small skin blister containing pus. Pustules may occur in a hair follicle or on ordinary skin, and may or may not be the result of infection; the pustules in *acne* are noninfective. A *stye* is a type of pustule that develops at the root of an eyelash.

## PUVA

A type of *phototherapy* used to treat certain skin conditions, especially *psoriasis*. PUVA combines the use of a *psoralen drug*, which sensitizes the skin to sunlight, and a controlled dose of long wavelength ultraviolet light. The abbreviation stands for psoralens and ultraviolet A.

## Pyelitis

See *Pyelonephritis*.

## Pyelography

A procedure for obtaining X-ray pictures of the urinary system. Also known as urography, the technique involves the introduction of a radiopaque, iodine-based dye into the kidneys, ureters, and bladder so that they show up well on X rays.

### WHY IT IS DONE

Pyelography is performed to help diagnose disorders of the urinary system. It is sometimes recommended for people who have recurrent urinary tract or kidney infections, *hematuria* (blood in the urine), or suspected urinary tract *calculi* (stones). The investigation may also be performed in young people who have *hypertension* (high blood pressure) to discover whether kidney disease is the cause.

P

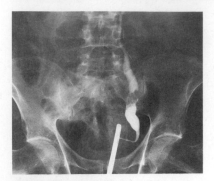

**Retrograde pyelogram**
The bright, rodlike object at bottom in this X ray is a cystoscope (viewing tube) that has been passed into the bladder. Via a catheter passed through the cystoscope, a radiopaque dye was introduced into the left ureter. As the dye filled the dilated ureter (bright area at right), X rays were taken. Part of the ureter did not fill with dye, indicating a tumor.

**HOW IT IS DONE**

**INTRAVENOUS PYELOGRAPHY (IVP)** Radiopaque dye is injected into the bloodstream via a vein in the arm; it travels from there to the kidneys and urinary tract. Before an IVP, the patient does not drink fluids for eight to 12 hours and is given a laxative to empty the bowel (to improve the quality of the X-ray films).

With the patient lying down, X rays of the complete abdomen are taken before the injection, immediately after it, and then five, 10, and 30 minutes later. Between the five- and 10-minute films, pressure may be applied to the abdomen to improve the definition of the central cavities of the kidneys. After the bladder has filled with dye, the patient is asked to urinate while another X ray is taken.

**RETROGRADE PYELOGRAPHY** Using an anesthetic, a cystoscope (viewing tube) is passed into the bladder (see *Cystoscopy*); a fine tube is threaded through the cystoscope and up the ureter to the kidney. A small quantity of dye is injected and X rays are taken.

**RESULTS**

The X rays obtained by IVP allow the radiologist to see the size, shape, and position of the kidneys, the course of the ureters, the size and position of the bladder, and whether there are any obvious obstructions in the ureters. The X ray taken after urination shows whether the bladder has emptied completely.

Retrograde pyelography shows up obstructions of the upper urinary outflow tract particularly clearly.

**COMPLICATIONS**

Pyelography is generally very safe, but must not be used in people who are sensitive to iodine. With retrograde pyelography, there is a risk of aggravating any infection that may be present in the urinary system.

## Pyelolithotomy

An operation performed to remove a *calculus* (stone) from the kidney. The surgeon approaches the kidney via a longitudinal incision to the right or left of the spine, the junction between the kidney and ureter is cut open, and the calculus is removed with a forceps.

Pyelolithotomy is being replaced by ultrasonic wave therapy as a means of dealing with kidney stones (see *Lithotripsy; Lithotriptor*).

## Pyelonephritis

Inflammation of the kidney, usually caused by a bacterial infection. Pyelonephritis may be acute, taking the form of a sudden attack, or chronic, in which repeated or inadequately treated attacks may cause permanent scarring of the kidney.

**ACUTE PYELONEPHRITIS**

Acute pyelonephritis is more common in women and more likely to occur in pregnancy. It usually results from *cystitis* (infection of the bladder) spreading up to the kidney.

Symptoms include a high fever, chills, and back pain. Treatment consists of *antibiotic drugs*, which may need to be given by intravenous infusion in severe cases. *Septicemia* (blood poisoning) is a possible complication.

**CHRONIC PYELONEPHRITIS**

Chronic pyelonephritis often starts in childhood. It is usually caused by *reflux* of urine from the bladder back into one of the ureters, often because the child has a congenital abnormality of the valve where the ureter enters the bladder.

Persistent reflux of urine causes repeated kidney infection, leading to inflammation and scarring, which, over a period of years, causes permanent kidney damage. Children in whom recurrent urinary tract infections develop require testing by a physician. A voiding *cystourethrogram* may help identify the presence of reflux so that the underlying abnormality can be corrected surgically.

Possible complications of chronic pyelonephritis include *hypertension* (high blood pressure) and *renal failure*.

## Pyloric stenosis

Narrowing of the pylorus (the lower outlet from the stomach) that obstructs the passage of food into the duodenum (the first part of the small intestine). Pyloric stenosis occurs in babies and in adults.

**CAUSES AND INCIDENCE**

In infants, the condition is caused by a thickening of the pyloric muscle that occurs, for unknown reasons, soon after birth; one in 4,000 are affected.

---

## PYLORIC STENOSIS IN INFANTS

In infantile pyloric stenosis, the muscle surrounding the outlet from the stomach is abnormally thickened, as shown in the enlarged drawing (below). The condition occurs more often in male than female babies and tends to run in families—infants of a woman who was affected with pyloric stenosis as a baby are liable to develop it.

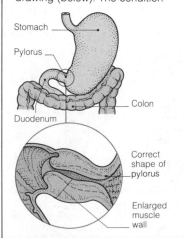

Stomach
Pylorus
Duodenum
Colon
Correct shape of pylorus
Enlarged muscle wall

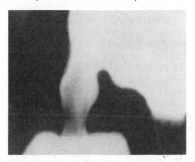

**Barium X ray of pylorus**
The X ray shows the blockage to the flow of the barium meal at the lower end of the stomach. Surgery is performed to cut through the thickened muscle around the outlet and relieve the blockage.

P

In adults, the narrowing is usually the result of scarring caused by a *peptic ulcer* or of a malignant tumor of the lower stomach (see *Stomach cancer*).

SYMPTOMS AND DIAGNOSIS

Three to four weeks after birth, an affected infant starts projectile vomiting (profuse, forceful vomiting in which the stomach contents may be ejected a distance of several feet) after feeding. Adults with the disorder vomit undigested food several hours after a meal.

In an infant, a physician can feel the thickened muscle through the abdominal wall, but a barium meal (see *Barium X-ray examinations*) may be required to confirm the diagnosis.

In adults, pyloric stenosis is diagnosed by a barium meal, which shows the narrowing, and by *gastroscopy* (examination of the stomach with a flexible viewing tube).

TREATMENT

Infant pyloric stenosis is sometimes treated with drugs. However, in most cases the only satisfactory treatment is an operation known as pyloromyotomy. While the patient is under a general anesthetic, the abdomen is opened and the obstruction relieved simply by making an incision along the length of the thickened muscle.

In adults, surgery is necessary to correct the underlying cause.

## Pyloroplasty

An operation in which the pylorus (the outlet from the stomach) is widened to ensure the free passage of food into the intestine. Pyloroplasty may be performed as part of the surgical treatment for a *peptic ulcer*; it prevents tightening of the pyloric muscles following *vagotomy* (cutting of the vagus nerve to reduce stomach acid production).

While the patient is under general anesthesia, a lengthwise incision is made across the pylorus. The beginning and end of the incision are pushed inward till they meet, and the opening, which is now at right angles to the original incision, is sewn up. This creates an extra wide passage for the movement of food.

## Pyo-

A prefix (py- is also used) that denotes a relationship to pus, as in pyuria, pus in the urine.

## Pyoderma gangrenosum

A rare condition characterized by ulcers, usually on the legs, that turn into hard, painful areas surrounded by discolored skin. It occurs as a complication in about 5 percent of people with *ulcerative colitis*.

## Pyrantel

An *antihelmintic drug* used to treat intestinal *worm infestations*. Possible adverse effects include nausea, loss of appetite, and abdominal pain.

## Pyrazinamide

A drug used in the treatment of *tuberculosis* when other drugs have not been effective. Pyrazinamide is prescribed in combination with other antituberculous drugs.

Possible adverse effects are nausea and an increased risk of gout. There may also be liver damage, resulting in loss of appetite and jaundice. Regular blood tests are performed during treatment with pyrazinamide to check liver function.

## Pyrexia

A medical term for *fever*.

## Pyrexia of uncertain origin

Persistent fever for which no cause is readily apparent despite extensive medical investigations. The cause is usually an illness that is difficult to diagnose or a common disease that presents itself in an unusual way.

Common causes include various viral infections; *tuberculosis*; cancer, particularly *lymphoma* (cancer of the lymphoid tissue); and *collagen diseases* such as systemic *lupus erythematosus*, *temporal arteritis*, and, in children, Still's disease (see *Rheumatoid arthritis, juvenile*).

Occasionally, fever of uncertain origin occurs as a reaction to a drug.

## Pyridostigmine

A drug used in the treatment of *myasthenia gravis* (an *autoimmune disorder* causing muscle weakness). Pyridostigmine significantly improves muscle strength in sufferers of myasthenia gravis but does not cure the condition.

Possible adverse effects of pyridostigmine include abdominal pain, nausea, diarrhea, and, rarely, an allergic skin rash.

## Pyridoxine

One of the $B_6$ group of vitamins (see *Vitamin B complex*). Pyridoxine is used to treat people with dietary deficiency, in cases of *neuritis* (nerve inflammation) caused by certain drugs, and to relieve the symptoms that occur in *premenstrual syndrome*.

## Pyrilamine

An *antihistamine drug* used to treat seasonal allergic *rhinitis* (hay fever) and *urticaria* (hives). Unlike some other types of antihistamines, pyrilamine rarely causes drowsiness.

## Pyrimethamine

A drug used to prevent and treat attacks caused by certain strains of *malaria* parasite and also to treat *toxoplasmosis*. It is usually given in combination with a *sulfonamide drug*.

Possible adverse effects include loss of appetite, vomiting, and, rarely, rash. Long-term use may reduce blood cell production by the bone marrow, causing *anemia*, abnormal bleeding, or susceptibility to infection.

## Pyrogen

A fever-producing substance. The term is usually applied to proteins that are released by white blood cells in response to bacterial or viral infections. These proteins act on the temperature-controlling center within the brain, causing the body temperature to increase.

The word pyrogen is also sometimes used to refer to chemicals released by the microorganisms themselves—such as bacterial *endotoxins*, which also have a temperature-raising effect on the body.

## Pyromania

A persistent impulse to set fires. The typical pyromaniac becomes fascinated with fires as a child, obtains relief of tension (or even pleasure) from setting fire to something and watching it burn, and has no other motive (such as money) for doing so. The disorder is more often diagnosed in males, and is associated with a low IQ, alcohol abuse, and *psychosexual disorder* (some people seem to be sexually aroused by fires). Pyromaniacs are often dangerous and difficult to treat; imprisonment is not unusual.

## Pyuria

The presence of white blood cells (pus cells) in the urine. Pyuria is usually an indication of infection and inflammation in the kidney or urinary tract.

Microscopic examination and *culture* of the urine are performed to look for a causative microorganism so that appropriate *antibiotic drugs* may be given. In some cases, pyuria occurs when no microorganisms are present and may indicate inflammation of the kidney due to another cause (e.g., interstitial *nephritis*).

P

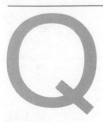

# Q fever

An uncommon illness with symptoms similar to *influenza*. Q fever occurs throughout the world; an effective vaccine is available.

The causative organism, *COXIELLA BURNETTI*, is a type of *rickettsia* harbored by farm animals. It occurs in the urine, feces, milk, flesh, and, particularly, placentas of infected animals. In dry areas, Q fever may be contracted by inhaling dust contaminated with feces, urine, or birth products. The disease may also, in rare cases, be spread by tick bites.

About 20 days after infection, the illness begins suddenly with a high fever (which may persist for up to two weeks), severe headache, muscle and chest pain, and cough. During the second week, a form of pneumonia develops. The patient then usually recovers. In some cases, however, the disease is prolonged; *hepatitis* develops in one third of these people and some suffer *endocarditis*. In less than 1 percent of cases, the illness is fatal unless treated.

A diagnosis of Q fever may be confirmed by a *blood test*. Treatment is with *antibiotic drugs*.

# Quackery

A false claim by someone to have both the ability and experience to diagnose and treat disease.

# Quadriceps muscle

A muscle with four distinct parts that is situated at the front of the thigh. The quadriceps muscle straightens the knee.

The most common disorder of the quadriceps is a *hematoma* (a collection of blood) caused by a direct blow. Bruising may follow a few days later; in rare cases, bone forms within the hematoma, restricting movement of the affected leg.

Sudden stretching of the leg may tear the muscle, especially in middle-aged or elderly people. Any knee disorder that brings on pain or swelling, limiting full extension of the leg,

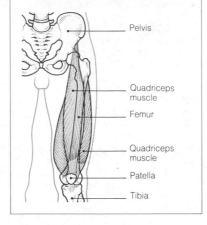

Pelvis

Quadriceps muscle

Femur

Quadriceps muscle

Patella

Tibia

causes the quadriceps muscle to begin wasting away within 48 hours, making the knee feel as though it is giving way when weight is placed on the affected leg.

# Quadriparesis

Muscle weakness in all four limbs and the trunk.

# Quadriplegia

*Paralysis* of all four limbs and the trunk. Quadriplegia is caused by damage to the spinal cord in the neck region. The condition results in loss of feeling and power in the affected parts. (See also *Paraplegia*.)

# Quarantine

Isolation of a person or persons recently exposed to a serious infectious disease. The aim is to prevent the spread of a disease by an infected, but symptomless, person.

Today, the reduced incidence of most serious infectious diseases and the widespread availability of *immunization* against many of them makes quarantine procedures rarely necessary. In some cases (principally to prevent the spread of yellow fever), quarantine has been replaced by compulsory vaccination for travel between certain countries. The contacts of people with highly infectious diseases (such as pneumonic *plague*) may have restrictions placed on their travel in addition to being given preventive immunization against the disease.

The principal remaining quarantine regulations apply to animals imported into countries that are free from *rabies*.

# Quickening

The stage of pregnancy when the movements of the fetus are first felt by the pregnant woman. Quickening usually occurs between 16 and 20 weeks of gestation.

# Quinacrine

A drug used during World War II to suppress malaria and now to treat *giardiasis*, an intestinal infection. Possible adverse effects include nausea, vomiting, and yellow discoloration of the skin and urine. Prolonged use can cause blood disorders or psychological disturbance.

# Quinestrol

A synthetic *estrogen drug* used to treat symptoms of the *menopause* (see *Hormone replacement therapy*).

# Quinidine

An *antiarrhythmic drug* used to treat irregular or abnormally fast heart beat. Quinidine may cause nausea, vomiting, diarrhea, and, occasionally, a dangerous drop in blood pressure or a worsening of the *arrhythmia*.

# Quinine

The oldest drug treatment for *malaria*. Quinine is now used mainly to treat strains of the disease that are resistant to other antimalarial drugs. Large doses are needed and there is a high risk of adverse effects, including headache, nausea, hearing loss, ringing in the ears, and blurred vision.

Quinine is frequently prescribed to help prevent painful leg cramps at night; low doses are used and adverse effects are rare.

# Quinsy

An abscess around the tonsil, usually occurring as a complication of *tonsillitis*. The infection causes a painful throat, high temperature, headache, impaired speech, drooling, and swollen, tender lymph glands in the neck. The uvula (the protuberance that hangs down from the soft palate at the back of the mouth) is displaced to the unaffected side of the throat.

*Antibiotic drugs* taken at an early stage sometimes clear up the infection. Otherwise, the abscess requires surgical incision and drainage. Once healing is complete, the tonsils are usually removed to prevent the infection from recurring.

# R

## Rabies

An acute viral infection of the nervous system, also known as hydrophobia. Rabies primarily affects animals, but it can be transmitted from a rabid animal to a human by a bite or by a lick over a break in the skin. The causative virus, present in the animal's saliva, travels from the wound along nerve pathways to the brain, where it causes inflammation that results in delirium, painful muscle spasms in the throat, and other severe symptoms. Once symptoms develop, human rabies is usually fatal.

### CAUSES AND INCIDENCE
The geographical distribution of rabies, and some important animal species affected, are shown on the map below.

Most human cases are the result of a bite from a rabid dog. However, the possibility of rabies must be considered whenever any mammal—domestic or wild—bites a human in a country where the rabies virus is present.

Worldwide, there are an estimated 15,000 cases of human rabies each year. Annually in the US, the number of human cases is generally less than five as a result of an intensive dog vaccination program and of prompt medical attention to animal bites.

### SYMPTOMS AND SIGNS
The incubation period between bite and appearance of symptoms ranges from nine days to many months (the average is four to eight weeks), depending largely on the site of the animal bite.

The initial symptoms are low-grade fever, headache, and loss of appetite leading to restlessness, hyperactivity, disorientation, and, in some cases, seizures. Often the victim has an intense thirst, but attempts to drink induce violent, painful spasms in the throat (hence the term hydrophobia). Eye and facial muscles may become paralyzed. Coma and death follow three to 20 days after the onset of symptoms.

### TREATMENT
Once symptoms have appeared, the features of the disease are treated with sedative drugs and analgesics (painkillers). A very small number of people with established rabies are reported as having survived as a result of intensive care aimed at maintaining breathing and the action of the heart. However, the main emphasis must be on preventing the disease.

### PREVENTION
In areas of the US where rabies exists in wild animals, domestic dogs are vaccinated annually and stray dogs are killed. All people with high-risk occupations (e.g., veterinarians and animal trappers) require regular vaccinations. Countries that are free from rabies impose strict quarantine regulations on the importing of dogs and other mammals.

Following any bite, the wound should be thoroughly cleansed (see *Bites, animal*). The wound should not be sutured (stitched). If the bite occurs in a country where rabies is present, medical opinion should be sought immediately on whether postexposure *immunization* is necessary. If there is any risk of rabies, passive immunization is given with human rabies immune globulin (ready-made antibodies against the rabies virus), and rabies vaccine is given by a course of injections lasting several weeks. (Because the vaccine has changed, these shots are no longer administered through the stomach.)

Passive immunization is omitted for persons who have been vaccinated before exposure. The vaccines used today have only mild side effects when compared with the ones used before the 1970s.

Every attempt is made to capture and confine the biting animal. If it appears rabid, it is killed and its brain examined for the presence of rabies inclusion bodies (microscopic findings in the nuclei of affected cells). If no evidence of antibodies can be found or if a healthy animal remains symptom-free after five days, treatment of the bitten person is stopped.

If immunization is given within two days of the bite, rabies is almost always prevented. The chances of prevention decrease with delay, but immunization can still be effective when given weeks or months after a bite.

## Rachitic
A term used to describe bony or other abnormalities associated with, or

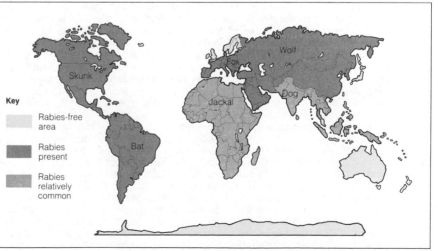

**GEOGRAPHICAL DISTRIBUTION OF RABIES**
In most rabies-affected areas, the disease circulates mainly among wild animals. Some of the principal animal "reservoirs" of rabies are shown at right, but other mammals may also be affected—e.g., raccoons and bats in North America. Most human cases result from the bite of a rabid dog. The dog may have acquired the virus through contact with a wild animal, but, in some areas, such as the Far East, stray dogs are themselves principal carriers. Vaccination of dogs can largely prevent human rabies.

Key
Rabies-free area
Rabies present
Rabies relatively common

suggestive of, *rickets* (the disease produced by a deficiency of vitamin D). Rachitic is also used to refer to people or populations that are particularly afflicted by rickets.

## Rad
A unit of absorbed dose of ionizing radiation (see the *Radiation* units box, opposite). Rad is an acronym for radiation absorbed dose.

## Radial nerve
A branch of the *brachial plexus*, the radial nerve is one of the main nerves of the arm, running down its full length into the hand. The radial nerve controls muscles that straighten the wrist so that the back of the hand is in line with the forearm. It also conveys sensation from the back of the forearm; from the thumb, second, and third fingers; and from an area at the base of the thumb.

### DISORDERS
The radial nerve winds around the shaft of the humerus (upper arm bone) and so may be damaged by a fracture of this bone. The nerve may also be damaged by persistent pressure on the armpit (e.g., from a crutch). Such damage may result in *wristdrop* (inability to straighten the wrist) and numbness in the areas of skin supplied by the radial nerve.

## Radiation
There are two main types of radiation—ionizing and nonionizing. Ionizing radiation is capable of forcibly ejecting one or more of the electrons that orbit the nucleus of an atom, thereby creating an entity called an *ion* that has an electrical charge and is capable of chemical combination with other ions. When ionization occurs in the atoms of molecules that play an important role in the body, it can lead to biological damage.

Nonionizing radiation has a different effect on molecules. It tends to cause excitation of the molecules' constituent atoms (somewhat like shaking them) but it does not impart enough energy to the atoms to displace electrons and form ions.

### IONIZING RADIATION
There are three types of ionizing radiation—*X rays*, gamma rays, and particle radiation. X rays are electromagnetic waves (i.e., they are part of the same continuous spectrum—the electromagnetic spectrum—that includes radio waves, infrared radiation, visible light, ultraviolet light, and gamma rays) of very short wavelength and very high frequency. X rays are produced by special electrical machines (X-ray generators). X rays have no mass and no electrical charge; their penetrating power depends on their energy, which, in turn, depends on the voltage used to generate them. X rays generated at a few tens of thousands of volts can penetrate only a few millimeters of tissue, whereas those generated at about 100,000 volts are just energetic enough to pass completely through the body and produce X-ray images. X rays used in *radiation therapy* are generated at several million volts and are sufficiently energetic to destroy deep-seated tumors.

Gamma rays have almost identical properties to X rays. The principal difference between the two is that gamma rays are produced by the spontaneous decay of radioactive materials rather than by a machine. They also tend to have shorter wavelengths and higher frequencies than X rays, although there is some overlap between the two.

Particle radiation—unlike X rays and gamma rays—has mass and may also have electrical charge. It represents parts of atoms, such as electrons (beta particles, which have a negative electrical charge and a very small mass), protons (positively charged particles, each with a mass about 1,800 times that of an electron), or neutrons (particles with the same mass as protons but no electrical charge). The nuclei of small atoms such as helium (helium nuclei are also known as alpha particles) and even larger atomic nuclei may be the source of particle radiation. Particle radiation may be produced during the decay of radioactive atoms or by machines.

### SOURCES OF IONIZING RADIATION
Ionizing radiation may originate from natural or man-made sources. One natural source is cosmic rays, which come from remote parts of the universe as well as from the sun. These rays consist largely of very high energy protons, along with a few atomic nuclei (principally helium nuclei). Cosmic rays are highly energetic and not only can irradiate people on the Earth's surface, but can also pass through many feet of soil and rock. The amount of cosmic rays an individual receives depends on the altitude at which he or she lives. A person who is living in Denver, Colorado, at an altitude of about 6,000 feet, receives more than twice the annual radiation dose of cosmic rays than a person living at sea level.

Secondary radiation is another natural source. It is generated in the upper atmosphere from cosmic rays and consists mainly of gamma rays and high-energy electrons. The annual dose from such secondary radiation varies with the latitude, being greatest at the Earth's poles and least at the equator.

The other principal natural source of radiation is radioactivity. Many minerals contain unstable atomic nuclei that spontaneously disintegrate (a process known as radioactive decay), thereby emitting alpha or beta particles and/or gamma rays. The naturally occurring radioactive isotope potassium 40 (isotopes are varieties of an element that are chemically identical but differ in some physical properties) is the principal source of radiation from within the body. Many other natural materials are radioactive and, in some areas, *radon* from soil, rocks, and/or building materials is a major contributor to the annual radiation dose.

Medical X rays—used to diagnose and/or treat numerous diseases and disorders—are the greatest artificial source of radiation to which the general public is exposed. In the US, the average yearly radiation dose from medical X rays is almost equal to that from all natural sources. Radioactive isotopes, also used in diagnosis and treatment, are another medical source of radiation (see *Radionuclide scanning*). Radioisotopes that emit gamma rays are most commonly used (although particle-emitting radioisotopes are also employed); the types selected are usually short-lived to reduce the dose to the patient.

Nuclear reactors are not only sources of direct radiation (such as gamma rays and neutrons, which are normally absorbed by thick reactor shielding to prevent them from escaping into the environment), but are also prolific producers of radioactive isotopes. *Uranium* is the most commonly used fuel, often enriched so that it contains more of the fissionable isotope uranium 235 than is present in natural uranium ores. In the reactor it undergoes fission (splitting), thereby producing heat and leaving behind a wide variety of radioactive isotopes. Radioisotopes of iodine, ruthenium, tellurium, and cesium are among those produced in the greatest amounts, although others of greater biological importance, such as *strontium* isotopes, are also produced. In fast-breeder reactors, *plutonium* is

R

used as the main fuel; uranium 238 is the source from which additional plutonium fuel is made.

Nuclear weapons, including atomic bombs of the types used at Hiroshima and Nagasaki (in which either uranium or plutonium undergoes rapid fission) and hydrogen bombs (which combine nuclear fission and fusion) are intense sources of man-made radiation. However, except for the relatively small battlefield weapons and the "radiation-enhanced" weapon (the so-called neutron bomb), the lethal effects from direct irradiation occur only comparatively near the point of explosion, whereas the lethal effects of blast and heat extend over a considerably larger area.

### NONIONIZING RADIATION

The most widespread type of nonionizing radiation is ultraviolet light, a component of sunlight (although much is absorbed by the atmosphere); it is also produced by sunlamps. This type of radiation can penetrate only superficial layers of body tissue but it damages the RNA (ribonucleic acid) and DNA (deoxyribonucleic acid) molecules in cells, which may lead to skin cancer.

Microwave ovens cook food by means of radio-frequency electromagnetic radiation, which can also heat body tissues and thereby damage them. This type of injury is unlikely to occur because modern appliances are shielded to prevent microwaves from escaping; they also have safety cutoffs that stop radiation emission when the door is opened. Radio and television transmissions are harmless forms of electromagnetic radiation.

The other types of nonionizing radiation to which people are subjected are magnetic fields and *ultrasound*. Weak magnetic fields are generated around all wires carrying electricity, and strong fields are used in medicine for magnetic resonance imaging (*MRI*). The effects of such fields are currently being studied, but they are not thought to be harmful; some authorities believe that they may even be beneficial. Ultrasound (inaudible high-frequency sound waves) is used in medicine for diagnosis and, on occasion, treatment. Its effects depend on the power used and the duration of exposure. The low power levels and relatively short durations used in medicine are harmless, but exposure to ultrasound at high power levels and/or for a long time may cause tissue damage. (See also *Radiation hazards; Radiation sickness*.)

## RADIATION UNITS

| | | |
|---|---|---|
| **Becquerel** | The SI unit of radioactivity. One becquerel (symbol Bq) is defined as one disintegration (or other nuclear transformation) per second. Although the number of becquerels is a measure of how strongly | radioactive a particular source is, it takes no account of the different effects of different types of radiation on tissue; for medical purposes, the sievert is generally more useful. |
| **Gray** | The SI unit of absorbed dose of ionizing radiation, the gray (symbol Gy) has superseded the rad. One gray is defined as an energy | absorption of 1 joule per kilogram of irradiated material. One gray is equivalent to 100 rads. |
| **Rad** | An acronym for radiation absorbed dose, the rad is a unit of absorbed dose of ionizing radiation. One rad is equal to an energy absorption of 100 ergs (an erg is a unit of work or | energy) per gram of irradiated material. The rad has been superseded by the gray (the corresponding SI unit); 1 rad is equivalent to 0.01 grays. |
| **Rem** | An acronym for roentgen equivalent man, the rem is the absorbed dose of ionizing radiation that produces the same biological effect as 1 rad of X rays or gamma rays. The rem was introduced as a result of the observation that some types of ionizing radiation, such as neutrons, produce a greater biological effect for an equivalent amount of absorbed energy than X rays or gamma rays. In short, the rem is a measure of the biological effectiveness of irradiation. For X rays and gamma rays, the rem is | equal to the rad. For other types of radiation, the number of rems equals the number of rads multiplied by a special factor (called the quality factor or relative biological effectiveness) that depends on the type of radiation involved. The rem has been superseded by the sievert in the SI system of units; 1 rem is equivalent to 0.01 sieverts. |
| **Sievert** | The SI unit of equivalent absorbed dose of ionizing radiation, the sievert (symbol Sv) has superseded the rem. One sievert is the absorbed dose of radiation that | produces the same biological effect as 1 gray of X rays or gamma rays. One sievert is equivalent to 100 rems. |

**Measurement of radiation levels**

In the SI system (the internationally agreed system of units), three main units are used to measure radiation levels—the becquerel, the gray, and the sievert. These three units are defined above, along with two other radiation units (the rad and rem) that have now been largely superseded but are still occasionally used for some purposes.

## Radiation hazards

Hazards from radiation may arise from exposure to external sources of radiation (such as X rays or gamma rays) and from internal irradiation from radioactive materials taken into the body (see *Radiation*). Two topics of particular public concern are whether there are any radiation hazards associated with visual display terminals (VDTs) or with the irradiation of food. In fact, there is no evidence that either of them poses such a hazard. VDTs do not emit significant amounts of penetrating radiation and food that has been irradiated does not itself become radioactive.

### TYPES OF HAZARDS AND THEIR EFFECTS

The effects of radiation depend critically on the dose received and the duration of exposure.

Some forms of radiation damage occur when the total radiation dose exceeds a certain threshold, usually 1 sievert or more (see *Radiation* units box above). Above the threshold, damage increases, including *radiation sickness* (an early reaction to radiation) and radiation *dermatitis*, *cataracts*, or failure of various organs, which may occur only many years after exposure. These hazards can be avoided by keeping the cumulative radiation exposure below the threshold dose.

R

For other radiation hazards, the severity of damage does not depend upon the specific radiation dose, but the risk that damage will occur increases with increasing doses. *Cancer* is the major example of this type of radiation damage. It usually occurs many years after exposure, typically five to 15 years for leukemia, and 40 years or longer for skin, lung, breast, and other cancers. Heritable genetic damage is another form of radiation damage.

The International Commission on Radiological Protection has concluded that the total risk factor for death from radiation-induced cancers is about one in 100 per sievert of radiation absorbed. The risk of a hereditary disorder occurring within the first two generations following irradiation of either parent is also thought to be about one in 100 per sievert, and the additional risk to subsequent generations is thought to be the same.

## Radiation sickness

The term applied to the acute effects of ionizing *radiation* on the whole, or a major part, of the body when the dose is greater than about 1 gray (1 Gy) of X rays or gamma rays, or 1 sievert (1 Sv) of other types of radiation (see previous page).

### SYMPTOMS

The effect of exposure to radiation depends critically on the dose and the time course over which it is received. Above acute exposures of 30 to 100 Gy, there is a rapid onset of nausea, vomiting (which may be repeated and severe), anxiety, and disorientation. Within a few hours, the victim usually loses consciousness and dies as a consequence of direct damage to the nervous system from the radiation, and to edema (accumulation of fluid) of the brain; these effects are known as the central nervous system syndrome.

People who have received radiation doses of 10 to 30 Gy also experience an early onset of nausea and vomiting, which tend to start within about two hours of exposure but disappear a few hours later. However, such individuals invariably die within four to 14 days of exposure as a result of radiation damage to the gastrointestinal tract—which causes severe and frequently bloody diarrhea (known as the gastrointestinal syndrome)—and overwhelming infection due to radiation damage to the *immune system*.

At doses of 1 to 10 Gy, transient nausea and occasional vomiting may occur, but these early symptoms usually disappear rapidly and are often followed by a two- to three-week period of relative well-being. However, by the end of this period, the effects of radiation damage to the bone marrow and immune system begin to appear, with repeated infections (which may be fatal unless treated with antibiotic drugs), and petechiae (pinpoint spots of bleeding under the skin). Some victims may be treated successfully by *bone marrow transplantation* or by isolation in a sterile environment until their own bone marrow recovers.

Radiation damage to other tissues, such as the skin and lining of the respiratory tract, may cause complications, but total-body doses of less than 2 Gy are unlikely to be fatal to an otherwise healthy adult. However, despite the most intensive medical care, few people survive doses of more than 6 Gy.

## Radiation therapy

Treatment of *cancer* (and occasionally other diseases) by X rays or other sources of radioactivity, both of which produce ionizing *radiation*. The radiation, as it passes through the diseased tissue, destroys or slows the development of abnormal cells. Provided the correct dosage of radiation is given, normal cells suffer little or no damage.

### WHY IT IS DONE

Radiation therapy has various applications in the treatment of cancer. In cancer of the larynx (see *Larynx, cancer of*), in certain kinds of *mouth cancer*, *basal cell carcinoma*, and *squamous cell carcinoma* (a type of skin cancer), in cancer of the cervix (see *Cervix, cancer of*), in cancer of the uterus (see *Uterus, cancer of*), in *Hodgkin's disease* (a cancer of lymphoid tissue), and in *leukemia* it may be used by itself in an attempt to destroy all the abnormal cells.

Radiation therapy is often used after surgical excision of a malignant tumor (such as in the treatment of *breast cancer*) to destroy any remaining tumor cells. It is also used to reduce the size of a tumor to relieve the symptoms of a cancer that is too far advanced to be curable. Examples of palliative treatment include relieving pressure from a tumor on the esophagus that prevents swallowing (see *Esophagus, cancer of*), relieving pain caused by bone cancer, and relieving headaches or paralysis caused by a *brain tumor*.

If the benefits of destroying diseased tissue far outweigh the risk of damage to healthy tissue, radiation therapy may be used to treat non-malignant diseases. A common example is the destruction of part of an overactive thyroid gland with radioactive iodine when it is producing severe symptoms (see *Thyrotoxicosis*).

### HOW IT IS DONE

Some of the main techniques of radiation therapy are shown opposite. Radiation is usually passed through diseased tissues by means of X rays (or sometimes electrons) produced by a machine called a linear accelerator. This device has largely supplanted apparatus containing radioactive cobalt, which has the drawback of producing ionizing radiation that is both less intense than that of X rays and incapable of being shut off.

Some malignant tumors are treated not by radiation from an external source, but by inserting radioactive material directly into the growth or surrounding tissue (see *Interstitial radiation therapy*) or into a body cavity (see *Intracavitary therapy*). Both procedures require an anesthetic.

Radiation used to treat thyrotoxicosis is given as a liquid form of radioactive iodine, which the patient drinks through a straw and which concentrates in the thyroid gland.

### COMPLICATIONS

Radiation therapy may produce unpleasant side effects, including fatigue, nausea and vomiting (for which *antiemetic drugs* may be prescribed beforehand), and loss of hair from irradiated areas. Rarely, there may be reddening and blistering of the skin, which can be alleviated by *corticosteroid drugs*.

### RESULTS

Radiation therapy cures most skin cancers and cancer of the larynx. The cure rate for other types of cancer varies depending on how early the treatment is begun, but the cure rate can be 80 percent or higher.

## Radical surgery

Extensive surgery aimed at eliminating a major disease by removing all affected tissue and any surrounding tissue that might be diseased.

In the past, radical surgery was commonly done in an attempt to cure cancer. Radical *mastectomy* for *breast cancer* involved removing the entire affected breast, along with chest muscles, underarm lymph nodes, and other tissue. Such operations are rarely performed today.

*Amputation*, usually to prevent the spread of *gangrene* (tissue death), is another form of radical surgery.

R

## RADIATION THERAPY

Before treatment, calculations are made of the doses of radiation needed and of the directions from which the rays should be aimed. The areas of the patient's body to be targeted are marked directly on the patient or on a plastic coat that he or she wears. The treatment is usually performed on an outpatient basis, with the patient receiving treatment several times a week.

### Radiation therapy machine in use

The patient lies on a table under the machine in a room designed to prevent radiation leakage. A radiation technologist operates the machine, which sends X rays, in the predetermined directions and amounts, through the diseased area of the patient's body. The procedure causes no discomfort and usually lasts just a few minutes.

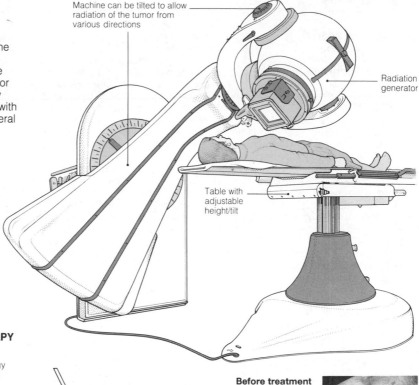

Machine can be tilted to allow radiation of the tumor from various directions

Radiation generator

Table with adjustable height/tilt

### EXAMPLES OF RADIATION THERAPY

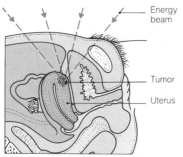

Energy beam

Tumor

Uterus

**Rays from different directions**
By targeting relatively low-energy rays coming from many directions at a tumor, a large enough dose is achieved in the locality of the tumor to destroy it. Tissues through which the rays pass are unharmed.

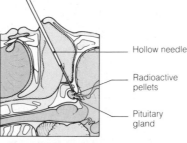

Hollow needle

Radioactive pellets

Pituitary gland

**Use of radioactive pellets**
Another technique is to insert a source of radiation, in the form of tiny radioactive pellets, directly into the tumor via a hollow needle. Pituitary tumors are sometimes treated in this way.

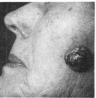

**Before treatment**
The patient has a malignant skin cancer.

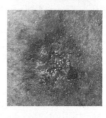

**After treatment**
The tumor is healing well after radiation therapy.

R

## Radiculopathy

Damage to the nerve roots that enter or leave the spinal cord. Radiculopathy may be caused by *disk prolapse*, spinal *arthritis*, thickening of the meninges (the membranes that cover the brain and spinal cord), and sometimes *diabetes mellitus* or ingestion of heavy metals, such as lead.

Symptoms are severe pain and, occasionally, loss of feeling in the area supplied by the affected nerves, and weakness, paralysis, and wasting of muscles supplied by the nerves.

Treatment is of the underlying cause if possible; otherwise, symptoms may be relieved by analgesics (painkillers), *physical therapy*, or, in some cases, surgery.

## Radioactivity

The emission of alpha particles or beta particles and/or gamma rays that occurs when the nuclei of certain unstable substances spontaneously disintegrate. Natural radioactivity is due to the disintegration of naturally occurring radioactive substances,

such as uranium ores. However, most elements can be induced to become radioactive by bombarding them with high-energy particles (such as neutrons)—so-called artificial radioactivity. (See also *Radiation*.)

## Radioimmunoassay

A very sensitive laboratory technique that employs radioactive isotopes to measure the concentration of specific proteins in a person's blood. Proteins that can be detected by radioimmunoassay include hormones, parts of microorganisms, and antibodies formed against microorganisms or allergens. (See *Immunoassay*.)

## Radioisotope scanning

See *Radionuclide scanning*.

## Radiologic technician

See *X-ray technician*.

## Radiologist

A physician (also known as a roentgenologist) who is specially trained and certified in the use of X rays, nuclear imaging devices, radioactive substances, ultrasound, and magnetic resonance to see into the body and diagnose and treat problems. In general, a radiologist (either at an outpatient clinic or in a hospital) is seen only on referral by another physician. Other specialists licensed by the nuclear regulatory agency may also use radioisotopes (radionuclides) for diagnosis and treatment.

## Radiology

The medical specialty that uses *X rays*, *ultrasound*, *MRI*, and *radionuclide scanning* for investigation, diagnosis, and treatment. Other specialists may also employ radionuclide scanning.

Radiologic tests can provide images of almost any organ, system, or part of the body in a *noninvasive* way so that diagnoses can be made and treatment planned or monitored frequently without the need for the patient to undergo exploratory surgery.

Radiologic techniques also enable instruments (such as needles and catheters) to be accurately guided into different parts of the body both for diagnosis and, increasingly, for treatment. This subspecialty is known as interventional radiology.

## Radiolucent

Almost transparent to radiation, especially to X rays and gamma rays (objects that are entirely transparent to radiation are radiotransparent). See also *Radiopaque*.

## Radionuclide scanning

A diagnostic technique based on the detection of radiation emitted by radioactive substances introduced into the body. Different radioactive substances, known as radionuclides, are taken up in greater concentrations by different types of tissue, so that specific organs can be studied. For example, the thyroid gland takes up more radioactive iodine than other parts of the body. The images pro-

vided by radionuclide scanning reflect the function of an organ better than other techniques, although they provide less anatomical detail.

### HOW IT WORKS

Radionuclide is swallowed or injected into the bloodstream and accumulates in the target organ. Radiation in the form of gamma rays (similar to X rays but of shorter wavelength) is emitted from the organ and detected by a "gamma camera." The camera contains a scintillation crystal that reacts to gamma rays by emitting minute quantities of light (photons). These are used to produce an image that can be displayed on a screen or in digital (numerical) form.

Using a principle similar to *CT scanning*, cross-sectional images (slices) can be constructed by a computer from radiation detected by a gamma camera that rotates around the patient. This specialized form of radionuclide scanning is known as SPECT (single photon emission computerized tomography).

It is also possible to create moving images with the aid of a computer by recording a series of images immediately following the administration of the radionuclide.

### WHY IT IS DONE

Radionuclide scanning can detect certain disorders earlier than other imaging techniques because changes in the functioning of an organ often occur before the structure is affected. For example, infection of bone results in increased activity of bone cells, resulting in radionuclide being taken up in greater amounts by diseased bone before structural changes show on conventional X rays. The technique is also useful for detecting disorders that affect only function (e.g., some *thyroid* disorders).

Moving images can provide information on functions such as blood flow, the movements of the heart walls, urine flow through the kidneys, and bile flow through the liver.

### RISKS

Radionuclide scanning is a safe procedure. It requires only minute doses of radiation and, since the radionuclide is ingested or administered by intravenous injection, it also avoids the risks associated with some X-ray procedures in which a radiopaque dye is administered by inserting a catheter into the organ (as in cardiac *catheterization* and coronary *angiography*). In addition, unlike radiopaque dyes, radionuclides carry virtually no risk of toxicity or allergy.

### OUTLOOK

Advances in radionuclide scanning depend on the continuing development of radionuclides specific to certain tissues. The fact that monoclonal antibodies (see *Antibody, monoclonal*) can now be produced for use against almost any antigen means that it should be possible to target almost any tissue. Experiments are being carried out using labeled antitumor monoclonal antibodies to assess tumor spread and recurrence.

## Radiopaque

Blocking the passage of radiation, especially X rays and gamma rays. Many body tissues are *radiolucent* to X rays (bones being a notable exception). Thus, in diagnostic X-ray imaging, it is sometimes necessary to introduce special radiopaque dyes into the body to make organs stand out more clearly. In intravenous *pyelography*, for example, radiopaque iodine compounds are excreted by the kidney into the lower urinary tract to make the structures clearly visible on X-ray photographs.

## Radiotherapy

See *Radiation therapy*.

## Radium

A rare radioactive metallic element that does not occur naturally in its pure form but is present as various compounds in *uranium* ores, such as pitchblende and carnotite. Radium has four naturally occurring isotopes (varieties of the element that are chemically identical but differ in some physical properties). In order of decreasing abundance they are radium 226, radium 228, radium 224, and radium 223. Artificial radium isotopes have also been produced.

The most important isotope is radium 226, which is produced by the decay of naturally radioactive elements of the uranium series. It is relatively long-lived (with a *half-life* of about 1,600 years), and itself decays to form the gas *radon*, which then decays further to form other, solid, radioactive decay products. During these decay stages, *radiation* is emitted in the form of alpha and beta particles and gamma rays. Radium 226 was once used to treat tumors but has now been superseded by other radioisotopes, such as cobalt 60 and cesium 137. It was also once used in some luminous paints until it was discovered that the radium caused leukemia and bone tumors in those using the paint.

R

## Radius

The shorter of the two long bones of the forearm; the other is the *ulna*. The radius is the bone on the thumb side of the arm.

The shaft of the radius has a broad base that articulates with the lower end of the ulna and with the upper bones of the wrist. The disk-shaped head of the radius, which is smaller than the base, articulates with the lower end of the *humerus* (the bone of the upper arm) to form part of the elbow joint.

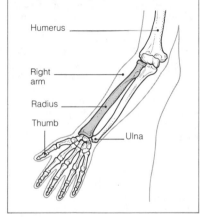

**LOCATION OF THE RADIUS**
The radius is the bone on the inside of the forearm with the palm facing down, or on the outside with the palm facing up.

Humerus

Right arm

Radius

Thumb

Ulna

The radius takes most of the strain when weight is placed on the wrist and is a common site of fractures (see *Radius, fracture of; Colles' fracture*). A fall or blow sometimes causes dislocation of the radius from the elbow joint along with fracture of the ulna, a condition known as *Monteggia's fracture*.

## Radius, fracture of

Fractures of the *radius* are among the most common of fractures and are usually caused by a fall on an outstretched hand.

Fracture of the radius just above the wrist is the most common of all fractures in people over 40. It is usually caused by falling on the palm, resulting in backward displacement of the wrist and hand (see *Colles' fracture*).

Fracture of the disk-shaped head of the bone just below the elbow joint is one of the most common fractures in young adults. Treatment consists of immobilizing the forearm (bent at a right angle to the upper arm) and the elbow in plaster to allow the fracture to heal. If the head of the bone is crushed or splintered, it may require removal by surgery before it is immobilized in a cast.

Fracture of the shaft of the radius often results in displacement of the bone ends. An operation is usually required to reposition the bone ends and fix them together with wires or plates and screws, but sometimes the bones can be externally manipulated back into position. In both cases, the limb is finally immobilized using a plaster cast.

## Radon

A colorless, odorless, tasteless, radioactive gaseous element produced by the radioactive decay of *radium*. Radon has three naturally occurring isotopes (varieties of the element that are chemically identical but differ in some physical properties)—radon 219, radon 220, and radon 222. Each of these is short-lived (radon 219 has a *half-life* of roughly 4 seconds, radon 220 of about 51 seconds, and radon 222 of about 3.8 days). They disintegrate—with the emission of *radiation* (in the form of alpha particles)—to form solid radioactive materials known as radon daughters, which themselves emit alpha and beta particles and gamma rays. In addition to radon's naturally occurring radioisotopes, more than a dozen artificial ones have been produced.

The parent sources of radon occur naturally in many materials, such as soil, rocks, and building materials, and the gas is released continually into the atmosphere. As a result, radon makes the largest single contribution to radiation doses received by humans from naturally radioactive materials. This fact has led some researchers to suggest that radon may be a significant causative factor in some cases of cancer (particularly lung cancer). However, this claim has yet to be tested scientifically.

## Ranitidine

An *ulcer-healing drug*, similar to *cimetidine* and *famotidine*, belonging to the *histamine-2 receptor antagonist* group of drugs. Ranitidine is used to prevent and treat *peptic ulcers* and to treat peptic *esophagitis*.

Ranitidine and famotidine are less likely to interact with other drugs or to produce any major side effects. Possible minor side effects include headache, skin rash, nausea, constipation, and lethargy.

## Rape

Forcible sexual intercourse with an unwilling partner.

Rape is a felony in every state. While the statutory definition may be expressed somewhat differently by the legislature of each state, the elements of the offense are essentially the same. Rape is defined as sexual intercourse by the use or threat of force or violence and against the victim's will or without the victim's consent.

In some states, the term aggravated sexual assault (including penetration of any body orifice without consent) is used instead of rape. In certain states, the law recognizes some forms of rape in marriage.

While rape has traditionally been considered to be an offense committed by a man against a woman, many states have amended their laws to remove the gender identification and to expand the scope of the law to include homosexual rape and other sexual offenses, such as incest.

Society, police, and the courts are attempting to do more for rape victims and there is generally a greater understanding of the traumatic effects the crime can have on the victim. Studies have clarified the nature of the crime, revealing that, contrary to popular belief, rape most often occurs between people who know each other, is not always accompanied by physical violence, and is not provoked by a girl or woman.

### INCIDENCE

In recent years, there has been a considerable increase in reported rape cases (see graph on next page). It is difficult to know whether these figures reflect a genuine increase in incidence or a greater willingness on the part of victims to report the crime. Nevertheless, rape is still one of the least reported of all crimes. It is estimated that 70 percent of rapes in the US are unreported due to the victim's shame, fear of family rejection, fear of reprisal by the rapist, or fear of the publicity and trauma associated with going through a trial.

### MOTIVES

Rape is a violent crime motivated by a need to dominate the victim. The rapist may use forcible sex as one of many forms of abusive, dehumanizing behavior, being motivated by a profound hostility toward women.

Rarely is rape sexually motivated; rape is a crime of dominance and anger, not of passion. There is also evidence of a significant link between alcohol abuse and rape.

**R**

## INCIDENCE OF REPORTED RAPE

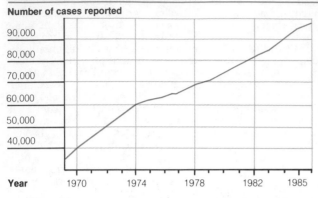

**Number of cases reported**

The graph shows the marked and alarming increase in rapes reported annually in the US since 1970. It is difficult to know whether the figures reflect a genuine increase in the incidence of rape or a greater willingness on the part of the victims to report the crime.

About 20 percent of rapists are reconvicted of sexual offenses; up to 80 percent subsequently commit other crimes and often have a long history of violent crime.

### EFFECTS

The rape victim may suffer a variety of physical injuries, usually as a result of beating or choking. Severe injury to the genitals is rare, but there may be swelling of the labia, bruising of the vaginal walls or cervix, and, occasionally, tearing of the anus or perineum (area between the genitals and the anus).

Even in the absence of physical injury, the psychological effects of rape are often severe, including significant *anxiety, depression,* or *posttraumatic stress disorder*. Nightmares or daytime flashbacks of the event may also occur.

### FORENSIC TESTS

The physician examining a rape victim performs a physical examination, noting signs of bruising or injury, particularly to the genital area. The examination includes inspection of the vaginal canal with a *speculum*. A woman is usually present to support the victim.

For laboratory analysis, the physician collects swabs from any suspected bite marks, from soiled areas of the body, and from the vagina, anus, or throat; fingernail scrapings or clippings; and any torn-out strands of head or pubic hair. These may be matched with samples of blood or saliva taken from suspects.

Clothing worn by the victim at the time of the assault is also retained for forensic examination.

### TREATMENT

Physical injuries are treated as required. If conception results from the rape, elective *abortion* may be considered. Treatment for sexually transmitted disease may be required in some cases.

For psychological trauma, rape crisis counseling is highly beneficial. Psychiatric support may also be needed. Help is readily available today, often from rape support groups in most community hospitals through the social work department.

### PREVENTION

There are a number of important ways to reduce the incidence of rape. First, rape cases should be moved quickly and effectively through the reporting, arrest, and trial process so that violent criminals are quickly removed from society. It must be clear to victims that they will be dealt with fairly and sympathetically by police and the court system. Rape victim advocacy groups have been established in many areas of the country to provide counseling and support to victims. Women's shelters can provide a temporary place to live, since many women need shelter from a current or previous partner who has become abusive.

Children should be told that there are people who may harm or hurt them due to their mixed-up sexual feelings. They should be instructed never to go into cars, alleys, or secluded places without permission.

True prevention may require more basic and complex changes. While society's emphasis on male machismo is no excuse for committing violent crimes, eliminating the concept of women as sexual objects (rather than as sexual partners) would help. There has also been a "blame the victim" mentality toward rape victims that must be eliminated; the onus must be placed solely on the perpetrator.

There is a place for assertiveness training and self-defense training for women. Although it is in no way the victim's fault that she is molested, learning assertive behavior patterns and even self-defense techniques can head off an attacker. Some of the best approaches teach women common-sense tips, such as how to recognize whether someone is testing you to see if you would make a good victim.

## Rash

A group of spots or an area of red, inflamed skin. A rash is usually temporary and only rarely is a sign of a serious underlying problem. It may be accompanied by itching or fever.

### TYPES

A rash may be localized (affecting only a small area of the skin) or generalized (covering the entire body). Physicians also describe rashes as blistering (either bullous or vesicular), macular,

**R**

## AGE WHEN VICTIMIZED BY RAPE

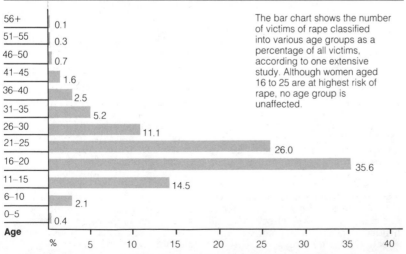

The bar chart shows the number of victims of rape classified into various age groups as a percentage of all victims, according to one extensive study. Although women aged 16 to 25 are at highest risk of rape, no age group is unaffected.

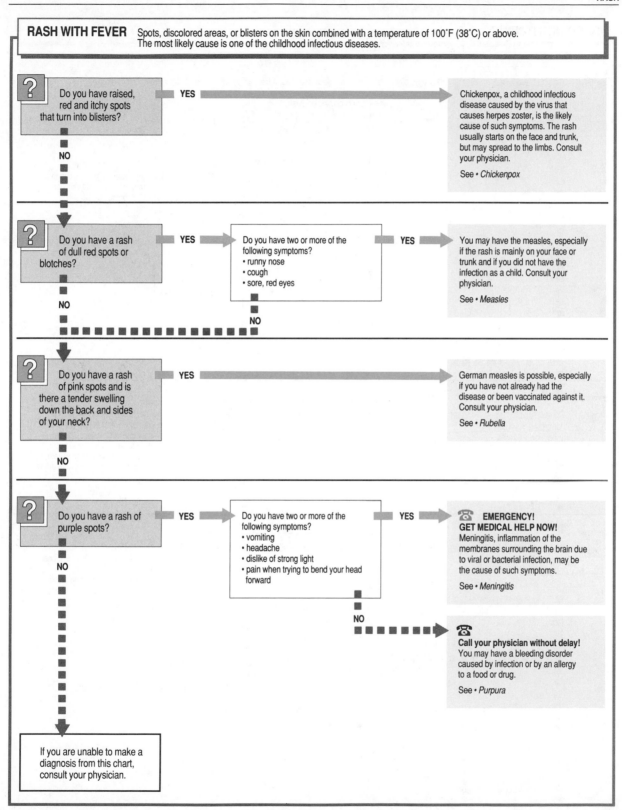

**RASH WITH FEVER** Spots, discolored areas, or blisters on the skin combined with a temperature of 100°F (38°C) or above. The most likely cause is one of the childhood infectious diseases.

Do you have raised, red and itchy spots that turn into blisters?

**YES** → Chickenpox, a childhood infectious disease caused by the virus that causes herpes zoster, is the likely cause of such symptoms. The rash usually starts on the face and trunk, but may spread to the limbs. Consult your physician.

See • *Chickenpox*

**NO**

Do you have a rash of dull red spots or blotches?

**YES** → Do you have two or more of the following symptoms?
• runny nose
• cough
• sore, red eyes

**YES** → You may have the measles, especially if the rash is mainly on your face or trunk and if you did not have the infection as a child. Consult your physician.

See • *Measles*

**NO**

**NO**

Do you have a rash of pink spots and is there a tender swelling down the back and sides of your neck?

**YES** → German measles is possible, especially if you have not already had the disease or been vaccinated against it. Consult your physician.

See • *Rubella*

**NO**

Do you have a rash of purple spots?

**YES** → Do you have two or more of the following symptoms?
• vomiting
• headache
• dislike of strong light
• pain when trying to bend your head forward

**YES** → ☎ **EMERGENCY!**
**GET MEDICAL HELP NOW!**
Meningitis, inflammation of the membranes surrounding the brain due to viral or bacterial infection, may be the cause of such symptoms.

See • *Meningitis*

**NO**

**NO** → ☎
**Call your physician without delay!**
You may have a bleeding disorder caused by infection or by an allergy to a food or drug.

See • *Purpura*

If you are unable to make a diagnosis from this chart, consult your physician.

R

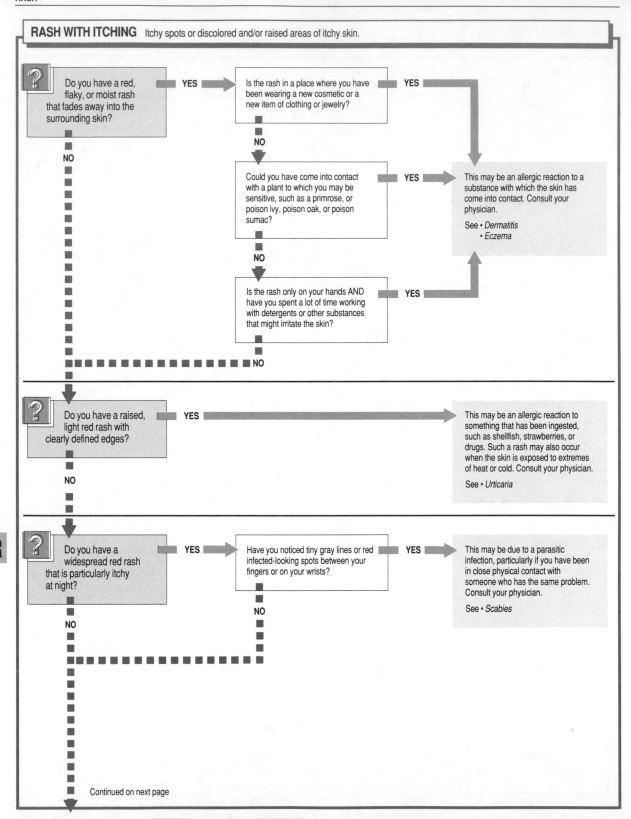

**RASH WITH ITCHING** Itchy spots or discolored and/or raised areas of itchy skin.

Do you have a red, flaky, or moist rash that fades away into the surrounding skin?

**YES** → Is the rash in a place where you have been wearing a new cosmetic or a new item of clothing or jewelry?

**YES** →

**NO** ↓

Could you have come into contact with a plant to which you may be sensitive, such as a primrose, or poison ivy, poison oak, or poison sumac?

**YES** →

**NO** ↓

Is the rash only on your hands AND have you spent a lot of time working with detergents or other substances that might irritate the skin?

**YES** →

This may be an allergic reaction to a substance with which the skin has come into contact. Consult your physician.

See • *Dermatitis*
  • *Eczema*

**NO** (from first question, dotted line down)

**NO** (bottom of third box)

---

Do you have a raised, light red rash with clearly defined edges?

**YES** →

This may be an allergic reaction to something that has been ingested, such as shellfish, strawberries, or drugs. Such a rash may also occur when the skin is exposed to extremes of heat or cold. Consult your physician.

See • *Urticaria*

**NO** ↓

---

R

Do you have a widespread red rash that is particularly itchy at night?

**YES** → Have you noticed tiny gray lines or red infected-looking spots between your fingers or on your wrists?

**YES** →

This may be due to a parasitic infection, particularly if you have been in close physical contact with someone who has the same problem. Consult your physician.

See • *Scabies*

**NO** ↓

**NO** ↓

Continued on next page

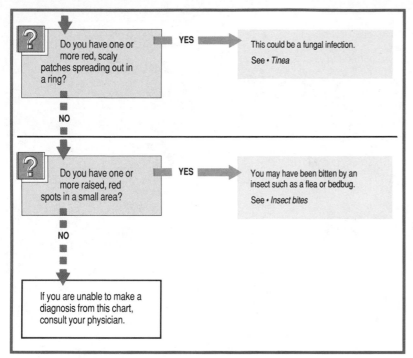

Do you have one or more red, scaly patches spreading out in a ring? — **YES** → This could be a fungal infection.
See • *Tinea*

**NO**

Do you have one or more raised, red spots in a small area? — **YES** → You may have been bitten by an insect such as a flea or bedbug.
See • *Insect bites*

**NO**

If you are unable to make a diagnosis from this chart, consult your physician.

nodular, papular, or pustular—according to the type of spots present.

**CAUSES**

A rash is the main sign of many childhood infectious diseases (such as *chickenpox* and *scarlet fever*) and of many other infections, ranging from ringworm (see *Tinea*) to *Rocky Mountain spotted fever*.

Rashes are a feature of many *skin disorders*, such as *eczema* and *psoriasis*. A rash may also indicate an underlying medical problem. Examples include the purple-red spots characteristic of *purpura* (a bleeding disorder); the rash of *scurvy* or *pellagra*, caused by vitamin deficiency; and the rashes appearing in *lupus erythematosus* and other *autoimmune disorders*.

The rashes of *urticaria* (hives) or of contact *dermatitis* may be caused by an allergic reaction to something that has been eaten or with which the skin has come in contact. Drug reactions, particularly to barbiturates and antibiotics, are also a common cause of rash.

**DIAGNOSIS AND TREATMENT**

The physician makes a diagnosis based on the appearance and distribution of the rash, the presence of any accompanying symptoms, and the possibility of allergy (e.g., to drugs).

Any underlying cause is treated if possible. An itching rash may be relieved by a soothing lotion or an *antihistamine drug*.

## RAST

An abbreviation for radioallergosorbent test. RAST is a type of radioimmunoassay and is used to detect antibodies to specific allergens. (See *Immunoassay*.)

## Rats, diseases from

 Rats are shy but potentially aggressive rodents that live close to human habitation; in many cities they outnumber humans. Rats damage and contaminate crops and food stores and can spread disease.

Various microorganisms harbored by rats can cause illness if spread to people. The organisms responsible for *plague* and one type of *typhus* are transmitted to humans by the bites of rat fleas. *Leptospirosis* (Weil's disease) is caused by contact with anything (usually water) contaminated with rat's urine. Rat-bite fever is a rare infection, transmitted directly by a rat bite. Either of two types of bacterium may be responsible. Symptoms may include inflammation at the site of the bite and of nearby lymph nodes and vessels, bouts of fever, a rash, and, in one type, painful joint inflammation. Antibiotics are effective in treating either type of infection.

Effective control of urban rat populations is important in the prevention of rat-borne epidemic diseases.

## Raynaud's disease

A disorder of the blood vessels in which exposure to cold causes the small arteries that supply the fingers and toes to contract suddenly. This action cuts off blood flow to the digits, which become pale. The fingers, usually on both hands, are more often affected than the toes. Young women are the most commonly affected.

When the symptoms develop with no known cause, the disorder is called Raynaud's disease. When symptoms are secondary to some other condition, the disorder is termed *Raynaud's phenomenon*; it may have more serious long-term consequences.

**SYMPTOMS AND SIGNS**

On exposure to cold, the digits turn white because of lack of blood. As sluggish blood flow returns, the digits become blue; when they are warmed and normal blood flow is re-established, they turn red. During an attack, there is often a feeling of tingling, numbness, or burning in the affected fingers or toes.

In rare cases, the walls of the arteries gradually thicken, permanently reducing blood flow and eventually leading to painful ulceration or even to *gangrene* (tissue death) at the tips of the affected digits.

**DIAGNOSIS AND TREATMENT**

The condition is diagnosed from the patient's history. A person with Raynaud's disease should keep the hands and feet as warm as possible. Cigarette smokers should stop because smoking further constricts the arteries. *Vasodilator drugs* may be prescribed to relax the walls of the blood vessels. *Sympathectomy* (an operation in which the nerves that control the caliber of the arteries are cut) has been tried in severe cases.

## Raynaud's phenomenon

A circulatory disorder affecting the fingers and toes marked by the same mechanism, symptoms, and signs as those of *Raynaud's disease* but resulting from a known underlying disorder.

Possible causes of the condition include arterial diseases (such as *Buerger's disease, atherosclerosis, embolism,* and *thrombosis*); connective tissue diseases (e.g., *rheumatoid arthritis, scleroderma,* and systemic *lupus erythematosus*); and various drugs (such as *ergotamine, methysergide,* and *beta-blocker drugs*). Raynaud's phenomenon is a recognized occupational disorder of people who use pneumatic drills, chain saws, or other vibrating machinery; it is sometimes seen in

R

## TYPES OF RECEPTOR

Sensory receptors (below) are the free endings of sensory nerve cells—or special structures forming the endings of these cells. They respond to specific stimuli (such as light of a certain wavelength) and send a signal indicating the presence of the stimulus to the spinal cord and/or the brain.

Cell surface or chemical receptors (right) are tiny structures on the outer surface of a cell. They allow certain chemicals to bind to the cell and trigger some change within it.

### Skin receptors
The skin contains many types of receptor that respond to stimuli such as pressure, cold, heat, and hair movement, allowing the sensations of touch, temperature, and pain. They include such structures as pacinian corpuscles and Merkel's disks and are all special types of nerve cell ending.

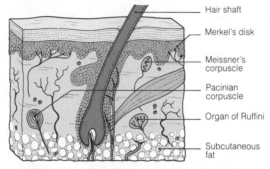

- Hair shaft
- Merkel's disk
- Meissner's corpuscle
- Pacinian corpuscle
- Organ of Ruffini
- Subcutaneous fat

### Receptors in tongue

Each taste bud (below) consists of many receptor cells. Each has surface receptors that respond to chemicals in food.

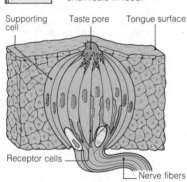

Supporting cell | Taste pore | Tongue surface

Receptor cells

Nerve fibers

### Receptors in eye

The retina, located at the back of the eye, contains receptor cells, called rods and cones, which are responsive to light.

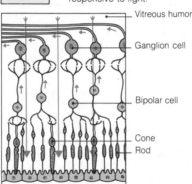

- Vitreous humor
- Ganglion cell
- Bipolar cell
- Cone
- Rod

### HOW CELL SURFACE OR CHEMICAL RECEPTORS WORK
Most cells have many surface receptors (only one is shown below). Their existence allows the activity of the cell to be influenced from outside.

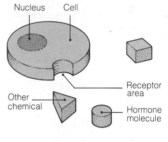

Nucleus | Cell

Other chemical

Receptor area

Hormone molecule

**1** A receptor allows only one specific chemical—which may be a hormone, or a neurotransmitter substance—to bind to it. The chemical must have a configuration that "fits" the receptor.

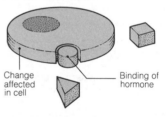

Change affected in cell

Binding of hormone

**2** The binding of chemical to receptor alters the outer cell membrane and triggers a change—such as contraction of a muscle cell or increased activity of an enzyme-producing cell.

typists, pianists, and others whose fingers suffer repeated trauma.

Treatment is the same as for Raynaud's disease, along with treatment of the underlying disorder.

## Reagent
A general term for any chemical substance that takes part in a chemical reaction. The term usually refers to a chemical (or mixture of chemicals) used in chemical analysis or employed to detect a biological substance.

## Receding chin
Underdevelopment of the lower jaw. The condition can be corrected by *cosmetic surgery* in one of three ways—lengthening each side of the jaw by inserting a wedge of bone into it, increasing the bulk of the bone at the front of the chin by a bone graft, or implanting a plastic bone substitute at the front of the chin.

## Receptor
A general term for any sensory nerve cell—that is, one that converts stimuli into nerve impulses (see box).

The term receptor is also used to refer to a specific area on the surface of a cell with a characteristic chemical and physical structure. Many natural body chemicals must bind to receptors on cells to exert their effects. For example, epinephrine binds to three different types of receptors (called alpha-, beta$_1$-, and beta$_2$-receptors) that are found on the cells of organs such as the heart and lungs.

## Recombinant DNA
A section of genetic material (*DNA*) from one organism that has been artificially spliced into the existing DNA of another organism, often a viral or bacterial cell. The new section may be the genetic code for a hormone such as insulin. If the recipient cell can be encouraged to multiply, large amounts of the hormone can be obtained. See also *Genetic engineering*.

## Reconstructive surgery
See *Arterial reconstructive surgery; Plastic surgery*.

## Recovery position
The correct position in which to place a casualty who is breathing, while waiting for help to arrive (see box).

## FIRST AID: THE RECOVERY POSITION

> **DO NOT:**
> ■ Leave an unconscious victim alone.
> ■ Put the victim into the recovery position if you suspect fractures to the neck or spine.

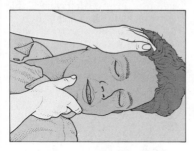

**1** Turn the victim's head toward you, tilting it back, to open the airway.

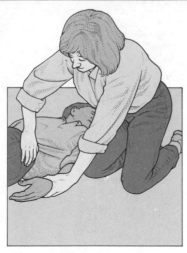

**2** Put the arm nearest you by the victim's side and slide it under his or her buttock.

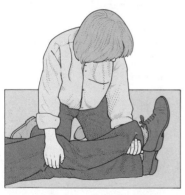

**3** Lay the other arm across the chest and cross the leg farthest from you over the near one at the ankle.

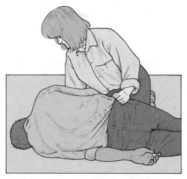

**4** Grasp clothing at the hip farthest from you with one hand and support the head with the other. Pull the victim toward you to rest against your knees.

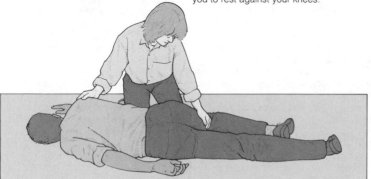

**5** Bend the uppermost arm and leg to support the body and stop the victim from rolling onto his or her face. The other arm should now be free. Readjust the head to make sure it is tilted well back and check to see if the airway is clear.

## Rectal bleeding

Bleeding from the rectum or anal canal. The blood may range from bright red to dark brown or black. It may be mixed with (or on the surface of) feces or passed separately and it may or may not be accompanied by pain. Rectal bleeding requires investigation by a physician.

**CAUSES**

The type of bleeding often gives a clue to its origin. *Hemorrhoids* are the most common cause of rectal bleeding in the form of small amounts of bright red blood found on the surface of the feces or on toilet paper. *Anal fissure, anal fistula, proctitis,* or *rectal prolapse* may also cause this type of bleeding.

Some disorders of the colon, such as *diverticular disease,* may cause dark red feces. Cancer of the intestine (see *Intestine, cancer of*), cancer of the rectum (see *Rectum, cancer of*), or polyps can also cause bleeding. Bloody diarrhea may be due to *ulcerative colitis, amebiasis,* or *shigellosis.*

Bleeding high in the digestive tract, usually from a *peptic ulcer,* may cause *melena* (black, tarry feces).

**DIAGNOSIS**

The physician may be able to make a diagnosis by *rectal examination. Proctoscopy, sigmoidoscopy, colonoscopy,* and air-contrast *barium X-ray examination* may also be performed.

## Rectal examination

Examination of the anus and rectum, performed to assess symptoms and to check for the presence of tumors of the rectum or prostate.

A rectal examination is performed as a part of a physical examination or when a person reports abdominal or pelvic pain, or a change in bowel habits. It may also be performed if a man complains of urological symptoms and, sometimes (along with a pelvic examination), if a woman has gynecological problems.

The patient usually lies on his or her left side, with the knees bent toward the chest. (The prostate may be examined while the patient stands bending at the waist.) The physician inserts a gloved, lubricated finger into the rectum to feel for any tenderness or abnormalities, such as ulcers or growths, and to examine the prostate or cervix, which can be felt through the rectum.

## Rectal prolapse

Protrusion outside the anus of the lining of the rectum, usually brought on by straining to defecate. The condition

R

causes discomfort, a discharge of mucus, and rectal bleeding.

In infants and young children, prolapse is usually temporary. In elderly people it tends to be permanent because of weakening of the tissues that support the *perineum*. Rectal prolapse may occur along with prolapsing *hemorrhoids*. If the rectal prolapse is large, leakage of feces may be a problem.

In younger people, a fiber-rich diet may be all that is necessary. Older people may undergo surgery, which is not uniformly successful.

## Rectocele

A protrusion into the back of the vaginal wall caused by the rectum pushing against weakened tissues in the vaginal wall. It is usually associated with a *cystocele* (protrusion of the bladder into the front wall of the vagina) or with a prolapsed uterus (see *Uterus, prolapse of*).

Depending on its size, a rectocele may cause no symptoms or may lead to constipation by interfering with muscle contraction in the rectum.

Exercises to strengthen the muscles of the pelvic floor may help relieve symptoms (see *Pelvic floor exercises*). If they do not, surgery may be attempted to tighten the tissues at the back of the vagina to improve support to the rectum.

## Rectum

A short, muscular tube that forms the lowest part of the large intestine and connects it to the *anus*. Feces collect in the rectum before defecation.

### STRUCTURE

Like the rest of the colon, the very first part of the rectum consists of four layers—the outermost serous layer; the muscular layer; the submucous layer; and the innermost mucous layer, which lubricates the rectum. There is no serous layer in the last 3 to 4 inches (8 to 10 cm) of the rectum.

### FUNCTION

The urge to defecate occurs when feces distend the rectum. Pressure on the rectal wall causes nerve impulses to pass to the brain, which, under voluntary control, sends messages to the muscles in the anus to relax, permitting defecation.

### DISORDERS

In rare cases, a baby is born with no rectum or anus (see *Anus, imperforate*).

Disorders of the colon may also affect the rectum. They include inflammation (see *Proctitis*), *polyps* (noncancerous, grapelike growths),

---

### STRUCTURE OF THE RECTUM

The rectum is 6 to 8 inches long. Its wall consists mainly of longitudinal and circular muscle; an inner, mucous layer provides lubrication.

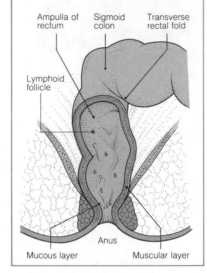

Ampulla of rectum   Sigmoid colon   Transverse rectal fold

Lymphoid follicle

Anus

Mucous layer   Muscular layer

---

familial *polyposis* (a condition characterized by numerous polyps that usually become cancerous), and cancer (see *Rectum, cancer of*).

The rectum can become obstructed as a result of narrowing caused by *radiation therapy*, *granuloma inguinale* (a sexually transmitted disease), or pelvic infection. Rarely, an ulcer develops in the rectum, causing bleeding and discharge. Similar symptoms may result from injury to the rectum due to anal intercourse or the insertion of foreign objects.

*Rectal prolapse* occurs when the lining of the rectum protrudes outside the anus. In a *rectocele*, the rectum and rear wall of the vagina are displaced downward into the vagina.

Rectal disorders are usually diagnosed by physical examination (see *Rectal examination*) and by *proctoscopy* or *sigmoidoscopy* (examination with a viewing tube).

## Rectum, cancer of

A malignant tumor in the muscular tube that forms the lower part of the colon (large intestine).

### CAUSES AND INCIDENCE

The cause of this cancer is unknown, but dietary and genetic factors are thought to play a part in its development (see *Intestine, cancer of*). Certain

---

diseases of the colon (e.g., familial *polyposis* and *ulcerative colitis*) increase the risk of colorectal cancer.

Colorectal cancer is responsible for about 20 percent of all cancer deaths in the US. Rectal cancer accounts for one fourth to one third of tumors of the large intestine; it is more common between the ages of 50 and 70.

### SYMPTOMS

The earliest symptom may be rectal bleeding during defecation; blood may appear in the feces. There may also be a change in bowel habits—diarrhea or constipation—and a sensation of incomplete emptying of the bowel. Later, pain may occur. Untreated, the cancer eventually may cause severe bleeding and pain and block the intestine, preventing the passage of feces. It may also spread to other organs in the pelvis and to other sites, such as the liver.

### DIAGNOSIS

A physician can often detect rectal cancer by an examination with a gloved finger. The diagnosis is confirmed by *proctoscopy* or *sigmoidoscopy* (examination of the rectum with a rigid or flexible viewing tube) and *biopsy* (removal of a sample of tissue for analysis).

### TREATMENT

In most cases surgery is performed. If the tumor is in the uppermost part of the rectum, the abdomen is opened, the upper rectum and descending colon are removed, and the two ends are sewn together. To promote healing of the joined bowel, a temporary *colostomy* (which diverts feces through a surgical opening in the abdomen) may be performed.

If the growth is in the lower rectum, the colon is cut through above the rectum, an incision is made around the anus, and the entire rectum and anus are removed. The wound is closed and, because there is no longer any outlet for the feces, a permanent colostomy is created.

Both operations take two to three hours to perform. Patients who have undergone surgery are examined at regular intervals to ensure that the tumor has not reappeared or spread to other parts of the body.

In elderly or generally sick people unable to undergo major surgery, *diathermy* (the application of high-frequency electric current) may be used to destroy the surface of the tumor and control local symptoms. Other forms of treatment when surgery is not possible are *radiation therapy* and, less commonly, *anticancer drugs*.

R

### OUTLOOK

The long-term outlook depends on how far the tumor has spread before treatment takes place. About 50 percent of all people operated on for rectal cancer are alive three years later and almost 40 percent ten years later. Survival rates are considerably higher when the disease is diagnosed and treated early.

## Red eye

Another name for *conjunctivitis.*

## Reducing

See *Weight reduction.*

## Reduction

The process of manipulating a displaced part of the body back to its original position. Reduction may be carried out to realign fractured bone ends (see *Fracture*), to replace a dislocated joint in its socket (see *Dislocation, joint*), or to treat a *hernia* by pushing the protruding intestine back through the abdominal wall.

## Referred pain

Pain felt in a part of the body at some distance from its cause. Referred pain occurs because some apparently remote parts of the body are served by the same nerve or the same nerve root (group of nerves that joins the spinal cord at one point). Nerve impulses reaching the brain from one of these areas may be misinterpreted as coming from the other (see *Pain*).

Common examples of referred pain are the pain down the inside of the left arm caused by *angina pectoris* or *coronary thrombosis*; the pain felt in the tip of the shoulder from irritation of the diaphragm; the pain felt in a testis when the ureter is stretched by a urinary tract *calculus*; and the pain felt in the leg or foot from compression in the spine by a *disk prolapse.*

## Reflex

An action that occurs automatically and predictably in response to a particular stimulus, independent of the will of the individual. Both the sensing of the stimulus and initiation of the action are carried out by components of the nervous system.

In the simplest reflex, a sensory nerve cell, perhaps at the skin surface, reacts to a stimulus such as heat or pressure. It sends a signal along its nerve fiber to the central nervous system (brain or spinal cord). There, the end of the fiber connects to another nerve cell, which becomes stimulated in turn. Activity in this second cell then causes a muscle to contract or a gland to increase its secretory activity. The passage of the nerve signal from original sensation to final action is called a reflex arc.

Sometimes the reflex is more complicated. Sensory signals may be sent from thousands of sensory receptors to groups of nerve cells within the central nervous system. Complex analysis of these signals may be carried out before responses are initiated.

### INBORN REFLEXES

Many reflexes are inborn, including those that control basic body functions. Examples include shivering automatically in response to cold, increased breathing in response to a rise in carbon dioxide in the blood, and contraction of the bladder to expel urine once it has filled beyond a certain point.

The part of the nervous system that is concerned with these processes is called the *autonomic nervous system.* Parts of the *brain stem* and the *hypothalamus* in the forebrain are processing centers for the system. Some autonomic system reflexes are under partial voluntary (willed) control—emptying of the bladder can be voluntarily delayed. Ultimately, however, reflex is stronger than will.

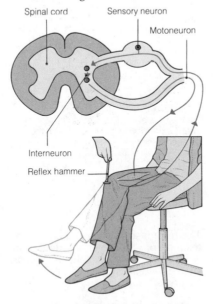

**Simple knee-jerk reflex**
A tap with a rubber hammer just below the kneecap stretches a tendon of one of the thigh muscles. A signal passes via a sensory neuron (nerve cell) to the spinal cord, activating a motor neuron, which contracts the muscle, jerking the lower leg upward.

Some inborn reflexes occur only in babies (see *Reflex, primitive*). An example is the grasp reflex when a finger is placed in the palm.

Any physical examination usually includes testing some simple, inborn reflexes, such as the knee jerk, plantar reflex (irritation of the sole of the foot causes the toes to curl), and pupil constriction in response to light. Changes in these reflexes may indicate damage to the nervous system. Part of a complete neurological examination may also include the testing of several other reflexes.

The examination of vital reflexes controlled by the brain stem is the basis for diagnosing *brain death.*

### CONDITIONED REFLEXES

Reflexes acquired (rather than inborn) as a result of experience are called conditioned reflexes. They result from the formation of new pathways and connections within the nervous system during life. The process by which these reflexes are acquired is called *conditioning*. One type, operant conditioning, is a particularly important process in *learning*. Once a satisfactory response to a new situation has been discovered (often by a process of trial and error) and repeated several times, it is eventually automatically elicited by that situation or stimulus and thus becomes a sort of reflex. For example, a person walking home from work may follow a familiar route without needing to make any conscious effort to do so.

## Reflex, primitive

An automatic movement in response to a stimulus; it is present in newborn infants but disappears during the first few months. Primitive reflexes are thought to represent actions that may have been important for survival in earlier stages of our evolution.

Because some of these reflexes can give an indication of the condition of an infant's nervous system, they are tested by the pediatrician at the first examinations after birth. Any abnormality of the primitive reflexes may indicate a nervous system disorder.

The main primitive reflexes are the grasp reflex, Moro's reflex, the tonic neck reflex, the walking or stepping reflex, and the rooting reflex (see chart on next page).

## Reflux

An abnormal backflow of fluid in a body passage due to failure of the passage's muscle to close fully. The most common types of reflux are

**R**

## TYPES OF PRIMITIVE REFLEX

**Grasping reflex**

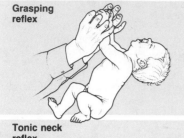

Certain automatic reflexes are present early in life before the baby becomes capable of voluntary movement. These reflexes disappear as the nervous system matures. For about the first four months, any object placed in the infant's palm will be firmly grasped.

**Tonic neck reflex**

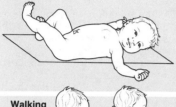

When the very young baby turns the head to one side, the arm and leg on that side are stretched out and the arm and leg on the opposite side bend. This reflex normally disappears after a few months, except in premature babies. A strong reflex suggests brain damage.

**Walking reflex**

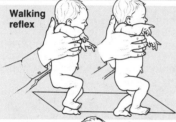

When the baby is held upright with the feet touching the ground, a forward stepping movement is made by each leg as the weight is placed on the other foot. This occurs during the first two months of life, and then is lost.

**Moro's reflex**

If the baby's head is momentarily left unsupported, the arms will be swung outward and then brought together in an embracing movement. At the same time the legs are extended and the baby cries. This symmetrical reflex should persist for three or four months.

**Rooting reflex**

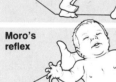

This reflex enables the baby to find the nipple; it is evoked by touching the baby's cheek with the fingertip near the corner of the mouth. The head turns so that the finger can enter the mouth. The reflex is best shown if tried near the normal feeding time.

R

regurgitation of acid fluid from the stomach into the esophagus (see *Acid reflux*) and the backflow of urine from the bladder into one or both ureters. Persistent urinary reflux may lead to kidney damage (see *Nephropathy*).

## Refraction

The bending of light rays as they pass from one substance to another. In the eye, refraction provides the mechanism by which an image is focused on the retina, thereby permitting vision.

The term is also used to describe the testing of the eye to determine whether there is any refractive error, such as *myopia*, *hyperopia*, or *astigmatism* (see *Vision tests*).

## Regenerative cell therapy

A treatment that claims to revitalize the skin. One such technique—developed in the 1930s and still popular—involves the injection of preparations made from a mixture of animal endocrine glands. Similar claims have been made for skin creams containing sex hormones or animal placentas. There is no evidence that any of these treatments works.

## Regression

A term used in *psychoanalytic theory* to describe the process of returning to a childhood level of behavior. Sigmund Freud suggested that humans progress psychologically through various stages of development from infancy to adulthood. Disturbed people, though superficially mature, may be unconsciously fixated at an earlier level. When frustrated or under stress, they undergo regression to immature forms of behavior, such as thumb-sucking or exposing the genitals. (See also *Fixation*.)

## Regurgitation

A backflow of fluid. The term is used in medicine to describe the return of swallowed food or drink from the stomach back into the mouth. Regurgitation is very common in babies immediately after feeding, when some of the milk is brought up with gas. Acid juices may also be regurgitated from the stomach into the mouth (see *Acid reflux*).

Regurgitation also describes the backflow of blood through a heart valve that has not closed fully because of a disorder such as *mitral insufficiency* or *aortic insufficiency*. (See also *Reflux*.)

## Rehabilitation

Treatment aimed at enabling a person to live an independent life following injury, illness, or drug or alcohol dependence (see *Alcohol dependence*; *Drug dependence*). Treatment may include *physical therapy*, *occupational therapy*, and *psychotherapy*.

Rehabilitation is often carried out in centers, some of which are residential, where people from different specialties work together to assess the severity of an individual's *disability* or dependence and develop a tailor-made treatment program. Industrial rehabilitation centers provide job retraining for people who are unable to return to their previous employment. Drug and alcohol rehabilitation centers help people through the period of withdrawal and provide psychological support to reduce the risk of relapse.

## Rehydration therapy

The treatment of *dehydration* by the administration of fluids and salts by mouth (oral rehydration) or by intravenous infusion. The amount of fluid necessary depends on the person's age, weight, and on the degree of dehydration (amount of fluids lost).

In mild dehydration (common in young children who have *diarrhea*), rehydration can usually be carried out with solutions given by mouth. Oral rehydration preparations are available commercially in liquid form, or in powder or tablet form to be added to water. The simplest products contain only sodium chloride and glucose; others also include salts containing potassium and bicarbonate. Any unused solution should be discarded 24 hours after preparation.

If commercial preparations are not available, a homemade oral rehydration solution may be prepared by adding one half teaspoon of salt, 2 teaspoons of sugar, and one quarter of a teaspoon of sodium bicarbonate (baking soda) to 1 pint (0.47 liter) of boiled water.

In severe dehydration, or if the patient is unable to take fluids by mouth because of nausea or vomiting, an intravenous infusion of saline (sodium chloride) solution, glucose solution, or a combination of both, sometimes supplemented with potassium chloride, may be given in the hospital. Additional treatment may be necessary depending on the underlying condition.

## Reimplantation, dental

Replacement of a tooth in its socket after an accident so that it can become reattached to supporting tissues. Front teeth are the most commonly involved. The alternative is to fill the gap with a false tooth or, if the jaws are still growing, to maintain the gap with an *orthodontic appliance*.

### HOW IT IS DONE

The dentist rinses the tooth in a sterile solution, replaces it in the socket, and maintains it with a splint (see *Splinting, dental*), often for several weeks.

### OUTLOOK

Successful reimplantation relies on replacing the tooth soon after the accident (ideally within 30 minutes). Keeping the tooth moist and sterile (for example, with saliva) also increases the chances of success.

## Reiter's syndrome

A condition in which there is a combination of *arthritis* and *urethritis*; there may also be *conjunctivitis*. Reiter's syndrome is more common in men and is the most common cause of arthritis in young men.

### CAUSES AND INCIDENCE

Reiter's syndrome usually develops after *nonspecific urethritis*; it affects about 2 percent of men with this disorder and may also occur after an attack of bacillary *dysentery*. Although Reiter's syndrome is induced by infection, it develops only in people with a genetic predisposition. About 80 percent of those with the syndrome have a certain tissue type (HLA-B27 positive; see *Histocompatibility antigens*).

### SYMPTOMS AND SIGNS

Reiter's syndrome usually starts with a urethral discharge followed by conjunctivitis and then arthritis. The arthritis seldom affects more than one or two joints and is often associated with fever and malaise. The affected joints, commonly the knee or ankle, are warm, painful, and stiff, and the inflammation persists for periods varying from a few days to several months. Tendons and ligaments (especially the Achilles tendon) may also become inflamed, as may fibrous tissue in the soles of the feet. Skin rashes are common.

### DIAGNOSIS AND TREATMENT

Diagnosis and treatment are based on the symptoms. *Analgesic drugs* and *nonsteroidal anti-inflammatory drugs* relieve pain and inflammation but may have to be taken for a long period. Antibiotics are of no value in treating the arthritis.

### OUTLOOK

Relapses occur in about one third of cases, especially after more episodes of nonspecific urethritis.

## Relapse

The recurrence of a disease after apparent recovery or the return of symptoms after a *remission*.

## Relapsing fever

An illness caused by infection with spirochetes (spiral-shaped bacteria) transmitted to humans by ticks or lice and characterized by high fever.

### CAUSES AND INCIDENCE

Ticks acquire the spirochetes by feeding on infected rodents. The spirochetes can survive in a population of ticks for years; they are transmitted to humans when the ticks bite. In the US, occasional cases of tick-borne relapsing fever occur in the southwestern and mountain states from Texas to Idaho. Louse-borne infection, transmitted from person to person, is rare in the US.

### SYMPTOMS AND SIGNS

Relapsing fever starts with a sudden high fever—up to 104°F (40°C)—accompanied by shivering, headache, muscle pains, nausea and vomiting. The symptoms persist for three to six days, culminating in a crisis, with a risk of collapse and death. The affected person then returns to normal but, seven to 10 days later, suffers another attack. In tick-borne fever, several of these relapses, each progressively milder, are common.

### DIAGNOSIS AND TREATMENT

A blood smear reveals the presence of the spirochetes. Relapsing fever can be effectively treated with an *antibiotic drug* (such as penicillin).

## Relaxation techniques

Methods of consciously releasing muscular tension and achieving a state of mental calm.

### WHY THEY ARE DONE

Relaxation techniques can benefit people who suffer from *anxiety* symptoms, can help to reduce *hypertension* (high blood pressure), and are a useful means of relieving the stress caused by a busy job or personal problems. They are taught in *prepared childbirth* classes to help pregnant women cope with the pain of labor.

### TYPES

Active relaxation consists of (in turn) tensing and then relaxing all the muscles in the body, usually starting with the head and moving down to the feet. Passive relaxation may also be used. It involves clearing the mind of everything to concentrate on a single phrase or sound. In both techniques, control of the breathing rate is emphasized (see *Breathing exercises*), since *hyperventilation* (rapid, shallow breathing) often brings on or worsens anxiety. Taped instructions or *biofeedback training* may help to reinforce learning. Once mastered, the techniques can be put into practice in potentially stressful situations.

Traditional methods of concentration, such as *yoga* and *meditation*, employ similar techniques.

### EFFECTIVENESS

Relaxation is a safe treatment; it may be useful in conjunction with other forms of therapy.

## Rem

A unit of equivalent absorbed dose of ionizing radiation (see *Radiation* units box). Rem is an acronym for roentgen equivalent man.

## Remission

A temporary diminution or disappearance of the symptoms of a disease, or the period during which this occurs.

R

Remissions occur in many long-term diseases; the most notable example is *multiple sclerosis*, which typically follows a pattern of alternating remissions and *relapses*. Initially, remissions may last months or years; however, they usually become shorter and may eventually disappear.

## Renal

The medical term for anything related to the *kidney*.

## Renal biopsy

A procedure in which a small portion of *kidney* tissue is removed and examined under a microscope. Renal *biopsy* is usually performed as part of the investigation and diagnosis of various kidney disorders, such as *glomerulonephritis*, *proteinuria*, *nephrotic syndrome*, or acute *renal failure*. It may also be used to assess the status of a *kidney transplant*. Percutaneous (through the skin) needle biopsy of the kidney may not be performed if the person has a bleeding disorder, only one functioning kidney, or chronic renal failure with small, contracted kidneys.

### HOW IT IS DONE

The procedure for performing a percutaneous needle biopsy of the kidney is shown at right.

If a percutaneous needle biopsy is not advisable, an open end renal biopsy may be performed. Using general anesthesia, the surgeon makes a small incision in the flank to visualize the kidney and then cuts a small wedge of renal cortex (the biopsy specimen).

In both cases, the renal tissue is sent to a pathologist for examination under a light microscope, electron microscope, or immunofluorescent microscope (see *Microscope*).

### RECOVERY PERIOD

The patient may have slight pain in the back for some hours after the biopsy and a small amount of blood may be passed in the urine. Provided there are no complications (such as severe bleeding), the patient can return home the following day.

## Renal cell carcinoma

The most common type of kidney cancer (see *Kidney cancer*).

## Renal colic

Intermittent spasms of severe pain on one side of the back, usually caused by a kidney stone (see *Calculus, urinary tract*). Each spasm usually lasts for several minutes.

## Renal disorders

See *Kidney* disorders box.

## Renal failure

The reduction in the ability of the *kidneys* to filter waste products from the blood and excrete them in the urine, to control the body's water and salt balance, and to regulate the blood pressure. The resultant buildup of waste products (and other chemical disturbances in the blood and tissues) leads to symptoms that vary in severity. This combination of symptoms is sometimes called uremia.

---

### PERCUTANEOUS RENAL BIOPSY

This procedure is performed with a local anesthetic injected into the skin and tissues over the kidney; it is virtually painless. There is a risk of bleeding from the kidney into the abdominal cavity.

**1** The kidney must be accurately located, usually by an ultrasound scan. Local anesthetic is then injected.

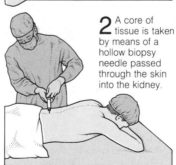

**2** A core of tissue is taken by means of a hollow biopsy needle passed through the skin into the kidney.

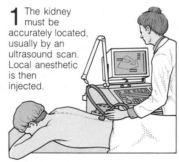

Kidney glomerulus (filtering unit) as seen under microscope

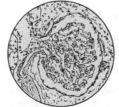

**3** The core of kidney tissue is embedded in wax and cut into thin slices, which are mounted on slides for staining and microscopic examination.

---

### TYPES AND CAUSES

Renal failure can be acute (of sudden onset) or chronic (developing more gradually). In acute renal failure, kidney function usually returns to normal once the underlying cause has been discovered and treated; in chronic failure, function is usually irreversibly lost.

Acute renal failure most often occurs in people who have suffered a severe injury or are seriously ill with some other underlying condition and are suffering from physiological *shock*. Severe bleeding or burns can reduce blood volume and pressure to the extent that the supply of blood to the kidneys is dramatically reduced. A *myocardial infarction* (heart attack) or acute *pancreatitis* can have a similar effect. The kidneys are particularly susceptible to reduced blood flow, which can cause damage to their filtering units.

Obstruction to urine flow as a result of a stone (see *Calculus, urinary tract*), *bladder tumor*, or enlargement of the prostate gland can also cause acute renal failure, as can certain rapidly developing types of kidney disease, such as *glomerulonephritis* and *hemolytic-uremic syndrome*.

Chronic renal failure can result from any disease that causes progressive damage to the kidneys, such as *hypertension* (high blood pressure), *diabetes mellitus*, polycystic kidney disease (see *Kidney, polycystic*), or *amyloidosis* (see also *Kidney* disorders box). It can also result from excessive use of *analgesics* (painkillers) over several years.

Chronic renal failure may progress over months or years to an advanced, life-threatening condition called end-stage renal failure.

### SYMPTOMS AND SIGNS

In acute renal failure, the most noticeable symptom may be a much reduced volume of urine. Production of less than a pint of urine per day is called *oliguria* and usually means that waste products are not being cleared effectively from the blood. Production of less than 50 ml (one ninth of a pint) in 24 hours is called *anuria* and results in a serious buildup of waste products. In some cases, however, the person passes normal amounts of urine despite the loss of the filtering and cleansing function; this is called nonoliguric acute renal failure. Within a short time of the development of acute renal failure, more symptoms (such as drowsiness, nausea, vomiting, and breathlessness) appear. In many cases, symptoms of the

R

underlying cause of failure (e.g., symptoms of shock such as pale skin and weak pulse) precede those of the renal failure itself.

Symptoms of chronic failure develop more gradually and may include nausea, loss of appetite, and weakness. Unless the progress of the kidney damage is slowed or arrested, symptoms of end-stage failure may appear (including severe lethargy, headache, vomiting, a furred tongue, unpleasant breath, intense, rashless skin itching, and, eventually, collapse, coma, and death).

**COMPLICATIONS**

Complications of acute renal failure may include infections such as pneumonia, bleeding into the stomach, and deep vein *thrombosis*. In chronic failure, complications may include high blood pressure (which is both a cause and result of kidney failure), *anemia, osteomalacia, hyperparathyroidism, neuropathy,* or *myopathy.* All result from various disturbances in blood chemistry.

**DIAGNOSIS**

A person with suspected renal failure should undergo *kidney function tests,* which include measuring the urea and creatinine (two waste products) in the blood; raised levels indicate renal failure. *Urinalysis* and blood pressure measurements are also performed. Unless there is an obvious cause of renal failure (such as severe bleeding), immediate testing is carried out to determine a cause. Techniques include examination of the urine sediment and the blood, intravenous *pyelography, renal biopsy, ultrasound scanning,* and *radionuclide scanning.*

**TREATMENT**

In acute renal failure, emergency treatment is given for any cause of shock, such as severe bleeding. Blood volume and pressure must be brought back to normal through saline *intravenous infusion* or *blood transfusions.* Surgery may be required for obstruction caused by stones or enlargement of the prostate gland. Treatment of other causes may be complex and sometimes controversial, but may include the use of *corticosteroid drugs* and other drugs (as is done for certain forms of *glomerulonephritis*). *Diuretic drugs* may also be given to improve urine flow and rid the body of excess fluid. In many cases of acute failure, temporary *dialysis* (artificial methods of removing waste products from the blood) may be required until the kidneys recover their function.

Dietary treatment is an important part of the treatment of all types of renal failure. The diet must be high in carbohydrates and low in protein (the main source of waste products) to reduce the work load on the kidneys; the salt content must also be controlled. Fluid intake is carefully balanced against urine output. If the patient has been taking certain drugs (whose breakdown products are removed from the blood by the kidneys), use of these drugs may be stopped or their dosages reduced.

If hypertension develops, drugs are prescribed to keep the blood pressure under control. In end-stage renal failure, long-term dialysis or, ideally, a *kidney transplant* is the only satisfactory form of treatment.

**OUTLOOK**

The outlook varies according to the cause of the failure and the patient's response to treatment. Most people with acute renal failure eventually make a full recovery, but some require a transplant or lifelong dialysis. In chronic failure, it may be several years before such measures are required. Well over half the people with end-stage renal failure that is treated by dialysis are able to lead comparatively normal lives for more than five years; a successful kidney transplant improves the outlook.

## Renal transplant
See *Kidney transplant.*

## Renal tubular acidosis
A condition in which the kidneys are unable to excrete normal amounts of acid generated by the body's *metabolism* (internal chemistry). In renal tubular acidosis, the blood is more acid than normal and the urine is less acid than normal.

The cause of the renal metabolism disorder is often unknown. Possible causes include kidney damage due to disease, drugs, or a genetic disorder. Renal tubular acidosis may lead to *osteomalacia* (softening of the bones), kidney stones (see *Calculus, urinary tract*), *nephrocalcinosis* (calcification of the kidney), and hypokalemia (an abnormally low level of potassium in the blood).

Sodium bicarbonate (to counteract the blood acidity) and potassium supplements may be prescribed.

## Renin
An enzyme involved in the regulation of blood pressure. When blood pressure falls, the kidneys release renin, which converts an inactive substance called angiotensinogen to the protein *angiotensin* I (also inactive). This protein is then rapidly converted to an active form, angiotensin II, which constricts blood vessels and so increases blood pressure. In addition, angiotensin II stimulates the release of the hormone *aldosterone,* which also increases blood pressure.

Blood pressure can be lowered by drugs that affect the renin-angiotensin system (e.g., *beta-blocker drugs,* which inhibit the production of renin, and *ACE inhibitor drugs,* which interfere with its actions).

## Renography
A type of *radionuclide scanning* used for investigation of the kidney. A radionuclide—either hippuran or pentetic acid—is injected into the bloodstream and passes through the kidney into the urine. Radiation counts are taken continuously during the procedure. The information is recorded graphically as a renogram (a curve of counts per second against time). Both kidneys are examined simultaneously so that a comparison can be made of their functions.

Renography is used when obstruction to the passage of urine is suspected. Normally, the radiation count rate increases rapidly for about 30 seconds after injection, rises more slowly for about five minutes, and then decreases as the radionuclide passes into the bladder. If obstruction is present, the radionuclide accumulates in the kidney and the count rate continues to rise, producing a differently shaped renogram.

Renography is performed quickly and painlessly; it utilizes only a small dose of radiation.

## Reportable diseases
Medical conditions that must be reported by the physician responsible for the affected person to the local health authorities who, in turn, report some of them to the national *Centers for Disease Control.*

The notification of certain potentially harmful infectious diseases is important because it enables public health officers to take the necessary steps to control the spread of infection (e.g., by isolation or by offering *immunization* to contacts). Reporting also provides valuable statistics on the *incidence* and *prevalence* of a disease; they may be used in formulating health policies such as immunization programs or improvements in sanita-

R

## INCIDENCE OF SOME REPORTABLE DISEASES IN US (per 100,000 population)

| Disease | 1950 | 1960 | 1970 | 1980 | 1985 |
|---|---|---|---|---|---|
| Diphtheria | 3.8 | 0.5 | 0.2 | 0.0 | 0.0 |
| Poliomyelitis | 22.0 | 1.8 | 0.0 | 0.0 | 0.0 |
| Measles | 211.0 | 245.4 | 23.2 | 6.0 | 1.2 |
| Rubella | . . . | . . . | 27.7 | 1.7 | 0.3 |
| Tuberculosis | 80.5 | 30.8 | 18.2 | 12.2 | 9.3 |
| Pertussis | 79.8 | 8.2 | 2.1 | 0.8 | 1.5 |
| Syphilis | 16.7 | 9.1 | 10.9 | 12.1 | 11.5 |
| Gonorrhea | 192.4 | 145.3 | 297.2 | 445.0 | 384.6 |
| Viral hepatitis, types A and B* | . . . | 23.1 | 31.9 | 21.2 | 20.9 |
| Salmonellosis (excluding typhoid) | . . . | 3.8 | 10.8 | 14.9 | 27.4 |

*Excluding New York City

Note the dramatic decline in the incidence of diphtheria, poliomyelitis, and measles since the 1950s, and the gentler decline of tuberculosis. The incidence of gonorrhea peaked in the late 1970s but may now be in decline. The incidence of pertussis has fluctuated in recent years around a low level. Meanwhile, other reportable diseases such as salmonellosis and AIDS have become more common.

tion. Examples of reportable infectious diseases are chickenpox, AIDS, hepatitis, tetanus, malaria, syphilis, and gonorrhea.

Some categories of disease other than infections must also be reported. These include some *birth defects* and certain types of *occupational disease*.

## Reproduction, sexual
The process of producing a new generation to continue the existence of the species by the fusion of two cells from different individuals; this is achieved in humans by the fusion of one *sperm* and one *ovum*. This fusion, called *fertilization*, is achieved by *sexual intercourse* or *artificial insemination*.

## Reproductive system, female
The organs that enable a woman to produce ova (eggs), to have *sexual intercourse*, to nourish a fertilized *ovum* until it has developed into a full grown *fetus*, and to give birth. Apart from the *vulva* (external genitalia), the female reproductive organs lie within the pelvic cavity.

Ova are released each month from the *ovaries*, two small egg-shaped glands. The glands also secrete sex hormones (see *Estrogen hormones*; *Progesterone hormones*), which control the reproductive cycle. Adjacent to each ovary is a *fallopian tube*, which carries ova to the *uterus*, a hollow, pear-shaped organ that is situated between the bladder and the rectum. If, on its journey along the fallopian tube, an ovum unites with a sperm, *fertilization* takes place.

Sperm travel upward through the *cervix* and uterus on their journey to the fallopian tubes. The cervix projects into the top of the *vagina*, a muscular passage that forms the lower part of the birth canal and that receives ejaculated sperm during sexual intercourse. Surrounding and protecting the opening of the vagina are the fleshy folds of the *vulva*.

Fertility, the normal functioning of the reproductive system, begins at *puberty* (when it is signaled by the onset of *menstruation*) and ceases at the time of the *menopause*.

## Reproductive system, male
The organs that enable a man to have *sexual intercourse* and to fertilize ova (eggs) with *sperm*. Sperm and male sex hormones (see *Androgen hormones*) are produced in the *testes*, a pair of ovoid glands suspended in a pouch known as the *scrotum*. From each testis, sperm pass into an *epididymis*, a long coiled tube behind the testis, where they slowly mature and are stored.

Shortly before *ejaculation*, sperm are propelled from the epididymis into a long duct called the *vas deferens*, which carries the sperm to the seminal vesicles, a pair of sacs that lies behind the bladder. These sacs produce seminal fluid, which is added to the sperm to produce *semen*.

Semen travels from the vesicles along two ducts to the urethra, a tube that acts as a passage for urine and semen. The ducts pass through the *prostate gland*, a chestnut-shaped organ lying beneath the bladder and surrounding the upper urethra. The prostate produces secretions that are added to the semen.

## TOP 20 REPORTABLE DISEASES IN US IN 1986

| | No. of cases reported |
|---|---|
| Gonorrhea | 900,868 |
| Chickenpox | 183,243 |
| Salmonellosis (excluding typhoid fever) | 49,984 |
| Syphilis | 27,883 |
| Viral hepatitis, type B* | 26,107 |
| Viral hepatitis, type A* | 23,430 |
| Tuberculosis | 22,768 |
| Shigellosis | 17,138 |
| AIDS | 12,932 |
| Viral meningitis | 11,374 |
| Mumps | 7,790 |
| Measles | 6,282 |
| Pertussis | 4,195 |
| Viral hepatitis, non-A non-B | 3,634 |
| Amebiasis | 3,532 |
| Meningococcus infections | 2,594 |
| Encephalitis, primary | 1,302 |
| Malaria | 1,123 |
| Legionnaires' disease | 948 |
| Rocky Mountain spotted fever | 760 |

*Excluding New York City.

## FEMALE REPRODUCTIVE SYSTEM

Each month an ovum from one ovary is carried along the fallopian tube. If fertilized, it begins to divide and implants into the lining of the uterus to develop into an embryo. At birth, the baby is forced out via the cervix, the usually narrow passage that forms the neck of the uterus.

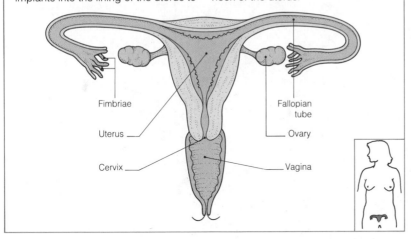

Fimbriae

Uterus

Cervix

Fallopian tube

Ovary

Vagina

At *orgasm*, semen is ejaculated from the urethra through the erect *penis*, which is placed in the woman's vagina during sexual intercourse.

## Resection

Surgical removal of all or part of a diseased or injured organ or structure. An anterior resection is an operation that removes part of the colon as a treatment for cancer.

## Reserpine

An *antihypertensive drug*, derived from an Indian plant, used alone or with a *diuretic drug* in the treatment of *hypertension* (high blood pressure). Reser-

pine is also used in the long-term treatment of *Raynaud's disease* (a circulatory disorder).

Possible adverse effects include nasal congestion, dry mouth, *bradycardia* (slow heart beat), depression, lethargy, and nightmares.

## Resident

A medical school graduate undergoing postgraduate training as a hospital staff member. A first-year resident used to be called an intern.

## Resistance

A term that has several different medical usages. Blood vessels exert a

dynamic resistance to the flow of blood. The resistance increases as the diameter of blood vessels decreases, whether due to normal physiological processes or narrowing as a result of disease. An increase in resistance leads to a rise in blood pressure backward from the narrowed vessels.

In *psychoanalysis*, resistance refers to the blocking off from consciousness of repressed material (e.g., memories or emotions). One task of the psychoanalyst is to help the patient break down this resistance.

Resistance may also refer to an ability to withstand attack from noxious agents (such as poisons, irritants, or microorganisms). A person's resistance to infection is called *immunity*; it varies according to age, nutritional and general health, the integrity of the person's *immune system*, and previous exposure to infective organisms.

Drug resistance refers to the ability of some microorganisms to withstand attack from previously effective drugs. Certain bacteria have acquired *genes* (units of hereditary material) that confer protection against specific antibiotics. Overuse of these antibiotics encourages the multiplication and spread of the resistant strains, which include some varieties of the organisms responsible for *gonorrhea*, *typhoid fever*, *salmonella* poisoning, *shigellosis* (bacterial dysentery), and other serious infections. In addition, some malarial parasites have become resistant to chloroquine, an important antimalarial drug.

When any dangerous infectious disease can no longer be treated with the established remedies, the situation is potentially serious. The development of new drugs has, to date, largely kept pace with the threat. Strategies to prevent the emergence of new resistant strains have included the cyclical use of different antibiotics to treat particular types of infection in hospitals (i.e., if a strain of bacteria resistant to one drug emerges, it is usually knocked out by the next drug in the cycle). Physicians are also learning to avoid indiscriminate use of antibiotic drugs, which encourages the emergence of resistance.

## Resorption, dental

Loss of substance from a tooth. Resorption may be external (affecting the surface of the root) or internal (affecting the wall of the pulp cavity).

**CAUSES AND INCIDENCE**

External resorption of tooth roots, which causes the teeth to become

## MALE REPRODUCTIVE SYSTEM

Sperm made in the testis pass via the vas deferens to the seminal vesicle. Secretions from the prostate increase the volume of the semen, which is ejaculated from the penis via the urethra during orgasm.

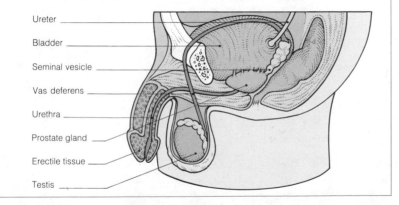

Ureter

Bladder

Seminal vesicle

Vas deferens

Urethra

Prostate gland

Erectile tissue

Testis

R

## RESPIRATION

The function of respiration is to provide the energy needed by body cells. Cells obtain this energy mainly by metabolizing glucose with oxygen, so they require a constant supply of oxygen. In addition, the waste products of the metabolic process—mainly carbon dioxide—must be carried away from the cells.

Respiration includes the breathing of air into the lungs, the transfer of oxygen from the air to the blood, the transport of oxygen in the blood to the body cells, the metabolism of glucose with oxygen in the cells, and the transport of carbon dioxide to the lungs to be breathed out.

During exercise, respiration increases to compensate for higher energy demands by muscle cells.

Artery

Vein

Alveolus

Network of capillaries

**1** Air, containing oxygen, is breathed into the lungs and enters the alveoli (tiny air sacs). Oxygen diffuses from the air into the blood vessels surrounding the alveoli.

Glucose    $C_6H_{12}O_6$

Oxygen $O_2$

Carbon dioxide $CO_2$

Water $H_2O$

Energy

**2** The oxygen-saturated blood passes from the lungs via the pulmonary veins to the left side of the heart.

$CO_2$  Carbon dioxide

$O_2$  Oxygen

Trachea

Lung

Alveoli

Pulmonary vein

Bronchiole

Aorta

Bronchus

Pulmonary artery

Left side of heart

Right side of heart

**3** From the left side of the heart, the oxygenated blood is pumped via the aorta to the body tissues. The oxygen is carried within the blood by red cells.

$O_2$

**6** Carbon dioxide is carried back in the blood to the heart, then to the lungs, where it diffuses into the alveoli and is breathed out of the body.

$CO_2$

**5** Within body cells, glucose and oxygen take part in a complex series of reactions, which provides energy to power the cells. During this cellular respiration (left), glucose is converted to carbon dioxide and water.

Oxygen

Glucose

Blood

Carbon dioxide

Water

Tissues

## BREATHING VOLUMES

One way the body copes with varied demands for oxygen is through changes in breathing volume. The tidal volume—the amount breathed into and out of the lungs at each breath—may vary from 0.5 liter at rest, up to 4.5 liters (near the maximum or vital capacity) during heavy exercise.

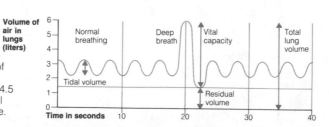

Volume of air in lungs (liters)

Normal breathing

Deep breath

Vital capacity

Total lung volume

Tidal volume

Residual volume

Time in seconds    10    20    30    40

**4** As the blood passes through tissue capillaries, it gives up oxygen (and nutrients such as glucose) to the body tissues and cells and picks up the waste products of cellular respiration—carbon dioxide and water.

R

loose, is part of the process by which *primary teeth* are shed. It is thought to be activated by pressure from the underlying *permanent teeth* as they erupt (see *Eruption of teeth*).

Some degree of external resorption, affecting the roots, occurs in most adults as part of the aging process. External resorption may also be caused by injury to a tooth, periapical *periodontitis* (inflammation of tissues around the root tip), or pressure from an *orthodontic appliance*, a tumor, or an impacted tooth. Completely impacted teeth occasionally undergo resorption of both the crown and the root.

The cause of internal resorption, which is a rare form of tooth resorption, occurring in about 1 percent of adults, is unknown. The condition sometimes spreads outward from the pulp cavity, producing a pink spot that shows through the crown.

**DIAGNOSIS AND TREATMENT**
Resorption is usually detected by taking *dental X rays*. Treatment of external resorption is of the underlying cause (such as removing an impacted tooth). Internal resorption can usually be successfully halted by *root-canal treatment*.

## Respiration
A term for the processes by which oxygen reaches body cells and is utilized by them in metabolism and by which carbon dioxide is eliminated.

The various stages in respiration are illustrated in the box opposite. (See also *Metabolism*; *Respiratory system*.)

## Respirator
See *Ventilator*.

## Respiratory arrest
Sudden cessation of breathing. Respiratory arrest results from any process that severely depresses the function of the respiratory center in the brain. Causes include prolonged *seizures*, an overdose of *narcotic drugs*, *cardiac arrest*, *electrical injury*, serious *head injury*, *stroke*, or *respiratory failure*.

Respiratory arrest leads to *anoxia* (lack of oxygen to tissues) and, if untreated, to cardiac arrest, brain damage, coma, and death. These effects may occur within a few minutes. The victim should be given *artificial respiration* or placed on a *ventilator* without delay. The underlying cause is treated if possible.

## Respiratory distress syndrome
A lung disorder that causes increasing difficulty in breathing; this results in a life-threatening deficiency of oxygen in the blood. The condition affects premature babies and adults whose lungs have been damaged by illness or injury. It is the most common cause of death in premature babies.

**CAUSES AND INCIDENCE**
Respiratory distress syndrome occurs in premature babies who are deficient in surfactant, a chemical that keeps open the *alveoli* in the lungs.

In adults, the disorder is caused by a stiffening of lung tissue associated with an increase of fluid in the interstitial (between the alveoli) part of the lungs. The many possible causes include severe *pneumonia*; inhaling vomit, an irritant gas (such as smoke or chlorine), or a high concentration of oxygen; partial drowning; an overdose of a narcotic drug, such as heroin or morphine; certain other drugs, among them nitrofurantoin; and certain *autoimmune disorders*.

**SYMPTOMS AND SIGNS**
The condition starts with an increase in breathing rate. Breathing then becomes labored and more rapid. Babies with respiratory distress syndrome make grunting noises and draw in the chest wall when they breathe. If the condition worsens, progressive deoxygenation of the blood makes the sufferer turn blue and eventually, if no treatment is given, death may result.

**DIAGNOSIS AND TREATMENT**
Respiratory distress syndrome is confirmed by listening to the lung with a stethoscope, by a *chest X ray*, and by analysis of *blood gases*. In adults, more tests may be needed to ensure that the heart is not malfunctioning.

Patients are treated in an *intensive-care* unit. In the early stages, oxygen is given by mask. If the condition does not worsen, this may be the only treatment required and is continued until the patient recovers. If respiratory distress increases, an *endotracheal tube* is inserted through the nose or mouth or a *tracheostomy* (insertion of a breathing tube into a hole made in the windpipe) performed; breathing is then maintained by a *ventilator*. Any underlying cause is treated if possible.

**OUTLOOK**
About 3 percent of premature babies die of respiratory distress syndrome. With modern intensive care, the survival rate for newborn babies with respiratory distress syndrome approaches 90 percent; for adults it is between 25 and 50 percent. However, some survivors are left with permanent lung damage.

## Respiratory failure
A condition in which there is a buildup of carbon dioxide and a fall in the level of oxygen in the blood (see *Hypoxia*). Respiratory failure may be caused by any disorder that disrupts the normal transfer of gases in the blood, including lung disorders (such as *emphysema*, severe *asthma*, or chronic *bronchitis*). Failure may also be due to damage to the respiratory center in the brain from an overdose of *narcotic drugs*.

Symptoms include breathlessness, cough, cyanosis (blue discoloration of the skin), shallow breathing, an increased respiratory rate, and, less commonly, a reduced respiratory rate.

Respiratory failure usually requires *oxygen therapy*, in which a carefully controlled dose of oxygen is given. In severe cases, the patient must be placed on a *ventilator*. The underlying cause is also treated.

## Respiratory function tests
See *Pulmonary function tests*.

## Respiratory system
The organs responsible for carrying oxygen from the air to the bloodstream and for expelling the waste product carbon dioxide.

Air passes from the nose or mouth, via various respiratory passages, to millions of balloonlike sacs, the alveoli, in the lungs. Oxygen in the warmed and moistened inhaled air

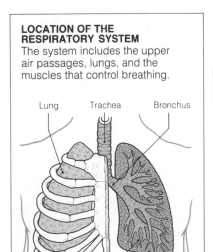

**LOCATION OF THE RESPIRATORY SYSTEM**
The system includes the upper air passages, lungs, and the muscles that control breathing.

Lung  Trachea  Bronchus

Bronchiole  Alveoli

R

passes through the thin walls of the alveoli into the bloodstream, and carbon dioxide passes from the blood into the alveoli to be breathed out (see *Respiration*).

Air is inhaled and exhaled by the actions of the chest muscles and diaphragm (see *Breathing*).

**DISORDERS**

Disorders of the respiratory system can affect the air passages (obstructing the passage of air into or out of the lungs) or the lung tissues (resulting in a poor exchange of oxygen and carbon dioxide). The functioning of the respiratory system can also be impaired by disorders, such as poliomyelitis, that affect the chest muscles and diaphragm and make it difficult to inflate the lungs. (See also articles on individual organs of the respiratory system; *Respiratory tract infection*.)

## Respiratory therapy

A paramedical discipline concerned with the maintenance of breathing capacity in people with impaired lung function or the prevention and treatment of pulmonary complications following surgery.

Working under the supervision of a physician, respiratory therapists treat severe respiratory diseases (such as chronic *bronchitis*) and care for the respiratory needs of patients who are on *ventilators* or recovering from major operations. Techniques include the administration of oxygen, drugs, or moisture to the lungs through a *nebulizer*; *postural drainage*; *percussion*; and *breathing exercises*.

Respiratory therapists must successfully complete the examination of the National Board for Respiratory Care (NBRC).

## Respiratory tract infection

Infection of the breathing passages, which extend from the nose to the alveoli. Most of these illnesses, which are classified as upper or lower respiratory tract infections, are caused by viruses or bacteria.

Upper respiratory tract infections affect the nose, throat, sinuses, and larynx. They are among the most common of all illnesses, especially in early childhood. The most familiar upper respiratory tract infections are the common *cold*, *pharyngitis*, *tonsillitis*, *sinusitis*, *laryngitis*, and *croup*.

Lower respiratory tract infections, which affect the trachea, bronchi, and lungs, include acute *bronchitis*, acute *bronchiolitis*, and *pneumonia*.

## Restless legs

A syndrome that features unpleasant tickling, burning, pricking, or aching sensations in the muscles of the legs. Symptoms tend to come on at night in bed, although prolonged sitting sometimes triggers the discomfort; relief may be obtained only by movement, such as walking.

Restless legs affects as many as 15 percent of the population, although many cases are very mild. It tends to run in families and is most common in middle-aged women, in people who consume a lot of caffeine, in smokers, and during pregnancy. The disorder often develops in people with rheumatoid arthritis.

The exact cause is unknown; there is no apparent nerve, muscle, or circulatory problem. Symptoms may be relieved by cold compresses or by keeping the legs warm.

## Restoration, dental

The process of reconstructing part of a tooth that has been damaged by disease or injury. Restoration also refers to the material or substitute part used to rebuild the tooth.

Small areas are usually repaired by first removing the decayed or diseased area and then *filling* the tooth with an inactive material. For more extensive repairs, it may be necessary to fit a dental *onlay*, *inlay*, or *crown*. They are constructed outside the mouth and then cemented into place. For repairing chipped front teeth the dentist may use a *bonding* technique, in which the surface of the tooth is etched with an acid solution and then plastic or porcelain material is attached to the roughened surface.

## Restricted growth

See *Short stature*.

## Resuscitation

See *Artificial respiration*; *Cardiopulmonary resuscitation*.

## Retainer

A type of *orthodontic appliance*.

## Retardation

See *Mental retardation*.

## Reticular formation

A network of nerve cells scattered throughout the *brain stem*.

## Reticulosarcoma

An obsolescent term for non-Hodgkin's lymphoma (see *Lymphoma, non-Hodgkin's*).

## Retina

The light-sensitive membrane that lines the inside of the back of the *eye* on which images are cast by the cornea and lens. The retina contains specialized nerve cells (the rods and cones) that convert light energy into nerve impulses. The retina also contains a network of connecting and integrating cells, some with very long fibers, that convey these impulses back along the *optic nerve* to the brain.

The rods are exceptionally sensitive, responding to very dim light. The cones are less sensitive but are responsible for color vision; different cones produce impulses that vary in strength with the color of the light striking them (see *Color vision*).

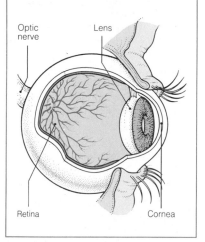

**LOCATION OF THE RETINA**
The retina is like the light-sensitive film in a camera. It forms a concave membrane over the back inner surface of the eye.

Optic nerve    Lens

Retina    Cornea

Near the center of the retina is the fovea. Here, retinal blood vessels are absent; the light-sensitive cells (almost all cones) are packed so that vision has the highest resolution.

## Retinal artery occlusion

Blockage of the main artery feeding blood to the *retina* or of one of its branches. Retinal artery occlusion is most commonly caused by a *thrombosis* (abnormal blood clot formation) or by an embolus (a clot or fatty deposit carried by the blood from another area).

If the main artery is blocked long enough, permanent blindness results in the affected eye. If a small branch is blocked, there is loss of part of the field of vision.

R

## DISORDERS OF THE RETINA

Despite its small size, the retina is subject to a wide variety of disorders, many of which seriously affect the vision or, in some cases, produce blindness.

### CONGENITAL AND GENETIC DISORDERS

Color blindness (see *Color vision deficiency*), an abnormality of retinal cones (color receptors in the retina), usually has a genetic basis. *Macular degeneration* (genetic predispositions leading to degeneration of the macula) may appear at any age. Other degenerative disorders of the retina with a genetic basis include *Tay-Sachs disease* and *retinitis pigmentosa*.

Retinopathy may result from exposure of a premature baby to excessive oxygen concentration. Abnormalities occur in the retinal vessels and *retrolental fibroplasia* may occur.

### INFECTION

*Toxoplasmosis* is a common infection of the retina. The infection is often acquired before birth and recurs later in life, with progressive damage to the retina. The parasite that causes toxoplasmosis is found in cat feces and raw beef.

*TOXOCARA CANIS* worm larvae may lodge in the retina and cause severe retinal destruction, producing a white mass resembling a tumor. *Onchocerciasis*, a worm infestation, may cause severe retinal damage. Bacterial and fungal infections elsewhere in the body can be carried by the blood to the retina. People whose immune systems are impaired are more susceptible to viral infections of the retina.

### TUMORS

*Retinoblastoma* is a malignant tumor that usually appears in the first three years of life. The affected eye may have visual loss and a visible whiteness in the pupil; *strabismus* often develops. The tendency to this cancer can be inherited. Secondary malignant tumors, spreading to the eye from primary tumors elsewhere in the body, can occur. A variety of benign tumors occurs in the retina. Malignant melanoma can arise from the *choroid* (layer beneath the retina) and spread throughout the body.

### INJURY

The retina may be torn (see *Retinal tear*) due to severe penetrating or nonpenetrating injury. Permanent damage may be caused by a retinal burn, sometimes caused by looking at an eclipse of the sun.

### METABOLIC DISORDERS

*Diabetes mellitus* may cause retinopathy with fluid leakage, tiny aneurysms of the capillaries, and hemorrhage into the retina. The growth of new, fragile blood vessels on the surface of the retina can be a feature of this type of retinopathy, and these vessels bleed readily. Hemorrhage into the vitreous gel may occur from blood vessels, and fibrous tissue can grow forward onto the gel in cases of proliferative retinopathy. This is a major cause of permanent loss of vision.

### IMPAIRED BLOOD SUPPLY

*Retinal vein occlusion* (or artery occlusion), a common cause of blindness, results from blockage of the central vein or artery of the retina. Hypertensive retinopathy is damage to the retina caused by high blood pressure, which leads to narrowing of the blood vessels of the retina. *Atherosclerosis* of the retinal arteries is common and frequently leads to retinal damage.

### POISONS

*Methanol* causes widespread and permanent destruction of certain retinal tissues, leading to blindness. A combination of heavy tobacco smoking, heavy alcohol intake, and poor nutrition may lead to visual loss. Both vitamin and lead poisoning may cause visual damage and loss.

### DRUGS

Many drugs can damage the retina. *Chloroquine*, used in large doses over a long period for the treatment of conditions such as rheumatoid arthritis, may damage the retina. *Phenothiazine drugs*, used to treat psychiatric disorders, may, in rare cases, damage vision.

### OTHER DISORDERS

Age-related macular degeneration, causing progressive loss of vision, is common in older people. *Retinal detachment* often occurs in the absence of injury and may be more common in people with severe *myopia* (nearsightedness).

### INVESTIGATION

Retinal disorders are investigated by checking the visual acuity and the visual fields (see *Vision tests*). After dilating the pupils with drops, the retinas are inspected by means of an *ophthalmoscope* and a camera. *Fluorescein* can be injected into a vein, where it is carried by the blood to the retina for investigation. Electrophysiologic tests may be performed to study certain retinal diseases. *Ultrasound scanning* can be used to study tumors in or under the retina.

R

---

## Retinal detachment

Separation of the light-sensitive inner surface of the back of the eye from the outer layers.

### CAUSES AND INCIDENCE

Retinal detachment is usually preceded by a break or tear in the retina (see *Retinal tear*), which may be due to natural degeneration or to pulling on the retina by contracting strands in the vitreous gel. Vitreous fluid collects between the delicate nerve membrane and the underlying pigment layer, thus separating them. Retinal detachment may occur after major injury to the eye, but in most cases the condition occurs spontaneously.

Detachment is more common in highly myopic (nearsighted) people who have thinned retinas with areas of degeneration and in those who have had cataract surgery.

### SYMPTOMS AND SIGNS

Retinal detachment is painless and the symptoms are exclusively visual. The first indication is the appearance of bright flashes of light, seen at the edge of the field of vision and accompanied by *floaters*. The flashes are caused by strong stimulation of the light-sensitive cells as the tear occurs, and the floaters by the release of blood or pigment into the vitreous gel.

These symptoms do not always occur; the affected person may be unaware of the detachment until a black "drape" obscures vision. This drape descends in a lower detachment, ascends in an upper detachment, enters from the right in a left detachment, and so on.

### TREATMENT

Retinal detachment is an emergency. An ophthalmologist must be consulted before the macula (the site of central vision) becomes detached. Once detachment has occurred, normal central vision may not be restored. With a lower detachment (descending drape), the affected person may safely stand in an upright position. If there is upper detachment, there is a risk that the accumulating fluid will strip off the macula and it is safer to lie flat on the back.

Treatment usually involves surgery, in which a soft silicone rubber sponge may be sewn in place on the outside of the sclera overlying the detachment. This indents the sclera and leads to absorption of the subretinal fluid, causing the retina to settle back into place. Cryopexy (involving the application of extreme cold) or a heating *diathermy* may be used to fix the retina in place by causing an inflammatory adhesiveness of the underlying tissues. If the macula has not been detached, the results can be excellent. If a retinal hole is found prior to retinal detachment, the hole may be sealed by laser or cryopexy.

## Retinal hemorrhage

Bleeding into the *retina* from one or more blood vessels. Retinal hemorrhage may be caused by *diabetes mellitus*, which leads to the formation of abnormal, small blood vessels that are fragile and bleed easily. Retinal hemorrhages also occur in *hypertension* and *retinal vein occlusion* (blockage of a vein that drains blood from the retina).

When the macula (site of central vision) is involved, vision is severely disturbed. Peripheral hemorrhages may pass unnoticed and may be detected only when the eye is examined with an ophthalmoscope.

## Retinal tear

The development of a split in the *retina*, usually caused by degeneration. Retinal tear is more common in people with severe *myopia* (nearsightedness). A retinal tear may also be caused by severe injury to the eye, especially a penetrating injury. *Retinal detachment* often follows a retinal tear.

## Retinal vein occlusion

Blockage of the main vein that carries blood away from the *retina* or of one of its branches, usually as a result of *thrombosis* (abnormal blood clot) formation in the vein. Retinal vein occlusion is more common in people who have *glaucoma* and usually causes disturbance of vision in the affected eye. Retinal vein occlusion may also cause glaucoma and can result in complete blindness.

## Retinitis

Inflammation affecting the *retina*. (See also *Retinopathy*.)

## Retinitis pigmentosa

A degeneration of the rods and cones of the *retina* in both eyes. The condition usually has a genetic basis, but seldom appears before a person reaches adolescence and may not appear until middle age.

The first symptom of retinitis pigmentosa is usually an awareness that vision in dim light is very poor (night blindness). Testing of the fields of vision shows a ring-shaped area of blindness that, over the course of years, gradually extends to destroy an increasing area of the field. The cones in the macula seem more resistant than the peripherally placed rods, so central vision is retained, often for many years. Progression and severity are variable.

Examination of the retinas by ophthalmoscopy shows numerous masses of branching black pigment distributed in areas corresponding to the areas of visual loss.

## Retinoblastoma

A malignant tumor (cancer) of the retina that affects babies and infants; the tendency to the disease is usually inherited. It occurs in approximately one baby in 20,000.

Retinoblastoma often first shows itself as a visible whiteness in the pupil. An affected eye may be blind and *strabismus* frequently develops. Retinoblastoma can spread from the eye to the orbit and along the optic nerve to the brain. Treatment is removal or *radiation therapy* of the affected eye. If both eyes are affected, the eye with the larger tumor may be removed and the other eye given radiation therapy.

In many instances retinoblastoma is inherited. If retinoblastoma runs in your family, genetic counseling and prompt and regular eye examinations of newborns are important.

## Retinoids

See *Vitamin A*.

## Retinol

The principal form of *vitamin A* found in the body.

## Retinopathy

Disease or disorder of the retina. The term is usually used to describe damage to the retina caused by persistent *hypertension* (high blood pressure) or *diabetes mellitus*. (See also *Retina* disorders box.)

## Retractor

A surgical instrument used to hold an incision open or hold back surrounding tissue so that the surgeon has free access to the underlying area being operated on. Some retractors are held by the nurse or an assisting physician; self-retaining retractors have a locking device that keeps them in position without support.

## Retrobulbar neuritis

Sudden total or partial loss of the central field of vision, usually in one eye, accompanied by pain during eye movement and a feeling of pressure in the eyeball.

The symptoms are caused by inflammation of the optic nerve, although the exact reason for the inflammation is often unknown. Sometimes, the condition is thought to be caused by a demyelination process in the nerve fibers similar to that which occurs in *multiple sclerosis*.

The visual loss usually lasts for about six weeks and, although recovery usually seems nearly complete, repeated attacks are likely to lead to permanent loss of some central vision. However, after recovering from one episode, a person may be free of further symptoms.

Although no treatment can affect the long-term outcome, *corticosteroid drugs* may sometimes be prescribed.

## Retrolental fibroplasia

Also called the retinopathy of prematurity, a condition that primarily affects the eyes of premature infants. Retrolental fibroplasia can occur when premature infants with a very low birth weight need to be given high concentrations of oxygen to treat *respiratory distress syndrome* and other effects of prematurity.

The tissues at the margin of the retina (as well as other immature tissues) respond to excess oxygen by shutting down their blood vessels.

R

When normal oxygen concentrations are resumed, these tissues can sometimes send out strands of new vessels and fibrous (scar) tissues into the vitreous gel behind the lens, which may seriously interfere with vision and lead to *retinal detachment*.

## Retroperitoneal fibrosis

Inflammation and scarring of tissues at the back of the abdominal cavity that occasionally leads to obstruction of both ureters. The resultant blockage of urine flow from the kidneys, if severe, causes *renal failure*.

Most cases of retroperitoneal fibrosis occur in middle-aged men and are of unknown cause. The condition may also be caused by long-term treatment with the drug *methysergide*.

## Retrosternal pain

Pain in the central region of the chest in the area of the sternum (breastbone). The most serious cause of such pain is a *myocardial infarction* (heart attack); it is more likely to be due to irritation of the esophagus or *angina pectoris*. (See also *Chest pain*.)

## Rett's syndrome

A recently discovered brain disorder that affects girls only. This rare condition was first described in the 1960s by an Austrian, Andreas Rett, but became medically recognized only during the 1980s. Rett's syndrome affects about one in every 15,000 female babies born and is thought to be caused by a *genetic disorder*.

The health and development of an affected baby appear normal until symptoms occur, usually when the child is 12 to 18 months old. Skills that had been acquired, such as walking and talking, gradually disappear and the girl becomes progressively handicapped and may appear autistic (see *Autism*). Odd, repetitive writhing movements of the hands and limbs are characteristic of the condition, and there are often inappropriate outbursts of crying or laughter.

There is no cure for Rett's syndrome; sufferers need constant care and attention because of the level of handicap. Parents of an affected child should receive *genetic counseling*.

## Reye's syndrome

A rare disorder characterized by brain and liver damage following an upper respiratory tract infection, chickenpox, or influenza. Reye's syndrome is almost entirely confined to children under age 15.

### CAUSES

Evidence suggests that Reye's syndrome is often (but not invariably) related to taking aspirin for a viral infection. Physicians recommend that children be given acetaminophen instead of aspirin for viral infections or fever of unknown origin.

### SYMPTOMS AND SIGNS

Reye's syndrome develops as the child is recovering from the infection, starting with uncontrollable vomiting, often with lethargy, memory loss, disorientation, or delirium. Swelling of the brain may cause seizures, deepening coma, disturbances in heart rhythm, and cessation of breathing. Jaundice indicates severe liver involvement.

### TREATMENT

Swelling of the brain is controlled by *corticosteroid drugs* and infusions of *mannitol*. *Dialysis* or *blood transfusions* may be carried out to correct the changes in blood chemistry caused by damage to the liver. If breathing stops, the patient is placed on a *ventilator*.

### OUTLOOK

With increasing knowledge of the condition, the death rate has dropped dramatically from about 60 percent to around 10 percent. The outlook is worse for those who have seizures, deep coma, and who stop breathing. Those who survive a serious attack may suffer brain damage.

## Rhabdomyolysis

Destruction of muscle tissue accompanied by the release of the oxygen-carrying red muscle pigment *myoglobin* into the blood. The most common cause is a severe, crushing muscle injury (see *Crush syndrome*). Other causes include *polymyositis* (a viral infection of muscles) and, rarely, excessive physical exercise.

Rhabdomyolysis usually causes temporary paralysis or weakness of the affected muscle. Unless the muscle is severely injured, it usually regenerates and the condition clears up without treatment.

## Rhabdomyosarcoma

A very rare, malignant tumor of muscle. Rhabdomyosarcoma may develop during infancy, usually affecting the throat, bladder, prostate gland, or vagina, or it may occur in old age, when it commonly affects a large muscle in the arm or leg. The tumor grows rapidly and spreads to other tissues. Treatment includes surgical removal, combined with *radiation therapy* and *anticancer drugs*.

## Rheumatic fever

A disease that causes inflammation in various tissues throughout the body. Rheumatic fever is very rare in most developed countries but has been reported to be on the increase again in parts of the US.

Joint inflammation occurs, but without crippling effect. Of importance is the frequency with which the disease permanently damages the heart. The nervous system may also be affected, causing *Sydenham's chorea*.

### CAUSES AND INCIDENCE

Rheumatic fever always follows a throat infection with certain strains of streptococcal bacteria. It is not caused by the presence of the bacteria in the affected tissues and is generally believed to be some form of *autoimmune disorder* (one in which the body's immune system attacks its own tissues) induced by streptococci. It can usually be prevented by prompt treatment of streptococcal throat infections with antibiotic drugs.

Children between 5 and 15 are the most commonly affected. In developed countries, the incidence of rheumatic fever has been dropping for many years. In the US, there are a few cases each year. However, in the poorer countries of Asia and Africa, rheumatic fever remains a common and significant cause of heart disease.

### SYMPTOMS AND SIGNS

There is fever with pain, inflammation, and swelling of one or more of the larger joints. As one joint improves, symptoms tend to develop in another, although sometimes several joints are affected simultaneously. If damage to the heart is to occur (it does not always occur), it develops insidiously; there may be no symptoms until years later. The heart may be affected in various ways, the most common and most serious being a thickening and scarring of the *heart valves*, leading to narrowing and/or leaking of valves (see *Mitral stenosis*; *Mitral insufficiency*). These effects are permanent and progressive. *Heart valve surgery* may be needed.

Sydenham's chorea in children occurs when rheumatic fever affects the nervous system. There are irregular, uncontrollable, aimless, jerky movements, and usually some emotional upset.

Pea-sized nodules situated beneath the skin (often over bony prominences) and a rash are other signs.

### DIAGNOSIS AND TREATMENT

There are no specific tests for rheumatic fever, but tests may be performed

**R**

to look for antibodies (proteins made by the *immune system*) directed against streptococci. The diagnosis may be suspected when arthritis moves from joint to joint, but the condition may be discovered only when late heart damage, with symptoms of *heart failure* or a heart *murmur*, is noted.

As soon as the diagnosis of acute rheumatic fever is made, penicillin is used to eradicate streptococci. Sodium salicylate (aspirin) is used to control the joint pain and inflammation and to try to minimize heart damage, but *corticosteroid drugs* may be needed. Sedative and tranquilizer drugs are helpful in treating Sydenham's chorea.

OUTLOOK

The outlook depends on the degree to which the heart has been affected and on whether recurrences can be avoided. The use of penicillin, taken daily for many months or years, may be necessary to prevent further infection with streptococci.

## Rheumatism

A popular term for any disorder that causes pain and stiffness in muscles and joints, including minor aches and twinges as well as disorders such as *rheumatoid arthritis*, *osteoarthritis*, and *polymyalgia rheumatica*.

## Rheumatoid arthritis

A type of *arthritis* (joint inflammation) in which the joints of the fingers, wrists, toes, or other joints in the body become painful, swollen, stiff, and, in severe cases, deformed.

The frequency of attacks, the number of affected joints, and the severity of symptoms are variable. The disease usually takes the form of recurring moderate attacks.

CAUSES AND INCIDENCE

Rheumatoid arthritis is an *autoimmune disorder* (in which the *immune system* attacks the body's own tissues). The disorder usually starts in early adulthood or middle age but can develop at any age (see *Rheumatoid arthritis, juvenile*). It affects two to three times more women than men.

SYMPTOMS AND SIGNS

The disease's onset is usually gradual, with mild fever and generalized aches and pains preceding specific joint symptoms. In some cases, joint inflammation develops suddenly.

Affected joints become swollen, red, warm, painful, and stiff. Structures around the joint may also become inflamed, resulting in weakness of the ligaments, tendons, and surrounding muscles.

## RHEUMATOID ARTHRITIS

One of the most serious forms of joint disease, rheumatoid arthritis may occur as a single episode or a succession of progressively severe attacks. It results from a disturbance in the body's defenses against infection, causing these defenses to attack various body tissues. In the worst cases, joints are completely destroyed, but modern treatment has reduced the incidence of severe disability.

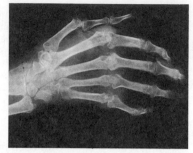

**X ray of the hand in rheumatoid arthritis**
Note the destructive changes in the joints and the way the finger bones curve away from the thumb side of the hand.

**Affected joints**
Rheumatoid arthritis can affect virtually any joint, but especially the fingers, wrists, shoulders, knees, hips, and spinal joints in the neck.

**Disease progression**
The synovium (membrane lining the capsule of an affected joint) becomes inflamed and thickened (right). Later, inflammation may spread to the cartilage and bone.

Bone
Inflamed synovium
Cartilage
Capsule

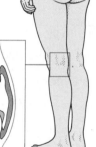

## TREATMENT OF RHEUMATOID ARTHRITIS

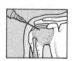

**Drug treatment** may include antirheumatic drugs to slow the progress of the disease, nonsteroidal anti-inflammatory drugs to relieve joint pain, and immunosuppressants to dampen the activity of the immune system.

**Occupational therapy** can help people who are disabled by rheumatoid arthritis. Sufferers are shown how to cope with everyday tasks, provided with aids for use in the home, and taught principles of joint protection.

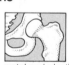

**Prostheses**
Many joints, such as the hip, can now be replaced with substitutes made from hard-wearing metal and plastic materials. Prostheses may be the only satisfactory solution if a joint becomes seriously damaged.

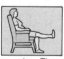

**Physical therapy** aids in the relief of pain and stiffness and helps sufferers to regain use of affected joints and muscles. The physician may recommend removable splints to relieve pain in the hands and wrists.

The finger joints are the most commonly affected, resulting in a weak grip. Swelling of the wrist and *carpal tunnel syndrome* (tingling and pain in the fingers caused by pressure on the median nerve) are also common. *Tenosynovitis* (inflamed painful tendon sheaths) may develop in the wrist and the fingers may turn white on exposure to cold, a condition known as *Raynaud's phenomenon*. Involvement of the feet causes pain in the ankles, arches, and toes. Some of the other joints affected are shown above.

In some cases, soft nodules develop beneath the skin over bony surfaces; in others, *bursitis* occurs, in which the fluid-filled sac around a joint becomes

R

inflamed. When the knee is affected, a fluid-filled swelling known as a *Baker's cyst* may develop behind it.

Many sufferers feel fatigued as a result of the *anemia* that usually accompanies the disease. Early morning stiffness is common, and sufferers may require help getting out of bed and dressing.

### DIAGNOSIS

The diagnosis is based on the patient's condition and history, the continuance of symptoms for at least six weeks, X rays of affected joints, and *blood tests* (including a check for specific antibodies known as rheumatoid factor). If rheumatoid factor is absent from a person who otherwise appears to have rheumatoid arthritis, the condition is known as seronegative rheumatoid arthritis.

### TREATMENT

Some of the main treatment options are outlined in the box opposite. *Nonsteroidal anti-inflammatory drugs* (NSAIDs) may be used to relieve joint pain and stiffness. *Antirheumatic drugs*, such as gold or penicillamine, may be used to arrest or slow the progress of the disease.

*Immunosuppressant drugs*, such as *corticosteroid drugs* or azathioprine, are given to suppress the body's immune system if antirheumatic drugs fail to control the disorder or if they produce severe side effects. Corticosteroid drugs may be injected into the joint to provide local pain relief.

*Physical therapy* and *occupational therapy* are often important.

Destroyed joints can sometimes be replaced with artificial substitutes (see *Arthroplasty*). Hip and knee replacements are the most common.

### COMPLICATIONS

In severe cases of rheumatoid arthritis, inflammation may also affect the covering of the heart (causing *pericarditis*), the small blood vessels (resulting in poor circulation and ulcers on the hands and feet), the lungs (leading to *pleural effusion* or *pulmonary fibrosis*), the eyes or mouth (making them dry; see *Sjögren's syndrome*), the lymph glands (producing tender swellings in the neck, armpit, and groin), and the spleen (causing *hypersplenism*).

### OUTLOOK

Most sufferers must take drugs for the rest of their lives, but effective control of symptoms usually allows a near-normal level of activity. Modern methods of treatment have reduced the incidence and severity of deformity and disability.

## Rheumatoid arthritis, juvenile

A rare form of *arthritis* (joint inflammation) that affects children and lasts more than three months. Juvenile arthritis occurs more often in girls than in boys, and most commonly starts between the ages of 2 and 4 or around puberty.

### TYPES AND SYMPTOMS

There are three main types of juvenile arthritis. Still's disease (systemic onset juvenile arthritis) starts with an illness characterized by fever, rash, enlarged lymph glands, abdominal pain, and weight loss. These symptoms last several weeks; joint pain, swelling, and stiffness may not begin for several months. A second type, called polyarticular juvenile arthritis, starts with pain, swelling, and stiffness in a number of joints. In the third type, pauciarticular juvenile arthritis, four or fewer joints are involved.

### DIAGNOSIS

Diagnosis is based on the symptoms and signs and the exclusion of other disorders that can cause joint symptoms in children, such as viral or bacterial infections, rheumatic fever, Crohn's disease, ulcerative colitis, hemophilia, sickle cell anemia, and leukemia. Blood tests may help identify the cause of the arthritis.

### COMPLICATIONS

Possible complications include short stature, anemia, pleurisy, pericarditis (inflammation of the outer lining of the heart), and enlargement of the liver and spleen.

*Uveitis* (inflammation of the iris and the surrounding muscles in the eye) may develop and, if untreated, may damage vision. Rarely, *amyloidosis* (deposition of a starchy substance in body organs) may occur; if the kidney is involved, *renal failure* may develop.

### TREATMENT

Joint pain and stiffness may be relieved by aspirin, *nonsteroidal anti-inflammatory drugs*, and, in very severe cases, *antirheumatic drugs* (such as gold, penicillamine, chloroquine, or azathioprine) or *corticosteroid drugs*.

Splints may be worn during the day to rest acutely inflamed joints and at night to reduce the risk of deformities. *Physical therapy* reduces the risk of muscle wasting and contractures. Excessive physical exercise should be avoided and special shoes worn to reduce the risk of foot deformity.

### OUTLOOK

In most children the arthritis disappears after several years. However, some are left with permanent stiffness and joint deformity.

## Rheumatoid spondylitis

See *Ankylosing spondylitis*.

## Rheumatologist

A physician who diagnoses and treats arthritis, rheumatism, and other afflictions of the joints, muscles, or connective tissues (see *Rheumatology*).

## Rheumatology

The branch of medicine concerned with the causes, development, diagnosis, and treatment of joint, muscle, and *connective tissue diseases*. Rheumatologists use a wide variety of investigative techniques, ranging from X rays of joints to tests of muscle function and blood analysis. Treatment is similarly varied; it includes courses of anti-inflammatory drugs or analgesics and rest.

## Rh incompatibility

A mismatch between the blood of a pregnant woman and that of her baby with respect to the Rh (Rhesus) *blood group*. In certain circumstances, this mismatch can lead to *hemolytic disease of the newborn*.

### CAUSE

Blood groups are determined by substances called factors on the surface of red blood cells, which differ among individuals. The best known grouping is the A,B,O system. The Rh system (first identified in Rhesus monkeys) was discovered early in this century. It consists of several factors, one of which (D factor) is the most important cause of Rh incompatibility. People can have blood that is Rh positive (carry the D factor in their blood) or Rh negative (do not carry it). Having a positive or negative blood type is determined by *genes* (i.e., it is an inherited trait).

Rh incompatibility can arise only when a woman's blood is Rh negative and her baby's blood is Rh positive. This can happen only if the baby's father's blood is also Rh positive. There are usually no problems during a woman's first pregnancy with a baby whose blood is Rh positive. However, as shown in the diagram (overleaf), the baby may sensitize the woman to Rh-positive blood; if she has a subsequent pregnancy with an Rh-positive baby, there is a risk of hemolytic disease of the newborn. A woman whose blood is Rh negative can also be sensitized if she is mistakenly given a transfusion of Rh-positive blood.

### INCIDENCE

Among white people in the US, about one person in six has Rh-negative

R

blood; in about one pregnancy in 11 the mother's blood is Rh negative and the baby's blood is Rh positive. In the past, hemolytic disease of the newborn was a common cause of stillbirth and of a severe fetal condition called erythroblastosis fetalis, in which destruction of fetal blood cells led to severe fetal disease or death. Hemolytic disease of the newborn due to Rh sensitization is becoming rare, primarily due to the development of *Rh₀(D) immune globulin*. When given by injection to a woman within 72 hours of delivery, it prevents 99 percent of Rh sensitization.

In addition, Rh₀(D) immune globulin is given to women after a miscarriage, elective abortion, amniocentesis, or any other procedure that might result in exposure of the mother to the fetal blood cells. Rh₀(D) immune globulin is also generally given to women with Rh-negative blood who are seven months pregnant.

The injection contains antibodies to Rh factor, which destroy any of the baby's blood cells that may have entered the woman before they have a chance to sensitize her.

Rh incompatibility is less common in black and Oriental families than in white families due to comparative rarity of the Rh-negative blood group in nonwhites.

### DIAGNOSIS AND TREATMENT

A pregnant woman's blood groups are checked at the first prenatal visit. Women who have Rh-negative blood are tested for the presence of Rh antibodies at this and subsequent visits. The management of the pregnancy and childbirth, if antibodies are present and there is a risk to the baby, is as described under *hemolytic disease of the newborn*.

## Rhinitis

Inflammation of the mucous membrane that lines the nose, usually manifested by some combination of nasal obstruction, nasal discharge, sneezing, and facial pressure or pain.

### TYPES

**VIRAL RHINITIS** A feature of the common cold (see *Cold, common*), rhinitis due to viral infection may lead to *sinusitis*.

**ALLERGIC RHINITIS** Also known as hay fever, this type may be seasonal, due to pollens, or year-round, due to house dust, molds, or pets (see *Rhinitis, allergic*). It most commonly occurs with vasomotor rhinitis.

**VASOMOTOR RHINITIS** This type of rhinitis is an intermittent or continual condition. The nose becomes overresponsive to stimuli, including pollutants such as tobacco smoke, temperature and humidity changes or extremes, certain foods, certain medicines, and/or certain emotions. The condition is common in pregnancy and in those taking the estrogen-progestogen contraceptive pill or other estrogen medication.

**HYPERTROPHIC RHINITIS** Repeated nasal infections can cause hypertrophic rhinitis, in which tissue in the nasal mucosa thickens and veins become chronically congested. This results in constant stuffiness, and sometimes impairment of the sense of smell. In extreme cases, part of the swollen tissue may be removed.

**ATROPHIC RHINITIS** This wasting of the mucous membrane can result from aging, chronic bacterial infections, or extensive nasal surgery. Other features of the disorder can include persistent nasal infection, a discharge that dries to a crust, loss of smell, and an unpleasant odor. Treatment is with *antibiotic* and *estrogen drugs*.

## Rhinitis, allergic

Inflammation of the mucous membrane that lines the nose due to an allergy to pollen, dust, or other airborne substances. Also known as hay fever, the disorder causes sneezing, a runny nose, and nasal congestion.

### CAUSES

In some people, inhaling particles of certain harmless substances provokes an exaggerated response by the *immune system*, which forms antibodies against them (see *Allergy*). The otherwise harmless substances, known as allergens, trigger the release of histamine and other chemicals that cause inflammation and fluid production in the lining of the nose and sinuses (air cavities around the nose). The most common of the allergens that cause allergic rhinitis are tree, grass, and weed pollens; molds; animal skin scales, hair, or feathers; house dust; and house-dust mites.

Pollen-induced allergic rhinitis is seasonal. Tree pollens are most prevalent in spring, grass pollens in summer, and weed pollens in summer and early fall. Sufferers are worst affected on days when the pollen count is high—that is, during hot and windy weather, especially in heavily vegetated, low-lying areas.

People affected by household allergens, such as dust, tend to have less severe symptoms but are affected throughout the year.

### INCIDENCE

Allergic rhinitis is a common complaint, affecting as many as 5 to 10 percent of the population. It is more common in people who have other allergies, such as asthma or eczema; like these disorders, it has a tendency to run in families. The condition usually develops before the age of 30 and affects more women than men.

### SYMPTOMS AND SIGNS

Exposure to the allergen produces an itching sensation in the nose, palate, throat, and eyes. This is followed by sneezing, stuffiness, a runny nose, and, usually, watering eyes. The eyes may also be affected by *conjunctivitis*, which makes them red and sore.

### PREVENTION AND TREATMENT

*Skin tests* help identify the allergen responsible for the disorder. Once the

**R**

## HOW Rh INCOMPATIBILITY OCCURS

Without preventive treatment, an Rh-negative woman who is exposed to D factor (a substance present only in Rh-positive blood) may develop antibodies that will attack the red blood cells of any future Rh-positive babies.

First pregnancy

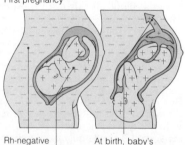

Rh-negative mother

Rh-positive baby

At birth, baby's blood enters mother's circulation

Subsequent pregnancies

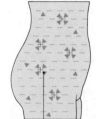

Antibodies against Rh-positive blood formed in mother

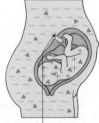

Antibodies cross placenta and destroy red blood cells of subsequent Rh-positive babies

allergen is known, exposure should be avoided or kept to a minimum, although this is difficult when the cause is pollens.

For mild attacks of allergic rhinitis, occasional use of a *decongestant* spray or drops may clear up symptoms, but use for more than three or four days can make the condition worse. For many sufferers, treatment is with *antihistamine drugs*. Antihistamines reduce the symptoms of itching and some degree of nasal congestion and runny nose, but many have the disadvantage of causing drowsiness. Treatment of allergic rhinitis may also include *corticosteroid drugs*, which can be used in the nose.

The drug cromolyn sodium, inhaled regularly throughout the pollen season, may help to prevent attacks by blocking the allergic response.

Desensitization to a particular pollen allergen by injecting gradually increasing amounts of it into the skin over a period of years can result in long-term relief of symptoms (see *Immunotherapy*).

## Rhinophyma

Bulbous deformity and redness of the nose occurring almost exclusively in elderly men. Rhinophyma is a complication of severe *rosacea* (a skin disorder of the nose and cheeks). The tissue of the nose thickens, small blood vessels enlarge, and the sebaceous glands become overactive, making the nose excessively oily.

Rhinophyma can be remedied by an operation. With the use of a general anesthetic, the swollen tissue is cut away until the nose is restored to a satisfactory shape. Skin grafting is not necessary, since the remaining tissue rapidly regenerates.

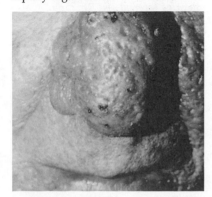

**Example of rhinophyma**
This disfiguring condition is remedied by paring away the excess tissue. The skin soon regenerates after treatment.

## Rhinoplasty

An operation that alters the structure of the nose to improve its appearance or to correct a deformity caused by injury or disease.

Incisions are made within the nose (to avoid visible scars) using either a local or a general anesthetic. The septum (the vertical wall of cartilage and bone that divides the nose) may be altered if breathing passages are blocked. Then the cartilage and bone of the nasal structure are reshaped. Occasionally, a bone or cartilage graft is used. The nose is splinted in position for about 10 days.

Rhinoplasty usually causes considerable bruising and swelling, and the results may not be clearly visible for weeks or months. Rare complications include recurrent nosebleeds due to persistent crusting at the incision sites and breathing difficulty due to narrowing of the nasal passages.

## Rhinorrhea

The discharge of watery mucus from the nose, usually due to *rhinitis* or to the flow of cerebrospinal fluid from the nose following a head injury. (See *Nasal discharge*.)

## Rh isoimmunization

The development of antibodies formed against Rh-positive blood in a person who has Rh-negative blood. (See *Rh incompatibility*; *Hemolytic disease of the newborn*.)

## Rh$_o$(D) immune globulin

An *antiserum* that contains antibodies against Rh (Rhesus) D factor (a substance present on the red blood cells of people who have Rh-positive blood). It is given to a woman who has Rh-negative blood after she has given birth to a baby whose blood is Rh positive or if she has had a miscarriage or elective abortion.

Rh$_o$(D) immune globulin is also given to a pregnant woman with Rh-negative blood after she has had amniocentesis or bleeding episodes or in other instances in which she might be exposed to fetal blood cells, as well as in the seventh month of pregnancy. The injected antibodies destroy any red cells from the fetus that have entered the woman's blood. This is important to prevent or reduce the risk of the woman forming her own antibodies against Rh-positive blood, which might adversely affect any subsequent pregnancies. (See *Rh incompatibility*; *Hemolytic disease of the newborn*.)

## Rhythm method

See *Contraception, periodic abstinence*.

## Rib

Any of the flat, curved bones that form a framework for the chest and a protective cage around the heart, lungs, and other organs.

There are 12 pairs of ribs, each joined at the back of the rib cage to a vertebra in the spine. Their arrangement is shown in the illustration on the next page. Between the ribs, and attached to them, are thin sheets of muscle that help to expand and relax the chest during breathing. The spaces between the ribs also contain nerves and blood vessels.

### DISORDERS
The ribs can easily be fractured by a fall or blow (see *Rib, fractured*).

A rib is one of the more common sites for a benign *bone tumor* or for a *metastasis* (a secondary malignant tumor that has spread from cancer elsewhere in the body).

In rare cases a person is born with one or more extra ribs lying above the uppermost normal rib. Known as *cervical ribs*, the additional ribs may press on nerves supplying the arm or cause other problems.

## Rib, fractured

Fracture of a rib is usually caused by a fall or blow, but occasionally it is caused by minor stress on the rib cage, such as that produced by prolonged coughing or even laughing.

The fracture causes severe pain that is made worse by deep breathing, and tenderness and swelling of the overlying tissue. The diagnosis is confirmed by *X rays*. Pain is relieved by *analgesics* (painkillers) or, occasionally, by an injection of a long-acting, local anesthetic drug.

Most rib fractures are undisplaced (i.e., the bone ends remain in alignment) and, in these cases, healing is usually spontaneous and straightforward. A displaced or splintered fracture may cause complications if the sharp ends or fragments rupture the *spleen* or pierce a lung, causing lung collapse (see *Pneumothorax*). Multiple rib fractures can result in *flail chest*.

Strapping is rarely used to aid healing because it hinders chest expansion and thus increases the risk of *pneumonia*. Instead, the patient is encouraged to take deep breaths while holding the injured side. If several ribs are fractured and displaced, an operation may be performed to wire them back in position.

R

## ANATOMY OF THE RIBS

There are seven true ribs attached to the sternum, three false ribs, each attached to a rib above, and two floating ribs on each side. They are joined to the spine and sternum so that, when pulled up by the intercostal muscles (between the ribs), they expand the chest, drawing air into the lungs. The front ends of the ribs are linked to the sternum by cartilages.

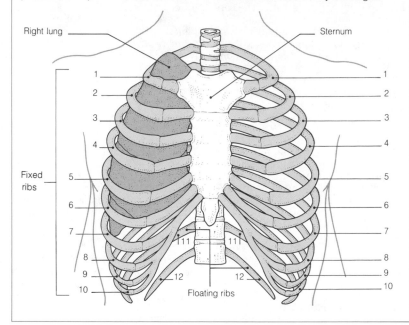

Right lung

Sternum

Fixed ribs

Floating ribs

## Riboflavin

The chemical name of vitamin $B_2$ (see *Vitamin B complex*).

## Rickets

A nutritional deficiency disease of childhood that affects the skeleton. Because inadequate amounts of calcium and phosphate are incorporated into an affected child's bones as they grow, the bones become deformed. In adults, a similar process leads to *osteomalacia*.

**CAUSES AND INCIDENCE**

The most common cause of rickets is deficiency of vitamin D, which is vital for the absorption of calcium from the intestines into the blood and for its incorporation into normal bone. Vitamin D is found in fat-containing animal substances, such as oily fish, butter, egg yolk, liver, and fish liver oils. There are also small amounts in human and animal milk. The vitamin is also made in the body through the action of sunlight on the skin.

Rickets occurs primarily in poor countries and in communities where babies receive inadequate vitamin D in the diet and simultaneously do not get enough sunlight. Breast milk alone cannot provide all a baby's needs for vitamin D, so a breast-fed baby who gets little sun should be given vitamin D supplements.

Rickets is now rare in the US and in other developed countries where vitamin D supplements are given to infants, where the vitamin is added to foods such as cow's milk, margarine, and breakfast cereals, and where most children and babies eat a varied diet and get adequate exposure to the sun. The disorder is seen only in vulnerable groups, such as premature babies, strict vegetarians, and some food faddists who avoid the foods rich in vitamin D listed above.

Rickets occasionally develops as a complication of an intestinal disorder that causes *malabsorption* (failure to absorb nutrients from the intestines). It also occurs in certain rare forms of kidney and liver disease and in children undergoing long-term therapy with *anticonvulsant drugs* (which interfere with the action of vitamin D).

**SYMPTOMS AND DIAGNOSIS**

The most striking feature of advanced rickets is deformity of the bones, especially of the legs and spine. Typically, there is bowing of the legs and, in infants, flattening of the head as a result of the softness of the skull. Infants with rickets often sleep poorly and show delay in crawling and walking. Other features include *kyphoscoliosis* (spinal curvature), enlargement of the wrists, ankles, and ends of the ribs, pelvic pain, a tendency to fractures, and muscle weakness.

**TREATMENT**

A child with rickets is treated with vitamin D supplements; he or she should also be given plenty of milk to provide calcium. Treatment continues until X rays show healing. The child should not be given excessive vitamin D supplements, however, as they can lead to *hypercalcemia*.

Treatment of other causes of rickets depends on the underlying disorder.

## Rickettsia

A type of parasitic microorganism. Rickettsiae resemble small bacteria, but they are able to multiply only by invading the cells of another life form; in this respect they are more like viruses.

Rickettsiae are primarily parasites of the arthropods (insects and insectlike animals), such as lice, fleas, ticks, and mites. However, these arthropods can transmit rickettsiae to larger animals (such as rodents, dogs, or humans) via the saliva of biting ticks or through their feces being deposited on the skin, with the rickettsiae passing to the blood via a small skin break.

Human diseases caused by different types of rickettsiae include *Rocky Mountain spotted fever*, *Q fever*, and the various forms of *typhus*.

## Rifampin

An *antibacterial drug* used in the treatment of *tuberculosis*. Rifampin is also used to treat *leprosy*, *endocarditis*, and *osteomyelitis*. It is also used to treat certain asymptomatic people who are *meningitis* bacteria carriers.

The drug is usually prescribed with other antibacterial drugs because some strains of bacteria quickly develop *resistance* to rifampin alone.

Rifampin causes harmless, orange-red discoloration of the urine, saliva, and other body secretions. Other side effects include muscle pain, nausea, vomiting, diarrhea, jaundice, flulike symptoms, rash, and itching.

## Rigidity

Increased tone in one or more muscles, causing them to feel tight; the affected part of the body becomes

R

stiff and inflexible. Causes of rigidity include injury to a muscle, arthritis affecting a nearby joint, a neurological disorder, such as Parkinson's disease or stroke, or the tightening of an abdominal muscle overlying an area of inflamed peritoneum (see *Peritonitis*). See also *Spasticity*.

## Rigor
Popularly called a chill, a violent attack of shivering, often associated with a fever. Rigor may also refer to stiffness or rigidity of body tissues, as in *rigor mortis*.

## Rigor mortis
The stiffening of muscles that occurs after death. It starts some three to four hours after death and is usually complete after about 12 hours; however, stiffness gradually disappears over the next 48 to 60 hours. The greater the amount of physical exertion before death, the sooner rigor mortis begins. Similarly, the sooner rigor mortis begins, the sooner it passes. These facts have important medicolegal implications and, along with other factors, are used to assess the time of death.

## Ringing in the ears
See *Tinnitus*.

## Ringworm
A popular name for fungal skin infections (commonly of the feet, groin, scalp, nails, or trunk). Ringworm is marked by ring-shaped, reddened, scaly, or blistery patches. (See *Tinea*.)

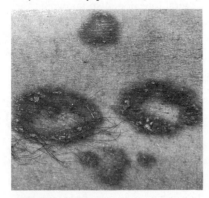

**Patch of ringworm**
The name arises from the tendency for certain skin fungus infections to spread uniformly outward, leaving normal skin inside the ring.

## Ritodrine
A drug used to prevent or delay premature labor (see *Prematurity*) by relaxing the muscles of the uterus.

Ritodrine causes an increased heart rate if given intravenously. Other side effects include tremor, palpitations, nausea, vomiting, chest pain, breathlessness, and nightmares.

## River blindness
See *Onchocerciasis*.

## RNA
 Ribonucleic acid, one of the two types of chemicals that carry the inherited, coded instructions within a cell for the cell's activities, or that assist in the decoding of these instructions; the other type is deoxyribonucleic acid (*DNA*). In all animal and plant cells, it is DNA that holds a permanent record of the instructions; RNA helps decode the instructions. In some viruses, the instructions for viral multiplication are held by RNA. (See also *Nucleic acids*; *Protein synthesis*.)

## Rocky Mountain spotted fever
 A rare, infectious disease caused by a rickettsia (a microorganism similar to a bacterium) and transmitted from rabbits and other small mammals by the bites of ticks. The disease occurs most commonly on the Atlantic seaboard (it was initially recognized in the Rocky Mountain states). Its incidence has risen steadily since 1980, and there are now more than 1,000 cases of Rocky Mountain spotted fever reported annually.

### SYMPTOMS AND SIGNS
About a week after the tick bite, mild fever, loss of appetite, and slight headache may develop gradually. However, sometimes symptoms (e.g., high fever, prostration, aching, tender muscles, severe headache, nausea, and vomiting) come on suddenly and are severe. Two to six days after the onset of symptoms, small pink spots appear on the wrists and ankles. The spots then spread over the body and darken, enlarge, and bleed.

The illness usually subsides after about two weeks; in untreated cases marked by extremely high fever, death may occur from pneumonia or heart failure.

### DIAGNOSIS AND TREATMENT
Diagnosis may be difficult because, initially, Rocky Mountain spotted fever resembles several other infections. Laboratory tests on blood and tissue samples can confirm the diagnosis. Treatment with the antibiotic drugs chloramphenicol or tetracycline usually cures the disease.

### PREVENTION
People living in tick-infested areas should use an insect repellent, examine the body daily for the presence of ticks, and gently pull away with forceps any ticks that are found.

## Roentgenography
See *X rays*; *Radiology*.

## Role-playing
The acting out of a role (the pattern of behavior expected of an individual in a given social situation). The conscious adoption of different roles is a useful technique for learning about oneself, other people, or particular situations.

The phrase "sick role" describes the type of passive behavior expected and allowed of a patient; people who have social or emotional problems may unconsciously adopt this role as a means of escaping from social obligations and of gaining the sympathy and understanding of others.

## Root-canal treatment
A dental procedure performed to save a tooth in which the pulp (the living tissue within a tooth) has died or become untreatably diseased, usually as the result of extensive *caries*.

### HOW IT IS DONE
The main steps in root-canal treatment are shown in the diagrams on the overleaf. X rays are taken to establish the length of the pulp cavity. A local anesthetic may be given. The tooth is isolated from the saliva with a *rubber dam* (a small sheet of rubber) to prevent infection. A hole is drilled in the crown of the tooth, the pulp is removed, and the crown is then sealed with a temporary filling.

About one week later the dentist removes the filling to ensure that the cavity is free of infection; if it is not, an antibiotic paste is applied and the tooth is resealed. When no infection can be detected, the cavity is filled and the chamber is sealed.

### COMPLICATIONS
If the pulp cavity has not been filled completely, bacteria may enter, leading to apical *periodontitis* (inflammation of the tissues around the root tips). It may then be necessary to make an opening in the gum and bone overlying the affected root to allow pus to drain. In some cases, a small portion of the root tip may be removed and the area filled with amalgam.

### RESULTS
Teeth whose pulp cavities have been filled may function well for as long as normal teeth. However, the teeth

R

## ROOT-CANAL TREATMENT

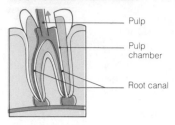

- Pulp
- Pulp chamber
- Root canal

**1** A hole is drilled into the crown so that all infected material can be removed from the pulp chamber. The root canals are then slightly enlarged and shaped with long, fine-tipped instruments.

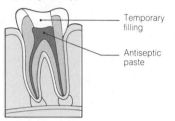

- Temporary filling
- Antiseptic paste

**2** Antibiotic paste is packed into the cavity and a temporary filling fitted. After a week or so, the filling is removed and the canals are checked for sterility.

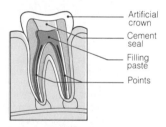

- Artificial crown
- Cement seal
- Filling paste
- Points

**3** The canals are filled with filling paste and/or tapering solid "points" made of gutta-percha resin mixed with zinc and bismuth oxides. The roots are then sealed with a cement and an artificial crown is fitted.

sometimes turn slightly gray; if this is unsightly, bleaching, a crown, or a facing can restore the appearance.

## Rorschach test

A test in which the subject reveals his or her attitude, conflicts, and emotions by responding to a set of inkblot pictures. The inkblot pictures are standardized, but of such a nature that the individual tends to project his or her unconscious attitude. The inkblot test was devised by the Swiss psychiatrist Hermann Rorschach early this century. (See also *Personality tests*.)

## Rosacea

A chronic skin disorder in which the nose and cheeks are abnormally red.

The exact cause of rosacea is unknown, but sometimes it is caused by overuse of *corticosteroid* creams in the treatment of other skin disorders. The condition affects about one in 500 people and is most common among middle-aged women.

Rosacea usually begins with temporary flushing, often after drinking a hot beverage or alcohol, eating spicy food, or entering a hot environment. It may then develop into permanent redness of the skin, sometimes accompanied by pustules resembling those of *acne*. In some elderly men, the condition leads to *rhinophyma* (bulbous swelling of the nose).

### TREATMENT

A lengthy course of the *antibiotic drug* tetracycline usually suppresses rosacea but it does not cure it. Rosacea may recur over a period of five to 10 years, after which the condition usually disappears on its own.

## Roseola infantum

A common infectious disease that primarily affects children aged 6 months to 2 years. Roseola infantum is probably caused by a virus and is characterized by the abrupt onset of irritability and a fever. The temperature may rise as high as 105°F (40.5°C). However, on the fourth or fifth day, it drops suddenly back to normal. At about the same time, a rash appears on the trunk, often spreading quickly to the neck, face, and limbs. The rash rarely lasts longer than a day or two. Other symptoms may include a sore throat and enlargement of lymph nodes in the head and neck.

Occasionally, a child may have a febrile *seizure* during the course of the fever, but the illness has no serious results or complications. There is no specific treatment other than to keep the child cool and give acetaminophen to reduce the fever.

## Rotator cuff

A reinforcing structure around the shoulder joint composed of four muscle tendons that merge with the fibrous capsule enclosing the joint.

The rotator cuff may be torn as the result of a fall. A partial tear may cause *painful arc syndrome* (pain when the arm is lifted in a certain arc away from the body). A complete tear seriously limits the ability to raise the arm and, in cases of severe disability, may require surgical repair.

## Roughage

See *Fiber, dietary*.

## Roundworms

Also known as nematodes, a class of elongated, cylindrically shaped worms. A dozen or so types are the main parasites of humans (the accompanying table summarizes the main ones). In many cases, the adult worms inhabit the human intestines, usually without causing symptoms unless there is a large number of worms. Sometimes, passage of worm larvae through various parts of the body is the main cause of symptoms. Most infestations are treated relatively easily with *antihelmintic drugs*.

In temperate areas, such as the US, the only common type of roundworm disease is *pinworm infestation* (which mainly affects children). *Ascariasis*, *whipworm infestation*, and *trichinosis* are also fairly common, although they often cause no symptoms. *Toxocariasis* occasionally occurs. In tropical countries, roundworm diseases are much more common; they include those mentioned above and *hookworm infestation, strongyloidiasis, guinea worm disease*, and different types of *filariasis*.

## Rubber dam

A rubber sheet used to isolate one or more teeth during certain dental procedures. The dam acts as a barrier against saliva and prevents the inhalation of debris or small instruments. To fit a dam, the dentist punches small holes in the sheet for the teeth to protrude, and secures the sheet with clamps and a frame.

## Rubella

A viral infection, also known as German measles (although the similarities to measles are few). Rubella causes a trivial illness in children and a slightly more troublesome one in adults. It is serious only when it affects a woman in the early months of pregnancy, when there is a chance that the virus will infect the fetus, which can lead to any of a range of severe birth defects, known as rubella syndrome.

### CAUSES AND INCIDENCE

Apart from mother-to-baby transmission, the rubella virus is spread from person to person in airborne droplets. Symptoms develop after an incubation period of two to three weeks.

Once common worldwide, rubella is now much less prevalent in most developed countries as a result of vaccination programs. The aim in the US has been to eradicate the virus by compulsory vaccination of all children before school entry; the results are encouraging. By 1986 the incidence in the US had been reduced to 551 reported cases of rubella and only 14 cases of rubella syndrome.

**SYMPTOMS AND COMPLICATIONS**
The infection usually occurs between the ages of 6 and 12 and is almost invariably mild. A rash appears on the face, spreads to the trunk and limbs, persists for a few days, and then disappears. There may be a slight fever and enlargement of lymph nodes at the back of the neck. In some cases, the entire infection passes unnoticed. In adolescents and adults, there may be more marked symptoms, such as headache before the rash appears and a more pronounced fever. The virus may be transmitted to others from a few days before the symptoms appear until a day after they disappear. Polyarthritis (inflammation affecting several joints) is an occasional short-lived complication, starting shortly after the rash has faded.

**CONGENITAL INFECTION**
Rubella is a risk to the unborn baby only if the mother is infected during the first four months of pregnancy. The earlier in pregnancy infection occurs, the more likely the infant is to be affected, and the more serious the abnormalities tend to be. In very early pregnancy, miscarriage may occur. An affected infant may have one or many defects. The most common abnormalities, in order of frequency, are *deafness*, congenital *heart disease*, *mental retardation*, *cataract* and other eye disorders, *purpura*, *cerebral palsy*, and bone abnormalities. About 20 percent of affected babies die in early infancy. An affected infant continues to harbor the virus and may infect others via his or her urine, stools, and saliva for a year or more after birth.

**DIAGNOSIS AND TREATMENT**
Rubella is easily confused with other conditions such as rashes caused by other viruses, drugs, and *scarlet fever*. It can be positively diagnosed only by laboratory isolation of the virus from a throat swab or by tests to look for antibodies to the virus in the blood. There is no specific treatment for rubella. Acetaminophen can be given to reduce fever. Treatment of rubella syndrome is of the defects exhibited.

**PREVENTION**
Rubella vaccine is highly effective in providing long-lasting immunity to the disease; it is given to all babies (usually combined with measles and mumps vaccine) at about 15 months of age. Reactions to the vaccine are usually negligible. Rubella infection itself also provides immunity.

## DISEASES CAUSED BY ROUNDWORMS (NEMATODES)

| Disease | Adult length | Distribution | How acquired |
|---|---|---|---|
| Ascariasis (common roundworm) | 6–15 inches | Worldwide | By swallowing worm eggs that have contaminated food or fingers |
| Enterobiasis (pinworm) | 0.1–0.5 inches | Worldwide | By swallowing worm eggs that have contaminated fingers |
| Trichuriasis (whipworm) | 1–2 inches | Worldwide | By swallowing worm eggs that have contaminated food or fingers |
| Ancylostomiasis (hookworm) | 0.5 inches | Tropics | By penetration of skin of feet by worm larvae in soil |
| Strongyloidiasis | 0.1 inches | Tropics | By penetration of skin of feet by worm larvae in soil |
| Toxocariasis | A few inches | Worldwide | By swallowing worm eggs from dirt or dog feces |
| Trichinosis (pork worm) | 0.05 inches | Worldwide | By eating undercooked pork containing encysted worm larvae |
| Filariasis | 1–20 inches | Tropics | By mosquito and other insect bites |

Any female of childbearing age (or approaching it) who is unsure whether she has been immunized or has had rubella, should have her immune status checked. If she is not immune, vaccination is performed only if there is no chance that she is pregnant because of the risk of the vaccine causing rubella in the fetus.

A nonimmune pregnant woman must avoid contact with anyone who has rubella; if such contact occurs, she should immediately seek a physician's advice. Passive immunization with immune globulin may help prevent infection of the fetus.

## Rubeola
Another name for *measles*.

## Running injuries
Many of the millions of people who jog or run to keep fit sustain a variety of injuries as a result. Most running injuries can be prevented by taking simple precautions.

**TYPES**
Common injuries include *tendinitis* (inflammation of a tendon); *stress fracture* of the tibia (shin), the fibula (the other long bone in the lower leg), or a bone in the foot; plantar *fasciitis* (inflammation of tissue in the sole of the foot); and other *overuse injuries*.

Tearing of the hamstring muscles at the back of the thigh is common in sprinting. Long-distance runners are more likely to suffer back pain due to jarring of the spine, tibial *compartment syndrome* (painful cramp in the lower leg caused by muscle compression), or *shin splints* (pain along the inner edge of the tibia).

**PREVENTION**
Shoes should fit snugly to provide stability but should not cramp the foot; they require insoles to cushion the jarring force on legs and spine. Shoes should not be allowed to become worn, since this can cause abnormal positioning of the foot during running, leading to foot strain.

Before running, warm-up exercises should be performed to reduce the risk of injury. Beginners should run short distances at first, and experienced runners should keep their running within sensible bounds.

Running should be done in an upright posture, with the trunk, neck, and arms relaxed. Long periods of running uphill, downhill, or along the side of a slope should be avoided because they increase stress on the ankle and knee.

## Rupture
See *Hernia*.

# S

## Sac
A pouch, or baglike organ or body structure. The amniotic sac is the thin, membranous, fluid-filled bag that surrounds the fetus.

## Saccharin
An *artificial sweetener*.

## Sacralgia
Pain in the *sacrum* (the triangular spinal bone below the lumbar vertebrae) caused by pressure on a spinal nerve in this area. Sacralgia is usually the result of a *disk prolapse*. In rare cases, however, it may be due to *bone cancer*. (See also *Back pain*.)

## Sacralization
Fusion of the fifth (lowest) lumbar vertebra with the upper part of the *sacrum* (the triangular spinal bone below the lumbar vertebrae). Sacralization may occur as a birth anomaly, in which case it usually produces no symptoms and is discovered only when an X ray of the back is taken for some other reason. Sacralization may also be performed as a surgical procedure to treat a *disk prolapse* or *spondylolisthesis*, in which a vertebra is displaced over the one below it. (See also *Spinal fusion*.)

## Sacroiliac joint
One of a pair of rigid joints between each side of the *sacrum* (the triangular spinal bone below the lumbar vertebrae) and each ilium (the largest of the bones that form the outer walls of the *pelvis*). The bony surfaces within the joint are lined with cartilage and have a small amount of synovial fluid (see *Synovium*) between them. Strong ligaments between the sacrum and ilium permit only minimal movement at the joint.
### DISORDERS
The sacroiliac joint may be strained (usually as a result of childbirth or overstriding when running), producing pain in the lower back and buttocks. It may also become inflamed, a condition called *sacroiliitis*.

## Sacroiliitis
Inflammation of the *sacroiliac joint* (one of a pair of joints between each side of the sacrum and each ilium). Sacroiliitis can be caused by *ankylosing spondylitis*, *rheumatoid arthritis*, or, in rare cases, by an infection that has spread through the bloodstream from elsewhere in the body.

The principal symptom is pain in the lower back, buttocks, groin, and back of the thigh. The pain may be accompanied by fever and malaise if the underlying cause is an infection. If the cause is ankylosing spondylitis, pain may be accompanied by stiffness in the back and hips that is worse after rest and alleviated by exercise.

Sacroiliitis is diagnosed by X rays and blood tests. If infection is suspected, fluid may be removed from the joint and checked for microorganisms. Treatment is with *nonsteroidal anti-inflammatory drugs* or, if the joint is infected, *antibiotic drugs*.

## Sacrum
The large triangular bone in the lower spine. Its broad upper part articulates with the fifth (lowest) lumbar vertebra, and its narrow lower part with the *coccyx* (tailbone). The sides of the sacrum are connected by *sacroiliac joints* to the iliums (the largest of the bones that form the *pelvis*). Thus, the sacrum sits like a wedge in the center of the back of the pelvis.

---

### STRUCTURE OF THE SACROILIAC JOINT
The joint forms an interface between the sacrum at the back of the pelvis and the ilium (hip bone) on each side of the body.

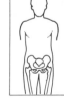

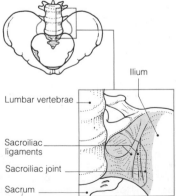

Ilium

Lumbar vertebrae

Sacroiliac ligaments

Sacroiliac joint

Sacrum

---

### STRUCTURE OF THE SACRUM
The sacrum consists of five vertebrae (spinal bones) that are fused together to form a single solid structure.

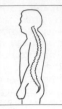

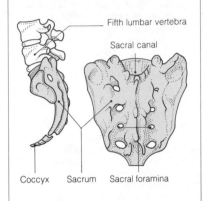

Fifth lumbar vertebra

Sacral canal

Coccyx    Sacrum    Sacral foramina

---

The sacrum is a strong bone and is rarely fractured. If a fracture does occur, it is usually a result of a fall or of a powerful direct blow to the bone. Other disorders include *sacralgia* (pain in the sacrum, sometimes due to a *disk prolapse*); *spondylolisthesis*, in which the fifth lumbar vertebra slips over the sacrum; and a birth anomaly in which the sacrum is fused to the fifth lumbar vertebra (see *Sacralization*). See also *Bone* disorders box; *Spine* disorders box.

## Sadism
A love of cruelty and inflicting pain on other people. The term is derived from the name of the French novelist the Marquis de Sade.

Sadism often refers specifically to the achievement of orgasm through hurting, humiliating, or torturing one's partner or other victim. It is more common in men and often accompanied by *masochism* (a desire to be abused). Sadistic activities include beating, whipping, and bondage, usually accompanied by verbal abuse. Sadists rarely inflict serious physical damage (the genuinely sadistic murderer is rare) but *rape* often has a sadistic basis. Only in rare cases do sadists seek help from a psychiatrist. (See also *Sadomasochism*.)

## Sadomasochism
Sexual arousal caused by inflicting pain or punishment (*sadism*) or by receiving abuse (*masochism*). Sadism

and masochism may be combined in a person, although one trait usually predominates. The sadomasochist is generally male and may practice other sexual *deviations*, such as *fetishism*.

Researchers have found sadomasochistic literature to be a common form of pornography. The practice may be more widespread than is generally known; biting is a common sex practice. In a broad sense, any relationship in which there is one very dominant and one submissive partner can be said to have sadomasochistic elements.

## SADS
Seasonal affective disorder syndrome, an incompletely studied and proved phenomenon in which mood changes are alleged to occur with the seasons.

## Safe period
See *Contraception, periodic abstinence.*

## "Safe" sex
A term used to describe preventive measures taken to reduce the risk of acquiring a sexually transmitted disease. "Safe" sex has been publicized recently because of the spread of *AIDS*, but the same principles apply to prevention of other sexually transmitted diseases, such as *hepatitis B, herpes,* and *gonorrhea.*

Sexual intercourse is completely safe only if you and your partner are monogamous (have not had sex with anyone else) and did not receive a blood product infusion before 1985, when blood products began to be tested for the AIDS virus. To reduce the risk of acquiring AIDS, casual sex and sex with multiple partners should be avoided. People with a higher risk of carrying AIDS include intravenous drug abusers, bisexual and homosexual men, prostitutes, promiscuous men or women, hemophiliacs and their partners, and people from areas where there is a very high incidence of AIDS (e.g., Central Africa and Haiti).

Antibody testing to show whether a person has been exposed to the AIDS virus is being used by dating organizations. Members are issued a "safe sex card" if their test results are negative; they are retested every six months. This procedure provides no guarantee against contracting AIDS. It can take six months to produce antibodies after exposure to the virus.

Known methods of transmitting the AIDS virus include vaginal intercourse, anal intercourse, oral sex, sharing sex aids such as vibrators, and any sexual activity that causes bleeding in the vagina or anus. Any sexual practice that involves contact with urine or feces also poses a risk. Sex during menstruation is particularly dangerous if the woman is a carrier. "Dry kissing," cuddling, caressing, massage, or mutual masturbation (providing there is no broken skin or ejaculation of semen near the vagina) are not believed to transmit the virus.

To reduce the risk of acquiring AIDS or any other sexually transmitted disease, a condom should be worn. If a condom fails to prevent transmission, the cause is most likely to be incorrect use or a torn condom (especially during anal intercourse).

## Salicylic acid
A *keratolytic drug* used in the treatment of skin disorders, including *dermatitis, eczema, psoriasis, ichthyosis, acne, warts,* and callosities (see *Callus, skin*). Salicylic acid is sometimes used to treat fungal infections.

Salicylic acid may cause inflammation and skin *ulcers* if used over a long period or applied to a large area.

## Saline
Salty, or consisting of or containing salt (sodium chloride). The term is also used to refer to a solution of salt, particularly one that has the same concentration as body fluids (known as physiological, or normal, saline). This solution, found in tears, is a component of contact lens solution.

Physiological saline may be given in large amounts (by injection or infusion into a vein) to replace body fluids in cases of dehydration. It is sometimes used in small quantities to dissolve drugs for injection.

## Saliva
The watery, slightly alkaline fluid secreted into the mouth by the *salivary glands* and the mucous membranes that line the mouth. Saliva contains the digestive enzyme amylase, which helps break down carbohydrates (see *Digestive system*). It also keeps the mouth moist, lubricates food to aid swallowing, and makes it possible to taste food (taste buds are stimulated only by dissolved substances). In addition to amylase, saliva contains chemicals, such as sodium, potassium, calcium, and chloride; pro-

## HOW TO USE A CONDOM
Using a condom is not a guarantee against transmission of HIV (the AIDS virus) or other sexually transmitted disease, but it does reduce the risks. Whether a condom is used to prevent disease transmission or to prevent conception, it should be used in conjunction with a spermicide preparation.

S

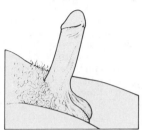

**1** The penis should be fully erect before the condom is put on. The condom should be in place before any vaginal or anal penetration by the penis and before oral sex.

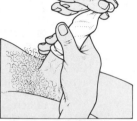

**2** Use a brand of condom that has been approved by a regulatory authority. Do not use a condom that has no teat, is time-expired, or appears defective.

**3** The teat-end should be squeezed free of air and the condom unrolled fully over the penis. Do not stretch the condom tightly; a tight condom is more likely to burst.

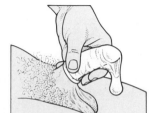

**4** The penis should be withdrawn soon after ejaculation. During withdrawal, the base of the condom should be held to prevent spilling the semen.

teins; mucin (the principal constituent of mucus); urea; white blood cells; and debris from the lining of the mouth.

## Salivary glands

Three pairs of glands that secrete *saliva*, via ducts, into the mouth. The largest pair, the *parotid glands*, lies over the angle of the jaw, just below and in front of the ears; the ducts of these glands run forward and inward to open inside the cheeks.

The sublingual glands are situated in the floor of the front of the mouth, where they form a low ridge on each side of the frenulum (the central band of tissue that attaches the underside of the tongue to the floor of the mouth). This ridge has a row of small openings through which saliva is secreted.

The submandibular glands lie toward the back of the mouth close to the sides of the jaw. Their ducts run forward to open under the tongue on two small swellings, one on either side of the frenulum.

### DISORDERS

Among the most common salivary gland disorders is infection of the parotid glands with the *mumps* virus. Another principal disorder is the formation of *calculi* (stones) in a duct or within the substance of a gland. A stone in a duct causes a swelling that enlarges during eating because of damming of the saliva flow; it may

also be painful. Surgical removal of a stone in a duct is straightforward, but a stone in a gland itself may necessitate removal of the entire gland.

Occasionally, the parotid glands are affected by *sarcoidosis*, which may cause considerable swelling. In rare cases, sarcoidosis also affects the facial nerve, which may result in *facial palsy*.

If oral hygiene is poor, the salivary glands may become infected by bacteria spreading from the mouth, which can lead to the development of an abscess in the affected glands.

Tumors of the salivary glands are rare, except for a type of parotid tumor that is usually slow-growing, painless, and benign (but which occasionally becomes malignant).

Insufficient secretion of saliva, causing a dry mouth (see *Mouth, dry*), may result from *dehydration* or *Sjögren's syndrome*. Certain drugs also decrease salivation as a side effect. (See also *Salivation, excessive*.)

## Salivation, excessive

The production of too much saliva occurs in numerous disorders, including mouth irritation caused by jagged teeth or dental *caries*, *toothache*, *gingivitis* (inflammation of the gums), *mouth ulcers*, any painful mouth injury, and *esophagitis* (inflammation of the esophagus).

A variety of conditions that affect the nervous system can also cause excessive salivation, among them *Parkinson's disease*, *rabies*, *mercury poisoning*, and overactivity of the parasympathetic division of the *autonomic nervous system* (which controls the salivary glands), usually due to disease or drugs.

## Salmonella

An important group of bacteria. One type of salmonella causes *typhoid fever*; others are a common cause of bacterial *food poisoning*.

## Salpingectomy

Surgical removal of one or both *fallopian tubes*. Salpingectomy may be performed if the tube has become infected (see *Salpingitis*), as a method of contraception (see *Sterilization, female*), or to treat an *ectopic pregnancy*. (See also *Salpingo-oophorectomy*.)

## Salpingitis

Inflammation of a *fallopian tube* (the tube that runs from the ovary to the top of the uterus), commonly caused by infection spreading upward from the vagina, cervix, or uterus.

### CAUSES AND INCIDENCE

Salpingitis may be a result of a *chlamydial infection* or a bacterial infection, especially *gonorrhea*. Although salpingitis usually results from a sexually transmitted disease, it may also follow childbirth, miscarriage, or elective abortion. Other causes include *peritonitis* (inflammation of the abdominal lining), or, rarely, a blood-borne infection, such as tuberculosis.

### SYMPTOMS AND SIGNS

Symptoms and signs include severe abdominal pain, fever, and frequent urination. The abdomen is very tender and the sufferer is usually most comfortable lying on her back with her legs bent at the knee. Vaginal examination is painful.

### DIAGNOSIS

The presence of infection may be confirmed by a blood test showing a high number of white blood cells. A culture of a swab sample of the vaginal discharge allows identification of the causative microorganism. *Laparoscopy* (examination of the inside of the abdominal cavity with a viewing tube) may be performed to confirm the diagnosis and to exclude the possibility of ectopic pregnancy or appendicitis, which can cause similar symptoms.

### COMPLICATIONS

Pus may collect within the fallopian tube itself (pyosalpinx), sometimes followed by fluid collection within the tube (hydrosalpinx). Pus collection within the abdominal cavity causes a pelvic abscess. Occasionally, the infection persists despite treatment and causes a variety of symptoms, such as persistent back pain that is worse before menstruation, frequent heavy periods, and pain during intercourse. If the infection damages the inside of the tubes, eggs may be unable to pass the blockage, resulting in *infertility* or an increased risk of *ectopic pregnancy*.

### TREATMENT

Treatment includes bed rest, fluids, *analgesics* (painkillers), and *antibiotic drugs*. Surgery is performed to drain a pyosalpinx, hydrosalpinx, or pelvic abscess. If infection persists despite antibiotics, the damaged tubes may be removed, sometimes with the uterus and most of the ovary. (See also *Salpingectomy*; *Salpingo-oophorectomy*.)

## Salpingography

See *Hysterosalpingography*.

## Salpingo-oophorectomy

Removal of one or both *fallopian tubes* and *ovaries*. Salpingo-oophorectomy may be performed to treat persistent

S

---

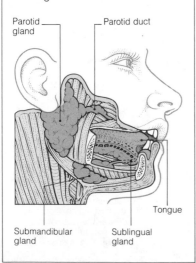

**ANATOMY OF THE SALIVARY GLANDS**

Each gland consists of thousands of saliva-secreting sacs. Tiny ducts carry the saliva into the main ducts leading to the mouth.

Parotid gland

Parotid duct

Tongue

Submandibular gland

Sublingual gland

*salpingitis* (inflammation of the fallopian tubes), cancer of the ovary (see *Ovary, cancer of*), cancer of the uterus (see *Uterus, cancer of*), or *choriocarcinoma* (a malignant tumor derived from placental tissue). The operation is often carried out with a *hysterectomy* (removal of the uterus and cervix).

Salpingo-oophorectomy is carried out using a general anesthetic. Removal of the fallopian tube or tubes is a brief, straightforward procedure and the short recovery period is usually problem-free.

## Salt

Any compound of an acid and a base. In general usage, the term usually refers specifically to one such compound—common table salt, known chemically as sodium chloride (see *Sodium*). The term salt may also be applied to a particular chemical salt or mixture of salts used medicinally (often as a purgative), as in magnesium sulfate and sodium sulfate. (See also *Saline*.)

## Salve

A term for a healing, soothing, often medicated, ointment.

## Sand-fly bites

Sand flies are tiny, delicate, long-legged flies that inhabit most warm parts of the world and, in some areas, transmit disease to humans via their bites. Sand flies are about one eighth of an inch (3 mm) long and can breed in a variety of habitats, including forests, sand, and city rubble.

In the US, sand flies are common in many areas, although they do not transmit disease. Elsewhere, diseases spread by these flies include various forms of *leishmaniasis* in tropical and subtropical regions and *bartonellosis* in the western Andes. Sand-fly fever is an influenzalike illness of short duration that is caused by a virus spread by the flies in parts of the Mediterranean and Asia.

Sand flies primarily bite after dusk. In areas where they are numerous, the best protection is to wear insect repellents and clothing that covers the arms and legs and is snug at the wrists and ankles (see *Insect bites*).

## Sanitary protection

Articles used to protect clothing from blood stains during *menstruation*. Disposable sanitary napkins or tampons are available in different absorbencies to meet individual needs.

## Sarcoidosis

A rare disease of unknown cause in which inflammation occurs in lymph nodes and other tissues throughout the body, usually the lungs, liver, skin, and eyes. The disorder occurs primarily in young adults.

### SYMPTOMS AND SIGNS

Acute sarcoidosis is associated with fever and generalized aches. It may also cause enlargement of lymph nodes in the neck and elsewhere, breathlessness, arthritis, or *erythema nodosum* (red-purple swellings on the legs). Chronic sarcoidosis can cause a variety of symptoms, including fever, a purple rash on the face, painful joints, a painful, bloodshot eye, and areas of numbness. Sometimes, the disease produces no symptoms.

Complications include scarring and thickening of the lung tissues (*fibrosis*) and *hypercalcemia* (an abnormally high calcium level in the blood), which may damage the kidneys.

### DIAGNOSIS AND TREATMENT

A diagnosis may be suggested from a chest X ray (which shows enlarged lymph nodes) and from the rash. A biopsy of the lung, skin, lymph gland, or liver confirms the diagnosis.

Many people with sarcoidosis are not seriously ill; the disease may resolve without treatment. About 90 percent of patients recover completely within two years, with or without treatment, but persistent, chronic disease develops in 10 percent.

*Corticosteroid drugs* are prescribed to treat persistent fever or persistent erythema nodosum, to prevent blindness in an affected eye, and to reduce the risk of permanent lung damage. *Chloroquine* is sometimes used to treat skin abnormalities.

## Sarcoma

A cancer of connective tissue (such as cartilage), blood vessels, or the fibrous tissue that surrounds and supports organs. Types of sarcoma include *osteosarcoma* and *chondrosarcoma* (both arising in bones), *Kaposi's sarcoma* (which mainly affects the skin and is common in people who have *AIDS*), and *fibrosarcoma*.

## Saturated fats

See *Fats and oils*.

## Scab

A crust that forms on the skin or on a mucous membrane at the site of a healing wound or infected area. A scab is composed of fibrin and serum that has leaked from the wound and

dried, along with skin scales, pus, and other debris. A similar term is eschar, used in connection with burns.

## Scabies

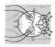

A skin infestation caused by the mite *SARCOPTES SCABIEI*, which burrows into the skin, where it lays eggs. Scabies is highly contagious. Hatched mites can pass from an infested individual to a person standing close beside him or her, although infestation is more likely through physical contact (such as sexual intercourse). The disorder is most common in infants, children, young adults, or in people who are institutionalized.

### SYMPTOMS

The openings of the mite's burrows can be seen on the skin as tiny, gray, scaly swellings, usually between the fingers, on the wrists and genitals, and in the armpits. Later, reddish lumps may appear on the limbs and the trunk. The infestation causes intense itching, particularly at night, and scratching results in the formation of scabs and sores.

### TREATMENT

The condition is treated by applying an insecticide lotion (such as *lindane*) to all skin below the sufferer's head. The lotion usually kills the mites, but itching may persist for up to two weeks. All members of the affected person's household (even if they show no signs of infestation) should be treated simultaneously.

## Scald

To burn with hot liquid or steam (see *Burns*).

## Scaling, dental

Removal of *calculus* (a hard, chalky deposit) from the teeth, performed to prevent or treat *periodontal disease* (disorders of the gums and other tissues supporting the teeth).

Scaling is carried out with an instrument called a scaler. It may have a sharp, scraping edge or be an ultrasonic model with a tip that vibrates at high speed to chip away the deposit. After scaling, the teeth are usually polished with a mild abrasive paste and motorized buffers.

## Scalp

The region of the skin and underlying tissue layers of the head that is normally covered with hair. Scalp skin differs from other areas of skin because it is tougher and it is attached to an underlying sheet of muscle

S

(called the epicranius) that extends from the eyebrows, over the top of the head, and to the nape of the neck. This muscle is only loosely attached (by connective tissue) to the skull, making it comparatively easy for areas of scalp to be torn off (e.g., as a result of catching the hair in machinery). Because the scalp is richly supplied with blood vessels, wounds bleed profusely.

The scalp may be affected by a variety of hair or skin disorders. The most common are *dandruff*; hair loss, particularly in men (see *Alopecia*); *sebaceous cysts*; *psoriasis*; fungal infections, such as ringworm (see *Tinea*); and parasitic infestations such as *lice*. *Cradle cap*, a harmless form of seborrheic *dermatitis* in which greasy, crusty patches appear on the scalp, is common in infants.

## Scalpel

A surgical knife for cutting tissue. Scalpels with steel blades are used for most operations, but in some cases (e.g., eye surgery) sharper diamond or ruby blades are used.

## Scanning techniques

Images of the body organs can be produced by a variety of scanning techniques that record, process, and (depending on the technique) analyze the sound waves, radio waves, or X rays that pass through or are generated by body tissues.

The scanning technique used most widely in medicine is *ultrasound*, in which inaudible, ultrahigh frequency sound waves are passed into the region being examined. These sound waves are reflected more strongly by some structures than others, and the pattern of reflections is detected by one or more transducers and displayed on a screen. Ultrasound was originally developed by the military for the detection of submarines beneath the sea. However, in the past 20 years, it has been refined and developed for the examination of a fetus and also the heart, liver, kidney, and other organs.

*CT scanning* uses X rays to measure variations in the density of the organ being examined; it compiles an image or picture by computer analysis.

*Radionuclide scanning* involves the injection into the body of radioactive substances that are taken up in different amounts by different organs. Radioactive iodine, for example, becomes concentrated in the thyroid gland. A radioactivity detector, such as a gamma camera, is positioned near the organ under study, and the pattern of radiation being emitted is recorded and displayed on a screen.

*MRI* (magnetic resonance imaging) uses a powerful electromagnet to align the nuclei of atoms of hydrogen, phosphorus, or other elements in the body. The nuclei are then knocked out of position by radio waves; in realigning themselves with the magnetic field, they produce a radio signal that can be detected and transformed into a computer-generated image. (See also *PET scanning*.)

## Scaphoid

One of the wrist bones. The scaphoid is the outermost bone on the thumb side of the hand in the proximal row of carpals (the row of wrist bones nearest the elbow).

A fracture of the scaphoid is one of the most common wrist injuries, usually occurring as a result of a fall on an outstretched hand. A characteristic symptom of this injury is tenderness in the space between the two prominent tendons at the base of the thumb on the back of the hand. This symptom may be a more positive indication of a scaphoid fracture than an X ray. Treatment consists of immobilizing the wrist in a cast.

An undiagnosed, untreated scaphoid fracture may not heal, which can lead to *osteoarthritis* or, in some cases, necrosis (death) of part of the bone. These complications may result in persistent pain in the wrist and restriction of its movement.

## Scapula

The anatomical name for the shoulder blade. The scapula is a flat, triangular bone situated over the back of the upper ribs. On its rear surface is a prominent spine (which can be felt under the skin) that runs diagonally upward and outward to a bony prominence (called the acromion) at the shoulder tip. The acromion articulates with the end of the *clavicle* (collarbone) to form the *acromioclavicular joint*. Just below the acromion is a socket (called the glenoid cavity) into which the head of the humerus (upper arm bone) fits to form the shoulder joint.

The scapula serves as an attachment for certain muscles and tendons of the arm, neck, chest, and back, and is involved with movements of the arm and shoulder.

Because the scapula is well padded with muscle, great force is required to fracture it. Treatment of a fracture consists of putting the shoulder in a *sling*

until the fracture has healed. *Physical therapy* may be needed to restore movement to the joint.

## Scar

Any mark left on damaged tissue after it has healed. Scar tissue forms not only on the skin but on all internal wounds (e.g., after a muscle tear or where surgery has been performed).

The body repairs a wound, ulcer, or other lesion by increasing production of the tough, fibrous protein *collagen* at the site of the damage. The collagen helps form new connective tissue, which covers the area of the lesion. If the edges of an incision are brought together when healing takes place, the resultant scar is narrow and pale; if the edges are left apart, the scar is more extensive (see *Healing*).

### ABNORMAL SCAR FORMATION

A hypertrophic scar is a large, unsightly scar that may develop at the site of a wound that has become infected. Some people have a family tendency toward hypertrophic scars for no apparent reason.

A *keloid* is a large, irregularly shaped scar that continues to grow in size as the body continues to produce extra collagen after a wound has healed; this type of scar is more common in black than in white people.

*Adhesions* are areas of scar tissue that form between unconnected parts of internal organs; they are a potential complication of intestinal surgery.

## Scarlatina

Another name for *scarlet fever*.

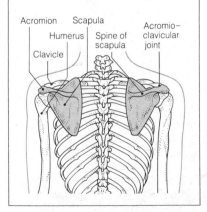

**LOCATION OF THE SCAPULAE**
The two scapulae are the prominent wing-shaped bones in the upper back. They facilitate many arm and shoulder actions.

Acromion   Scapula
Humerus   Spine of scapula   Acromio-clavicular joint
Clavicle

S

# Scarlet fever

An infectious disease of childhood that is caused by a strain of streptococcal bacteria. Characterized by a sore throat, fever, and rash, scarlet fever is far less common and dangerous than it once was.

### CAUSES AND SYMPTOMS

The bacteria are spread in droplets coughed or breathed into the air. After an incubation period of two to four days, a sore throat, headache, and fever develop in an infected child. A rash soon appears, caused by a toxin released by the bacteria. The rash begins as a mass of tiny red spots on the neck and upper trunk and spreads rapidly. The face is flushed (except for an area around the mouth) and a white coating with red spots may develop on the tongue. After a few days the coating peels to reveal a bright red appearance. Soon afterward, the fever subsides, the rash fades, and there is frequently some skin peeling, especially on the hands and feet.

As with other types of sore throat caused by streptococci (see *Strep throat*), there is a risk of *rheumatic fever* or *glomerulonephritis* (inflammation in the kidneys) if the infection is not treated promptly.

### DIAGNOSIS AND TREATMENT

The physician diagnoses scarlet fever from the symptoms and signs and, if necessary, by *culture* of the bacteria from a throat swab.

Treatment is with *antibiotic drugs*, usually penicillin (or erythromycin if the person has a penicillin allergy). Treatment usually leads to a rapid recovery. During the illness, the child should rest, drink plenty of fluids, and be given acetaminophen to relieve discomfort and reduce fever.

# Schistosome

 A type of fluke (flattened worm). Three types of schistosomes are parasites of humans, causing the disease *schistosomiasis* in tropical regions of the world.

# Schistosomiasis

A parasitic disease, also known as bilharziasis, that occurs in most tropical countries and afflicts over 200 million people worldwide.

### CAUSES AND INCIDENCE

The disease is caused by any of three species of flukes called schistosomes and is acquired from bathing in infested lakes and rivers in the tropics. Forms of schistosome (cercariae) penetrate the bather's skin and develop within the body into adult flukes (see life-cycle diagram at right). Eggs produced by the adult females provoke inflammatory reactions, which in turn may cause symptoms.

The infestation causes bleeding, ulceration, and *fibrosis* (scar tissue formation) in the bladder or intestinal walls; infestation may also cause inflammation and fibrosis in other organs, such as the liver.

### SYMPTOMS

Symptoms vary considerably. Some infested people have no symptoms, others become severely ill and suffer serious complications.

The first symptom is usually tingling and an itchy rash where the cercariae have penetrated the skin. Many weeks later, when the adults start producing eggs, an influenzalike illness may develop. Sometimes severe, the illness is marked by high fever, chills, aching, and pains. Subsequent symptoms may include blood in the urine or feces, abdominal or low back pain, and enlargement of the liver and/or spleen. Complications of long-term infestation may include liver *cirrhosis*, *bladder tumors*, and *renal failure*.

### DIAGNOSIS AND TREATMENT

The diagnosis is made from a special blood test for antibodies to the parasites (see *Immunoassay*) and from microscopic examination of a sample of urine or feces to detect eggs.

Since the early 1980s, treatment has been revolutionized by a new drug (praziquantel), a single dose of which kills the flukes and thus prevents, or limits, damage to internal organs.

### PREVENTION

Since no vaccine is available against the disease, visitors to areas where schistosomiasis is present (i.e., much of the tropics) should regard all lakes and rivers as unsafe for swimming.

Control of the disease rests on the provision of latrines and their regular use by the population. The Chinese claim to have achieved some success through measures directed against snails and through imposing strict sanitary regulations.

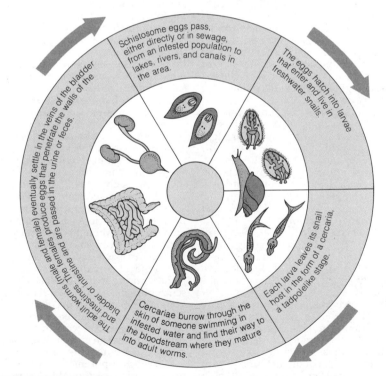

Schistosome eggs pass, either directly or in sewage, from an infested population to lakes, rivers, and canals in the area.

The eggs hatch into larvae that enter and live in freshwater snails.

Each larva leaves its snail host in the form of a cercaria, a tadpolelike stage.

Cercariae burrow through the skin of someone swimming in infested water and find their way to the bloodstream where they mature into adult worms.

The adult worms (male and female) eventually settle in the veins of the bladder and intestines. The females produce eggs that penetrate the walls of the bladder or intestine and are passed in the urine or feces.

**Cycle of schistosomiasis**
The disease affects a large proportion of the population in some parts of the world, such as the Nile valley in Egypt. Many methods have been tried to break the cycle of the disease in affected areas, with varying success. Methods used have included strict sanitary regulations and measures to eradicate freshwater snails.

S

## Schizoid personality disorder

Inability to relate socially to other people. People with this trait, which is apparent from childhood, are often described as "loners" and have few, if any, friends. They are markedly eccentric, seem to lack warmth or concern for others, and may be vague and detached from day-to-day activities. Psychoanalysts believe the condition results from an impoverished mother-child relationship.

*Schizophrenia* develops in about 10 percent of people diagnosed as having a schizoid personality. However, not all schizophrenics initially have schizoid personalities.

Although the marital and employment prospects for schizoid people are severely impaired, some succeed in socially isolated occupations. (See also *Avoidant personality disorder*.)

## Schizophrenia

A general term for a group of psychotic illnesses characterized by disturbances in thinking, emotional reaction, and behavior. Schizophrenia is sometimes referred to as "split personality" because the sufferer's thoughts and feelings do not relate to each other in a logical fashion. However, the disorder should not be confused with *multiple personality*. Schizophrenia is a disabling illness with a prolonged course that almost always results in chronic ill health and some degree of personality change.

### PREVALENCE

Schizophrenia is the most common form of psychotic illness. It has an average lifetime prevalence throughout the world of just under 1 percent. Approximately 1.5 million US citizens are currently affected. For reasons that are not understood, the disorder is more common in certain geographic areas (e.g., Western Ireland and inner-city populations).

Onset is usually between the ages of 15 and 25, being, on average, five years later in women than in men; otherwise, males and females are equally affected.

### CAUSES

Inheritance has been shown to play a role in the development of schizophrenia. First-degree relatives (parents, children, or siblings) of schizophrenics have a 10 percent chance of the illness; more distant relatives have a lower risk. If both parents are schizophrenic, one in three of their children becomes ill, and, if schizophrenia develops in one identical twin, the other twin has

approximately a one in two chance of being affected. However, factors other than genetics must also play a part or the illness would inevitably develop in both twins.

Biological studies have shown that certain forms of brain damage (such as temporal lobe epilepsy, tumors, and encephalitis) tend to be related to schizophrenic symptoms. Brain imaging techniques, especially *CT scanning* and *PET scanning*, have revealed abnormalities of structure and function in the brains of schizophrenics. It has also been demonstrated that certain drugs, such as amphetamines, can cause a schizophrenic illness and that drugs blocking the action of the brain chemical dopamine often relieve schizophrenic symptoms.

It seems likely that schizophrenia is possibly worsened by stress in the individual's personal life.

### SYMPTOMS

Schizophrenia may begin insidiously, with the individual becoming slowly more withdrawn and introverted, and losing his or her drive and motivation. The change may not be noticed for months or years, until it becomes apparent that the individual is suffering from *delusions* (false ideas that do not respond to reasoned argument) or *hallucinations* (a sensory experience in the absence of an external stimulus). In other cases, the illness comes on more suddenly, usually in response to some external stress.

Delusions may take a variety of forms, ranging from single ideas, such as the belief that one is Jesus Christ or Napoleon, to elaborate delusional systems in which special significance is attached to everyday objects or events. In paranoid schizophrenia, the illness is dominated by delusions of grandeur, persecution, or jealousy.

Hallucinations frequently are experienced as voices that comment on behavior or thoughts, occasionally in the form of conversations in which the sufferer is referred to as he or she. This type of auditory third person hallucination occurs exclusively in schizophrenia. True visual hallucinations are rare in Western cultures, but distortions of visual perception do occur; faces or objects may look sharper or change shape. Bodily sensations, such as tingling, are common.

Most schizophrenics also suffer from a variety of thought disorders, which impair concentration or clear thinking. Sufferers describe their thoughts as being blocked, or inserted into or withdrawn, from their

minds by some outside force. They may also feel that their thoughts are being broadcast to others; in rare cases, the thoughts are experienced as echoes inside the head.

Disordered thinking is reflected in muddled and disjointed speech. Disturbance of association results in the schizophrenic jumping between subjects that are seemingly unrelated. Inability to think in abstractions often leads to bizarre responses to questions. For example, when a girl was asked why she was turning in a circle, she said she felt she was in a knot and was trying to unravel herself. In some cases, speech disintegrates, becoming a "word salad" of odd phrases, *neologisms* (made-up words), and detached syllables.

In a rare form of schizophrenia, catatonia may occur, in which sufferers adopt prolonged rigid postures or engage in outbursts of repeated movement.

Symptoms of *manic-depressive illness* may accompany schizophrenia, especially in the early stages. However, as the illness progresses, emotions usually become severely blunted, there is increasing detachment from other people, and there is a loss of interest in hobbies or occupations. Behavior becomes more eccentric and self-neglect is common.

### DIAGNOSIS

For a diagnosis of schizophrenia to be made by current US standards, the individual must have continuous signs of a profound break with reality and evidence of fragmentation (disorganization) of the personality for at least six months during some time in his or her life. This six-month period must include at least one phase when there are symptoms of hallucinations, delusions, or marked thought disorders.

### TREATMENT

The main form of treatment consists of *antipsychotic drugs* (such as chlorpromazine), some of which can be given as long-acting *depot injections*, which reduces the symptoms and makes the person more amenable to *psychotherapy*. Drug treatment is effective in suppressing the more obvious symptoms, such as hallucinations, but may result in side effects, particularly *dyskinesia* (abnormal muscular movements) and tremor.

Schizophrenics may be treated initially in the hospital; once the major symptoms are controlled, most return to the community. Adequate provision of day centers, decent housing,

S

and vocational opportunities can do much to further control symptoms, improve the sufferer's self-reliance, prevent relapse, and reduce the stigma attached to mental illness. If the patient is to live at home, the family needs to be provided with support and guidance, since some schizophrenics may be difficult to live with. A certain number relapse, especially if they do not take their medication regularly.

**OUTLOOK**

While some 10 percent of those in whom schizophrenia develops remain severely impaired for life, the majority can return to varying degrees of independence. About 30 percent return to normal lives and occupations.

The particular form of the illness is important in determining the outlook. Individuals who have schizophrenia combined with manic-depressive symptoms often recover fully, as do many with catatonia. Paranoid schizophrenics, because of the preservation of their personalities, are often able to function well, albeit as somewhat eccentric members of the community. Schizophrenia that comes on slowly, starting around puberty, often causes significant impairment.

Although drugs have improved the outlook for most schizophrenics, inadequate community care frequently results in relapse, neglect, vagrancy, or imprisonment.

## Schönlein-Henoch purpura

Inflammation of the blood vessels, causing leakage of blood into the skin, joints, kidneys, and intestine. The disease is most common among young children, especially boys, and often occurs after an infection such as a sore throat. The precise cause of Schönlein-Henoch purpura is unknown, although some experts believe it is due to an abnormal allergic reaction in response to an infection.

**SYMPTOMS**

The main symptom is a slightly raised, purplish rash on the buttocks and backs of the legs and arms. The joints are often painful, the hands and feet may be swollen, and the child may complain of colicky abdominal pain. Infrequently, bleeding from the intestine occurs, which gives rise to blood in the feces. The kidneys may become inflamed, resulting in *hematuria* (blood in the urine).

**DIAGNOSIS AND TREATMENT**

The condition must be distinguished from blood-clotting disorders by performing *blood-clotting tests*.

No specific treatment is required other than bed rest and mild *analgesics* (painkillers). Most children recover within a month, although complications may arise if *nephritis* (inflammation of the kidneys) persists. In severe cases, the physician may prescribe *corticosteroid drugs*.

## Sciatica

Pain that radiates along the *sciatic nerve*. The pain sometimes extends from the buttock down the leg to the foot, although usually only part of this area is affected (usually the buttock and thigh). In severe cases, the pain may be accompanied by numbness and/or weakness in the affected area.

**CAUSES**

The most common cause of sciatica is a prolapsed intervertebral disk pressing on a spinal root of the nerve (see *Disk prolapse*). Less commonly, it may be caused by pressure on the nerve from a tumor, abscess, or blood clot, or simply from sitting in an awkward position. Any disorder that involves nerves (such as certain infections, *diabetes mellitus*, or *alcohol dependence*) may affect the sciatic nerve and produce sciatica.

**TREATMENT**

Treatment is directed toward the underlying cause, but in many cases the cause is not identified. Thus, treatment consists of measures to relieve the pain, including taking *analgesics* (painkillers) and resting in bed. With such treatment, the pain usually disappears within a few days. In severe cases, the pain may persist for several weeks. Sciatica tends to recur.

## Sciatic nerve

The primary nerve of the leg and the largest nerve in the body. The sciatic nerve is a branch of the sacral plexus (nerve network) in the pelvis, and is formed from several lumbar and sacral *spinal nerves*. From the sacral plexus, the sciatic nerve passes below the sacroiliac joint (at the back of the pelvis, near the sacrum) and backward to the buttock, from where it passes behind the hip joint and runs down the back of the thigh. Above the back of the knee, the sciatic nerve divides into two main branches, called the tibial nerve and the common peroneal nerve.

The upper part of the sciatic nerve, above the point of division, supplies the hip joint, many of the thigh muscles, and the skin on the back of the thigh. The lower part—the tibial and peroneal nerves—supplies the

**LOCATION OF THE SCIATIC NERVE**
The diagram below shows the nerve in a cutaway of the right thigh and knee, as seen from behind.

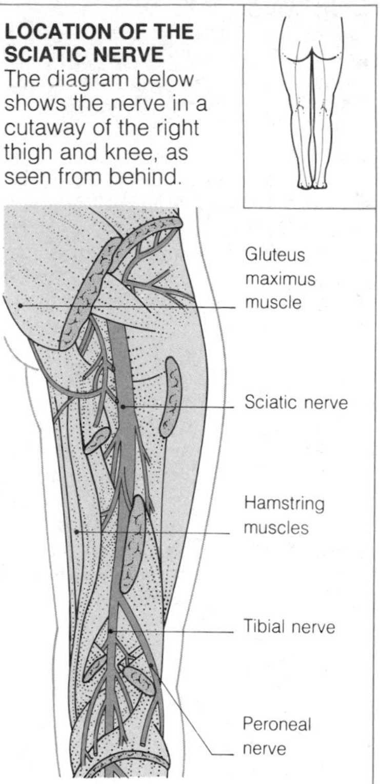

- Gluteus maximus muscle
- Sciatic nerve
- Hamstring muscles
- Tibial nerve
- Peroneal nerve

knee and ankle joints, all the muscles of the lower leg and foot, and most of the skin below the knee.

**DISORDERS**

Probably the most common disorder of the sciatic nerve is *sciatica*, which is often due to a prolapsed intervertebral disk pressing on a spinal root of the nerve (see *Disk prolapse*). The upper part of the nerve may also be damaged by dislocation of the hip joint, which, in severe cases, may result in paralysis of muscles below the knee and widespread numbness of the skin in that part of the body.

Damage to the peroneal nerve, often due to a fracture of the upper *fibula* (the outer bone of the lower leg), may produce *footdrop* and numbness of the skin at the side of the lower leg and back of the foot.

The tibial nerve is deeply buried in body tissues and thus is rarely injured. However, it is sometimes damaged by dislocation of the knee, which may cause paralysis of the lower leg and foot, and numbness in the sole of the foot.

## Scintigraphy

A less common, alternative name for *radionuclide scanning*.

**S**

## Scirrhous

A medical term meaning hard and fibrous. The word is usually applied to malignant tumors that have dense, fibrous tissue within them.

## Sclera

The white outer coat of the *eye*, visible through the transparent *conjunctiva*. The sclera is composed of dense, fibrous tissue formed from *collagen*, which is strong and protects the inner structures of the eye from injury. It may, however, be penetrated by sharp objects.

Disease of the sclera is uncommon, but *scleritis* (inflammation of the sclera) may occur, usually with a *collagen disease* such as *rheumatoid arthritis*. The healthy sclera sometimes shows a blue tinge from the underlying choroid. If the sclera is exceptionally thin, which occurs in *osteogenesis imperfecta*, this blue appearance is striking.

**LOCATION OF THE SCLERA**
The sclera is about one seventieth of an inch thick and continuous with the cornea at the front of the eye. It is extremely tough.

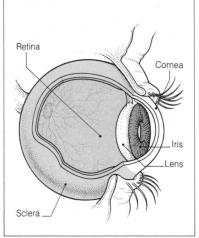

Retina
Cornea
Iris
Lens
Sclera

## Scleritis

Inflammation of the *sclera* (white of the eye). Scleritis usually accompanies a *collagen disease*, such as rheumatoid arthritis. It also occurs in *herpes zoster ophthalmicus*, and in Wegener's granulomatosis, when it may lead to areas of local thinning and possible perforation of the sclera.

Scleritis is persistent, but often responds well to *corticosteroid* eye drops. In severe cases, these drugs may increase the risk of perforation.

## Scleroderma

A rare condition, also known as systemic sclerosis, that can affect many organs and tissues in the body, particularly the skin, arteries, kidneys, lungs, heart, gastrointestinal tract, and joints. Scleroderma is an *autoimmune disorder* (in which the body's immune system attacks its own tissues). Scleroderma is twice as common in women and is most likely to appear between the ages of 40 and 60.

**SYMPTOMS AND SIGNS**

The number and the severity of symptoms varies dramatically. The most common symptom is *Raynaud's phenomenon*, a painful, three-color (white, red, blue) response of the hands and/or feet to cold exposure; it may be present for many years without any other symptoms.

Also common are changes in the skin (especially of the face and fingers), which becomes shiny (as if it had been waxed), tight, and thickened. There is often puckering around the mouth, giving the sufferer a characteristic masklike appearance. The pulled skin often leads to difficulty performing certain maneuvers, such as bending the fingers or opening the mouth.

In some people, other parts of the body are affected, leading to problems such as difficulty swallowing, shortness of breath, palpitations, high blood pressure, joint pain, stiffness, and muscle weakness. There are wide variations from person to person in the degree to which different parts of the body are involved and the rate at which the disease progresses. Progression is often rapid in the first few years and then slows down or even stops. In a small number of people, degeneration is rapid, usually leading to death from *heart failure*, *respiratory failure*, or *renal failure*.

**DIAGNOSIS AND TREATMENT**

A physical examination is usually sufficient to confirm the diagnosis, but a blood test and a skin *biopsy* (removal of tissue for microscopic examination) may be performed.

There is no cure for scleroderma, but treatment can relieve symptoms and associated problems. *Vasodilator drugs* and avoiding exposure to cold can relieve Raynaud's phenomenon. *Physical therapy* may be recommended for joint problems. *Antihypertensive drugs* may be given to treat high blood pressure and *dialysis* may be undertaken for renal failure. *Corticosteroid drugs* are sometimes prescribed if the muscle is involved.

## Scleromalacia

Softening of the *sclera* (the white portion of the eye). Scleromalacia is frequently a complication of *scleritis* (inflammation of the sclera), especially when the scleritis is caused by rheumatoid arthritis.

Scleromalacia perforans is a rare, severe form of the condition in which the entire thickness of sclera is involved; the underlying choroid bulges through and sometimes perforates the sclera.

## Sclerosis

A medical term for hardening of a body tissue. It is usually used to refer to hardening of blood vessels, as in *atherosclerosis* (hardening of arteries), or to hardening of nerve tissue due to deposition of abnormal connective tissue, which occurs in the later stages of *multiple sclerosis*.

## Sclerotherapy

A method of treating *varicose veins* (distended, tortuous veins), especially in the legs. *Hemorrhoids* (varicose veins in the anus) and *esophageal varices* (swollen veins at the bottom of the esophagus that may bleed) are sometimes treated this way.

The vein is injected with a strongly irritating solution (called a sclerosant). This causes inflammation in the lining of the vein, blocking it, and eventual fibrosis (scar tissue formation), which leads to the vein's obliteration. For a varicose vein in the leg, the process is assisted by first emptying the vein of blood. After injection, firm pressure is applied so that the walls of the vein are pressed together. Compression is maintained by tight bandaging.

## Scoliosis

A deformity in which the spine is bent to one side. The thoracic (chest) or lumbar (lower back) regions are the most commonly affected.

**TYPES AND CAUSES**

Scoliosis usually starts in childhood or adolescence and progressively becomes more marked until the age at which growth stops. In many such cases, another part of the spine curves toward the opposite side of the body to compensate for the scoliotic curvature, resulting in the spine becoming S-shaped. The cause of juvenile scoliosis is unknown; if the condition is not corrected, it may lead to severe deformity.

More rarely, scoliosis develops as a result of a congenital abnormality of the vertebrae, *poliomyelitis* that has

S

weakened the spinal muscles on one side of the body, or tilting of the pelvis due to one leg being shorter than the other. Occasionally, a spinal injury (such as a *disk prolapse* or ligament sprain) causes temporary scoliosis. In such cases, the spinal curvature appears suddenly and is accompanied by back pain and *sciatica*.

### DIAGNOSIS AND TREATMENT

Scoliosis is diagnosed by a physical examination of the spine, hips, and legs, along with X rays of the spine.

If the cause of the condition is known, treatment is directed toward that cause (e.g., bed rest for a disk prolapse or wearing an orthopedic shoe with a raised heel to correct a pelvic tilt due to unequal leg lengths).

Scoliosis of unknown cause may not require treatment if the curvature is slight. However, regular measurement of the spine is necessary to assess the progress of the condition. If it seems to be worsening—or if the curvature is already marked—it may be treated by immobilization of the spine in a hinged plaster jacket or adjustable metal brace, followed by surgery and bone grafting to fuse the affected spinal vertebrae in a straight line (see *Spinal fusion*). A steel rod with hooks or some other metal device may be used to keep the spine straight until the bones become fused.

## Scopolamine

An *antispasmodic drug* used to treat *irritable bowel syndrome*, nausea, and *motion sickness*. Scopolamine is also a *premedication* (drug given to prepare a person for surgery). Adverse effects may include drowsiness, dry mouth, and blurred vision.

## Scorpion stings

 Scorpions are eight-legged creatures with flexible tails ending in a poison reservoir and a sharp stinger. They are present in most warm regions of the world and are nocturnal, spending the day in dark crevices under rocks and in the loose bark of trees. Sometimes scorpions enter human habitation and crawl into shoes or clothing. If accidentally disturbed, a scorpion is likely to sting, which is achieved by arching its tail over its back.

Some highly venomous species are found in Mexico, North Africa, South America, parts of the Caribbean, and India. About 40 species exist in the US, but only one, found in southern states, is dangerous to humans.

### SYMPTOMS

The effects of many types of scorpion stings are little worse than a bee sting, with mild to moderate pain and tingling or burning at the site of the puncture wound. With more dangerous species, there may be sweating, restlessness, diarrhea, and vomiting (caused by stimulation of the *autonomic nervous system*) in addition to severe pain. The venom may also affect the rhythm and strength of the heart's contractions. Fatalities are uncommon in adults; young children and the elderly are at greater risk.

### TREATMENT

Any person stung by a scorpion should seek immediate medical attention. For children, or if there are symptoms other than pain, admission to the hospital is advisable.

If pain is the only symptom, mild *analgesics* (painkillers) and cold compresses may be all that is needed. In severe cases, local anesthetics and powerful painkillers may be required, and an *antivenin* to deactivate the venom may be given by intravenous infusion. Antivenins active against the venoms of local, dangerous types of scorpions are available in most parts of the world where such species exist.

### PREVENTION

In areas where scorpions are common, clothes and footwear should be shaken out before being put on. Scorpions can be discouraged from entering a house by barriers, such as a porch elevated at least 8 inches above the ground.

## Scotoma

An area of abnormal vision within the *visual field*.

## Screening

The testing of apparently healthy people with the aim of detecting disease at an early, treatable stage. The ideal screening test is reliable, with a low rate of false-positive results (the results of the test are positive even though the people tested do not in fact have the disease) and a low rate of false-negative results (the results of the test are negative even though the people tested have the disease). An ideal test is also inexpensive, simple, and acceptable to people, causing neither discomfort nor danger. For a screening test to be of practical use, people found to have the disease must benefit from early diagnosis.

Screening for unsuspected diabetes is of no use since there is no evidence that the late complications of the

disease are lessened by diagnosis before symptoms develop. (See also *Cancer screening*.)

## Scrofula

*Tuberculosis* of the lymph nodes in the neck, often those just beneath the angle of the jaw. Scrofula was once a common disorder, usually caused by the drinking of contaminated milk. Abscesses would form in the lymph nodes and, after bursting through the skin, leave scars on the neck.

Today scrofula is rare in developed countries. It occasionally develops in Asian or African immigrants in whom the infection has spread from tuberculosis elsewhere in the body. *Antibiotic drugs* clear up the condition in most cases.

## Scrotum

The pouch that hangs below the penis and contains the *testes*. The scrotum consists of an outer layer of thin, wrinkled skin over a layer of muscle-containing tissue.

Swelling of the scrotum may be caused by an inguinal *hernia*, a swelling of one of the testes, a *hydrocele* (a fluid-filled sac around one of the testes), or, in severe heart failure, *edema* (fluid retention).

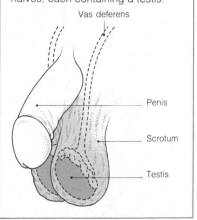

**LOCATION OF THE SCROTUM**
The scrotum has oil-secreting glands and thinly scattered hairs on its surface. Internally it is divided by a membrane into two halves, each containing a testis.

Vas deferens

Penis

Scrotum

Testis

## Scuba-diving medicine

A minor medical specialty concerned with the physiological hazards of underwater diving with self-contained underwater breathing apparatus (S.C.U.B.A.).

## THE MAIN HAZARDS

Most diving hazards stem from the increase in pressure with depth. At a depth of 33 feet (10 m), the total pressure is twice the surface pressure. At 99 feet (30 m), it is four times the surface pressure.

## MECHANICAL EFFECTS OF PRESSURE CHANGE

During descent, divers must introduce gas into their middle-ear cavities and facial sinuses to prevent damage as the pressure mounts. This mounting pressure is what airline passengers experience during descent and repressurization (see *Barotrauma*).

Whatever depth they attain, divers must be supplied with breathing mixtures at a pressure equal to the external water pressure. Thus, at 99 feet (30 m), a diver breathes gas at four times the surface pressure. During ascent, gas in the lungs expands and can rupture the lung tissues if the diver panics and inadvertently holds his or her breath—a serious condition known as pulmonary barotrauma (burst lung). Symptoms may include coughing up blood, inability to urinate, breathing difficulties, and unconsciousness.

## TOXIC EFFECTS OF GASES

Amateur divers breathe compressed air, which consists mainly of nitrogen and oxygen. These gases are harmless at surface pressures (oxygen is essential to life), but they become toxic at high pressure. Nitrogen impairs the nervous system when air is breathed at depths from about 80 feet (24 m) downward, causing slowed mental functioning and other symptoms that mimic alcohol intoxication (nitrogen narcosis). Oxygen becomes toxic when air is breathed at about 260 feet (80 m), when it can cause convulsions or lung damage.

To attain greater depths without risking nitrogen and oxygen poisoning, professional divers use gas mixtures other than air. A typical mixture consists of helium, with only small amounts of oxygen and nitrogen; the helium is relatively nontoxic.

## THE BENDS

At depth, divers accumulate in their tissues excess quantities of any inert gas they are breathing (nitrogen, if air is being breathed). If pressure is released too quickly (i.e., the diver ascends too fast) and if a large amount of gas has accumulated because the diver remained at depth for too long, this gas can no longer be held in the tissues and may form bubbles, causing *decompression sickness*.

## OTHER HAZARDS

Additional hazards include *hypothermia* (dangerous chilling) due to immersion in cold water, bites or stings from marine animals (see *Bites, animal; Venomous bites and stings*), and risk of *drowning*.

## ACCIDENT PREVENTION AND TREATMENT

Any person taking up scuba diving should first receive a medical checkup and undergo thorough training at a recognized diving school.

Pressure-related accidents, such as burst lung and decompression sickness, are treated by recompression of the diver in a special pressure chamber so that any bubbles or pockets of gas in the blood or tissues are reabsorbed. This is followed by slow release of the pressure.

Treatment of other accidents (such as hypothermia and near drowning) is as for nondivers.

## Scurvy

A disease caused by inadequate intake of *vitamin C*. Scurvy is rare today in developed countries as a result of increased consumption of fresh fruit and vegetables. Body stores of vitamin C give protection against scurvy for about three months.

## CAUSES AND SYMPTOMS

Inadequate supplies of vitamin C disturb the body's normal production of *collagen* (connective tissue). Collagen continues to be produced but it is unstable, causing weakness of small blood vessels and poor healing in wounds. Hemorrhages may occur anywhere in the body. They are most obvious in the skin, where they result in widespread bruising. Bleeding from the gums and loosening of the teeth are common; bleeding into muscles and joints also occurs in scurvy, causing pain.

Scurvy is especially serious in children because bleeding into the membranes surrounding the long bones may cause separation of the growing ends of the bones and interference with growth. Major, and sometimes fatal, hemorrhages into and around the brain can occur.

Scurvy is often associated with other vitamin deficiencies and *anemia* is common.

## PREVENTION AND TREATMENT

A modest intake of fruit (particularly citrus fruit) and vegetables provides the body with sufficient vitamin C to

---

## RECOMPRESSION CHAMBER FOR DIVING ACCIDENTS

Divers suffering from the bends or other pressure-related accidents are often treated in a recompression chamber. The patient is usually accompanied in the recompression chamber by a physician.

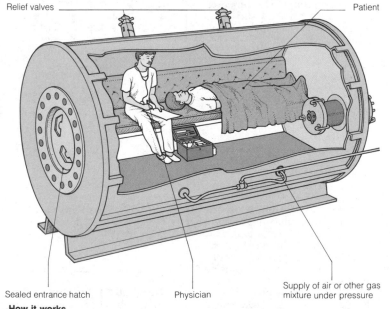

Relief valves

Patient

Sealed entrance hatch

Physician

Supply of air or other gas mixture under pressure

### How it works

A gas mixture (usually air) is pumped into the chamber. As pressure increases, bubbles (pockets of gas) in the diver's tissues are reabsorbed, and symptoms disappear. Once all symptoms have gone, the pressure is slowly released.

S

prevent scurvy. Other sources are milk, liver, kidneys, and fish.

Scurvy is treated with large doses of vitamin C. Bleeding stops in 24 hours, healing resumes, and muscle and bone pain quickly dissipate.

## Sealants, dental
Plastic materials applied to the chewing surfaces of the molars and premolars to help prevent decay. Back teeth have minute surface grooves in which food debris and bacteria can collect and cause decay (see *Caries, dental*). Sealing the teeth stops harmful material from getting into the grooves. Sealants are of the most benefit to children and should be applied as soon as possible after the permanent teeth have erupted.

Teeth to be sealed often require no drilling or anesthesia. The tooth surface may be acid-etched to roughen it so that the sealant will adhere better (see *Bonding, dental*). The semiliquid sealant is then applied and is usually hardened by directing a narrow beam of intense light at the treated tooth for a few seconds. Some sealants are premixed with a chemical activator that causes them to set.

## Seasickness
A type of *motion sickness*.

## Seasonal affective disorder syndrome
See *SADS*.

## Sebaceous cyst
A nonspecific term for a large, smooth nodule under the skin (also called a wen when it is on the scalp). The most common sites of sebaceous cysts are the scalp, face, ear, and genitals.

Although harmless, sebaceous cysts may grow very large and sometimes become infected by bacteria, in

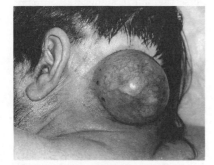

**Massive sebaceous cyst**
Cysts rarely grow as large as this one, located on the back of the neck. Cysts are harmless and easily removed surgically.

which case they are very painful. Large cysts or cysts that have been infected should be removed using local anesthetic. The physician makes a small incision in the skin and removes the cyst. If the entire cyst wall is removed, recurrence is rare.

## Sebaceous glands
Minute glands in the skin that secrete a lubricating substance called *sebum*. Sebaceous glands either open into hair follicles or discharge directly onto the surface of the skin. They are most numerous on the scalp, face, and anus; they do not occur on the palms of the hands or soles of the feet. The production of sebum by the sebaceous glands is partly controlled by *androgen hormones* (male sex hormones).

Disorders of the sebaceous glands may lead to *seborrhea*, seborrheic *dermatitis*, or *acne* vulgaris.

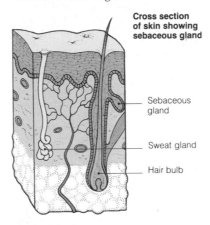

**Cross section of skin showing sebaceous gland**

Sebaceous gland

Sweat gland

Hair bulb

## Seborrhea
Excessive secretion of *sebum*, causing increased oiliness of the face and a greasy scalp. The exact cause is uncertain, although *androgen hormones* (male sex hormones) are known to play a part. The condition is most common in adolescent boys.

Seborrhea usually disappears by adulthood without treatment. However, people with seborrhea are more likely than the average to have other skin conditions, particularly seborrheic *dermatitis* and *acne* vulgaris.

## Seborrheic dermatitis
See *Dermatitis*.

## Sebum
The oily secretion produced by the *sebaceous glands* of the skin. Sebum is composed of fats and waxes; it lubricates the skin, keeps it supple, and protects it from becoming sodden

when immersed in water or cracked when exposed to a dry atmosphere. Sebum also protects the skin from invasion by bacteria and fungi.

Oversecretion causes a greasy skin, called *seborrhea*. It may lead to seborrheic *dermatitis* or *acne* vulgaris.

## Secobarbital
A *barbiturate drug* sometimes used as a *premedication* (drug given to prepare a person for surgery) because of its sedative effect. Secobarbital is seldom used today as a sleeping drug because of its short-lived action and the risk of *drug dependence*. Other possible adverse effects include daytime drowsiness, clumsiness, dizziness, confusion, and rash.

## Secondary
A term applied to a disease or disorder that results from or follows another disease (which is called the *primary* disease). For example, secondary *hypertension* (high blood pressure) occurs as a result of some underlying primary disorder, such as a hormonal or kidney disease. The term secondary is also used to refer to a *metastasis* (a malignant tumor that has spread from a primary cancer to affect another part of the body).

## Secretion
The manufacture and release by a cell, gland, or organ of chemical substances (such as *enzymes* or *hormones*) that are needed for metabolic processes elsewhere in the body. In contrast, *excretion* is the production and release of waste products. The term secretion is also used to refer to the secreted substances themselves.

The secretions of *exocrine glands* (e.g., the salivary glands) are carried away in ducts; the secretions of *endocrine glands* (e.g., the thyroid) are released directly into the bloodstream.

## Security object
A significant item, such as a special blanket, an old garment, or a favorite soft toy, that provides comfort and reassurance to a young child. In many cases, a child settles down to sleep more easily if his or her security object is near. Some children are unable to sleep without their security objects.

Sometimes referred to as transitional objects, these items represent to the child something partway between a person and a thing. The child may become deeply attached to the object and may become highly distressed if an attempt is made to remove it.

Security objects are often important during the toddler stage and may be used for several years. Most children grow out of the need for such an item by the time they are 7 or 8 years old, but close attachments to special toys may persist. There is no evidence that security objects are in any way harmful. (See also *Thumb-sucking*.)

## Sedation

The use of a drug to calm a person. Sedation is used to reduce excessive *anxiety* and occasionally to control dangerously aggressive behavior. It may also be used as part of *premedication* to produce relaxation before an operation or before an uncomfortable procedure such as *gastroscopy*. (See also *Sleeping drugs*.)

## Sedative drugs

A group of drugs used to produce *sedation* (calmness). Sedative drugs include *sleeping drugs*, *antianxiety drugs*, *antipsychotic drugs*, and some *antidepressant drugs*. A sedative drug is often included in a *premedication* (drug given to prepare a person for surgery).

## Seizure

A sudden episode of uncontrolled electrical activity in the brain. If the abnormal activity remains confined to one area, the person may experience tingling or twitching of only a small area of the body, such as the face or an extremity.

Other possible symptoms include hallucinations or intense feelings of fear or familiarity (*déjà vu*). If the abnormal electrical activity spreads

Each numbered trace shows changes in electric potential between two points on the skull surface.

Normal traces        Abnormal traces during seizure

**EEG changes during a seizure**
The traces are recordings of electrical activity in a patient's brain, obtained from electrodes placed at various locations on the scalp and linked to an EEG machine. They show the change in activity at the onset of a seizure.

throughout the brain, consciousness is lost and a *grand mal* seizure results. Recurrent seizures are called *epilepsy*.

Seizures may be caused by many different neurological or medical problems, including *head injury*, infection, cerebrovascular accident (*stroke*), brain tumor, metabolic disturbances, or *alcohol* (withdrawal or hereditary intolerance of alcohol).

## Seizure, febrile

Twitching or jerking of the limbs with loss of consciousness occurring in a child after a rapid rise in temperature. Febrile seizures are common; about one child in 20 experiences one or more attacks. The seizures tend to run in families, are usually not serious, and occur mainly in children between 6 months and 5 years.

### CAUSES AND SYMPTOMS

Febrile seizures are caused by a disturbance in the normal electrical activity in the brain, but in most cases there is no underlying brain disorder. The fever that triggers the seizure usually develops with an acute infectious illness, such as *tonsillitis* or *otitis media* (inflammation of the middle ear).

The child loses consciousness and his or her arms and legs twitch uncontrollably for a few minutes. After regaining consciousness, the child may be drowsy.

### TREATMENT

During a seizure, objects that could be harmful should be moved out of the child's way. Biting the tongue is rare and absolutely no attempt should be made to prevent it by wedging the mouth open. This can cause cuts and broken teeth. Once the seizure is over, the child should be placed in the *recovery position*.

If the child has not had a seizure before, a physician should be consulted; if the seizure lasts for more than five minutes, an ambulance should be called.

If something other than a fever is suspected of causing the seizure, the physician may perform investigative tests, such as a *lumbar puncture* to determine whether *meningitis* is the cause. No treatment is needed for the seizure, but treatment may be given for the underlying infection.

### PREVENTION AND OUTLOOK

If an infectious illness develops in a susceptible child, parents can prevent further seizures by reducing the child's temperature. Acetaminophen should be given immediately at the first signs of fever at the full dose for the child's weight given on the

package. The dose can be repeated every four hours. Bedclothes should be removed and a fan directed toward the child. Sponging the child's face and body with lukewarm water may be comforting but is of dubious value in lowering temperature.

Most children who have one or more febrile seizures are completely normal and suffer no ill effects from the attacks. A second febrile seizure occurs in about 30 to 40 percent of cases, usually within the following six months. Recurrences are more likely if the child is abnormally mentally developed, if there was a complex or prolonged (longer than 15 minutes) first febrile seizure, and if there are family members with *epilepsy*. Children with all of these handicaps have about a one in 10 chance of having epilepsy develop. In healthy children, the risk of epilepsy is small.

## Selenium

A *trace element* that helps preserve the elasticity of body tissues, thereby slowing the aging process. Selenium also improves the oxygen supply to the heart and helps form prostaglandins (substances that help prevent abnormal blood clotting and high blood pressure).

A balanced diet supplies the minute amount of selenium required by the body. The richest dietary sources are meat, fish, whole grains, and dairy products. The selenium content of vegetables depends on the amount of the mineral in the soil in which they were grown.

### DEFICIENCY AND EXCESS

Neither deficiency nor excess of selenium usually has any effect on health. However, prolonged selenium deficiency—as a result of a poor diet or subsistence on vegetables grown in selenium-poor soil—may possibly cause premature aging, muscle pain, and, eventually, heart disease.

Excessive intake as a result of taking supplements or, rarely, from eating vegetables grown in soil with an abnormally high selenium content (as is found in some intensively irrigated areas) may cause baldness, loss of nails and teeth, fatigue, vomiting, and, with massive doses, death.

### MEDICAL USES

Selenium is a constituent of some *multivitamin* and *mineral* preparations. Selenium sulfide is used in some anti-dandruff shampoos.

## Self-help organizations

See special section at back of book.

## Self-image

An individual's view of his or her personality. Some psychologists believe that neurosis stems from incongruity between self-image and how others see one (as occurs in an *inferiority complex*). *Psychotherapy* treats neurosis by bringing about a change in the person's perception of the self.

## Self-mutilation

The act of deliberately injuring oneself. Self-mutilation usually takes the form of cutting the wrists or burning the forearms with cigarettes. It most often occurs in young adults with *personality disorders*, many of whom are also drug or alcohol abusers, and is three times more common in women. Self-mutilators often have had a violent upbringing and may also suffer from *mental retardation*. The reasons self-mutilators give for their behavior include aggressive impulses, relief of tension, and sadomasochistic fantasies.

More unusual forms of self-harm, such as gouging out the eyes or mutilating the genitals, are almost always due to *psychosis*.

Self-destructive biting is a feature of Lesch-Nyhan syndrome, a rare metabolic disorder that causes gout and mental retardation.

## Semen

Fluid produced by the male on *ejaculation*. Semen is composed of fluid from the seminal vesicles (which produce the greatest part of the semen volume), fluid from the *prostate gland*, and *sperm*.

An important constituent of the fluid from the seminal vesicles is fructose (a sugar), which stimulates the sperm to become mobile. The concentration of fructose, the production of sperm, and the volume of the semen is dependent on the presence of the male sex hormone *testosterone*.

*Semen analysis* is performed as part of the investigation of male *infertility*.

## Semen analysis

A method of determining the concentration, shape, and motility (ability to move) of sperm. Semen analysis is important in the investigation of male *infertility*. It is also performed some weeks after *vasectomy* (male sterilization) to ensure that the semen no longer contains sperm.

The semen specimen is produced by masturbation and should be as fresh as possible for successful analysis in the laboratory. The volume of semen is measured and the specimen examined under the microscope.

Normal semen contains from 20 million to 200 million sperm per milliliter. Semen analysis may show a deficiency in the number of sperm (*oligospermia*), a complete absence of sperm (*azoospermia*), altered shape, or diminished motility.

## Semen, blood in the

A harmless condition, also called hemospermia, in which a small amount of blood is present in the semen. The blood, which is usually seen as a darkish stain in the semen at *ejaculation*, usually comes from small blood vessels in the region of the prostate gland or seminal vesicles. In the majority of cases, no cause is found.

## Seminoma

See *Testis, cancer of*.

## Senile dementia

See *Dementia*.

## Senility

Changes in mental ability caused by old age. Most people over age 70 suffer from some degree of impaired memory and reduced ability to concentrate. With age, there is an increasing risk of *dementia*, which affects about one in five of those over 80. Depressive illness (see *Depression*) and *confusion* due to physical disease are also common, but there is a reduced prevalence of neurotic illness.

## Senna

A *laxative drug* obtained from the leaves and pods of the Arabian shrubs *CASSIA ACUTIFOLIA* and *CASSIA ANGUSTIFOLIA*. Senna stimulates bowel contraction and is used to treat severe *constipation*; it may color the urine yellow-brown or red.

## Sensate focus technique

A method taught to couples who are experiencing sexual difficulties caused by psychological rather than organic factors. The aim of the technique is to make each partner more aware of his or her pleasurable bodily sensations as well as those of the partner, and to reduce anxiety about performance.

Sensate focus technique is particularly useful in treating loss of sexual desire, failure to become sexually

S

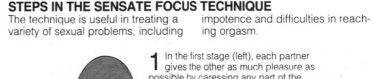

### STEPS IN THE SENSATE FOCUS TECHNIQUE

The technique is useful in treating a variety of sexual problems, including impotence and difficulties in reaching orgasm.

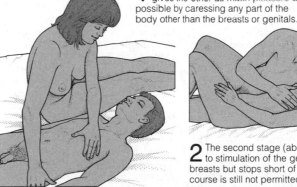

**1** In the first stage (left), each partner gives the other as much pleasure as possible by caressing any part of the body other than the breasts or genitals.

**2** The second stage (above) progresses to stimulation of the genitals and breasts but stops short of orgasm. Intercourse is still not permitted at this stage.

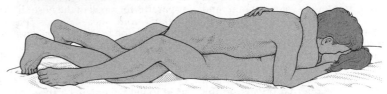

**3** The final stage consists of sexual intercourse. Both partners concentrate on enjoyment rather than on orgasm, which is not the main goal.

## PRINCIPAL SENSORY PATHWAYS INTO THE BRAIN

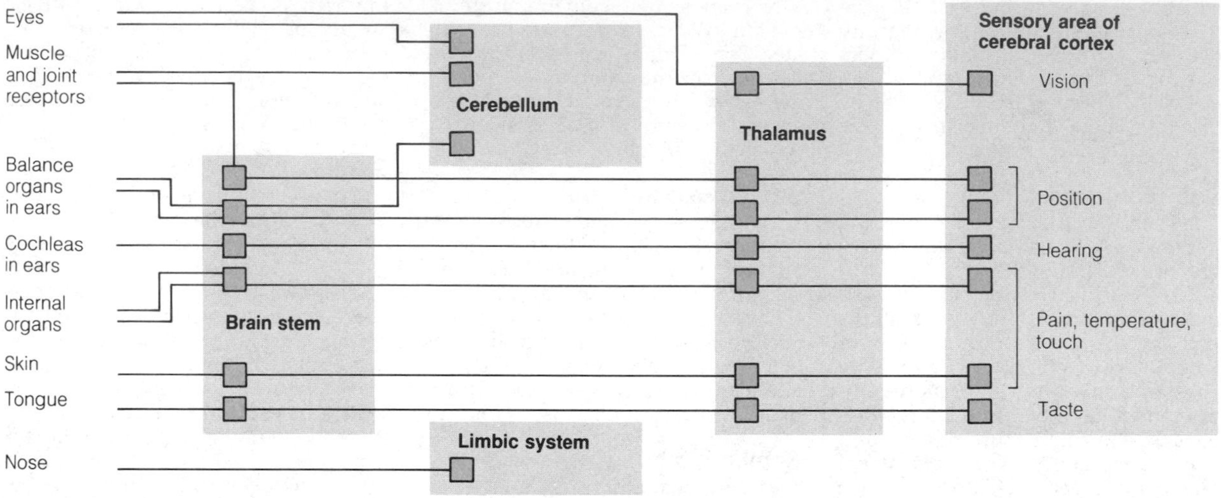

Eyes
Muscle and joint receptors
Cerebellum
Sensory area of cerebral cortex
Vision
Thalamus
Balance organs in ears
Position
Cochleas in ears
Hearing
Internal organs
Brain stem
Pain, temperature, touch
Skin
Tongue
Taste
Limbic system
Nose

**Destinations of sensory information**
Some of the information entering the brain passes via the brain stem and/or thalamus to the cerebral cortex (outer surface of the brain), where sensations are perceived. Other information does not lead to conscious sensation. This includes certain data about body posture, processed in the cerebellum, and about internal body functioning, processed in the brain stem.

aroused (see *Sexual desire, inhibited*), or inability to achieve orgasm (see *Orgasm, lack of*), and in helping overcome *impotence* or premature ejaculation (see *Ejaculation, disorders of*).

### HOW IT IS DONE
The technique, which should ideally be practiced in a relaxed, romantic or erotic setting, has three stages (see illustrated box on previous page). If premature ejaculation is a problem, one of the techniques to prevent it can be used (see *Sex therapy*).

### EFFECTIVENESS
The sensate focus technique has an extremely high success rate—between 80 and 98 percent, depending on the sexual problem.

## Sensation
A feeling or impression (such as a sound, an odor, touch, or hunger) that has entered consciousness. The senses are the faculties by which information about the external environment and about the body's internal state is collected and brought to the central nervous system (brain and spinal cord).

### SENSORY RECEPTORS
Information is collected by millions of microscopic structures (called *receptors*) throughout the body. Receptors are found in the skin, muscles, and joints, in the internal organs, in the walls of blood vessels, and in special sense organs, such as the eye and inner ear. Receptors are attuned to a particular stimulus, such as light of a particular wavelength, chemical molecules of a certain shape, vibration, or temperature. They fire (send an electrical signal) when excited.

Some receptors are the terminals (free nerve endings) of long nerve cell fibers, others are specialized cells that connect to such fibers. When a receptor fires, a signal passes along the appropriate nerve fiber to the spinal cord, to the brain, or to both.

The principal pathways and destinations of sensory information entering the brain are shown in the diagram above. Only a proportion of this information reaches sensory areas of the cerebral cortex (outer surface of the brain) and is consciously perceived (see *Sensory cortex; Brain*).

### THE SPECIAL SENSES
The special senses include *vision, hearing, taste,* and *smell*. The receptor cells for these senses are collected into special organs—the retina in the eyes, the auditory apparatus in the ears, the taste buds in the tongue, and the apparatus for smell in the nose. Information from these organs passes directly to the brain via *cranial nerves*. Much of the information passes to the cerebral cortex, although some goes to other areas of the brain (e.g., from the eyes to the cerebellum, where it is used to help maintain balance).

### INTERNAL AND TOUCH SENSES
These senses include the pain, proprioception (position), pressure, and temperature sensations. Proprioception relies on receptors in the muscles and joints to provide information on the position in space of parts of the body. Pain is one of the most primitive senses; it warns of noxious stimuli through receptors at the skin surface and inside.

Many types of receptors are found in the skin. Some are sensitive to pressure, others to the movement of hairs, others to temperature change. Skin receptors are made up of the terminals of nerve fibers, which are wrapped around the roots of hairs, formed into disks, or surrounded by a series of membranes to form onionlike structures (called pacinian corpuscles). Different patterns of stimulation of these receptors give rise to such sensations as pain, tickling, firm or light pressure, heat or cold. Certain skin areas (the lips, palms of the hands, and genitals) have a particularly high concentration of receptors.

Most of the signals from these receptors pass, via the cranial or spinal nerves and tracts in the brain or spinal cord, to the thalamus and then to two regions of the sensory cortex called the somatosensory cortices. Sensations perceived at certain points within these regions correspond to the parts of the body from which the signals originated. Much larger areas of cortex are devoted to sensations originating from the hands and lips than from less sensitive parts.

## Sensation, abnormal

Unpleasant, dulled, or otherwise altered sensations without obvious stimulus (e.g., a burning sensation when there is no heat). Abnormal sensations result from damage to, or pressure on, sensory nerve pathways.

### TYPES AND CAUSES

The most common types are *tinnitus* or *numbness* and/or a *pins and needles sensation*, sometimes combined with *pain* and, in some cases, with coldness or burning sensations. *Neuralgia* is characterized by pain with a stabbing, brief, repetitive quality.

More unusual disturbances include the feeling that fluid is trickling down the skin, that part of the body is being constricted by a tight band, or that insects are crawling over the skin (formication). The special senses can also be impaired or altered by damage to the relevant sensory apparatus or nerve tracts (see *Vision, disorders of*; *Smell*; *Deafness*; *Tinnitus*).

*Neuropathy* (damage to peripheral nerves) from thiamine deficiency in alcoholics, from *diabetes mellitus*, or from heavy metal (such as lead) poisoning is a common cause of abnormal sensation. The sufferer may complain of tingling or a feeling of walking on cotton. The peripheral nerves may also be damaged or irritated by infections such as *herpes zoster* (shingles) or by a tumor pressing on a nerve, often causing severe pain. *Spinal injury*, *head injury*, *stroke*, and *multiple sclerosis* are other causes of damage or degeneration of nerve pathways in the brain or spinal cord.

Damage to the thalamus (a relay station for sensory pathways in the center of the brain) can produce particularly unpleasant results, such as a spreading sensation resembling an electric shock that occurs after a simple pinprick. Damage to the parietal lobe in the brain can lead to loss of the ability to locate or recognize objects by touch.

### DIAGNOSIS AND TREATMENT

Many tests (including tests of sensation, testing of *reflexes*, *blood tests*, *urinalysis*, and *CT scanning* or *angiography*) may be required to discover the cause of abnormal sensation.

Pressure on or damage to nerves can sometimes be relieved by surgery or by dietary or other treatments to remove or treat the underlying cause. In other instances, severe intractable pain or other abnormal sensation can be relieved only by cutting the relevant sensory nerve fibers or by giving injections to chemically block the transmission of signals along them.

## Senses

See *Sensation*.

## Sensitization

The initial exposure of a person to an allergen or other substance recognized as foreign by the body's *immune system*, which leads to an immune response. On second and subsequent exposures to the same substance, there is a much stronger and faster immune reaction. This action forms the basis of *allergy* and other types of *hypersensitivity* reaction.

## Sensory cortex

A region of the outer part of the *cerebrum* (the main mass of the brain) in which sensory information comes to consciousness. The sensory cortex contains several layers of interconnected neurons (nerve cells) with complex interconnections.

Pressure, pain, and temperature sensations from the skin, muscles, joints, and internal organs are perceived in regions of the parietal lobe (upper side part of the cerebrum) on both sides of the brain. These regions are called the somatosensory cortices. Taste sensations are also perceived in the parietal lobes. Light, color, shape, and other visual sensations are perceived in the occipital lobes at the back of the cerebrum; sounds are perceived in the temporal lobes at the sides.

## Sensory deprivation

Removing the normal sights, sounds, and physical feelings from a person. Sensory deprivation can produce a variety of mental changes, demonstrated by studies in which volunteers lie immobile in bed (or in a tub of warm water) wearing masks and gloves in a sound-deadened room. After long periods, reported effects generally include feelings of unreality, difficulty thinking, and hallucinations; EEG recordings show a slowing of brain activity.

Prisoners kept in solitary confinement experience similar symptoms, and infants deprived of the companionship and presence of others tend to be disturbed in later life. (See also *Bonding*; *Emotional deprivation*.)

## Separation anxiety

The feelings of distress that a young child experiences when parted from his or her parents or home. Separation anxiety is a normal aspect of infant behavior that increases in intensity until about 2 years of age, but is often minimal by 3 to 4 years. When threatened with separation, the child usually reacts by crying, clinging to the parent, and demanding to be cuddled. Such signs are indicative of *bonding*, which is considered essential to a child's emotional development.

Separation anxiety disorder is a childhood illness in which the reaction to separation is greater than that expected for the child's level of development. The anxiety may manifest itself in the form of headaches, nausea, toothaches, dizziness, or difficulty sleeping. When separated, the child may worry that he

---

### NEUROLOGIC SENSORY TESTING

**Light touch**
With the patient's eyes closed, a piece of cotton is brushed lightly across the face.

**Pinprick**
The prick tests pain sensation and may be repeated at different locations on the patient's body.

**Pain pinch**
Pain sense may be further tested by pinching the Achilles tendon at the back of the heel.

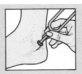

**Vibration**
A vibrating tuning fork is held against a prominent bone, such as the ankle bone or mastoid bone.

**Position sense**
The patient, with eyes closed, tells in which direction his or her finger is moved.

**Two-point discrimination**
Measures ability to distinguish two pinpricks from a single prick.

**Standard tests**
When examining a patient's nervous system, a physician usually includes several standard tests of touch, position, pain, and vibration senses, such as those above.

**S**

or she will never be reunited with the parents or that they will be killed. Some children refuse to visit friends or attend school. Separation anxiety disorder may be a feature of *depression*.

## Sepsis

Infection of a wound or body tissues with bacteria that leads to the formation of pus (see *Suppuration*) or to multiplication of the bacteria in the blood. If the blood becomes infected with bacteria that the *immune system* can eradicate entirely or prevent from multiplying excessively, the condition is known as *bacteremia*. However, if bacteria that form toxins are present in the blood in large numbers and are multiplying rapidly, the condition (as a result of the toxemia and bacteremia) is called *septicemia* (blood poisoning). See also *Septic shock*.

## Septal defect

A heart abnormality, developed before birth, in which there is a hole in the septum (partition) between the left and right sides of the heart. Commonly known as a hole in the heart, septal defect varies in its effects according to the size and position of the defect.

### TYPES

When the hole is in the septum separating the two ventricles (lower chambers of the heart), the abnormality is known as a ventricular septal defect; when it is in the septum between the two atria (upper chambers), it is called an atrial septal defect. In both types, the hole allows some of the freshly oxygenated blood in the left half of the heart (which supplies tissues throughout the body) to flow into the right half, mix with deoxygenated blood, and recirculate through the lungs. If the hole is large, the misdirection of blood results in a greatly reduced oxygen supply to the tissues and excessive blood flow through the lungs.

Some children are born with both atrial and ventricular septal defects; either type may be accompanied by one or more other heart abnormalities and/or other birth defects.

### CAUSES AND INCIDENCE

The precise cause of this defect is unknown in most cases. (For information on factors influencing the development of congenital heart abnormalities, see *Heart disease, congenital* and *Birth defects*.)

Ventricular septal defects are the most common type of congenital heart abnormality, occurring in about 30 percent of all cases of congenital heart disease and affecting about 200 babies in every 100,000. Atrial septal defects occur in about 8 percent of cases (50 babies per 100,000).

### SYMPTOMS AND SIGNS

A small defect of either kind produces little or no effect. With a large ventricular hole, *heart failure* may develop six to eight weeks after birth, causing breathlessness, feeding difficulties, pallor, and sweating. With large atrial defects, however, heart failure may not develop for many years or may not develop at all.

With both types of defect, *pulmonary hypertension* (high blood pressure in the arteries supplying the lungs) may develop. This is more likely, and occurs at an earlier age, in large ventricular defects.

With ventricular defect there is also a slight risk of *endocarditis* (inflammation of the lining of the heart); in atrial septal defect, *atrial fibrillation* (rapid, irregular beating of the atria) may occur after age 30.

### DIAGNOSIS

The diagnosis is made by a physician who hears, through a stethoscope, a heart *murmur* (a type of abnormal heart sound made by turbulent blood

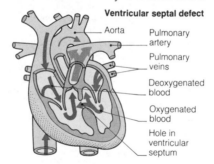

**Ventricular septal defect**

- Aorta
- Pulmonary artery
- Pulmonary veins
- Deoxygenated blood
- Oxygenated blood
- Hole in ventricular septum

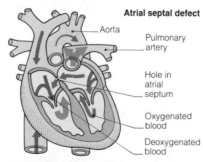

**Atrial septal defect**

- Aorta
- Pulmonary artery
- Hole in atrial septum
- Oxygenated blood
- Deoxygenated blood

**Two types of septal defect**
In both cases, oxygenated blood is forced from the left to the right side of the heart through the hole in the septum. Too much blood passes to the lungs (via the pulmonary artery) and too little to the body tissues (via the aorta).

flow through the hole). Diagnosis also includes chest X rays and an ECG. The diagnosis can be confirmed by Doppler *echocardiography*.

### TREATMENT

Atrial septal defects are repaired only if they cause symptoms or if examination and tests suggest that complications may develop.

As the child grows, small ventricular holes often become smaller, or even close, on their own. If a large ventricular defect is causing heart failure, it is treated with *diuretic drugs* and with *digitalis drugs* in babies. If the hole does not close spontaneously, it is repaired by *open heart surgery*, usually before the child reaches school age. The operation has an extremely high safety and success rate.

### OUTLOOK

Modern surgery is so effective in dealing with large septal defects that it enables most affected people to lead normal lives.

## Septicemia

Rapid multiplication of bacteria and the presence of their toxins in the blood, a condition commonly known as blood poisoning. As distinct from *bacteremia* (in which bacteria are present in the blood but do not always multiply), septicemia is always a serious, life-threatening condition.

### CAUSES

Septicemia usually arises through escape of bacteria from a focus of infection somewhere in the body (such as from an abscess or from a urinary tract or intestinal infection, or because of pneumonia or meningitis). Septicemia is more likely in people whose natural resistance to infection has been lowered by an *immunodeficiency disorder* or by *immunosuppressant drugs*, allowing the bacteria to multiply unchecked.

### SYMPTOMS AND SIGNS

A person in whom septicemia develops suddenly becomes seriously ill, with a high fever, chills, rapid breathing, headache, and often clouding of consciousness. Skin rashes or jaundice may occur and sometimes the hands are unusually warm. In many cases, especially when large amounts of toxins are produced by the circulating bacteria, the person passes into a state of *septic shock*, a life-threatening condition.

### DIAGNOSIS AND TREATMENT

A diagnosis of septicemia can be confirmed, and the infective bacteria identified, by growing a *culture* of the organisms from a blood sample.

S

Treatment is started as soon as septicemia is suspected by giving an *intravenous infusion* (slow introduction into a vein) of *antibiotic drugs* and of glucose and/or saline solution.

The focal site of infection is sought immediately and may be surgically removed. Provided the infection is recognized and treated promptly, there is usually a full recovery.

## Septic shock

A highly dangerous condition in which there is tissue damage and a dramatic drop in blood pressure as a result of *septicemia* and *toxemia* (the multiplication of bacteria and the presence of their toxins in the blood).

In many cases, the toxins are the main cause of trouble because they can cause damage to cells and tissues throughout the body, promote clotting of blood in the smallest blood vessels, and seriously interfere with the normal blood circulation. Damage occurs especially to tissues in the kidneys, heart, and lungs. The toxins may cause leakage of fluid from blood vessels and a reduction of the ability of the vessels to constrict, leading to a drop in blood pressure.

### CAUSES AND INCIDENCE

Septic shock is most common in people hospitalized with such major disorders as *diabetes mellitus*, *cancer*, or liver *cirrhosis* and who have a focus of infection somewhere in the body (often the intestines or urinary tract) that has led to septicemia. Progression to septic shock is especially likely in people who have an *immunodeficiency disorder*, in people taking *immunosuppressant drugs* for cancer, or in people given prolonged and inappropriate antibiotic treatment. Newborn infants are also particularly susceptible if septicemia develops.

### SYMPTOMS AND SIGNS

The symptoms vary with the extent and site of major tissue damage. Broadly, they are the same as in septicemia, with additional symptoms including cold hands and feet, often with *cyanosis* (blue-purple coloration) due to slowed blood flow, a weak, rapid pulse, and markedly reduced blood pressure. There may be vomiting and diarrhea. A poor output of urine may indicate that damage to the kidneys is occurring and that there is a risk of *renal failure*. *Heart failure* and abnormal bleeding may also develop.

### TREATMENT

Septic shock requires immediate treatment, including the use of *antibiotic drugs* and sometimes surgery to remove the focus of infection. Rapid fluid replacement by infusion and the maintenance of urine flow to prevent the effects of renal failure are other essential procedures. Measures are also taken to raise the blood pressure and to promote better blood supply to tissues. These measures include *intravenous infusions* and *oxygen therapy*.

Despite treatment, septic shock remains a grave condition; survival rates are no better than 50 percent.

## Septum

A thin dividing wall within or between parts of the body. The nasal septum is the sheet of cartilage and bone that separates the nostrils.

## Sequela

A condition that results from or follows a disease, disorder, or injury. The term is usually used in the plural (sequelae) to refer to the complications of a disease. The sequelae of a common cold may include *bronchitis*, *sinusitis*, and *otitis media* (inflammation of the middle ear).

## Sequestration

A term used in medicine to refer to a portion of diseased or necrotic (dead) tissue being separated from, or joined abnormally to, surrounding healthy tissue. The term usually refers to a complication of *osteomyelitis* (bone infection) in which part of a bone dies and becomes separated from healthy bone. Sequestration may also refer to a rare congenital abnormality of the lungs in which part of a lobe is not directly connected to a bronchus (airway) but may be connected to surrounding alveoli (air sacs).

## Serology

A branch of laboratory medicine concerned with analysis of the contents of blood *serum* (the clear fluid that separates from clotted blood).

Various serological techniques are extremely useful in the diagnosis of infectious diseases. If a person has been exposed to a particular infectious organism, *antibodies* (proteins with a role in immunity) directed specifically against the organism appear in that person's serum some days after exposure. Their presence or absence in the blood can be detected by such laboratory techniques as *immunoassay*, including the ELISA test and radioimmunoassay. The absence of specific antibodies detected by serology may allow a physician to exclude a particular infection as the cause of the illness; a rising level of antibody may give good evidence that a particular infection is present.

In other cases, serological techniques are used to identify parts of infectious organisms (*antigens*) by studying the reaction between the antigens (obtained by *culture* of a specimen taken from a patient) and serum samples known to contain certain antibodies. A series of tests may be carried out in which the unknown antigen is added to various *antiserums* (preparations containing specific antibodies) in test tubes; a positive reaction is sometimes revealed by a color change.

In addition to devising and carrying out such diagnostic tests, serologists may be involved in developing antiserums for passive *immunization*.

Serologists may also test blood samples for various genetically determined protein markers, including substances that determine blood groups. Such tests can help resolve paternity suits (see *Paternity testing*) or cases in which blood left at the scene of the crime can be compared with blood taken from suspects.

## Serotonin

A substance found in many tissues, particularly blood platelets, the lining of the digestive tract, and the brain. Serotonin has a variety of effects in the body. It is released from platelets at the site of bleeding, where it constricts small blood vessels, thus reducing blood loss. In the digestive tract, it inhibits gastric secretion and stimulates smooth (involuntary) muscles in the intestinal wall. In the brain, it acts as a *neurotransmitter* (a chemical involved in the transmission of nerve impulses between nerve cells). Serotonin is thought to be involved in controlling states of consciousness and mood; its action in the brain is disrupted by certain hallucinogenic drugs, notably *LSD*.

## Serum

The clear fluid that separates from blood when it clots. Serum does not contain blood cells or the protein (fibrinogen) in blood that helps form clots. Serum does contain salts, glucose, and other proteins (including various *antibodies* formed by the body's *immune system* to protect against infection).

Serum prepared from the blood of a person (or animal) who has been infected with a microorganism usually

S

contains antibodies that can protect against that organism if the serum is injected into someone else. This is called an *antiserum*, and its use forms the basis of passive *immunization*.

## Serum sickness

A short-lived illness that may develop about 10 days after injection with an *antiserum* of animal origin (e.g., antirabies serum equine, obtained from horses). Serum sickness is a type of *hypersensitivity* reaction similar to an allergy. A similar illness can occur after taking certain drugs.

### CAUSES

Antiserums are preparations obtained from human or animal blood containing specific *antibodies* (substances with a role in immunity). Antiserums are sometimes given to protect against dangerous infections. When an antiserum is prepared from animal blood, a protein in the serum may be misidentified by the body's *immune system* as a potentially harmful foreign substance (*antigen*). In serum sickness, the immune system produces antibodies that combine with the antigen to form particles called immune complexes. They are deposited in various tissues, stimulate more immune reactions, and lead to inflammation and symptoms.

Certain drugs can cause a similar response, though the drug molecules probably combine with a protein in the blood or tissues before they are misidentified as antigens. Penicillin is the most important drug capable of causing serum sickness.

Serum sickness is different from *anaphylactic shock*, another type of hypersensitivity reaction that can also develop in response to antiserums, drugs, and other substances. Anaphylactic shock is a more severe, immediate reaction.

### SYMPTOMS AND TREATMENT

A week or two after exposure to the antiserum or drug, symptoms appear. There may be an itchy rash, pain in the joints, fever, and enlargement of lymph nodes. In severe cases, a state similar to *shock*, with low blood pressure, develops. All symptoms usually clear up within a few days provided (in the case of a drug) that its use is stopped.

Soothing lotions can help relieve itching. The physician may prescribe a *nonsteroidal anti-inflammatory drug* to relieve joint pain and an *antihistamine drug* to shorten the duration of the illness. In severe cases, a *corticosteroid drug* may be prescribed.

People who have had serum sickness or anaphylactic shock should note the name of the injection or drug to which they are sensitive. Mention should also be made in the medical records to warn health care personnel against future use of the drug.

## Sex

Another term for gender and a commonly used term for *sexual intercourse*.

## Sex change

Radical surgical procedures, usually combined with sex hormone therapy, that alter a person's anatomical gender. Sex change operations are performed on transsexuals (see *Transsexualism*) or on people with ambiguous genitalia (see *Pseudohermaphroditism*; *Hermaphroditism*).

### WHY IT IS DONE

Sex change operations on transsexuals are performed to give the person a physical appearance that he or she believes coincides with his or her psychological *gender identity*.

Sex change operations on people with ambiguous genitalia (i.e., with external sex organs resembling those of the opposite sex) are performed to modify or improve the anatomical gender and thus provide a more defined sexual identity.

### HOW IT IS DONE

**TRANSSEXUALS** Sex change involves a series of major operations on the genitourinary tract carried out after hormone therapy and counseling.

The male-to-female sex change is the more common procedure. Prosthetic breasts may be implanted to augment the breast growth that has resulted from hormone therapy. An operation removes the erectile tissue of the penis and repositions the urethra. The skin of the penis is used to make the lining for a vagina, which is created in the *perineum*. The testes are removed and the skin of the scrotum is used to make the labia.

In the female-to-male sex change, a mastectomy is performed to remove the breasts. Afterward, removal of the uterus and ovaries is carried out. This may be followed by a penile graft, which involves constructing a new urethra by grafting an abdominal skin flap over a catheter; the graft and the surrounding skin are then separated to make a penis. The upper end is inserted into the perineum and the lower end is detached.

**AMBIGUOUS GENITALIA** Operations are usually carried out in infancy. Babies with ambiguous genitalia are assigned

a sex as soon as possible after birth, given appropriate surgical and hormonal treatment, and reared as a member of the assigned sex.

Operations on adults who have ambiguous genitalia are uncommon today. In general, they are similar to those performed on transsexuals, with variations depending on specific anatomical problems.

### OUTLOOK

The degree to which transsexuals adjust to their new gender varies. Some make a complete adjustment but others are left with serious psychological problems. Hormone therapy may need to be continued for life to maintain secondary sexual characteristics such as body shape, hair distribution, and voice change. Female transsexuals can have intercourse but cannot conceive. Males cannot impregnate or ejaculate; they achieve an erection only with mechanical aids (e.g., *penile implants*).

## Sex chromosomes

A pair of chromosomes that determines gender. Sex chromosomes are found in each of a person's cells along with 44 other chromosomes (autosomes). In women, the sex chromosomes are of similar appearance and are called X chromosomes. In men, one sex chromosome is an X and the other, a smaller chromosome, is a Y. Thus, the normal sex chromosome complement for women is XX, and for men, XY.

### FUNCTION

Like all chromosomes, the X and Y chromosomes exert their effects in the body through the activities of their constituent *genes*. These genes contain the coded instructions for chemical processes within cells and aspects of growth and development within the body as a whole.

The X and Y chromosomes differ in one fundamental way. Genes on the Y chromosome are concerned solely with gender. Their presence ensures a male, their absence a female. The X chromosome, which is common to both sexes, contains many genes vital to general body development and functioning. Absence of the X chromosome is incompatible with life.

The presence of a single X chromosome and 44 autosomes appears to provide the blueprint for general body functioning and development, which seems to have an underlying female pattern. This is demonstrated in people with *Turner's syndrome*, who

S

have only one sex chromosome, an X. Although full female sex characteristics never develop, these people are nevertheless unmistakably female in appearance and identity. Full female sex characteristics develop only in the presence of a second X chromosome. Addition of a Y chromosome converts the female to the male pattern.

## Sex determination

The factors that determine biological sex. The underlying determinants are the *sex chromosomes* in a person's cells—two X chromosomes in females, and one X and one Y chromosome in males. During early life in the embryo, these chromosomes cause the development of different gonads (primary sex organs)—the testes in males and the ovaries in females. In males, the testes then produce hormones that cause the development of a male reproductive tract, including a penis. In females, absence of these male hormones leads to a different pattern of development, with the formation of fallopian tubes, uterus, and vagina. Many years after birth, another surge of hormones from the gonads leads to the development of secondary *sexual characteristics*, such as facial hair in males and breasts in females.

Defects can arise in this process, leading, in some cases, to ambiguous sex. Some people acquire an abnormal complement of sex chromosomes (see *Chromosomal abnormalities*) and all the characteristics of one sex do not develop. In some female fetuses, a metabolic defect causes the production of large amounts of male hormones (see *Adrenal hyperplasia, congenital*), causing masculinization of the female genitals (such as enlargement of the clitoris to form an appendage resembling a penis). Conversely, in some male fetuses, male hormones are not produced or they are produced but fail to cause masculinization; the child's genitals are feminized to some degree (the extreme case of this is called *testicular feminization syndrome*). Finally, there are very rare cases of true *hermaphroditism*, in which a child is born with both testicular and ovarian tissue and may have both a vagina and a penis.

These ambiguities are different from *transsexualism*, in which a person's biological sex is not in doubt, although it conflicts with his or her psychological disposition.

When an infant is born with ambiguous genitals, the cause of the ambiguity is investigated and the child is assigned the sex believed to offer the best chance for a healthy life. The decision depends on the possibilities for establishing one sex or another through hormonal and/or surgical treatment. In most cases, a satisfactory male or female appearance and sexual capacity can be achieved. Full reproductive potential (ability to have children) can be achieved in some cases.

## Sex hormones

Hormones that control the development of primary and secondary sexual characteristics and regulate various sex-related functions in the body, such as the menstrual cycle and the production of eggs or sperm. There are three main types of sex hormones—*androgen hormones* (male sex hormones), *estrogen hormones* (female sex hormones), and *progesterone hormones* (which have the specialized function of preparing for and maintaining *pregnancy*).

## Sex-linked

Pertaining to a trait or a disorder determined by the *sex chromosomes* in a person's cells or by the *genes* carried on those chromosomes.

Most people carry two sex chromosomes in their cells. Disorders caused by an abnormal number of sex chromosomes include *Turner's syndrome* (which affects females only and is caused by a missing X chromosome) and *Klinefelter's syndrome* (which affects males only and is caused by one or more extra X chromosomes).

Most other sex-linked traits or disorders are caused by recessive genes on the X chromosome (see *Genetic disorders*). These traits or disorders, which almost exclusively affect males, include such conditions as *hemophilia*, Duchenne *muscular dystrophy*, and *color vision deficiency*.

## Sex therapy

Counseling for and treatment of *psychosexual dysfunction* (sexual difficulties not due to a physical cause). Sex therapy is usually undertaken in conjunction with *marital* (or relationship) *counseling*.

It is estimated that at least 50 percent of couples experience some form of sexual problem at some stage in their relationships; in most cases, the problem is psychological in origin. Sex therapy can help by changing the general attitude of one or both partners toward sex, by increasing each person's understanding of his or her sexual needs and those of the partner, and by teaching techniques to deal with specific problems at home. Both partners attend the therapy sessions, but individual sex therapy may also be useful.

### TECHNIQUES

In the *sensate focus technique*, the couple explores pleasurable, relaxed, sensual rather than sexual, bodily sensations. The goal of this technique is to reduce anxiety about sexual performance and increase individual awareness of how to give and receive pleasure for at least 15 minutes.

To prevent premature ejaculation (see *Ejaculation, disorders of*), the most common sexual difficulty in men, two techniques are taught. One is the squeeze technique (see illustration below). The other technique requires both partners to stop thrusting a moment before ejaculation is imminent. In both cases, once the man has achieved control of this reflex, sexual activity is resumed. The techniques can be repeated as many times as required. They can be learned and are highly successful.

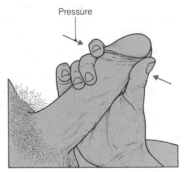

**THE SQUEEZE TECHNIQUE**
This technique is used for treating and preventing premature ejaculation in men.

Pressure

**Method**
Either partner squeezes the penis when the man is about to ejaculate, pressing just beneath the glans (head of the penis) using the thumb and two fingers.

Women who rarely or never experience orgasm (see *Orgasm, lack of*) or who have *vaginismus* (spasm of the vaginal muscles, preventing intercourse) may be treated individually, conjointly, or at group therapy sessions. The woman is encouraged to come to terms with her sexuality. She is taught exercises for relaxing and tightening the pelvic muscles and

**S**

to stimulate the clitoris to achieve orgasm (through masturbation) as a preliminary to intercourse.

RESULTS

Sex therapy has proved successful for many sexual problems, with particularly effective results in treating vaginismus, premature ejaculation, lack of orgasm, impotence, and failure to consummate marriage.

## Sexual abuse

The subjection of a person to sexual activity that is likely to cause physical or psychological harm. There is a federal law mandating that child-adult sexual contact be reported to a child protection agency. (See also *Child abuse; Rape*.)

## Sexual characteristics, secondary

Physical features appearing at *puberty* that indicate the onset of adult reproductive life.

In girls, the earliest secondary sexual characteristic is enlargement of the nipples and breasts. Soon thereafter, pubic and underarm hair appears, and body fat increases around the hips, stomach, and tops of the thighs to produce the female body shape.

In boys, enlargement of the testes is the first change, followed by thinning of the skin of the scrotum and enlargement of the penis. Pubic, facial, and other body hair appears, the voice deepens, and muscle bulk and bone size increase.

## Sexual desire, inhibited

Lack of sexual desire or of the ability to become physically aroused during sexual activity (see *Sexual intercourse*). Either form of the condition may be physical or psychological.

CAUSES

LACK OF DESIRE  A high proportion of women and some men experience loss of sexual desire at some point in their lives. Common physical causes include fatigue, ill health, and vaginal tenderness after childbirth. Certain drugs can also reduce sexual desire, including sleeping pills, antidepressants, antihypertensives, oral contraceptives, and alcohol. Psychological factors include *depression*, anxiety, severe stress, a conflictual relationship with or grief at the death of a sexual partner, or an unwanted pregnancy, an abortion, or a traumatic sexual experience such as *rape* or *incest*.

LACK OF PHYSICAL AROUSAL  It is rare for a woman or a man to be incapable of physical sexual arousal. The most

common reason for failure is the partner's poor or insensitive sexual overtures or technique, although hostility, anxiety, guilt about the sex act, or fear of sexual inadequacy may contribute to the problem. In rare cases, an individual is simply unable to respond to a particular partner but can respond to another, making the sexual problem selective.

TREATMENT

Problems that have a psychological basis or that are caused by the partner's sexual technique can often be successfully treated by *sex therapy* or *marital* (relationship) *counseling*. Sexual problems with a physical or chemical cause often improve once the underlying condition is resolved.

## Sexual deviation

See *Deviation, sexual*.

## Sexual dysfunction

See *Psychosexual dysfunction*.

## Sexual intercourse

The act in which a man's penis is inserted into a woman's vagina with her consent and cooperation. Sexual intercourse provides pleasurable sensations that may result in *orgasm* for one or both partners. The ejaculation of the man's *sperm* into the woman's reproductive tract is the usual means by which reproduction is achieved.

Couples bring many variations to the sexual act in terms of emotions, positions, and techniques used. However, for most, kissing, tenderness, and foreplay precede penetration. During sexual intercourse, a series of physiological responses occurs.

PHASES OF INTERCOURSE

Physiologically, intercourse can be divided into four phases—arousal, plateau, orgasm, and resolution.

DISORDERS

Problems with intercourse may have physical or psychological origins. (See also *Intercourse, painful; Psychosexual dysfunction; Sexual problems*.)

## Sexuality

A general term for the capacity, behavior patterns, impulses, emotions, and sensations connected with reproduction and the use of the sex organs. In biology, sex refers specifically to the anatomical differences between male and female. Sexual attraction, distraction, control, and expression make sexuality a powerful factor in the workplace, as a marketing tool, and in the pursuit of personal or mutual gratification.

*Heterosexuality* is sexuality directed toward the anatomically opposite sex; in *homosexuality* the attraction is toward the same sex. The term *bisexuality* refers to people who experience sexual attraction to members of either sex. (See also *Gender identity*.)

## Sexually transmitted diseases

Infections transmitted primarily, but not exclusively, by sexual intercourse.

HISTORY AND INCIDENCE

Also known as venereal diseases, sexually transmitted diseases (STDs) are acquired more often by people who have many new sex partners each year. Some of the major STDs are also transmitted by blood and thus occur in drug addicts who share needles.

Until about 25 years ago, STDs were thought to be limited to *syphilis, gonorrhea, chancroid*, and *lymphogranuloma venereum*. Today, however, these four diseases account for only 10 to 15 percent of all STDs seen in STD clinics. The most common conditions are *chlamydial infections, trichomoniasis*, genital herpes (see *Herpes, genital*), *pubic lice*, genital warts (see *Warts, genital*), and *AIDS*. Some other diseases, including viral *hepatitis, scabies, candidiasis*, and *molluscum contagiosum*, can also be transmitted by sexual intercourse, but they are not usually classified as STDs.

During the second world war, STDs became more prevalent in the US and Europe; they declined when the introduction of penicillin provided a cure for syphilis and gonorrhea. In the 1960s and 1970s, however, STDs increased again with the introduction of oral contraception. The birth-control pill led not only to women having more sex partners, but also to fewer couples using barrier contraceptives, which provide some protection against infection in addition to preventing pregnancy.

Also in the 1970s, genitourinary physicians recognized that so-called *nonspecific urethritis* was usually due to chlamydia. By the early 1980s a diagnosis of nonspecific urethritis was being made in about 25 percent of all people who visited STD clinics; in most of these people, careful laboratory testing showed evidence of chlamydial infection.

Throughout the 1970s and the early 1980s, most patients with an STD could expect a rapid cure with an antibiotic. In the late 1970s, however, it became apparent that certain STDs (notably herpes and hepatitis B) could not be cured by drugs and that herpes

S

## SEXUAL INTERCOURSE

The term sexual intercourse usually refers to the act during which the male penis is inserted into the female vagina. However, some people use the term more broadly to refer to a much wider range of sexual activity. Physiologically, intercourse falls into four main stages—arousal (which generally includes a period of foreplay), a plateau phase (during which penetration usually occurs), orgasm, and resolution. The duration of each stage of intercourse varies.

### Arousal in men
Sexual thoughts, the sight and feel of his partner's body, and foreplay may sexually arouse a man. Blood enters the penis so that it becomes firm and erect.

### Plateau phase in men
Vaginal penetration usually takes place during this phase and thrusting movements begin. The penis reaches maximum size and the testes elevate.

### Orgasm in men
Muscular contractions in the ducts connecting the testes, prostate, and penis force semen out of the penis, accompanied by intensely pleasurable sensations.

### Resolution in men
The penis returns to half its fully erect size and the testes descend.

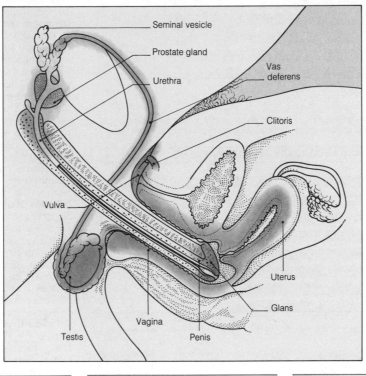

### Arousal in women
Similar factors lead to arousal in women as in men, though foreplay may be more important. The clitoris lengthens, the vagina enlarges, and its walls secrete a lubricating fluid.

### Plateau phase in women
Muscular contractions in the walls of the vagina help grip the penis. The uterus rises, and the clitoris pulls back beneath its hood of skin.

### Orgasm in women
The walls of the outer part of the vagina contract rhythmically and strongly several times and an intense sensual feeling spreads from the clitoris and throughout the body.

### Resolution in women
The clitoris subsides and, more gradually, the vagina relaxes and the uterus falls.

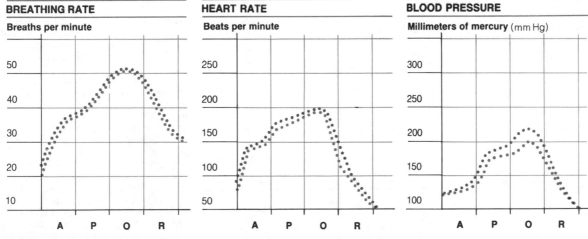

**Key** ••• Men ••• Women **A** = arousal **P** = plateau **O** = orgasm **R** = resolution

### Breathing rate
Both men and women breathe faster and louder as sexual excitement builds. The rate rises gradually, peaking at about twice the normal rate at orgasm.

### Heart rate
Intercourse provides vigorous exercise for the heart. The heart rate increases rapidly during arousal, peaks as high as 200 beats per minute at orgasm, then drops.

### Blood pressure
Systolic blood pressure rises in a similar pattern to heart rate, peaking at orgasm. The rise may be more marked in men than in women.

S

## INCIDENCE OF GONORRHEA IN THE US

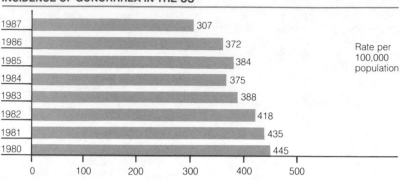

Rate per 100,000 population

| Year | Rate |
|------|------|
| 1987 | 307 |
| 1986 | 372 |
| 1985 | 384 |
| 1984 | 375 |
| 1983 | 388 |
| 1982 | 418 |
| 1981 | 435 |
| 1980 | 445 |

**Gonorrhea**
The incidence of gonorrhea peaked in the 1970s but has shown an almost uninterrupted decline in the 1980s. It remains, however, the most common of all reportable diseases.

## INCIDENCE OF PRIMARY AND SECONDARY SYPHILIS IN THE US

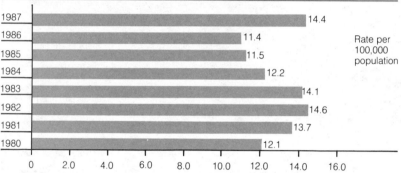

Rate per 100,000 population

| Year | Rate |
|------|------|
| 1987 | 14.4 |
| 1986 | 11.4 |
| 1985 | 11.5 |
| 1984 | 12.2 |
| 1983 | 14.1 |
| 1982 | 14.6 |
| 1981 | 13.7 |
| 1980 | 12.1 |

**Syphilis**
Syphilis is uncommon in the US today. Its incidence increased in the late 1970s and early 1980s, then declined in the middle 1980s—possibly helped by a move toward "safe" sex after the appearance of AIDS. There was an unexpected increase in 1987

## INCIDENCE OF NEW CASES OF AIDS IN THE US

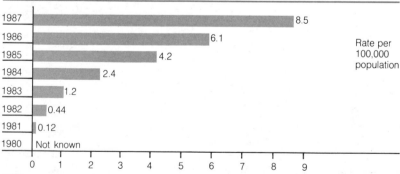

Rate per 100,000 population

| Year | Rate |
|------|------|
| 1987 | 8.5 |
| 1986 | 6.1 |
| 1985 | 4.2 |
| 1984 | 2.4 |
| 1983 | 1.2 |
| 1982 | 0.44 |
| 1981 | 0.12 |
| 1980 | Not known |

**AIDS**
New cases of AIDS roughly doubled each year from 1982 to 1985, but it was two years before cases doubled again. This may reflect a reduction in the rate of spread of the virus from about 1982 onward, due to greater awareness of the disease.

could become chronic and hepatitis could be fatal. With the recognition of AIDS in 1982, STDs became a threat to life. Promiscuous sex is now a high-risk activity.

**DIAGNOSIS AND TREATMENT**
Diagnosis and treatment are given at special STD clinics or from specialists in genitourinary medicine and infectious disease. The physician deter-mines which STDs are present (there may be more than one) and then assesses the sensitivity of the infection to various antibiotics. Once drugs have relieved the symptoms, tests are performed to ensure that the patient is no longer infectious.

**PREVENTION AND OUTLOOK**
To prevent transmitting infection, treatment is made available to all recent sexual partners. The confidential tracing and treatment of contacts is an essential part of the management of STDs (see *Contact tracing*).

The incidence of most STDs (with the exception of AIDS) fell in the middle 1980s. There were 372 new cases of gonorrhea per 100,000 in 1986 compared with 470 cases in 1976. However, a resurgence of penicillin-resistant gonorrhea in 1988 suggested that efforts to educate people on *"safe"* sex measures had yet to take effect.

## Sexual problems

Sexual problems are a common reason for consultation with physicians, psychiatrists, marital guidance counselors, and sex therapists. A sexual problem may be perceived by both partners in a relationship, by one partner who is affected by a disorder that lies primarily with the other, or by a person worried about his or her sexual identity or behavior.

**CAUSES**
Many problems affecting a person's sexual performance or behavior are partly or wholly psychological in origin because of inhibitions, lack of knowledge, anxieties, or a couple's conflicts (see *Psychosexual dysfunction; Deviation, sexual; Transvestism*).

Sometimes, sexual problems are due to organic disease, such as blood flow or hormonal problems. Disorders of the sexual organs may cause pain during intercourse (see *Intercourse, painful*). Some types of chemicals can affect sexual performance; examples include alcohol, *antihypertensive drugs*, and *oral contraceptives*.

People with disabilities may have sexual problems that often go unrecognized. Normal sexual desire may be present but gratification may be difficult to achieve because of physical difficulty with mobility for intercourse or because the disabled person may be avoided sexually by other people.

The mentally handicapped and cognitively impaired may not show normal personal control of their sexual behavior. Sexual molestation and pregnancy may occur.

S

### TREATMENT
Many sexual problems disappear when the underlying cause is treated. In other cases, people may benefit from sex education and counseling.

## Sézary syndrome
A rare condition in which there is an abnormal overgrowth of lymphoid cells (*lymphocytes*) in the skin, liver, spleen, and lymph nodes. Sézary syndrome primarily affects middle-aged and elderly people.

The first symptom is the appearance of red, scaly patches on the skin that spread to form a severe, flaky, itchy rash. There may also be an accumulation of fluid beneath the skin, baldness, and distorted nail growth; *leukemia* may also be associated with Sézary syndrome. Treatment includes *anticancer drugs* and *radiation therapy*.

## Shellfish poisoning
See *Food poisoning*.

## Shigellosis

An acute infection of the intestine by bacteria belonging to a group called shigella. Also known as bacillary dysentery, shigellosis causes diarrhea and abdominal pain.

### CAUSES AND INCIDENCE
The source of infection is the feces of infected people. The causative bacteria may be spread by an infected person failing to wash his or her hands after defecation and then handling food, or by flies in areas of inadequate sanitation. Endemic in some countries, shigellosis occurs in isolated outbreaks in the US, where about 15,000 cases are reported annually. It is particularly prevalent in children's day-care centers, institutions for the elderly, and mental hospitals.

### SYMPTOMS AND SIGNS
The disease usually starts suddenly, with watery diarrhea, abdominal pain, nausea, vomiting, generalized aches, and fever. After a few days, the need to defecate becomes frequent and urgent, and small, watery feces containing pus and blood are passed. Persistent diarrhea may cause *dehydration*, especially in babies and older people. Occasionally, toxemia (the presence of bacterial poisons in the blood) develops, resulting in a high fever and sometimes delirium.

The illness usually subsides after a week or so, but in severe cases may last several weeks. Death is rare, usually occurring only in dehydrated babies and older people.

### DIAGNOSIS AND TREATMENT
The diagnosis is confirmed by growing a *culture* of the causative bacteria from a sample of feces.

Dehydration is treated by *rehydration therapy*. Solid food should not be eaten for 24 to 48 hours after the onset of symptoms. In certain cases, *antibiotic drugs* may be prescribed. Infected people should be cared for in isolation until their feces are found to be free of the causative bacteria.

## Shingles
See *Herpes zoster*.

## Shin splints
A condition characterized by pain in the front and sides of the lower leg that develops or worsens during exercise. There may also be tenderness over the shin and edema (accumulation of fluid) of the surrounding tissues. Shin splints are a common problem in runners.

### CAUSES
Shin splints may be caused by various disorders, including *compartment syndrome* (buildup of pressure in a muscle as a result of exercise), *tendinitis* (inflammation of a tendon), *myositis* (inflammation of a muscle), a muscle tear, or *periostitis* (inflammation of the outer layer of a bone).

### DIAGNOSIS AND TREATMENT
Diagnosis is based on the symptoms, along with an X ray or radionuclide bone scan (see *Bone imaging*) to exclude the possibility of a stress fracture of the tibia (shin bone), which produces similar symptoms.

In most cases, shin splints clear up after a week or two of rest. However, if the pain is severe or recurrent, other treatment may be necessary, such as a course of *nonsteroidal anti-inflammatory drugs* or *corticosteroid drugs*; infrequently, a surgical operation is performed to alleviate excessive pressure in a muscle. Some people benefit from *physical therapy* instruction that includes stretching and strengthening exercises for the legs.

## Shivering
Involuntary trembling of the entire body caused by the rapid contraction and relaxation of muscles. Shivering is the body's normal automatic response to cold; it also occurs in association with *rigors* and fever.

When the body becomes cold, temperature-sensitive nerve cells in the *hypothalamus* (part of the brain) act as a thermostat, initiating the shivering reflex. This causes muscles to contract, generating heat. Shivering caused by cold usually disappears as soon as the body is warmed.

Shivering during rigors and fever is caused by the release of certain substances by the white blood cells. The substances effectively "reset" the thermostat at a higher point, causing the body to shiver when it needs to lose, rather than retain, heat. The trigger for this release is usually an infection, but fever also occurs in some metabolic, autoimmune, and malignant diseases, and as a side effect of certain types of drugs.

## Shock
A dangerous reduction of blood flow throughout the body tissues that, if untreated, may lead to collapse, coma, and death. Shock in this sense is physiological shock—different from the mental distress (*posttraumatic stress disorder*) that may follow a physically or emotionally traumatic experience. Reduced blood pressure is, in most cases, a major factor in causing physiological shock and is one of its main features.

### CAUSES
Shock is a common accompaniment to severe injury or illness. It may develop in any situation in which blood volume is reduced (through blood or fluid loss), in which blood vessels are abnormally widened, in which the heart's action is weak, in which blood flow is obstructed, or through a combination of these factors. Causes include severe *bleeding* or *burns*, persistent *vomiting* or *diarrhea*, *myocardial infarction* (heart attack), *pulmonary embolism* (blockage of blood flow to the lungs), *peritonitis* (inflammation of the abdominal cavity, often due to perforation of an organ), *spinal injury*, and some types of *poisoning*. *Septic shock* results from bacteria multiplying in the blood and releasing toxins. *Anaphylactic shock* is a type of severe *hypersensitivity* or allergic reaction to an injected substance, such as insect venom or sometimes a drug. Shock is made worse by pain and anxiety.

### SYMPTOMS AND TREATMENT
Symptoms of all types of shock include rapid, shallow breathing; cold, clammy skin; rapid, weak pulse; dizziness; weakness; and fainting.

First aid for shock after an injury includes measures to arrest bleeding (see *Bleeding, treatment of*), maintenance of an open airway, keeping the victim flat, reducing heat loss with blankets, and reassurance. A physician or ambulance should be called

## FIRST AID: SHOCK

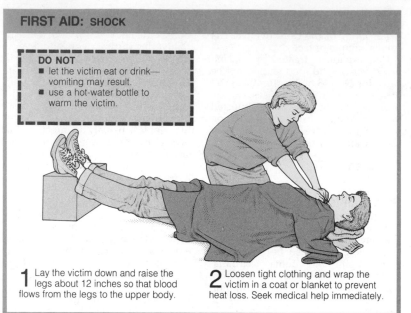

**DO NOT**
- let the victim eat or drink—vomiting may result.
- use a hot-water bottle to warm the victim.

**1** Lay the victim down and raise the legs about 12 inches so that blood flows from the legs to the upper body.

**2** Loosen tight clothing and wrap the victim in a coat or blanket to prevent heat loss. Seek medical help immediately.

immediately; in the interim, no alcohol or food should be given. Emergency treatment in the hospital involves an *intravenous infusion* of fluid or a blood transfusion, *oxygen therapy*, and, if necessary, morphine or similar powerful painkillers. Further treatment depends on the underlying cause. (See also *Toxic shock syndrome; Shock, electric*.)

## Shock, electric

The sensation caused by an electric current passing through the body and its effects and aftereffects. A mild shock may produce a sense of having been slightly shaken. A current of an appreciable size and duration can cause loss of consciousness, cardiac arrest (cessation of the heart beat), respiratory arrest, burns, and tissue damage. (See *Electrical injury*.)

## Shock therapy

The use of electricity or other agents to produce a sudden and severe disturbance in the nervous system as a means of treating mental illness, particularly severe *depression*. The mechanism of action is unknown.

Only *ECT* (electroconvulsive therapy) is regularly used today. Insulin coma therapy (in which coma was induced by repeated injections of insulin) was a form of shock therapy used in the 1940s and 1950s; it was abandoned because of the risk of permanent, severe brain damage. Another earlier method, involving

the use of drugs to stimulate the nervous system, was abandoned because patients often suffered injuries due to violent seizures.

## Short stature

A height markedly below the average for a person's age.

### CAUSES

In developed countries, restricted growth in children is usually due to heredity factors or to slow bone growth that eventually speeds up, resulting in normal development. Much less commonly, short stature has an abnormal cause, such as a specific growth disorder. The most common types are *growth hormone deficiency*; thyroid hormone deficiency (see *Hypothyroidism*), which also affects brain development; and *achondroplasia*, a hereditary disorder in which primarily the ends of the long bones fail to grow, resulting in disproportionately short limbs.

In certain other disorders, restricted growth occurs as one of several features. Such disorders include those that impair absorption of nutrients, vitamins, or minerals, such as *cystic fibrosis* and *celiac sprue*; chronic infections, such as *tuberculosis*; chronic *asthma*; chromosomal disorders, such as *Down's syndrome* and *Turner's syndrome*; and metabolic disorders, such as *phenylketonuria*.

Other causes of restricted growth in children include certain drugs, particularly *corticosteroid drugs* and *anti-*

*cancer drugs*. Undernourishment and emotional deprivation, both common in abused or neglected children, can also cause short stature.

### INVESTIGATION

The physician takes into account the parents' height and looks for signs of any possible underlying disease.

Most importantly, the child's growth rate is determined by means of regular measurements of height plotted on a chart. If the growth rate is normal, it indicates that the child's short stature is probably due to heredity or to temporary slow skeletal development. Slow growth rate suggests that short stature has an abnormal cause. A sudden drop in growth rate can indicate the onset of disease such as a glandular disorder (e.g., of the thyroid gland).

Other tests may include *X rays* to determine bone age (see *Age*) and *blood tests* to measure hormone levels. More testing is done to ascertain whether the cause is *failure to thrive*.

### TREATMENT

Any underlying disorder is treated. Growth hormone is given not only for growth hormone deficiency but also to treat short stature due to Down's syndrome or Turner's syndrome; it is sometimes given in combination with the anabolic steroid *oxandrolone*. (See also *Growth, childhood*.)

## Shoulder

The area of the body where the arm attaches to the trunk. The rounded bony surface at the front of the shoulder is the upper part of the *humerus* (upper arm bone); the bony surfaces that form the top and back of the shoulder are parts of the *scapula* (shoulder blade). The *clavicle* (collarbone) articulates with the acromion (the bony prominence at the outer top part of the scapula) at the *acromioclavicular joint* and extends across the top of the chest to the *sternum* (breastbone), to which it is attached at the sternoclavicular joint.

Just below the acromion, on the outer wall of the scapula, is a socket (called the glenoid cavity) into which the head of the humerus fits to form the shoulder joint. A *bursa* (fluid-filled sac) under the acromion reduces friction at the joint. The shoulder joint is a ball-and-socket joint with a wide range of movement produced by part of the *biceps muscle*, several small muscles that make up the *rotator cuff*, various muscles in the chest wall, and the *deltoid* muscle (the muscle at the top of the upper arm and shoulder).

S

## STRUCTURE OF THE SHOULDER

Three bones meet at the shoulder—the scapula (shoulder blade), clavicle (collar bone), and humerus (upper arm bone). The shoulder is an example of a ball-and-socket joint.

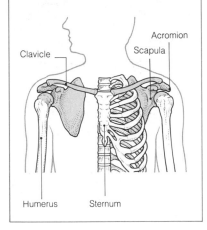

Clavicle

Acromion

Scapula

Humerus     Sternum

### DISORDERS

Shoulder injuries are relatively common, including dislocation of the shoulder joint (see *Shoulder, dislocation of*) or acromioclavicular joint, and *fractures* of the clavicle or the upper part of the humerus. Fractures of the scapula are less common.

The shoulder joint may be affected by any joint disorder, including *arthritis* and *bursitis* (inflammation of a bursa). In severe cases, a joint disorder may lead to *frozen shoulder* (in which movements at the joint are extremely restricted). Movement of the shoulder may also be painful and/or restricted as a result of *tendinitis* (inflammation of a tendon) that affects the tendons of the shoulder muscles. (See also *Bone* disorders box; *Joints*; *Painful arc syndrome*.)

## Shoulder blade

The common name for the *scapula*.

## Shoulder, dislocation of

Displacement of the head of the humerus (upper arm bone) out of the shoulder joint. The most common type of dislocation is a forward and downward displacement, caused by a fall onto an outstretched hand or onto the shoulder itself. A backward dislocation may occur as a result of a powerful direct blow to the front of the shoulder or as a result of violent twisting of the upper arm (such as that caused by an electric shock or seizure).

Either type of dislocation may be accompanied by a fracture, usually of the humerus (see *Humerus, fracture of*).

### SYMPTOMS AND DIAGNOSIS

The main symptom is pain in the shoulder and upper arm that is made worse by movement. A forward dislocation often produces obvious deformity of the shoulder; a backward dislocation usually does not.

A dislocation is diagnosed by X rays, which also reveal whether there is an accompanying fracture.

### TREATMENT

Treatment consists of reduction (maneuvering the head of the humerus back into the joint socket), which is usually performed using an anesthetic. After reduction, X rays are taken to ensure the head of the humerus has been correctly repositioned; the shoulder is then immobilized in a sling for about three weeks. When the humerus has been fractured, treatment is usually the same, although the arm may require a longer period of immobilization.

### COMPLICATIONS

A dislocation may damage nerves, which may cause weakness and numbness in the shoulder. Such nerve damage is usually temporary, with full recovery occurring within two to three months. Occasionally, a dislocation damages one of the arteries in the upper arm, causing pain and discoloration of the arm and hand. In severe cases, *arterial reconstructive surgery* may be necessary.

A violent dislocation may damage the muscles that support the shoulder, resulting in the joint being susceptible to recurrent dislocation after only minor injuries. These cases can often be successfully treated by a surgical operation to tighten one of the supporting muscles.

## Shoulder-hand syndrome

Pain and stiffness in the shoulder and hand of one side of the body; the affected hand may also become hot, sweaty, and swollen. Because of the pain and stiffness, the arm cannot be used properly and the arm muscles may wither as a result of lack of use.

The precise cause is unknown, but it may occur as a complication of *myocardial infarction* (heart attack), *stroke*, *herpes zoster* (shingles), or a burn or other injury to the shoulder.

In most cases spontaneous recovery occurs within about two years. This period may be shortened by *physical therapy* and treatment with *corticosteroid drugs*. In rare cases, a cervical

## DISLOCATION OF SHOULDER

In this injury, the rounded head of the humerus (upper arm bone) has been forced out of its socket just beneath the acromion (tip of the shoulder blade).

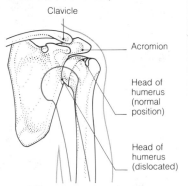

Clavicle

Acromion

Head of humerus (normal position)

Head of humerus (dislocated)

**Forward dislocation of left shoulder**
A forward and downward dislocation, as shown above, is the most common type.

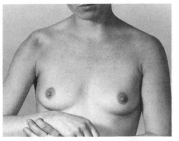

**Backward dislocation**
A pit can be seen in this woman's right shoulder where the head of the humerus is normally situated.

*sympathectomy* (severing of nerves of the sympathetic nervous system on one side of the neck) is performed.

## Shunt

An operation performed to relieve abnormal fluid pressure from excess fluid around the brain in *hydrocephalus* or in the portal veins in *portal hypertension*. A shunt between an artery and a vein is installed to provide easy access to the bloodstream for hemodialysis (see also *Arteriovenous fistula*).

### SHUNT FOR HYDROCEPHALUS

The shunt for hydrocephalus consists of two catheters and a valve to prevent backflow. The first catheter is inserted through the skull to drain fluid from the ventricles of the brain. The second is passed into another body cavity, usually the abdominal cavity or the right atrium of the heart, where the excess fluid is absorbed.

S

Problems with this procedure include the need to replace the catheter as a child grows and the need to revise the operation two or three times in the first 10 years. The shunt also may become blocked or infected.

**SHUNT FOR PORTAL HYPERTENSION**

A variety of surgical procedures is used to reduce pressure in the portal system (the veins that carry blood from the digestive organs and spleen to the liver) and thus reduce the risk of bleeding from *esophageal varices*. Shunts are made by creating a direct link between the portal system and the vena cava. Shunt operations prevent bleeding but do not improve liver function and, in fact, may worsen it. The operation itself carries a fairly high mortality that is related to the severity of the disease. Although bleeding is controlled, it is questionable whether survival is prolonged.

## Shy-Drager syndrome

A rare degenerative condition that causes progressive damage to the *autonomic nervous system*. The cause of Shy-Drager syndrome is unknown. It begins gradually, affecting people between the ages of 60 and 70, and occurs in more men than women.

The main symptoms are postural *hypotension* (dizziness and fainting when arising or after standing still for a long time), urinary incontinence, reduced ability to sweat, impotence, and *parkinsonism* (muscle tremor, rigidity, and slow movements). The condition worsens over several years, leading to disability and sometimes premature death.

Although there is no cure and no means of slowing the inevitable degeneration, many of the symptoms, particularly the parkinsonism and low blood pressure, can be relieved by drug treatment.

## SIADH

An abbreviation for syndrome of inappropriate antidiuretic hormone (secretion). SIADH is a rare condition in which there is excessive production of *ADH*, resulting in retention of water and a low level of sodium in the body.

**CAUSES**

SIADH may be associated with various underlying disorders, including cancers such as small cell carcinoma of the lung (see *Lung cancer*), cancer of the pancreas or duodenum, or *Hodgkin's disease*; certain lung diseases, such as *pneumonia* or chronic obstructive lung disease (see *Lung disease, chronic obstructive*); or brain dis-

orders, such as *encephalitis*, a brain hemorrhage, or brain damage that results in the pituitary gland overproducing ADH. In addition, certain drugs (such as *chlorpropamide* or *oxytocin*) may increase ADH production and lead to SIADH.

**SYMPTOMS AND DIAGNOSIS**

The symptoms of SIADH include weakness, tiredness, confusion, and weight gain due to excessive *edema*. The condition is diagnosed from the symptoms and from the results of tests that measure the level of ADH in the blood and compare the concentration of sodium in the blood and the urine.

**TREATMENT**

Treatment includes restriction of water intake, *diuretic drugs* to increase water loss, and saline infusions to increase the concentration of sodium in the body. However, these measures treat only the symptoms; the underlying cause must be treated successfully to bring about a cure.

## Siamese twins

Two babies that are born physically joined. Also called conjoined *twins*, they are named for the first recorded pair, Chang and Eng, who were born in Thailand (formerly Siam) in 1811 and lived for 63 years joined at the hip. Siamese twins are essentially identical twins that fail to develop normally from a single fertilized egg. The cause is unknown.

Siamese twins range from two well-developed individuals, connected only by skin and superficial tissue, to a person with only one extra body part (such as one leg) as evidence of the second twin. Between these extremes are Siamese twins with two heads and two trunks joined at the waist but with only two legs. In some cases one of the twins is very small and poorly developed. The internal organs and brains may be separate, or some or all may be shared.

**TREATMENT**

If the twins survive birth, and if each one is sufficiently developed to function independently, complete separation by surgery may be possible.

## Sibling rivalry

A term that describes the intense competition that is normal between siblings (brothers and/or sisters). An obvious example occurs after the birth of a new baby, when an older sibling constantly seeks to command the parents' attention. Feelings of rivalry may persist through life.

## Sick building syndrome

A collection of symptoms sometimes reported by people who work in modern office buildings; the symptoms include loss of energy, headaches, and dry, itching eyes, nose, and throat.

The cause of the syndrome is unknown, although it has been attributed to air conditioning, fluorescent lighting, loss of natural ventilation and light, and psychological factors, especially frustration at being unable to control physical conditions (such as temperature and ventilation) in the working environment. Some authorities believe that many outbreaks of sick building syndrome may be *pseudoepidemics* (conditions without physical causes that are thought to be a form of *hysteria*).

Treatment using environmental agents, such as ionizers, has been unsuccessful. Modification to the building may be the only solution if a large proportion of the work force is affected and the syndrome is thought not to be a pseudoepidemic.

## Sickle cell anemia

 An inherited blood disease that occurs primarily in blacks and, less commonly, in individuals of Mediterranean origin. In sickle cell anemia, the red cells are abnormal, resulting in a chronic, very severe form of *anemia* (reduced oxygen-carrying capacity of the blood).

**CAUSE**

The red cells of affected people contain an abnormal type of *hemoglobin* (oxygen-carrying pigment) called hemoglobin S. In the blood capillaries, where blood is less oxygenated, the deficiency of oxygen causes hemoglobin S to crystallize, distorting the red cells into a sickle shape. This makes the cells fragile; they are easily destroyed, leading to hemolytic anemia. Also, the abnormal cells are unable to pass easily through tiny blood vessels, so they may intermittently block blood flow to various organs, causing sickle cell crises.

Sickle cell anemia occurs in a person who has inherited hemoglobin S from both parents. If hemoglobin S is inherited from one parent, the person has sickle cell trait and is usually free of symptoms. If two such carriers have a child, there is a 1 in 4 chance that the child will have sickle cell anemia, a 2 in 4 chance that the child will have sickle cell trait, and a 1 in 4 chance that the child will have neither.

S

## INCIDENCE

In the US, about 150 black children in every 100,000 suffer from sickle cell anemia. About one in 12 blacks has sickle cell trait.

## SYMPTOMS AND SIGNS

The symptoms of sickle cell anemia usually first appear after 6 months of age. Chronic hemolytic anemia causes fatigue, headaches, shortness of breath on exertion, pallor, and *jaundice*. Sickle cell crises are sometimes brought on by an infection, cold weather, or dehydration caused, for example, by prolonged vomiting and diarrhea. However, the crises may also occur for no apparent reason. They start suddenly and attack or damage various parts of the body. The sufferer may experience pains (especially in bones), blood in the urine (from kidney damage), or damage to the lungs or intestines. The brain may also be affected, leading to *seizures*, a *stroke*, or unconsciousness.

In some children, the spleen enlarges and traps red cells at a particularly high rate, causing a severe, life-threatening form of anemia. From adolescence onward, the spleen usually shrivels and ceases to function; as a result, the person is at risk of *septicemia* (blood poisoning) if infected by certain types of bacteria.

Children with sickle cell anemia have an increased risk of pneumococcal *pneumonia*, for which prophylactic penicillin has been beneficial. There is also an increased risk of *gallstones*.

## DIAGNOSIS

The diagnosis is made from examination of a specially treated *blood smear* for the presence of sickle-shaped red cells and from *electrophoresis* to check for the presence of hemoglobin S.

## TREATMENT

There is no cure for the disease. Chronic hemolytic anemia is treated with a lifelong course of folic acid supplements. Affected children should be immunized with pneumococcal vaccine and adolescents and adults may be advised to take penicillin to guard against septicemia.

Because sickle cell crises can be life-threatening, they require prompt treatment. *Intravenous infusions* of fluids are given for dehydration, *antibiotic drugs* are given to treat and prevent infections, *oxygen therapy* is carried out to increase blood oxygenation, and *analgesic drugs* are given to relieve severe pain.

If a severe crisis does not respond to the above measures, an exchange *blood transfusion* may be performed to effect a temporary replacement of hemoglobin S. This may be done regularly for people who suffer frequent severe crises. Exchange transfusions may be carried out during pregnancy to reduce the risk of a crisis (with possibly fatal consequences for mother and child) and before surgery, since anesthesia presents a hazard to patients who have sickle cell anemia (and, to a lesser degree, to those with sickle cell trait).

## OUTLOOK

Until about 30 years ago, sickle cell anemia usually proved fatal in childhood. Today, although the mortality is still high in those under 5, improving methods of treatment have enabled more sufferers to survive into adulthood; some are having children.

Blacks and relatives of anyone with sickle cell anemia are advised to have a blood test to determine whether or not they carry the sickle cell gene. A couple, both of whom have sickle cell anemia and/or trait, should obtain *genetic counseling* before starting a family. Tests can be performed in early pregnancy to determine whether a fetus has inherited a double dose of the sickle cell gene.

# Sick sinus syndrome

Abnormal function of the sinoatrial node (the heart's pacemaker) that leads to episodes of *bradycardia* (slow heart rate), alternating bradycardia and *tachycardia* (fast heart rate), or very short episodes of cardiac arrest (complete stoppage of the heart beat). The most common cause of sick sinus syndrome is *coronary heart disease*, but the condition can also be caused by a *cardiomyopathy*.

Symptoms include light-headedness, dizziness, fainting, and, occasionally, palpitations (awareness of the heart beat). The diagnosis is confirmed by a 24-hour *ECG* (*Holter monitor*) recording.

# Side effect

A reaction or consequence of medication or therapy that is additional to the desired effect. The term usually (although not always) refers to an unwanted or adverse effect. It is not usually applied to the toxic effects produced by a drug overdose, but to a secondary effect of a normal dose.

A side effect may occur as a result of the primary object of therapy continuing beyond its desired limits (e.g., when bleeding results from treatment with *anticoagulant drugs*). Alternatively, the side effect may be com-pletely unrelated, such as when drowsiness results from *antihistamine drugs* prescribed to alleviate allergic *rhinitis* (hay fever). However, an unwanted side effect in one circumstance may be a desired effect in another (drowsiness is the desired effect when antihistamines are used as sedatives).

The aforementioned unwanted side effects are examples of predictable effects; that is, they are expected from the known actions of a particular drug and occur in most patients taking that drug. These side effects are known as type I effects. Type II side effects occur in a minority of patients and are usually unpredictable—until the physician discovers the connection between a particular drug and a patient's idiosyncratic response to it. Type II effects may be caused by factors in the patient, such as a genetic disorder (e.g., the lack of a specific enzyme that usually inactivates the drug) or an allergic reaction. Common type II side effects include a rash, swelling of the face, or jaundice. The occurrence of a type II side effect usually necessitates withdrawal of the drug. (See also *Drug*.)

# Siderosis

Any of a variety of conditions in which there is too much iron in the body. Excess iron in the blood or tissues without associated damage is usually called *hemosiderosis*.

# SIDS

An abbreviation for *sudden infant death syndrome*.

# Sievert

The SI unit of equivalent absorbed dose of ionizing radiation (see *Radiation* units box).

# Sight

See *Vision*.

# Sight, partial

Loss of vision short of total *blindness*. Partial sight may involve a loss of *visual acuity*, of *visual field*, or of both.

# Sigmoid colon

Also known as the pelvic colon, the S-shaped part of the *colon* in the lower abdomen that extends from the brim of the pelvis, usually down to the third segment of the *sacrum* (the triangular bone immediately below the lumbar vertebrae). The sigmoid colon is connected to the descending colon above and the rectum below.

S

## Sigmoidoscopy

Examination of the rectum and the sigmoid colon (last part of the large intestine) with a viewing instrument called a sigmoidoscope or proctosigmoidoscope (see *Endoscopy*).

**WHY IT IS DONE**

Sigmoidoscopy is performed to investigate symptoms such as bleeding from the rectum or lower colon and to inspect the passage for evidence of disorders such as polyps (small benign growths), *ulcerative colitis*, or cancer (see *Intestine, cancer of*). Attachments on the end of the instrument allow the physician to perform a *biopsy* (removal of a small sample of tissue for analysis) if necessary.

Sigmoidoscopy is usually performed as a followup to a rectal examination, in which the physician examines the rectum by inserting a gloved finger. Sigmoidoscopy may also be preceded by *proctoscopy* (examination of the anal canal and rectum with a viewing instrument).

**HOW IT IS DONE**

The procedure for sigmoidoscopy, along with a typical view through a sigmoidoscope, is shown in the illustrated box at right.

## Sign

An objective indication of a disease or disorder (e.g., *jaundice*) that is observed or detected by a physician, as opposed to a *symptom* (e.g., pain), which is noticed by the patient.

## Silicone

Any of a specific group of silicon compounds. Silicones are defined as polymeric (long-chain), organic (carbon-containing) compounds of silicon and oxygen. They exist and are used medically in the form of oils, greases, plastics, or rubbers.

Synthetic silicones are widely used as implants in *cosmetic surgery* because they are resistant to body fluids, permeable to oxygen, and are not rejected by the body. Silicone oil in a silicone rubber bag is used in breast reconstruction or breast enlargement (see *Mammoplasty*).

## Silicosis

A lung disease caused by the inhalation of dusts containing silica—a common mineral found in sand, quartz, and various types of rock. (See *Pneumoconiosis*.)

## Silver nitrate

An *astringent* used to prevent a serious form of *conjunctivitis* in the newborn (ophthalmia neonatorum). Silver nitrate may also be used on dressings for burns and wounds.

Silver nitrate may cause irritation or pain and, if used over long periods, may result in a permanent blue-black discoloration of the skin.

## Silver sulfadiazine

An *antibacterial drug* applied in a cream to prevent infection in burns or after *skin graft*. Possible adverse effects are an allergic reaction, causing a burning sensation, rash, or itching. In rare cases, long-term use may produce serious blood disorders (symptoms of which may include sore throat, fever, or jaundice) or kidney damage.

## Simethicone

A drug used on its own or combined with *antacid drugs* to relieve *flatulence*. Simethicone is also used to disperse gas bubbles in the stomach before *gastroscopy* (examination of the stomach with a viewing tube) is performed by a physician. There are no known adverse effects.

## Sinew

A common nonmedical term for a *tendon*, a tough fibrous cord that joins a muscle to a bone.

## Singers' nodes

Small, grayish-white lumps that develop on the vocal cords as the result of constant voice strain. They occur in singers, schoolteachers, politicians, and other people who use their voices excessively, causing hoarseness or loss of voice.

A *biopsy* (removal of a small sample of tissue for microscopic examination) may be performed to rule out a malignant tumor (see *Larynx, cancer of*). Treatment consists of removal of the nodules and voice training.

---

## PROCEDURE FOR SIGMOIDOSCOPY

This is an office procedure taking less than half an hour and needing no anesthetic. Either a rigid or a flexible endoscope (viewing tube) may be used. An *enema* may be used beforehand. The patient lies on the left side with knees drawn up. The entry of the lubricated instrument causes little discomfort.

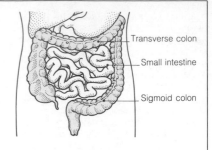

Transverse colon

Small intestine

Sigmoid colon

**View through sigmoidoscope**

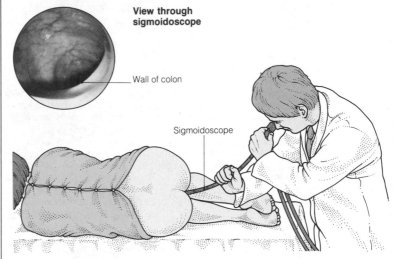

Wall of colon

Sigmoidoscope

**Value of sigmoidoscopy**

If the bowel is properly cleared of feces beforehand and distended by air pumped in through the instrument, a good view of the lining of the rectum and lower colon may be obtained. This area is often affected by benign growths, ulcers, or cancer. Direct observation of disorders allows early diagnosis and treatment.

S

## Sinoatrial node

The heart's natural pacemaker. The sinoatrial node consists of a cluster of specialized muscle cells within the wall of the right atrium (upper chamber) of the heart. Without any external influence, these cells emit electrical impulses at a rate of 100 per minute, which initiate the contractions (beats) of the heart. Various hormones and nervous system activity can affect the node, causing it to emit impulses at a different rate, thus slowing down or speeding up the heart. (See also *Heart rate*.)

## Sinus

A cavity within a bone, in particular one of the mucous membrane-lined, air-filled spaces in the bones surrounding the nose (see *Sinus, facial*).

The term sinus also refers to any wide channel that contains blood, such as the venous sinuses in the outermost covering of the brain.

Sinus is also a term for an abnormal, often infected, tract.

## Sinus bradycardia

A slow, but regular, heart rate (less than 60 beats per minute). Sinus bradycardia is caused by reduced electrical activity in the sinoatrial node (the heart's pacemaker). Unlike *heart block*, there is no impairment to the transmission of electrical impulses through the heart.

Sinus bradycardia is normal in athletes and in people who exercise regularly; it can be achieved by relaxation techniques.

Sinus bradycardia may also be caused by *hypothyroidism*, a *myocardial infarction* (heart attack), or drugs such as beta-blockers or digoxin.

## Sinus, facial

Any of the mucous membrane-lined, air-filled cavities in the bones surrounding the nose. The facial sinuses comprise the two frontal sinuses in the frontal bone of the forehead just above the eyebrows; the two maxillary sinuses in the cheekbones; the two ethmoidal sinuses, honeycomblike cavities in bones that lie between the nasal cavity and the eye sockets; and the sphenoidal sinuses, a collection of air spaces in the large, winged bone behind the nose that forms the central part of the base of the skull. Mucus drains from each sinus along a narrow channel that opens into the nose.

Infection, usually spreading from the nose, may cause *sinusitis* (inflammation of the lining of the sinuses).

### LOCATION AND FUNCTION OF THE SINOATRIAL NODE

The sinoatrial (SA) node is a small mass of muscle cells in the right atrium of the heart. It sends out impulses at an inherent rate of over 100 impulses per minute. External control, mainly by the vagus nerve, reduces the rate to about 70 per minute at rest.

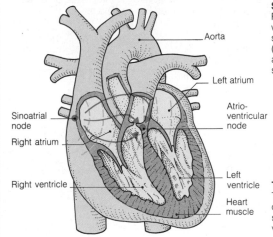

**Spread of the impulse**
From the SA node, the waves of contraction spread over both atria (pink area) and then to the atrioventricular node serving the ventricles.

Wave of excitation spreading over atria

Excitation spreading over ventricles

**The electrocardiogram**
The spread of excitation over the two atria is fairly slow; the spread over the ventricles is rapid.

## Sinusitis

Inflammation of the membrane lining the facial *sinuses* (the air-filled cavities in the bones surrounding the nose) caused by infection. The ethmoidal sinuses, between the eyes, and the maxillary sinuses, in the cheekbones, are commonly affected.

**CAUSES AND INCIDENCE**
Most sinusitis is caused by infection spreading to the sinuses from the nose along the narrow passages that drain mucus from the sinuses into the nose. The disorder is usually the result of a bacterial infection that develops as a complication of a viral infection, such

### LOCATION OF SINUSES

The air spaces, or sinuses, in the skull bones lighten the skull and improve the resonance of the voice. The sinuses surround and drain into the nose, although the position of the outlets is not always ideal for free drainage.

**Cross section through skull**

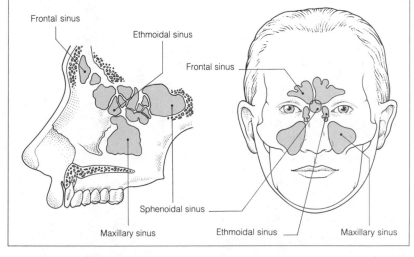

S

as the common *cold*. Less commonly, infection may arise from an abscess in an upper tooth (see *Abscess, dental*), from infected water being forced into the sinuses when a person jumps feet first into water without covering the nose, or from a severe facial injury.

Sinusitis is extremely common; many people suffer an attack after every common cold. It seems that once the tendency to sinus infection is established, recurrence is more likely with each cold.

### SYMPTOMS AND SIGNS

Sinusitis usually causes a feeling of tension or fullness in the affected area and sometimes a throbbing ache. It may also result in fever, a stuffy nose, and loss of the sense of smell.

A common complication is the formation of pus in the affected sinuses, causing pain and a nasal discharge. Other rare complications include orbital cellulitis (see *Orbit*), *osteomyelitis*, and *meningitis*.

### DIAGNOSIS AND TREATMENT

X rays are sometimes taken to determine the location and extent of the disorder; a *culture* may be grown from a lavage (washing) of the maxillary sinus to identify the infective bacteria.

*Antibiotic drugs* are given immediately to combat the infection, but the antibiotic chosen may be changed after the result of the culture is known. *Decongestant* drops or a spray, by reducing inflammation of the mucous membranes, restores drainage of the sinuses. Steam inhalations moisten the secretions and are helpful in removing them. If sinusitis persists, surgical drainage of the affected sinuses (by creating a new opening in them) may be performed.

## Sinus tachycardia

A fast, but regular, heart rate (more than 100 beats per minute). Sinus tachycardia is caused by increased electrical activity in the sinoatrial node (the heart's pacemaker). It is normal during sudden stressful or anxious moments and during (and for a short time after) exercise. Persistent sinus tachycardia at rest may be caused by fever, *hyperthyroidism*, and other disorders. (See *Tachycardia*.)

## Situs inversus

An unusual condition in which the internal organs are situated in the mirror image of their normal positions. No treatment is required unless there is an associated abnormality of any of the organs, in which case surgery may be necessary. (See also *Dextrocardia*.)

S

## BONES OF THE SKELETON

There are two main parts to the skeleton—the axial and appendicular skeletons (shown below). Some parts, such as the skull and pelvis, consist of several fused or associated bones. The function of the skeleton is not merely mechanical; bones are active living structures that are constantly producing blood cells and interchanging minerals with the blood.

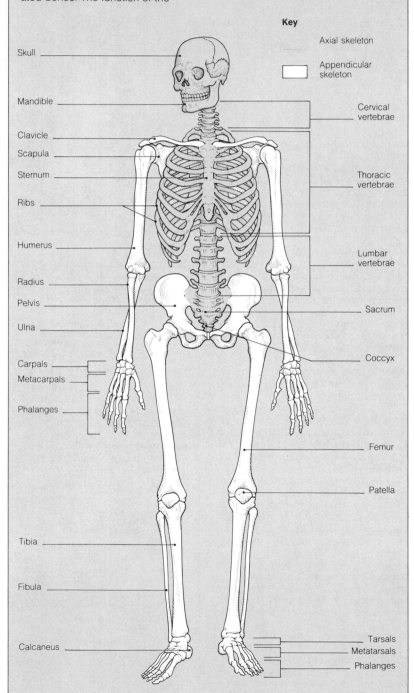

Key

Axial skeleton

Appendicular skeleton

Skull

Mandible

Clavicle

Scapula

Sternum

Ribs

Humerus

Radius

Pelvis

Ulna

Carpals

Metacarpals

Phalanges

Tibia

Fibula

Calcaneus

Cervical vertebrae

Thoracic vertebrae

Lumbar vertebrae

Sacrum

Coccyx

Femur

Patella

Tarsals

Metatarsals

Phalanges

## Sjögren's syndrome

A condition in which the eyes, mouth, and vagina become excessively dry. Sjögren's syndrome tends to occur with certain *autoimmune disorders*, such as *rheumatoid arthritis* or systemic *lupus erythematosus*. The exact cause is unknown. However, because the body's defense system is upset with the autoimmune disorder, it begins to destroy the glands that produce lubricating secretions.

Ninety percent of sufferers are women—mostly middle-aged and often postmenopausal.

The most characteristic and troublesome feature of the condition is *keratoconjunctivitis sicca* (dry eye), which causes itching and burning of the eyes and creates the sensation of a foreign body under the eyelid. Artificial tears can be used to moisten the eye. Lack of saliva leads to an increased risk of dental caries; good oral hygiene and dental care are therefore essential. A water-soluble lubricating jelly may be used to facilitate sexual intercourse.

## Skeleton

The average human adult skeleton has 206 *bones* joined with *ligaments* and tendons to form a protective and supportive framework for the attached muscles and underlying soft tissues of the body. In some people, however, there may be a variation in the number of vertebrae or there may be additional small bones (called sesamoids) in tendons around the joints.

### STRUCTURE

The skeleton consists of two main parts, known as the axial and appendicular skeletons. The axial skeleton comprises the *skull*, *spine*, *ribs*, and *sternum* (breastbone). Together, they represent a total of 80 bones—29 in the skull (including the *hyoid* bone and three pairs of auditory *ossicles*), 26 in the spine (seven cervical, 12 thoracic, and five lumbar *vertebrae*, the *sacrum*, and the *coccyx*), and 25 in the chest (12 pairs of ribs and the sternum).

The appendicular skeleton consists of the two limb girdles (the *shoulder* and *pelvis*) and their attached limb bones. The appendicular skeleton includes 126 bones, 64 in the shoulders and upper limbs and 62 in the pelvis and lower limbs. There are two bones in each shoulder—the *clavicle* (collarbone) and *scapula* (shoulder blade); three in each arm—the *humerus* (upper arm bone) and the *radius* and *ulna* (forearm bones); eight carpals in each *wrist*; five *metacarpals* in each palm; and 14 *phalanges* in the digits of each hand (two in each thumb and three in each finger).

The pelvic girdle consists of two innominate (hip) bones, and each of the lower limbs has 30 bones—a *femur* (thigh bone), *patella* (kneecap), and *tibia* and *fibula* (lower leg bones) in each leg; seven tarsals in the *ankle*, heel (see *Calcaneus*), and back part of the foot; five *metatarsals* in the middle of each foot; and 14 phalanges in the toes (two in each big toe and three in each other toe).

There are only minor differences between the skeletons of men and women. In general, men's bones tend to be slightly larger and heavier than the corresponding bones in women; the female pelvic cavity is wider to facilitate childbirth.

The individual bones of the skeleton are connected by three types of *joints*, which differ in the amount of mobility they permit through the various planes and ranges of movement.

### FUNCTION

The skeleton plays an indispensable role in movement by providing a strong, stable, yet mobile, framework on which the muscles can act. In effect, it consists of a series of independently movable internal levers on which the muscles can pull to move different parts of the body.

The skeleton also supports and protects body organs, notably the brain and spinal cord (which are encased in the skull and spine) and the heart and lungs (which are protected by the ribs). The ribs also make breathing possible by supporting the chest cavity so that the lungs are not compressed, and by helping in the breathing movements themselves.

The skeleton is not an inert frame, however. It is an active organ that produces blood cells (formed in bone marrow) and acts as a reservoir for minerals such as calcium, which can be drawn on, if required, by other parts of the body.

## Skin

The outermost covering of body tissue, which protects the internal organs from the environment. The skin is the largest organ in the body. Its cells are continually being replaced as they are lost by wear and tear.

### STRUCTURE

The skin consists of a thin outer layer (the epidermis) and a thicker inner layer (the dermis). Beneath the dermis is the subcutaneous tissue, which contains fat. The *hair* and *nails* are extensions of the skin and are composed mainly of *keratin*, which is the main constituent of the outermost part of the epidermis.

---

## STRUCTURE OF SKIN

The skin consists essentially of two layers—dermis (true skin), which contains most of the living elements, and epidermis, which is a protective and disposable covering with a dead outer layer.

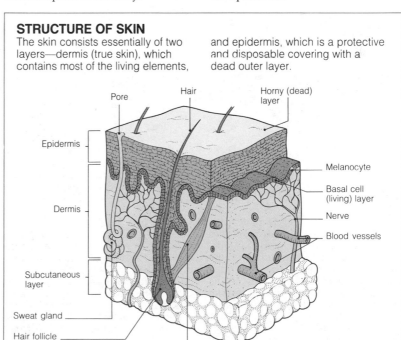

Pore · Hair · Horny (dead) layer · Epidermis · Dermis · Subcutaneous layer · Sweat gland · Hair follicle · Hair erector muscle · Melanocyte · Basal cell (living) layer · Nerve · Blood vessels

## DISORDERS OF THE SKIN

The skin is the largest and most vulnerable organ of the body. Although skin conditions are seldom life-threatening, many can be severely debilitating and cause psychological problems.

### CONGENITAL DISORDERS

A *birthmark* is a type of *nevus* (pigmented skin blemish) present from birth. Nevi include moles, freckles, *Mongolian spots*, and *hemangiomas*, such as port-wine stains and strawberry marks.

### INFECTION AND INFLAMMATION

Viral infections of the skin include *cold sores, warts, chickenpox, molluscum contagiosum,* and *herpes zoster* (shingles). Bacterial infections include *boils, cellulitis, erysipelas,* and *impetigo.* Fungal infections, such as *tinea,* cause *athlete's foot* and ringworm.

Inflammation of the skin occurs in *dermatitis* and *eczema;* it may be caused by an allergic reaction to a substance (such as nickel), a detergent, a plant, or a drug. *Psoriasis* is a common and persistent skin disease of unknown cause that consists of large, red patches with silvery, scaly surfaces. *Prickly heat* is an irritating rash that is caused by blockage of the sweat glands.

### TUMORS

Benign (noncancerous) tumors of the skin are extremely common; these include seborrheic *keratoses* and most types of nevi. *Bowen's disease* is a skin disorder that may slowly become cancerous. Three common forms of skin cancer are *basal cell carcinoma, squamous cell carcinoma,* and malignant melanoma (see *Melanoma, malignant*). Less common skin cancers include *Paget's disease of the nipple, mycosis fungoides,* and *Kaposi's sarcoma.*

### INJURY

The skin is vulnerable to many minor injuries, including cuts and bites (see *Bites, animal; Insect bites*) as well as more serious *wounds.* Burns can be among the most serious of all skin injuries and may cause extensive scarring or death.

### HORMONAL DISORDERS

*Acne* is partially related to the action of *androgens* on the sebaceous glands; it is common among adolescents.

### NUTRITIONAL DISORDERS

Deficiency of vitamins B and C can cause *rashes.*

### IMPAIRED BLOOD SUPPLY

*Leg ulcers,* which are particularly common in the elderly, may be caused by poor blood flow to the skin as a result of *atherosclerosis,* by poor drainage of blood through *varicose veins,* or by the leg swelling associated with heart failure.

### DRUGS

Many drugs, including antibiotics, barbiturates, and sulfonamides, may cause a rash. Some cause *urticaria* (hives), others cause *eczema* or a rash similar to the measles rash, and some cause *photosensitivity.*

### RADIATION

All forms of radiation are potentially damaging to the skin. Overexposure to sunlight (ultraviolet radiation) causes premature aging of the skin and increases the risk of skin cancer (see *Sunlight, adverse effects of*). High doses of other forms of radiation, such as X rays, may cause severe injury to the skin and may lead to cancer.

### AUTOIMMUNE DISORDERS

These disorders include *lupus erythematosus,* a disorder that may affect the skin alone or the skin and other organs; *vitiligo,* characterized by pure white patches and caused by destruction of the skin's pigment cells; *dermatomyositis,* which is characterized by a specific skin rash and muscle weakness; *morphea* and *scleroderma,* in which there is progressive hardening of the skin and other tissues; and *pemphigoid* and *pemphigus,* in which large blisters develop on the skin.

### OTHER DISORDERS

A *keloid* is an abnormally large and protruding *scar* caused by the continuing production of scar tissue long after healing would usually be complete. *Striae* (stretch marks) often develop during pregnancy and may also develop as a side effect of treatment with *corticosteroid drugs.*

*Erythema* simply means redness and has many possible causes. *Petechiae* are pinpoints of blood in the skin; in certain conditions, petechiae give rise to *purpura* or larger bruises.

*Xanthelasma* are yellowish patches that tend to occur on the eyelids; they are a result of the deposition of cholesterol.

### INVESTIGATION

Most skin disorders can be diagnosed from their physical characteristics. A skin *biopsy* (removal of a tissue sample for microscopic analysis) may also be performed, usually to aid in the diagnosis of a skin problem or to exclude skin cancer.

**EPIDERMIS** The epidermis is made up of flat cells that resemble paving stones when viewed under the microscope. Its thickness varies depending on the part of the body, being thickest on the soles and palms and very thin on the eyelids. It is generally thicker in men than in women and normally becomes thinner with age.

The outermost part of the epidermis is composed of dead cells, which form a tough, horny, protective coating. As these dead cells are worn away, they are replaced. The new cells are produced by rapidly dividing living cells in the innermost part of the epidermis. Between the outer and inner parts is a transitional region that consists of both living and dead cells.

Most of the cells in the epidermis are specialized to produce keratin, a hard protein substance that is the main constituent of the tough, outermost part of the epidermis. Some of the cells produce the protective pigment *melanin,* which determines skin color.

**DERMIS** The dermis is composed of connective tissue interspersed with various specialized structures, such as hair follicles, *sweat glands,* and *sebaceous glands,* that produce an oily substance called *sebum.* The dermis also contains blood vessels, lymph vessels, and nerves.

### FUNCTION

The skin's most important function is to protect. It acts as the main barrier between the environment and the internal organs of the body, shielding

S

them from injury, the harmful rays of sunlight, and invasion from infective agents, such as bacteria.

The skin is a sensory organ containing many cells that are sensitive to touch, temperature, pain, pressure, and itching. It also plays a role in keeping body temperature constant. When the body is hot, the sweat glands produce perspiration (which cools the body) and the blood vessels in the dermis dilate to dissipate the heat; if the body gets cold, the blood vessels in the skin constrict, which conserves the body's heat.

The epidermis contains a unique fatty substance that makes the skin waterproof—thus making it possible to sit in a bath without soaking up the water like a sponge. The outer epidermis also has an effective water-holding capacity, which contributes to its elasticity and serves to maintain the body balance of fluid and electrolytes. If the water content drops below a certain level, the skin becomes cracked, reducing its efficiency as a barrier.

## Skin allergy

A large number of substances can provoke an allergic reaction through direct contact with the skin of a susceptible person. However, the substance first must have sensitized the person's *immune system* during a previous contact or contacts. If the skin reaction is truly an allergic one, the causative substance produces symptoms only in susceptible people. Many substances that cause skin reactions (fiberglass spicules, for example) are irritant by nature, rather than allergenic, and can affect anyone, not just a sensitive few.

There are two main types of allergic skin reactions. Contact allergic *dermatitis* consists of red, itchy patches, which may blister or form crusts. The patches correspond to the area of contact with the causative substance and develop between a few hours and two days of contact. Substances that can produce such a reaction are adhesives, poison ivy, elastic, nickel in jewelry, some cosmetics, and chromium salts used in hat and shoe manufacture.

Contact *urticaria* (red, itchy, raised areas on the skin) may develop within a few minutes to half an hour of skin contact with some medications, chemicals, plants, insect saliva (from an insect bite), and foods such as shellfish. Urticaria can also be a symptom of an allergic reaction to something eaten, but the majority of cases of urticaria are probably not

allergic in origin. Many drugs can cause skin eruptions, some of which resemble urticaria. However, not all of them are allergic in nature (see *Rash*).

Atopic *eczema* is an itchy skin condition that is most common in babies and children, particularly those with a family history of allergic-type illnesses such as asthma. It does not seem to be caused by skin contact with an allergen, but in some cases may be the result of a food allergy.

In many skin allergies, the causative substance is obvious and contact with it should be minimized. In other cases, it may be difficult to know which ingredient (e.g., of a cosmetic) is the cause of allergy. The causative agent may be discovered only through exhaustive tests in which the skin is challenged by exposure to various suspected substances (see *Skin tests*).

## Skin and muscle flap

A surgical technique in which a section of skin and underlying tissue, sometimes including muscle, is

moved to cover an area from which skin and deeper tissue have been lost or damaged.

**WHY IT IS DONE**

Unlike a *skin graft*, a flap retains its blood supply—either by remaining attached at one end to the donor site or through reattachment of its blood vessels to vessels at the new site. This makes a flap particularly useful for covering an area (such as exposed bone or tendon) that has lost its blood supply and on which a graft would not "take." Flaps are also used for regions that require thick covering to protect them (e.g., bony prominences such as the hip). In addition, because flaps are less likely to contract than skin grafts, they are useful for releasing tension from scarred areas. Skin flaps may be preferable to skin grafts because healing is more reliable and cosmetic results are better.

**HOW IT IS DONE**

When the area to be covered is relatively small and there is sufficient skin nearby, the flap may be left

---

### TECHNIQUE FOR MOVING A SKIN AND MUSCLE FLAP

A flap of skin and muscle can be moved to a new site to replace tissue loss; if its blood supply is maintained, the flap will adhere well. Microsurgery to rejoin blood vessels facilitates the technique.

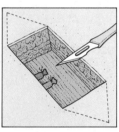 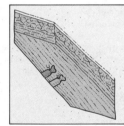 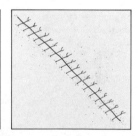

**1** The donor area needs a good blood supply if muscle is to be taken.

**2** The ends of the donor area need to be tapered to allow satisfactory closure.

**3** The skin may have to be undercut and freed before the wound is closed.

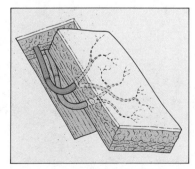 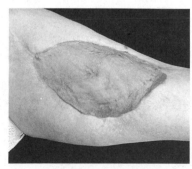

An artery and a vein of suitable size must be available at the recipient site to be joined to blood vessels in the flap.

Skin and muscle flaps are useful when there has been much loss of deep tissue. The results are usually excellent.

S

attached at one end and moved by stretching, rotating, or transposing it. Otherwise, the flap is removed from another area of the body and its vessels are attached to new arteries and veins at the site of the graft using microsurgical techniques (see illustrated box on previous page). The area left bare by cutting the flap is closed with stitches or, if necessary, by a skin graft. (See also *Microsurgery*.)

## Skin biopsy

Removal of a portion of diseased skin for laboratory analysis. Skin *biopsy* may be performed when *skin cancer* is suspected or to confirm the diagnosis of certain skin disorders (such as *pemphigus* or *dermatomyositis*).

Using a local anesthetic, the skin is removed with a *scalpel* or a *curet*. When a highly malignant condition (such as *melanoma*) is suspected, all of the affected area is cut away with skin around and beneath it. Otherwise, only a small portion of tissue is removed. The wound usually requires minimal stitching and leaves little or no scar.

## Skin cancer

A malignant tumor in the skin. Skin cancer is one of the most common forms of cancer.

*Basal cell carcinoma, squamous cell carcinoma,* and malignant *melanoma* are common forms of skin cancer related to long-term exposure to sunlight. *Bowen's disease,* a rare skin disorder that can become cancerous, also may be related to sunlight exposure.

Less common types of skin cancer include *Paget's disease of the nipple* and *mycosis fungoides*; both produce inflammation similar to that of eczema. *Kaposi's sarcoma* is a type of skin cancer commonly found in patients with *AIDS* (although elderly patients may have Kaposi's sarcoma and not have AIDS).

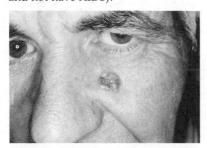

**Basal cell carcinoma**
This is the most common form of skin cancer. Also called rodent ulcer, it develops most often on the face.

Even though most skin cancers can be easily cured if treated early, many people die because they delay seeking treatment, especially from squamous cell carcinoma and malignant melanoma. Changed or new growths should be reported to a physician.

## Skin graft

A technique used in plastic surgery to repair areas of lost or damaged skin. A piece of healthy skin is detached from one part of the body and transferred to the affected area. New cells grow from the graft and cover the damaged area with fresh skin.

Skin taken from an identical twin can be used for a graft, but skin from another person or an animal is soon rejected by the recipient's body (although it may provide useful temporary cover).

**WHY IT IS DONE**
A skin graft is performed because the area is too large to be repaired by stitching or because natural healing would result in scarring that might be unsightly or restrict movement.

**TYPES**
There are two basic types of skin graft—split-thickness and full-thickness (see illustrated box below).

---

### TYPES OF SKIN GRAFT

The two main types of skin graft are split-thickness (in which less than the full thickness of skin is removed) and full-thickness. There are advantages to each of these types.

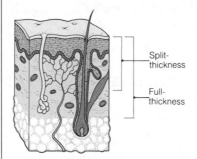

Split-thickness

Full-thickness

**Split-thickness graft**
When large areas need to be covered, such as after burns, split-thickness grafts are used and the donor sites are left to regenerate, which they do in a few days. Such sites can be repeatedly harvested.

**Full-thickness graft**
Full-thickness skin grafts are usually preferred for the face because they more closely approximate the appearance of normal skin. However, donor sites are limited and must be sutured (stitched).

---

### HOW A FULL-THICKNESS GRAFT IS DONE

Most skin grafts are performed using general anesthesia. Full-thickness grafts are easily cut with a scalpel. Subcutaneous fat is avoided and any bleeding at the recipient site prevented.

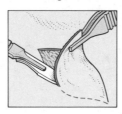 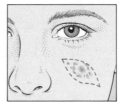 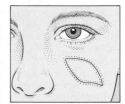

**1** Skin for a full-thickness graft is often taken from behind the ear.

**2** The graft must be larger than the area to be covered, to allow for shrinkage.

**3** Precise fitting and firm pressure are needed to ensure there is a satisfactory "take."

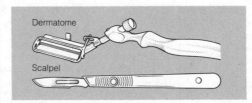

Dermatome

Scalpel

**Instruments**
Split-skin grafts are cut, usually from the abdomen or thigh, with an instrument called a dermatome. If necessary, the skin can be expanded into a trellislike mesh on the donor site.

S

In some cases, underlying muscle is removed with the full thickness of skin (see *Skin and muscle flap*).

**HOW IT IS DONE**

Most grafts are done by removing skin from the donor site and transferring it to the recipient site (see box).

**RESULTS**

All grafts leave scars. Full-thickness grafts yield more natural color and texture and contrast less than split-thickness grafts. However, full-thickness grafts are less likely to take.

## Skin infections

See *Skin* disorders box.

## Skin peeling, chemical

A cosmetic operation to remove freckles, acne scars, delicate wrinkles, or other surface skin blemishes. A paste containing phenol (carbolic acid) or some other caustic agent is applied to the skin, left for a half hour, and then scraped off. The outer layers of the skin peel away with the paste, thus removing the blemishes.

Because of *photosensitivity*, the raw area must not be exposed to sunlight until new skin layers have fully grown. Permanent discoloration of the skin is common; it may be improved by wearing makeup.

## Skin tag

A small, brown or flesh-colored, protruding flap of skin caused by unsatisfactory healing of a wound or occurring spontaneously. Anal tags often occur as a complication of *anal fissures* or hemorrhoids. Skin tags usually can be removed.

## Skin tests

Procedures for determining the body's reaction to various substances by injecting a small quantity of the substance underneath the skin or by applying it to the skin.

Patch tests are widely used in the diagnosis of contact allergic *dermatitis* (a type of skin allergy). Various suspected substances are applied by means of adhesive patches to the skin. After a specific period of time, the patches are removed and the reactions observed. If one substance has caused reddening or blistering, the person is probably allergic to the substance and should avoid it in the future.

Substances injected under the skin may help identify allergens responsible for *asthma*, allergic *rhinitis* (hay fever), or other allergic-type illnesses, even though skin symptoms are not one of the primary features of these conditions. The tests may also be used to test immunity to certain infectious diseases (such as in the *tuberculin test*).

## Skin tumors

A growth on or in the skin that may or may not be cancerous (see *Skin cancer*).

Very common types of benign (noncancerous) skin tumors include *keratoses* (wartlike growths caused by overproduction of keratin) and squamous *papillomas* (small, raised, flesh-colored growths).

Other benign skin tumors include *sebaceous cysts*, cutaneous *horns* (hard protrusions from the skin), *kerato-acanthomas* (rapidly growing, flesh-colored nodules), and *hemangiomas* (birthmarks formed by a collection of blood vessels in the skin).

## Skull

The bony skeleton of the head. The skull has several functions. It encases and protects the brain, houses organs of the special senses, provides points of attachment for muscles of the head and neck, and helps form the first parts of the respiratory and digestive tracts. Many of the bones are hollow, reducing the weight of the skull and adding to the resonance of the voice.

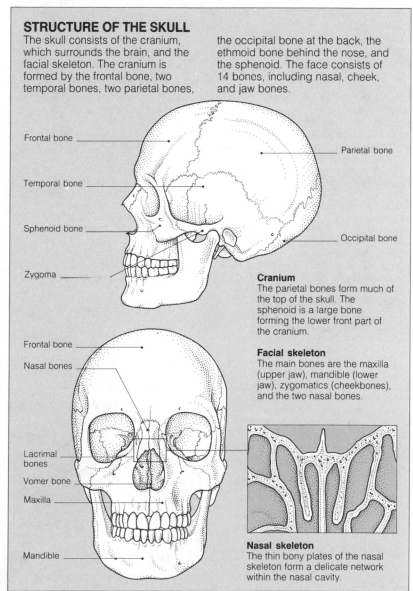

**STRUCTURE OF THE SKULL**

The skull consists of the cranium, which surrounds the brain, and the facial skeleton. The cranium is formed by the frontal bone, two temporal bones, two parietal bones, the occipital bone at the back, the ethmoid bone behind the nose, and the sphenoid. The face consists of 14 bones, including nasal, cheek, and jaw bones.

Frontal bone
Temporal bone
Sphenoid bone
Zygoma
Parietal bone
Occipital bone

Frontal bone
Nasal bones
Lacrimal bones
Vomer bone
Maxilla
Mandible

**Cranium**
The parietal bones form much of the top of the skull. The sphenoid is a large bone forming the lower front part of the cranium.

**Facial skeleton**
The main bones are the maxilla (upper jaw), mandible (lower jaw), zygomatics (cheekbones), and the two nasal bones.

**Nasal skeleton**
The thin bony plates of the nasal skeleton form a delicate network within the nasal cavity.

S

## STRUCTURE

The arrangement of the bones in the skull is shown in the illustrated box on the previous page. All the skull bones, except the mandible, are fixed to each other by immovable joints called sutures. The mandible articulates with the temporal bones at the freely movable temporomandibular joints.

Closely associated with, but not strictly part of, the skull are the hyoid (a small bone in the back of the tongue) and the auditory ossicles (the three tiny bones in each middle ear).

The skull contains several cavities, including the cranial cavity (which houses the brain), the nasal cavity (which is involved in smell and breathing), and the orbits (which house the eyeballs and their associated muscles). Part of the mouth is also formed by the skull.

Several of the skull bones, notably the maxillas, sphenoid bone, frontal bone, and ethmoid bone, contain *sinuses* (air-filled spaces); these sinuses are called the paranasal sinuses. In addition, there are spaces in the temporal bones that house the structures of the middle and inner ear.

In the cranium are many holes (called foramens) for the passage of nerves and blood vessels. Passing through are the *cranial nerves* (which supply most of the sensory structures and muscles of the head and neck) and blood vessels such as the *carotid arteries* and *jugular veins* (which carry blood to and from the brain). The largest of the holes, the foramen magnum, is situated in the occipital bone (which forms part of the base and back of the cranium); this hole allows the brain stem to enter the spinal canal, where it continues as the spinal cord.

The skull rests on the first cervical vertebra (called the atlas), a ring-shaped bone that articulates with the occipital bone and permits nodding movements of the head. Turning the head is a function of the joint between the atlas and the second cervical vertebra (axis). The occipital bone, atlas, and axis are connected by numerous small muscles.

## DISORDERS

The skull may be affected by any bone disorder (see *Bone* disorders box) that involves the skeleton, such as *Paget's disease*, but the most common disorder is injury. A blow to the head may cause a fracture (see *Skull, fractured*), which may result in damage to the brain, and, if a foramen is involved, in damage to a blood vessel or cranial nerve. (See also *Head injury*.)

# Skull, fractured

A break in one or more of the skull bones caused by a head injury. Because the skull is extremely strong, most fractures are closed and cause no complications. Closed fractures are also called simple fractures—that is, the bone is cracked without any displacement of the broken pieces. However, severe injury to the head may result in an open (also called depressed) fracture in which the bone fragments are displaced, usually inward. In this case, the blood vessels in the *meninges* (the membranes that cover the brain) may be ruptured, resulting in an epidural hemorrhage (bleeding into the space between the skull and the outer membrane) or a *subdural hemorrhage* (bleeding into the space between the outer and middle membranes). The resultant blood clot may press on and displace brain tissue. Less commonly, all the meninges may be torn, and the brain itself may be damaged.

## SYMPTOMS AND SIGNS

The degree of brain injury does not always correlate with damage to the skull. Severe brain injury can occur with no skull fracture and, in some cases of closed fracture, little or no brain injury may occur. The symptoms and signs of skull fractures (see *Head injury*) depend mainly on the degree of brain damage sustained. Leakage of cerebrospinal fluid (the liquid that bathes the brain and spinal cord) through the nose or ears indicates rupture of the meninges by an open fracture of the base of the skull.

## DIAGNOSIS AND TREATMENT

Any person who has suffered a significant blow to the head—particularly one that has caused unconsciousness—should consult a physician even if there are no symptoms. If the physician suspects a hemorrhage, *CT scanning* may be performed.

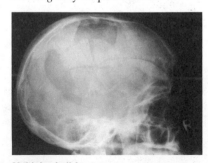

**Multiple skull fracture**
This side-view X ray shows the cranium smashed into several pieces. Some pieces have been surgically removed.

A person with a closed fracture is hospitalized and observed closely for 12 to 24 hours for signs of complications. If no signs develop, treatment is generally not necessary because the fracture usually heals by itself.

An open fracture often requires treatment by a neurosurgeon. A hemorrhage may necessitate a *craniotomy* to drain the blood and repair damaged vessels. When deeply depressed fractures have penetrated the meninges and brain tissue, an operation is performed to raise or remove the pieces of fractured bone and repair the damaged tissue. After such an operation, there can be some degree of skull distortion.

*Antibiotic drugs* are given for all open fractures because of the risk of infection of the meninges (see *Meningitis*) or of the brain itself (see *Encephalitis*).

# Skull X ray

A technique for providing images of the skull.

## WHY IT IS DONE

A skull X ray is usually taken after a *head injury* to look for a fracture (see *Skull, fractured*) or locate any foreign bodies in the soft tissues.

A normal skull X ray does not rule out significant brain injury. If such an injury is suspected, or if a skull fracture is found, *CT scanning* of the brain is also performed.

Skull X rays are also useful in evaluating a variety of conditions that affect the bones of the skull, such as *pituitary tumors* or metabolic disorders (such as *hyperparathyroidism*), and in evaluating tumors that have spread to the bones of the skull.

## HOW IT IS DONE

A skull X-ray examination is a procedure performed by an *X-ray technician*. It is not uncomfortable and, depending on the number of views taken, takes about 20 minutes. The films are interpreted by a *radiologist*.

# SLE

The abbreviation for the disorder systemic *lupus erythematosus*.

# Sleep

The natural state of lowered consciousness and reduced *metabolism*. Sleep consumes about one third of an average person's life.

## PHYSIOLOGY

*EEG* recordings of the electrical impulses produced by the brain during sleep show that there are two distinct types of sleep, known as REM (rapid eye movement) and NREM

S

(nonrapid eye movement) sleep. They alternate in cycles lasting roughly 90 minutes throughout the sleep period. NREM sleep, which accounts for the major part of sleep, starts with drowsiness; brain waves become increasingly deeper and slower until brain activity and metabolism fall to their lowest level. Dreams are infrequent.

In REM sleep, the brain suddenly becomes more electrically active (with a wave pattern resembling that of an awake person) and its temperature and blood flow increase. The eyes move rapidly and *dreaming*, often with elaborate story lines, occurs. REM sleep, also known as paradoxical sleep, periodically interrupts NREM sleep. The first REM period usually takes place 90 to 100 minutes after the onset of sleep and lasts about five to 10 minutes. REM sleep periods grow progressively longer as sleep continues; the last of a night's four or five REM sleep periods may last about an hour. REM sleep occupies about one half of sleep time in babies and about one fifth of sleep time in adults.

### FUNCTIONS OF SLEEP
Sleep is a fundamental human need, as is shown by the detrimental effects of *sleep deprivation*. However, it is not understood exactly in what way sleep is beneficial, or why a few, extremely rare individuals sleep very little yet suffer no ill effects. Apart from the obvious theory that the brain and metabolic processes require periodic rest to function efficiently, it has been suggested that dreaming is necessary to enable the brain to sort out information gathered during waking hours.

### SLEEP REQUIREMENTS
The need for sleep decreases with age. A 1-year-old baby requires about 14 hours of sleep a day, a child of 5 about 12 hours, and adults about seven to eight hours. These amounts can vary from person to person. Some adults need to sleep 10 hours or more a day, others function efficiently on half that amount or less. As people age, their ability to sustain sleep generally declines; the elderly get less sleep at night but doze more during the day than younger adults.

### SLEEP DISORDERS
More than 100 disorders of sleeping and waking have been identified. They are divided into four main categories—problems with falling or staying asleep (the *insomnias*), problems with staying awake, problems with adhering to a consistent sleep/wake schedule, and problems with sleep-disruptive behaviors.

Problems with falling or staying asleep trouble one in three adults in the US. Insomnias are classified as transient—lasting up to several nights, usually resulting from excitement or minor stress; short-term—lasting up to two or three weeks, related to major stress or illness; and chronic—frequent or continued poor sleep, a complex disorder with many causes, including physical illnesses, psychological factors, a poor sleeping environment, and life-style. Insomnia is not a disease; it is a symptom warranting medical attention.

Problems with staying awake are the prime reason people seek help at sleep disorders centers, of which more than 200 now exist in the US. The primary causes of this symptom are *sleep apnea*, a potentially life-threatening disorder in which breathing intermittently stops during sleep, and *nar-colepsy*, a disorder in which REM sleep intrudes into wakefulness, causing sudden daytime sleep "attacks."

Problems with a consistent sleep/wake schedule involve difficulty sleeping and difficulty staying awake as a result of disruptions of the internal clocks that regulate sleeping and waking. A common example is *jet lag*, in which body clocks are desynchronized by rapid travel across several time zones. Shift workers on rotating schedules, who frequently change their hours for work and sleep, commonly suffer "occupational jet lag." Shift workers, particularly those working at night, complain more about poor sleep and daytime drowsiness than do day workers.

Behaviors that interfere with sleep include *sleepwalking*, *night terrors* (partial awakening from sleep in a terrified state), and *enuresis* (bed-wetting).

---

## SLEEP PATTERNS

The brain does not rest when a person is sleeping, but there is some reorganization of activity within it.

EEGs (electroencephalograms) and other recordings reveal cyclical patterns to this activity.

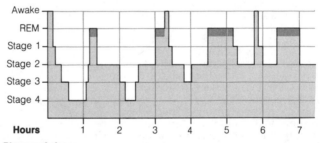

**Key**
REM sleep
NREM sleep

**Phases of sleep**
There are two types of sleep, REM (rapid eye movement) and NREM (nonrapid eye movement). They can be distinguished by the presence or absence of REMs and by EEGs or other recordings. The chart shows how a sleeper passes in cycles between the four stages of NREM sleep during the night, with bursts of REM sleep.

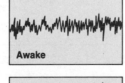
Awake

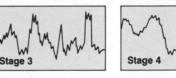
Stage 1

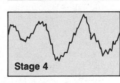
Stage 3

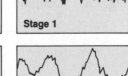
Stage 4

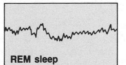
REM sleep

**REM sleep**
The EEG (left) shows high-frequency, low-voltage waves. People awakened during REM sleep often report dreams.

**NREM sleep**
This is sometimes called orthodox sleep; in adults it makes up about 80 percent of the sleeping pattern. It has four stages of progressively greater "depth" of sleep, characterized by EEG waves (left) of increasingly larger voltage (amplitude) and slower frequency (number of waves per second). People awakened during NREM sleep often report they were "thinking" about everyday matters but rarely report dreams.

S

# Sleep apnea

Episodes of cessation of breathing, lasting 10 seconds or longer, during sleep. Failure to breathe triggers the brain to reinitiate breathing. The wakeful arousals are so brief that they generally go unremembered in the morning. Rather than complaining of restless nights, people with severe sleep apnea typically complain of excessive sleepiness during the day. The sleepiness may be so profound that it disrupts work and social life, causing sleep at inappropriate times and contributing to motor vehicle accidents. Difficulty with concentration and memory also may occur.

Severe sleep apnea may induce high blood pressure, heart failure, heart attack, and stroke.

### INCIDENCE AND CAUSES

The most common and severe form of sleep apnea, obstructive sleep apnea, affects an estimated one in 100 men aged 30 to 50, most often overweight, heavy snorers. However, sleep apnea occurs in both sexes and all ages. It has been implicated in some cases of *sudden infant death syndrome* and becomes increasingly common with age.

In obstructive sleep apnea, the most frequent reason for difficulty is excessive relaxation during sleep of muscles of the soft palate at the base of the throat and the uvula (the small, conical, fleshy tissue hanging from the center of the soft palate). These sagging muscles obstruct the airway, making breathing labored and causing extremely loud snoring. If a complete blockage occurs, breathing stops and the sleeper falls silent. Pressure to breathe makes muscles of the diaphragm and chest work harder; opening of the blockage is signaled by a gasp and a brief arousal as breathing restarts. Obstructive sleep apnea may also be caused by enlarged tonsils and adenoids or individual anatomic differences such as a large tongue or small airway opening.

In another form of sleep apnea, central sleep apnea, the airway remains open but the diaphragm and chest muscles fail to work. Snoring may not occur. The fault is believed to lie in a disturbance in the brain's regulation of breathing during sleep.

People with sleep apnea commonly experience mixed apnea, in which a brief period of central apnea precedes a longer period of obstructive apnea. In mixed apnea, snoring is common.

### TREATMENT

Weight reduction helps those who are overweight, as is the case in the majority of people with severe sleep apnea. Alcohol should not be consumed within two hours of bedtime and *sleeping drugs* generally should not be used; both drugs slow the activity of breathing muscles and may contribute to a worsening of the disorder.

An effective treatment developed in recent years, continuous positive airway pressure, involves wearing a mask over the nose and mouth during sleep. Air from an air compressor is forced through the mask into nasal passages and into the airway to keep it open. Supplemental oxygen and the drug protriptyline benefit some people. Surgical procedures helpful in some cases include removal of excess tissue at the back of the throat, removal of enlarged tonsils or adenoids, and creation of an opening in the windpipe (*tracheostomy*), which permits air to flow directly to the lungs during sleep, bypassing the obstructed upper airway.

# Sleep deprivation

An insufficient amount of *sleep*. Studies of sleep-deprived volunteers have shown that irritability and a shortened attention span may occur after a night in which there was less than three hours' sleep.

After longer periods without sleep, individuals become increasingly unable to concentrate and their performance of tasks deteriorates as they continually slip into short periods of "microsleep." People with epilepsy are more prone to *seizures* after sleep deprivation. Three days or more without sleep may lead to visual and auditory *hallucinations* and, in some cases, *paranoia*.

Sleep deprivation has been employed in torture, to extract confessions, and as a brainwashing technique.

# Sleeping drugs

| COMMON DRUGS |
| --- |
| Barbiturates |
| *Secobarbital* |
| |
| Benzodiazepines |
| *Flurazepam Temazepam Triazolam* |
| |
| Others |
| *Chloral hydrate* |
| *Diphenhydramine* |
| *Glutethimide* |

A group of drugs used in the treatment of *insomnia*. Prescription sleeping drugs include *benzodiazepine drugs, barbiturate drugs, antihistamine drugs, antidepressant drugs,* and *chloral hydrate*. Certain antihistamines are sold as nonprescription sleep aids.

### WHY THEY ARE USED

Sleeping drugs are given to reestablish the habit of sleeping after self-help measures (e.g., a warm bath or drinking hot milk at bedtime) have not worked and after causes of insomnia, such as breathing disorders or abnormal leg muscle activity, have been ruled out. These drugs promote sleep by reducing nerve cell activity within the brain.

### HOW THEY ARE USED

Sleeping drugs always should be taken in the smallest effective dose for the shortest period of time. Generally, this means taking the drugs for no longer than three weeks and, preferably, not every night.

### POSSIBLE ADVERSE EFFECTS

The morning after a sleeping drug has been taken, a hangover effect (drowsiness and unsteadiness) may occur. It may impair concentration and the ability to operate machinery.

A sleeping drug may be dangerous if the person awakens during the night and gets out of bed. This poses a special danger to elderly people, who are more prone to falls than others. Use of sleeping drugs may induce *tolerance* and *dependence*.

Sleeping drugs may interact dangerously with alcohol and adversely with other drugs, including those used in the treatment of duodenal ulcers, heart disease, and depression. No sleeping drugs have been determined as safe for use in pregnancy.

# Sleeping sickness

A serious infectious disease of tropical Africa caused by the protozoan (single-celled) parasite *TRYPANOSOMA BRUCEI*. Sleeping sickness is spread by the bites of tsetse flies, which transmit the protozoa to people and animals. Within humans, the parasites multiply and spread to the bloodstream, lymph nodes, heart, and, eventually, the brain.

There are two forms of sleeping sickness. One, occurring in West and Central Africa, is spread primarily from person to person. The other occurs in East Africa and mainly affects wild animals, but is occasionally transmitted to humans.

Sleeping sickness is controlled by eradication measures directed against the tsetse fly. Nevertheless, tens of thousands of Africans—and some visitors to safari parks—still contract the disease each year.

S

## SYMPTOMS AND SIGNS

With both forms of sleeping sickness, a painful nodule develops at the site of the tsetse fly bite. In the West African form, the disease then takes a slow course, with bouts of fever and lymph gland enlargement. After months or years, spread to the brain occurs, causing headaches, confusion, and, eventually, severe lassitude. The victim may become completely inactive, have drooping eyelids, and a vacant expression (hence, sleeping sickness). Without treatment, coma and death follow. The East African form runs a faster course. A severe fever develops within a few weeks of infection; effects on the heart may be fatal before the disease has spread to the brain.

## DIAGNOSIS, TREATMENT, AND PREVENTION

Microscopic examination of the blood, lymph fluid withdrawn from a lymph gland, or cerebrospinal fluid obtained by a *lumbar puncture* reveals the presence of the parasites.

Drugs are effective against the parasites but may cause severe side effects. In most cases, a complete cure can be achieved, although there may be residual brain damage if the infection has already spread to the brain.

To avoid sleeping sickness, visitors to rural parts of Africa should take measures to protect themselves against tsetse fly bites (see *Insect bites*).

## Sleep paralysis

The sensation of being unable to move at the moment of going to sleep or when waking up. The experience may be accompanied by *hallucinations*, which often are frightening. Sleep paralysis most often occurs in people with *narcolepsy*, but occasionally it affects otherwise healthy people. Although alarming, the sensation rarely lasts for more than a few seconds. (See also *Cataplexy*.)

## Sleep terror

See *Night terror*.

## Sleepwalking

Walking while sleeping. Sleepwalking, also known as somnambulism, occurs during NREM (nonrapid eye movement) *sleep* and does not represent the acting out of dreams. It affects perhaps 5 percent of adults; probably 75 percent of children, especially boys, walk in their sleep at least once. Some people show a regular tendency to sleepwalk.

Usually the child calmly gets out of bed, wanders around aimlessly for a few minutes, and then goes back to

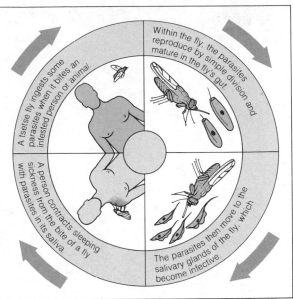

**CYCLE OF SLEEPING SICKNESS**
The life cycle of the trypanosomes that cause sleeping sickness is shown. They multiply in a person's blood and lymph vessels and may spread to the brain or heart with serious effects.

A tsetse fly ingests some parasites when it bites an infested person or animal.

Within the fly, the parasites reproduce by simple division and mature in the fly's gut.

A person contracts sleeping sickness from the bite of a fly with parasites in its saliva.

The parasites then move to the salivary glands of the fly, which become infective.

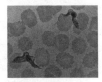

**Trypanosomes**
The parasites are shown here in blood.

bed. Sometimes sleepwalking arises from a *night terror*, in which case the child's behavior is more frantic and may involve shrieking or thrashing. The child sometimes talks (usually simple words or phrases) during the sleepwalk or urinates in an inappropriate place and may get into the wrong bed. Waking the child is difficult and unnecessary; steer him or her gently back to bed. Take precautions, such as blocking off the stairs, to avoid injury.

Sleepwalking in children is seldom associated with psychological problems; although it may be aggravated by anxiety, it tends to disappear naturally with age. Sleepwalking in adults may be related to anxiety. It may be associated with sleeping pill use, especially in the elderly.

## Sling

A device used to immobilize, support, or elevate an upper limb. A sling is usually made from a triangular *bandage*, although an emergency sling can be created from a belt, tie, or scarf.

An arm sling may be used as a first-aid measure to support the arm following a fracture, sprain, or other injury (see illustrated box overleaf). It may also be used to provide relief during infection or after an operation on the hand or arm.

An elevation sling is used in first aid to hold the hand in a well-raised position to control bleeding or to prevent movement of the arm and shoulder if the clavicle (collarbone) is broken.

This type of sling is applied in a similar fashion to an arm sling, except the victim's arm is placed across the chest with the fingers nearly touching the opposite shoulder.

## Slipped disk

See *Disk prolapse*.

## Slipped femoral epiphysis

See *Femoral epiphysis, slipped*.

## Slit lamp

An illuminated microscope used to examine the internal structures of the front part of the eye. When special contact lenses are applied, the slit lamp may be used to examine the retina. (See also *Eye, examination of*.)

## Slough

Dead tissue that has been shed from its original site. Examples of sloughing include the loss of dead skin cells from the skin's surface and the shedding of the lining of the uterus during menstruation. Sloughing also occurs as part of the healing process of wounds and ulcers.

## Slow virus diseases

A group of diseases of the central nervous system (brain and spinal cord) that occurs many months or years after infection with a virus. The diseases take a slow course in which there is gradual widespread destruction of nerve tissue. This causes progressive loss of brain function and, at present, a fatal outcome.

**S**

## FIRST AID: ARM SLING

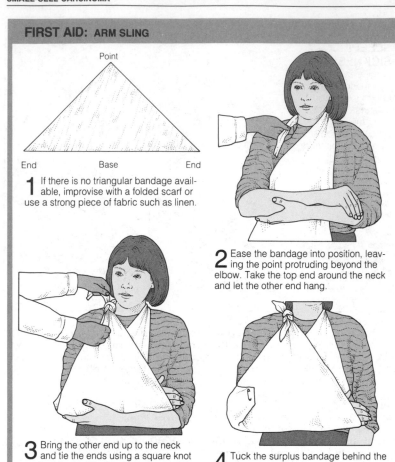

Point

End    Base    End

**1** If there is no triangular bandage available, improvise with a folded scarf or use a strong piece of fabric such as linen.

**2** Ease the bandage into position, leaving the point protruding beyond the elbow. Take the top end around the neck and let the other end hang.

**3** Bring the other end up to the neck and tie the ends using a square knot on the injured side. The knot should sit in the hollow above the collarbone.

**4** Tuck the surplus bandage behind the elbow and bring the point forward, securing it with a pin.

The group of slow virus diseases includes *Creutzfeldt-Jakob syndrome*, *kuru*, possibly one form of *Alzheimer's disease*, subacute sclerosing panencephalitis (a very rare complication of measles), and possibly the brain disease that occurs in some people infected with the *AIDS* virus.

## Small-cell carcinoma
The most dangerous and rapidly spreading form of lung cancer. Also called oat-cell carcinoma, this type of tumor accounts for about 25 percent of lung cancers. Most small-cell carcinomas reach an inoperable stage by the time a diagnosis is made. Life extension from surgery is achieved in about 10 percent of cases, but, even in these cases, the outlook is poor. Spread to other parts of the body is almost inevitable.

Treatment is usually with *anticancer drugs* with or without *radiation therapy*.

Because this treatment must be given in very high doses, bone marrow transplants are being tried.

## Smallpox
A highly infectious viral disease, common in the nineteenth century and before, with the distinction of having been totally eradicated by a successful worldwide vaccination campaign. The World Health Organization declared smallpox extinct in 1980.

Smallpox was transmitted from person to person; it was characterized by an illness resembling influenza and a rash that spread over the body and eventually developed into pus-filled blisters. The blisters became crusted and would sometimes leave deeply pitted scars. Complications included blindness, pneumonia, and kidney damage. There was no effective treatment for the disease, which killed up to 40 percent of its victims.

Eradication was achieved through the cooperative international use of a highly effective vaccine. Eradication was possible because smallpox affected only humans, cases of infection were easily recognized, and victims of the disease were infectious to others only for a short time. These characteristics are shared by some other diseases (e.g., measles, another possible candidate for eradication).

Smallpox vaccination certificates are no longer required for travel abroad, and most countries have discontinued vaccination because the risk of the disease is zero and because there is a risk of encephalitis from the vaccine. The virus responsible for smallpox is still maintained at laboratories at the Centers for Disease Control in Atlanta and at a research institute in Moscow.

## Smear
A specimen for microscopic examination prepared by spreading a thin film of the cells to be examined onto a glass slide. Common examples are a *blood smear* and a *cervical smear test*.

## Smegma
An accumulation of sebaceous gland secretions beneath the foreskin in an uncircumcised male, usually as a result of poor hygiene.

Fungal or bacterial infection of smegma may cause *balanitis* (inflammation of the glans). In a child with *phimosis* (tight foreskin), smegma occasionally hardens into a small stone, known as a smegma pearl. The higher incidence of cancer of the penis in uncircumcised men who smoke may be due to the buildup of cancer-inducing substances in the smegma.

An uncircumcised man should regularly wash his penis with the foreskin retracted to prevent a buildup of smegma.

## Smell
One of the five senses. The mechanisms by which smell is perceived are shown in the illustrated box opposite.
### DISORDERS
Disturbance of the sense of smell may consist of anosmia (loss of the sense of smell, which may be complete or partial, temporary or permanent) or dysosmia (abnormal smell perception). Because the senses of smell and taste are so closely connected, disturbances of smell usually result in disturbances of taste.

Temporary partial anosmia frequently results from conditions in which the nasal mucous membrane

**S**

becomes inflamed, such as the common *cold, influenza,* and several forms of *rhinitis,* notably allergic rhinitis (hay fever). Cigarette smoking also commonly causes anosmia. In hypertrophic rhinitis, the mucous membrane thickens, burying and sometimes distorting the olfactory nerve endings, which may cause permanent anosmia unless the condition is treated. In atrophic rhinitis, the nerve endings waste away, causing some degree of permanent anosmia; there is also a foul-smelling discharge that may overpower other odors.

The olfactory nerves can be torn in a head injury. If both nerves are torn, complete, permanent anosmia results; during recovery from less severe damage, dysosmia, in the form of illusory bad smells, may occur.

Rarely, anosmia is caused by a *meningioma* (tumor of the meninges, the membranes that surround the brain) or a tumor behind the nose (see *Nasopharynx, cancer of*).

Dysosmia, in the form of illusory, unpleasant odors, may occur as a feature of various psychological disorders, such as *depression* or *schizophrenia*. It may also occur in some forms of *epilepsy* and during "drying out" periods in severe *alcohol dependence*. A person with dysosmia may believe the source of the smell is his or her body and, despite reassurance to the contrary, may wash excessively and tend to avoid others.

## Smelling salts
A preparation of *ammonia* that causes a person to withdraw from the pungent substance. Smelling salts were once used to prevent fainting or to revive a person who had fainted.

---

## THE SENSE OF SMELL
The smell receptors are specialized nerve cell endings situated in a small patch of mucous membrane lining the roof of the nose. The axons (fibers) of these sensory cells pass up through tiny perforations in the overlying bone to enter the two elongated olfactory bulbs lying on top of the bone. These bulbs are swellings at the ends of the olfactory nerves; the nerves contain millions of nerve fibers and enter the brain on its lower surface. The olfactory nerves carry sensory information to smell centers situated within the brain.

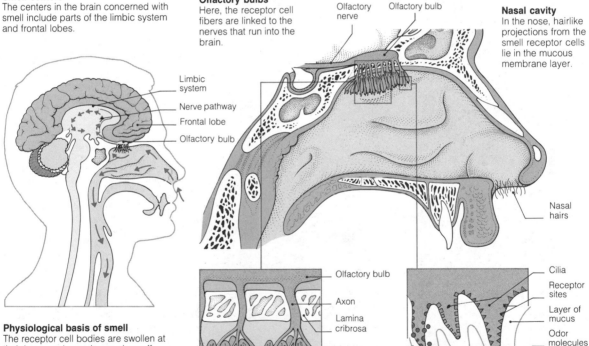

**Smell centers**
The centers in the brain concerned with smell include parts of the limbic system and frontal lobes.

Limbic system
Nerve pathway
Frontal lobe
Olfactory bulb

**Olfactory bulbs**
Here, the receptor cell fibers are linked to the nerves that run into the brain.

Olfactory nerve
Olfactory bulb
Olfactory bulb

**Nasal cavity**
In the nose, hairlike projections from the smell receptor cells lie in the mucous membrane layer.

Nasal hairs

**Physiological basis of smell**
The receptor cell bodies are swollen at their lower ends; each one gives off several cilia that extend down to the surface of the mucous membrane. The cilia contain the receptor sites at which stimulation by the molecules of odorous substances gives rise to nerve impulses passing up to the brain. We know that we are able to distinguish several thousand different odors, but the exact basis of this high degree of specificity is uncertain. No microscopic difference can be detected among different receptors.

Olfactory bulb
Axon
Lamina cribrosa
Receptor cell
Supporting cell
Cilia

**Probable mechanism**
The smell process probably is based on a physical "fit" between the odor molecules and the receptor sites. For example, the receptors on some cells may fit only with ether molecules, others with molecules of bleach.

Cilia
Receptor sites
Layer of mucus
Odor molecules

Ether
Garlic
Bleach

The molecules must dissolve in the mucus before they can stimulate the receptors. The sensitivity of the system is remarkable; as few as four molecules can give a recognizable smell.

S

## VENOMOUS SNAKES IN THE US

The distribution of eight of the more dangerous or commonly biting poisonous snakes in the US is shown below. Apart from the eastern coral snake, all are pit vipers. These snakes have stout bodies, broad heads, retractable front fangs, slitlike eyes, and are 2 to 8 feet in length. Heat-sensitive pits between the eyes and nostrils help them locate warmblooded prey in the dark.

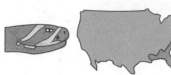

**Eastern diamondback rattlesnake**
A brown snake, up to 8 feet long, with a diamond pattern on its body. Like all rattlesnakes, it has a rattle on its tail.

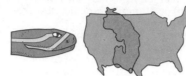

**Prairie rattlesnake**
This rattler, found in the Great Plains, is greenish-gray to brown in color, and 3 to 4 feet long.

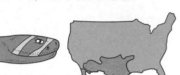

**Western diamondback rattlesnake**
Similar to the eastern species, but often reddish in color with less distinct diamonds. Widespread in dry habitats.

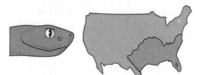

**Water moccasin (cottonmouth)**
This snake lives in or near water. When alarmed, its mouth opens to show a white interior. It has no tail rattle.

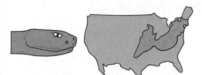

**Timber rattlesnake**
This snake lives in forests, swamps, and rocky hillsides. It has a pale brown body with black bands and a black tail.

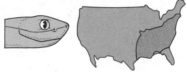

**Copperhead**
This species has a russet-colored body with dark bands and a yellowish top to its head. It vibrates its tail when angry.

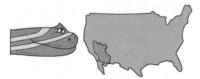

**Sidewinder rattlesnake**
This smaller, desert-living snake has a pale brown body and distinctive hornlike "eyelash" scales above the eyes.

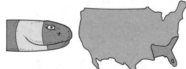

**Eastern coral snake**
This snake is up to 4 feet long and slender, with a yellow-black-yellow-red recurring ring pattern.

### AVOIDING SNAKEBITES

Anyone working, camping, or walking in areas known to be inhabited by venomous snakes should take these precautions:

- Wear long pants and boots
- Keep to cleared tracks when hiking through the brush
- If moving large rocks or logs, use a stick
- Never sleep on the ground
- Never disturb a snake or try to kill one. Move quietly away
- Burn garbage, which attracts rodents, which in turn attract snakes

## Smoking

See *Tobacco smoking.*

## Snails and disease

Snails act as host to various types of parasitic flukes (flattened, wormlike animals), which, at different stages in their life cycles, infest people. The flukes include *liver flukes* and the parasites responsible for *schistosomiasis* and various other tropical diseases. Control of snail populations can be important in combating these diseases. There is no risk to eating thoroughly cooked snails anywhere in the world.

## Snakebites

Every year, hundreds of thousands of people worldwide are bitten by snakes. However, the chance of death or even serious injury occurring from a bite is relatively small. The majority of bites are by non-poisonous species; in only a proportion of bites by poisonous snakes is venom actually injected. Furthermore, modern medical treatment is effective in treating most serious cases, provided the victim is transported to the hospital quickly. It takes hours or days, not minutes or seconds, for even the most powerful snake venom to kill.

Venomous snakes are found throughout North America, except in Maine, Alaska, and northern Canada. In the US each year, about 45,000 people are bitten by snakes, including 1,500 by poisonous species. The number of deaths annually is less than 20.

**VENOMOUS AND NONVENOMOUS SPECIES**
Three quarters of the 3,000 types of snakes worldwide belong to the colubrid family. They have slender, tapered bodies and are mostly nonvenomous. Most North American snakes are harmless colubrids.

In the US, most venomous bites are caused by pit vipers, which are widespread. The pit vipers, which belong to the crotalid family, include the copperhead, water moccasin (cottonmouth), and about 30 different species of rattlesnake. Rattlesnakes carry a horny rattle on the tail that they vibrate when disturbed. If disturbed, any pit viper is likely to bite, striking quickly and withdrawing at once.

The only other venomous snake in the US is the coral snake. It belongs to a group of snakes called the elapids, which have slender, tapering bodies, narrow heads, round eyes, and small

S

nonretractable fangs. Other members of the group are the cobras, kraits, and mambas of Africa and Asia. Coral snakes are about 4 feet (1.2 m) long, and decorated with black and brightly colored bands. Their colors are mimicked by other, nonvenomous, species, but the coral snakes have red bands bordered by yellow or white; the mimic snakes have red bands bordered by black.

Other venomous snakes include the true vipers, which are not found in North America, and sea snakes, which rarely bite humans.

### EFFECTS OF A BITE

The effects of a venomous bite vary considerably and depend on the species of snake, its size, the amount of venom injected, and the age and health of the victim.

Rattlesnakes and other pit vipers make two distinct puncture wounds in the skin. There is an immediate burning pain at the site of the wound and swelling of the bitten limb. Over the next 20 minutes the pain increases in severity and the victim becomes dizzy, nauseated, pale, and sweaty. Blood pressure falls and there is an increase in heart rate. Thirst, headache, and a pins and needles sensation are other common symptoms.

The venom may prevent the blood from clotting, causing bleeding from the fang wounds and bruises beneath the skin. There may also be bleeding into the urine or from the mouth, rectum, or vagina. Internal bleeding further lowers the blood pressure. There is also widespread tissue destruction around the wound.

Coral snakes and other elapids typically make two small puncture wounds with their fangs; they may also chew the skin, producing several wounds. A bite from a coral snake usually causes little pain or swelling. The venom primarily affects the nervous system. Serious symptoms develop from 10 minutes to eight hours after the bite and may include drooping eyelids, slurred speech, and double vision. The victim becomes drowsy or delirious and may have convulsions. Eventually, if treatment is not given, respiratory paralysis causes death.

### TREATMENT

Any person accompanying a victim of a snakebite should administer first aid (see box) and then obtain medical help. Antibiotics and injections of tetanus antitoxin are given for all bites, whether venomous or not, to prevent bacterial infection or tetanus.

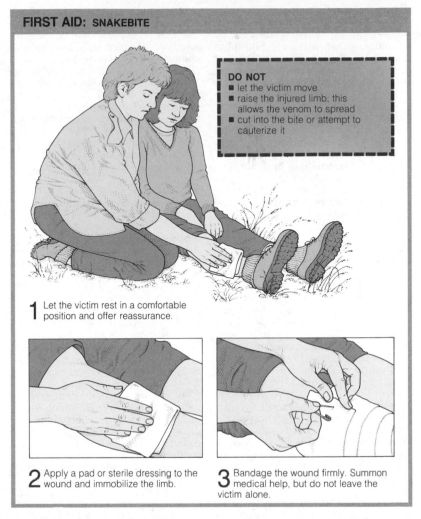

**FIRST AID: SNAKEBITE**

**DO NOT**
- let the victim move
- raise the injured limb; this allows the venom to spread
- cut into the bite or attempt to cauterize it

**1** Let the victim rest in a comfortable position and offer reassurance.

**2** Apply a pad or sterile dressing to the wound and immobilize the limb.

**3** Bandage the wound firmly. Summon medical help, but do not leave the victim alone.

For a severe venomous bite, the victim is given a highly effective injection of *antivenin* (a serum containing antibodies against the poison). In the US, one antivenin is available to treat a bite by any pit viper and another is available for coral snakebites.

In the most severe cases, kidney *dialysis* to treat *renal failure* or artificial *ventilation* to overcome respiratory paralysis may be required.

Modern treatment of venomous snakebites is so advanced that almost all victims who receive prompt medical care survive and do so with minimal aftereffects.

## Sneezing

The involuntary, convulsive expulsion of air through the nose and mouth as a result of irritation of the upper respiratory tract. The irritation may be caused by inflammation of the tract, which occurs in the common *cold*, *influenza*, and allergic *rhinitis* (hay fever); by mucus; or by inhaling an irritant (e.g., dust or pepper).

## Snellen's chart

A standard method of measuring *visual acuity* used during *vision tests*. Snellen's chart, bearing rows of letters of standard, decreasing size, is set at a distance of 20 feet (6 m) from the patient. One eye is covered and the patient is asked to read as far down the chart as possible. The procedure is repeated with the other eye.

Normal vision (20/20 vision) requires that all the letters in a line near the bottom of the chart be read correctly. If the person being tested can read only the letters twice as large as those on the 20/20 line (which a normal eye would be able to read at 40 feet), the acuity is said to be 20/40.

S

## Snoring

Noisy breathing through the open mouth during sleep, produced by vibrations of the soft palate. Snoring is usually caused by any condition that hinders breathing through the nose, such as a common *cold*, allergic *rhinitis*, or enlarged *adenoids*. It is more common while sleeping on the back, when the lower jaw tends to drop open. In some people who snore because of upper airway obstruction, snoring alternates with *sleep apnea* (temporary cessation of breathing).

A sometimes effective way to prevent snoring is to sew an object into the pajama top near the small of the back, thus making it uncomfortable to sleep on the back.

## Snuff

A preparation of powdered tobacco (often with other substances) for inhalation into the nose; it is also made into a wad for chewing. Snuff is irritating to the nasal lining, which may waste as a result of prolonged snuff inhalation. Also, because it contains *nicotine*, snuff is addictive.

The increased use in North America and northern Europe of "smokeless" tobacco has provoked interest in its carcinogenic (cancer-causing) effects. Chewing tobacco and snuff are carcinogens. There is a direct proportion between the amount used, the period over which it is used, and the likelihood of cancer. Carcinogens are also present in betel nut and in pan (which is a combination of betel nut, lime, and tobacco).

Among practicing Mormons (who use neither tobacco nor alcohol), *squamous cell carcinomas* of the head and neck are uncommon. In contrast, the majority of people with head and neck cancers have a history of heavy alcohol and tobacco use.

Cultural differences in the way tobacco is used have led to great variation in the location of cancers, in accordance with the principle that increased exposure to heavy concentrates of tobacco carcinogens results in an increased risk of tumor development in the tissue exposed.

A striking example of this has been observed among the women of a certain area of India, where carcinoma of the hard palate (roof of the mouth), which is rare in the rest of the world, has a high incidence. It is correlated with the local custom of reverse chutta smoking, in which the lit end of a slow-burning cigarette is held in the mouth and seldom removed.

Similarly, about one half of all cancer in Bombay, India, is cancer of the buccal mucosa (cheek pouch), which is associated with the custom of chewing pan. Pan is held in the user's cheek throughout the day and sometimes kept in place during sleep. The majority of tumors develop in the place in the mouth where the pan is stored. The practice of dipping snuff among the women of North Carolina has been shown to increase the risk of cancers of the cheek and gum 50 times more than the population at large.

## Sociopathy

An outdated term for *antisocial personality disorder*.

## Sodium

A mineral that, along with potassium and other substances, regulates the body's water balance, maintains normal heart rhythm, and is responsible for the conduction of nerve impulses and the contraction of muscles.

The body of an average-sized person contains about 2 ounces (55 grams) of sodium. The level of sodium in the blood is controlled by the kidneys, which eliminate any excess of the mineral in the urine.

Almost all foods contain sodium naturally or as an ingredient added during processing or cooking. The principal forms of sodium in food are sodium chloride (table salt) and sodium bicarbonate (baking soda). Apart from table salt, the main dietary sources of sodium are processed foods, cheese, breads and cereals, and smoked, pickled, or cured meats and fish. Pickles and snack foods contain large amounts; sodium is also present in water treated with water softeners.

DEFICIENCY AND EXCESS
Because most foods contain sodium, deficiency is very rare. In fact, most Western diets contain too much sodium. While many nutritionists suggest a daily intake of only 0.04 to 0.1 ounces (1 to 3 grams), the average consumption is 0.1 to 0.25 ounces (3 to 7 grams) per day. There is no official recommended daily allowance.

Sodium deficiency is usually the result of excessive loss of the mineral through prolonged or excessive treatment with *diuretic drugs*. It may also be caused by persistent diarrhea or vomiting or by profuse sweating. Rarely, deficiency is due to *cystic fibrosis*, underactivity of the adrenal glands, or certain kidney disorders. Symptoms of deficiency include tiredness, weakness, muscle cramps, and

dizziness. In severe cases, there may be a drop in blood pressure, leading to confusion, fainting, and palpitations. Treatment consists of taking sodium supplements. In very hot conditions, supplements may also help prevent exhaustion that occurs as a result of sodium loss from excessive sweating.

Excessive sodium intake is thought to be a contributory factor in the high incidence of *hypertension* (high blood pressure) in Western countries. In people whose blood pressure is already raised, excessive sodium may increase the risk of heart disease, *stroke*, and kidney damage. Another adverse effect is fluid retention, which, in severe cases, may cause dizziness and swelling of the legs.

## Sodium bicarbonate

An over-the-counter *antacid drug* used to relieve *indigestion*, *heartburn*, and pain caused by a *peptic ulcer*.

Sodium bicarbonate often causes belching and abdominal discomfort. Long-term use may cause swollen ankles, muscle cramps, tiredness, weakness, nausea, and vomiting. Sodium bicarbonate should not be taken by people with *heart failure* or a history of kidney disease.

## Sodium salicylate

An *analgesic drug* used to relieve minor musculoskeletal pain and reduce inflammation.

## Soft-tissue injury

Damage to one or more of the tissues that surround bones and joints (e.g., to a *ligament*, *tendon*, or *muscle*). Soft-tissue injuries include ligament *sprain*, *tendinitis* (inflammation of a tendon), and muscle tears (see *Strain*). See also *Sports injuries*.

## Soiling

The accidental passing of soft, unformed feces into the clothes after the age at which bowel control is usually achieved (about age 3 or 4). More than half the children with this problem also wet the bed (see *Enuresis*). Soiling is distinct from *encopresis* (the deliberate passing of normal feces in inappropriate places).

Causes of soiling include slowness in developing bowel control, long-standing *constipation* (in which fecal liquid leaks around hard feces blocking the large intestine), poor *toilet-training*, and psychological stress (such as starting school). Soiling is usually distressing to the child, who may hide the messy clothes.

S

Soiling due to constipation usually responds to treatment. If there is no physical cause, it may pass after a discussion involving the child, the parents, and the physician; if not, *psychotherapy* may be used.

## Solar plexus

The largest autonomic *plexus* (nerve network) in the body (see *Autonomic nervous system*). Also known as the celiac plexus, the solar plexus is situated behind the stomach, where it surrounds the celiac artery and lies between the adrenal glands. The solar plexus incorporates the greater and lesser splanchnic nerves (part of the sympathetic nervous system) and branches of the *vagus nerve*, the most important component of the parasympathetic nervous system. The solar plexus sends out branches to the stomach, intestines, and most other abdominal organs.

## Solvent abuse

The practice of inhaling the intoxicating fumes given off by certain volatile liquids. Glue sniffing is the most common form of solvent abuse, but many other substances are used, especially those containing toluene or acetone. The usual method of inhalation is from a plastic bag containing the solvent, but sometimes aerosols are sprayed into the nose or mouth.

### INCIDENCE

Solvent abuse is common among boys in poor urban areas. It is usually a group activity that is indulged in for no more than a few months. Solitary abuse over a longer period is frequently associated with a disturbed family background and delinquency.

### EFFECTS

Inhaling solvent fumes produces an effect similar to that of becoming drunk or getting high on drugs, sometimes including hallucinations. If carried on for any length of time, it can bring about headache, vomiting, stupor, confusion, and coma. Occasionally, death occurs as the result of a direct toxic effect on the heart, a fall, choking on vomit, or asphyxiation due to a clinging plastic bag.

Long-term harmful effects include erosion of the membrane lining the nose and throat and damage to the kidneys, liver, and nervous system.

### DIAGNOSIS AND TREATMENT

The signs of solvent abuse include intoxicated behavior, a flushed face, ulcers around the mouth, a smell of solvent, and personality changes, such as moodiness and nervousness.

Solvent abusers should be warned of the serious risks to health. Professional counseling may be needed. Acute symptoms resulting from solvent abuse, such as vomiting or coma, require urgent medical attention.

## Somatic

A term that means related to the body (soma), as opposed to the mind (psyche), or related to body cells, as opposed to germ cells (eggs and sperm). The term somatic also refers to the body wall, in contrast to the viscera (internal organs).

## Somatization disorder

A condition in which the individual complains over several years of various physical problems for which no physical cause can be found. The disorder, previously classified as *hysteria*, usually begins before age 30 and leads to numerous tests by many physicians. Unnecessary surgery and other treatments often result.

This disorder may be slightly more prevalent in women, many of whom have a family history of *antisocial personality disorder* in male relatives. Symptoms most commonly complained of are neurological (e.g., double vision, seizures, weakness), gynecological (painful menstruation, pain on intercourse), and gastrointestinal (abdominal pain, nausea). Associated features may include *anxiety* and *depression*, threats of *suicide*, and various forms of substance abuse.

These physical symptoms are caused by underlying emotional conflicts, anxiety, and depression that the person is unable to confront and which are unconsciously displaced onto the body. It is thought that it is easier for the person to view the problem as physical than face the emotional conflicts from which he or she is trying to escape. (See also *Conversion disorder*; *Hypochondriasis*.)

## Somatoform disorders

A group of conditions in which there are physical symptoms for which no physical cause can be found, and for which there is definite or strong evidence that the underlying cause is psychological. Somatoform disorders include *conversion disorder*, *hypochondriasis*, and *somatization disorder*.

## Somatotype

The physical build of an individual. A variety of attempts have been made to classify people according to body type and to identify corresponding personality traits.

In the 1920s, the German psychiatrist Ernst Kretschmer divided people into three types, each of which he

---

## BODY TYPES AND PERSONALITY

The idea that the features of the psyche (mind) are related to those of the soma (body) is not always borne out in practice. Even so, there is a very general relationship between the two.

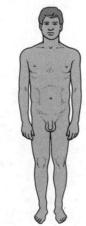

**Endomorph**
Tends to be sociable, easygoing, pleasure-loving, relaxed, and convivial.

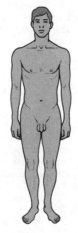

**Mesomorph**
Is often physically active, strong, athletic, ready for action, and aggressive.

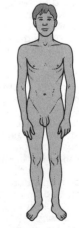

**Ectomorph**
Is more sensitive, selfconscious, restrained, introspective, and quiet.

S

thought was more prone to certain types of mental illness—asthenic (thin) types seemed more likely to have a schizoid personality or schizophrenia; pyknic (stocky) types were more prone to manic-depressive illness; athletic (muscular) types were not associated with any single disorder, but there was more delinquency within this group.

An American psychologist, working in the 1940s, believed that people did not fit into rigid categories of body type. Instead he identified three structural tendencies (each associated with certain personality traits), which everyone had in different proportions. They were ectomorphic—a tall, thin physique, with light bones and muscles, linked with a restrained, self-conscious personality; endomorphic—a heavy physique, with poorly developed bones and muscles, associated with a sociable, loving personality; and mesomorphic—strong, well-developed bones and muscles, paired with a physical, adventurous personality.

## Somatrem

A preparation of human *growth hormone*. Somatrem is given to children to treat *short stature* caused by growth hormone deficiency. A year's treatment with somatrem costs between $10,000 and $20,000.

## Somnambulism

See *Sleepwalking*.

## Sore

A term used to describe an ulcer, septic wound, or any disrupted area of the skin or mucous membranes. The word is also used to describe an area that is tender or painful.

## Sore throat

A rough or raw feeling in the back of the throat that causes discomfort, especially when swallowing.

Sore throat is an extremely common symptom that is usually caused by *pharyngitis*, and occasionally by *tonsillitis*. It may also be the first symptom of the common *cold*, *influenza*, *laryngitis*, infectious *mononucleosis*, and many common childhood viral illnesses, including *chickenpox*, *measles*, and *mumps*.

A *streptococcal infection* produced by the beta-hemolytic streptococcus produces a sore throat that must be diagnosed. Left untreated, this type of sore throat may result in acute *glomerulonephritis* or *rheumatic fever*.

Treatment consists of gargling with salt water or, for adults, taking aspirin. If a sore throat persists for more than 48 hours or a *rash* develops, a physician should be consulted. (See also *Strep throat*.)

## Space medicine

A minor medical specialty concerned with the physiological and pathological effects of spaceflight.

During lift-off, there is a large upward acceleration that makes the astronaut feel many times heavier. There is also a tendency for blood to pool downward. To prevent loss of consciousness as a result of blood draining from the brain, the astronaut must lie in a reclining seat and wear a special suit that exerts pressure on certain parts of the body (such as the limbs) and helps redistribute the flow of blood toward the head.

Once in orbit, the effects of gravity (which pulls spacecraft and astronaut toward Earth) and velocity (which is vertically opposed to this pull) combine to make the astronaut feel weightless. One effect of weightlessness is on the body's balance mechanisms. The brain may be unable to make sense of the lack of signals from the balance organ in the inner ear; one manifestation is *motion sickness*.

Changes also occur in the cardiovascular system (heart and blood vessels) because, in the absence of weight, body fluids are redistributed toward the head. Other effects may include loss of bone and muscle tissue. Such effects could ultimately limit space travel, unless a means can be found to recreate weight within spacecraft. (See also *Aviation medicine*.)

## Spasm

An involuntary, often powerful, muscle contraction. A spasm may affect one or more muscles and may occur once or more; pain is not necessarily an accompanying feature.

Examples include *hiccups* (in which the diaphragm goes into spasm), muscle cramps (which often affect the muscles in the calves), and *tics* (which frequently affect facial muscles).

Less commonly, a spasm may be the result of an abnormality in the central nervous system or a symptom of a muscle disorder. Spasms caused by disease of the nervous system include *myoclonus* and *chorea*. Conditions characterized by spasm include *trigeminal neuralgia* (which affects the muscles of the face and head), *tetany* (spasm caused by a drop of the

calcium level in the blood), and *tetanus* (an infectious disease). Rare causes of widespread spasm are *rabies*, *strychnine poisoning*, and the bite of the black widow spider.

Other types of muscle spasm include *bronchospasm* (contraction of muscles in the small airways of the lungs), which occurs in asthma, and vasospasm (tightening of the muscles in the blood vessels).

## Spasticity

Increased rigidity in a group of muscles, causing stiffness and restriction of movement. Spasticity can occur with or without *paralysis* or muscle weakness. *Cerebral palsy* causes spasticity and paralysis; *Parkinson's disease* and *multiple sclerosis* may cause spasticity without paralysis. *Tetanus* causes spasticity, initially of the muscles in the face and neck (lockjaw) and then of other body muscles.

## Spastic paralysis

The inability to move a part of the body accompanied by rigidity of the muscles; the immobilized parts are frozen in one position. Causes of spastic paralysis include *stroke*, *cerebral palsy*, and *multiple sclerosis*. (See also *Paralysis*.)

## Spatulate

Shaped like a spatula (i.e., with a broad, blunt, flattened, spoonlike end). Spatulate fingers are normal and do not indicate disease.

## Specialist

A physician with advanced training and knowledge in a particular branch of medicine or surgery. A nephrologist is a specialist in the function and disorders of the kidneys. (See also individual entries, e.g., *Cardiologist*; *Gastroenterologist*; *Pediatrician*.)

## Specific gravity

Also called relative density, the ratio of the *density* of a substance to that of water. Materials with a relative density of less than 1 are less dense ("lighter") than water; those with a relative density of more than 1 are denser ("heavier") than water. The specific gravity of urine shows if it has a large amount of material dissolved in it (near 1.030) or if it is almost water (near 1.010).

## Specimen

A sample of tissue, body fluids (such as blood), waste products (such as urine), or an infective organism taken for the purpose of examination, identification, analysis, and/or diagnosis. The term is also applied to a sample of a tissue or organism specially prepared for examination under a *microscope*. (See also *Blood tests; Urinalysis*.)

## SPECT
The abbreviation for single photon emission computerized tomography, a type of *radionuclide scanning*.

## Spectacles
See *Glasses*.

## Speculum
A device designed to hold open a body orifice (opening), enabling a physician to perform an examination. A speculum is made of plastic or metal.

### TYPES
There are many types of speculum designed for use on different parts of the body. The speculum used to examine the eardrum is funnel-shaped, with a narrow end inserted into the ear canal and a wide end attached to an *otoscope*. The speculum used to hold open the walls of the vagina during a pelvic examination may be shaped either like a duck's bill, with wide, smooth, curved edges and a self-retaining lock to hold them in position, or like a shoehorn bent at both ends at an angle of 90 degrees.

## Speech
The most frequently used method of human communication.

### LANGUAGE AND SPEECH
The terms "speech" and "language" are often used interchangeably, but have different meanings. Language is the representation of objects and ideas by strings of symbols, which form words. These symbols may be speech sounds, written characters, or hand signals. There are two main facets of language ability—understanding the meaning of words (comprehension) and generating words, in grammatical order, to express something meaningful (expression).

Speech is just one method by which language can be communicated to others. Writing and hand signals are others. Each method relies on sequences of muscle movements. Speech involves the muscles used in breathing, the larynx, tongue, palate, lips, jaw, and face.

### LANGUAGE CENTERS
Language comprehension and expression take place in two areas of the cerebral cortex (the outer layer of the cerebrum and main mass of the brain)

### LANGUAGE AND SPEECH DEVELOPMENT IN CHILDHOOD

| 3 months | Period of babbling begins. The child produces strings of sounds for pleasure. Babbling is important in building movement sequences, which will be used | later to produce meaningful speech sounds. |
|---|---|---|
| 9 months | Child echoes the speech of others, but words are not yet used with meaning. By listening to and copying adults, the child learns that clusters of sounds | refer to specific objects, people, or situations. |
| 12 to 18 months | The child begins to utter simple words with meaning, often accompanied by gestures. Examples are "bye-bye," "dog," "hot," and "daddy." Only single | words are used, with vocabulary gradually increasing from two or three words initially. |
| 18 to 24 months | The child begins to combine concepts to form two-word sentences (e.g., "Hello John" or "That hot!"). By age 2, the child | may be using 100 or more different words. |
| 2 to 3 years | The child's sentences expand in length (e.g., "I like cake" or "Peter hit Mary"). He or she begins to incorporate adjectives and adverbs into sentences (e.g., "That's daddy's old coat" or "I want lunch now"). By 3 | years, average sentence length is four words, Most sounds have developed, with "th," "r," "j," "ch," and "sh" possible exceptions. |
| 3 years and up | More elaborate sentences with several nouns, verbs in past and future tenses, and linked phrases begin to be used—for example "We went to Amy's and we had milk and cookies" or "I think mommy went downstairs." | However, mistakes are often made, such as "What did you played?", reflecting the child's linguistic immaturity. Language skills continue to develop throughout childhood. |

called Wernicke's and Broca's areas. Both are in the dominant cerebral hemisphere (the left hemisphere in most people). In Wernicke's area, incoming messages (heard or read) are scanned and compared with information held in the memory to extract meaning. In Broca's area, words and sentences are composed from vocabulary and from grammatical rules stored in the memory.

### SPEECH PRODUCTION
The movement sequences for speech sounds originate from two regions of the cerebral cortex on either side of the brain. These regions are linked to the center for language expression (Broca's area). The signals for movement pass down nerve pathways to the muscles controlling the larynx, tongue, and other parts involved in speech. The cerebellum (a region at the back of the brain) plays a part in coordinating these movements.

Air from the lungs is vibrated by opening and closing the vocal cords in the larynx. This produces a noise, which is amplified in the hollow cavities of the throat, nose, and sinuses. The sound of vibrated or nonvibrated air is modified by movements of the tongue, mouth, jaw, and lips to produce speech sounds. Vibrated air blown through top teeth resting on lower lips gives "v" or, if the air is not vibrated, "f." Consonants are produced mainly by contact among the tongue, roof of the mouth, teeth, and lips; vowels are produced by changing the shape of the mouth cavity.

### LANGUAGE AND SPEECH DEVELOPMENT
Normal development of language and speech in a child depends on maturation of the nervous system and muscles, on the child's exploration of his or her environment (which should be stimulating), and on interaction with adults. Through play, the child

S

acquires many concepts (sets of ideas) about different aspects of the world. From adults, the child acquires the verbal labels for objects and concepts that are vital to language development. Normal hearing is, therefore, essential. Language and speech are learned through listening to the speech of others and monitoring one's own speech.

Stages in the development of language and speech in a child, with the significance of each, are shown in the table (see previous page).

## Speech disorders

Defects or disturbances can arise in various parts of the nervous system, muscles, and other apparatus involved in *speech*, leading to an inability to communicate effectively. Some of these disorders are, strictly, disturbances of language rather than of speech, since they result from an impaired ability to understand or to form words in the language centers of the brain, rather than from any fault of the apparatus of speech production.

### DISORDERS OF LANGUAGE

Damage to the language centers of the brain (usually as a result of a *stroke*, *head injury*, or *brain tumor*) leads to a disorder known as *aphasia*. Both children and adults can be affected. The ability to speak and write and/or to comprehend written or spoken words is impaired, depending on the site and extent of the damage.

Delayed development of language in a child is characterized by slowness to understand speech and/or slow growth in vocabulary and sentence structure. Delayed development has many causes, including hearing loss, lack of stimulation, or emotional disturbance (see *Developmental delay*).

### DISORDERS OF ARTICULATION

Articulation is the ability to produce speech sounds; a defect of articulation is sometimes referred to as *dysarthria*. Damage to nerves passing from the brain to muscles in the larynx (voice box), mouth, or lips can cause speech to be slurred, indistinct, slow, or nasal. The sources of such damage are similar to those that cause aphasia (e.g., stroke, head injury, tumors, *multiple sclerosis*, *Parkinson's disease*) but the affected regions of the brain are different. Damage to the cerebellum, for example, produces a characteristic form of slurred speech. Structural abnormalities of the mouth, such as cleft palate (see *Cleft lip and palate*) and malaligned teeth, can also cause poor articulation.

Delayed development of articulation, characterized by an inability to make sounds at appropriate ages, may cause incomprehensible speech. Causes are hearing problems or slow maturation of the nervous system.

### DISORDERS OF VOICE PRODUCTION

These disorders include hoarseness, harshness, inappropriate pitch or loudness of the voice, and abnormal nasal resonance. In many cases, the cause is a disorder affecting closure of the vocal cords (see *Larynx* disorders box). A voice pitched too high or low or that is too loud or soft may be caused by a hormonal or psychiatric disturbance or by severe hearing loss.

Abnormal nasal resonance is caused by too much air (hypernasality) or too little air (hyponasality) flowing through the nose during speech. Hypernasality may result from damage to the nerves supplying the palate (roof of the mouth) or be a result of cleft palate. It causes a deterioration in the intelligibility of speech. Hyponasality is caused by blockage to the nasal airways by excess mucus and has the sound of someone speaking with a cold.

### DISORDERS OF FLUENCY

Nonfluent speech is marked by repetitions of single sounds or whole words and by blocking of speech; the underlying cause is not understood (see *Stuttering*).

## Speech therapy

A form of therapy that attempts to help people with a variety of communication problems.

### WHY IT IS DONE

Any person with a disturbance of language or a disorder of articulation, voice production, or fluency of speech (see *Speech disorders*) may be helped by speech therapy. These problems may occur as part of a broader problem, such as a physical handicap, learning difficulty, or hearing loss. Speech therapists work with all age groups.

### HOW IT IS DONE

The therapist—a person trained in the causes, assessment, and treatment of speech and language problems—usually begins by taking a history from the client or from a relative or friend, asking how and when the difficulties developed. Relevant medical details are also sought from the client's physician, if necessary.

The client may be asked to provide a sample of speech (which may be recorded) or of writing for detailed analysis. An examination of the physical structures of speech and a hearing

test may be performed. The therapist may also assess language comprehension by observing the client's reaction to written or spoken requests.

After making an assessment, the therapist decides on the form of treatment, which is carried out in two parts. A program of exercises is started to improve a specific aspect of language ability or speech performance (e.g., a technique to improve speech fluency). Also, the therapist works with the people most involved with the client (e.g., family, teachers, or friends), explaining to them the nature of the difficulties and how they can help. The aim of therapy is to create a climate that will provide the client with opportunities for effective communication.

## Sperm

 The male sex cell, also known as spermatozoon (singular) or spermatozoa (plural), responsible for *fertilization* of the female ovum. Sperm are microscopically tiny, measuring 0.002 inch (0.05 mm) in length.

Sperm are produced within the seminiferous tubules of the *testes* by a process known as spermatogenesis. The production and development of sperm is dependent on the male sex hormone *testosterone* and on *gonadotropin hormones* produced by the *pituitary gland*. Sperm production commences at *puberty*.

The original cell from which a sperm develops contains 46 chromosomes, including the XY pair of male sex *chromosomes*. By a process of *cell division*, the number of chromosomes in the sperm is halved to 23, including either the X or the Y from the original pair of sex chromosomes. This X or Y is responsible for determining the sex of an embryo that develops after fertilization of the ovum by the sperm (see *Sex determination*).

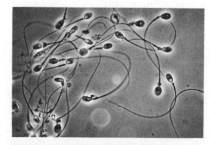

**Human sperm magnified 350 times**
Each sperm consists of a head that contains the hereditary material and a long, whiplike tail that propels it along.

S

The final stage of spermatogenesis takes place in the *epididymis*, where the sperm grow tails that will propel them through the woman's reproductive tract after *ejaculation* during sexual intercourse.

## Spermatocele

A harmless cyst of the *epididymis* (the tube that transmits sperm from the testis) that contains fluid and sperm. If the spermatocele grows to a large size or becomes uncomfortable, it is usually removed surgically. Although the operation is straightforward, it may result in an interruption of the passage of sperm, which may render the testis on the affected side infertile.

## Spermatozoa

See *Sperm*.

## Spermicides

Contraceptive preparations that kill sperm. Spermicides are usually recommended for use with a barrier device, such as a condom or diaphragm, to increase the final contraceptive effect (see *Contraception, barrier methods*).

Some spermicides, such as nonoxynol, may protect against the organisms that cause various *sexually transmitted diseases*, including *gonorrhea* and *AIDS*.

A possible adverse effect is irritation of the genitals of either partner.

## Sphenoid bone

The bat-shaped bone in the center of the base of the cranium (the part of the *skull* that encases the brain). The central body of the bone contains the sphenoidal sinus (air space) and, in the upper surface, a depression in which the *pituitary gland* is situated. The wings support part of the temporal lobe of the brain (see *Cerebrum*) and form part of the back and side walls of the orbits (eye sockets). There are various canals and foramens (holes) in the wings to enable the optic and other cranial nerves to pass through.

## Spherocytosis, hereditary

An inherited disorder so named because of the large number of unusually small, round, red blood cells (spherocytes) in the circulation. These cells have an abnormal membrane (outer envelope), which makes them fragile, and a much reduced life span because they are readily trapped, broken up, and consumed when blood passes through

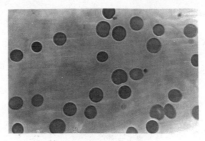

**Spherocytes in blood**
A person with hereditary spherocytosis has a large number of these unusually small, round, fragile, red cells in the blood.

the *spleen*. At times, the rate of hemolysis (red cell destruction) exceeds the rate at which new cells can be made in the bone marrow, leading to *anemia* (reduced level of the oxygen-carrying pigment *hemoglobin* in the blood due to lack of red cells).

### INCIDENCE

Hereditary spherocytosis is the most common form of inherited hemolytic anemia in people of northern European extraction. About one person in 4,500 in the US has the condition. The disorder is inherited in autosomal dominant fashion (see *Genetic disorders*). Each of an affected person's children has a 50 percent chance of inheriting the defective gene responsible for the abnormality.

### SYMPTOMS, DIAGNOSIS, AND TREATMENT

Symptoms of anemia, such as tiredness, shortness of breath on exertion, and pallor, may develop at any age. Other symptoms include *jaundice* (caused by the high rate of blood cell destruction) and enlargement of the spleen. Occasionally, there are crises (triggered by infections) when all the symptoms worsen. *Gallstones*, also caused by the high rate of bilirubin release, are a frequent complication.

The diagnosis is made from the presence of spherocytes in the blood of someone with anemia and from tests to ascertain the structure of the red cell membrane.

The treatment is *splenectomy* (removal of the spleen). The red cells remain abnormally shaped, but the rate at which they are destroyed drops markedly, leading to a striking, and usually permanent, improvement in the patient's health.

## Sphincter

A ring of muscle around a natural opening or passage that acts like a valve, regulating inflow or outflow. For example, the outlet of the stomach into the duodenum is called the

pyloric sphincter. It controls the stomach's outflow. The anal sphincter at the rectal outlet is partly under voluntary control, permitting us to decide when to empty the bowel.

## Sphincter, artificial

A surgically created valve or other device used to treat or prevent urinary or fecal *incontinence*.

An artificial urinary sphincter consists of an inflatable cuff that is inserted around the base of the bladder or upper part of the urethra. When inflated, the cuff prevents urine from leaking from the bladder. The patient deflates the cuff by using a pump, which is usually situated in the scrotum in males or adjacent to the labia in females.

An artificial sphincter to prevent fecal incontinence may be created after removal of the colon and rectum. This operation, an alternative to a conventional *ileostomy*, involves using a loop of ileum to create a pouch in which bowel contents collect. Evacuation of feces is controlled by an artificial sphincter, surgically fashioned from a section of ileum.

A similar "continent ileostomy" may be provided for a person whose bladder has been removed to treat cancer and whose ureters are then joined to a segment of ileum that is formed into a pouch. This procedure is still under development and considered experimental, as are other methods of continent *urinary diversion*.

## Sphincterotomy

A surgical procedure that involves cutting the muscle that closes a body opening or that constricts the opening between body passages. In rare cases, sphincterotomy is performed on the anal sphincter to treat an *anal fissure*. It is also performed on the ampulla of Vater (the opening of the common bile duct into the duodenum) to release an impacted *gallstone*.

## Sphygmomanometer

An instrument for measuring blood pressure. It consists of a cuff with an inflatable bladder that is wrapped around the upper arm, a rubber bulb to inflate the bladder, and a device that indicates the pressure of blood. This pressure device may consist of a calibrated glass column filled with mercury, a spring gauge and dial, or, in more modern instruments, a digital readout display. (For an explanation of how a sphygmomanometer is used, see *Blood pressure*.)

S

## Spider bites

Nearly all spiders produce venom, which they inject, via a pair of fangs, to paralyze and kill their prey. However, only a few species are harmful to humans. In the US, the two most dangerous types are the black widow spider (*LATRODECTUS MACTANS*) and the brown recluse spider (*LOXOSCELES RECLUSA*).

The black widow is a small, shiny black spider, less than half an inch (1 cm) long but with a leg span of up to 2 inches (5 cm). It has a red hourglass-shaped marking on its underside. This spider can be found in most parts of the US in woodpiles, sheds, and the bowls of outside toilets, from which it may deliver a bite to a person's buttocks or genitals.

A bite from a black widow can cause severe pain and muscle spasms (starting near the site of the bite and spreading), heavy sweating, stomach cramps, nausea, vomiting, tightness in the chest, breathing difficulty, and a sharp rise in blood pressure. These symptoms may continue for several days. Deaths from *cardiac arrest* or *respiratory failure* occur occasionally in children or the elderly, but are uncommon in adults. Treatment consists of *analgesics* (painkillers) and an intravenous injection of a solution of calcium gluconate, which relieves the muscle cramps. If symptoms are very severe, or if the patient is a young child, an *antivenin* active against the spider venom may also be given.

Recluse spiders are brown or brown-yellow. They occur in southern and southwestern states, where they inhabit crevices in or around houses. Their bite causes severe pain, reddening, blistering, and death of tissue at the site of the wound, followed by a deep ulcer. Treatment consists of analgesics, care of the wound to prevent infection, and measures to deal with complications, which can include hemolytic *anemia* and *renal failure*. Fatalities have occurred in children.

Other dangerous spiders include relatives of the black widow spider, and the "funnel web" spider of Australia. The hairy tarantula of southern Europe is relatively harmless, although its bite is painful.

## Spider nevus

A discolored patch of skin that takes the form of a red, raised dot the size of a pinhead with small blood vessels radiating from this dot. Also called telangiectasia, spider nevi represent

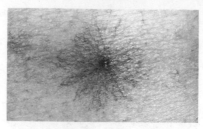

**Typical spider nevus**
The nevus consists of a tiny, red, raised dot from which widened blood capillaries radiate outward in all directions.

the outward appearance of a dilated arteriole (small artery) and its connecting capillaries.

Small numbers of spider nevi are common in children and pregnant women. However, in larger quantities, spider nevi may be a sign of an underlying disorder, such as advanced *cirrhosis* of the liver. Lesions resembling multiple spider nevi (but without the "spider legs") may be a sign of hereditary hemorrhagic telangiectasia, a disorder of the blood vessels that causes bleeding and iron-deficiency anemia.

## Spina bifida

A congenital defect in which part of one (or more) *vertebrae* fails to develop completely, leaving a portion of the *spinal cord* exposed. Spina bifida can occur anywhere on the spine but is most common in the lower back. The severity of the condition depends on how much nerve tissue is exposed.

**CAUSES AND INCIDENCE**
The cause of spina bifida remains unknown; it is thought that many factors are involved.

The incidence is about one case per 1,000 babies born. The incidence increases with either very young or old maternal age. A woman who has had one affected child is ten times more likely than the average of having another affected child.

**TYPES**
There are four known distinct forms of spina bifida.

**SPINA BIFIDA OCCULTA** This is the most common and the least serious form. There is little external evidence of the defect apart from a dimple or a tuft of hair over the area of the underlying abnormality. Spina bifida occulta often goes completely unnoticed in otherwise healthy children, although occasionally there are accompanying abnormalities of the lower part of the spinal cord. Symptoms, which include leg weakness, cold and blue

feet, and urinary incontinence, may be present from birth or may develop later in life.

**MYELOCELE** Also known as meningomyelocele, this is the most severe form of spina bifida. The nature of the defect is shown in the illustrated box on the opposite page.

A child with myelocele is usually severely handicapped. The legs are partially or completely paralyzed, with loss of sensation in all areas below the level of the defect; hip dislocation and other leg deformities are common. *Hydrocephalus* (excess cerebrospinal fluid within the skull) is common and may result in brain damage. Associated abnormalities include *cerebral palsy, epilepsy, mental retardation*, and visual problems. Paralysis of the bladder leads to urinary incontinence or urinary retention, repeated urinary tract infections, and eventual kidney damage. The anus may be paralyzed, causing chronic constipation and leakage of feces.

**MENINGOCELE** This form is less severe than myelocele. The nature of the defect is shown in the box opposite.

**ENCEPHALOCELE** This is a rare type of spina bifida in which the protrusion occurs through the skull. There is usually severe brain damage.

**DIAGNOSIS**
Closure of the vertebral canal usually occurs within four weeks of conception, meaning that meningomyelocele can often be diagnosed at an early stage in the pregnancy by *ultrasound scanning*. High levels of *alpha-fetoprotein* in the amniotic fluid or maternal blood may indicate spina bifida.

After birth, spina bifida is easy to recognize if there is a protruding sac. Spina bifida occulta can be diagnosed only by spinal X ray.

**TREATMENT**
In cases that are not severe, surgery may be performed to close the defect and thus prevent further damage to the spinal cord. Ideally, the operation should be performed in the first few days of life. If the abnormality is serious, surgery may allow the child to survive, although he or she may have gross physical and mental handicap.

If hydrocephalus develops, a *shunt* (tube) is inserted into the brain to relieve the buildup of fluid. Retention or incontinence of urine is relieved by an indwelling catheter (which is changed every four to six weeks); in older children, self-catheterization can be taught (see *Catheterization, urinary*). Laxatives or enemas may be needed for constipation.

**S**

## TYPES OF SPINA BIFIDA

There are different forms of spina bifida. In one type (spina bifida occulta), the only defect is a failure of the fusion of the bony arches behind the spinal cord. When the bone defect is more extensive, there may be a meningocele, with protrusion of the meninges (the membranes surrounding the cord) or, more seriously, a myelocele, with change in the spinal cord itself.

### MENINGOCELE

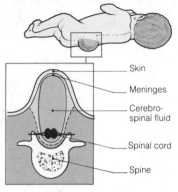

Skin
Meninges
Cerebro-
spinal fluid
Spinal cord
Spine

**Meningocele**
In this type, the nerve tissue of the spinal cord is usually intact; there is skin over the bulging sac and there are therefore usually no functional problems. However, repairs are necessary early in life.

### MYELOCELE

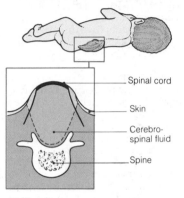

Spinal cord
Skin
Cerebro-
spinal fluid
Spine

**Myelocele**
In this type, the baby is born with a raw swelling over the spine. It consists of malformed spinal cord, which may or may not be contained in a membranous sac. The child is likely to be very handicapped.

*Physical therapy* encourages mobility and independence; for the more severely affected, wheelchairs and other walking aids may be required. Depending on the degree of disability, special schooling and training for employment may be needed.

#### PREVENTION
Parents who have had one child with spina bifida should undergo *genetic counseling* if they are considering another pregnancy.

## Spinal accessory nerve

The eleventh *cranial nerve*. The spinal accessory nerve differs from the other cranial nerves in that only a small part of it originates from the brain; most of the nerve comes from the spinal cord.

The part of the nerve originating from the brain supplies many muscles of the palate, pharynx (throat), and larynx (voice box). Damage to this part of the nerve may give rise to dysphonia (difficulty speaking) and dysphagia (difficulty swallowing).

The spinal part of the nerve supplies some large muscles of the neck and back, notably the sternomastoid (which runs from the breastbone to the side of the skull) and the trapezius (a large, triangular muscle of the upper back, shoulder, and neck). Damage to the spinal fibers of the nerve paralyzes these muscles. Such damage usually occurs as a result of surgery for cancer in which lymph nodes in the neck are removed.

## Spinal anesthesia

A method of blocking pain sensations before they reach the central nervous system by injecting an anesthetic into the cerebrospinal fluid in the spinal canal. The technique is primarily used to accompany surgery on the lower abdomen and legs. Operations on the hip and prostate gland are commonly performed using spinal or *epidural anesthesia*. The decision as to which anesthesia to use is made after discussion among the patient, anesthesiologist, and surgeon.

The procedure is performed by inserting a delicate needle between two vertebrae in the lower part of the spine (see *Lumbar puncture*) and introducing anesthetic into the cerebrospinal fluid surrounding the spinal cord and its terminal nerve roots. Because the nerves emerging from the spinal cord are bathed in cerebrospinal fluid, they absorb the anesthetic. The position of the injec-

tion and subsequent controlled spread of the local anesthetic solution determines the area that is anesthetized.

After spinal anesthesia, a headache may develop in between 1 and 5 percent of patients.

## Spinal cord

A cylinder of nerve tissue, about 18 inches long and roughly the thickness of a finger, that runs down the central canal in the *spine*. It is a downward extension of the brain. The spinal cord and brain can be considered parts of a single unit—the central nervous system (CNS).

#### STRUCTURE
At the core of the spinal cord is a region with a butterfly-shaped cross section, called the gray matter. It contains the cell bodies of neurons (nerve cells) along with glial (supporting) cells. Some of the nerve cells are motor neurons, whose axons (long, projecting fibers) pass out of the spinal cord in bundles within the *spinal nerves* and extend to glands or muscles in the trunk and limbs. Others are interneurons (nerve cells contained entirely within the central nervous system), which act to convey messages between other neurons. Also entering the gray matter are the axons of sensory neurons (which have their cell bodies outside the spinal cord). These axons connect with the motor neurons or interneurons.

Surrounding the gray matter are areas of white matter, which consist of bundles of nerve cell axons running lengthwise through the cord.

Sprouting from the spinal cord on each side at regular intervals are two nerve bundles—the spinal nerve roots, which contain the fibers of motor and sensory nerve cells. They combine to form the spinal nerves, which emerge from the spine and are the communication cables between the spinal cord and all regions of the trunk and limbs.

The whole of the spinal cord is bathed in *cerebrospinal fluid* and surrounded by a protective sheath, a continuation of the *meninges* that protect the brain.

#### FUNCTION
The nerve tracts that make up the white matter of the spinal cord act mainly as highways for sensory information passing upward toward the brain (ascending tracts) or motor signals passing downward (descending tracts). However, the cord is also capable of handling some of the sensory information itself and of provid-

S

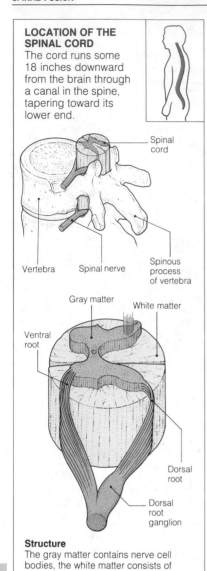

**LOCATION OF THE SPINAL CORD**
The cord runs some 18 inches downward from the brain through a canal in the spine, tapering toward its lower end.

Spinal cord

Vertebra    Spinal nerve    Spinous process of vertebra

Gray matter    White matter

Ventral root

Dorsal root

Dorsal root ganglion

**Structure**
The gray matter contains nerve cell bodies, the white matter consists of tracts of nerve fibers. Spinal nerves join the cord at regular intervals.

ing appropriate motor responses without recourse to the brain. Many *reflex* actions (such as the knee jerk reflex) are controlled in this way by the spinal cord.

**DISORDERS**

The spinal cord may be injured as a result of trauma to the spine (see *Spinal injury*). If an ascending or descending tract is severed, it interrupts communication between the brain and parts of the body served from parts of the cord below the injury. This can lead to a variety of patterns of paralysis and/or loss of sensation, which are usually permanent because

nerve cells and fibers within the cord do not regenerate. However, reflexes controlled by the spinal cord are usually maintained.

Pressure on the cord (e.g., by a blood clot, an abscess, or tumor) can similarly affect movement and sensation. However, the effects of pressure can often be relieved by surgery.

Infections of the spinal cord (including *poliomyelitis*) are relatively rare but can cause serious damage. In *multiple sclerosis*, a degenerative disease, there is patchy loss of the insulating sheaths around nerve fibers.

## Spinal fusion

A major surgical procedure to join two or more adjacent vertebrae, the bones that make up the spine.

**WHY IT IS DONE**

Spinal fusion is performed if abnormal movement between adjacent vertebrae (as revealed by X rays) causes severe back pain or may damage the spinal cord. Such abnormal movement may be due to various spinal disorders, including *spondylolisthesis*, dislocated facet joints (the movable joints that connect vertebrae), *scoliosis*, *osteomyelitis*, a tumor or injury destroying one or more vertebrae, or *osteoarthritis* that causes degeneration of spinal joints.

**HOW IT IS DONE**

Using a general anesthetic, the affected vertebrae are exposed. *Arthrodesis* (joint fusion) is then carried out, sometimes with a *bone graft*, using bone chips taken from the pelvis. A temporary fixation is made with a plate or screws.

The recovery period includes bed rest for up to six weeks. When mobility is resumed, the patient may initially need to wear a plaster jacket. Full fusion of the vertebrae takes up to six months.

Results are usually good, but fusing the vertebrae may place greater strain on the rest of the spine and cause more back pain. The potential gain must be weighed against the risks.

## Spinal injury

Damage to the *spine* and sometimes to the *spinal cord*, in which case the injury may cause loss of sensation and muscle weakness or paralysis.

**CAUSES**

Spinal injury is usually caused by one of three types of severe force—longitudinal compression, hinging, and shearing. Longitudinal compression, usually due to a fall from a height, crushes the vertebrae (seg-

ments of spine) lengthwise against each other. Hinging, which can occur in a whiplash injury suffered in an automobile accident, subjects the spinal column to sudden, extreme bending movements. Shearing, which may occur when a person is knocked over by a motor vehicle, for example, combines both hinging and rotational (twisting) forces.

Any of these forces can dislocate the vertebrae, fracture them, or rupture the ligaments that bind them together. In severe dislocations and fractures, the vertebrae, accumulated fluid, or a blood clot may press on the spinal cord, or the cord may be torn or even severed. In all of these cases the function of the spinal cord is impaired or destroyed. An unstable injury is one in which there is the possibility that vertebrae will shift and cause damage, possibly severing the spinal cord. Other injuries are called stable.

**SYMPTOMS AND SIGNS**

Damage to the vertebrae and ligaments usually causes severe pain and swelling of the affected area. Damage to the spinal cord results in loss of sensation and/or motor function below the site of injury. Injuries below the neck may cause *paraplegia* (weakness or paralysis of the legs and sometimes part of the trunk); damage to the cord in the neck may result in *quadriplegia* (weakness or paralysis of all four limbs and the trunk) or may be fatal. Weakness or paralysis is often accompanied by loss of bladder or bowel control, resulting in urinary or fecal incontinence or retention.

Pressure on the spinal cord may cause motor abnormalities, such as muscle weakness or paralysis. It may also cause abnormalities of sensation, such as pain, tingling, or burning sensations.

**DIAGNOSIS AND TREATMENT**

After an accident in which a spinal injury may have occurred, the victim should be moved only by someone trained in all aspects of first aid. *X rays* of the spine are carried out to determine whether the spine has been injured and the extent of any damage.

In a stable injury, the patient must rest in bed until comfortable movement is possible; he or she may then need to wear an orthopedic *collar* or *corset* for support or to relieve pain in the injured area.

The priority in an unstable injury is to stabilize the affected bones. If they are dislocated, the surgeon usually manipulates them back into position using a general anesthetic. Some unstable fractures are treated by skeletal *traction* to align the bone ends and hold them in position until healing occurs (which may take up to three months). Other unstable fractures require an operation to fasten the bone ends together permanently with a metal plate or wires.

Surgical repair of damaged nerve tracts in the spinal cord is not possible. Treatment is directed toward preventing the development of problems secondary to the main symptoms. For example, the patient is turned regularly in bed to prevent *bedsores* from forming as the result of immobility and lack of sensation in the skin. *Physical therapy* is carried out to stop joints from locking and muscles from contracting as the result of paralysis. Retention of urine or feces may require catheterization (see *Catheterization, urinary*) or *enemas*.

**OUTLOOK**
Recovery is usually complete when the spinal cord has not been damaged, although there may be some residual pain and stiffness. When there has been pressure on the spinal cord, surgery to remove the source of the pressure can bring variable improvement in symptoms. Even when there is damage to the cord, some improvement may occur for up to 12 months. In such cases, the patient's recovery can be aided by a program of *rehabilitation*. This may include forms of physical and occupational therapy, which can help morale and independence.

# Spinal nerves

A set of 31 pairs of nerves that connects to the spinal cord.

**STRUCTURE**
The spinal nerves emerge in two rows from either side of the spinal cord and leave the spine through gaps between adjacent vertebrae (segments of spine). Because the spinal cord runs only two thirds of the way down the canal in the center of the spine, the lowest nine pairs of nerves must travel some distance down the canal before finally leaving the backbone. They form a spray of nerves in this area known as the cauda equina.

The distribution and branching of the spinal nerves ensures that all parts of the trunk, arms, and legs are supplied with a network of sensory and motor nerve twigs.

**FUNCTION**
Like all nerves, the spinal nerves consist of bundles of the axons (long fibers) of individual neurons (nerve cells). Some of these fibers carry information from sensory receptors in the skin, muscles, and elsewhere toward the spinal cord; other motor fibers carry signals from the spinal cord to muscles and glands. Just before it connects to the spinal cord, each spinal nerve splits into two bundles, one of which carries only sensory fibers and the other of which carries only motor fibers. These bundles are sometimes called spinal nerve roots.

**DISORDERS**
Damage to the shock-absorbing disk of cartilage between two vertebrae sometimes leads to pressure on a spinal nerve root, causing pain (see *Disk prolapse*). Injury to a spinal nerve may lead to loss of sensation and movement in a part of the body. Damage or degeneration from such causes or from infection, diabetes, vitamin deficiency, and poisoning can lead to neurological symptoms such as pain, numbness, or twitching (see *Nerve injury*; *Neuropathy*).

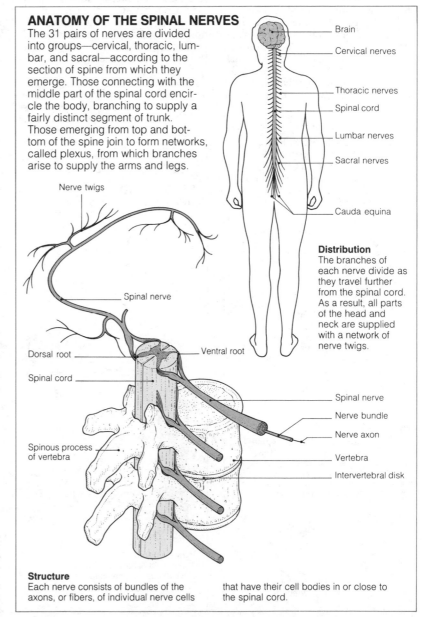

## ANATOMY OF THE SPINAL NERVES
The 31 pairs of nerves are divided into groups—cervical, thoracic, lumbar, and sacral—according to the section of spine from which they emerge. Those connecting with the middle part of the spinal cord encircle the body, branching to supply a fairly distinct segment of trunk. Those emerging from top and bottom of the spine join to form networks, called plexus, from which branches arise to supply the arms and legs.

Brain
Cervical nerves
Thoracic nerves
Spinal cord
Lumbar nerves
Sacral nerves
Cauda equina

Nerve twigs
Spinal nerve
Dorsal root
Ventral root
Spinal cord
Spinous process of vertebra
Spinal nerve
Nerve bundle
Nerve axon
Vertebra
Intervertebral disk

**Distribution**
The branches of each nerve divide as they travel further from the spinal cord. As a result, all parts of the head and neck are supplied with a network of nerve twigs.

**Structure**
Each nerve consists of bundles of the axons, or fibers, of individual nerve cells that have their cell bodies in or close to the spinal cord.

S

## Spinal tap
See *Lumbar puncture*.

## Spine
The column of bones and cartilage that extends from the base of the skull to the pelvis, enclosing and protecting the *spinal cord* and supporting the trunk and head.

#### STRUCTURE AND FUNCTION
The spine is made up of 33 roughly cylindrical bones called *vertebrae*. Each pair of adjacent vertebrae is connected by a joint, called a facet joint, which both stabilizes the vertebral column and allows movement in it. Between each pair of vertebrae lies a disk-shaped pad of tough fibrous cartilage with a jellylike core (nucleus pulposus) called an intervertebral disk (see *Disk, intervertebral*). These disks act to cushion the vertebrae during movements such as running or jumping.

The whole of the spine encloses the spinal cord, a column of nerve tracts running from the brain. Peripheral nerves (see *Peripheral nervous system*) branch off from the spinal cord to every part of the body, their roots passing between the vertebrae.

The vertebrae are bound together by two long, thick ligaments running the length of the spine and by smaller ligaments between each vertebra.

Several groups of muscles are attached to the vertebrae. These muscles control movements of the spine and also help to support it.

In a normal spine the cervical section curves forward, the thoracic section backward, the lumbar section forward (particularly in women), and the pelvic section backward.

## Spirochete
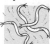
A spiral-shaped bacterium. Spirochetes cause *syphilis*, *pinta* and *yaws* (both related to syphilis), and *leptospirosis*, *relapsing fever*, and *Lyme disease*.

## Spirometry
A *pulmonary function test* used to help diagnose or assess a lung disorder or to monitor treatment.

The procedure is shown in the illustrated box below. The spirometer records the total volume of air breathed out, known as the forced vital capacity (FVC). It also records the volume of air breathed out in 1 second, known as the forced expiratory volume in 1 second (FEV$_1$).

In obstructive lung disease (such as *asthma*, *emphysema*, and chronic bronchitis), the FEV$_1$/FVC ratio is reduced because the airways are narrowed, thus slowing expiration. In a restrictive lung disease (such as *interstitial pulmonary fibrosis*), the FVC and FEV$_1$ are reduced almost equally with little change in the ratio. This is because lung expansion is limited but the airways are not narrowed.

## Spironolactone
A potassium-sparing *diuretic drug*. Combined with thiazide or loop diuretics, spironolactone is given to treat

---

### STRUCTURE OF THE SPINE
The spine is made up of a column of 33 roughly cylindrical bones called vertebrae. Running through the center of this bony structure is the spinal cord.

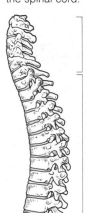

**Cervical spine**
Seven vertebrae, the topmost of which supports the skull.

**Thoracic spine**
Twelve vertebrae that run down the rear wall of the chest. A pair of ribs is attached to each vertebra.

**Lumbar spine**
Five vertebrae. This section is the one under the most pressure during lifting.

**Sacrum**
Five fused vertebrae.

**Coccyx**
Four fused vertebrae.

---

### SPIROMETRY
This technique is used to assess certain lung conditions and the patient's response to treatment. It records the rate at which a patient exhales air from the lungs and the total volume exhaled.

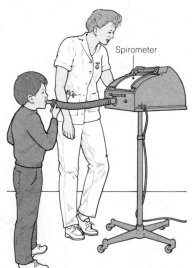

Spirometer

**How it is done**
The patient exhales forcibly through a mouthpiece into the spirometer. This causes the spirometer to produce a graph like that shown at right.

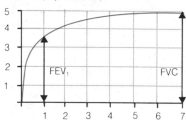

**Volume** (expired liters)

FEV$_1$    FVC

**Time** (seconds)

**Normal**
FEV$_1$ (forced expiratory volume of the first second) is the volume of air exhaled in the first second and is normally 60 to 80 percent of FVC (forced vital capacity), the total volume exhaled.

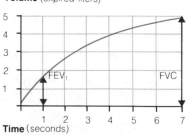

**Volume** (expired liters)

FEV$_1$    FVC

**Time** (seconds)

**Asthma**
A patient with asthma cannot exhale air as fast as normal, due to narrowing of the airways, so FEV$_1$ is reduced in comparison with FVC.

S

## DISORDERS OF THE SPINE
Many disorders of the spine, despite their different causes, result in just one symptom—*back pain.*

### CONGENITAL DISORDERS
Some children are born with a gap in the vertebrae that leaves part of the spinal cord exposed. This condition (*spina bifida*) results in leg paralysis and incontinence.

### INFECTION
*Osteomyelitis* (infection of bone and bone marrow) may in rare cases affect a vertebra, destroying both bone and disk. The most common cause is the spread of an infection, such as tuberculosis, from elsewhere in the body.

### INFLAMMATION
In *ankylosing spondylitis*, and in some cases of *rheumatoid arthritis*, the joints in the spine become inflamed and later fuse, causing permanent stiffness. *Osteochondritis juvenilis* (inflammation of the growing area of bone in children and adolescents) can affect the vertebrae, when the disease may cause deformity of the spine.

### INJURIES
Lifting heavy objects, twisting suddenly, or adopting bad posture can cause any of the following spinal injuries—a sprained ligament, torn muscle, *spondylolisthesis* (dislocated vertebrae), dislocated facet joint, or *disk prolapse* (rupture of the tough outer layer of the disk).

A direct blow, a fall from a height, or sudden twisting can result in fracture of one or more vertebrae. Overexercising the spine can have the same effect (see *Stress fracture*).

### TUMORS
Tumors of the spine are usually malignant; in most cases, they have spread from cancer elsewhere in the body (see *Bone cancer*).

### DEGENERATION
*Osteoarthritis* (degeneration of joint cartilage due to wear and tear) affects the joints in the spines of virtually everyone over 60, particularly people who do heavy manual work or people whose spines have already been affected by disease or injury.

*Osteoporosis* (thinning and softening of bone), which is most common in older women, can weaken the vertebrae. Under the weight of the trunk, the vertebrae may then fracture.

### OTHER DISORDERS
In some people the spine becomes abnormally curved. The excessive curvature may be inward in the lower back (see *Lordosis*), outward in the upper back (see *Kyphosis*), or to one side (see *Scoliosis*). Causes include infection, osteoporosis, congenital spine disorder, and muscle disorders.

### INVESTIGATION
Spinal disorders are investigated by *X rays, CT scanning*, and *myelography.* Other *bone imaging* techniques, including *MRI*, may sometimes be performed, as may other tests.

---

*hypertension* (high blood pressure) and *edema* (fluid retention).

Spironolactone may cause numbness, weakness, nausea, and vomiting. Less common adverse effects include diarrhea, lethargy, impotence, rash, and irregular menstruation in women. High doses of spironolactone may cause abnormal breast enlargement in men.

## Spleen
An organ that removes and destroys worn-out red blood cells and helps fight infection. Weighing about 7 ounces (200 grams), the spleen is a fist-sized, spongy, dark purple organ lying in the upper left abdomen behind the lower ribs.

### STRUCTURE
The spleen is covered with a capsule from which many fibrous bands run inward to give the organ a spongelike structure. The spaces between the bands are filled with lymph tissue, composed of *lymphocytes* and *phagocytes* (cells that ingest other cells or foreign particles), and red blood cells. Blood is supplied to the spleen by a large artery that branches extensively within the organ.

### FUNCTION
One of the two main functions of the spleen is to control the quality of circulating red blood cells. It accomplishes this by removing and breaking down all worn-out red cells approximately 120 days after they have been produced in the bone marrow and by destroying other red cells that are misshapen or defective.

The other role of the spleen is to help fight infection by producing some of the *antibodies*, phagocytes, and lymphocytes that destroy invading microorganisms.

In the fetus, the spleen produces red blood cells. After birth, this function is taken over by the bone marrow. However, in certain diseases that affect cell production in the bone marrow (such as *thalassemia*), the spleen may resume production.

Despite its functions, the spleen is not an essential organ. If it is removed, its activities are largely taken over by other parts of the lymphatic system, although the individual is more susceptible to infection.

### DISORDERS
The spleen enlarges in many diseases, including infections such as *malaria*, *infectious mononucleosis* (glandular fever), *schistosomiasis*, *tuberculosis*, and *typhoid fever*; in *leukemia* and thalassemia; in some diseases that cause hemolytic *anemia* (such as *sickle cell anemia*); and in tumors of the spleen. The enlargement, which can often be felt as a swelling in the upper left abdomen, is sometimes accompanied by *hypersplenism*.

*Lymphomas* (tumors of lymphoid tissue) may develop in the spleen and elsewhere in the lymphatic system.

The spleen is sometimes ruptured by a severe blow to the abdomen, usually in an automobile crash or by a fall from a height. A rupture is much more likely if the spleen is enlarged or if overlying ribs are fractured. Rupture can cause severe bleeding, which may be fatal. For this reason, the injury requires an emergency operation to remove the spleen and tie off the artery supplying it (see *Splenectomy*).

## Splenectomy
Surgical removal of the *spleen.*

### WHY IT IS DONE
Splenectomy is usually performed after the spleen has been seriously injured, causing severe hemorrhage.

S

The organ is removed because it is difficult to repair and because, in an adult, its absence has virtually no known ill effects. Its function is largely taken over by other parts of the lymphatic system and by the liver.

The spleen is also removed to treat primary *hypersplenism* and certain types of anemia, such as hereditary *spherocytosis*. Splenectomy may be performed during *laparotomy* (surgical exploration of the abdomen) as part of a process (called staging) to assess the extent of *Hodgkin's disease*.

#### HOW IT IS DONE
Using a general anesthetic, a vertical or horizontal incision is made in the upper left abdomen, exposing the spleen. After attachments to other tissues have been cut and blood vessels leading into and out of the spleen have been clamped and severed, the organ is removed. The operation takes about an hour.

#### RECOVERY PERIOD AND OUTLOOK
Patients usually leave the hospital six to 10 days after the operation. Complications, such as infection of the operation site, are rare.

In an adult, absence of the spleen slightly increases the risk of contracting infections; children become markedly more susceptible, particularly to pneumococcal pneumonia. A child who has undergone a splenectomy should be immunized with pneumococcal vaccine and given long-term *antibiotic drugs*. Healthy fragments of a removed spleen are occasionally reimplanted in a child immediately after splenectomy; in some cases, these fragments regenerate to form an efficient new spleen.

## Splint
A device used to immobilize part of the body. Splints may be made of acrylic, polyethylene foam, plaster of Paris, or aluminum. Ambulances may carry inflatable splints. In an emergency, a splint can be constructed from a piece of wood or a rolled magazine or newspaper that is secured to the extremity.

## Splinting
The application of a *splint*. Splinting is used as a first-aid measure (see illustrated box) to prevent movement of a fractured limb or to immobilize a suspected fracture of the spine; this is especially important when the victim is being moved.

Splinting is sometimes required for leg fractures that are being treated by *traction*. Other uses of splint-ing include treatment of finger injuries, such as fracture or *baseball finger*, and of rheumatic disorders affecting the fingers, such as *tenosynovitis* (inflammation of tendon linings) and *rheumatoid arthritis*.

## Splinting, dental
The mechanical joining of several teeth to hold them firmly in place while an injury heals or *periodontal disease* is treated.

Splints may be used to secure teeth that have been fractured (see *Fracture, dental*) or loosened (see *Luxated tooth*). They may also be used after a tooth has been reimplanted (see *Reimplantation, dental*). Occasionally, teeth loosened by periodontal disease may be splinted to adjacent, firmer teeth. Splints may also be required after *orthognathic surgery*.

Splints are fashioned directly in the mouth with a variety of materials, such as wire, quick-setting plastic, and plastic crowns that can be bonded together. (See also *Wiring of the jaws*.)

## Split personality
A term used to describe two distinct disorders—*multiple personality*, in which an individual has two or more personalities, each of which dominates at different times, and *schizophrenia*, in which the sufferer's feelings and thoughts are not logically related to each other.

## Spondylitis
Inflammation of the joints between the vertebrae in the spine. Spondylitis is usually caused by a rheumatic disorder, such as *ankylosing spondylitis* or *rheumatoid arthritis*. In rare cases, spondylitis is due to a bacterial infection that has spread from elsewhere in the body.

### FIRST AID: SPLINTS

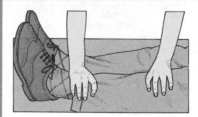

**1** If help is coming, do not move the victim but support the limb by placing one hand above the fracture and the other below it.

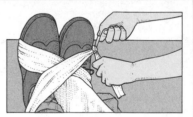

**3** Tie the victim's ankles and feet together with a figure-of-eight bandage. Secure the bandage on the victim's uninjured side.

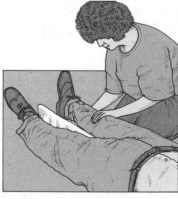

**2** If the ambulance is delayed or if the victim must be moved out of danger, first immobilize the leg. Place soft padding, such as a roll of cotton rolled around a splint, between the victim's knees and ankles and gently bring the uninjured leg to the injured one.

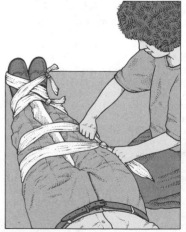

**4** Tie bandages around the knees, thighs, and legs, being careful to avoid the fracture site. Tie all knots on the uninjured side.

S

## Spondylolisthesis

The slipping forward (or occasionally backward) of a vertebra over the one below it. A forward slippage of the fifth (lowest) lumbar vertebra over the top of the sacrum is the most common form of the condition, but it may also occur between the fourth and fifth lumbar vertebrae or between two cervical (neck) vertebrae.

**CAUSES AND SYMPTOMS**
Lumbar spondylolisthesis, which involves two lumbar vertebrae or the fifth lumbar vertebra and the sacrum, is usually due to *spondylolysis* (in which the bony arch of a lumbar vertebra is abnormally soft and thus liable to slip under stress) or to *osteoarthritis* of the spine (in which the joints between the vertebrae become worn and unstable).

The principal symptoms of lumbar spondylolisthesis include pain in the back that is worse when standing and *sciatica*.

Cervical spondylolisthesis may be caused by a neck injury, congenital abnormality of the cervical spine, or *rheumatoid arthritis* (in which the supporting ligaments of the cervical spine are weakened or the joints between the vertebrae become worn). The main symptoms are pain and stiffness in the neck and, in severe cases, pain, numbness, or weakness in the sufferer's hands and arms.

**DIAGNOSIS AND TREATMENT**
Spondylolisthesis is diagnosed by X rays of the spine. Treatment may include *traction*, immobilization of the affected area in a plaster jacket or cervical collar, and *physical therapy*. In severe and rare cases (in which there is nerve compression damage or severe back pain), an operation to fuse the affected vertebrae may be necessary (see *Spinal fusion*).

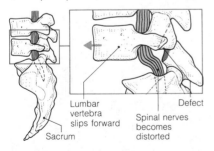

Lumbar          Defect
vertebra
slips forward   Spinal nerves
                becomes
Sacrum          distorted

Normal spine          Spondylolisthesis

**Lumbar spondylolisthesis**
If the lowest lumbar vertebra slips forward on the sacrum, it may distort or press on a spinal nerve, causing symptoms such as backache or sciatica.

## Spondylolysis

A spinal disorder in which the arch of the fifth (or, rarely, the fourth) lumbar vertebra consists of relatively soft fibrous tissue instead of normal bone. As a result, the arch is weaker than normal and is more likely to be deformed or damaged under stress, which may produce *spondylolisthesis* (forward slippage of a vertebra over the one below it). Otherwise, spondylolysis is usually symptomless.

## Sponge, contraceptive

A disposable, circular piece of polyurethane foam impregnated with *spermicide* that is inserted into the vagina as a method of birth control. (See *Contraception, barrier methods*.)

## Sporotrichosis

A chronic infection caused by the fungus *SPOROTHRIX SCHENCKII*, which grows on moss and other plants. The infection is most often contracted through a skin wound; gardeners and florists are particularly vulnerable. An ulcer develops at the site of the wound and is followed by the formation of nodules (which can be seen as a chain of protuberances beneath the skin) in lymph channels around the site. Potassium iodide solution taken by mouth usually clears up the infection.

Rarely, in people whose resistance to disease has been lowered, sporotrichosis spreads to the lungs, joints, and other parts of the body. This condition may require prolonged treatment with the *antifungal drug* amphotericin B.

## Sports, drugs and

The use of drugs to improve athletic performance has been universally condemned by authorities because it endangers the health of athletes and gives users of drugs an unfair advantage. Random urine tests to detect drug abuse are performed in most sports, both during competition and at other times during the season.

Certain drugs may be taken legitimately by athletes for medical disorders such as asthma or epilepsy. Care should be used, however, when taking a drug to treat diarrhea, nasal congestion, or cough because some common medications contain prohibited substances.

**TYPES OF DRUGS ABUSED**
Four types of drugs are abused to enhance physical or mental condition.
**STIMULANTS** Drugs of this group are taken to prevent fatigue and to increase self-confidence. However,

they also impair judgment and may cause excessive aggression, which increases the risk of injury to the user or an opponent.

Stimulants, such as *amphetamine drugs*, carry the risk of causing *arrhythmias*; prolonged use may cause *heart failure* (reduced pumping efficiency) and increase the risk of a *brain hemorrhage*. Some cold and cough remedies contain low doses of prohibited drugs and should be avoided before competition.

*Caffeine* contained in coffee, tea, and cola drinks, and available in tablets, is another popular stimulant. Most authorities only prohibit the use of caffeine in high doses.

**HORMONES** Two types of hormone drugs may be abused—anabolic steroids (see *Steroids, anabolic*) and growth hormone.

Anabolic steroids are substances similar to the male sex hormone testosterone. They are used because they speed the recovery of muscles after strenuous exercise. This permits a more demanding training schedule and causes an increase in muscle bulk and strength. Anabolic steroids are used primarily by weight lifters, field event athletes, and bodybuilders.

Risks of anabolic steroids include liver damage, liver tumors, and adrenal gland damage. In men they may cause infertility and impotence; in women they may cause *virilization*. If taken during childhood, anabolic steroids may cause short stature by affecting the growing areas of bones.

*Growth hormone* is abused to stimulate growth of muscle; it is likely to cause *acromegaly* (excessive bone growth leading to deformity of the face, hands, and feet) and may cause *diabetes mellitus*.

**PAINKILLERS** Only narcotic *analgesics* are prohibited but the use of any painkiller (even a weak analgesic such as acetaminophen) may aggravate an injury or lead to permanent damage by allowing the individual to participate with his or her pain masked.

**BETA-BLOCKER DRUGS** *Beta-blocker drugs* are taken to reduce tremor in sports in which a steady hand is vital. Many authorities now prohibit these drugs in the absence of a specific medical disorder that requires them.

## Sports injuries

Any injury that arises during participation in sports. Most sports injuries are not actually specific to sports; they can also occur as the result of other activities.

S

The wide range of sports injuries includes all types of *fracture, head injury* (including *concussion*), muscle tear (see *Strain*), ligament *sprain* or tears, *tendinitis* (inflammation of a tendon) or tendon rupture, joint *dislocation* or *subluxation* (partial dislocation), or injury to a specific organ (such as an *eye injury*).

Injuries specific to sports activities are mostly comparatively trivial. Examples include *joggers' nipple* (nipple soreness caused by friction) and *baseball finger* (tendon rupture in a finger caused by the ball striking the end of the finger).

Many injuries are given a sports prefix to their names, but can also be caused by injury unrelated to sports. *Tennis elbow* (painful inflammation of the bony prominence on the outside of the elbow) is a type of *overuse injury* that may occur from playing tennis, but more commonly results from an activity such as sawing wood.

Treatment of a sports injury depends on the body part involved and the severity of the damage. Recovery is not complete until the damaged area is free of pain during exercise. Exercises under the guidance of a sports physician or physical therapist may be required to ensure full recovery of movement, balance, and coordination of the injured part and to restore general fitness to reduce the likelihood of further injury.

## Sports medicine
The branch of medicine concerned with assessment and improvement of *fitness* and the treatment and prevention of medical disorders related to sports. Sports medicine physicians give advice about exercises that improve endurance, strength, and flexibility; perform fitness tests; offer nutritional advice to improve performance; regulate the abuse of drugs by athletes (see *Sports, drugs and*); and provide on-site medical care at sporting events.

Preventive work in sports medicine includes advising the individual on footwear, clothing, and protective equipment to reduce the likelihood of injury, and on fluid requirements to prevent dehydration. In addition, the sports physician advises professional athletes on immunization requirements before competition abroad, on coping with *jet lag*, and on changes in altitude and climate. In conjunction with the physical therapist (see *Physical therapy*), a sports physician diagnoses and treats *sports injuries*.

## Spouse abuse
Repeated deliberate physical injury inflicted by one spouse on the other, most often by a man on a woman.
### PREVALENCE
About one third of all reported assaults are by males on their female partners, and about one third of women filing for divorce describe physical abuse. There is little doubt that in addition to reported cases of spouse abuse many cases go unreported. In about 20 percent of reported cases the abuse continues for more than 10 years.
### CAUSES
Men who abuse their spouses have usually learned domestic violence from their parents' behavior, have an immature personality and low self-esteem, and acquire macho attitudes from their peer groups. Aggravating factors including *alcohol dependence, drug abuse, stress,* and obsession with the partner's sexual fidelity (see *Jealousy, morbid*).

Abused women in many cases stay with their partners for a combination of reasons, the most common of which are feelings of personal inadequacy, a sense of guilt leading to the belief that the violence is justified, fear of the social stigma involved in telling others about the abuse, underlying love for the partner, financial dependence, unwillingness to break up the family, social isolation, and depression (producing apathy).
### MANAGEMENT OF THE PROBLEM
Shelters have been opened in some areas to provide a temporary refuge for abused women and their children. More effective means of enforcing alimony payments by the courts would provide women with the financial resources needed to leave their partners. *Marital counseling* also has a role, provided the couple wishes to address the problem openly.

The best long-term approach to reducing the scale of the problem probably lies through education and a downgrading of the traditional macho view of acceptable male behavior.

## Sprain
Tearing or stretching of the ligaments that hold together the bone ends in a joint, caused by a sudden pull. The fibrous capsule that encloses the joint may also be damaged. The most commonly sprained joint is the ankle; it is usually sprained as a result of "going over" the outside of the foot so that the complete weight of the body is placed on the ankle.

A sprain causes painful swelling of the joint, which cannot be moved without increasing the pain. There may also be spasm (involuntary contraction) of surrounding muscles.
### TREATMENT
An X ray of the joint is usually performed to exclude the possibility of fracture. Treatment consists of applying an ice pack to reduce swelling, wrapping the joint with a compression bandage, resting it in a raised position until the pain and swelling begin to subside, and taking *analgesics* (painkillers) to relieve pain. Once the joint is no longer painful, it should be gently exercised.

If ligaments are badly torn, *nonsteroidal anti-inflammatory drugs* may be prescribed to speed healing. In extremely severe cases, surgical repair may be necessary.

## Sprue
A disorder of the intestines that causes failure to absorb nutrients from food. There are two forms of sprue. One occurs mainly in tropical regions (see *Sprue, tropical*); the other, *celiac sprue*, occurs more widely and is due to sensitivity to the wheat protein gluten.

## Sprue, tropical
A disease characterized by chronic *malabsorption* (impaired absorption of nutrients from the diet by the small intestine) and, as a result, *malnutrition*. As in *celiac sprue*, villi (frondlike projections) on the lining of the intestine become flattened, decreasing their surface for absorption.
### CAUSE AND INCIDENCE
The cause of tropical sprue is unknown, but it may result from an infection of the intestine. The disease occurs in tropical regions (e.g., the Caribbean, Far East, and India).
### SYMPTOMS AND TREATMENT
Symptoms include loss of appetite, weight loss, megaloblastic *anemia* (caused by a deficiency of folic acid and vitamin $B_{12}$), an inflamed mouth, sore tongue, and greasy diarrhea.

The diagnosis is confirmed by a jejunal *biopsy* (removal of a small sample of tissue from the upper small intestine for analysis). The disease responds well to treatment with *antibiotic drugs* and dietary supplements of folic acid, vitamin $B_{12}$, and other vitamins and minerals if necessary.

## Sputum
Mucous material produced by the cells lining the respiratory tract. Also known as phlegm, sputum is released

S

## FIRST AID: SPRAINS

> **WARNING**
> A severe sprain may be indistin-
> guishable from a broken bone. If
> in doubt, treat as a *fracture*.

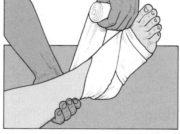

**1** The victim may not be able to move the affected joint or stand up if the knee or ankle is injured. Help the victim into a comfortable position and raise the injured body part.

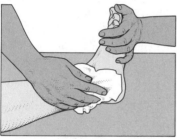

**2** If the sprain is recent, apply a cold compress to the affected area and leave for about 30 minutes. This will reduce blood flow and swelling.

**3** Cover the area with a roll of cotton and secure with a bandage. Make two turns around the foot, bring it across the top, and around the ankle..

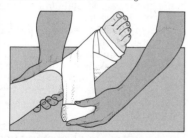

**4** Continue figure-of-eight turns, with each turn of the bandage overlapping the last turn by three fourths of its width.

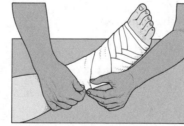

**5** Bandage until the foot (not toes), ankle, and lower leg are covered. Secure the loose end. Seek medical aid—an X ray may be necessary.

from glands in the walls of the bronchi (airways) and from cells lining the nose and sinuses.

Sputum production may be increased by infection (see *Respiratory tract infection*), by an allergic reaction (see *Asthma; Rhinitis, allergic*), or by inhalation of irritants, such as tobacco smoke (see *Cough, smokers'*). The presence of sputum in the bronchi triggers a reflex *cough*.

The character of sputum varies. A bacterial infection usually causes yellow or green sputum, an allergic reaction normally produces colorless sputum, and pulmonary *edema* (fluid retention in the lungs) may result in frothy, pink sputum. *Hemoptysis* (blood in the sputum) may be caused by infection or *lung cancer*.

Sputum may be examined under a microscope or prepared to *culture* any bacteria that might be present.

## Squamous cell carcinoma

One of the three most common types of skin cancer; the others are *basal cell carcinoma* and malignant *melanoma*.

**CAUSES AND INCIDENCE**
Squamous cell carcinoma arises from flattened, scalelike cells in the skin, usually areas that have been exposed to strong sunlight for many years and that may already have developed actinic or solar *keratoses*. This cancer is most common in pale-skinned, fair-haired people older than 60. The incidence is also higher in people whose work has exposed them to compounds such as arsenic, tar, coal, paraffin, or heavy oils.

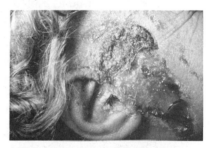

**A squamous cell carcinoma**
This tumor has spread slowly to cover much of the area in front of the patient's ear. It can be treated by radiation therapy.

**SYMPTOMS AND SIGNS**
The tumor starts as a small, firm, painless lump or patch (usually on the lip, ear, or back of the hand) and slowly enlarges, often resembling a wart or ulcer. If untreated, it may spread to other parts of the body and prove fatal. All suspicious skin lesions should be reported to a physician.

**DIAGNOSIS AND TREATMENT**
The diagnosis is based on a skin *biopsy* (removal of a small sample of tissue for analysis). The tumor is either removed surgically or destroyed by *radiation therapy* or *cryosurgery* (application of extreme cold). Treatment with *anticancer drugs* may also be necessary.

Any person who has had a squamous cell carcinoma should limit his or her exposure to sunlight. A follow-up examination is required to check for recurrence.

**S**

## Squint

See *Strabismus*.

## Stable

Unmoving, fixed, resistant to change, or in a state of equilibrium. A patient's condition is described as stable when it is neither deteriorating nor improving; a stable personality is one that is not susceptible to abnormal behavioral excesses or mental illness. In chemistry, a stable substance is one that is resistant to changes in its chemical composition or physical state, or is not radioactive.

## Stage

A term used in medicine to refer to a period or phase in the course of a disease, particularly in the progression of *cancer*. In assessing most types of cancer, a method (staging) is used to determine how far the cancer has progressed. The cancer is described in terms of how large the main tumor is, the degree to which it has invaded surrounding tissue, and the extent to which it has spread to lymph glands or other areas of the body. In *Hodgkin's disease*, staging also takes into account whether the lymph nodes on both sides of the diaphragm are affected, and whether the spleen is involved.

Staging not only helps to assess outlook (in general, the more advanced the stage, the worse the outlook) but also the most appropriate treatment. For example, a cancer at a particular stage may respond better to radiation therapy than to surgery.

## Staining

The process of dyeing specimens of cells, tissues, or microorganisms so that they are clearly visible or easily identifiable under a *microscope*. Staining is also sometimes carried out to detect or identify certain chemical substances in cells.

Before a specimen can be examined under a microscope, it must be preserved and then sliced (or smeared) extremely thinly. After these procedures, most specimens are almost transparent, so staining is necessary to make them easily visible. In *cytology* (the study of cells), cells are most commonly stained by the Papanicolaou (Pap) method; in *histology* (the study of tissues), the most commonly used stain is hematoxylin-eosin, a double stain that colors nuclei blue and cytoplasm pink.

Many other stains can be used to identify particular structures or products within cells. These stains may be used in addition to hematoxylin-eosin to clarify a diagnosis or to identify a particular microorganism in tissues.

In bacteriology, *Gram's stain* is widely used to identify and differentiate between groups of bacteria. A more recent development is the use of special fluorescent dyes that stain specific chemical constituents of cells or tissues; when illuminated with ultraviolet light, the stained constituents glow.

Another widely used technique called immunoperoxidase staining involves labeling (washing) the cells with antibodies to various cell components or cell chemicals. The antibodies are tagged with a dye that can be seen under the microscope as red-brown, enabling the observer to identify certain components if they are present within the cell.

## Stammering

See *Stuttering*.

## Stanford-Binet test

A type of *intelligence test*.

## Stanozolol

A steroid drug (see *Steroids, anabolic*).

## Stapedectomy

An operation to treat hearing loss caused by *otosclerosis*. In this disorder, the base of the *stapes* (the innermost of the three sound-conducting bones in the middle ear) becomes fixed to the entrance of the inner ear by an overgrowth of spongy bone. As a result, the stapes can no longer move freely to transmit sound to the inner ear. This form of deafness, often familial, is helped by a hearing aid but is curable only by surgery.

### HOW IT IS DONE

Using a local or general anesthetic, an incision is made in the ear canal and the eardrum is folded forward. All or most of the stapes is removed and a plastic or metal prosthesis is inserted into the entrance to the inner ear; the other end is attached to the incus (the middle auditory ossicle). In this way, sound can once again be successfully transmitted to the inner ear. The eardrum is then repaired.

### OUTLOOK

The operation improves hearing considerably in more than 90 percent of cases. However, in about 1 percent of patients, hearing deteriorates or is lost altogether. Because of this risk, a stapedectomy is usually carried out on only one ear at a time, although otosclerosis usually affects both ears.

## Stapes

Also known as the stirrup because of its shape, the stapes is the innermost of the three tiny, sound-conducting bones in the middle ear called auditory ossicles (see *Ear*); it is the smallest bone in the body. The head of the stapes articulates with the incus (the middle auditory ossicle) and its base fits into the oval window in the wall of the inner ear.

Overgrowth of bone that causes the stapes to become fixed in position (*otosclerosis*) can cause deafness.

## Staphylococcal infections

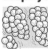 A group of infections caused by bacteria of the staphylococcus family. Staphylococci, which grow in grapelike clusters, are a common cause of skin infections but can also cause serious internal disorders.

Staphylococcal bacteria are present harmlessly on the skin of most people. If the bacteria become trapped within the skin by a blocked sweat or sebaceous gland, they may cause superficial skin infections, such as *pustules*, *boils*, *abscesses*, *styes*, or *carbuncles*. Infection of deeper tissues may result if the skin is broken (see *Wound infection*). In newborn babies, toxins released by bacteria on the skin can cause a severe, blistering rash called the scalded skin syndrome (see *Necrolysis, toxic epidermal*).

Staphylococcal bacteria are also harmlessly present in the membranes that line the nose and throat. When mucus is not cleared from the lungs, such as after a viral infection, organisms may accumulate in the lungs and cause *pneumonia*.

In menstruating women (particularly those using highly absorbent tampons), toxin-producing staphylococci may colonize the mucous membranes lining the vagina, causing *toxic shock syndrome*. A different type of staphylococcus can cause *urinary tract infection*.

Sometimes staphylococci enter the bloodstream as a result of spread from a skin infection or as a result of introduction from a needle, leading to *septic shock*, infectious *arthritis*, *osteomyelitis*, or bacterial *endocarditis*.

Staphylococcal *food poisoning* is caused by ingestion of toxins produced by the bacteria. A common source of contamination is a pustule on the skin of a food handler.

## Starch

See *Carbohydrates*.

## Starvation

A condition caused by lack of food over a long period, resulting in weight loss, changes in *metabolism* (body chemistry), and extreme hunger. (See also *Anorexia nervosa; Fasting; Nutritional disorders*.)

## Stasis

A reduction or cessation of flow. For example, in venous stasis there is diminution or complete stoppage of blood flow through one or more veins.

## Statistics, medical

The science of medical statistics has grown rapidly in recent years as physicians feel increasing pressure from insurance companies and the public to evaluate and choose among the numerous medical treatments available. As a result, all medical research institutions today employ statisticians to advise on the design and interpretation of medical trials, and on the interpretation of data obtained from such trials.

For example, when two treatments are to be compared (or the results of surgical treatment are to be compared with not operating), the statistician advises on how many patients are required in the trial to establish a valid conclusion. He or she also advises on other aspects of methodology, including how to allocate patients to various treatment groups, how frequently to take measurements of the outcomes of the treatments, and how to analyze the mathematical results.

In addition to assessing treatments, statisticians are involved in the analysis of other medical data, which may be as diverse as the *incidence* and *prevalence* of various disorders and diseases, infection rates after surgery, waiting times in outpatient clinics, and the frequency of side effects from drugs. (See also *Statistics, vital*.)

## Statistics, vital

Assessment of the health of a country's population, which relies on the collection of data on birth and death rates and the causes of death (see *Mortality*). In most Western countries today, all deaths are certified (usually by a medical practitioner) and recorded in a national register. They are then classified by cause and analyzed according to factors such as age, sex, occupation, social class, and ethnic group. Particular attention is paid to deaths associated with childbirth (see *Maternal mortality; Infant mortality*) or with factors that cause public concern, such as alcohol or drug abuse, accidents, violence, or diseases such as AIDS, coronary heart disease, and cancer.

Comparison of the vital statistics of different countries (or regions within a country) gives a measure of the relative health of their populations as a whole. A detailed comparison may also show variations between social classes or ethnic groups. (See also *Life expectancy; Statistics, medical; Centers for Disease Control*.)

## Status asthmaticus

A severe and prolonged attack of *asthma*. Status asthmaticus is a serious and potentially life-threatening condition that requires urgent treatment.

## Status epilepticus

Prolonged or repeated epileptic seizures without any recovery of consciousness between attacks. Status epilepticus is a medical emergency that may be fatal if not treated promptly. It is more likely to occur if *anticonvulsant drugs* are taken erratically or if they are withdrawn suddenly. (See *Epilepsy*.)

## STDs

See *Sexually transmitted diseases*.

## Steatorrhea

The presence of excessive fat in the feces. Steatorrhea causes diarrhea characterized by offensive-smelling, bulky, loose, greasy, pale-colored feces, which tend to float in the toilet and are difficult to flush away. Steatorrhea is a symptom of diseases that interfere with the breakdown and absorption of fat in the diet (notably *pancreatitis* and *celiac sprue*) and of the removal of large segments of small intestine. It is also a side effect of some lipid-lowering drugs.

## Stein-Leventhal syndrome

See *Polycystic ovary*.

## Stenosis

Narrowing of a duct, canal, passage, or tubular organ, such as a blood vessel or the intestine. *Aortic stenosis* is narrowing of the aortic valve opening from the left ventricle (lower chamber of the heart); *pyloric stenosis* is narrowing of the pylorus (the lower outlet from the stomach).

## Stereotaxic surgery

Brain operations carried out by inserting delicate instruments through a surgically created hole in the skull and guiding them, using *X rays* or *CT scanning*, to a specific area.

**WHY IT IS DONE**
Stereotaxic procedures are used in the treatment of pituitary gland tumors, in which the gland is cut out or a radioactive implant is inserted into the gland to destroy it.

Other uses include a brain *biopsy* (taking a small sample of tissue for analysis), insertion of permanent stimulating wires to control otherwise intractable pain, and destruction of areas of the brain to treat disabling neurological disorders, such as severe *depression* (see *Psychosurgery*) or, in rare cases, *temporal lobe epilepsy*. Stereotaxic surgery is also occasionally used to treat people with *Parkinson's disease* in whom severe tremor has not responded to drugs.

**HOW IT IS DONE**
With the use of a general or local anesthetic, an adjustable metal frame is attached to the skull with screws. The area to be treated is located by X rays or CT scanning and the best position for inserting the instrument is calculated mathematically. The skull is then entered by means of a *burr hole* or *craniotomy*, and the angle of the frame is adjusted to hold and guide a hollow tube into the brain at the correct angle. The required instrument (a needle for biopsies, a scalpel or diathermy probe for cutting or destroying areas) is then inserted through the tube and the operation is performed; more X rays or scans may be taken during the procedure.

## Sterility

The state of being germ-free, or a term for permanent *infertility*.

## Sterilization

A term that refers to the complete destruction or removal of living organisms or to any procedure that renders a person unable to reproduce (see *Sterilization, female; Vasectomy*).

The elimination of microorganisms is vitally important in preventing the spread of infection. It may be achieved by various physical or chemical means, such as by boiling, steaming, or autoclaving (steaming under high pressure); irradiation with ultraviolet light or X rays; or applying *antiseptics* or *disinfectants*. Sometimes, more than one method is used (e.g., bed linen may be disinfected and then autoclaved). Liquids can also be sterilized by passing them through extremely fine filters that trap microorganisms as tiny as viruses.

## Sterilization, female

A usually permanent method of *contraception* in which the fallopian tubes are sealed or cut to prevent the male sperm from reaching the ova.

Sterilization is a common method of contraception; nearly 10 percent of women over the age of 30 and one fourth of women with five or more children have been sterilized.

### WHY IT IS DONE

Women who have completed their families or do not plan to have children may choose to be sterilized to avoid the inconvenience or side effects of other methods of contraception. Sterilization may also be chosen by a woman in whom a pregnancy would be a serious threat to health, or in whom there is an unacceptably high risk of children being affected by a serious hereditary disease.

### HOW IT IS DONE

The illustrated box shows common procedures for female sterilization, performed using *laparoscopy*.

Alternatively, the surgeon may work directly through a small incision just below the navel. Known as a minilaparotomy, this procedure is carried out in the first few weeks after a woman has delivered a baby, when the uterus is high in the abdomen and the fallopian tubes can be reached easily. In other cases, the surgeon may approach the fallopian tubes via the vagina. The tubes are cut and tied off.

Surgical removal of the uterus, fallopian tubes, or ovaries to treat specific disorders also results in sterilization. These operations are performed through a larger abdominal incision and today are considered too drastic to be performed only for sterilization.

In an investigational method, a hysteroscope (a type of endoscope) is passed through the vagina into the uterus; the exits to the fallopian tubes are plugged from the inside.

Most sterilization techniques are performed on an outpatient basis. Surgical removal of the uterus (see *Hysterectomy*) or fallopian tubes and ovaries (see *Salpingo-oophorectomy*; *Oophorectomy*) requires a hospital stay.

### OUTLOOK

Sterilization has a small failure rate; if pregnancy does occur after sterilization, the chance of an *ectopic pregnancy* is 10 times greater than the normal rate. Although sterilization should be considered permanent, microsurgical techniques may be successful in restoring fertility; 70 to 75 percent of women who undergo such surgery later achieve pregnancy.

## Sterilization, male

See *Vasectomy*.

## Sternum

The anatomical name for the breastbone, the long, narrow, flat plate of bone that forms the central part of the front of the chest. The sternum consists of three main parts—an upper, triangular portion, called the manubrium; a long, narrow middle part, the body; and, at the lower end, a small, slightly flexible, leaf-shaped projection, the xiphoid process. The upper part of the manubrium articulates with the inner ends of the two *clavicles* (collarbones); attached to the sides of the manubrium and body are the seven pairs of costal cartilages that join the sternum to the *ribs*. Between the manubrium and body is a type of joint known as a *symphysis*. It allows slight movement between these two parts of the sternum when the ribs rise and fall during breathing.

The sternum is very strong and requires great force to fracture it. The principal danger of such an injury is not the fracture itself, but the possibility that the broken bone may be driven inward and damage the heart (which lies behind the sternum).

## Steroid drugs

### COMMON DRUGS

*Nandrolone Oxandrolone Stanozolol*

A group of drugs that includes the *corticosteroid drugs*, which are similar to hormones produced by the cortex of the *adrenal glands*, and the anabolic steroid drugs (see *Steroids, anabolic*), which have an effect similar to that of the hormones produced by the male sex organs.

## Steroids, anabolic

Drugs that have an anabolic (protein-building) effect similar to *testosterone* and other male sex hormones.

---

### FEMALE STERILIZATION

Laparoscopic sterilization (below) is the most common method. Both fallopian tubes must be cut, sealed, or otherwise obstructed so that eggs and sperm cannot meet for fertilization to occur.

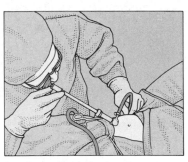

**Laparoscopic sterilization**
An endoscope (viewing tube) and an operating instrument are passed through separate small incisions in the abdomen.

**Instruments**
The trocar is a sharp-pointed inner stylus surrounded by a close-fitting tube, the cannula. The instrument can be passed through the abdominal wall. After insertion, the trocar is removed, leaving the hollow cannula in place. Other instruments are passed through the hollow cannula.

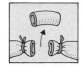

**Cutting**
A small loop of the fallopian tube may be drawn up, secured by a tight ligature, and then cut off.

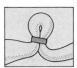

**Constriction**
The loop is constricted by a tight band. Reversal is possible with this sterilization technique.

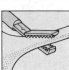

**Clipping**
A plastic or metal clip may be applied to obstruct egg passage. In theory, this method is also reversible.

**Cautery**
Electrocoagulation (diathermy) can be used to burn through and thus seal the fallopian tube.

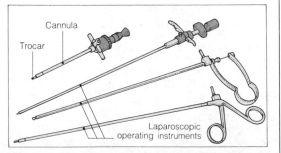

Cannula

Trocar

Laparoscopic operating instruments

S

## LOCATION OF THE STERNUM
The sternum, or breastbone, is joined to the ribs and clavicles by flexible couplings that allow adequate freedom of the chest while breathing in and out.

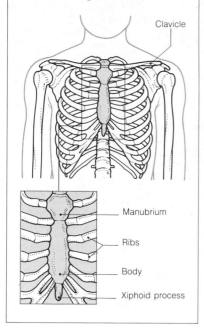

Clavicle

Manubrium

Ribs

Body

Xiphoid process

### WHY THEY ARE USED
Anabolic steroids, by mimicking the anabolic effects of testosterone, build tissue, promote muscle recovery following injury, and help strengthen bones. They are given to treat some types of *anemia* and, infrequently, to treat postmenopausal women who have *osteoporosis*.

### ABUSE
Anabolic steroid drugs have been widely abused by athletes despite the serious risks to health (see *Sports, drugs and*).

### POSSIBLE ADVERSE EFFECTS
Adverse effects include acne, *edema*, liver and adrenal gland damage, infertility, impotence in men, and *virilization* in women.

## Stethoscope
An instrument for listening to sounds in the body, particularly those made by the heart or lungs.

The standard stethoscope consists of a Y-shaped flexible plastic tube with an earpiece at the end of each arm of the Y, and a sound-detecting device at the base. One side of this device consists of a thin plastic diaphragm; the other side has a concave bell that has a

hole in its center. A physician presses the diaphragm against a patient's chest or back to hear high-pitched sounds. The concave bell side is placed in gentle contact with the skin to hear low-pitched sounds.

## Stevens-Johnson syndrome
A rare skin condition characterized by severe blisters and bleeding in the mucous membranes of the lips, eyes, mouth, nasal passage, and genitals. Stevens-Johnson syndrome is a severe form of *erythema multiforme*.

## Sticky eye
A common description of one of the symptoms of *conjunctivitis* (inflammation of the conjunctival membrane) in which the eyelids become stuck together with discharge.

## Stiff neck
A very common symptom, usually due to spasm (involuntary contraction) in muscles at the side or back of the neck. In most cases, the spasm occurs suddenly and for no apparent reason. It is usually first noticed as a stiff neck upon waking and is called *torticollis*, or wryneck. Torticollis is thought to occur as a result of a minor neck injury—such as a ligament *sprain* or *subluxation* (partial dislocation) of a cervical (neck) joint—that has passed unnoticed but has caused irritation of the cervical spinal nerves; this, in turn, leads to spasm of the neck muscles. A stiff neck due to muscle spasm may also be caused by a *disk prolapse* or by a *whiplash injury* in the cervical spine.

A relatively rare, but potentially serious, cause of a stiff neck is *meningitis* (infection of the meninges, the membranes that surround the brain and spinal cord). In such cases, the stiffness is usually accompanied

### STETHOSCOPE

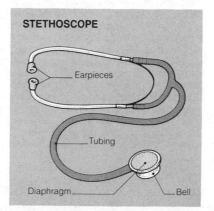

Earpieces

Tubing

Diaphragm

Bell

by headache, vomiting, fever, photophobia (abnormal sensitivity to light), and intense pain when bending the neck.

## Stiffness
A term used to refer to difficulty in moving a joint, to restriction of movement in a joint, or to difficulty stretching a muscle.

Causes of joint stiffness include *arthritis* (inflammation of joint surfaces) and *capsulitis* (inflammation of the joint lining). In *rheumatoid arthritis*, severe joint stiffness may last up to two hours after waking. Causes of muscle stiffness include *cramp* and *spasticity* (increased rigidity).

## Stillbirth
A baby born dead after the 28th week of *pregnancy*. Stillbirth is also called late fetal death. Stillbirths must be reported and the cause of death recorded on the death certificate.

### INCIDENCE
The incidence of stillbirth has decreased dramatically in developed countries over the last 50 years. In the US the incidence fell from 19.2 stillbirths per 1,000 total births (i.e., live births plus stillbirths) in 1950 to 9.2 stillbirths per 1,000 total births in 1980. In general, stillbirths are more common in poor communities, among older women, and when good prenatal and obstetric care are lacking.

### CAUSES
The precise cause of stillbirth is unknown in at least one third of cases. Severely malformed babies, particularly those with *anencephaly*, *spina bifida*, or *hydrocephalus*, account for at least one fifth of stillbirths.

A maternal disorder, such as *antepartum hemorrhage*, *hypertension* (high blood pressure), or any other condition affecting the function of the *placenta*, may result in stillbirth, often because the fetus is deprived of oxygen. Another cause is *Rh incompatibility* between mother and baby.

Some infectious diseases (including measles, chickenpox, influenza, toxoplasmosis, rubella, cytomegalovirus, herpes simplex, syphilis, and malaria) may harm the fetus if contracted during pregnancy. In general, the more severe the infection, the greater the risk of stillbirth. A pregnant woman who is exposed to an infectious disease to which she is not immune should consult her physician.

### PSYCHOLOGICAL EFFECTS
The loss of a baby is deeply distressing. The bereaved parents usually

**S**

experience a sense of loss that is just as intense as if any other loved person had died, and often they experience feelings of depression, guilt, anger, and inadequacy. Emotional support from friends, relatives, and self-help groups is useful, as is counseling by a medical professional.

## Still's disease

See *Rheumatoid arthritis, juvenile*.

## Stimulant drugs

| COMMON DRUGS |
| --- |

Nerve stimulants
*Caffeine Dextroamphetamine*
*Methylphenidate*

Respiratory stimulants
*Doxapram Nikethamide*

Drugs that increase nerve activity in the brain by initiating the release of *norepinephrine* from nerve endings (see *Neurotransmitter*).

### TYPES

There are two main groups of stimulant drugs—nerve stimulants (including *amphetamine drugs*), which reduce drowsiness and increase alertness by their action on the reticular activating system in the *brain stem*, and respiratory stimulants (see *Analeptic drugs*), which act on the respiratory center in the brain stem.

### WHY THEY ARE USED

Nerve stimulants are given to treat *narcolepsy* (characterized by excessive sleepiness). Paradoxically, they have also been found useful in the treatment of *hyperactivity* in children. Nerve stimulants also suppress the appetite but their use in the treatment of *obesity* has decreased because of their adverse effects.

Despite the risk of adverse effects, nerve stimulants are sometimes abused because they prevent fatigue, increase alertness, and may improve self-confidence. The use of nerve stimulants by athletes is widely condemned by physicians and sports organizations (see *Sports, drugs and*).

### POSSIBLE ADVERSE EFFECTS

Effects include shaking, sweating, palpitations, nervousness, sleeping problems, hallucinations, paranoid delusions, and seizures. Long-term use may lead to *tolerance* (the need for greater amounts to have the same effects) and *drug dependence*.

## Stimulus

Anything that evokes a response (i.e., an agent or event that directly results in a change in the activities of the body

as a whole or of any individual part). For example, the sight and smell of food stimulate salivation. Certain nerve cells (known collectively as *receptors*) are specialized to respond to specific stimuli. One example of such nerve cell specialization is the rods and cones in the retina of the eye that respond to light.

## Stings

Stinging animals include scorpions and some insects (such as bees and wasps), jellyfish and related marine animals (such as anemones and corals), and some fish (such as stingrays). There are marked differences among these groups in the way the sting is delivered and its effects. (See *Insect stings; Scorpion stings; Jellyfish stings; Venomous bites and stings*.)

Nettles and some other plants carry minute stinging hairs that hold an irritant liquid. The hairs penetrate and break off in the skin; the liquid enters the wound and has an immediate irritant effect, which rarely lasts more than an hour or two. Washing the affected area and applying calamine lotion can provide relief. Contact with poison ivy and related plants may result in a more severe allergic reaction, sometimes requiring medical attention (see *Plants, poisonous*).

## Stitch

A temporary, sudden, sharp pain in the abdomen or side that occurs during severe or unaccustomed exercise, usually running. The cause of a stitch is unknown.

Stitch is also commonly used to refer to a suture used to close a wound (see *Suturing*).

## Stokes-Adams syndrome

Recurrent episodes of temporary loss of consciousness caused by insufficient blood flow from the heart to the brain. This deficient blood supply is due to very rapid or very slow arrhythmia (see *Arrhythmia, cardiac*), which markedly reduces the pumping efficiency of the heart, or to complete *heart block* (abnormally slow conduction of electrical impulses through the heart muscle), resulting in temporary cessation of the heart beat.

### SYMPTOMS AND TREATMENT

In a typical attack, the person faints suddenly and turns blue if the period of unconsciousness is prolonged. The breathing rate increases and a very slow pulse can be felt. Occasionally, lack of oxygen supply to the brain may cause a *seizure* (convulsion).

In most cases, the heart soon starts beating again, the skin flushes, and consciousness is regained. If this fails to happen, *cardiopulmonary resuscitation* should be carried out promptly to prevent brain damage.

Most sufferers are fitted with a *pacemaker* to maintain normal heart beat and prevent future attacks.

## Stoma

A term meaning mouth or orifice. A stoma in the abdomen acts as an artificial anus; it may be temporary (diverting feces from a healing wound in the intestine) or permanent (because part of the intestine has been removed). See also *Colostomy; Ileostomy*.

## Stomach

A hollow, saclike organ of the *digestive system* that is connected to the esophagus and the duodenum (the first part of the small intestine). The stomach lies in the left side of the abdomen under the diaphragm.

### STRUCTURE

The stomach is flexible, allowing it to expand when food is eaten; in an adult, the average capacity is about 3

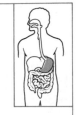

**LOCATION OF THE STOMACH**
Food enters the stomach from the esophagus and exits into the duodenum. The stomach lining secretes gastric juice and protective mucus.

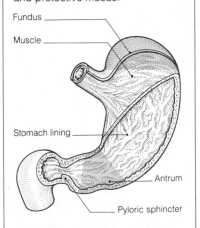

Fundus

Muscle

Stomach lining

Antrum

Pyloric sphincter

**Parts of the stomach**
The fundus and antrum are two of the main stomach parts; the lower esophageal segment and pyloric sphincters control entry and exit of food.

# DISORDERS OF THE STOMACH

Disorders of the stomach have a variety of causes. Because the stomach is a reservoir, disorders in the process of emptying the stomach contents occur. Other problems relate to the stomach's role in the preparation of ingested food for digestion.

## INFECTION

The large amount of hydrochloric acid secreted by the stomach protects the stomach from some infections by destroying many of the bacteria, viruses, and fungi that are taken in with food and drink. When the protective power is insufficient, a variety of gastrointestinal infections may occur.

## TUMORS

*Stomach cancer* causes about 15,000 deaths annually in the US. Early symptoms are often mistaken for *indigestion* and diagnosis is often delayed until it is too late for a cure. Any change in the customary functioning of the digestive system is important, especially after fifty. A persistent feeling of fullness, or pain before or after meals, should never be ignored. Unexplained loss of appetite or frequent nausea should always be reported. A tumor in the upper part of the stomach, near the opening of the esophagus, can cause obstruction and difficulty in swallowing. Sometimes a stomach tumor remains "silent" and the first signs are due to the appearance of secondary growths elsewhere in the body.

Benign (noncancerous) *polyps* can also develop in the stomach.

## ULCERATION

The acid and other digestive juices secreted by the stomach sometimes attack the stomach lining. The healthy stomach is prevented from digesting itself mainly by the protective layer of mucus secreted by the lining and by the speed with which damaged surface cells are replaced by the deeper layers. Many influences can upset this delicate balance. One of the most important is excessive acid secretion. The resulting *peptic ulcers* are probably the most common serious stomach disorder. Peptic ulcers are sometimes caused by stress, or by severe injury, such as major burns, accidents, and after surgery and severe infections; often they occur for no apparent reason. The stomach lining can be damaged by large amounts of aspirin or alcohol, sometimes causing *gastritis* (inflammation of the stomach lining). This may lead to ulceration of the stomach lining.

## AUTOIMMUNE DISORDERS

*Pernicious anemia* is caused by the failure of the stomach lining to produce intrinsic factor, a substance whose role is to facilitate the absorption of vitamin $B_{12}$. Failure to produce the intrinsic factor occurs if there is atrophy of the stomach lining, which also causes failure of acid production. Tests that determine a person's ability to absorb vitamin $B_{12}$ are important in the investigation of this condition. Pernicious anemia is usually due to an *autoimmune disorder*.

## OTHER DISORDERS

Enlargement of the stomach may be caused when scarring from a chronic peptic ulcer occurs at the stomach outlet. It may also be a complication of *pyloric stenosis*, a rare but serious condition caused by narrowing of the stomach outlet. Rarely, the stomach may become twisted and obstructed, a condition called *volvulus*.

## INVESTIGATION

Stomach disorders are investigated primarily by *barium X-ray examinations* and/or *gastroscopy*. Occasionally, a *biopsy* (removal of a tissue sample for microscopic analysis) is performed.

pints (1.5 liters). The stomach wall consists of layers of longitudinal and circular muscle, lined by special glandular cells that secrete gastric juice, and supplied by blood vessels and nerves. A strong muscle at the lower end of the stomach forms a ring called the pyloric sphincter that can close the outlet leading to the duodenum.

## FUNCTION

Although the main function of the stomach is to continue the breakdown of food that is started in the mouth and completed in the small intestine, it also acts as a storage organ, enabling food to be eaten only two or three times a day. Food would have to be eaten every 20 minutes or so if storage were not possible.

The sight and smell of food and the arrival of food in the stomach stimulate gastric secretion. The gastric juice secreted from the stomach lining contains pepsin (an enzyme that breaks down protein), hydrochloric acid (which kills bacteria taken in with the food and which creates the most suitable environment for the pepsin to work in), and intrinsic factor (which is essential for the absorption of vitamin $B_{12}$ in the small intestine). The stomach lining also contains glands that secrete mucus, which helps provide a barrier to prevent the stomach from digesting itself.

The layers of muscle produce rhythmic contractions about every 20 seconds that churn the food and gastric juice; the combined effect of this movement and the action of the digestive juice convert the semisolid food into a creamy fluid. This process takes varying lengths of time, depending on the nature of the food. Generally, however, the richer the meal, the longer it takes to be emptied from the stomach. The partially digested food is squirted into the duodenum at regular intervals by the contractions of the stomach and relaxation of the pyloric sphincter.

## Stomach cancer

A malignant tumor that arises from the lining of the stomach, also called gastric cancer.

### CAUSES AND INCIDENCE

The cause of stomach cancer remains uncertain but evidence suggests that an environmental factor, probably diet, plays a part. Recent speculation has centered on an association between stomach cancer and eating quantities of salted, pickled, or smoked foods. Certain other factors, such as megaloblastic *anemia*, partial *gastrectomy*, and belonging to blood group A, seem to increase the risk of this cancer developing.

S

Stomach cancer rarely affects people under the age of 40 and is twice as common in men as in women. There is marked geographic variation—with a very high rate of 80 to 90 cases per 100,000 people in Japan compared with fewer than 10 per 100,000 in the US, where it causes around 15,000 deaths per year. There has been a dramatic decrease in the worldwide incidence of stomach cancer over the past 50 years.

##### SYMPTOMS AND SIGNS

The symptoms of stomach cancer (if any) are often indistinguishable from those of *peptic ulcer*. In the advanced stages, there is usually loss of appetite, the sensation that the stomach is filling up quickly, nausea and vomiting, and weight loss.

##### DIAGNOSIS AND TREATMENT

The condition is suggested by *barium X-ray examination* and confirmed by *gastroscopy* (examination of the stomach by a flexible viewing tube). A *biopsy* of the stomach lining (removal of a tissue sample for microscopic examination) may also be performed using a gastroscope.

The only effective treatment is gastrectomy. However, only about 20 percent of patients are able to undergo such surgery; in the rest, the tumor has spread too widely at the time of diagnosis. In inoperable, advanced cases, *radiation therapy* and *anticancer drugs* may be used.

##### OUTLOOK

If the cancer is detected at a very early stage (before it has spread beyond the stomach lining), a high cure rate is possible. In Japan, where mass screening by gastroscopy is performed, 85 percent of people are still alive five years after treatment by surgery. In advanced disease, however, the outlook is not good, with less than 10 percent of patients surviving longer than five years.

## Stomach imaging

See *Barium X-ray examinations*.

## Stomach pump

See *Lavage, gastric*.

## Stomach ulcer

A raw area in the stomach lining, also called a gastric ulcer. If nonmalignant, it is a *peptic ulcer*.

## Stomatitis

Any form of inflammation or ulceration of the mouth. Examples include *mouth ulcers*, *cold sores*, *candidiasis* (thrush), and *Vincent's disease*.

## Stones

Small, hard aggregates of solid material within the body. Also called calculi, they are formed from substances that are present to excess in fluids such as urine or bile. (See *Calculus, urinary tract*; *Gallstones*.)

## Stool

Another word for *feces*.

## Stork bite

A small, flat, harmless, pinkish-red skin blemish found in 30 to 50 percent of newborn babies. Such marks, which are also called salmon patches, are a type of *hemangioma* usually found around the eyes and at the nape of the neck. Stork bites around the eyes usually disappear within the first year; those at the base of the neck may persist indefinitely.

## Strabismus

A condition in which there is abnormal deviation of one eye in relation to the other. Strabismus, also known as squint, may be convergent (cross-eye), in which one eye is directed too far inward, or divergent (walleye), in which one eye is directed outward. Occasionally, one eye is directed upward or downward relative to the other (vertical strabismus).

##### CAUSES

Strabismus usually starts in early childhood because of a failure in the

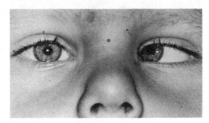

**Convergent strabismus**
This boy is using his right eye (note the light reflection in the center of the pupil). Left visual development has stopped.

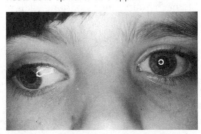

**Divergent strabismus**
Simultaneous perception with both eyes would cause double vision, so the brain suppresses the image from the deviating eye.

proper development of the mechanisms that align the two eyes. A common contributory factor is *hyperopia* (farsightedness), which forces the child to *accommodate* (focus to see clearly) excessively and causes the eyes to turn inward.

In children who are acquiring the capacity to see simultaneously with two eyes, strabismus causes double vision and noncorresponding, different images from the malaligned eyes. Because of the double vision, the brain rapidly suppresses the image from the deviating eye. Strabismic *amblyopia* (visual loss) may occur.

In adults, strabismus may occur as a result of various disorders of the brain, of the nerves controlling the eye muscles, or of the eye muscles themselves. It may be a symptom of *stroke*, *diabetes mellitus*, *multiple sclerosis*, tumor, or thyroid eye disease. Strabismus that develops in adults causes double vision; although untreated strabismus may disappear, treatment is usually needed.

##### TREATMENT

Treatment in young children may include covering the normal eye with a patch to force the child to use the weak (amblyopic) eye. This treatment attempts to allow development of normal vision in the affected eye by establishing the functional connections between the eye and the brain. Glasses and/or surgery can be used to try to correct the deviation of the eyes. Patching to try to improve the poor vision in the weak eye may be tried until age 10; surgery can be performed later to improve appearance.

Strabismus acquired later in life always causes double vision and requires medical investigation of the underlying cause. If the strabismus does not clear up, then special glasses or surgery may be tried.

## Strain

Tearing or stretching of muscle fibers as a result of suddenly pulling them too far. There is bleeding into the damaged area of muscle, causing pain, swelling, and muscle spasm; a bruise usually appears a few days after the injury. Muscle strain of the back is a common cause of nonspecific *back pain*. Strains are most common in athletes.

Treatment consists of applying an ice pack to the affected area to reduce swelling, wrapping it with a compression bandage, and resting the limb in a raised position for 48 hours. Analgesics (painkillers) may also be

S

taken to relieve pain. After resting the muscle, *physical therapy* involving stretching exercises should be started to prevent possible shortening of the muscle as a result of scar tissue forming in it. In some cases, *nonsteroidal anti-inflammatory drugs* may be prescribed to speed healing.

The risk of muscle strain can be reduced by performing warm-up exercises before any sports activity.

## Strangulation
The constriction, usually by twisting or compression, of a tube or conduit in the body, blocking blood flow and interfering with the function of the affected organ. This may occur with a *hernia* or after twisting of the testis (see *Testis, torsion of*).

Strangulation of the neck with the hands or with a ligature, such as a cord or scarf, may be deliberate or accidental. The primary lethal effect arises from compression of the jugular veins in the neck. This prevents blood from flowing out of the brain and head, where it stagnates and its oxygen content is quickly used up. In addition, compression of the windpipe restricts breathing and impairs oxygenation of the blood. The victim's face becomes congested with blood and takes on a livid purple-blue coloration. He or she loses consciousness and, some minutes later, brain damage and death occur from lack of oxygen.

Any constricting ligature must be removed as quickly as possible and medical help summoned. If the victim is not breathing, *artificial respiration* should be performed until an ambulance or physician arrives.

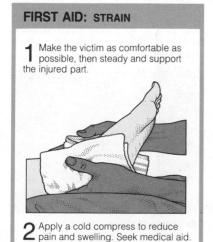

### FIRST AID: STRAIN

**1** Make the victim as comfortable as possible, then steady and support the injured part.

**2** Apply a cold compress to reduce pain and swelling. Seek medical aid.

To prevent accidental strangulation, a child's environment should be kept free of potential ligatures—such as cords on toys or clothing or dangerous restraining apparatus. Children should be discouraged from playing with lassos.

## Strangury
A symptom characterized by a painful and frequent desire to empty the bladder, although only a few drops of urine can be passed. Causes of strangury include *prostatitis* (inflammation of the prostate gland), *cystitis*, and bladder cancer (see *Bladder tumors*).

## Strapping
The application of adhesive tape to part of the body to exert pressure and hold a structure in place. Strapping is used to reduce pain and swelling caused by soft tissue injuries, such as sprains and muscle tears. It may also be applied to joints to prevent injury due to excessive movement, or to strengthen a joint that has been injured to help prevent recurrence.

## Strawberry nevus
A bright red, raised birthmark that is a type of *hemangioma*.

## Strep throat
An infection of the throat caused by certain bacteria of the streptococcus group. Strep throat is most common in children and is spread by droplets (containing the bacteria) that are coughed or breathed into the air.

In some people, the bacteria cause few or no symptoms, but a proportion suffer a sore throat, fever, general malaise, and enlarged lymph nodes in the neck. In some cases, toxins released by the bacteria lead to a rash, a condition known as *scarlet fever*.

The diagnosis is usually made by identifying the bacteria in a culture grown from a throat swab. The infection is treated with penicillin or with another antibiotic drug if the person is allergic to penicillin.

An untreated strep throat infection may lead to the serious complications of *glomerulonephritis* (inflammation in the kidneys) or *rheumatic fever*.

## Streptococcal infections
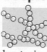
A group of infections caused by bacteria of the streptococcus family. Streptococci are spherical bacteria that grow like strung beads; they are among the most common disease-causing bacteria in humans.

Certain types of streptococci are present harmlessly in most people's mouths and throats. If the bacteria gain access to the bloodstream (sometimes after dental treatment), they are usually destroyed. However, in some people with heart valve defects there is a risk of the bacteria settling in the heart to cause bacterial *endocarditis*. Another type of streptococcus is present harmlessly in the intestines but can spread, via the urethra, to cause a *urinary tract infection*.

Other types of streptococci cause *tonsillitis*, *strep throat*, *otitis media* (middle-ear infection), *pneumonia*, *erysipelas*, or wound infections.

Beta-hemolytic streptococcal infection may be the cause of any of the aforementioned, or may result in *scarlet fever* (characterized by a rash).

Infections from these same streptococci may also give rise to the serious complications of *rheumatic fever* and *glomerulonephritis*. These infections are prevented through prompt treatment with *antibiotic drugs* (most often penicillin).

People in whom rheumatic fever has developed are advised to take an antibiotic drug before, during, and after dental treatment and certain diagnostic and surgical procedures.

## Streptokinase
A *thrombolytic drug* used to dissolve blood clots in *myocardial infarction* (heart attack) and *pulmonary embolism*. Streptokinase is most effective in dissolving newly formed clots. Given by injection in the early stages of a heart attack, streptokinase may limit the amount of damage that is caused to the heart muscle.

Treatment with streptokinase is strictly supervised because of the risk of allergic reaction or excessive bleeding. Other adverse effects include rash, fever, wheezing, and *arrhythmias* (irregularities of the heart beat).

## Streptomycin
An *antibiotic drug* used to treat a number of uncommon infections, including *tularemia*, *plague*, *brucellosis*, and *glanders*. Streptomycin is sometimes given with a *penicillin drug* to treat *endocarditis* (inflammation of the lining of the heart and heart valves).

Once used to treat a wide range of other infections, streptomycin has now been largely superseded by newer, more effective drugs with less serious side effects. Discovered in the 1940s, streptomycin was the first effective drug treatment for *tuber-*

S

culosis; it is still sometimes used to treat resistant strains.

**POSSIBLE ADVERSE EFFECTS**

Most seriously, streptomycin may damage nerves in the inner ear, disturbing balance and causing dizziness, ringing in the ears, and deafness. Other possible adverse effects include numbness of the face, tingling in the hands, headache, malaise, nausea, and vomiting.

## Stress

Any interference that disturbs a person's healthy mental and physical well-being. A person may experience stress in response to a wide range of physical and emotional stimuli, including physical violence, internal conflicts, and significant life events (e.g., death of a loved one, the birth of a baby, or divorce). Some people are more susceptible than others to stress-related medical problems.

**EFFECTS**

When faced with a stressful situation, the body responds by increasing production of certain hormones, such as *cortisol* and *epinephrine*. These hormones lead to changes in heart rate, blood pressure, metabolism, and physical activity designed to improve overall performance. However, at a certain level, they disrupt an individual's ability to cope. Less than 20 percent of people are effective in crises such as fires or floods.

Continued exposure to stress often leads to mental and physical symptoms, such as *anxiety* and *depression*, *dyspepsia*, palpitations, and muscular aches and pains. *Posttraumatic stress disorder* is a direct response to a specific stressful event. (See also *Relaxation techniques*.)

## Stress fracture

A *fracture* that occurs as a result of repetitive jarring of a bone. Common sites include the metatarsal bones in the foot (see *March fracture*), the tibia or fibula (lower leg bones), the neck of the femur (thigh bone), and the lumbar region of the spine. Stress fractures are most common among runners, particularly those who run on hard surfaces with inadequate footwear (see *Sports injuries*).

The main symptoms include pain and tenderness at the fracture site. Diagnosis is by X rays, although sometimes a stress fracture does not show up on an X ray until it has started to heal. Occasionally, a radionuclide bone scan (see *Bone imaging*) may be performed to confirm the diagnosis.

Treatment consists of resting the affected area for four to six weeks. In some cases, it is also necessary to immobilize the fracture in a plaster cast. After recovery, modification of exercise routines and the use of suitably cushioned footwear may help to prevent a recurrence.

## Stress ulcer

An acute *peptic ulcer* that sometimes develops after shock, serious burns, severe injuries, or during a major illness. Stress ulcers are usually multiple and are most common in the stomach; they differ from chronic peptic ulcers in that the raw area does not spread deep into the stomach lining.

The exact cause is unknown. Treatment is primarily preventive; patients in intensive-care units are commonly given *antacid drugs* and/or *histamine*-2 *receptor antagonists*.

## Stretcher

A frame covered with fabric that is used in first aid for carrying the sick, injured, or deceased.

Many stretchers are available, including the standard stretcher, which consists of canvas stretched between two long poles on each side, and the trolley bed, a more sophisticated, adjustable stretcher on wheels that is carried in ambulances.

Stretchers can be improvised by passing two poles through holes made in the corners of canvas bags, or by rolling up poles in parallel sides of a strong rug or blanket. An overcoat may also be used. Ideally, stretchers should be fairly rigid. The ends of a loaded stretcher should be lifted simultaneously.

## Stretch mark

The common name for *stria*.

## Stria

Commonly called a stretch mark, a line on the skin caused by thinning and loss of elasticity in the dermis (underlying skin layer). Striae first appear as red, raised lines. Later they become purple, eventually flattening and fading to form shiny streaks, usually between a quarter of an inch and a half inch wide.

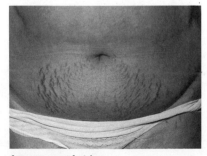

**Appearance of striae**
Commonly known as stretch marks, striae often develop on the abdomen, thighs, and breasts of pregnant women.

S

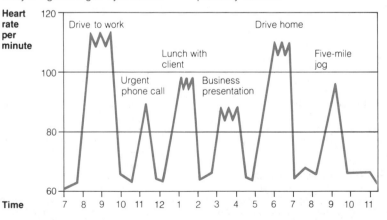

## STRESS AND HEART RATE

The graph shows how a person's heart rate varies over a typical day. Exercise and stress both activate the body's "fight or flight" system and increase heart rate, but repeated alerting of the system without accompanying physical activity is probably harmful.

**Stress levels through the day**
Although the home and workplace both present stress, for many city dwellers the most taxing parts of the day are those spent commuting.

## USING A STRETCHER

Stretchers are used to carry injured or seriously ill people to avoid the risk of further injury. Any type of stretcher should be fairly rigid and should always be tested for strength before use.

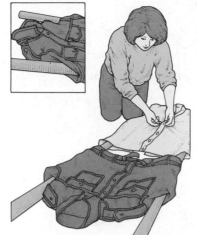

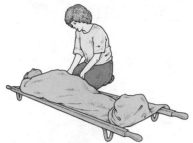

**Keeping the victim warm**
Place a blanket diagonally on the stretcher. Lift the victim carefully onto the blanket and tuck in the corners.

**Improvising a stretcher**
Turn the sleeves of two coats inside out. Pass two strong poles through the sleeves and button the coats.

Striae often develop on the hips and thighs during the adolescent growth spurt, especially in athletic girls. They are a common feature of pregnancy, developing in about 75 percent of pregnant women, and tend to occur on the breasts, thighs, and lower abdomen. Purple striae characteristically develop in people with *Cushing's syndrome*.

Striae are possibly caused by an excess of *corticosteroid hormones*, which are known to suppress fiber formation in the skin and to cause collagen in the skin to waste away. There is no effective means of prevention or treatment.

## Stricture

Narrowing of a duct, canal, or other passage in the body. A stricture may result from infection and inflammation; damage to and subsequent formation of scar tissue in or around a passage; the development of a tumor; spasm of muscles in a passage wall; or excessive growth of tissue around a passage, which occurs in *prostatism* when the enlarged prostate gland constricts the urethra (the passage between the bladder and outside). In some cases, a stricture is *congenital*.

## Stridor

A noisy, high-pitched breathing sound caused by abnormal narrowing of the *larynx* or *trachea*.

Stridor is most common in young children. It usually occurs in *croup*, which is caused by a viral infection of the upper airways. A less common, but more serious, cause is the bacterial infection *epiglottiditis*. Other causes of stridor include an inhaled *foreign body* and certain disorders of the *larynx*, such as tumors, vocal cord paralysis, and laryngomalacia (softening of the cartilage of the larynx).

## Stroke

Damage to part of the brain caused by interruption to its blood supply or leakage of blood outside of vessel walls. Sensation, movement, or function controlled by the damaged area is impaired. Strokes are fatal in about one third of cases and are a leading cause of death in developed countries.

**CAUSES**
The main types and causes of stroke are shown in the box overleaf.

Certain factors increase the risk of having a stroke. The two most important are *hypertension* (high blood pressure), which weakens the walls of arteries, and *atherosclerosis* (thickening of the lining of arterial walls, which narrows arteries.

Other factors that increase the risk of a stroke include *atrial fibrillation* (a type of irregular heart beat), a damaged *heart valve*, and a recent *myocardial infarction* (heart attack). All of these conditions can cause blood clots in the heart that may break off and migrate to the brain. *Polycythemia* (a raised level of red cells in the blood), *hyperlipidemia* (a high level of fatty substances in the blood), *diabetes mellitus*,

and smoking also increase the risk of stroke by increasing the risk of hypertension and/or atherosclerosis. Oral contraceptives increase the risk of stroke in women under 50.

**INCIDENCE**
In the US, the overall incidence of stroke is about 200 people per 100,000 population annually. The incidence rises steeply with age and is higher in men than in women.

**SYMPTOMS AND SIGNS**
Damage to a specific area of the brain impairs bodily sensation, movement, or function controlled by that part of the brain. Some of the possible symptoms and signs are shown in the illustrated box overleaf. A stroke that affects the dominant of the two cerebral hemispheres in the brain (usually the left hemisphere) may cause disturbance of language and speech (see *Aphasia*).

Movement on one side of the body is controlled by the cerebral hemisphere on the opposite side. Thus, damage to areas controlling movement in the right cerebral hemisphere results in weakness or paralysis on the left side of the body. Such one-sided weakness or paralysis, known as *hemiplegia*, is one of the most common effects of a serious stroke.

When symptoms last for less than 24 hours and are followed by full recovery, the episode is known as a *transient ischemic attack*. Such an attack, which usually lasts for only a few minutes, is a warning signal that a sufficient supply of blood is not reaching part of the brain.

About a third of major strokes are fatal, a third result in a permanent handicap, and a third result in no lasting ill effects.

**COMPLICATIONS**
Possible complications of a major stroke include *pneumonia* and the formation of blood clots in the veins of the leg (see *Thrombosis, deep vein*), which may travel to the artery supplying the lung to cause a potentially fatal *pulmonary embolism*.

**DIAGNOSIS**
If someone is thought to have had a stroke, a physician or ambulance should be summoned immediately. In about two thirds of cases, symptoms are serious enough to require admission to the hospital.

*CT scanning* of the brain is performed to determine whether the symptoms are caused by a stroke or by some other disorder, such as a *brain tumor, brain abscess, subdural hemor-*

S

## TYPES AND CAUSES OF STROKE

Stroke may be caused by any of three mechanisms (below). Thrombosis and embolism both lead to cessation of the blood supply to part of the brain and thus to infarction (tissue death). Rupture of a blood vessel in or near the brain may cause an *intracerebral hemorrhage* or a *subarachnoid hemorrhage*. Any part of the brain may be affected by a stroke; accordingly, the symptoms vary considerably.

### CEREBRAL THROMBOSIS

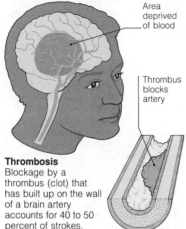

Area deprived of blood

Thrombus blocks artery

**Thrombosis**
Blockage by a thrombus (clot) that has built up on the wall of a brain artery accounts for 40 to 50 percent of strokes.

### CEREBRAL EMBOLISM

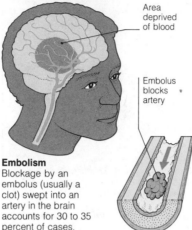

Area deprived of blood

Embolus blocks artery

**Embolism**
Blockage by an embolus (usually a clot) swept into an artery in the brain accounts for 30 to 35 percent of cases.

### HEMORRHAGE

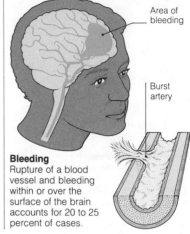

Area of bleeding

Burst artery

**Bleeding**
Rupture of a blood vessel and bleeding within or over the surface of the brain accounts for 20 to 25 percent of cases.

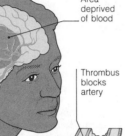

**Tissue death within brain**
The photograph at left shows a vertical slice through the brain of someone who died of a stroke. A large region of tissue death (dark area), caused by bleeding and oxygen deprivation, can be seen on one side.

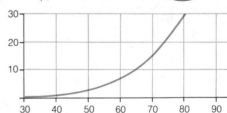

**Estimated incidence per 1,000 population**

**Age**

**Incidence with age**
Strokes are rare to uncommon under the age of 60, but thereafter the chances of one occurring increase rapidly.

## SYMPTOMS

The symptoms of a stroke usually develop over minutes or hours, but occasionally over several days. Depending on the site, cause, and extent of damage, any or all of the symptoms at right may be present, in any degree of severity. The more serious cases lead to rapid loss of consciousness, coma, and death or to severe physical or mental handicap, but some strokes cause barely noticeable symptoms.

**Hemiplegia**
Weakness or paralysis on one side of the body is one of the more common effects of a serious stroke.

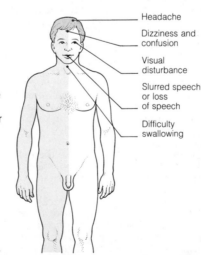

Headache

Dizziness and confusion

Visual disturbance

Slurred speech or loss of speech

Difficulty swallowing

## RISK FACTORS

Age

High blood pressure

Atherosclerosis (narrowed artery channels)

Heart disease

Diabetes mellitus

Smoking

Polycythemia

Hyperlipidemia

Use of estrogens

S

*rhage* (bleeding into the space between the outermost and middle membranes covering the brain), or *encephalitis* (inflammation of the brain). A *lumbar puncture* may be necessary to exclude the possibility of *meningitis* (inflammation of the membranes covering the brain and spinal cord).

To further examine the cause and extent of brain damage, investigations may include an *ECG, chest X rays, blood tests, angiography,* and *MRI.*

### TREATMENT
In the hospital, patients who are unconscious or semiconscious require a clear airway, feeding by means of *intravenous infusion* or a *nasogastric tube,* and regular changing of position to avoid bedsores or pneumonia. Any *edema* (accumulation of fluid) within the brain caused by the stroke may be treated with *corticosteroid drugs* or *diuretic drugs.*

When a stroke has been caused by an *embolism, anticoagulant drugs* may be prescribed (in many cases for the rest of the patient's life) to help prevent recurrences. In other instances, aspirin is prescribed or vascular surgery performed to reduce the risk of subsequent stroke.

Every effort is made to restore any lost movement or sensation by *physical therapy* and to remedy any speech disturbance by *speech therapy.*

### OUTLOOK
About half of patients recover more or less completely from their first stroke. Many people paralyzed by a stroke learn to walk again. Any intellectual impairment, however, is often permanent. Survivors left with some form of permanent handicap may require *occupational therapy* and aids in the home. About 5 percent require long-term institutional care.

## Stroma
The tissue that forms the framework of an organ, as distinct from the functional tissue (called the *parenchyma*) and the fibrous outer layer that holds the organ together. The stroma of the ovaries is the supporting tissue in which the ovarian follicles (the parenchyma) are embedded. The ovarian stroma consists of fibrous tissue, smooth muscle cells, spindle-shaped cells, and a rich supply of blood vessels.

## Strongyloidiasis
An infestation of the intestines by a tiny parasitic worm, STRONGYLOIDES STERCORALIS. The disease is widespread in the tropics, especially the Far East. In the US, it is occasionally found in Vietnam War veterans and refugees, but is otherwise rare.

Strongyloidiasis is contracted in affected areas by walking barefoot on soil contaminated with feces. Worm larvae penetrate the skin of the feet and, via the lungs and throat, migrate to the small intestine. There they develop into adults, which burrow into the intestinal wall to produce larvae. Most larvae are passed in the feces, but some enter the bloodstream to begin a new cycle. Thus, an infestation may persist in one person for many years.

### SYMPTOMS AND TREATMENT
The larvae cause itching and raised red patches where they enter the skin. In the lungs they may cause bleeding (resulting in the coughing up of blood) or pneumonia. Intestinal infestation may produce no symptoms but, if heavy, causes discomfort, a swollen abdomen, and diarrhea. Occasionally, an infested person dies of complications, such as *septicemia* or *meningitis,* many years after contracting the infection. Pneumonia may occur more readily in a person whose immune system has been compromised.

The disease is diagnosed from microscopic examination of a sample of feces. Strongyloidiasis is treated with an *antihelmintic drug,* which eradicates the worms.

## Strontium
A metallic element that does not occur naturally in its pure form but is present as various compounds in certain minerals (notably strontianite and celestite), seawater, and marine plants. It is also found in food and, although not essential to the body, is metabolized in a manner similar to calcium and incorporated into bone.

In addition to the compounds, there are several radioisotopes (radioactive varieties) of the element, of which strontium 90 is medically the most important. It does not occur naturally, but is produced in relatively large amounts during nuclear fission reactions and is also present in the fallout from some nuclear bomb explosions. Strontium 90 emits *radiation* (in the form of beta particles) for a comparatively long time (the *half-life* of this radioisotope is about 28 years), and accumulates in bone, where the radiation may cause *leukemia* and/or *bone tumors.*

Other radioisotopes of strontium have also been used in medicine to diagnose and treat bone tumors.

## Strychnine poisoning
 Strychnine is an extremely poisonous chemical found in the seeds of species of STRYCHNOS, a group of tropical plants. Although once used as a tonic and general stimulant, strychnine is no longer used therapeutically. Its principal use today is as an ingredient in some rodent poisons; most cases of strychnine poisoning occur in children who accidentally eat such poisons. However, the extremely bitter taste of strychnine and its lack of easy availability makes this form of poisoning rare.

### SYMPTOMS AND TREATMENT
The symptoms of poisoning begin soon after strychnine has been eaten. If untreated, death may occur. Initial symptoms include restlessness, stiffness of the face and neck, and increased sensitivity of sight, hearing, taste, and smell. These symptoms are followed by alternating episodes of seizures and floppiness. Eventually, death occurs from respiratory arrest.

The primary objectives of treatment are to prevent seizures and maintain breathing. The victim is given intravenous injections of a tranquilizer or barbiturate, which counteract the effects of strychnine and thus help prevent seizures. To maintain breathing, the victim may be placed on a ventilator. With prompt medical treatment, recovery usually occurs within about 24 hours.

## Stuffy nose
See *Nasal congestion.*

## Stump
The end portion of a limb that remains after *amputation.*

## Stupor
A state of almost complete *unconsciousness* from which a person can be aroused only briefly and only by vigorous external stimulation. (See also *Coma.*)

## Sturge-Weber syndrome
A rare, congenital condition that affects the skin and the brain. Characteristically, a large purple *hemangioma* (a birthmark caused by abnormal distribution of blood vessels) extends over one side of the face, including the eye. A similar malformation of blood vessels in the brain may cause some degree of weakness on the opposite side of the body, progressive *mental retardation,* and *epilepsy. Glaucoma* (increased pressure within the eyeball)

S

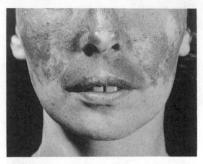

**Appearance of Sturge-Weber syndrome**
The characteristic birthmark, shown here on the lower part of the face, extends over the left eye and temple.

may develop in the affected eye, leading to a partial or complete loss of vision.

The birthmark can be disguised with masking creams; seizures can usually be controlled with *anticonvulsant drugs*. In severe cases, surgery on the affected part of the brain may need to be performed.

## Stuttering

A speech disorder in which there is repeated hesitation and delay in uttering words or in which sounds are unusually prolonged. Stuttering, also known as stammering, usually starts in childhood, beginning before age 8 in 90 percent of sufferers.

### INCIDENCE

Stuttering occurs in about 1 percent of the adult population. It is also fairly common temporarily in children aged 2 to 4. About half the children whose stutter persists until age 5 continue to stutter in adult life. The problem is more common in boys, twins, and left-handed people.

### SYMPTOMS

People who stutter have problems with different words and sounds. The severity of the stutter is also related to circumstances. Some people find that the stuttering is worse when they are anxious (such as during public speaking or when using the telephone), while others experience more difficulty when relaxed. Problems rarely occur during singing or reading in unison (possibly because less communication is involved). Some stutterers also have *tics* and *tremors*.

### CAUSES

The cause of stuttering is uncertain, although it tends to run in families. Some researchers believe that stuttering is due to a subtle form of brain damage; others regard it as a primarily psychological problem.

### TREATMENT

Stuttering can often be improved by *speech therapy*, which may include teaching the person to give equal weight to each syllable. Electronic aids to mask the speaker's voice or to relay speech back to the speaker via headphones are also employed.

## St. Vitus' dance

An outdated term for the disorder now called *Sydenham's chorea*.

## Stye

Also called a hordeolum, a small, pus-filled *abscess* near the eyelashes caused by infection. If the stye is painful, warm compresses may help the pus to discharge. Antibiotic eye ointment can help prevent recurrence.

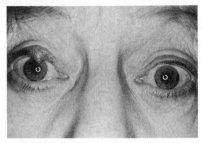

**Stye on upper eyelid**
A stye most often forms near the inner corner of an eye but may develop at the base of any of the eyelashes.

## Subacute

A medical term applied to a disease that runs a course in time between *acute* and *chronic*. In subacute *meningitis*, the symptoms persist over a period of several weeks; in the acute form, the entire illness may last several days or a couple of weeks.

## Subarachnoid hemorrhage

A type of brain hemorrhage in which blood from a ruptured blood vessel spreads over the surface of the brain.

### CAUSES AND INCIDENCE

The most common cause of subarachnoid hemorrhage is a burst *aneurysm* (bulge in a weakened wall of an artery), frequently on the circular arrangement of blood vessels at the base of the brain, less commonly a ruptured *angioma* (abnormal proliferation of blood vessels within the brain). Bleeding takes place in the space between the arachnoid and the pia mater (the middle and the innermost of the three *meninges* that cover the brain). This space also contains *cerebrospinal fluid*, which becomes mixed with blood.

Subarachnoid hemorrhage usually occurs spontaneously, without any head injury, although it may follow unaccustomed physical exercise. In the US each year, about five to 10 people per 100,000 suffer a subarachnoid hemorrhage. It is somewhat less common than *intracerebral hemorrhage* (another form of *stroke*), in which bleeding occurs within the brain itself. Subarachnoid hemorrhage is particularly common between the ages of 35 and 60.

### SYMPTOMS

An attack may cause immediate loss of consciousness or a sudden violent headache, often followed by loss of consciousness. If the person remains conscious, other symptoms such as *photophobia* (dislike of bright light), nausea, vomiting, drowsiness, and stiffness of the neck may develop. Unconscious patients may recover, but attacks during the ensuing day or weeks are common and often fatal.

### DIAGNOSIS

The diagnosis is confirmed by *CT scanning* and by the presence of large amounts of blood in the cerebrospinal fluid following *lumbar puncture*. The site of the burst blood vessel is investigated by *angiography* (injection of a radiopaque substance into the bloodstream followed by X rays), which may not be performed until the patient's condition has stabilized.

### TREATMENT

Treatment consists of general life-support procedures, bed rest, and measures aimed at reducing the risk of recurrence—principally, control of high blood pressure. In some cases, a burst aneurysm is surgically accessible. Angiomas can also sometimes be surgically removed, blocked off, or obliterated. Surgery is usually delayed some weeks after the acute attack.

About one third of patients make a full recovery; another one sixth recover but have some residual disability, such as paralysis, mental deterioration, or epilepsy. The remaining patients (about half) die due to the initial or a recurrent attack.

## Subclavian steal syndrome

Recurrent attacks of blurred or double vision, loss of coordination, or dizziness caused by reduced blood flow to the base of the brain when one arm (usually the left) is moved. The underlying cause is narrowing of the major arteries that carry blood to the arms (usually due to *atherosclerosis*). The left subclavian artery is particularly affected. Blood supply to the

S

affected arm is weak, but it is sufficient providing the arm is kept at rest. When the arm is moved, its muscles require an increased amount of blood, which must be diverted from the base of the brain.

A physician confirms the diagnosis by finding a weak pulse and low blood pressure in the affected arm. *Angiography* (injection of radiopaque dye into the blood vessels followed by X rays) establishes the site of the narrowed artery. Treatment is by *arterial reconstructive surgery*.

## Subclinical

A medical term applied to a disorder that produces no symptoms or signs because it is so mild or because it is in the early stages of development. A subclinical infection may not produce any symptoms, but may cause damage to organs such as the liver.

## Subconjunctival hemorrhage

Bleeding under the *conjunctiva* (transparent membrane covering the white of the eye). The small blood vessels of the conjunctiva are fragile, poorly supported, and frequently leak. Subconjunctival hemorrhage may occur spontaneously or after coughing or vomiting, which increases pressure in the veins. Subconjunctival hemorrhage is usually harmless and only rarely signals a serious disorder.

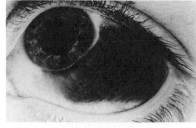

**Subconjunctival hemorrhage**
The bleeding causes a bright red area to appear in the white of the eye. This may look alarming but is usually harmless.

Subconjunctival blood disappears without treatment, usually within 10 to 14 days. Recurrences sometimes occur as a result of local weakness in a conjunctival blood vessel.

## Subconscious

A term describing mental events (e.g., thoughts, ideas, or feelings) that one is temporarily unaware of but that can be recalled under the right circumstances. In *psychoanalytic theory*, the subconscious refers to that part of the

mind through which information passes on its way from the *unconscious* to the conscious mind.

## Subcutaneous

A medical term meaning beneath the skin, as in a subcutaneous injection, one in which a drug is injected into the tissue under the skin.

## Subdural hemorrhage

Bleeding into the space between the dura mater, the tough outer layer of the *meninges* (coverings of the brain) and the arachnoid (middle meningeal layer). The trapped blood slowly forms a large hematoma (enlarging blood clot) within the skull. The most common cause is torn veins on the inside of the dura mater following a blow to the head. Subdural hemorrhage most often affects elderly or alcoholic people who have fallen.

### SYMPTOMS

The bleeding occurs slowly; it may be weeks or months before the hematoma enlarges sufficiently to cause symptoms by raising pressure within the skull and displacing and pressing on brain tissue. The symptoms, which tend to fluctuate, consist of headache, episodes of confusion and drowsiness, and the development of one-sided weakness or paralysis.

Any person in whom such symptoms develop should consult a physician immediately. Because the symptoms are similar to those of a *stroke*, it is important that mention be made of any head injury that occurred within the previous few months.

### DIAGNOSIS AND TREATMENT

The diagnosis is confirmed, and the location of the hematoma investigated, by means of *angiography* (injection of a radiopaque dye into the bloodstream followed by X rays) and *CT scanning*.

Surgical treatment is by drilling burr holes into the skull (see *Craniotomy*), drainage of the blood clot, and repair of damaged blood vessels, which usually allows a full recovery if carried out soon enough. (See also *Head injury*; *Extradural hemorrhage*.)

## Sublimation

The unconscious process by which primitive, unacceptable impulses are redirected into socially acceptable forms of behavior. Aggression, for example, may be channeled into sports. *Psychoanalytic theory* regards sublimation as a healthy process, characteristic of mature personalities.

## Subluxation

Incomplete *dislocation* of a joint—that is, displacement of the bony surfaces in a joint so that they no longer face each other exactly but remain in partial contact. In a dislocation, the joint surfaces are displaced so that there is total loss of contact between them. In general, subluxation causes less damage to the joint and surrounding tissues than a dislocation.

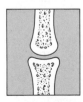

**Normal**
The diagram at left shows the normal position of the bony surfaces in a simple joint, such as the joint in the middle of a finger.

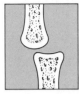

**Subluxation**
In a subluxation, the surfaces of the bones are slightly displaced from their normal positions relative to each other but are still in contact.

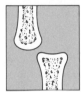

**Dislocation**
Here, there is almost complete loss of contact between the bone surfaces and usually considerable damage to surrounding tissues.

## Submucous resection

An operation to correct a deviated *nasal septum* (the central partition inside the nose) when it is causing breathing difficulty. With the use of a local anesthetic, an incision is made in the mucous membrane covering the septum; displaced cartilage and bone are then cut away. The membrane is closed with absorbable stitches, which do not require removal. Because some deviation is normal, a second opinion is often recommended.

## Subphrenic abscess

An *abscess* under the diaphragm.

## Substrate

A substance on which an *enzyme* acts. The digestive enzyme amylase acts on the substrate starch (a polysaccharide) and breaks it down into smaller saccharide (sugar) units.

## Sucking wound

An open wound in the chest wall through which air passes, causing the lung on that side to collapse (see *Lung, collapse of*). The mediastinum (central

S

partition of the chest) may also shift to the other side, causing partial collapse of the other lung.

A sucking wound causes severe breathlessness and a life-threatening lack of oxygen. Emergency first-aid treatment is vital. Cover the wound with your hand (or first cover it with a piece of impermeable material, such as a plastic bag). The wound must be kept tightly sealed until medical attention is obtained.

## Sucralfate

An *ulcer-healing drug* used to treat *peptic ulcer*. Sucralfate forms a protective barrier over the ulcerated stomach or duodenal lining and thus protects it from further attack by the digestive juices and allows an ulcer to heal.

*Antacid drugs* should not be taken within an hour of taking sucralfate as they may reduce its effectiveness.

Constipation is an adverse effect. Sucralfate may interfere with the absorption of drugs, such as tetracycline and digoxin. Prolonged treatment may impair the absorption of certain vitamins.

## Suction

The removal of unwanted fluid or semifluid material from the body with a syringe and hollow needle or with an intestinal tube and a mechanical pump. Among the many uses of suction is cleaning secretions from the throats of newborn babies and from surgical patients after an operation using general anesthesia. Suction is also used to drain blood and other fluids from the abdominal cavity during or after surgery.

## Suction lipectomy

See *Body contour surgery*.

## Sudden death

Death that occurs unexpectedly in a person who previously seemed healthy and who had not complained of any symptoms of illness (deaths due to *accidents* are excluded).

The most common cause of sudden death is *cardiac arrest*. People older than about 35 who die from cardiac arrest are frequently found at autopsy to have had *coronary heart disease*; younger victims are often found to have had a congenital heart abnormality. Sudden death may also occur in people suffering from unsuspected *myocarditis* or as a result of a *stroke*.

To reduce the risk of sudden death from heart disease, any person about to begin an exercise program after a period of inactivity should consult a physician for a checkup, especially if exertion causes chest pain, breathlessness, extreme fatigue, or palpitations, or if he or she is overweight, smokes, or has a family history of coronary heart disease. (See also *Sudden infant death syndrome*.)

## Sudden infant death syndrome

The sudden, unexpected death of an infant, which often cannot be explained even after an autopsy. Such deaths, also known as crib deaths, typically occur in apparently healthy babies who seem well when put to sleep but later are found dead.

### CAUSES AND INCIDENCE

In developed countries, sudden infant death syndrome (SIDS) is the most common form of death between the ages of 1 month and 1 year; three quarters of these occur in babies under 6 months old. SIDS is slightly more common among boys, among second children, and in winter. More deaths seem to occur between midnight and 9 AM and on weekends.

Much of the research has been focused on possible risk factors. They include *prematurity* and low birth weight; bottle-feeding; cold weather; young, single mothers; smoking, drug addiction, or anemia in the mother; poor socioeconomic background; the death of a sibling as a result of SIDS; and so-called "near miss" infants who have been found near death and have been resuscitated just in time.

Most experts believe there is no single cause of SIDS. It seems probable that some babies die of a sudden overwhelming respiratory infection and others of undetected inborn errors of metabolism (see *Metabolism, inborn errors of*). Most deaths are thought to be caused by some abnormality in the breathing and heart rate. Abnormal breathing rhythms may be due to a fault in the brain stem, the lungs may have abnormally sensitive airway reflexes, or there may be an abnormality of surfactant (a substance that prevents the air sacs of the lungs from collapsing).

Even though most deaths seem to occur without warning, it is becoming clear that some babies may have been suffering from minor symptoms (such as a cold with a stuffy nose) for several days before death or have shown an inexplicable weight loss.

### PREVENTION

Possible preventive measures include good *prenatal care*, avoidance of smoking and unnecessary taking of drugs during pregnancy, good obstetric care, breast-feeding, and close observation of the baby for several days after a minor illness.

Parents of a child who has died from SIDS and parents of "near miss" infants may be reassured by use of an alarm that sounds if the baby stops breathing. However, there is no evidence that the use of such alarms lowers the risk of death, and the number of false alarms that occurs may increase, rather than allay, the parents' anxiety.

### EFFECTS

The death of an infant from SIDS is a highly distressing experience.

Grief may manifest itself in a variety of ways, ranging from withdrawal and anger to physical symptoms. There may be feelings of intense guilt; family relationships may be badly strained by misplaced blame and by severe and persistent grief. The family should be prepared for a visit from the coroner's office and the local police.

Parents may lose confidence in their ability to properly care for any other children. They should be reassured that they did not cause the death of their babies.

Siblings are also affected by the death; their grief may be expressed through misbehavior, nightmares, bedwetting, or regression to habits long outgrown. Sometimes siblings fear they will die in the same way.

Professionals, such as the pediatrician, family physician, social worker, and minister, can provide support. Group therapy with other parents who have been through the experience can provide great comfort.

## Sudeck's atrophy

Swelling and loss of use of a hand or foot after a fracture or other injury.

Pain, swelling, and stiffness (especially in the joints) develop in the affected hand or foot about two months after the original injury, usually after the plaster cast has been removed. The nails may stop growing normally and hair on the affected limb may fall out. Despite physical therapy and attempts to start using the hand or foot again, the pain, swelling, and stiffness persist.

The condition is diagnosed by X rays, which usually show thinning of the bones (see *Osteoporosis*).

Treatment of Sudeck's atrophy includes elevation of the affected hand or foot, gentle exercise, and different forms of heat. A full recovery is usually made within about four months. However, if pain persists, a *nerve block* may be tried and, if this procedure proves temporarily successful, *sympathectomy* may be attempted.

## Suffocation

A condition in which there is a lack of oxygen due to an obstruction to the passage of air into the lungs. Suffocation may be caused by blockage of the nose and mouth, by blockage of the pharynx or larynx, or by blockage of the trachea. (See also *Asphyxia; Choking; Strangulation.*)

## Sugar

See *Carbohydrates.*

## Suicide

The act of intentionally killing oneself. In the US, suicide accounts for about 35,000 deaths (about 1 percent of all deaths) each year.

---

### FIRST AID: SUFFOCATION

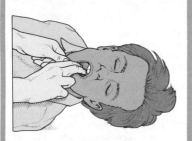

**1** Immediately remove any obstruction and move the victim into fresh air.

**2** If the victim is conscious, offer reassurance. If unconscious but breathing normally, place in the *recovery position.*

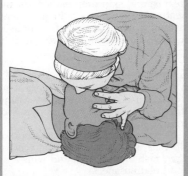

**3** If breathing is difficult or has stopped, begin *artificial respiration* immediately.

---

### CAUSES

More than 90 percent of suicides occur as the result of a psychiatric illness. Among people who take their own lives are about 15 percent of people suffering from severe *depression*, about 10 percent of those with *schizophrenia* (particularly young males in the early stages of the illness), about 7 percent of those suffering from *alcohol dependence*, about 5 percent of those with an *antisocial personality disorder*, and a smaller percentage of people suffering from some form of *neurosis*. An underlying depression is also associated with these disorders.

Suicide results from a person's reaction to a perceived overwhelming problem, such as social isolation, death of a loved one (especially a spouse), a broken home in childhood, serious physical illness, growing old, unemployment, financial problems, and drug abuse.

### INCIDENCE

The incidence of suicide shows wide variation from one country to another (see table). Published figures may not reflect the true number of suicides in some countries, especially where there are poor systems of reporting deaths or where suicide is considered to be sinful or shameful.

In the US the average age of suicide is 49.3 years, with the highest rate among the elderly. However, in recent years there has been a steady increase in the suicide rate among young people. Over the last 30 years, suicide has tripled in those aged 15 to 19; suicide is now the third most common cause of death in students, after accidents and homicide.

More men than women commit suicide, although women attempt the act more often (see *Suicide, attempted*). Marital status is also a factor. Suicide is most common in divorced people, less so in the single and widowed, and least common in those who are married. For unknown reasons, the peak months for suicide are May and June.

### METHODS

The most common method of committing suicide is poisoning, usually by taking an overdose of analgesics (painkillers) or sleeping tablets or by inhaling car exhaust fumes. Violent methods of committing suicide, such as shooting, are far more common in men than in women.

### PREVENTION

One myth about suicide is that only people who are not serious about suicide talk about it beforehand. In fact, many people who commit suicide

### SUICIDE RATES (per 100,000 population, age standardized to world population)

| Country | Year | Rate |
| --- | --- | --- |
| Hungary | 1986 | 35.2 |
| Finland | 1986 | 22.6 |
| Austria | 1986 | 22.3 |
| Denmark | 1985 | 22.0 |
| Belgium | 1984 | 18.4 |
| Switzerland | 1986 | 18.1 |
| France | 1985 | 17.5 |
| Japan | 1986 | 16.4 |
| Czechoslovakia | 1985 | 15.7 |
| Sweden | 1985 | 14.5 |
| West Germany | 1986 | 14.0 |
| Norway | 1985 | 12.5 |
| Bulgaria | 1985 | 12.1 |
| Poland | 1986 | 11.8 |
| Canada | 1985 | 11.3 |
| US | 1984 | 10.7 |
| Australia | 1985 | 10.4 |
| The Netherlands | 1985 | 9.3 |
| New Zealand | 1985 | 9.3 |
| Portugal | 1986 | 7.4 |
| England and Wales | 1985 | 7.1 |
| Italy | 1983 | 5.7 |
| Greece | 1985 | 3.2 |

**Suicide rates compared**
This table is a comparison of suicide rates in selected countries. The suicide rate in the US is less than one third that in Hungary, which has by far the highest national suicide rate in the world.

repeatedly threaten to take their own lives; relatives and friends should always take such threats seriously. Suicidal people usually feel desperately lonely, and the opportunity to talk to a sympathetic, understanding listener is sometimes enough to prevent the despairing act. It was for this reason that suicide prevention centers were established to provide 24-hour telephone counseling service for suicidal people.

A psychiatrist should be consulted immediately so that the person's depression can be treated. Hospitalization (or frequent sessions with the psychiatrist) may be necessary to provide enough support to help the sick person through the risky period.

Following a suicide threat, family or friends should remove any obvious tools for committing the act and should watch the person closely.

## Suicide, attempted

Any deliberate act of self-harm that is or is believed to be life-threatening but that in effect proves nonfatal. Most attempted suicides, or parasuicides, are carried out in a setting that makes rescue possible. They must therefore be viewed as cries for help by people in extreme distress.

S

## CAUSES AND INCIDENCE

People who attempt suicide constitute a sociologically different group from those who actually kill themselves (see *Suicide*), although there is some overlap between the two. Parasuicide is three times more common in women than in men and is most common in the 15-to-30 age group and in single and divorced people. The rate is highest among people who have personality disorders, those who live in deprived urban areas, and those who have problems with alcohol or drugs. Common precipitating factors include an argument with a relative or sexual partner, recent death of a loved one, financial worries, or severe loss of any kind that results in depression.

Suicide attempts far outnumber actual suicides and, since the 1950s, have become one of the primary reasons for hospital admission. The most common method used is to take an overdose of drugs, most often analgesics (painkillers) or sleeping tablets, often with alcohol.

## TREATMENT AND PREVENTION

If someone is discovered to have taken a drug overdose, emergency help should be summoned; if the person is unconscious or not breathing, first-aid measures should be carried out (see *Drug poisoning*). In other cases, appropriate measures depend on the victim's condition.

All suicide attempts should be treated seriously. Twenty to 30 percent of people who attempt suicide repeat their attempt within a year, and 10 percent eventually kill themselves, especially socially isolated men in whom a physical or mental illness has developed.

The most important aspect of treatment is for the person to see a psychiatrist as soon as possible to help resolve the underlying depression.

# Sulfacetamide

A *sulfonamide*-type *antibacterial drug* used in the treatment of *conjunctivitis*. Sulfacetamide is also sometimes given to treat chronic *blepharitis* (inflammation of the eyelids) and to prevent infection after an eye injury or the removal of a foreign body.

Sulfacetamide may cause stinging of the eye. Itching, redness, and swelling of the eyelids are occasionally caused by an allergic reaction.

# Sulfamethoxazole

A *sulfonamide*-type *antibacterial drug* used to treat *conjunctivitis* and ear infections. Sulfamethoxazole combined with *trimethoprim* (another antibacterial drug) is also given to treat a variety of respiratory tract infections (including *pneumocystis pneumonia*), urinary tract infections, *gastroenteritis*, and *gonorrhea*.

Possible adverse effects include rash, nausea, vomiting, diarrhea, and, rarely, headache, dizziness, muscle pain, and joint pain.

# Sulfasalazine

A drug used to relieve inflammation in the intestinal disorders *ulcerative colitis* and *Crohn's disease*.

Sulfasalazine may cause nausea, vomiting, headache, abdominal pain, and loss of appetite. An allergic reaction, causing fever and rash, occasionally occurs. Prolonged treatment may cause *folic acid* deficiency, resulting in *anemia*.

# Sulfinpyrazone

A drug used to treat *gout* (a metabolic condition associated with an excessive level of uric acid in the blood, sometimes causing painful arthritis and kidney stones). Sulfinpyrazone does not relieve the symptoms of gout but does reduce the frequency of attacks.

Sulfinpyrazone is also given to reduce *hyperuricemia* (raised levels of uric acid in the blood) caused by certain drugs, such as thiazide *diuretic drugs* and some *anticancer drugs*. Sulfinpyrazone reduces the amount of uric acid in the blood by increasing the amount excreted in the urine.

## POSSIBLE ADVERSE EFFECTS

Adverse effects include nausea, vomiting, headache, flushing, cloudy or bloodstained urine, rash, itching, wheezing, and breathlessness.

# Sulfisoxazole

A *sulfonamide*-type *antibacterial drug* used in the treatment of urinary tract and eye infections. Given with a *penicillin drug*, sulfisoxazole is used to treat ear and chest infections resistant to penicillin alone.

Sulfisoxazole may cause nausea, vomiting, loss of appetite, diarrhea, headache, dizziness, or rash.

# Sulfonamide drugs

| COMMON DRUGS |
| --- |
| *Sulfacetamide  Sulfamethoxazole* |
| *Sulfisoxazole* |

A group of *antibacterial drugs*. Before the advent of *penicillin drugs*, sulfonamide drugs were widely used to treat infectious diseases. Today, they are used mainly to treat urinary tract infections. Often prescribed in combination with *trimethoprim*, sulfonamide drugs are sometimes used to treat *bronchitis*, certain types of *pneumonia*, skin infections, and infections of the middle ear.

# Sulfur

A mineral that plays several important roles in the body. Sulfur is a constituent of vitamin $B_1$ and of several essential amino acids (building blocks of proteins). In particular, sulfur is necessary for the manufacture of *collagen* (which helps to form bones, tendons, and connective tissue) and is a constituent of *keratin* (the chief component of hair, skin, and nails).

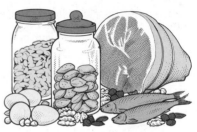

**Sulfur-rich foods**
The main sources of sulfur in the diet are protein-rich foods such as eggs, fish, lean meat, nuts, and dried beans.

## DEFICIENCY AND EXCESS

A balanced diet contains enough sulfur for the body's needs; only people who eat little protein (such as those on extremely restricted vegetarian diets) are likely to suffer from sulfur deficiency. People deficient in sulfur have the symptoms of general protein deficiency, such as weakness and tiredness.

## MEDICAL USES

Sulfur is used in some ointments, creams, and skin preparations for the treatment of various skin disorders, including acne, dandruff, psoriasis, scabies, diaper rash, and certain fungal infections.

# Sulindac

A *nonsteroidal anti-inflammatory drug* (NSAID) used to relieve joint pain and stiffness caused by various types of *arthritis*.

Adverse effects are typical of other NSAIDs, including indigestion, *peptic ulcer*, rash and itching, and wheezing and breathlessness.

# Sunburn

Inflammation of the skin caused by overexposure to the sun. The ultraviolet rays in sunlight destroy cells in the outer layer of the skin and damage tiny blood vessels beneath.

Sunburn is most common in fair-skinned people, whose skin produces only small amounts of the protective pigment *melanin*, and in people attempting to acquire a tan in strong sunlight too quickly. The affected skin turns red and tender and may become blistered. In severe cases, the sunburn may be accompanied by symptoms of sunstroke—such as vomiting, fever, and collapse. Several days later the dead skin cells are shed by peeling.

Repeated overexposure to sunlight can age the skin prematurely, producing yellowish, wrinkled skin through which capillary vessels may be seen. Overexposure can also increase the risk of skin cancer (see *Sunlight, adverse effects of*).

### PREVENTION
Exposure to strong sunlight should be limited to 15 minutes on the first day, particularly if the person has fair skin, and should be increased very gradually. This applies even if conditions are hazy. Until a tan is acquired, the skin should be protected with a high protection factor *sunscreen*.

### TREATMENT
Calamine lotion or a sunburn cream should be applied to soothe the burned skin, which should be protected from further sun exposure until healing takes place. *Analgesic drugs* (painkillers) may be required to relieve tenderness. A person with severe sunburn should consult a physician, who may prescribe a cream containing *corticosteroid drugs* to speed healing.

## Sunlight, adverse effects of
Some exposure to ultraviolet radiation from the sun is necessary for the body to produce vitamin D. Overexposure can have various harmful effects, particularly in fair-skinned people, who produce only small amounts of the protective skin pigment *melanin*.

Short-term overexposure causes *sunburn* and, in intense heat, can result in *heat exhaustion* or *heat stroke*. Repeated overexposure over a long period can cause premature aging of the skin and the production of wartlike growths called solar *keratoses*. Most seriously, it considerably increases the risk of *skin cancer*.

*Photosensitivity* (skin rash resulting from abnormal sensitivity to sunlight) may be triggered by taking certain drugs. The condition may also occur in people who have systemic *lupus erythematosus* or *porphyria*.

## Sunscreens

---
**WARNING**
Some suntanning preparations do not contain a sunscreen and therefore provide no protection against sunburn.
---

Preparations that protect the skin from the harmful effects of sunlight (see *Sunlight, adverse effects of*). Sunscreens are used mainly to prevent *sunburn*. They are also used to treat rash caused by *photosensitivity*.

Most sunscreens, including the very common *para-aminobenzoic acid* (PABA), work by absorbing ultraviolet rays. Some, such as titanium dioxide, reflect the sun's rays.

Sunscreen products are labeled with a sun protection factor (SPF), with the highest factor affording the greatest protection. Choice of product should depend on skin type (see box). A sunscreen with a lower SPF may be used once the skin tans. During prolonged sunbathing, sunscreens should be reapplied at regular intervals and also after swimming.

Some people are allergic to sunscreen chemicals and a skin rash develops. This is more common with preparations containing PABA.

## Sunstroke
The most common type of *heat stroke*, usually brought on by overexposure to direct sun in a person who is unaccustomed to a hot climate.

## Suntan
Darkening of the skin after exposure to sunlight. Specialized cells in the outer layer of the skin respond to the ultraviolet rays in the sunlight by producing more of the protective pigment *melanin*. People who spend a lot of time in the sun are likely to experience premature aging and wrinkling of the skin and run a greatly increased risk of skin cancer. (See also *Sunlight, adverse effects of*; *Sunburn*.)

## Superego
The part of the personality, described in *psychoanalytic theory*, that is responsible for maintaining an individual's standards of behavior. Popularly termed a person's "conscience," the superego arises as a result of the child incorporating the ideals and moral views of those in authority (usually parents). The superego can create feelings of guilt and anxiety by criticizing the *ego* (the conscious "I") when the ego gives way to the primitive impulses of the *id* (the pleasure-seeking part of the personality).

An excessively strong superego is said to be the cause of severe, puritanical personality types and of *obsessive-compulsive behavior*. By contrast, failure to develop an appropriate superego leads to impulsive and immoral behavior.

In psychoanalytic theory, a harsh, self-punishing superego is said to result from childhood experience with a harsh parent.

## Superficial
Situated near the surface, as in the superficial blood vessels (the capillaries that lie near the surface of the skin and play an important role in the regulation of body temperature and blushing).

## Superinfection
A second infection that occurs during the course of an existing infection. The term usually refers to an infection by a microorganism that is resistant to drugs being used against the original infection. The second microorganism may be a resistant strain of the first infection, a different pathogen (disease-causing microorganism), or a member of the body's normal flora (microorganisms that are normally present in the body without producing ill effects) that has proliferated excessively because other microorganisms that normally keep it in check have been killed by drug

S

### SAFE EXPOSURE TIMES USING SUNSCREENS OF DIFFERENT STRENGTHS

| Protection factor | 4 | 8 | 15 |
|---|---|---|---|
| Skin type | Safe exposure time | | |
| Fair | 10 minutes | 40 to 80 minutes | 1.5 to 2 hours |
| Medium | 50 to 80 minutes | 2 to 2.5 hours | 5 to 5.5 hours |
| Dark | 1.5 to 2 hours | 3.5 to 4 hours | all day |
| Black | 4 hours | all day | all day |

therapy. For example, tetracycline therapy may result in superinfection of the mouth, vagina, and/or anus with the fungus that causes candidiasis (thrush).

## Superiority complex
An exaggerated and unrealistic belief that one is better than other people. *Adlerian theory* suggests that a superiority complex develops in some people in response to the natural feelings of inferiority that everyone is born with. In more modern psychoanalytic terms, a superiority complex is a compensation for unconscious feelings of inadequacy or low self-esteem.

## Supernumerary
More than the normal number, as in supernumerary nipples, additional nipples that are not usually associated with underlying glandular tissue; they develop along a line that extends from the armpit to the groin. (See also *Supernumerary teeth*.)

## Supernumerary teeth
One or more teeth in excess of the usual number (20 deciduous and 32 permanent). An extra tooth may be a duplicate of an existing tooth or it may have an abnormal shape and position (usually appearing as a small conical protrusion from the gum above the existing teeth in the upper front jaw).

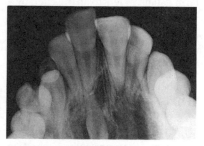

**Supernumerary (extra) tooth**
This X ray of the upper jaw shows a supernumerary incisor tooth on the roof of the mouth behind the normal incisors.

Supernumerary teeth may interfere with the proper *eruption of teeth* and are usually extracted.

## Supination
The act of turning the body to a supine (lying on the back with the face upward) position or the hand to a palm forward position. Movements in the opposite direction to supination are called *pronation*.

## Suppository
A solid, cone- or bullet-shaped object containing a drug and an inert (chemically inactive) substance, usually derived from cocoa butter or another type of vegetable oil. The suppository is placed in the vagina or rectum and melts at body temperature, releasing the active ingredient.

Vaginal suppositories are used to treat vaginal disorders, such as *candidiasis* (thrush) or *trichomoniasis*, or to introduce contraceptive *spermicides* into the vagina.

Rectal suppositories are used to treat rectal disorders, such as *hemorrhoids* or *proctitis*. They may also be used to soften feces and stimulate a bowel movement. A rectal suppository is also used to administer a drug into the general circulation via blood vessels in the rectum if vomiting is likely to prevent absorption or if the drug would cause irritation of the stomach lining.

Drugs given by suppository include antifungal drugs, local anesthetics, corticosteroid drugs, nonsteroidal anti-inflammatory drugs, antibiotic drugs, and antiemetic drugs.

## Suppuration
The formation or exudation of *pus*. Suppuration occurs at the site of bacterial infection, where the pus may accumulate, forming an *abscess* in solid tissue or a *boil* or *pustule* on the skin. Open sores often suppurate, particularly when they are slow to heal, because the exposed underlying tissue tends to become repeatedly infected with bacteria.

## Suprarenal glands
Another name for the *adrenal glands*.

## Supraspinatus syndrome
See *Painful arc syndrome*.

## Supraventricular tachycardia
An abnormally fast but regular heart rate of between 140 and 180 beats per minute (or, rarely, of up to 300 beats per minute in certain arrhythmias) that occurs in intermittent episodes lasting for several hours or days. Supraventricular tachycardia is caused by abnormal electrical impulses arising within the atria (upper chambers) of the heart taking over control of the heart beat from the *sinoatrial node* (the heart's pacemaker).

Symptoms may include palpitations, breathlessness, chest pain, or fainting (see *Stokes-Adams syndrome*). Diagnosis of the condition is made by an *ECG* (electrocardiogram). An attack can sometimes be terminated by *Valsalva's maneuver* or by drinking cold water. Recurrent attacks are treated with *antiarrhythmic drugs*. Rarely, the condition may require treatment by electrical conversion of the heart rhythm (by applying an electric shock to the heart).

## Surfactant
A wetting agent (i.e., a substance that reduces surface tension). Soaps, detergents, and emulsifiers are surfactants. Pulmonary surfactant is a substance secreted by the alveoli (air sacs) in the lungs that prevents them from collapsing during exhalation.

## Surfers' nodules
Multiple *exostoses* (bony outgrowths) occurring on bones in the foot and on the tibial tubercle (the bony prominence below the knee at the top of the shin). Surfers' nodules are caused by the repeated banging of the surfboard against the knees and tops of the feet as the surfer kneels to paddle the board. They can be avoided by paddling in a lying position.

## Surgeon
A physician who performs operations that involve cutting body tissue. Surgery may be done to diagnose illness, remove diseased tissue and organs, repair injuries, or correct malfunctioning parts. General surgeons perform a variety of operations on almost all parts of the body. Other surgeons operate only on particular parts of the body. (See also *Surgery*.)

## Surgery
The treatment of disease, injury, or other disorders by direct physical intervention, usually with instruments. The term is also used to denote those aspects of medical practice that deal with the study, diagnosis, and management of all disorders treated by operative surgery (as distinct from those treated by drugs, diet, or modification of life-style).

Operative surgery involves incision (cutting) into the skin or other organ, inspection, removal of diseased tissues or organs, relief of obstruction, replacement of structures to their normal position, redirection of body channels, transplantation of tissues or whole organs, and implantation of mechanical or electronic devices.

Surgery may be minor or major. Minor operations are usually, but not always, performed using local

**S**

anesthesia. Major operations are usually performed using general anesthesia, although local anesthesia is sometimes used. Neurosurgeons and ophthalmologists, for instance, often operate using local anesthesia.

Surgery has for many years been divided into specialties, such as orthopedic surgery, neurosurgery, obstetrics and gynecology, ophthalmology, gastrointestinal surgery, and plastic surgery. In recent years there has been an increasing trend toward further subspecialization; some surgeons now confine their practices to such narrow limits as surgery of the hand, the cornea, the small blood vessels, or the skin.

## Surrogacy

The agreement by a woman to become pregnant and give birth to a child with the understanding that she will surrender the child after birth to the contractual parents. Surrogacy became publicized with the advent of *in vitro fertilization*, in which the egg and sperm are brought together in the laboratory. The fertilized egg can be transferred to the uterus of any woman who is at the appropriate stage of the menstrual cycle.

Another means of accomplishing surrogacy is through the *artificial insemination* of the surrogate mother with the contracting father's sperm.

The ethical and legal aspects of surrogacy have yet to be resolved. In most countries a woman who wishes to act as a surrogate for her infertile sister can be helped to do so. Surrogacy for financial reward has been forbidden by law in some countries but not in others. In the US (in 1988), the issue was still before the courts. If surrogacy-for-money agreements were deemed illegal, it would not be possible for either party to go to the courts to enforce a contract.

## Susceptibility

A total or partial vulnerability to an infection, disease, or disorder. In *AIDS*, the immune system is impaired and the sufferer is vulnerable to a wide range of infections and diseases.

## Suture

A type of *joint* (found only between the bones of the *skull*) in which the adjacent bones are so closely and firmly joined by a thin layer of fibrous connective tissue that movement between them is impossible. The term suture is also used to refer to a surgical stitch (see *Suturing*).

## METHODS OF SUTURING

Suturing is carried out using a general or local anesthetic. The type of stitch used depends on the nature of the wound or incision (two types are shown below). In all cases the surgeon sews the wound edges together to produce minimal distortion of tissue.

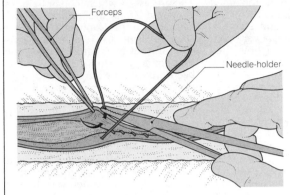

Forceps

Needle-holder

**Technique**
The surgeon grasps the edge of the wound with forceps held in one hand and, with the other hand, inserts the needle through the skin. In this illustration, the surgeon is shown using a needle-holder, which gives greater control for very fine stitches. In other cases, the needle may be held in the hand.

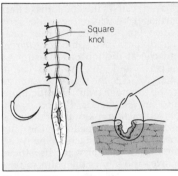

Square knot

**Standard interrupted sutures**
The needle is passed into one skin edge, through the full depth of the wound, and out the other skin edge. Each stitch is tied at the side using a square knot.

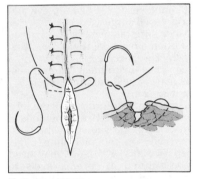

**Mattress sutures**
For deeper wounds, the needle is passed through the wound twice: first shallowly, close to the skin edges, and then more deeply, farther from the edges.

## OTHER METHODS OF CLOSURE

Alternatives to suturing include removable staples and clips (staples are also used internally) and adhesive tape.

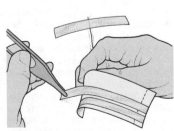

**Adhesive tape**
When the wound is shallow, tape may be applied directly. For deeper wounds, absorbable stitches are first inserted just below the skin.

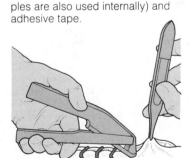

**Inserting staples**
The wound edges are held up with forceps and equally spaced staples are inserted using an automatic stapling device.

S

## Suturing

The closing of a surgical incision or a wound by sutures (stitches) to promote healing.

### MATERIALS USED

A variety of sterile materials is used as sutures, including catgut (obtained from sheep intestines); linen, silk, or synthetic fiber thread; and stainless steel wire. These materials vary considerably in the length of time they retain their strength, the reaction they provoke in tissues, and the likelihood of their allowing minute pockets of infection to form. In addition, certain materials, such as catgut, are absorbable (i.e., they eventually dissolve in the body). The choice of which material to use for an operation is made by the surgeon. The thickness of sutures varies from almost 0.04 inch (1 mm), used for the repair of major injuries, to a barely visible 0.004 inch (0.01 mm), used for delicate eye and blood vessel surgery.

Most surgical needles are curved and often have a point with a cutting edge. The needle is held in a tweezerlike instrument; larger needles may be held with the fingers.

### HOW IT IS DONE

The method of suturing a typical incision, and some alternative methods of skin closure, are shown in the illustrated box on the preceding page. Deep incisions or wounds may need to be sutured at several levels to achieve full closure throughout the depth of tissue, thus preventing collection of blood below the surface.

Internal sutures, made of absorbable material, are left in place permanently. Skin sutures are removed painlessly after one to two weeks.

## Swab

A wad of absorbent material used in surgery or to obtain a sample of bacteria from an infected patient.

One type of swab, a surgical sponge, is commonly a folded piece of cotton gauze held in the hand or in a clamp. It is used to apply cleansing and antiseptic solutions to the skin before an incision is made and to soak up blood and other fluids during an operation. The swab often contains material opaque to X rays to enable it to be detected if it is accidentally left in the body, an occurrence that is usually prevented by a "sponge count" made before the operation begins and again before the patient is stitched up.

A bacteriological swab consists of a twist of cotton at the end of a thin stick that is sealed in a container and sterilized. It is applied to an infected area of the body to absorb pus or mucus, from which a *culture* can be grown to identify bacteria.

## Swallowing

The process by which food or liquid is conveyed from the mouth to the stomach via the esophagus. The first stage is voluntary (under conscious control), but is so familiar that little thought is given to it. Once food has been well chewed and mixed with saliva (which greatly facilitates swallowing), the tongue pushes it to the back of the mouth and the voluntary muscles in the palate push the food into the pharynx (throat).

The rest of the swallowing act is involuntary (automatic), brought about by a series of *reflexes*; once started, it is rapid, powerful, and difficult to stop. Entry of food into the pharynx causes the epiglottis (a flap of cartilage) to close over the larynx (voice box) leading to the trachea (windpipe). A sphincter (circular muscle) at the top of the esophagus relaxes, and the muscles of the pharynx seize the food and squeeze it in the form of a bolus (rounded lump) into the esophagus. Powerful waves of contraction then pass down the esophagus, propelling the food toward the stomach. Finally, the muscle at the entry to the stomach relaxes and allows the bolus to pass.

## Swallowing difficulty

A fairly common symptom with a wide variety of causes, known medically as dysphagia.

### CAUSES

Temporary swallowing difficulty may be caused by a foreign object (such as a fish bone) lodging at the back of the throat or in the esophagus. Most foreign objects are able to pass on to the stomach, but a scratch in the lining of the throat or esophagus may cause discomfort. Swallowing difficulty may also result from insufficient production of saliva (see *Mouth, dry*).

Disorders of the esophagus that may disrupt normal swallowing include *esophageal spasm* (uncoordinated contractions of the esophagus), *esophageal stricture* (narrowing) caused by scar or tumor (see *Esophagus, cancer of*), *esophagitis* (inflammation), *achalasia* (abnormal contraction of the muscles at the lower end of the esophagus), or a *pharyngoesophageal diverticulum* (hernia of part of the esophagus through a weak area in the surrounding muscle).

*Esophageal atresia* (closure or failure of the esophagus to open) can cause feeding problems in the newborn.

Difficulty swallowing may also be caused by a nervous system disorder (e.g., *myasthenia gravis*, *stroke*, or, rarely, *poliomyelitis*).

Pressure on the outside of the esophagus may obstruct the passage of food. In rare instances, pressure is exerted by a *goiter*, an aortic *aneurysm*, or cancer of the bronchus.

### DIAGNOSIS AND TREATMENT

Any person who experiences persistent swallowing difficulty should be examined without delay. Investigations may include *esophagoscopy* (examination of the esophagus with a viewing tube) or barium swallow (see *Barium X-ray examinations*). Treatment depends on the cause.

## Sweat glands

Minute structures deep within the skin that produce sweat. Each gland is made up of a coiled tube, in which the sweat is secreted, and a narrow passageway, which carries the sweat to the skin surface. The average person has about 3 million sweat glands.

### TYPES

There are two types of sweat glands—eccrine and apocrine. Eccrine glands are the most common, especially on the palms and soles; these glands open directly to the skin surface. Apocrine glands, which develop at puberty, occur only in hairy areas, particularly the armpits, pubic region, and around the anus. These glands produce cellular material as well as sweat; they open into a hair follicle before reaching the skin surface.

### FUNCTION

Sweat is composed mainly of water (99 percent) and minute quantities of dissolved substances, including sodium chloride (salt).

The activity of the sweat glands is controlled by the *autonomic nervous system*. Usually the glands are stimulated to produce sweat to keep the body cool, in which case sweating is heaviest on the forehead, upper lip, neck, and chest. Sweating can also be caused by anxiety or fear, in which case sweat appears mainly on the palms and soles and in the armpits. Sweating also occurs in many illnesses in which fever is a feature.

Sweat is odorless until bacteria act upon it, producing body odor.

### DISORDERS

The most common problem affecting the sweat glands is *prickly heat*, an intensely irritating skin rash caused by blockage of the glands with debris and sweat. Less common disorders of the sweat glands include *hyperhidrosis* (excessive sweating), *hypohidrosis* (reduced sweating), and abnormal or excessive skin odor.

## Sweating

The process by which the body cools itself. Sweating also occurs as a response to psychological stress or fear. (See *Sweat glands; Heat disorders.*)

## Sweeteners, artificial

See *Artificial sweeteners.*

## Swimmers' ear

A common name for *otitis externa.*

## Sycosis vulgaris

Inflammation of the beard area, also called barbers' itch. The condition is caused by infection of hair follicles, usually with *STAPHYLOCOCCUS AUREUS* bacteria contracted from infected razors and towels. Pus-filled blisters or boils develop around the follicles, sometimes resulting in severe scarring unless treated.

Treatment is usually with *antibiotic drugs*; growing a beard may help prevent a recurrence.

## Sydenham's chorea

A childhood disorder of the central nervous system, once called St. Vitus' dance. The condition is characterized by involuntary, irregular, jerky movements and usually follows an attack of *rheumatic fever.*

Sydenham's chorea is rare in the US today but remains a common disorder in developing countries.

Restlessness and irritability usually precede the chorea, which affects the head, face, limbs, and fingers. The involuntary fidgets are random and

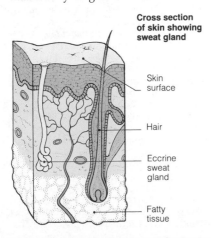

**Cross section of skin showing sweat gland**

Skin surface

Hair

Eccrine sweat gland

Fatty tissue

unrepetitive. Voluntary movements are clumsy and the limbs are often floppy. Early signs are slurred speech and deteriorating handwriting.

Treatment is bed rest and antibiotics. Sedation is sometimes necessary if the fidgeting is extreme. The condition usually clears up after two to three months and has no long-term adverse effects. Thereafter, the person may be given antibiotics before surgical or dental treatment to prevent heart disease.

## Sympathectomy

An operation in which the ganglia (nerve terminals) of sympathetic nerves are destroyed to interrupt the nerve pathway and thus improve blood supply to a limb or relieve chronic pain.

### WHY IT IS DONE

The sympathetic nerves form part of the *autonomic nervous system* and control involuntary activities in the body, including the caliber of blood vessels. In *peripheral vascular disease* (narrowing of blood vessels in the legs and sometimes the arms), stimulation from the sympathetic nerves produces spasms in the blood vessels that worsen constriction. Sympathectomy prevents spasms from occurring and thus may improve blood supply to the affected area. Sometimes this response is limited only to the vessels of the skin when it is the blood flow to the muscles that needs to be improved.

The sympathetic nerves also play an important part in producing the sensation of pain. In some cases of *causalgia* (a persistent severe pain usually caused by nerve injury), sympathectomy offers the only prospect of relieving the pain.

### HOW IT IS DONE

The surgeon may first perform a trial procedure, injecting local anesthetic into the nerves that supply the affected area. If this provides considerable temporary relief of the symptoms, a sympathectomy is usually performed.

Destruction of the nerve ganglia, which lie near the spinal cord, can be accomplished by injecting a sclerosing solution, which causes inflammation and subsequent degeneration of the nerves. Symptoms in the upper part of the body are controlled by an injection into the cervicodorsal sympathetic nerves at the base of the neck. To treat disorders of the lower part of the body, sclerosing solution is injected into the lumbar sympathetic nerves in the middle of the back.

Alternatively, nerve ganglia may be destroyed surgically while using a general anesthetic. In a cervicodorsal sympathectomy, this is done through an incision made in the armpit; in a lumbar sympathectomy, the incision runs horizontally from the spine in the lower back almost to the navel.

### RESULTS

Sympathectomy performed to widen blood vessels is variable in its results. Results generally depend on the disease for which it is being performed. In controlling severe pain, however, the operation usually proves successful. Lumbar sympathectomy in men occasionally results in inability to ejaculate.

## Sympathetic nervous system

One of the two divisions of the *autonomic nervous system*. In conjunction with the other division (the parasympathetic nervous system), this system controls many of the involuntary activities of the glands, organs, and other parts of the body.

## Sympatholytic drugs

A group of drugs that blocks the action of the *sympathetic nervous system*. Sympatholytic drugs include *beta-blocker drugs*, *guanethidine*, *hydralazine*, and *prazosin*. They work either by reducing the release of the stimulatory *neurotransmitter* norepinephrine from nerve endings, or by occupying the receptors that the neurotransmitters epinephrine and norepinephrine normally bind to, thereby preventing their normal actions.

## Symphysis

An anatomical term for a type of joint in which two bones are firmly joined by tough, fibrous cartilage. Such joints occur between the bodies of the vertebrae (the parts of the bones that are separated by the intervertebral disks), between the two pubic bones at the front of the *pelvis*, and between the manubrium (upper part) and body (middle part) of the *sternum*.

## Symptom

An indication of a disease or disorder (such as pain) that is noticed by the sufferer. Presenting symptoms are those that prompt a person to obtain medical advice, but they are not necessarily the first to appear. The indications that a physician notes are called signs. The overall clinical picture (syndrome), including the symptoms and signs, helps the physician to identify a disease.

S

The distinction between symptoms and signs is not always clear. For example, fever is felt by the patient and observed by the physician. Similarly, in *appendicitis*, pain is a cardinal symptom; tenderness, which is pain felt only when pressure is applied, is a sign generally elicited by the physician, but it may also be elicited by the patient pressing on his or her own abdomen.

In some conditions, an accurate recollection and description of symptoms is extremely important. For example, because physical signs are often absent in *angina pectoris*, diagnosis of this condition may depend almost entirely on the patient's description of the chest pain.

## Symptothermal method
See *Contraception, periodic abstinence*.

## Synapse
A junctional connection between two neurons (nerve cells) across which a signal can pass. A single neuron may form thousands of these connections with adjacent nerve cells.

A typical neuron has one long fiber (axon) that projects from its cell body; it splits into several smaller branches and twigs, each ending in a terminal that forms a synapse, usually close to the cell body of an adjacent neuron. At a synapse, the two neurons do not come directly into contact; their surface membranes are separated by a gap called the synaptic cleft. When an electrical signal passes along a neuronal axon and reaches a synapse, it cannot bridge the cleft directly; instead, it causes the release of a chemical, called a *neurotransmitter*. The chemical travels across the cleft and is received at the surface membrane of the next neuron, where it changes the electrical potential of the membrane.

The axonal membrane from which the neurotransmitter is released is called the presynaptic membrane; the neuronal membrane at which it is received is called the postsynaptic membrane. Signals can be transmitted across a synapse in one direction only—from presynaptic to postsynaptic membrane.

A synapse may be excitatory or inhibitory. When a neurotransmitter passes across an excitatory synapse, the effect is to excite the postsynaptic membrane, making it more likely that the receptor neuron will "fire" and propagate an electrical impulse in turn. Inhibitory synapses decrease the excitation of the next neuron.

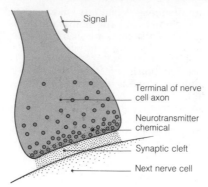

**Structure of a synapse**
When a signal arrives at the terminal of a nerve cell axon, it causes release of a neurotransmitter, which crosses the synaptic cleft and affects the next cell.

Most drugs affecting the nervous system work through their effects on synapses. They may modify neurotransmitter release or may modify the effects of neurotransmitters on postsynaptic membranes.

## Syncope
The medical term for *fainting*.

## Syndactyly
A congenital (present at birth) defect in which two or more fingers or toes are joined. The toes of one or both feet are more frequently affected. Often inherited and more common in boys, syndactyly is caused by incomplete development of the digits at the embryo stage, or by constriction of the digits by tissue within the uterus later in fetal development.

In mild cases, only the skin between the affected fingers or toes is joined. More seriously, the bones of adjacent digits are fused, as is the overlying skin, and there may be only one nail.

Treatment is usually by one or more operations during early childhood to separate the affected digits.

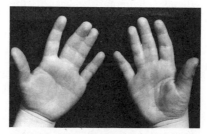

**Syndactyly**
In this case, the middle and ring fingers in both hands are partly joined. Sometimes, syndactyly occurs in association with other birth defects.

## Syndrome
A group of symptoms and/or signs that, occurring together, constitutes a particular disorder. For example, *irritable bowel syndrome* is characterized by a combination of any or all of the following—intermittent pain in the lower abdomen (usually relieved by bowel movement or passing gas), abdominal swelling, irregular bowel movements (often with a sense of incomplete evacuation of the bowel afterward), mucus in the feces, excessive gas, and worsening of symptoms after eating.

## Synovectomy
Surgical removal of the *synovium* (thin membrane lining a joint capsule) to treat recurrent or persistent *synovitis* (inflammation of the synovium), usually in sufferers from severe *rheumatoid arthritis*. The operation is usually performed only if the condition is severely disabling and has not responded to injections of *corticosteroid drugs* or to the taking of *nonsteroidal anti-inflammatory drugs* or *antirheumatic drugs*.

The joint may be opened while using a general anesthetic and the synovium cut away, or the operation may be performed by means of *arthroscopy*. After the operation, the joint is kept mobile to inhibit scarring. Synovectomy is a temporary expedient that usually improves symptoms for no more than about two years; further surgery may then be required.

## Synovitis
Inflammation of the *synovium* (thin membrane lining a joint capsule). The condition may be acute (of sudden onset and short duration), in which case it is usually caused by infection, injury, or overuse of the joint, or chronic (recurrent or persistent), as in a disorder such as *rheumatoid arthritis*.

The inflammation causes the synovium to secrete an abnormal amount of lubricating fluid, which makes the joint swollen, painful, and often warm and red. To determine the cause of the condition, an arthrocentesis (removal of fluid from a joint) or a *biopsy* (removal of a sample of the synovium) may be required.

Symptoms are relieved by rest, supporting the joint with a splint or cast, *analgesics* (painkillers), *nonsteroidal anti-inflammatory drugs*, and, occasionally, an injection of *corticosteroid drugs*. Any causative infection is treated with *antibiotic drugs*. Chronic

S

synovitis that does not respond to drug treatment or injection may be treated by *synovectomy* (surgical removal of the synovium).

## Synovium

A thin membrane that lines the fibrous capsule surrounding a movable joint. The synovium also forms a sheath for certain tendons of the hands and feet, lining the fibrous or bony tunnels through which they glide. The membrane secretes synovial fluid, a clear, sticky liquid resembling egg white that lubricates the joint or the tendon. The synovium can become inflamed; in a joint lining this is known as *synovitis*, in a tendon sheath it is known as *tenosynovitis*.

---

**LOCATION OF SYNOVIUM**

Every movable joint is enclosed within a fibrous capsule. The inner lining of the capsule is known as the synovium.

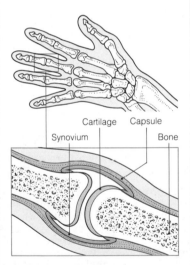

Cartilage   Capsule

Synovium   Bone

**Function**

The membrane secretes a thick fluid that lubricates the joint; it may accumulate and cause pain if the joint is injured.

---

## Syphilis

A sexually transmitted or *congenital* (existing at birth) infection of worldwide distribution, first recorded as a major epidemic in Europe in the last decade of the 15th century following the return of Columbus from America. Today, infection is transmitted almost exclusively by sexual contact. Congenital syphilis, once very common, is now rare.

**CAUSES**

Syphilis is caused by *TREPONEMA PALLIDUM*, a spirochete (spiral-shaped bacterium) that penetrates broken skin or *mucous membranes* in the genitalia, rectum, or mouth during sexual intercourse. Infection may be acquired by kissing or by intimate bodily contact with an infected person. The risk of infection during a single contact with an infected person is about 30 percent. After gaining access, the organism passes quickly by way of the bloodstream and lymphatic system to all parts of the body; within hours, the organism has spread beyond hope of local treatment.

**INCIDENCE**

The incidence of syphilis in the US increased during the late 1970s and early 1980s, especially in homosexual men, but has demonstrated a marked decrease since 1982. This decrease may be attributed to changes in sexual practices since *AIDS* was first publicized. However, a resurgence of penicillin-resistant *gonorrhea* in 1988 suggested that efforts to educate people on the avoidance of sexually transmitted diseases had yet to take effect.

**SYMPTOMS AND SIGNS**

Untreated syphilis usually passes through the following stages.

**PRIMARY** The first symptom is a primary sore (chancre) that usually appears three to four weeks after contact. The chancre is a painless ulcer with a hard, wet base that is covered with serum teeming with spirochetes. The usual site is the genitals but may be the anus, mouth, rectum, or fingers. Often, the chancre is inconspicuous and may be missed. The lymph nodes connected with the area containing the chancre become painlessly enlarged and rubbery but are not tender. The chancre heals in four to eight weeks.

**SECONDARY** Six to 12 weeks after infection, the secondary stage begins. The most obvious feature is a skin rash, which may be transient, recurrent, or may last for months. In whites, the rash is conspicuous, with crops of pinkish or pale red, round spots; in blacks, the rash is pigmented and appears darker than the normal skin color. The rash is associated with extensive lymph node enlargement; there is often headache, aches and pains in the bones, loss of appetite, fever, and fatigue. Meningitis may occur. The hair may fall out in clumps and, in moist skin areas, thickened, gray or pink patches called con-

dylomata lata may develop. They are highly infectious. The secondary stage may persist for about a year.

**LATENT** During this stage, which may last for a few years or for the rest of the person's life, the infected person appears normal. However, about 30 percent of untreated cases proceed, eventually, to tertiary syphilis.

**TERTIARY** This stage usually starts within ten years of infection, but may appear as early as three years or as late as 25 years. The effects are varied. Tissue destruction, by a process called gumma formation, may involve the bones, palate, nasal septum, tongue, skin, or almost any organ of the body. Among the more serious effects are cardiovascular syphilis, which affects the aorta (the main artery of the body) and leads to aneurysm formation and heart valve disease; neurosyphilis, with progressive brain damage and general paralysis (once called "general paralysis of the insane"); and tabes dorsalis, which affects part of the spinal cord.

**DIAGNOSIS**

Primary syphilis can be readily diagnosed by microscopic demonstration of the active spirochetes in the chancre serum. Confirmation is given by tests such as the Venereal Disease Research Laboratory (VDRL) test or the fluorescent treponemal antibody absorption test. Secondary, latent, and tertiary syphilis give strongly positive results with these and similar tests. In

S

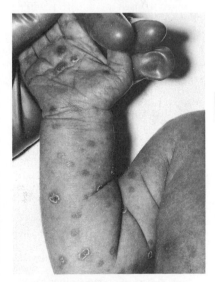

**Congenital syphilis**

This baby's mother had syphilis during pregnancy. A rash and other signs of infection developed in the baby early in life. Congenital syphilis is very rare today.

neurosyphilis, it may be necessary to perform these tests on a sample of cerebrospinal fluid.

**TREATMENT**

The significance of the disease has been altered since the introduction of penicillin. It remains the drug of choice for all forms of the disease. Early syphilis can often be cured by a single large *depot injection*; later forms of syphilis require a longer course of treatment. Although penicillin is, in general, a very safe drug, the treatment of syphilis is not without danger. More than half of those treated suffer a severe reaction within six to 12 hours, caused by the body's response to the sudden killing of large numbers of spirochetes. Organ damage already caused by the disease cannot be reversed.

**PREVENTION**

Promiscuous and frequent heterosexual or homosexual intercourse inevitably involves a risk of infection with syphilis. Infection can be avoided by maintaining monogamous relationships. Condoms offer some measure of protection but do not offer absolute protection (see *"Safe" sex*). People with syphilis are infectious in the primary and secondary stages but not in the late latent and tertiary stages.

## Syringe

An instrument for injecting fluid into, or withdrawing fluid from, a body cavity, blood vessel, or tissue. Most syringes consist of a barrel with a plunger at one end and, at the other, a nozzle to which a hollow needle can be attached. The barrel is calibrated to enable the correct dosage of medication to be given. Most modern syringes are disposable plastic instruments that are presterilized and packed in sealed bags.

A hypodermic syringe is, strictly, one used for giving injections just beneath the skin. However, identical instruments are used for intramuscular (into a muscle) and intravenous (into a vein) injections. Thus, the term hypodermic syringe (or sometimes simply syringe) is used for all types.

## Syringing of ears

A procedure for removing excessive *earwax* or, less commonly, a foreign body from the outer-ear canal (see *Ear, foreign body in*).

The physician first examines the ear to see if there is a condition (e.g., perforated eardrum) that indicates syringing should not be done. If there is no such indication, any hard wax

may first require softening by putting drops of oil in the ear. The earwax is then washed out using the procedure shown in the illustrated box below. Afterward, the canal is dried, sometimes with the help of alcohol drops. As an alternative to flushing out, wax and other debris may be removed by suction or by small instruments.

Ear syringing may be an uncomfortable procedure. Sudden acute pain or dizziness may indicate a perforation of the eardrum and the need to stop the procedure.

## Syringomyelia

A very rare, usually congenital condition in which a cavity forms in the brain stem or at neck level in the spinal

---

**EAR SYRINGING**

This procedure should be carried out only by a physician or nurse; amateur attempts can damage the eardrum.

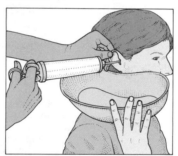

**1** The nozzle of a large syringe is placed just inside the ear canal, which is straightened out by pulling the external ear upward and backward.

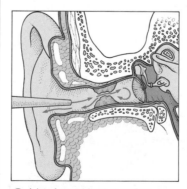

**2** A jet of warm water or sodium bicarbonate solution is directed along the upper wall of the patient's ear canal in order to dislodge the blockage.

---

cord. The cavity gradually expands, filling with cerebrospinal fluid, eventually causing damage to nerve fibers.

The first symptoms usually appear in early adulthood. Affected persons are unable to feel pain or temperature changes in the neck, shoulders, arms, and hands, causing them to suffer burns and injure themselves without realizing it. The muscles in the same region gradually become weak, wasted, and cold, and there is some loss of the sensation of touch.

In people with advanced syringomyelia, there is spasticity (abnormal stiffness and rigidity) in the legs, nasal speech, and sometimes difficulty swallowing. Many severely affected people are confined to wheelchairs.

No drug treatment is available. In some cases, surgical treatment to relieve pressure in the affected region (see *Decompression, spinal canal*) may arrest what is otherwise an inevitably progressive disease.

## System

A group of interconnected or interdependent organs that acts to perform a common function. For example, the different parts of the *digestive system* (the mouth, salivary glands, esophagus, stomach, intestines, gallbladder, pancreas, and liver) act together to ingest, break down, absorb, and excrete food.

The term system may also be applied to a method of classification, as in the ABO system for classifying *blood groups*.

## Systemic

A term applied to something that affects the whole body rather than a specific part of it. For example, fever is a systemic symptom, whereas swelling is a localized symptom. The term systemic is also applied to the part of the blood circulation that supplies all parts of the body except the lungs.

## Systemic lupus erythematosus

See *Lupus erythematosus*.

## Systole

A period of muscular contraction of a chamber of the heart that alternates with a resting period, called *diastole*. With each heart beat, the atria (upper chambers) contract first (atrial systole), squeezing blood into the ventricles (lower chambers). The ventricles then contract (ventricular systole), pumping blood out of the heart into the arteries.

**S**

# T

## Tabes dorsalis

A complication of *syphilis*, once common but now rare, that affects the spinal cord, causing abnormalities of sensation, sharp pains, incoordination, and incontinence. Symptoms appear several years after infection.

## Tachycardia

A heart rate of over 100 beats per minute in an adult. Most people have a rate of between 60 and 100 beats per minute, with an average of 72 to 78 beats. Tachycardia occurs in healthy people during exercise, when the heart is stimulated to work faster and thus increase blood flow to muscles. Tachycardia at rest may be caused by *fever*, *hyperthyroidism*, *coronary heart disease* or any other cause of heart disease or heart failure, a high intake of caffeine, or treatment with an *anticholinergic drug* or some *decongestant drugs*. Types of tachycardia include *atrial fibrillation*, *sinus tachycardia*, *supraventricular tachycardia*, and *ventricular tachycardia*.

Symptoms of tachycardia may include *palpitations*, *breathlessness*, and lightheadedness, depending on how fast the heart is beating and on how effectively it is pumping blood.

## Tachypnea

An abnormally fast rate of breathing. Tachypnea may be caused by exercise, anxiety, a lung disorder (such as emphysema), or a cardiac disorder (such as heart failure).

## T'ai chi

A Chinese exercise based on a series of more than 100 postures between which many slow, continuous, deliberate movements occur. T'ai chi is characterized by outer movement and inner stillness; its purpose is to exercise the muscles and achieve integration of mind and body. Devotees believe that continuous flow of movement is important in performing the exercises because it prevents "blockage" of the internal flow of chi—the essential life energy.

## Talipes

A congenital deformity in which the foot is twisted out of shape or position. There are many different varieties of talipes, all of which are commonly labeled clubfoot. The causes are not fully understood, but there is a genetic factor (relatives of affected people have a higher incidence of the disorder).

The most common, and serious, form of talipes is an equinovarus deformity in which the heel is turned inward and the rest of the foot is bent downward and inward. The arch of the foot is higher than normal and there may be underdevelopment of the muscles in the lower leg above the affected foot.

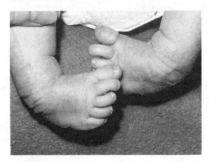

**Talipes equinovarus**
This birth defect affects about one baby in 1,500. Treatment is by gentle manipulation, repeated several times a day.

### TREATMENT

Treatment of talipes equinovarus, which should begin soon after birth, consists of repeated manipulations of the foot and ankle over several weeks. Between manipulations, the foot is held in the corrected position by a plaster cast, metal splint, or adhesive strapping. If this procedure is not effective, an operation to cut the tight ligaments and tendons is performed and the foot is then immobilized in a plaster cast for at least three months. Treatment undertaken after age 2 cannot restore the foot to normal, but function can be improved by transferring a tendon from one bone to another (see *Tendon transfer*) or by lengthening a tendon.

Other types of talipes can usually be corrected by repeated stretching of the foot into a normal position. Occasionally, immobilization in a plaster cast is required.

## Tamoxifen

An *anticancer drug* used in the treatment of certain types of *breast cancer*. Tamoxifen is also sometimes effective in the treatment of other cancers, such as those of the prostate.

In women of childbearing age, tamoxifen stimulates *ovulation* (egg release) and is therefore under investigation as a treatment for certain types of *infertility*.

Tamoxifen works by blocking *estrogen hormone* receptors. It has fewer adverse effects than most anticancer drugs, but may cause hot flashes, nausea, vomiting, swollen ankles, and irregular vaginal bleeding.

## Tampon

A plug of absorbent material, such as cotton, that is inserted into a wound or body opening to soak up blood or other secretions. The term usually refers to a sanitary tampon that is inserted into the vagina to absorb menstrual blood.

## Tamponade

Compression of the heart. Tamponade may occur in *pericarditis* (inflammation of the outer lining of the heart) due to fluid collecting under the lining; it may also result from blood and blood clots surrounding the heart after heart surgery or a penetrating injury of the chest.

Symptoms include breathlessness and, sometimes, collapse because the heart is unable to pump blood efficiently to the lungs and brain. The diagnosis may be best made by using *echocardiography*.

Treatment involves immediate removal of any fluid that is pressing on the heart via a hollow needle guided through the chest wall. If blood clots are present, a *thoracotomy* is usually performed to open the chest wall and remove them.

## Tan

See *Suntan*.

## Tannin

Also known as tannic acid, an organic chemical that occurs in many plants, particularly in oak gallnuts, the barks of oak, sumac, and mangrove trees, and tea.

Tannin has been used in medicine to stop bleeding, to control diarrhea, and as an antidote to plant poisons. It is no longer used therapeutically because more effective agents are available and because it can cause liver damage. Although tea contains significant amounts of tannin, drinking moderate amounts is unlikely to lead to liver damage. However, it may cause constipation.

## Tantrum

An outburst of bad temper, common in toddlers, usually indicating frustration and anger. Tantrums occur in many children between 15 months and 4 years, but are especially likely in 2 year olds.

During a tantrum, the child may scream, cry, yell, kick, bang feet and fists, roll on the floor, go red in the face, spit, and bite. In some cases, the toddler develops the habit of holding his or her breath during tantrums, and may even turn blue and, in rare cases, lose consciousness momentarily (see *Breath-holding attacks*).

### CAUSES

Tantrums occur at the age when a child starts to gain independence and becomes frustrated by restraints imposed by others, but is not yet able to express these feelings verbally. The outbursts are more likely when the child is tired, and are often brought on by a disagreement between child and parents. Tantrums may start with the birth of another baby, when the child may believe the baby is getting all the parents' attention.

Most children have occasional tantrums; frequent outbursts may indicate a *behavioral problem*, sometimes due to emotional strain or to a communication problem.

### TREATMENT

Try to ignore tantrums as much as possible; becoming angry only excites the child further. Firm and consistent treatment is essential. Do not punish the child and then give in to his or her demands. With calm, quick thinking you can often divert your child's attention to a game or project. This often works better than trying to argue with a 2 year old. Most children grow out of tantrums as they develop the ability to express their feelings through speech, which should be encouraged.

If parents are unable to cope with the tantrums, or the child does not seem to be growing out of them, a physician should be consulted. *Child guidance* may be necessary.

## Tapeworm infestation

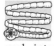 Tapeworms, also called cestodes, are ribbon-shaped parasitic worms that live in human or animal intestines. They are typically acquired from eating undercooked meat or fish. Each adult tapeworm bears suckers or hooks on its head, by which it attaches itself to the intestinal wall. The rest of the worm consists of a chain of flat segments.

### CAUSES, TYPES, AND INCIDENCE

Human tapeworms have life cycles that usually also involve another animal host. A typical life cycle is shown in the illustration below.

Three large types of tapeworm, acquired by eating undercooked, infected beef, pork, and fish, all have life cycles of this type. The adults may grow to 20 or even 30 feet (6 to 9 meters) long. All occur worldwide, but, in developed countries, infestations are largely prevented by measures such as adequate meat inspection and sanitary disposal of sewage. In the US, the pork tapeworm is extremely rare and the beef and fish tapeworms are uncommon.

The much smaller dwarf tapeworm, which is only 1 inch (2.5 cm) long, has a different life cycle. An infested person may directly cause an infestation of someone else through accidental transfer of worm eggs from feces to fingers to mouth. The dwarf tapeworm is found worldwide, but especially in the tropics; it primarily affects children.

Humans may act as intermediate host to the larvae of a tapeworm for which dogs are the main host. The larvae grow and develop into cysts in the liver and lungs, a condition called *hydatid disease*.

### SYMPTOMS, DIAGNOSIS, AND TREATMENT

Despite their size, beef, pork, and fish tapeworms rarely cause symptoms, except mild abdominal discomfort or diarrhea. However, segments of the worm may detach and emerge through the anus or may appear in the feces. In rare cases, fish tapeworms cause *anemia*. Dwarf tapeworms can cause diarrhea and abdominal discomfort.

Tapeworm infestation is diagnosed by a physician finding worm segments and/or eggs excreted in the feces; infestation is treated by drugs (such as niclosamide) which effectively kill the worms.

Treatment of pork tapeworm must be carried out carefully because there is a risk of worm eggs being released and regurgitated into the stomach. The patient may then accidentally become the host to the worm larvae, which burrow into the tissues and form cysts. This leads to a condition called cysticercosis, the symptoms of which may include muscle pains and convulsions. Cysticercosis is treated with drugs such as praziquantel.

## Tarsalgia

Pain in the foot at the point where it forms the ankle joint, usually associated with *flatfoot*.

## Tarsorrhaphy

An operation in which the upper and lower eyelids are sewn together.

### WHY IT IS DONE

Tarsorrhaphy may be performed as part of the treatment of *corneal ulcer*. The eyelids act as a bandage to promote healing of the cornea. Frequently, tarsorrhaphy is used to protect the corneas in people who cannot close their eyelids because of

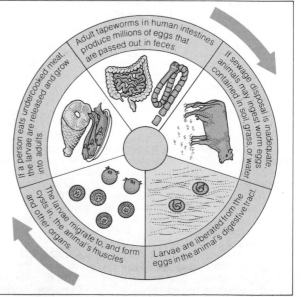

**LIFE CYCLE OF TAPEWORM**
Many tapeworms have life cycles in which the adult and larval worms infest different hosts. In the cycle at right, the adult worms infest humans and the larvae infest cattle (called the intermediate hosts). Pigs and fish may also act as intermediate hosts to human tapeworms, and humans may act as intermediate hosts to dog and pig tapeworms.

Adult tapeworms in human intestines produce millions of eggs that are passed out in feces.

If sewage disposal is inadequate, animals may ingest worm eggs contained in soil, grass, or water.

Larvae are liberated from the eggs in the animal's digestive tract.

The larvae migrate to, and form cysts in, the animal's muscles and other organs.

If a person eats undercooked meat, the larvae are released and grow into adults.

nerve or muscular disorders or scarring. Tarsorrhaphy is also occasionally performed to protect the cornea in people with *exophthalmos*.

**HOW IT IS DONE**

A strip of tissue is removed from the upper and lower lid edges. The raw surfaces of the lids are then stitched together. By about two or three weeks after the operation, the eyelids have grown together and the stitches can be removed. The eyelids are cut apart and allowed to open when the original abnormality subsides.

## Tartar

See *Calculus, dental*.

## Taste

One of the five special senses. Alone, taste is a relatively crude sense, able to distinguish only between sweet, salty, sour, and bitter. In practice, however, many different flavors can be distinguished because of the combination of the sense of taste and the much more discriminating sense of *smell*. This combination explains why loss of the sense of smell (caused by a common cold, for example) also apparently causes loss of taste (see *Taste, loss of*). The full sensory appreciation of food also involves other factors, such as the appearance of food (which helps stimulate saliva-tion) and the consistency and temperature of the food. The mechanisms and structures on the tongue involved in taste are illustrated below.

## Taste, loss of

Loss of *taste* usually occurs as a result of loss of the sense of *smell* (usually due to a common cold or influenza), which contributes greatly to taste.

Loss of taste without loss of smell is relatively rare. A possible cause is any condition that results in a dry mouth (see *Mouth, dry*), because taste buds can detect the substances responsible for flavors only when those substances are dissolved in saliva.

---

## THE SENSE OF TASTE

Tastes are detected by special structures called taste buds, of which everyone has some 10,000, mainly on the tongue, with a few at the back of the throat and on the palate. These taste buds surround pores within papillae (protuberances) on the tongue surface and elsewhere. Four types of taste buds exist—sensitive to sweet, salty, sour, and bitter chemicals. All tastes are formed from a mixture of these four basic elements.

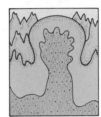

**Fungiform papillae**
These mushroom-shaped papillae occur in small numbers at random over the tongue surface, mainly in the middle.

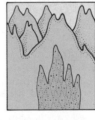

**Filiform papillae**
These smaller peak-shaped protuberances occur in large numbers over all except the back of the tongue's upper surface, and on the palate.

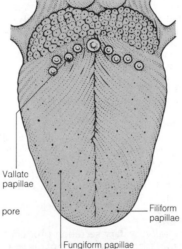

Vallate papillae

Filiform papillae

Fungiform papillae

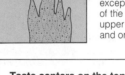

Olfactory bulb

Tongue

Glosso-pharyngeal nerve

Vallate papillae

Taste pore

Taste bud

**How a substance is tasted**
Chemicals in food or drink dissolve in saliva and enter pores in the papillae on the tongue. Around these pores are groups of taste receptor cells—the taste buds. The chemicals stimulate hairs projecting from the receptor cells, causing signals to be sent from the cells along nerves to taste centers in the brain.

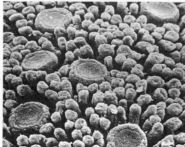

**Magnified photograph of tongue surface**
The photograph shows large (fungiform) and small (filiform) papillae. Taste buds are arranged around pores in the surface of the papillae.

**Taste centers on the tongue**
Taste buds sensitive to sweet, salty, sour, and bitter chemicals tend to be grouped into particular areas on the surface of the tongue.

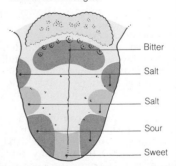

Bitter

Salt

Salt

Sour

Sweet

T

Complete or partial loss of taste may result from damage to the taste buds themselves as a result of *stomatitis* (inflammation of the mouth), *mouth cancer* or *radiation therapy* (which also eliminates salivation by damaging the salivary glands) to treat mouth cancer, the side effects of certain drugs, or, most commonly, the natural degeneration of the taste buds with age.

Loss of taste may also be caused by damage to the cranial nerves that convey taste sensations to the brain. Nerve damage may occur as a result of a head injury, a tumor of the brain or of the cranial nerves associated with taste, or surgery on the head or neck. In these cases, loss of taste is usually accompanied by facial paralysis.

Disturbances of taste occur in some psychiatric disorders, usually taking the form of taste hallucinations rather than true loss of taste.

## Tattooing

The introduction of permanent colors under the surface of the skin, usually to create a picture. Practiced for thousands of years, tattooing was originally used as a means of identification. Today it is almost always carried out for decorative purposes.

Tattooing, even by professionals, is potentially dangerous; if the tattooist does not follow strict sterile procedures, *hepatitis* and *AIDS* may be transmitted through the needles used to introduce the dyes.

Removal of a tattoo is usually difficult and unsatisfactory; a scar almost always results. Small tattoos are best treated by complete removal of the colored area of skin and the stitching together of the edges of the wound. Larger tattooed areas can sometimes be removed by *dermabrasion* or *laser treatment*.

## Tay-Sachs disease

A serious inherited brain disorder that results in very early death. Tay-Sachs disease was formerly known as amaurotic familial idiocy.

### CAUSES AND INCIDENCE

Tay-Sachs disease is caused by a deficiency of hexosaminidase, a certain *enzyme* (a protein essential for regulating chemical reactions in the body). Deficiency results in a buildup of a harmful substance in the brain.

The disease is most common among Ashkenazi Jews. The incidence in this group is around one in 2,500, which is 100 times higher than in any other ethnic group. The gene for Tay-Sachs disease is recessive and an Ashkenazi Jew has a one in 25 chance of carrying it. If two carriers marry, there is a one in four chance that they will have an affected child.

### SYMPTOMS AND SIGNS

Signs of the illness, which appear during the first six months of life, are blindness, dementia, deafness, seizures, and paralysis. An exaggerated startle response to sound is an early sign. Symptoms progress rapidly and the affected child usually dies before age 3.

### DIAGNOSIS

The diagnosis is based on family history and physical examination; it is confirmed by enzyme analysis of any tissue sample—tears, serum, blood cells, or hair roots.

### TREATMENT AND PREVENTION

There is no treatment for Tay-Sachs disease. Programs for detecting carriers of the gene have been introduced in some countries. Carriers and those with an affected child or relative should receive *genetic counseling* before starting a family or planning another pregnancy. If *prenatal screening* shows that a fetus may be affected, the parents may choose to have an abortion.

## TB

An abbreviation for *tuberculosis*.

## T cell

One of the two main classes of *lymphocytes* (a type of white blood cell). T cells play an important role in the body's *immune system* (defenses against infection and against cancer cells).

## Tears

The salty, watery secretion produced by the lacrimal glands, part of the *lacrimal apparatus* of the *eye*. The tear film over the *cornea* and the *conjunctiva* consists of three layers—an inner, mucous layer secreted by glands in the conjunctiva; an intermediate layer of salt water; and an outer, oily layer secreted by the meibomian glands.

A deficiency in tear production causes *keratoconjunctivitis sicca* (dry eye). Excessive tear production may cause *watering eye*.

## Tears, artificial

Preparations used to supplement inadequate production of tears in *keratoconjunctivitis sicca* and other conditions causing dryness of the eyes. To be effective, artificial tears must be applied at frequent intervals. Artificial tears may also be used to relieve discomfort caused by irritants, such as smoke or dust, but provide only temporary relief.

Many preparations contain a preservative that can irritate the eyes. Contaminated preparations may cause serious eye infections.

## Technetium

A radioactive metallic element that does not occur naturally either in its pure form or as compounds; technetium is produced during nuclear fission reactions. It was the first element to be made artificially (in 1937). Several isotopes (varieties of the element that are chemically identical but differ in some physical properties) have been synthesized, of which the most important medically is a form known as technetium 99m. This radioisotope, incorporated in various chemical substances, is used in *radionuclide scanning* of numerous organs, including the brain, heart, lungs, liver, kidneys, and bones.

## Teeth

Hard structures set in the jaw that are used for *mastication* (chewing) of food. The teeth also give shape to the face and help people to speak clearly. In humans, there are two sets of teeth—the *primary teeth* (of which there are 20) and the *permanent teeth* (of which there are 32). The primary teeth usually erupt between the ages of 6 months and 3 years and start to be replaced by the permanent teeth at about age 6 (see *Eruption of teeth*). In some people, the teeth fail to grow in the correct relationship to each other, resulting in *malocclusion* (incorrect bite). The arrangement of the teeth is shown in the box opposite.

Although the enamel that covers the crown of each tooth is the hardest substance in the body, it can be eroded by acid created when bacteria in the mouth break down the carbohydrates in food, resulting in *caries* (decay). To help prevent decay, good *oral hygiene* is essential, consisting of daily *toothbrushing* and flossing (see *Floss, dental*). See also *Gum*.

## Teeth, care of

See *Oral hygiene*.

## Teething

The period when a baby cuts his or her first set of teeth. The primary teeth usually begin to erupt at about 6 or 7 months (see *Eruption of teeth*). On average, the first set of teeth is complete soon after the second birthday.

## STRUCTURE AND ARRANGEMENT OF TEETH

At the heart of each tooth is the living pulp, which contains blood vessels and nerves. A hard substance called dentin surrounds the pulp. The part of the tooth above the gum, the crown, is covered by enamel. The roots of the tooth, which fit into sockets in the jawbone, are covered by a sensitive, bonelike material, the cementum. The periodontal ligament connects the cementum to the gums and to the jaw. It acts as a shock absorber and prevents jarring of the teeth and skull when food is being chewed.

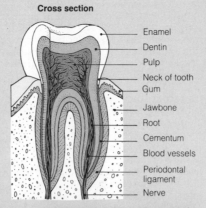

**Cross section**

- Enamel
- Dentin
- Pulp
- Neck of tooth
- Gum
- Jawbone
- Root
- Cementum
- Blood vessels
- Periodontal ligament
- Nerve

Central and lateral incisors (7 to 9 years)

First and second premolars (10 to 12 years)

Second molars (11 to 13 years)

Third molars (17+ years)

First molars (6 to 7 years)

Canines (12 to 14 years)

**The permanent teeth**
The illustration above shows the arrangement in the jaw of the permanent teeth—eight incisors, four canines, eight premolars, and 12 molars. The ages when these teeth erupt are indicated.

**X ray of teeth**
The panoramic X ray at left shows all the teeth of the upper and lower jaw (there are no wisdom teeth) and their surrounding structures. The tooth roots, buried in the jaw bones, can be clearly seen; several teeth have been filled.

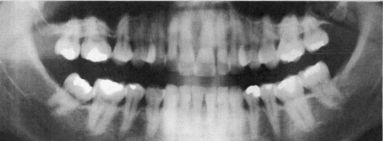

Molars | Premolars | Canines | Incisors | Canines | Premolars | Molars

Third | Second | First

**Molars**
The molars are large, strong teeth, efficient at grinding food. The third molars, or wisdom teeth, are the last to erupt; in some people, the wisdom teeth never appear.

**Premolars**
Also known as bicuspids, because of their two distinct edges, the premolars are concerned with grinding food. There are no premolars among the baby teeth.

**Incisors**
These teeth have a chisel-shaped, sharp cutting edge ideal for biting. The upper incisors overlap the lower incisors slightly when the jaws are closed.

**Canines**
The canines are sharp, pointed teeth, ideal for tearing food. They are larger and stronger than the incisors, with very long roots. The upper canines are often known as eye teeth.

**SYMPTOMS AND SIGNS**
While teeth are erupting, a baby may be irritable, fretful, clinging, have difficulty sleeping, and may cry more than usual. Extra saliva may be produced, resulting in dribbling, and the baby tends to chew on anything that he or she can hold.

Before a tooth comes through, the overlying gum may become red and swollen and the erupting tooth can be felt through the gum as a hard lump.

When molars erupt, the cheek may feel warm and red on the affected side.

Teething should never be considered the cause of a very high temperature, vomiting, diarrhea, prolonged loss of appetite, earache,

T

convulsions, cough, or diaper rash. These are symptoms of illness and a physician should be consulted.

### TREATMENT
Give the baby something firm to chew on, such as a piece of apple, or rub the swollen gum with a finger to ease the irritation. A small dose of a simple analgesic, such as acetaminophen, may be necessary if the child is very uncomfortable. Painkilling dental creams or gels are also available to rub on the gums.

## Telangiectasia
An increase in the size and number of the small blood vessels in an area of skin, causing redness. Telangiectasia is most common on the nose and cheeks. It is often a result of overexposure to sunlight or long-term high alcohol consumption.

**Appearance of telangiectasia**
Although sometimes referred to as broken veins, the blood vessels are in fact simply more numerous and larger than usual.

Telangiectasia is a feature of *rosacea* and also of *lupus erythematosus*, *dermatomyositis*, and *psoriasis*. A common, localized form of telangiectasia is the *spider nevus*. Hereditary hemorrhagic telangiectasia is a rare condition in which frequent bleeding occurs from small, rounded patches of widened blood vessels around the mouth and nose or elsewhere in the skin or gastrointestinal tract.

## Temazepam
A *benzodiazepine drug* used in the short-term treatment of *insomnia*.

## Temperature
For the body to function optimally, its temperature must be maintained within narrow limits. The generally accepted figure for the average normal body temperature (measured in the mouth) is 98.6°F (37°C). However, in practice, body temperature varies not only among individuals, but also in the same person, being affected by

factors such as exercise, sleep, eating and drinking, time of day (lowest at about 3 AM and highest at about 6 PM), and, in women, the stage of the menstrual cycle (lowest at menstruation and highest at ovulation). In most people, body temperature varies between 97.8°F (36.5°C) and 99°F (37.2°C). The temperature is higher in the rectum, by about 0.5 to 0.7°F (0.3 to 0.4°C), and lower in the armpit, by about 0.3 to 0.5°F (0.2 to 0.3°C).

### TEMPERATURE REGULATION
Body temperature is maintained within optimal limits by the *hypothalamus*, an area of the brain that acts like a thermostat, constantly monitoring blood temperature and automatically activating mechanisms to compensate for changes.

When body temperature falls, the hypothalamus sends nerve impulses to stimulate *shivering* (which generates heat by muscle activity) and to constrict blood vessels in the skin, which reduces heat loss. Conversely, when body temperature rises, the hypothalamus stimulates *sweating* and dilates blood vessels in the skin to increase heat loss.

A variety of factors—such as infections, certain disorders (notably those of the thyroid gland), unusual symptoms of a tumor, and overexposure to cold or extreme heat—may disrupt the body's heat-regulating system, resulting in *fever, heat stroke*, or *hypothermia*.

## Temperature method
See *Contraception, periodic abstinence*.

## Temporal arteritis
An uncommon disease of elderly people in which the walls of the arteries that pass over the temples in the scalp become inflamed. Other arteries in the head and neck may also be affected, as may the aorta (the large artery that carries oxygenated blood from the heart) and its main branches. The inflamed blood vessels become narrowed, and blood flow through them is reduced. The disease is also known as giant cell arteritis.

### CAUSES AND INCIDENCE
The cause of temporal arteritis is unknown, but it is often associated with *polymyalgia rheumatica* (pain and stiffness in the muscles of the hips, thighs, shoulders, and neck).

In the US, about 10 cases of temporal arteritis are diagnosed per 100,000 population each year. Nearly all patients are over 50, and more women than men are affected.

### SYMPTOMS AND SIGNS
The most common symptom is a headache, usually severe, on one or both sides of the head. The temporal artery (located at the side of the head above the earlobe) may be prominent and the scalp may be tender. In nearly one half of sufferers, the ophthalmic arteries supplying the eyes may become affected, resulting in partial loss of vision or even sudden blindness.

Other symptoms and signs of temporal arteritis include low fever, poor appetite, and lethargy.

Involvement of the aorta or its main branches results in circulatory disorders, such as intermittent *claudica-*

---

**TEMPORAL ARTERITIS**
In this disorder, the temporal artery and other arteries in the head are inflamed. Early reporting of symptoms is vital, since, in untreated cases, there is a risk of sudden blindness.

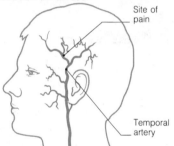

Site of pain

Temporal artery

**Telltale symptoms**
If the temporal artery is inflamed, it is usually prominent and there is a persistent severe headache and scalp tenderness in the area shown.

Normal blood flow

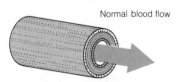

**Normal artery**
A normal artery has a smooth lining, and blood flow is sufficient to meet the needs of the tissues it supplies.

Reduced blood flow

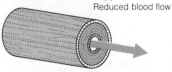

**Inflamed artery**
In arteritis, the walls of the artery become disrupted and thickened, and blood flow is markedly reduced.

*tion* (pain in the legs on walking) or *Raynaud's phenomenon* (pallor in the fingers on exposure to cold).

**DIAGNOSIS AND TREATMENT**

Early reporting of symptoms to a physician is essential because of the risk of blindness. The diagnosis is made by a *biopsy* (removal of a small sample of tissue for analysis) of the temporal artery and *blood tests* to detect the presence of a raised *ESR* (erythrocyte sedimentation rate).

The disease responds rapidly to a *corticosteroid drug*, which is initially given in high doses to prevent blindness. Most people need to take the drug, at a reduced dosage, for one or two years. If the disease fails to respond to the corticosteroid, or if the drug causes serious side effects, *immunosuppressant drugs* (such as azathioprine) may be given.

**OUTLOOK**

With treatment, the disease usually clears up within two years. Most people are not left with any lasting disability. However, if one or both eyes become blind before treatment has become effective, the blindness may be permanent.

## Temporal lobe epilepsy

A form of *epilepsy* in which abnormal electrical discharges in the brain are confined to a localized region on one side, the temporal lobe. The seizures therefore differ from the generalized disturbances that occur in a grand mal seizure or in an absence seizure (petit mal).

**LOCATION OF THE TEMPORAL LOBE**

The temporal lobe forms much of the lower side of each half of the cerebrum (main mass of the brain).

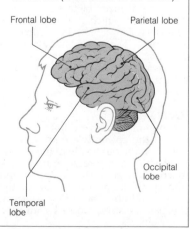

Frontal lobe  Parietal lobe
Occipital lobe
Temporal lobe

**CAUSE**

There is usually an area of damage within one of the temporal lobes that acts as a focus for the abnormal development of electrical discharges in attacks. Damage may be caused by a *birth injury, head injury, brain tumor, brain abscess,* or *stroke*. The temporal lobes are concerned with such functions as smell, taste, hearing, visual associations, and some aspects of memory. Abnormal electrical activity in a lobe may thus cause peculiarities in any of these functions.

**SYMPTOMS AND SIGNS**

People affected by temporal lobe epilepsy suffer dreamlike states that range from partial loss of awareness to total disregard. The person may have unpleasant hallucinations of smell or taste. Also common during attacks is the perception of an illusory scene or the phenomenon of *déjà vu*. There may also be facial grimacing, rotation of the head and eyes, and often sucking and chewing movements.

The affected person may perform tasks with no memory of them after the attack. An attack may last for minutes or hours before full consciousness returns.

In some cases a temporal lobe seizure progresses after several seconds or minutes to a generalized grand mal seizure.

**DIAGNOSIS AND TREATMENT**

The principles of investigation and drug treatment for temporal lobe epilepsy are the same as for other types of epilepsy. Surgery has been used with success in some cases of temporal lobe epilepsy. The operation is designed to remove the part of the lobe containing the irritating focus for the attacks. Operations are performed only in severe cases that have not responded to drug treatment because of the possible effects on other important functions of the brain.

## Temporomandibular joint syndrome

Pain and other symptoms affecting the head, jaw, and face that are believed to result when the temporomandibular joints (jaw joints) and the muscles and ligaments that control and support them do not work together correctly.

**CAUSES**

The most common cause of the temporomandibular joint syndrome is spasm of the chewing muscles. Frequently, this is due to habits such as clenching or grinding the teeth, usually as a result of emotional ten-

**LOCATION OF THE TEMPOROMANDIBULAR JOINT**

The head of the mandible (jawbone) fits into a hollow on the underside of the temporal bone of the skull at the joint.

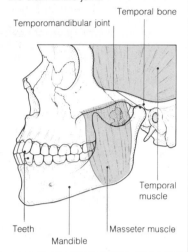

Temporal bone
Temporomandibular joint
Temporal muscle
Teeth
Mandible
Masseter muscle

sion. An incorrect bite, which places additional stress on the muscles, may be a contributing factor.

Temporomandibular joint problems may also be caused by displacement of the joint as a result of jaw, head, or neck injuries. In rare cases, *osteoarthritis* is a cause.

**SYMPTOMS**

Headaches, tenderness of the jaw muscles, and dull, aching facial pain with severe exacerbation in or around the ear are common symptoms of temporomandibular joint syndrome. Other symptoms may include clicking or popping noises when the mouth is opened or closed, difficulty opening the mouth, jaws that "lock" or get stuck, or pain brought on by yawning, chewing, or opening the mouth wide.

**TREATMENT**

In most cases, treatment is aimed at eliminating muscle spasm and relieving pain. This may be done by applying moist heat to the face, taking muscle-relaxant drugs, massaging the muscles, eating soft, nonchewy foods, or using a bite splint (a device that fits over the teeth at night to prevent clenching or grinding). Counseling, *biofeedback training*, and *relaxation exercises* may also help.

The bite may need to be corrected by selective grinding of teeth or by the use of braces or other *orthodontic appliances*. In severe cases, surgery on the jaw joint is required.

## Tenderness

Pain or abnormal sensitivity in a part of the body when it is pressed or touched during medical palpation (examination by touch) or contact with objects in daily living. Tenderness is usually a sign of *inflammation*. For example, *appendicitis* (inflammation of the appendix) causes tenderness of the abdomen; *arthritis* (joint inflammation) causes tenderness around the affected joint. Tenderness is usually associated with swelling, redness, and warmth of the affected part.

## Tendinitis

Inflammation of a tendon, usually caused by injury. Symptoms include pain, tenderness, and, occasionally, restricted movement of the muscle attached to the affected tendon. A common example is *painful arc syndrome*, which causes pain in the shoulder when the arm is raised above a certain angle.

Treatment of tendinitis may include *nonsteroidal anti-inflammatory drugs* (NSAIDs), *ultrasound treatment*, or an injection of *corticosteroid drugs* around the tendon.

## Tendolysis

An operation performed to free a tendon from *adhesions* (fibrous bands) that surround it and limit its free movement. The adhesions are usually caused by *tenosynovitis* (inflammation of the inner lining of a tendon sheath).

The procedure consists of making a skin incision over the tendon and then splitting open its fibrous sheath. The adhesions are cut away from the tendon surface and the incisions in the sheath and the skin are stitched. Despite surgery, symptoms of tenosynovitis sometimes recur because adhesions form again.

## Tendon

A fibrous cord that joins muscle to bone or muscle to muscle. Tendons are extremely strong, flexible, and inelastic. Most are cylindrical, but some, such as those attached to the flat muscles of the abdominal wall, consist of wide sheets of fibers known as aponeuroses.

Tendons are made up principally of bundles of collagen (a white, fibrous protein) and contain some blood vessels. The larger tendons (but not the aponeuroses) also have a nerve supply. Squeezing the tendon hard causes pain; stretching it triggers a *reflex* contraction of the adjoining muscle (e.g., the quadriceps jerk).

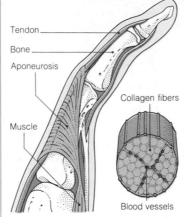

**FINGER TENDONS**
Finger bending and extension are controlled by tendons on either side of the finger; the tendons originate from forearm muscles.

Tendon

Bone

Aponeurosis

Muscle

Collagen fibers

Blood vessels

**Internal structure**
A cross section of a tendon (inset) shows that it consists of numerous parallel bundles of collagen fibers along with some blood vessels.

The tendons in the hands, wrists, and feet are enclosed in synovial sheaths (fibrous capsules) and bathed in a lubricating fluid secreted by the lining of the sheath. These tendons require this additional protection because they do not move in a straight line and, without the fluid, might be subjected to excessive friction.

**DISORDERS**
Rupture of the *Achilles tendon* can occur during sprinting and jumping as a result of sudden contraction of the calf muscles stretching the tendon. Rupture of a tendon on the back of a finger, resulting in deformity of the fingertip, may be caused by a direct blow to the end of the finger (see *Baseball finger*). In many cases, however, because tendons are so strong, severe stress pulls off a piece of bone where the tendon is attached to it rather than tearing the tendon itself.

The long tendon of the biceps muscle in the upper arm may become weakened as a result of repeated rubbing against the humerus (upper arm bone) and may rupture under even moderate stress. Rupture of tendons in the hands can occur as a complication of *rheumatoid arthritis*.

Tendons in the hand are commonly severed by a deep cut with a knife or piece of glass; *tendon repair*, using a graft taken from a tendon elsewhere in the body, may be required.

*Tendinitis*, inflammation of a tendon, may follow an injury. *Tenosynovitis*, inflammation of the inner lining of a tendon sheath, usually results from overuse; it affects tendons in the hands and wrists. If the outer wall of a tendon sheath is inflamed, the gliding movement of the tendon through the sheath may be restricted (as in *trigger finger*).

## Tendon release
See *Tendolysis*.

## Tendon repair
An operation to join the cut or torn ends of a *tendon* or to replace a damaged tendon.

If the cut or torn ends can easily be brought together, they are stitched together with sutures. If the ends are widely separated or contained within a sheath, it may be necessary to insert a tendon graft. Tendons for grafting are taken from elsewhere in the body, usually the foot.

## Tendon transfer
An operation to reposition a *tendon* so that it causes a muscle to perform a different function. Tendon transfer may be used to restore function impaired by a deformity, such as *talipes* (clubfoot), or by permanent muscle injury or paralysis.

To perform the transfer, the tendon is cut away from its original point of attachment and reattached elsewhere. Tendon transfer causes the muscle to which the tendon is attached to lie in a different position and thus to produce a different body movement when the muscle contracts.

## Tenesmus
A feeling of incomplete emptying of the bowel in which the urge to pass feces is accompanied by ineffective straining. Tenesmus may be a symptom of disease of the rectum, such as polyps or cancer, or of severe inflammation caused by *ulcerative colitis* or *dysentery*.

## Tennis elbow
A condition caused by inflammation around the epicondyle (bony prominence) on the outer side of the elbow, to which certain forearm muscles are attached by *tendons*. It causes pain and tenderness at the outer side of the elbow and in the back of the forearm. The pain is made worse by lifting a heavy object.

T

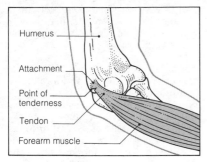

**Site of tennis elbow**
Pulling of the forearm muscles where they attach to the humerus causes tenderness on the outer side of the elbow.

Tennis elbow is caused by overuse of the muscles that straighten the wrist and fingers. Inflammation occurs as a result of constant tugging of the tendons at their point of attachment. Activities that can cause the condition include home decorating, gardening, or playing tennis (or other racket sports) with a faulty grip.

**TREATMENT**
Treatment consists of resting the arm, applying *ice packs*, and taking *analgesic drugs* (painkillers) and/or *nonsteroidal anti-inflammatory drugs* (NSAIDs). *Ultrasound treatment* may help reduce the inflammation. If the pain is severe or persistent, injection of a *corticosteroid drug* may be required.

If the pain has occurred after playing a racket sport, it is wise to take a break from the sport for a week or two to prevent recurrence. It is also useful to consult a professional about your playing technique and the size of the grip on your racket.

## Tenosynovitis
Inflammation of the thin inner lining of the sheath that surrounds a *tendon*. Tenosynovitis is usually caused by excessive friction due to overuse; it is often brought on by using a badly designed tool or working in an awkward position to do a job that involves repetitive movements. A rare cause of tenosynovitis is a bacterial infection, such as tuberculosis. The tendons in the hand and wrist are the most commonly affected.

Symptoms include pain, tenderness, and swelling over the tendon. There is also occasionally *crepitus* (a grating noise or sensation) when the tendon is moved. Persistent or recurrent tenosynovitis may lead to restricted movement as a result of *adhesions* (fibrous bands) forming between the tendon and its sheath.

**TREATMENT**
If infection is the cause, *antibiotic drugs* are prescribed. Otherwise, treatment usually consists of *nonsteroidal anti-inflammatory drugs* (NSAIDs) or an injection of *corticosteroid drugs* around the tendon. The hand and wrist may need to be immobilized in a splint for a few weeks. If the condition does not improve, surgery may be required to release adhesions (see *Tendolysis*).

## Tenovaginitis
Inflammation or thickening of the fibrous wall of the sheath that surrounds a *tendon*. The cause is unknown. Tenovaginitis that affects the sheath of one of the tendons that bends a finger results in *trigger finger*.

## TENS
The abbreviation for *transcutaneous electrical nerve stimulation*.

## Tension
A feeling of mental and physical strain associated with anxiety. Sufferers feel unpleasantly keyed up, cannot relax, and may have feelings of bottled-up anger. Muscle tension accompanies the mental symptoms and may result in headaches and muscular stiffness and pain, particularly in the back and shoulders. Persistent tension is related to *generalized anxiety disorder*. (See also *Stress*.)

## Teratogen
An agent that causes physical abnormalities in a developing embryo or fetus. Examples of teratogens include the *rubella* virus and the drug *thalidomide*. For a drug to be categorized as teratogenic, there must be evidence that taking the drug during pregnancy causes an increased incidence of congenital abnormalities that cannot be explained by other factors. Many chemicals that are known to be teratogenic in some species (such as rats) have not been proved to be teratogenic in humans. Drug-regulating agencies usually refuse to license drugs for use during pregnancy if they have been found to be teratogenic for any species.

## Teratoma
A primary tumor consisting of cells that bear no resemblance to those normally found in that part of the body. For example, teratomas that develop in the ovary—one of the most common sites for this type of tumor—often form cysts (called *dermoid cysts*) that may contain skin, hair, teeth, or

bone. Other common sites include the testes, the pineal gland in the brain, and the *mediastinum*.

## Terbutaline
A *bronchodilator drug* used in the treatment of *asthma*, chronic *bronchitis*, and *emphysema*. Terbutaline also relaxes the muscles of the uterus, making it useful for the prevention of premature labor (see *Prematurity*). Terbutaline is under investigation as a treatment for *heart failure*.

Adverse effects include tremor, nervousness, restlessness, nausea, and, in rare cases, palpitations.

## Terfenadine
An *antihistamine drug* used to treat allergic *rhinitis* (hay fever) and allergic skin conditions, such as *urticaria* (hives). Terfenadine has little sedative effect and is therefore useful for people who need to avoid drowsiness. Possible adverse effects include nausea, loss of appetite, and rash. In addition, potentially life-threatening changes in heart rhythm have occurred in people taking terfenadine along with ketoconazole or erythromycin.

## Terminal care
See *Dying, care of the*.

## Testicle
See *Testis*.

## Testicular feminization syndrome
A rare inherited condition in which, despite having the external appearance of a female, the affected individual is genetically a male with internal testes. Testicular feminization syndrome is a form of *intersex* and is the most common form of male *pseudohermaphroditism*.

**CAUSE**
Testicular feminization syndrome is caused by a defective response of the body's tissues to *testosterone* (male sex hormone), even though a normal male level of the hormone is produced. The genes for testicular feminization syndrome are transmitted on the X chromosome (see *Genetic disorders*); thus, females can carry the genes and transmit them to their sons.

**SYMPTOMS AND SIGNS**
Affected individuals appear to be girls throughout childhood; female secondary *sexual characteristics* develop in most at puberty. People with testicular feminization syndrome tend to be taller than average and are of normal intelligence. However, menstruation

does not occur because there is no uterus and the vagina is short and blind-ending.

**DIAGNOSIS, TREATMENT, AND OUTLOOK**

The condition may be diagnosed before puberty if a girl is found to have an inguinal *hernia* or a swelling in the labia that turns out to be a testis. Otherwise, the diagnosis is usually made at puberty during investigations for *amenorrhea* (failure to menstruate).

The diagnosis is made by *chromosome analysis*, which shows the normal male chromosomal status, and by blood tests, which indicate male levels of testosterone.

Treatment involves the surgical removal of the testes (because of an increased risk of testicular cancer) and hormonal therapy with *estrogen drugs*. An affected individual can never be fertile, but can lead an otherwise normal life as a woman.

## Testis

One of two male sex organs, also called testicles, that produce *sperm* and the male sex hormone *testosterone*.

The testes are formed within the abdomen near the kidneys early in the growth of the male fetus. In response to hormones produced by the mother and to hormones produced in the testes themselves, the testes gradually descend through the inguinal canal (a tunnel in the groin). At birth, they have usually reached the surface of the body, where they hang suspended in a pouch of skin called the *scrotum*.

**STRUCTURE**

Within each of the testes are the seminiferous tubules, delicate coiled tubes that produce sperm. The seminiferous tubules lead via the vas efferens (small ducts) to the *epididymis*, a structure lying behind the testis in which the newly formed sperm mature. Interstitial cells between the seminiferous tubules produce the male sex hormone testosterone, which passes into small blood vessels in the testis and then into the circulation.

Each testis is protected by a tough, fibrous capsule, the tunica albuginea, and is attached by the spermatic cord, composed of the *vas deferens* (the tube that transports sperm from the epididymis to the urethra) and a number of blood vessels and nerves.

**DISORDERS**

A direct blow sometimes tears the wall of the testis, resulting in severe pain and bleeding into the scrotal tissue. An operation may be required to drain the blood and repair the testis.

---

**LOCATION OF THE TESTIS**

Each testis is suspended in the scrotum by a spermatic cord, which contains the vas deferens, and the arteries, veins, and nerves that supply the testis.

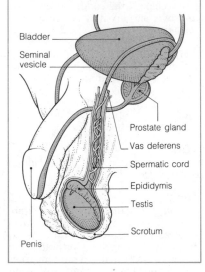

Bladder

Seminal vesicle

Prostate gland

Vas deferens

Spermatic cord

Epididymis

Testis

Scrotum

Penis

---

Occasionally, a testis fails to develop completely, does not descend fully into the scrotum (see *Testis, undescended*), or descends into an abnormal position (see *Testis, ectopic*). This may lead to reduced or absent sperm production or, if both testes are affected, *infertility*.

Inflammation of the testis, known as *orchitis*, usually results from infection with the mumps virus. Inflammation of the testis and the epididymis occurs in *epididymo-orchitis*, which is usually caused by a bacterial infection.

Painless swelling of the tissues surrounding the testis usually results from *hydrocele* (collection of fluid in the scrotum). Other causes of testicular swelling include *varicocele* (swollen veins within the scrotum), *epididymal cyst* (fluid-filled swelling of the epididymis), and *spermatocele* (a sperm-filled swelling of the epididymis).

Torsion of the testis occurs when the spermatic cord becomes twisted, cutting off the blood supply to the testis; it is most common around puberty (see *Testis, torsion of*).

In rare cases, the testis is affected by cancer (see *Testis, cancer of*).

## Testis, cancer of

Malignant growth of the *testis*. Cancer of the testis is rare. It occurs most commonly in young to middle-aged men,

---

and is very rare before puberty or in old age. The risk is higher in men with a history of undescended testis (see *Testis, undescended*).

**TYPES**

The most common types of testicular cancer are seminomas and teratomas. Seminomas are made up of a single type of cell (probably developing from the cells that produce sperm). Teratomas consist of several different types of cell. Other cancers affecting the testis are extremely rare and develop from testicular tissue or from lymphatic tissue (see *Lymphoma*) within the testis.

**SYMPTOMS AND SIGNS**

Testicular cancer most commonly appears as a firm, painless swelling of one testis. In some cases there may be pain and inflammation.

**DIAGNOSIS**

The physician first examines the testis and may perform tests to exclude other causes of testicular swelling (see *Testis, swollen*).

The diagnosis of testicular cancer can be confirmed only by *orchiectomy* (surgical removal of the testis) and microscopic examination of the testicular tissue. This confirms the presence of cancer and also shows the

---

**SELF-EXAMINATION OF THE TESTIS**

A lump that can be felt in the testis must be considered potentially malignant until surgical exploration proves otherwise. Cancers are usually firm to the touch and not tender or painful when pressed.

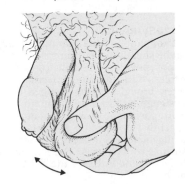

**Procedure**

Only regular self-examination can detect a tumor early enough to provide assurance of cure. The entire surface of both testes should be felt. The skin over the testes moves freely, making palpation easy.

T

type of cancer that is present. In addition, other tests (including *CT scanning, ultrasound scanning,* and *blood tests*) are performed to look for any signs that the cancer has spread to other parts of the body.

**TREATMENT**

Orchiectomy may be sufficient to cure testicular cancer in its early stages. However, *radiation therapy* on the remaining testis and on the lymph glands is also usually carried out, even if there are no signs that the disease has spread to these areas. Cancer that has spread beyond the testis is usually treated with *anticancer drugs* in addition to orchiectomy; occasionally, surgery may be needed to remove cancerous tissue from the abdomen.

**OUTLOOK**

The outlook, which varies according to the type of cancer and how advanced it was when first discovered, is generally good. The cure rate for early testicular cancer is 95 to 97 percent; the cure rate for advanced disease is 80 to 85 percent. Treatment with radiation therapy or anticancer drugs may not cause infertility in the remaining testis.

## Testis, ectopic

A *testis* that is absent from the scrotum because it has descended into an abnormal position, usually in the groin or at the base of the penis. An ectopic testis is most often discovered soon after birth during a routine physical examination. Treatment involves an *orchiopexy*, which places the testis in the scrotum.

## Testis, pain in the

Even mild injury to the testis may result in pain. Usually, no damage is caused, but a direct blow such as a kick may tear the wall of the testis. In this case, the pain is particularly severe, and an operation may be required to drain any accumulated blood and repair the testis.

Severe pain and swelling are a feature of *orchitis* (inflammation of the testis), *epididymo-orchitis* (inflammation of the testis and epididymis), and torsion of the testis (see *Testis, torsion of*). Cancer of the testis (see *Testis, cancer of*) does not usually cause pain.

Occasionally, pain that seems to come from the testis is actually caused by a small kidney stone lodged in the ureter (see *Calculus, urinary tract*). Sometimes a physician can find no cause for testicular pain; in most of these cases the problem disappears without treatment.

## Testis, retractile

A testis that is drawn up high into the groin by a pronounced muscle reflex in response to cold or touch. Retractile testis is normal in young children but usually disappears by puberty. Failure to feel the testis in the scrotum sometimes causes the condition to be confused with undescended testis (see *Testis, undescended*).

## Testis, swollen

Swelling of the testis or its surrounding tissues in the scrotum may or may not be accompanied by pain. Most scrotal swellings are harmless and the testis itself is usually not affected. However, swelling of a testis should always be reported to a physician to rule out the possibility of a serious underlying disorder.

**PAINLESS SWELLINGS**

There are several types of harmless, painless swelling, the most common of which is *hydrocele* (a collection of fluid in the scrotum). Other usually painless swellings include *epididymal cyst* (fluid-filled swelling of the epididymis), *spermatocele* (sperm-filled swelling of the epididymis), *varicocele* (varicose veins in the scrotum), and hematocele (swelling that contains blood and results from injury).

Cancer of the testis (see *Testis, cancer of*) may also cause a painless swelling and requires prompt treatment.

**PAINFUL SWELLING**

Painful swelling of the scrotum may be caused by a sudden event, such as twisting of the spermatic cord (see *Testis, torsion of*) or a direct blow. When associated with fever, the swelling is usually due to infection of the testis (see *Orchitis*) or of the testis and epididymis (see *Epididymo-orchitis*). In rare cases, a painful swelling is due to cancer of the testis.

## Testis, torsion of

Twisting of the spermatic cord, causing acute, severe pain and swelling of the *testis*. Unless treated within a few hours, the testis is damaged permanently and sperm production ceases.

Torsion of the testis is most common around puberty, but may also occur in infants or in young adults. The condition is more likely to occur if the testis is unusually mobile within its covering in the scrotum.

**SYMPTOMS AND SIGNS**

Pain develops rapidly and is occasionally accompanied by abdominal pain and nausea. The testis becomes swollen and very tender, and the scrotal skin becomes discolored.

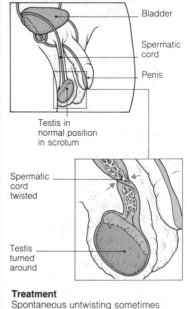

**TORSION OF THE TESTIS**

If a testis rotates, veins in the spermatic cord become obstructed and there is severe swelling and pain. Torsion of the testis most commonly occurs around puberty.

Bladder

Spermatic cord

Penis

Testis in normal position in scrotum

Spermatic cord twisted

Testis turned around

**Treatment**

Spontaneous untwisting sometimes occurs but unrelieved torsion is dangerous. Torsion must be treated urgently by manipulation or surgery.

**DIAGNOSIS AND TREATMENT**

A provisional diagnosis is made from a physical examination; *ultrasound scanning* may also be performed.

Treatment is by surgery. An incision is made in the skin of the scrotum and, if the diagnosis is confirmed, the testis can be immediately untwisted. If blood flow resumes, the testis is anchored in the scrotum with small stitches to prevent torsion from recurring. If irreversible damage exists, *orchiectomy* is performed.

In all cases, the other testis is also anchored to the scrotum to prevent torsion on that side.

**OUTLOOK**

Recovery from the operation is rapid. If treatment was prompt, the testis recovers completely. Even if one testis was removed, the other is usually capable of maintaining fertility.

## Testis, undescended

A *testis* that has failed to complete its normal passage from within the abdomen to the scrotum. Not all testes that

T

are absent from the scrotum are undescended (see *Testis, ectopic; Testis, rectractile*). Undescended testis is found in 2 percent of full-term and in up to 10 percent of premature male babies. Usually, only one testis fails to descend. In many cases, the testis descends of its own accord within several months of birth.

CAUSES AND SYMPTOMS

The final descent of the testis through the inguinal canal to the scrotum is controlled by hormones from the mother and from the testis itself. If these stimuli do not have an effect, the spermatic cord (which carries the vas deferens and the blood vessels to the testis) fails to lengthen sufficiently to allow full descent. Alternatively, a normal testis may be prevented from reaching the scrotum by the presence of fibers that interrupt its route and cause it to remain in the groin.

An undescended testis does not develop normally and is not capable of normal sperm production. If both testes are undescended, *infertility* results. A testis that fails to descend normally is at increased risk of testicular cancer (see *Testis, cancer of*).

DIAGNOSIS AND TREATMENT

The diagnosis is made during examination of the newborn or later in infancy. It is rare for the condition to remain unnoticed into adult life.

Treatment is by *orchiopexy*, an operation in which the undescended testis is lowered into the scrotum. Surgery within the first few years of life gives the testis the best chance of developing normally. If the testis is very poorly developed (and the other testis is normal) the undescended testis is removed.

## Test meal

A portion of food or a small meal given to determine the functioning of some part of the digestive tract. The meal may contain standardized amounts of various types of food, portions of which are removed at intervals from the stomach. Isotope-labeled food may be given and scanned.

Another type of meal contains a substance that allows the digestive tract to be revealed on an X ray (see *Barium X-ray examinations*).

## Testosterone

The most important of the *androgen hormones* (male sex hormones). Testosterone stimulates bone and muscle growth and sexual development. It is produced by the testes and in very small amounts by the ovaries.

DRUG THERAPY

Synthetic or animal testosterone is used to stimulate *puberty* or treat *infertility* in males suffering from deficiency caused by disorders of the testes or *pituitary gland*. Testosterone was once used to treat *breast cancer*, but is rarely used today for this purpose.

Testosterone given to stimulate puberty may interfere with normal growth or cause overrapid sexual development. In males, testosterone may cause *priapism* (painful, persistent erection). In females, high doses of testosterone may cause deepening of the voice, excessive hair growth, or hair loss. Treatment with some oral forms of testosterone may cause liver damage.

## Tests, medical

About 10 billion medical tests are carried out each year in the US—about 45 for each man, woman, and child.

### TYPES OF MEDICAL TESTS

| | | |
|---|---|---|
| **Brain and nervous system** | EEG<br>Evoked responses<br>Hearing tests<br>Vision tests<br>Lumbar puncture<br>Intelligence tests | Myelography<br>Brain imaging<br>   CT scanning<br>   MRI<br>   PET scanning |
| **Skin, bones, and muscles** | EMG<br>Biopsy | Bone imaging<br>X rays |
| **Endocrine system and metabolism** | Thyroid function tests<br>Thyroid scanning | Blood tests<br>Urinalysis |
| **Blood and immune system** | Lymphangiography<br>Blood tests | Skin tests<br>Bone marrow biopsy |
| **Heart and circulation** | Heart imaging<br>   Chest X ray<br>   Angiography<br>   Echocardiography<br>   Venography | ECG<br>Catheterization, cardiac<br>Cardiac stress test |
| **Lungs** | Pulmonary function tests<br>   Blood gases<br>   Peak flow meter<br>   Spirometry | Chest X ray<br>Bronchoscopy |
| **Biliary system** | Liver function tests<br>Liver imaging<br>   Ultrasound scanning<br>Cholangiography | Cholecystography<br>ERCP<br>Liver biopsy |
| **Gastrointestinal tract** | Endoscopy<br>   Colonoscopy<br>   Gastroscopy | Barium X-ray examinations<br>Jejunal biopsy<br>Occult blood, fecal |
| **Urinary tract** | Kidney imaging<br>   Pyelography<br>   Ultrasound scanning | Kidney function tests<br>Cystoscopy<br>Urinalysis |
| **Reproductive system** | Hysterosalpingography<br>Mammography<br>Ultrasound scanning<br>Laparoscopy<br>Pregnancy tests | Amniocentesis<br>Cervical smear test<br>Chorionic villus sampling<br>Chromosome analysis<br>Semen analysis |

The table above lists some commonly performed medical tests, classified according to the body system they are used to study. Each test listed in the table has its own encyclopedia entry. Only some of the most important imaging techniques for each body organ have been included; a complete list appears in the appropriate imaging article.

T

Medical tests are usually used to investigate the cause of a person's symptoms to establish a *diagnosis*. In addition, tests are performed on apparently healthy people to find disease at an early stage; this is known as *screening*. The yield from screening is considered small by some, and many unnecessary follow-up procedures may be performed to investigate a falsely positive test result.

To be of value, a medical test must be reasonably accurate in identifying or excluding the presence of a particular disease. The degree of accuracy is based on three factors—sensitivity, specificity, and predictive value.

Sensitivity is the ability of a test to show a positive (abnormal) value when the disease being tested for is actually present. A test that always detects a specific disease is said to have 100 percent sensitivity. One that shows positive results in only 80 people out of a hundred who have the disease is said to have 80 percent sensitivity; the 20 percent of the cases missed on the test reflect the false-negative test results.

The specificity is the extent to which a test shows false-positive results in healthy people. For example, a test that shows false results in 20 percent of the people tested has 80 percent specificity.

Sensitivity and specificity may vary with the controls (known standards) used in different laboratories and with the criteria for normal values.

The third measure of a test's accuracy is its predictive value. It is determined by a mathematical formula that includes the number of times the test is accurate (the true-negative test results plus the true-positive test results) and the total number of tests performed. The predictive value thus determines the probability that a patient with a positive test result actually has the disease or, conversely, that a patient who has a negative test result does not have the disease. The predictive value is dependent on the prevalence of the disease in the group being tested; when a disease is rare, a positive result is much more likely to be significant.

There is tremendous variation in accuracy among tests. For example, the fecal occult blood test (see *Occult blood, fecal*) used to detect cancer of the stomach or intestine is very sensitive; a person whose test results are negative (normal) is unlikely to have the disease. However, the test is not highly specific and many people whose test results are positive (abnormal) do not have the disease. More tests are required to confirm the diagnosis before treatment is performed.

An *ECG* to diagnose acute myocardial infarction (heart attack) is reasonably specific. A person whose test results are positive is almost definitely affected and is admitted to an intensive-care unit for treatment. However, the test is not sensitive; about half the people with severe chest pain who have negative test results may also need treatment.

The best tests have both high specificity and high sensitivity, and therefore high predictive value. Today's tests for syphilis have almost 100 percent predictive value. They almost always show a positive result in someone who has the disease and a negative result in someone who does not have the disease.

## Tetanus

A serious, sometimes fatal, disease of the central nervous system caused by infection of a wound with spores of the bacterium CLOSTRIDIUM TETANI.

**CAUSES AND INCIDENCE**

The spores live mainly in soil and manure, but are also found in the human intestine and elsewhere. If, through a wound, spores enter tissues that are poorly supplied with oxygenated blood, they multiply and produce a toxin that acts on the nerves controlling muscle activity.

About half a million cases of tetanus occur worldwide each year; in the US only about 100 cases are reported annually. All occur in nonimmunized people, mostly in those over age 50. In developing countries, tetanus often causes death in newborn infants as a result of spores contaminating the umbilical stump.

**PREVENTION**

*DPT vaccination*—combined immunization against diphtheria, pertussis (whooping cough), and tetanus—is given routinely in the US during childhood, after which tetanus immunization booster shots are needed every 10 years. Any wound, particularly a deep or dirty one, should be cleaned and treated with an antiseptic.

**SYMPTOMS AND SIGNS**

The most common symptom is *trismus* (stiffness of the jaw, commonly known as lockjaw), which makes it difficult to open the mouth. Other symptoms include stiffness of abdominal and back muscles, and contraction of facial muscles, producing a fixed, mirthless smile. There may also be a fast pulse, slight fever, and profuse sweating. Eventually, painful muscle spasms develop. If they affect the larynx or chest wall, asphyxia may result. The spasms usually subside after 10 to 14 days.

**DIAGNOSIS AND TREATMENT**

The diagnosis is made from the patient's symptoms and signs, and a course of tetanus antitoxin injections is started. Severe cases may require a *tracheostomy* (insertion of a breathing tube into the windpipe) and maintenance of the person's breathing with a *ventilator*. Given prompt treatment, most people recover completely.

## Tetany

Spasms and twitching of the muscles, most commonly those in the hands and feet, although the face, larynx (voice box), or spinal muscles may also be affected. Initially, the spasms are painless; if the condition persists, they tend to become increasingly painful. In some cases, muscle damage eventually results if the underlying cause is not treated. (Tetany, which is a symptom of a biochemical disturbance in the body, should not be confused with *tetanus*, which is an infection.)

The most common cause of tetany is hypocalcemia (a low level of *calcium* in the blood), sometimes due to a diet lacking in vitamin D. Other causes include hypokalemia (a low blood level of *potassium*), which is commonly a result of prolonged diarrhea or vomiting; *hyperventilation* (abnormally deep or rapid breathing), which is most often a result of anxiety; or, more rarely, *hypoparathyroidism* (underactivity of the parathyroid glands). The latter two are also associated with hypocalcemia.

## Tetracaine

A local anesthetic (see *Anesthesia, local*). Tetracaine is used to anesthetize the eye before minor surgical procedures; it is also used to facilitate dental treatment, throat examinations, and procedures in which a tube is passed down the throat. Tetracaine is occasionally used for *spinal anesthesia* or *epidural anesthesia* during *childbirth*, and to relieve pain, itching, and inflammation in anal disorders.

**POSSIBLE ADVERSE EFFECTS**

Tetracaine may cause a localized allergic reaction, which includes burning discomfort, redness, itching, and swelling. Eye preparations may cause dryness or watering of the eyes. High doses may cause anxiety, dizziness, and drowsiness.

T

# Tetracycline drugs

COMMON DRUGS

*Minocycline Oxytetracycline Tetracycline*

A group of *antibiotic drugs* commonly used to treat conditions including *acne, bronchitis, syphilis, gonorrhea, nonspecific urethritis*, and certain types of *pneumonia*. Tetracyclines are also prescribed for some less common infections, such as *cholera, Rocky Mountain spotted fever*, and *brucellosis*.

Possible adverse effects include nausea, vomiting, diarrhea, and, less commonly, rash and itching. Tetracyclines may discolor developing teeth and are therefore not usually prescribed for children under the age of 12 or for pregnant women. Tetracyclines may worsen the condition of the kidneys in people with poor kidney function.

## Tetrahydroaminoacridine

A drug under investigation for use in the treatment of *Alzheimer's disease*. In a small clinical trial with the drug, memory loss improved in people with Alzheimer's disease. A large clinical trial intended to establish the effectiveness of tetrahydroaminoacridine was underway until the frequency of adverse drug effects (impaired liver function) became too high.

In Alzheimer's disease, the level of the brain chemical *acetylcholine* is abnormally low. It is thought that tetrahydroaminoacridine increases the production of this chemical. However, the drug does not halt degeneration of brain tissue and thus cannot cure Alzheimer's disease.

Tetrahydroaminoacridine can impair liver function during treatment; the risk of permanent damage from long-term treatment is unknown.

## Tetrahydrozoline

A *decongestant drug* used to relieve *sinusitis*, allergic *rhinitis* (hay fever), and the common *cold*. Tetrahydrozoline is also given to relieve redness of the eyes that is caused by minor irritation.

Long-term use may worsen congestion. Other possible adverse effects include headache, restlessness, and palpitations. Eye drops may occasionally cause blurred vision and oversensitivity to light.

## Tetralogy of Fallot

A form of congenital *heart disease*, consisting of four coexisting heart anomalies, present from birth (see dia-

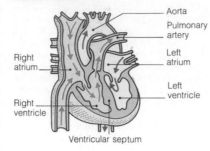

**NORMAL HEART**

Aorta
Pulmonary artery
Right atrium
Left atrium
Left ventricle
Right ventricle
Ventricular septum

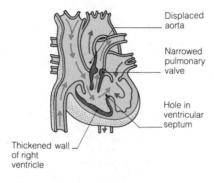

**TETRALOGY OF FALLOT**

Displaced aorta
Narrowed pulmonary valve
Hole in ventricular septum
Thickened wall of right ventricle

**Defects in tetralogy of Fallot**
The four defects are shown above. Insufficient blood passes to the pulmonary artery and lungs to be oxygenated, and the large volume of blood pumped to the body via the aorta is therefore lacking in oxygen.

gram). The result of the defects is that blood pumped to the body from the heart is insufficiently oxygenated, which leads to *cyanosis* (blue-purple coloration) and breathlessness. Tetralogy of Fallot occurs in about 50 out of 100,000 babies born.

**SYMPTOMS AND SIGNS**
Affected infants appear normal at birth, although turbulence in the heart can be detected as murmurs by a physician using a stethoscope. There is usually a gradual increase in the degree of cyanosis and breathlessness. Other symptoms include difficulty feeding, failure to gain weight, and poor development.

In older children who remain untreated, *clubbing* of the fingers and toes is usually evident. Another feature in older children is the adoption, after exertion, of a squatting position, with the knees on the chest, to help them recover from breathlessness.

**DIAGNOSIS, TREATMENT, AND OUTLOOK**
The condition is suspected on the basis of the child's symptoms and a

physical examination. A chest *X ray* shows a characteristic shape of the heart. An *ECG*, echocardiogram (see *Echocardiography*), and in some cases cardiac *catheterization* are performed to determine the extent of the abnormality.

Surgery is necessary for permanent correction of the disorder. The optimal time for surgical repair is before the child starts school. A temporary procedure is usually performed first. A duct is created between the aorta and pulmonary artery so that some of the blood pumped into the aorta is diverted to the lungs. Subsequently, a corrective operation is performed in the course of *open heart surgery*. The narrowed pulmonary artery is widened and the hole in the heart is closed. If successful, no other operation should be necessary.

## Thalamus

A structure consisting of two egg-shaped masses of nerve tissue, each about the size of a walnut, deep within the brain. The thalamus sits at the top of the brain stem and is connected by many tracts to all parts of the brain.

**FUNCTION**
The thalamus is an important relay center for sensory information flowing into the brain. Different clusters of nerve cells within the thalamus receive information from different sense organs (e.g., from the eyes, ears, and, via the spinal cord, from

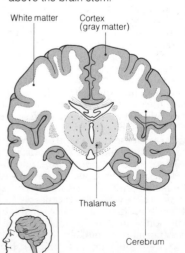

**LOCATION OF THE THALAMUS**
The thalamus lies deep within the brain, its two lobes located just above the brain stem.

White matter
Cortex (gray matter)
Thalamus
Cerebrum

T

touch and pressure receptors in the skin). Some basic sensations, such as pain, may actually reach consciousness within the thalamus. Other types of sensory information are processed and relayed to parts of the cerebral cortex (outer layer of the brain), where the sensations are perceived.

The thalamus seems to act as a filter, selecting only information of particular importance from the mass of sensory signals entering the brain. This is important for the ability to concentrate on a particular task. Certain centers within the thalamus may also play a part in long-term memory.

### DISORDERS

Damage to the thalamus due to *stroke* or *brain tumor* usually causes loss of sensation, but sometimes causes heightened sensitivity to pain, temperature, and other sensory stimuli.

## Thalassemia

A group of inherited disorders in which there is a fault in the production of *hemoglobin*, the oxygen-carrying substance that is synthesized in the bone marrow for incorporation into red blood cells. Many of the red cells produced are fragile and rapidly hemolyzed (broken up), leading to hemolytic *anemia*.

Thalassemia is prevalent in the Mediterranean region, the Middle East, and Southeast Asia, and in families originating from these areas.

### CAUSES, TYPES, AND INCIDENCE

The hemoglobin of healthy people contains two pairs of globins (protein chains), known as alpha chains and beta chains. In thalassemia, synthesis of either the alpha or the beta chains is reduced, causing an imbalance between alpha and beta chains in much of the hemoglobin produced.

Abnormal hemoglobin production in thalassemia is caused by inheritance of a defective *gene*. Most commonly, it is the production of beta chains that is disturbed, leading to beta-thalassemia. This condition is inherited in an autosomal recessive pattern (see *Genetic disorders*). If a person inherits one defective gene for the disease, he or she is said to have beta-thalassemia minor, or thalassemia trait (which is never severe). If two defective genes are inherited—one from each parent—the result is a much more severe condition called beta-thalassemia major, or Cooley's anemia. If two people with the minor trait have offspring, each child has a one in four chance of suffering from beta-thalassemia major.

Alpha-thalassemia is much less common than the beta type. If there is a severely reduced production of alpha chains, the lack of normal hemoglobin is incompatible with life and an affected infant dies within a few hours of birth. Lesser degrees of alpha-thalassemia also occur.

### SYMPTOMS

Beta-thalassemia major produces the symptoms of hemolytic anemia, including fatigue and shortness of breath with jaundice and spleen enlargement due to the rapid break up of red blood cells. These symptoms first appear three to six months after birth. In untreated cases, the bone marrow expands greatly (to compensate for the reduced life span of red cells), which can cause bones to grow abnormally. This leads to an enlargement of the skull in untreated patients. Normal body growth is arrested and, without treatment, death occurs during early childhood.

In the forms of alpha-thalassemia compatible with life, there are also symptoms of anemia but they are generally less severe.

### DIAGNOSIS AND TREATMENT

The diagnosis of beta-thalassemia major is made from microscopic examination of the blood, which shows many small, pale red blood cells, and from other blood tests that show reduced levels of adult hemoglobin in the blood.

Treatment is with blood transfusions, which can allow an affected child to grow normally. In addition, the spleen may be removed when the child is older (see *Splenectomy*). However, as each blood transfusion is administered, some iron is absorbed and eventually the internal organs become overloaded with iron. This can lead to liver *cirrhosis*, to gland disorders such as *diabetes mellitus*, and to *heart failure*, which is a frequent cause of death in young adults with the disease.

Research is helping to reduce the iron overload with compounds called *chelating agents*. Efforts have been made to cure the disease with a bone marrow transplant.

### OUTLOOK

Parents or other relatives of a child with thalassemia, and any person known to have beta-thalassemia minor (thalassemia trait), may benefit from *genetic counseling*. Beta-thalassemia major can now be diagnosed by *prenatal screening* techniques; parents may choose to have the pregnancy terminated.

## Thalidomide

A *sleeping drug* never approved by the FDA for sale in the US. It caused limb deformities in many of the babies born to women who were given this drug during pregnancy.

Thalidomide is currently under investigation for use in treating certain types of *leprosy*.

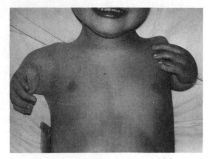

**Thalidomide child**
Phocomelia (seal-limb) was a common result of the action of thalidomide on the fetus at an early stage of development.

## Thallium

A rare metallic element that does not occur naturally in its pure form but is present (in minute amounts) as various compounds in certain ores of zinc and lead. Thallium 201 (an artificial radioactive isotope of the element) is sometimes used in *radionuclide scanning* of the heart. In this role, it reveals areas of heart muscle that have a poor blood supply or that have been damaged by a *myocardial infarction* (heart attack).

## THC

The abbreviation for tetrahydrocannabinol (dronabinol), the active ingredient in *marijuana*. This drug is used to treat the nausea and vomiting of cancer patients undergoing radiation therapy and/or chemotherapy.

## Theophylline

A *bronchodilator drug* used primarily in the treatment of *asthma* and to prevent attacks of *apnea* (cessation of breathing) in premature infants. The drug may be used to treat *heart failure* because it stimulates heart rate and increases urine excretion.

Possible adverse effects include dizziness, nausea, vomiting, diarrhea, palpitations, and seizures.

## Therapeutic

A term meaning "related to treatment." The therapeutic dose of a drug is the amount required to have a beneficial effect.

T

## Therapeutic community

A method of treating antisocial behavior in which patients live together as a group in a nonhospital environment under the supervision of medical staff. Therapeutic communities are used for treating *drug dependence*, *alcohol dependence*, and certain *personality disorders*.

Staff and patients share all decisions at regular group meetings, and unacceptable behavior and its effects are confronted and discussed openly. All aspects of day-to-day activity thus provide a focus for learning appropriate social and interpersonal skills.

## Therapy

The treatment of any disease or abnormal physical or mental condition. Examples of therapy include *radiation therapy* for cancer and *psychotherapy* for psychiatric disorders.

## Thermography

A technique in which temperature patterns on the surface of the skin are recorded in the form of an image.

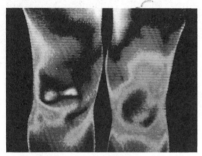

**Thermographic image of knees**
Areas that have different surface temperatures show up as different shades in the thermographic image.

**WHY IT IS DONE**
Thermography provides clues to the presence of diseases and abnormalities of the skin that alter the temperature of the skin, such as circulation problems, inflammation, and tumors. However, because so many conditions affect skin temperature, further examination and tests are necessary to confirm the underlying cause.

**HOW IT IS DONE**
Two techniques are used in thermography to detect skin temperature. In one, a special camera or scanner picks up infrared radiation naturally emitted from the skin. In the other, sheets of special temperature-sensitive liquid crystals are applied to the skin; they change color in response to changes in temperature.

**RESULTS**
Thermography is a safe technique. Results are not sufficiently reliable for thermography to fulfill hopes that it might prove useful as an early screening test for breast cancer.

## Thermometer

An instrument used to measure *temperature*. A traditional clinical thermometer consists of a glass capillary (very fine bore) tube sealed at one end and with a mercury-filled bulb at the other. When the bulb is placed in the mouth, the mercury expands up the capillary tube. The thermometer is removed from the mouth and the body temperature—indicated by the level of the mercury—is then read against a scale on the glass. There is a small kink in the capillary tube just above the bulb to prevent the mercury from moving down the tube when the thermometer is removed from the mouth. Before the thermometer can be used again, the mercury must be shaken back down into the bulb.

The capillary tube has a very narrow bore to make the thermometer sensitive to small temperature changes. In addition, the wall of the tube is thickened on one side to form a cylindrical lens that makes the mercury easier to see. Clinical thermometers may be calibrated in *Celsius* (centigrade) or *Fahrenheit* (or sometimes both); different styles may be used in the mouth, armpit, and rectum. A modern version of the traditional clinical thermometer uses an electronic probe connected to a digital readout display.

Recently, there has been a trend toward using disposable skin thermometers that employ heat-sensitive chemicals that change color at specific temperatures. These thermometers are generally less accurate than the mercury or digital types because they are more likely to be affected by external factors, such as the temperature of the environment.

## Thiabendazole

An *antihelmintic drug* used to treat *worm infestations*, including *strongyloidiasis*, *trichinosis*, and *toxocariasis*.

Thiabendazole may cause dizziness, loss of appetite, nausea, vomiting, headache, drowsiness, and diarrhea. In rare cases, an allergic reaction may occur.

## Thiamine

See *Vitamin B complex*.

## Thiopental

A *barbiturate drug* widely used as a general anesthetic (see *Anesthesia, general*). Thiopental, which is given by intravenous injection, quickly produces unconsciousness. However, because it has a relatively short-lived effect, a different anesthetic agent is used to maintain anesthesia.

## Thioridazine

An *antipsychotic drug* used to treat *schizophrenia*, *mania*, and *dementia*. Although thioridazine does not cure the underlying disorder, its tranquilizing effect suppresses abnormal behavior, reduces aggression, and helps relieve *anxiety* and *depression*, rendering the person more amenable to psychotherapy.

Thioridazine may cause dyskinesia (abnormal movements) but is less likely to do so than some other antipsychotic drugs. Drowsiness, dry mouth, muscle stiffness, and dizziness may occur. High doses of the drug taken over long periods may damage the retina.

## Thiothixene

An antipsychotic drug similar to *trifluoperazine*.

## Thirst

The desire to drink. Thirst is one means by which the amount of water in the body is controlled (the other is the volume of urine that is produced by the kidneys).

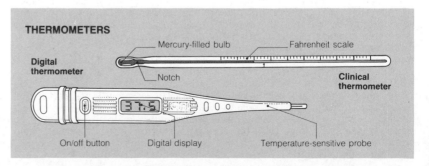

**THERMOMETERS**

Digital thermometer

Mercury-filled bulb — Fahrenheit scale

Notch

Clinical thermometer

On/off button — Digital display — Temperature-sensitive probe

37.5

T

Thirst is stimulated by an increase in the concentration of salt, sugar, or certain other substances in the blood. Particle concentration of the serum (the liquid portion of blood) rises if fluid intake falls or if dietary intake of certain substances (most commonly salt) increases. As the concentrated blood passes through the hypothalamus in the brain, special nerve receptors are stimulated, inducing the sensation of thirst.

Thirst is also stimulated if the volume of blood decreases as a result of sweating, vomiting, diarrhea, severe bleeding, or extensive burns.

In addition, although thirst causes a dry mouth, dryness may also cause thirst, even when a person is adequately hydrated; in such cases, thirst can usually be relieved merely by moistening the mouth.

Damage to the hypothalamus (e.g., as a result of a head injury) may cause loss of the desire to drink and consequent *dehydration*.

## Thirst, excessive

A strong and persistent need to drink, most commonly due to *dehydration*. Excessive thirst is a symptom of untreated *diabetes mellitus* and *diabetes insipidus*. Other causes of excessive thirst include *renal failure*, treatment with certain drugs (such as phenothiazine derivatives), and severe blood loss. Abnormal thirst may also be psychological in origin, a condition known as psychogenic polydipsia.

## Thoracic outlet syndrome

A condition in which pressure on the *brachial plexus* (the nerve roots that pass into either arm from the neck) causes pain in the arms and shoulders, a pins and needles sensation in the fingers, and weakness of grip and other hand movements.

Pressure on the brachial plexus may result from drooping shoulders; it is made worse by lifting and carrying heavy loads or by an increase in body weight. Severe symptoms are usually caused by a *cervical rib* (an extra rib above the first rib), which is linked to the first rib by a fibrous band of tissue that presses on the brachial plexus.

Treatment usually involves exercises to improve posture. Sometimes *nonsteroidal anti-inflammatory drugs* and *muscle-relaxant drugs* are helpful. Severe cases may be treated by surgical removal of the first rib. Women with large breasts should wear a bra that provides good support.

## Thoracic surgeon

A surgeon who specializes in operations on organs within the chest cavity, excluding the heart. These organs include the lungs, esophagus, and trachea (windpipe). Patients generally see a thoracic surgeon only on referral by another physician.

## Thoracotomy

An operation in which the thorax (chest) is opened.

### WHY IT IS DONE

A thoracotomy is usually performed to allow a surgeon to operate on a diseased heart, lung, or other organ in the chest cavity. It may also be carried out as an emergency procedure following a severe chest injury.

### HOW IT IS DONE

There are two types of thoracotomy—lateral and anterior. Both are performed using general anesthesia.

A lateral thoracotomy provides access to the lungs, major blood vessels, and esophagus. A curved incision is made from between the shoulder blades, around the side of the trunk beneath the armpit, to just below the nipple. The underlying muscles are divided to expose the ribs, which are gently spread apart; occasionally, part of a rib is removed. The necessary operation is then performed. Afterward, a drainage tube is inserted into the pleural cavity (the space between the membrane covering the lung and the membrane lining the chest wall) to allow fluid to drain and to prevent the lung from collapsing. The muscles and overlying skin are then closed with stitches.

An anterior thoracotomy provides access to the heart and coronary arteries. A vertical incision is made from between the clavicles (collarbones) at the base of the neck to the lower end of the sternum (breastbone). The sternum is divided with a saw and gently pried apart. The heart is then exposed and the necessary surgery performed. Following insertion of a drainage tube into the pleural cavity, the sternum is closed with strong stitches (sometimes wire) and the overlying skin sewn up.

### RECOVERY PERIOD

Despite drainage, secretions in the air passages often cause breathing problems after surgery. To clear the passages, the patient is encouraged to breathe deeply and cough and is given *respiratory therapy*. Within 48 hours after surgery, the drainage tube is usually removed and the patient can begin to move.

## Thorax

The medical name for the chest. The thorax extends from the base of the neck to the *diaphragm muscle* and is supported and protected by the *ribs*, *sternum* (breastbone), and vertebrae (see *Spine*). The main structures in the thorax are the *heart, lungs, esophagus*, and large blood vessels such as the *aorta* and pulmonary arteries. (See illustrated box, overleaf.)

## Thought

A mental activity that enables humans to reason, form judgments, and solve problems. The essential features of thought are the substitution of symbols (in the form of words, numbers, or images) for objects, the formation of these symbols into ideas, and the arrangement of ideas into a certain order in the mind. A person's thoughts are represented to others by speech, writing, and behavior.

Aspects of thought that can be examined or tested include speed and efficiency, content of ideas, and the logical relationship among ideas. (See also *Thought disorders*.)

## Thought disorders

Abnormalities in the structure or content of *thought* as reflected in a person's speech, writing, or behavior.

In the thought disorder characteristic of *schizophrenia*, sometimes referred to as formal thought disorder, associations lose their logical connection. The individual may jump from one subject to another that is apparently unrelated, or may make indirect associations or clang associations (relating words that sound the same rather than connect logically).

Other thought disorders that occur in schizophrenia include inventing new words (*neologisms*), thought blocking (sudden interruption in the train of thought), experiencing thoughts as being inserted into or withdrawn from the mind by some outside force, and auditory *hallucinations*, in which a voice dictates or repeats the subject's thoughts.

An inability to think clearly and coherently occurs in all types of *confusion*, including *dementia* and delirium. Rapidly jumping from one idea to another ("flight of ideas") as a result of loosening of associations is characteristic of *hypomania* and *mania*. In *depression*, the opposite occurs; thinking becomes slow, there is a lack of ideas and associations, and a tendency to dwell in great detail on trivial subjects. Recurrent ideas that seem to

T

## ANATOMY OF THE THORAX

The heart, lungs, and large blood vessels, such as the aorta, occupy almost the whole of the thoracic cavity. The extra protection that is afforded to these organs by the rib cage, which also allows breathing movements, reflects their vital importance.

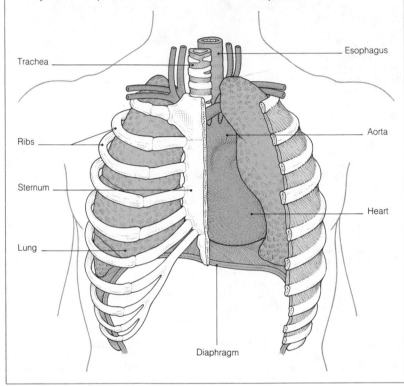

Trachea
Ribs
Sternum
Lung
Esophagus
Aorta
Heart
Diaphragm

come into a person's mind involuntarily are characteristic of *obsessive-compulsive behavior*.

*Delusions* (false beliefs that do not respond to reasoned argument), which occur in schizophrenia and other psychotic illnesses, may be an expression of distorted thinking.

### Threadworm infestation
See *Pinworm infestation*.

### Thrill
A vibrating sensation felt when the flat of the hand is held against the front of the chest. It is caused by abnormal blood flow in the heart as a result of a diseased heart valve or due to some form of congenital *heart disease*. An audible heart murmur always coexists.

### Throat
A popular term for the *pharynx*, the passage running down from the back of the mouth and nose to the upper part of the *esophagus* and the opening into the *larynx* (voice box). The term is also used popularly to refer to the front of the neck. (See also *Sore throat*.)

### Throat cancer
See *Pharynx, cancer of*.

### Throat, lump in the
See *Globus hystericus*.

### Thrombectomy
The removal of a thrombus (blood clot) that is partially or completely blocking a blood vessel.

Thrombectomy may be performed as an emergency procedure if a thrombus is blocking a major artery (such as one supplying blood to the brain, lungs, or intestines). It may also be performed as a precautionary measure if there is a risk of a fragment (an embolus) breaking off from a thrombus and being carried into the bloodstream to block an artery.

Before surgery, the site of the thrombus is established by *angiography* and the patient is given *anti-coagulant drugs* (drugs that prevent the blood from clotting). Incisions are made (with the use of a general anesthetic) to uncover the affected blood vessel, which is opened, and the thrombus is aspirated (sucked out). The incision is then closed with delicate stitches.

### Thromboangiitis obliterans
Another name for *Buerger's disease*.

### Thrombocytopenia
A reduction in the number of *platelet* cells in the blood. Because platelets play a vital role in the arrest of bleeding (by plugging any small breaks that develop in the walls of blood vessels), thrombocytopenia causes a tendency to bleed, especially from the smaller blood vessels. The result may be abnormal bleeding into the skin and from other parts of the body (thrombocytopenic purpura).

**CAUSES AND SYMPTOMS**
Thrombocytopenia may be caused by a reduced rate of production of platelets by the bone marrow or by a fast rate of destruction of the platelets.

In some cases, the underlying cause of the thrombocytopenia is not apparent (idiopathic thrombocytopenia). However, the condition frequently follows a viral infection and may be an *autoimmune disorder* in which the infection triggers destruction of the platelets by the immune system. Idiopathic thrombocytopenia occurs mainly in children and young adults; it usually runs a brief course of a few days to a few weeks before clearing up, although sometimes, particularly in adults, the bleeding tendency recurs from time to time.

The symptoms may include purple bruises or bleeding points in the skin, nosebleeds, *hematuria* (blood in the urine), bleeding in the mouth, and *menorrhagia* (heavy periods). There is a small risk of a *brain hemorrhage*, the warning signs for which are headache and dizziness.

Thrombocytopenia and associated bleeding can also occur as a feature of *leukemia, lymphoma*, some types of *anemia*, systemic *lupus erythematosus*, or *hypersplenism* (overactivity of the spleen). It may also occur after exposure to X rays or radiation, in severe fevers, and as a reaction to certain drugs, such as quinine.

**DIAGNOSIS AND TREATMENT**
Thrombocytopenia is diagnosed from the patient's symptoms and the presence of low numbers of platelets when a *blood count* is performed. A diagnosis

of idiopathic thrombocytopenia is made by excluding possible causes.

If thrombocytopenia is due to some other disease, treatment is of the underlying disease. If a drug is responsible, it is withdrawn. Children with idiopathic thrombocytopenia may not require treatment, but adults are generally given *corticosteroid drugs*. If the condition persists for many weeks or becomes recurrent, *splenectomy* (removal of the spleen) is often performed, giving a lasting cure in about three quarters of the cases.

## Thromboembolism

The blockage of a blood vessel by a fragment that has broken off and been carried from a thrombus (blood clot) elsewhere in the circulation. (See also *Thrombosis*; *Embolism*.)

## Thrombolytic drugs

A group of drugs, also known as fibrinolytic drugs, used to dissolve blood clots in *thrombosis, embolism*, and *myocardial infarction* (heart attack). Thrombolytic drugs work by increasing the blood level of plasmin (an enzyme that dissolves fibrin, the main constituent of blood clots).

Treatment is carefully monitored because of the risk of bleeding. An allergic reaction, causing rash and breathing difficulty, may also occur.

## Thrombophlebitis

Inflammation of part of a vein, usually near the surface of the body, along with clot formation in the affected segment. Thrombophlebitis can occur after minor injury to a vein (such as after an injection or intravenous infusion) and is particularly common in intravenous drug abusers. It can develop as a complication of *varicose veins* and also in blood vessel disorders such as *Buerger's disease*.

There is obvious swelling and redness along the affected segment of vein, which is extremely tender to the touch. Fever and malaise often occur. Serious complications are uncommon, although sometimes more serious clot formation develops in deeper veins (see *Thrombosis, deep vein*).

Treatment is by gentle support using a crepe bandage and by the use of a *nonsteroidal anti-inflammatory drug* and sometimes *antibiotic drugs* if infection of the vein is suspected.

## Thrombosis

The formation of a blood clot (thrombus) within an intact blood vessel. Clotting is a normal response that pre-

vents bleeding when a blood vessel wall is injured. Thrombus formation is abnormal if it occurs when a vessel wall has not been cut or punctured.

A thrombus within an artery may eventually grow to block the artery, preventing blood and oxygen from reaching the organ or tissue supplied by the artery. Thrombi of this type are an important cause of death and disability in the US and other developed countries. A thrombus that forms within one of the arteries supplying the heart muscle (coronary thrombosis) is the usual cause of a *myocardial infarction* (heart attack). A thrombus within one of the arteries supplying the brain (cerebral thrombosis) is a common cause of *stroke*.

Thrombi may similarly block the blood supply to the legs, kidneys, retinas, intestines, and other organs, sometimes causing severe damage and symptoms such as pain and loss of function. Another danger is that a fragment of thrombus—an embolus—may break off and be carried in the bloodstream to block an important blood vessel some distance from its site of origin.

Thrombi may also form in veins—either in inflamed veins near the surface (a condition called *thrombophlebitis*) or in deeper veins (see *Thrombosis, deep vein*). In deep vein thrombosis, the risk of large emboli breaking off and being carried to the heart and lungs is particularly serious.

**CAUSES**
In the blood there is a fine balance between the mechanisms that encourage and discourage clotting, so there is neither a tendency to bleed nor a tendency to form clots (see *Blood clotting*). Thrombosis can occur if there is an upset in favor of clotting.

In arteries, the clotting process may be encouraged by a buildup of atheroma (fatty deposits) on blood vessel walls. Any of the factors that encourage *atherosclerosis*—such as smoking, obesity, *diabetes mellitus*, or *hypertension* (high blood pressure)—is similarly associated with an increased tendency to form clots. Damage to blood vessel walls from inflammation (which occurs in *arteritis* and phlebitis) may also encourage clot formation, as may spread of infection to blood vessels locally or in *septicemia* (spread and multiplication of bacteria through the blood).

A clotting tendency can result from an increase in the level of coagulation factors in the blood; this tendency can occur in pregnancy or when using oral

contraceptives. It can result from liver disease that leads to deficient production of antithrombin, an anticlotting factor. It can also result from any cause that slows down blood flow to a certain area (e.g., inactivity during long airplane flights, or general anesthesia induced for a surgical operation).

**SYMPTOMS AND DIAGNOSIS**
An arterial thrombus may cause no symptoms until it impairs the blood flow through a blood vessel. At this point it may cause reduced function of the organ or tissue supplied by the blood vessel and, in some cases, severe pain. Venous thrombosis may also cause pain and swelling.

When thrombosis is a suspected cause of symptoms, it is investigated by *angiography* or by *venography* (X rays of blood vessels after injection of a radiopaque substance).

**TREATMENT**
Treatment may include the use of *anticoagulant drugs*, which discourage clotting, or *thrombolytic drugs*, which help break down clots that have already formed. *Nonsteroidal anti-inflammatory drugs* are often given to relieve the inflammation of thrombophlebitis. Other treatment, such as *antibiotic drugs* if infection is the cause of thrombosis, may be necessary. In cases where a clot is life-threatening, surgical removal may be required (see *Thrombectomy*).

## Thrombosis, deep vein

Clotting of blood within deep-lying veins, usually in the legs. *Thrombophlebitis* is a condition affecting superficial veins (nearer the surface) when they become inflamed.

**CAUSES AND INCIDENCE**
Deep vein thrombosis is generally caused by a combination of sluggish blood flow through one part of the body and some factor that increases the tendency of the blood to clot.

Sluggish blood flow occurs when a person lies or sits still for long periods. An increase in the level of coagulation factors in the blood, which occurs after an operation or injury, during pregnancy, and in women taking the birth-control pill, causes an increased tendency for the blood to clot.

An increased tendency to form clots can also occur as a result of *polycythemia* (increased numbers of red cells in the blood), severe infection, liver disease, and certain types of cancer. Deep vein thrombosis is common in people with *heart failure* and in those who have had a *stroke* or who are immobilized for long periods. Other

T

causes include injury to the veins or an extension of thrombophlebitis to deeper veins. Age and obesity both predispose to thrombosis.

**SYMPTOMS AND COMPLICATIONS**

If the thrombosis is not in a leg, there are often no symptoms. Clots in the leg veins may cause symptoms such as pain, tenderness, swelling, discoloration, and ulceration of the skin, depending on the site of the clots and how extensive they are.

Deep vein thrombosis is not always of serious significance; occasionally, if the clots are extensive, part of a clot may break free and be carried up to the heart and from there to the lungs, where it may block an artery. This is called a *pulmonary embolism* and is always a serious condition.

**DIAGNOSIS**

The presence and extent of deep vein thrombosis is diagnosed by *venography*

(introduction of a radiopaque substance into the veins followed by X rays) and by a type of *radionuclide scanning* called the radioactive fibrinogen test. Doppler *ultrasound scanning* is also sometimes used to help detect certain thrombi.

**TREATMENT**

Treatment depends on the site and extent of the blood clots. If they are small, confined to the calf, and the patient is mobile, treatment may be unnecessary, as the clots often break up spontaneously. In some cases, *anticoagulant drugs* may be given to prevent extension of the clots. In other cases, *thrombolytic drugs*, which actively dissolve the clots, may be given. If there is a high risk of a clot breaking off and causing a pulmonary embolism, *thrombectomy* may be performed to remove the clot surgically from the vein.

**PREVENTION**

The incidence of deep vein thrombosis has been reduced by encouraging people to get up as soon as possible after an operation or childbirth. If a person is immobilized for a long period, he or she should wiggle the toes and flex the ankles and knees to keep the blood moving. Blood flow in the legs of an immobilized person may also be stimulated by putting the legs in plastic bags, which are pumped up with air and then deflated.

When an operation is performed on someone thought to be particularly susceptible to deep vein thrombosis, anticoagulant drugs may be given.

## Thrombus

A blood clot that has formed inside an intact blood vessel—as distinct from one that has formed to seal the wall of a blood vessel after injury.

---

## DEEP VEIN THROMBOSIS

Thrombi, or clots, tend to form when blood flow is sluggish and in circumstances such as pregnancy where there is a rise in the level of coagulation factors in the blood. Once a clot has formed, it may provide a site for further clotting, so that a long, snaky clot may grow along the length of a vein. Thrombi form most commonly in the leg veins and may interfere with the drainage of blood from a leg (below right), causing signs and symptoms of varying severity.

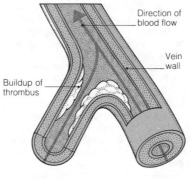

Direction of blood flow

Vein wall

Buildup of thrombus

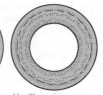

Partly blocked vein     Healthy vein

**Normal and obstructed vein**
Thrombi tend to form at points where a vein lining is damaged and may then grow to obstruct blood flow. The big danger is that a piece of clot will detach and be carried to the heart and lungs to cause a potentially fatal obstruction.

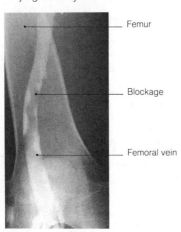

Femur

Blockage

Femoral vein

**Example of deep vein thrombosis**
This venogram shows a thrombus blocking the femoral vein just above the knee.

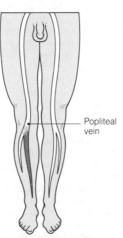

Popliteal vein

**Calf vein thrombosis**
When clots are localized to the calf and popliteal veins, there is usually some pain in the calf but there may be little swelling.

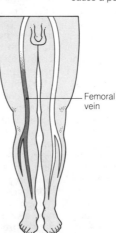

Femoral vein

**Femoral vein thrombosis**
If clots are present in the femoral vein as well as calf veins, there is usually pain and swelling up to the region above the knee.

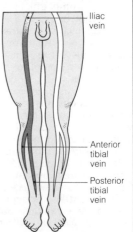

Iliac vein

Anterior tibial vein

Posterior tibial vein

**Iliofemoral vein thrombosis**
Clots in the iliac vein may affect drainage of blood from the whole leg, causing severe pain and swelling.

T

A thrombus is life-threatening if it grows to obstruct the blood supply to an organ such as the heart or brain. Even a thrombus in a less vital blood vessel can be dangerous because it may produce gangrene in part of the organ or extremity served, or a fragment of it (an embolus) may break off and be carried to obstruct the blood circulation elsewhere. (See also *Blood clotting*; *Thrombosis*; *Embolism*.)

## Thrush
A common name for the fungal infection *candidiasis*.

## Thumb-sucking
A common habit in young children. For the young child, thumb-sucking provides comfort (especially before falling asleep), oral gratification, amusement if the child is bored, and reassurance, especially during periods of stress, such as the birth of a new baby in the family.

Thumb-sucking tends to decrease after the age of about 3. Only a few children do not grow out of the habit by 6 or 7. In general, it is best for parents to ignore the habit; constant reprimands increase anxiety and may make thumb-sucking worse.

**COMPLICATIONS**
In most cases, there is no evidence that thumb-sucking is harmful. However, *malocclusion* (incorrect bite) of the second teeth may develop if the habit continues after about age 6. The effect on the teeth is usually only temporary; their position improves considerably or even completely after thumb-sucking stops. In severe cases of malocclusion, repositioning of the displaced teeth with an *orthodontic appliance* may be recommended.

## Thymoma
A tumor of the *thymus* gland. Thymomas are rare and are classified according to the type of thymus tissue from which they arise. An epithelial thymoma, arising from *epithelium*, is a slow-growing tumor that rarely spreads to other parts of the body. A lymphoid thymoma arises from lymphoid tissue, eventually resulting in generalized non-Hodgkin's *lymphoma*. A granulomatous thymoma consists of a mixture of epithelial and lymphoid tissue, and closely resembles *Hodgkin's disease*. The other main type of thymoma is a thymic *teratoma* (a tumor consisting of tissue that is not normally found in the thymus), which is usually benign in women but malignant in men.

Thymomas may affect function of the *immune system*, causing increased susceptibility to infection. They are commonly associated with *myasthenia gravis* (an autoimmune disease), which sometimes can be cured by removal of the thymoma.

## Thymus
A gland that forms part of the *immune system*. The thymus is situated in the upper part of the chest, behind the breastbone, and consists of two lobes that join in front of the trachea. Each lobe is made up of lymphoid tissue consisting of tightly packed *lymphocytes*, *epithelium*, and fat.

The thymus plays a part in the body's immune response from about the 12th week of gestation until puberty. The gland gradually enlarges until puberty, when it begins to shrink. Lymphoid and epithelial tissues are gradually replaced by fat, although some glandular tissue remains until after middle age.

The function of the thymus is to cause lymphocytes to become T cells. These T cells play an important part in the body's defense against viruses and other infections.

**DISORDERS**
Abnormal enlargement of the thymus sometimes occurs in several conditions, including *myasthenia gravis*, *acromegaly*, *thyrotoxicosis*, and *Addison's disease*. Myasthenia gravis is also sometimes associated with *thymomas*

**LOCATION OF THE THYMUS**
At full size, the thymus lies partly in the neck and partly in the chest. It shrinks later in life.

Thymus

Trachea

Lungs

(tumors of the thymus). In children, *immunodeficiency disorders* may arise as a result of abnormal development of the thymus.

## Thyroglossal disorders
Congenital defects arising from failure of the thyroglossal duct to disappear during embryonic development. In the embryo, this duct runs from the base of the tongue to the thyroid gland in the neck. Abnormal development may cause the duct to persist in its entirety or partially as a cyst.

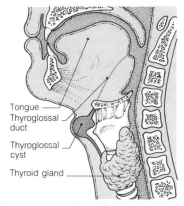

Tongue
Thyroglossal duct
Thyroglossal cyst
Thyroid gland

**Thyroglossal duct and cyst**
The thyroglossal duct, lying between the tongue and the thyroid, sometimes persists after fetal life, and a cyst may form.

A thyroglossal cyst almost always becomes infected and swollen, a condition that may be mistaken for an abscess. Infection may lead to formation of a thyroglossal fistula (abnormal passage between the cyst and the surface of the neck).

Because of the danger of repeated infection, a thyroglossal cyst or fistula should be completely removed surgically, along with any remaining parts of the thyroglossal duct.

## Thyroid cancer
Cancer of the *thyroid gland* is relatively rare, accounting for only about 1 percent of all cases of cancer. In most cases, the cause of the condition is unknown, although it is one of the cancers associated with exposure to radioactive fallout. Thyroid cancer has one of the highest cure rates of all cancers.

**SYMPTOMS**
A thyroid cancer is usually first noticed as a single, firm nodule in the neck, which, on initial physical examination, cannot be distinguished from a benign (noncancerous) mass. For this reason, all single thyroid

T

nodules are imaged (see *Imaging techniques*), sometimes examined with needle *biopsy*, and, when necessary, removed surgically for microscopic examination. If there are several nodules, they are likely to be benign rather than cancerous. The three cell types are papillary (the most common), follicular, and medullary (which secretes *calcitonin*).

Cancerous tumors may grow slowly or rapidly, depending on their type and the age of the patient (growth tends to be slower in younger people). However, in most cases, the cancer spreads to the lymph nodes at an early stage. Advanced cancers are usually hard and irregularly shaped and are often firmly attached to adjacent structures in the neck.

In many cases, thyroid cancers are painless; symptoms arise when they press on other structures in the neck. Such symptoms may include severe hoarseness or loss of voice from pressure on the nerves to the larynx or difficulty swallowing due to pressure on the pharynx (throat).

### TREATMENT
Treatment is usually by surgical removal of the entire gland (total thyroidectomy); occasionally, it is necessary to remove surrounding tissues. The loss of thyroid tissue results in a lack of natural *thyroid hormones*, and patients usually need to take hormone supplements for the rest of their lives. Such supplements may also help to control *metastases* (secondary growths).

In virtually all cases, treatment with radioactive iodine is used after surgery. Because it is selectively taken up and concentrated in the thyroid, radioactive iodine has the advantage of destroying any residual cancers while leaving normal body tissue undamaged, minimizing any side effects. This treatment may need to be repeated at one- to five-year intervals if any residual tissue is detected.

If thyroid cancer is diagnosed and treated at an early stage (even if local spread has occurred), the outlook is generally excellent. Papillary cancer is highly treatable; follicular cancer is only slightly less so. Medullary cancer has a less favorable outlook.

## Thyroidectomy
Surgical removal of all or part of the thyroid gland.
### WHY IT IS DONE
Thyroidectomy is performed to treat *thyroid cancer*, cases of *thyrotoxicosis* (an abnormally high blood level of thyroid

### SUBTOTAL THYROIDECTOMY
This operation entails removal of only part of the thyroid. The parathyroids (at the rear of the gland) are left intact.

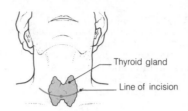

Thyroid gland

Line of incision

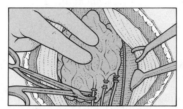

**1** After administration of a general anesthetic, an incision is made in the neck. Layers of skin and muscle are then drawn aside to expose the thyroid gland underneath.

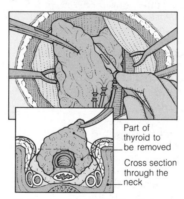

Part of thyroid to be removed

Cross section through the neck

**2** Once the front of the gland has been detached from its blood supply, much of it is cut away (with care taken not to damage nearby nerves), and bleeding vessels are sealed.

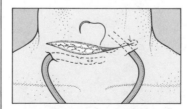

**3** Tubes are sometimes placed in the site of the removed gland to drain blood that accumulates. The muscle and skin layers are replaced and the incision closed with sutures or clips.

hormone) that cannot be controlled by drugs, *goiter* that is causing breathing or swallowing difficulties or unsightly swelling, or a benign tumor.
### HOW IT IS DONE
The operation to remove part of the thyroid (subtotal thyroidectomy) is shown in the illustration at left.
### RECOVERY PERIOD
The wound usually heals quickly. The stitches and drainage tube can usually be removed within a few days of the operation, after which the patient leaves the hospital.

Removal of all—or a large part—of the thyroid gland necessitates lifelong thyroid hormone replacement therapy with thyroxine.
### COMPLICATIONS
There is a very small risk of damage to structures close to the thyroid gland. Injury to the nerve supplying the vocal cords can lead to hoarseness; damage to the *parathyroid glands* can result in a low calcium level in the blood and tetany (painful muscle spasms in the hands, feet, and face). After the operation, careful monitoring is required to ensure that hormone levels are in the normal range.

## Thyroid function tests
A group of procedures used to evaluate the function of the *thyroid gland* and to detect or confirm any disorder of the gland.

Thyroid function can be measured by carrying out *blood tests* to determine the level of thyroxine ($T_4$) and triiodothyronine ($T_3$) in the blood. A sample of blood is taken from the patient's vein and the serum (liquid part of the blood) is tested.

The main function of the thyroid gland is to convert tyrosine (an amino acid) and iodine into $T_4$ and $T_3$. One way of measuring thyroid function is therefore to measure the rate at which iodine is accumulated by the gland. This can be done by introducing into the body a radioactive isotope of iodine (or technetium, which behaves in a similar way to iodine) and measuring the level of radioactivity in the gland (see *Thyroid scanning*).

The thyroid secretes $T_4$ and $T_3$ into the bloodstream under the direct control of thyroid-stimulating hormone (TSH) from the pituitary gland. Thus measurement of the amount of TSH produced by the pituitary provides a sensitive means of diagnosing thyroid malfunction. Various indices created by ratios of $T_3$ and $T_4$ enable the specialist to more accurately diagnose the condition.

T

## Thyroid gland

An important organ of the *endocrine system*. The thyroid gland is situated in the front of the neck, just below the larynx (voice box). It consists of two lobes, one on each side of the trachea (windpipe), joined by a narrower portion of tissue called the isthmus.

### STRUCTURE

Thyroid tissue is composed of two types of secretory cells—follicular cells and parafollicular cells (or C cells). Follicular cells make up most of the gland. They are arranged in the form of hollow, spherical follicles, and secrete the iodine-containing hormones thyroxine ($T_4$) and triiodothyronine ($T_3$). The space inside the follicles is filled with a semifluid, colloid material that is essential for the production of $T_4$ and $T_3$.

Parafollicular cells occur singly or in small groups in the spaces between the follicles. They secrete the hormone *calcitonin*. Also between the follicles are numerous blood capillaries, small lymphatic vessels, and connective tissue. The entire thyroid gland is encased in a thin outer layer of connective tissue.

### FUNCTION

$T_4$ and $T_3$ play an important role in controlling body *metabolism*. Calcitonin acts in conjunction with parathyroid hormone to regulate calcium balance in the body. (See also *Thyroid gland* disorders box; *Thyroid hormones*.)

---

### LOCATION OF THYROID GLAND

This major gland lies at the base of the neck just in front of the trachea (windpipe).

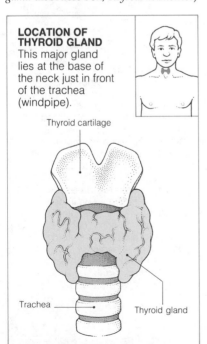

Thyroid cartilage

Trachea

Thyroid gland

## Thyroid hormones

The hormones thyroxine ($T_4$), triiodothyronine ($T_3$), and *calcitonin*, produced by the *thyroid gland*.

### FUNCTION

$T_4$ (the hormone produced in greatest amounts by the thyroid gland) and $T_3$ regulate *metabolism* (the chemical activity in cells that releases energy from nutrients or uses energy to create other substances, such as proteins). In children, these hormones are also essential for normal physical growth and mental development.

Calcitonin acts in conjunction with parathyroid hormone (secreted by the *parathyroid glands*) to regulate the level of calcium in the body.

### REGULATION

**$T_4$ AND $T_3$** The secretion of $T_4$ and $T_3$ by the thyroid is controlled by a hormonal feedback system involving the *pituitary gland* and *hypothalamus*.

**CALCITONIN** The secretion of calcitonin by the thyroid is regulated directly by the level of calcium in the blood. Raised blood calcium stimulates calcitonin secretion, stimulating deposition of calcium in bone and thereby reducing the calcium level; decreased blood calcium inhibits calcitonin output to help increase the calcium level. This regulation occurs independently of the pituitary gland or hypothalamus.

### DEFICIENCY AND EXCESS

Insufficient thyroid hormone production is known as *hypothyroidism*. Symptoms include tiredness, dry skin, hair loss, weight gain, constipation, and sensitivity to cold. In childhood, deficiency may cause severe growth retardation.

Overproduction of thyroid hormones (*hyperthyroidism*) causes symptoms including fatigue, anxiety,

---

### CONTROL OF THYROID HORMONE PRODUCTION

(Raised blood levels of thyroid hormones)

**Bloodstream**
If blood levels of the thyroid hormones $T_3$ and $T_4$ rise, they decrease the sensitivity of the pituitary to thyrotropin-releasing hormone (TRH), secreted by the hypothalamus.

**Hypothalamus**
Secretes TRH.

**Pituitary gland**
The pituitary becomes less sensitive to TRH, so it secretes less thyroid-stimulating hormone (TSH).

**Thyroid gland**
In response to lowered TSH stimulation, the thyroid reduces its production of the hormones $T_3$ and $T_4$.

**Bloodstream**
The blood levels of $T_3$ and $T_4$ thus gradually fall back to normal.

(Reduced blood levels of thyroid hormones)

**Bloodstream**
If blood levels of the thyroid hormones $T_3$ and $T_4$ fall, the hypothalamus is stimulated to produce more TRH.

**Hypothalamus**
Increases secretion of TRH.

**Pituitary gland**
In response to stimulation by TRH, the pituitary increases production of TSH.

**Thyroid gland**
In response to increased TSH stimulation, the thyroid increases its production of $T_3$ and $T_4$.

**Bloodstream**
The blood levels of $T_3$ and $T_4$ thus gradually rise back to normal.

### Why control is necessary

The blood levels of the hormones $T_3$ (triiodothyronine) and $T_4$ (thyroxine) produced by the thyroid must be kept within narrow limits, otherwise hyperthyroidism or hypothyroidism may result. The control systems above exist to achieve this balance but certain disorders may interfere with the system.

T

# DISORDERS OF THE THYROID GLAND

The function of the thyroid gland is controlled by both the pituitary gland and the hypothalamus, so thyroid disorders may be due not only to defects in the gland itself, but also to disruption of the hypothalamic-pituitary hormonal control system. Thyroid disorders may cause symptoms due to overproduction of thyroid hormones (*hyperthyroidism*), underproduction of these hormones (*hypothyroidism*), or enlargement or distortion of the gland. Idiopathic (of unknown cause) *goiter* (enlargement of the gland), *Graves' disease*, and *Hashimoto's thyroiditis* are the common disorders of thyroid function. Goiter sometimes occurs without any accompanying abnormality of thyroid function.

## CONGENITAL DEFECTS

In rare cases, the thyroid gland is missing completely at birth, producing severe *cretinism*. However, congenital thyroid deficiency more often takes the form of underdevelopment or maldevelopment, in which there is sufficient hormone-producing thyroid tissue to avoid cretinism but insufficient tissue to produce normal amounts of hormones. If untreated, this may lead to juvenile *myxedema*.

Sometimes the thyroid develops in an abnormal position in the neck; in rare cases, this causes difficulty swallowing or breathing.

## GENETIC DISORDERS

A genetic disorder may impair the thyroid's ability to secrete hormones. The low blood level of thyroid hormones results in greatly increased secretion by the pituitary gland of thyroid-stimulating hormone (TSH), which, in turn, causes the thyroid to enlarge in an effort to produce more hormone. This is one way in which a goiter may develop.

## INFECTION

Thyroid infection is uncommon, but sometimes occurs as a complication of infection elsewhere in the body. The resulting *thyroiditis* may require treatment with antibiotics. If an abscess forms, a minor operation may be necessary to open and drain it. Viral infection of the thyroid can cause temporary hyperthyroidism as well as an extremely painful gland.

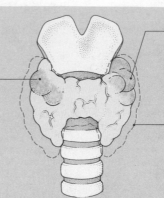

**Tumors**
Lumps in the thyroid are usually benign and some cancers are not highly malignant. Stone-hard, rapidly growing lumps suggest thyroid cancer.

**Autoimmune disease**
This is the most common cause of thyroid disorders. In Hashimoto's disease, much of the glandular tissue is replaced by masses of lymphocytes.

**Goiter**
Gland swelling (goiter) is common at puberty due to hormonal disturbance or may be due to autoimmune disease or, rarely, to iodine deficiency.

## TUMORS

Thyroid tumors may be benign or malignant. Thyroid *adenomas* are benign tumors that may secrete thyroid hormone, sometimes in sufficient amounts to cause hyperthyroidism. *Thyroid cancers* vary greatly in their malignancy and rate of growth. They are relatively rare but may be suspected if only a single firm or hard lump can be felt in the gland. One particular type of thyroid tumor secretes the hormone calcitonin.

## AUTOIMMUNE DISORDERS

Graves' disease is a form of thyroid overactivity whose chief feature is hyperthyroidism. The disease is thought to be due to the body producing an "autoantibody" that stimulates the thyroid to secrete excessive amounts of hormones. Autoantibodies are also believed to be associated with certain other thyroid disorders, notably Hashimoto's thyroiditis, in which the antibodies damage glandular cells.

## MYXEDEMA

Deficiency of thyroid hormone (hypothyroidism) may be associated with Hashimoto's thyroiditis or atrophy of the thyroid or be a consequence of treatment for hyperthyroidism. A possible result is myxedema, wherein the skin becomes dry and thickened and facial features become coarse. Constipation, cold intolerance, and fatigue are other common symptoms. In many cases, the cause of myxedema is not known.

## HORMONAL DISORDERS

Hormonal changes during puberty or pregnancy are a relatively common cause of a minor degree of goiter, which usually subsides when hormone levels return to normal.

Hyperthyroidism due to excessive production of TSH by the pituitary gland is rare but can occur as a result of a pituitary tumor.

## NUTRITIONAL DISORDERS

Because iodine is necessary for the production of thyroid hormone, deficiency of this mineral may lead to enlargement of the thyroid gland (goiter). Severe iodine deficiency in children may cause myxedema. These problems can be avoided by using table salt that contains iodine.

## RADIATION

Irradiation of the head or neck (e.g., for acne or enlarged tonsils or thymus gland) increases the likelihood of malignant thyroid tumors, although it may be 25 years or more until such tumors develop.

## INVESTIGATION

Suspected disturbances of thyroid function are investigated initially by the taking of a medical history and the performance of a physical examination. Blood samples may also be taken for *thyroid function tests*, in which the levels of thyroid or pituitary hormones are measured, and the gland itself may be imaged by various *thyroid scanning* techniques. In some cases, such as a suspected thyroid tumor, a fine-needle *biopsy* may be carried out to obtain a sample of thyroid tissue for examination under the microscope.

T

palpitations, sweating, weight loss, diarrhea, and intolerance of heat.

**DRUG THERAPY**

The most commonly used thyroid hormone drugs are the synthetic thyroid hormone preparations levothyroxine and liothyronine. These drugs are used to treat hypothyroidism, to prevent hypothyroidism and reduce thyroid enlargement in certain types of *goiter*, and to treat *thyroid cancer*.

Because a sudden increase in the body's thyroid hormone level may strain the heart, levothyroxine and liothyronine are usually prescribed in low doses that are gradually increased. Since too high a dose may cause symptoms of hyperthyroidism, regular visits to the physician are essential; when necessary, blood tests are carried out to monitor the thyroid hormone level.

Calcitonin is used to treat *Paget's disease, osteoporosis,* and *hypercalcemia* (see *Calcitonin*).

## Thyroiditis

The medical term for inflammation of the thyroid gland. The condition can be caused by a variety of factors, and occurs in several different forms. The most common form is *Hashimoto's thyroiditis,* an autoimmune disorder causing *hypothyroidism* (underactivity of the thyroid gland).

Subacute thyroiditis is a less common form in which the thyroid becomes tender and painful. Pain, which may be referred (see *Referred pain*) to the jaw, ears, or back of the head, may be accompanied by fever, weight loss, and a general feeling of illness. The condition may persist for several months, but in most cases eventually subsides on its own. In severe cases, treatment with *corticosteroid drugs* may be utilized to reduce the inflammation.

Thyroiditis due to infection is rare; when it does occur, it is usually as a result of an infection that has spread from elsewhere in the body. In some such cases, an abscess forms in the gland, which may require surgical drainage. Rarer still is a condition known as Riedel's thyroiditis (Riedel's struma), in which deposits of dense, fibrous tissue form in the gland and surrounding tissues, resulting in a hardening of the entire area.

## Thyroid scanning

Techniques used to provide information about the location, anatomy, and function of the *thyroid gland. Radionuclide scanning* is the method

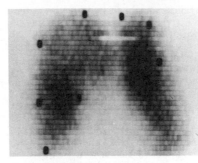

**Radionuclide thyroid scanning**
In this case, one area of the thyroid has taken up so much of the radioisotope that a diagnosis of a thyroid *adenoma* is likely.

available for investigating thyroid disorders, but *ultrasound scanning* can be useful in some cases.

**HOW IT IS DONE**

For radionuclide scanning, an injection or an oral dose of a radioisotope substance is given, followed after an interval by the recording of images on a gamma camera. The radioisotope substance usually contains a tiny dose of specially prepared technetium or radioiodine, both of which are taken up avidly by thyroid tissue, but hardly at all by other body tissues.

For the ultrasound scanning, a transducer producing high-frequency sound waves that penetrate tissue is moved back and forth across the skin over the thyroid gland. Echoes of the sound waves are picked up by the transducer and transformed electronically into an image.

**WHY IT IS DONE**

Radionuclide scanning reveals the position of any functioning thyroid tissue and is therefore useful in showing whether the gland is abnormally located or absent. The scan also shows the amount of the radioisotope substance that is taken up by the gland, thus allowing *hyperthyroidism* (overactivity) or *hypothyroidism* (underactivity) to be detected.

A radionuclide scan may suggest whether a thyroid nodule or tumor is benign or malignant and can show whether it is active or inactive. It can also detect malignant thyroid tissue that has spread to other parts of the body, therefore playing an important part in planning and evaluating the treatment of *thyroid cancer.*

Ultrasound scanning is of more limited use because it can show only the structure of thyroid tissue. It can be useful in showing whether a *goiter* is solid, cystic (fluid-filled), or a mixture of the two.

## Thyrotoxicosis

A term for any toxic condition that results from *hyperthyroidism* (overactivity of the thyroid gland). The term thyrotoxicosis is often used as a synonym for *Graves' disease.*

## Thyroxine

The most important *thyroid hormone* produced by the *thyroid gland*. Its symbol is $T_4$.

## Tibia

The inner and thicker of the two long bones in the lower leg, also called the shin. The tibia is the supporting bone of the lower leg. It runs parallel to the other, narrower bone, the *fibula*, to which it is attached by ligaments.

The front surface of the tibia lies just beneath the skin and is easily felt. The upper end articulates with the femur (thigh bone) to form the *knee* joint and the lower end forms part of the *ankle joint*. On the inside of the ankle, the tibia is widened and protrudes to form a large bony prominence called the medial malleolus.

**FRACTURE**

The tibia is one of the most commonly fractured bones. It may break across the shaft as a result of a direct blow to the front of the leg, or at the upper end from a blow to the outside of the leg below the knee. Fracture of the lower end of the tibia may accompany dislocation of the ankle and fracture of

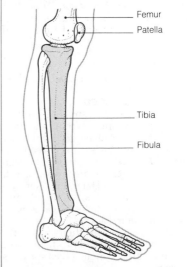

**LOCATION OF THE TIBIA**
Also called the shin, the tibia is easily felt beneath the skin of the lower leg.

- Femur
- Patella
- Tibia
- Fibula

the fibula in a *Pott's fracture*, caused by violent twisting of the ankle. Prolonged running or walking on hard ground may cause a *stress fracture* of the tibia.

Some fractures of the shaft heal satisfactorily if the leg is immobilized in a plaster cast, usually for about six to eight weeks. If the bone ends are displaced or unstable, an operation may be needed to fasten them together with a nail or screw.

## Tic

A repeated, uncontrolled, purposeless contraction of a muscle or group of muscles, most commonly in the face, shoulders, or arms. Typical tics include pointless blinking, mouth twitching, and shoulder shrugging.

Tics are often a sign of a usually minor psychological disturbance. Most develop in childhood, occurring in as many as a quarter of children and affecting three times more boys than girls. Tics are made worse by stress or by drawing attention to them, but often disappear when the child is deeply absorbed or asleep.

Tics usually stop within a year of onset but in some cases persist into adult life. Most can be controlled for short periods of time by will. However, such control is of questionable value because tics appear to release emotional tension.

In rare cases, tics become so severe that they require treatment with *benzodiazepine drugs* or *antipsychotic drugs*. Examples include involuntary contractions of the diaphragm (the muscle that separates the chest from the abdomen), resulting in grunting noises, and *Gilles de la Tourette's syndrome*, a disorder that is characterized by widespread tics and involuntary noises.

## Tic douloureux

Another name for *trigeminal neuralgia*.

## Ticks and disease

Ticks are small, eight-legged animals that can attach themselves to human or animal skin to feed on blood. They are about one eighth of an inch long; when bloated with blood, they may grow much larger. There are two broad categories called soft and hard ticks (hard ticks have a hard shield on their backs). Soft ticks are nocturnal and visit their hosts for relatively short periods to feed; hard ticks may attach themselves for days or weeks.

Ticks may be picked up when a person walks through or reclines in various rural habitats, such as long grass, scrub, woodland, or caves. Ticks can also be brought into the home by dogs. An attached tick may not be noticed for hours; others cause irritation, pain (which is sometimes severe), or bruising.

For walking through tick-infested areas, wear boots and long pants and examine your body afterward. If a tick has attached itself to your skin, remove it by grasping the tick with tweezers as close to its mouth as possible. Gently but firmly remove the whole tick. If a tick is pulled off forcibly, its mouthparts may be left behind and can cause infection. The bite wound should then be washed with soap and water.

Ticks in various parts of the world can spread infectious organisms from animals to humans via their bites. Soft ticks spread *relapsing fever* in parts of North America, South America, and Africa. Hard ticks spread *Rocky Mountain spotted fever, Q fever, Lyme disease, tularemia*, and certain types of viral *encephalitis*, all of which can be contracted in the US.

The prolonged bite of certain female ticks can cause a condition called tick paralysis, in which a toxin in the tick saliva affects the nerves that control movement. In extreme cases, this can lead to paralysis of the respiratory muscles and can be fatal to a young child or elderly person.

## Tietze's syndrome

Chest pain localized to an area on the front of the chest wall, usually made worse by movement of the arms or trunk or pressure from the fingers. Tietze's syndrome is caused by inflammation of one or several rib cartilages on their inside edges where they join the sternum (breastbone) or on their outside edges where they join the bony part of the rib. Symptoms may persist for several months.

Treatment is with *analgesic drugs* (painkillers) and *nonsteroidal anti-inflammatory drugs*.

## Timolol

A *beta-blocker drug* used in tablet form to treat *hypertension* (high blood pressure) and *angina pectoris* (chest pain due to inadequate blood supply to the heart muscle). Timolol is also among the beta blockers given after a *myocardial infarction* (heart attack) to prevent further damage to the heart muscle. It is also used in eye-drop form to treat *glaucoma*.

Possible adverse effects are typical of other beta-blocker drugs. Eye drops may cause irritation, blurred vision, and headache.

## Tinea

Any of a group of common *fungal infections* of the skin, hair, or nails. Most infections are caused by a group of fungi called the dermatophytes and are often called ringworm. Tineal infections may be acquired from another person, from an animal, from soil, or from an inanimate object such as a chair, shower stall, or carpeting.

Physicians commonly use the word tinea followed by the Latin term for the part of the body affected; tinea pedis affects the feet and tinea cruris affects the groin.

### TYPES AND SYMPTOMS

The appearance and symptoms of tinea vary according to the site. The most common type is tinea pedis, also called *athlete's foot*. It causes cracking and itching between the toes.

Tinea corporis (ringworm of the body) is characterized by itchy patches on the body that are usually circular with a prominent edge. Tinea cruris (also commonly called jock itch) produces a reddened, itchy area spreading from the genitals outward over the inside of the thigh. It is more common in males.

Tinea capitis (ringworm of the scalp) causes one or several round, itchy, patches of hair loss on the scalp; it occurs mainly in children and is more common in large cities and overcrowded conditions. Ringworm of the nails, also called tinea unguium or onychomycosis, is often accompanied by scaling of the soles or palms. The nails become thick and white or yellow.

### DIAGNOSIS AND TREATMENT

Most types of tinea are diagnosed by a physician from their appearances. However, sometimes the diagnosis must be confirmed, and the type of fungus identified, by culture of the organisms in a laboratory. Some scalp infections exhibit fluorescence under a filtered ultraviolet light (Wood's light), but most do not.

For most types of tinea, treatment is with *antifungal drugs* in the form of skin creams, lotions, or ointments. However, for widespread infections or those affecting the hair or nails, an antifungal drug in tablet form (usually griseofulvin) may be taken.

Treatment may be continued for some time after symptoms have subsided to eradicate the fungi and pre-

T

vent recurrence. For mild infections on the skin surface, there may be four to six weeks of treatment; for toenail infections, treatment may continue for up to one or two years.

## Tinea versicolor

A common skin condition that produces patches of white, brown, or salmon-colored finely flaking skin over the trunk and neck. Also known as pityriasis versicolor, it is caused by colonization of the dead outer layer of skin by a fungus that exists unnoticed on most people's skin as a yeast. The condition primarily affects young and middle-aged adults and is more common in men. It is not contagious.

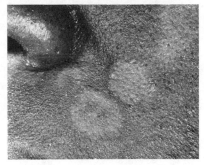

**Appearance of tinea versicolor**
This fungal infection causes patches of color change in the skin and is particularly common in tropical and subtropical areas.

The condition is usually noticed because of the contrast in color between the affected and surrounding skin. Exposure to sunlight can make it more or less noticeable.

Treatment consists of applying an antifungal cream or lotion at night and washing underclothes and nightclothes thoroughly. It is important to treat the entire trunk, neck, arms, and upper legs (ears to knees) each time the antifungal preparation is applied. Otherwise, a spot may be missed and the fungus will recur. This treatment usually clears the condition, but the spots may take many months to return to normal skin color.

## Tingling
See *Pins and needles sensation*.

## Tinnitus

A ringing, buzzing, whistling, hissing, or other noise heard in the ear in the absence of environmental noise.
### CAUSES
In tinnitus, the acoustic nerve transmits impulses to the brain not as the result of vibrations produced by

external sound waves but, for reasons not fully understood, as the result of stimuli that originate inside the head or within the ear itself. The condition is almost always associated with hearing loss, particularly *presbycusis*.

Tinnitus can occur as a symptom of many ear disorders, including *labyrinthitis, Meniere's disease, otitis media, otosclerosis, ototoxicity*, and blockage of the outer-ear canal with *earwax*. In rare cases, it is a symptom of an *aneurysm* or a tumor pressing on a blood vessel in the head.
### SYMPTOMS
The noise in the ear may sometimes change in nature or intensity. In most cases it is present continuously but the sufferer's awareness of it is usually intermittent. Tolerance of tinnitus varies considerably from one person to another and is largely determined by the sufferer's personality. Many people learn to accept the condition without distress, but some find it almost intolerable.
### TREATMENT
Any underlying disorder is treated if possible. Many sufferers make use of a radio, television, tape player, or headphones to block out the noise in their ears. Some find a tinnitus masker—headphones that play white noise (sounds produced by frequencies throughout the auditory field)—particularly effective.

## Tipped uterus
See *Uterus, tipped*.

## Tiredness

A common complaint that is usually the result of overwork or lack of sleep. In some people, persistent tiredness is caused by depression or anxiety. Tiredness may be due to a more serious condition, such as anemia or cancer, but usually there are accompanying symptoms.

## Tissue

A collection of *cells* specialized to perform a particular function. Examples of tissues include muscle tissue, which consists of cells that are specialized to contract; epithelial tissue, which forms the *skin* and *mucous membranes* that line the respiratory and other internal tracts; nerve tissue, comprising cells specialized to conduct electrochemical nerve impulses; and connective tissue, which includes blood, adipose tissue (fat), and the various fibrous and elastic tissues (such as tendons and cartilage) that hold the body together.

## Tissue fluid

The watery liquid present in the tiny spaces between body cells, also known as interstitial fluid. Tissue fluid is one component of extracellular fluid, which is any body fluid outside the cells, including blood and lymph.

To reach cells, oxygen and nutrients must pass from the blood vessels and into the tissue fluid. Similarly, there is a reverse movement of carbon dioxide and other waste products from the cells into the tissue fluid, and then into the bloodstream.

In addition to nutrients and wastes, tissue fluid also contains *ions*. This fluid contains a much higher level of sodium ions, and a much lower level of potassium ions, than intracellular fluid. It is this difference in ion levels that helps control the movement of water into and out of cells by *osmosis*; ion levels also play a role in the transmission of electrical impulses through nerves and muscles.

Tissue fluid is formed by the filtration of liquid out through the walls of the first part of blood capillaries (that is, the part nearest an arteriole), where it is forced out by the high blood pressure. In the last part of capillaries (nearest to a venule), blood pressure is much lower, and tissue fluid passes back into the capillaries; some tissue fluid is also drained away into the lymphatic vessels. Thus, there is a continual flow that keeps the amount of tissue fluid constant. Various disorders—such as congestive *heart failure*—may disrupt the balance between formation and drainage of tissue fluid, leading to *edema* (excess fluid in tissues).

## Tissue-plasminogen activator

A substance produced by body tissues that prevents abnormal blood clotting. Also called TPA, it is produced in small amounts by the inner lining of blood vessels and by the muscular wall of the uterus.
### DRUG THERAPY
TPA can be prepared artificially by *genetic engineering* techniques for use as a *thrombolytic drug* (a drug that dissolves blood clots). It is used in the treatment of *myocardial infarction* (heart attack), of severe progressive *angina pectoris* (chest pain caused by inadequate blood supply to the heart muscle), and of arterial *embolism* (blockage of an artery), including *pulmonary embolism*.

Given by *intravenous infusion*, TPA dissolves blood clots by converting plasminogen (a chemical in the blood)

**T**

to the enzyme plasmin. Plasmin in turn breaks down fibrin, the main constituent of a blood clot.

**POSSIBLE ADVERSE EFFECTS**

Bleeding or the formation of a *hematoma* (collection of blood) may occur at the site of injection. TPA may also cause bleeding elsewhere in the body but such bleeding can usually be controlled because TPA has a short-lived action. Allergic reaction may occur, although this effect is less likely than with other thrombolytic drugs. (See also *Fibrinolysis*.)

## Tissue-typing

The investigation of certain characteristics of the tissues of prospective organ donors and recipients.

**WHY IT IS DONE**

Tissue-typing is necessary to help match recipient and donor tissues for *transplant surgery*, thus minimizing the risk of rejection of a donor organ by the recipient's *immune system*.

The main features by which a person's immune system distinguishes his or her own tissues from those of other people are called *histocompatibility antigens*. The most important members of this group are called HLAs (human leukocyte antigens), which are present on the surface of the person's cells. A person's set of HLAs is inherited and unique to that person (except for identical twins, who have the same set). Hence, perfect tissue matching is achieved only between identical twins. Nevertheless, close relatives often have closely matching HLA types.

**HOW IT IS DONE**

A person's tissue type, or HLA "fingerprint," is established by tests in the laboratory on cells from a sample of the person's blood. There are many different possible HLAs and the presence or absence of each must be tested individually.

In one of the simpler methods of tissue-typing, an *antiserum* containing *antibodies* (substances that react with a particular antigen—in this case, a particular HLA) is added to the test specimen. If the antigen is present, it is detected by an observable color or other change.

For organ transplantation, once a recipient has been tissue-typed, a selection is made of a donor whose HLA grouping best matches that of the recipient. This helps reduce the chances of organ rejection after transplantation. It is easiest to find such donors among close relatives, such as brothers or sisters.

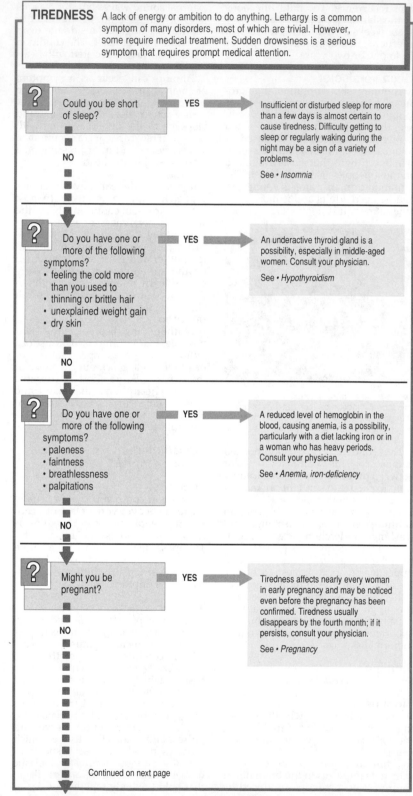

**TIREDNESS** A lack of energy or ambition to do anything. Lethargy is a common symptom of many disorders, most of which are trivial. However, some require medical treatment. Sudden drowsiness is a serious symptom that requires prompt medical attention.

**Could you be short of sleep?**

YES → Insufficient or disturbed sleep for more than a few days is almost certain to cause tiredness. Difficulty getting to sleep or regularly waking during the night may be a sign of a variety of problems.

See • *Insomnia*

NO ↓

**Do you have one or more of the following symptoms?**
- feeling the cold more than you used to
- thinning or brittle hair
- unexplained weight gain
- dry skin

YES → An underactive thyroid gland is a possibility, especially in middle-aged women. Consult your physician.

See • *Hypothyroidism*

NO ↓

**Do you have one or more of the following symptoms?**
- paleness
- faintness
- breathlessness
- palpitations

YES → A reduced level of hemoglobin in the blood, causing anemia, is a possibility, particularly with a diet lacking iron or in a woman who has heavy periods. Consult your physician.

See • *Anemia, iron-deficiency*

NO ↓

**Might you be pregnant?**

YES → Tiredness affects nearly every woman in early pregnancy and may be noticed even before the pregnancy has been confirmed. Tiredness usually disappears by the fourth month; if it persists, consult your physician.

See • *Pregnancy*

NO ↓

Continued on next page

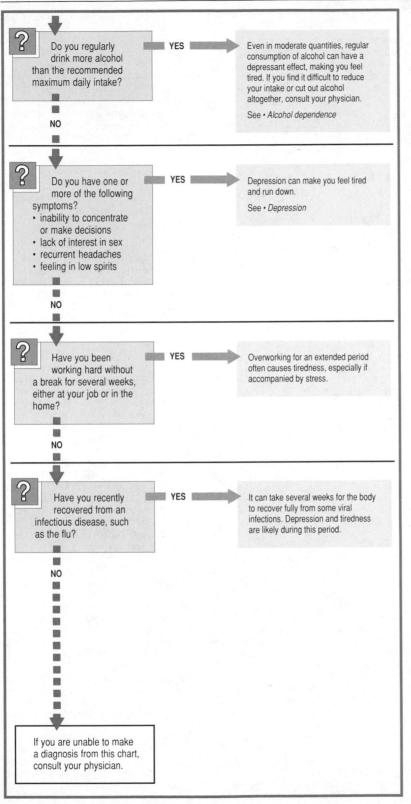

Do you regularly drink more alcohol than the recommended maximum daily intake?

**YES** → Even in moderate quantities, regular consumption of alcohol can have a depressant effect, making you feel tired. If you find it difficult to reduce your intake or cut out alcohol altogether, consult your physician.

See • *Alcohol dependence*

NO

Do you have one or more of the following symptoms?
• inability to concentrate or make decisions
• lack of interest in sex
• recurrent headaches
• feeling in low spirits

**YES** → Depression can make you feel tired and run down.

See • *Depression*

NO

Have you been working hard without a break for several weeks, either at your job or in the home?

**YES** → Overworking for an extended period often causes tiredness, especially if accompanied by stress.

NO

Have you recently recovered from an infectious disease, such as the flu?

**YES** → It can take several weeks for the body to recover fully from some viral infections. Depression and tiredness are likely during this period.

NO

If you are unable to make a diagnosis from this chart, consult your physician.

## Titanium dental implants

Posts surgically embedded in the jaw to form a framework for the attachment of false teeth. Titanium or other synthetic materials that form a bond with the jaw may be used.

Implants are useful for people who have lost all their teeth and who either are unable to tolerate a *denture* or have lost so much tooth-bearing tissue through injury or disease that a denture would not be stable.

**FITTING**

The procedure for fitting dental implants and attaching a prosthesis is shown in the box on the next page. Some prostheses can be removed only by the dentist; others can be removed by the patient.

## TMJ syndrome

See *Temporomandibular joint syndrome*.

## Toadstool poisoning

See *Mushroom poisoning*.

## Tobacco chewing

See *Snuff*.

## Tobacco smoking

Despite its practice in Western countries for more than 400 years—and for much longer in other parts of the world—tobacco smoking has only relatively recently been recognized as a major health hazard. Much of what is known today about the harmful effects of tobacco on the lungs concerns cigarette smoking because cigarette smokers have been studied in much greater depth than pipe or cigar smokers.

**HARMFUL EFFECTS**

*Lung cancer* is probably the best known harmful effect of smoking. More than 30 studies in 10 countries have demonstrated a direct link between smoking and lung cancer, a condition that is difficult to treat successfully and which causes about 8 percent of all deaths in men and 4 percent of all deaths in women in the US. Because pipe and cigar smokers tend not to inhale tobacco smoke, they have a slightly lower risk of lung cancer, although the risk is still significantly greater than for nonsmokers. The risk of developing lung cancer begins to diminish as soon as a person stops smoking.

Pipe and cigar smokers have a higher risk of cancer of the oral cavity and upper respiratory tract; tobacco chewers and those who use snuff risk cancer of the oral cavity (see *Nasopharynx, cancer of*).

T

## FITTING DENTAL IMPLANTS

Replacement of missing teeth is sometimes carried out by surgically implanting posts into the jaw and then attaching a dental prosthesis to the posts. When all the teeth in the jaw are missing, six posts are usually implanted (below). The procedure is carried out in several stages, with pain prevented by means of a local anesthetic.

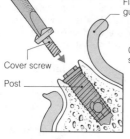

Flap of gum tissue

Cover screw

Post

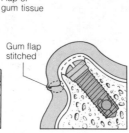

Gum flap stitched

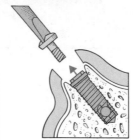

**1** Flaps of gum tissue are cut and raised. Holes are drilled in the jaw, posts are inserted, and cover screws fitted.

**2** The gum is stitched back over the posts and left for several months to allow time for healing to take place.

**3** After the healing period, incisions are made to expose the posts. The cover screws are then removed.

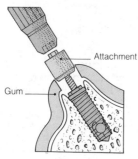

Attachment

Gum

Screw

Dental prosthesis

Attachment

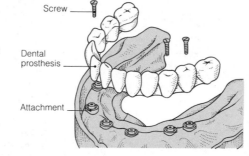

**4** Attachments that protrude above the gum are screwed into the posts. The cut edges of the gum are stitched.

**5** Several weeks later, when the gums have healed, measurements are taken for the prosthesis. The appliance, which is similar to a *bridge*, is manufactured in the laboratory and then screwed onto the protruding attachments over the posts.

---

The other important respiratory diseases associated with smoking are chronic *bronchitis* and *emphysema* and combinations of the two. These diseases, features of which include increasing breathlessness and coughing up sputum, account for tens of thousands of deaths annually in the US from respiratory failure. In addition, smoking also increases the risk of *mouth cancer*, *lip cancer*, and throat cancer (see *Pharynx, cancer of*).

The most significant harmful effect of smoking is *coronary heart disease*, which is the most common cause of death in middle-aged men in Western countries. The risk of coronary heart disease in a young man who smokes 20 cigarettes a day is about three times that of a nonsmoker, and the risk increases proportionally with the number of cigarettes smoked.

In addition to its effects on the coronary arteries, smoking damages arteries that supply other parts of the body and also raises blood pressure. Smoking seriously affects the arteries of the legs, leading to *peripheral vascular disease*; in severe cases of peripheral vascular disease, painful *neuropathy*, or *gangrene*, amputation may be necessary. Also affected by smoking are the arteries of the brain, which may result in a *stroke*.

Smoking is extremely harmful during pregnancy. The babies of women who smoke are smaller and less likely to survive than those of nonsmoking mothers. Even after birth, there are hazards for the children of parents who smoke. These children are more likely to suffer from *asthma* or other respiratory diseases and are more likely to become smokers themselves.

There is also evidence that anybody in the vicinity of a smoker is at increased risk of tobacco-related disorders. These "passive smokers" also suffer considerable immediate discomfort in the form of coughing, wheezing, and watering eyes.

### HOW SMOKING CAUSES HARM

Tobacco contains a variety of different noxious substances, but the dangers of three of them are particularly important.

*Nicotine* is the substance that causes addiction to tobacco. It acts as a tranquilizer, but also stimulates the release of *epinephrine* into the smoker's bloodstream, which may explain why some smokers have raised blood pressure.

Tar in tobacco produces chronic irritation of the respiratory system and is a major cause of lung cancer.

Carbon monoxide passes from the lungs into the bloodstream, where, in competition with oxygen, it easily combines with hemoglobin and thus interferes with oxygenation of tissues. In the long term, persistently high levels of carbon monoxide in the blood—which occur in smokers—lead to hardening of the arteries, which increases the risk of *coronary thrombosis*.

### STOPPING SMOKING

The most important prerequisite for successfully stopping smoking is an absolute commitment to giving up the habit. The slightest doubt over genuinely wanting to stop is likely to sabotage your efforts. For this reason, simply cutting down the number of cigarettes smoked rarely works; you must decide whether you will continue to smoke or will become a complete nonsmoker.

If you decide to stop smoking, there are many tools that may be helpful. Groups that emphasize behavior modification are effective and may utilize adjuncts such as nicotine-containing chewing gum, *acupuncture*, and *hypnosis*. Those who miss the oral sensation of smoking may find that sucking sweets or chewing gum or toothpicks helps.

Many people worry that they will gain weight as a result of stopping smoking. There is a risk that this will occur, because smoking tends to increase the metabolic rate (the rate at which the body "burns" food) and because many people eat more after they stop smoking. However, most physicians agree that being moderately overweight is far less hazardous to health than smoking.

T

## TOBACCO SMOKING

Smoking is a sure way to damage your health; it contributes to about one death in seven in the US. The main harmful effects come from nicotine, carbon monoxide, and tar. The first two contribute to heart disease, while tar causes lung disease and cancer.

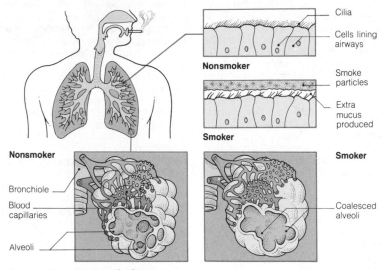

**How smoking damages the lungs**

Smoke particles irritate the lung airways, causing excess mucus production (top right). They also indirectly destroy the walls of the lungs' alveoli, which coalesce (above left and right). Both factors reduce lung efficiency. In addition, tar in tobacco smoke has a direct cancer-causing action.

**SMOKERS AS A PROPORTION OF US ADULT POPULATION**

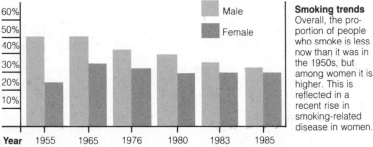

**Smoking trends**
Overall, the proportion of people who smoke is less now than it was in the 1950s, but among women it is higher. This is reflected in a recent rise in smoking-related disease in women.

**SMOKING-RELATED DEATHS BY SEX AND DISEASE IN US IN 1982**

|  | Total | Male | Female |
|---|---|---|---|
| Cancer | 139,000 | 103,000 | 36,000 |
| Cardiovascular disease | 123,000 | 84,000 | 39,000 |
| COAD | 52,000 | 35,000 | 17,000 |
| Total deaths from smoking | 314,000 | 222,000 | 92,000 |

**Major killers**

Most of the deaths result from coronary heart disease (a cardiovascular disease), lung cancer, and chronic obstructive airways disease, or COAD (i.e., chronic bronchitis and emphysema). Male smoking-related deaths far outnumber female deaths because, until recently, many more men than women smoked.

## Tobramycin

An *antibiotic drug* used to treat *peritonitis, meningitis*, and severe infections of the lungs, skin, bones, and joints. It is given by injection, usually in combination with a *penicillin drug*. Tobramycin eye drops or ointments are sometimes used to treat *conjunctivitis* and *blepharitis* (inflammation of the eyelids).

High doses given by injection may cause kidney damage, deafness due to inner-ear damage, nausea, vomiting, and headache. Any preparation that contains tobramycin may cause rash and itching.

## Tocainide

An *antiarrhythmic drug* that is used to prevent and treat certain ventricular arrhythmias (heart beat irregularities; see *Arrhythmia, cardiac*).

There is a high risk of adverse effects, including nausea, dizziness, tremor, loss of appetite, diarrhea, confusion, and hallucinations. Prolonged treatment may cause blood disorders, such as *thrombocytopenia*.

## Tocography

An obstetric procedure for recording the muscular contractions of the uterus during *childbirth*. Tocography is performed in conjunction with *fetal heart monitoring* to assess the quality of labor by measuring the frequency of contractions.

## Tocopherol

See *Vitamin E*.

## Toe

One of the digits of the foot. Each toe has three phalanges (bones), except for the hallux (big toe), which has two. The phalanges join at hinge joints, which are moved by muscle tendons that flex (bend) or extend (straighten) the toe. A small artery, vein, and nerve run down each side of the toe. The entire structure is enclosed in skin with a nail at the top.

The main function of the toes is to maintain balance during walking. People without hands often learn to use their toes to perform tasks usually performed with the fingers.

**DISORDERS**

Congenital disorders include *polydactyly* (extra toes), missing toes, *syndactyly* (fused toes), or *webbing* (skin flaps between the toes).

Injuries to a toe are fairly common, particularly a bruise under the skin or a fracture. Inflammation of one or several toe joints, causing stiffness,

T

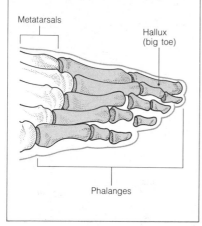

**ANATOMY OF THE TOES**
Each hallux, or big toe, has two bones called phalanges, which are connected by hinge joints. All the other toes have three phalanges.

Metatarsals

Hallux
(big toe)

Phalanges

pain, swelling, and deformity, may be caused by *osteoarthritis* or *rheumatoid arthritis* as well as other forms of arthritis (e.g., gout).

Infections occur under the nail as a complication of an *ingrown toenail*.

Impaired blood supply, usually due to *peripheral vascular disease* (narrowing of arteries in the legs), causes pain and blueness of the toes and can eventually lead to *gangrene*. Numbness and a pins and needles sensation in the toes may be caused by damage to peripheral nerves, which is common in *diabetes mellitus*.

A common deformity of the big toe is *hallux valgus*, in which the joint at the base projects outward and the top of the toe turns inward. The condition often results in a *bunion* (a firm, fluid-filled swelling over the joint). Abnormality of a tendon in one of the toes may cause the main joint to bend upward (see *Hammer toe*).

## Toenail, ingrown
See *Ingrown toenail*.

## Toilet-training
The process of teaching a young child to acquire complete bowel and bladder control and make appropriate use of toilet facilities.

### WHEN TO START
There is no reason to start toilet-training until the child's nervous system is sufficiently mature. Up to the age of about 18 months, emptying of the bladder and bowel is a totally automatic reaction. The child is not yet able to connect the actions of defecation and urination with their results, and does not have the ability to control these actions at will.

At around 18 months, a child is able to indicate that he or she has passed urine or a bowel movement, but is not yet aware that he or she is about to do so. At this stage, the child is not quite ready to use the potty, but he or she should become familiar with it, be told what it is for, and practice sitting on it. Around the second birthday, the child becomes aware that he or she is about to pass urine or a bowel movement, and says so. At this stage, the child is ready to start using the potty.

### USING THE POTTY AND TOILET
Toilet-training should be approached in a relaxed, unhurried manner. The child may rebel if the potty is introduced too early or if he or she is forced to sit on it. Boys initially urinate sitting on the potty but soon learn to urinate standing up.

When the child has gained proficiency using the potty, he or she should be introduced to the toilet. A useful intermediate step is to place the potty near the toilet. The child continues to use the potty for a while, but is taught to wipe with toilet paper and to flush the toilet. When reasonable control has been achieved, the child can be taken out of diapers during the day. However, diapers should continue to be worn at night until the child awakens dry most mornings.

Children vary in the age at which they become toilet-trained and more so in the age at which they are dry both by day and night. A child is unlikely to be completely toilet-trained or be able to empty the bladder on demand before the third birthday. Accidents are common up to age 5, particularly wetting, because a young child can hold on for only several minutes after the urge to urinate starts. Also, children who are toilet-trained may revert to soiling or wetting when anxious or under stress. (See also *Encopresis*; *Enuresis*; *Soiling*.)

## Tolazamide
An oral hypoglycemic drug (see *Hypoglycemics, oral*) used to treat non-insulin-dependent *diabetes mellitus*. Tolazamide has a mild diuretic action and is therefore useful in treating people with diabetes who have a tendency to retain water.

## Tolbutamide
An oral hypoglycemic drug (see *Hypoglycemics, oral*).

## Tolerance
The need to take increasingly higher doses of a *drug* to continue producing the same physical or mental effect. Tolerance develops as the result of taking a drug over a period of time and is usually caused either by the liver becoming more efficient at breaking down the drug or by the body tissues becoming less sensitive to it. The most familiar example of tolerance occurs in heavy drinkers who become so tolerant of *alcohol* that they are capable of drinking amounts that would render occasional drinkers unconscious. (See also *Alcohol dependence*; *Drug dependence*.)

## Tolmetin
A *nonsteroidal anti-inflammatory drug* (NSAID) used to relieve pain, stiffness, and inflammation in *osteoarthritis*, *rheumatoid arthritis*, and *ankylosing spondylitis*. Tolmetin is also given to treat pain caused by minor injuries, such as a ligament *sprain*.

## Tolnaftate
An *antifungal drug* used to treat and sometimes prevent the recurrence of types of *tinea*, including *athlete's foot*. Tolnaftate, which is available over-the-counter as a cream, powder, or aerosol, may in rare cases cause skin irritation or rash.

## Tomography
An *X-ray* technique that produces a cross-sectional image ("slice") of an organ or part of the body. In tomography, the X-ray camera and film are positioned so that tissue is in focus at one depth only. All background and foreground structures appear blurred.

By taking a series of tomograms it is possible to build an outline image of a part of the body that, on an ordinary X-ray film, would be hidden by other structures. For example, tomography is often used during intravenous *pyelography* to obtain a clear outline of the kidneys (when they would otherwise be obscured by gas or fecal matter in the intestines).

Most tomography today is performed using computerized techniques (see *CT scanning*), which produce extremely accurate, highly detailed pictures.

## -tomy
A suffix denoting the operation of cutting or making an incision, as in thoracotomy, a surgical operation in which the thorax (chest) is opened.

T

## Tone, muscle

The natural tension in the fibers of a muscle. At rest, all muscle fibers are maintained in a state of partial contraction by nerve impulses from the spinal cord. This resting muscle tone helps control posture, keeps the eyes open, and allows muscles to contract more efficiently.

Abnormally high muscle tone causes *spasticity*, rigidity, and an increased resistance to movement. Abnormally low muscle tone causes floppiness of the body part.

## Tongue

A muscular, flexible organ that occupies the floor of the mouth.

### STRUCTURE AND FUNCTION

The tongue is composed of a mass of muscles covered by mucous membrane. These muscles are attached to the mandible (lower jaw) and to the hyoid bone above the larynx. Minute nodules called papillae project from the upper surface of the tongue, giving it a rough texture. Situated between the papillae at the sides and base of the tongue are minute sensory organs called taste buds, which are responsible for the sense of *taste*.

Apart from being an organ of taste, the tongue is essential for breaking down food (see *Mastication*), *swallowing*, and *speech*.

---

### ANATOMY OF THE TONGUE

The tongue consists mainly of muscle; on its surface, it has various types of papillae that contain the taste buds.

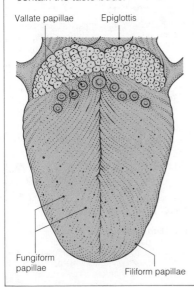

Vallate papillae    Epiglottis

Fungiform papillae

Filiform papillae

---

### DISORDERS

A large tongue is a feature of *Down's syndrome*, *cretinism*, and *acromegaly*. Temporary swelling occurs in *glossitis*.

Fissures on the tongue are common and usually cause no trouble, but in some cases they are so deep that food particles collect in them, causing discomfort. Unnatural smoothness of the tongue, accompanied by redness and soreness, is a feature of pernicious anemia (See *Anemia, megaloblastic*), iron-deficiency anemia (see *Anemia, iron-deficiency*), *syphilis*, and *glossitis*.

In rare cases, the papillae on the tongue become elongated and turn black or brown, a condition known as black tongue. The disorder, of which the cause is unknown, is harmless but persistent. The unsightly discoloration can be removed by cleaning the tongue twice a day with a toothbrush dipped in an antiseptic mouthwash.

The tongue can be a site for *mouth ulcers* and *leukoplakia* (thickened white or gray patches), a condition that occasionally becomes cancerous (see *Tongue cancer*). Any ulcer or lump on the tongue that does not disappear within about three weeks should be reported to a physician because of the risk of cancer.

## Tongue cancer

The most serious type of *mouth cancer* because of its rapid spread. Tongue cancer is one of the two most common types of mouth cancer (the other being *lip cancer*). It primarily affects people over 40. It is usually associated with tobacco smoking and heavy consumption of alcohol; poor oral hygiene is a contributing factor.

### SYMPTOMS AND SIGNS

The edge of the tongue is most commonly affected. The first sign may be a small ulcer with a raised margin, a white patch of thickened tissue known as *leukoplakia*, a deep fissure with hard edges, or a raised, hardened mass. Pain is rare until the cancer is advanced, when there is also excessive salivation, stiffness of the tongue, difficulty swallowing, and sometimes offensive breath.

The tumor may become very large, obstructing the throat and occasionally causing asphyxia. It spreads rapidly, to any or all of the following: the gums, the lower jaw, and the lymph nodes in the floor of the mouth and the neck.

### DIAGNOSIS AND TREATMENT

Any physical change in the tongue that does not clear up within two or three weeks should be reported to a

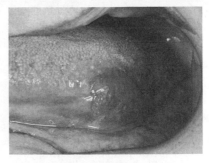

**Appearance of tongue cancer**
The cancer often starts at the edge of the tongue. It may appear (as here) as a raised mass or as a fissure or an ulcer.

physician. Cancer is diagnosed by means of a tongue *biopsy* (removal of a small sample of tissue for microscopic examination).

Small tumors, especially those at the tip of the tongue, are usually removed surgically. Larger tumors or tumors that have spread often require *radiation therapy*. If a tumor is very large and has spread to lymph nodes, the whole tongue, the lymph nodes, and sometimes the lower jaw must be removed. The disease may also be treated with *anticancer drugs*.

### OUTLOOK

Unless the cancer is detected very early, its spread makes the outlook poor. In about half of all sufferers, the lymph nodes are involved by the time of diagnosis. About half of affected women but only a quarter of men survive for five years or more.

## Tongue depressor

A flat wooden or metal instrument for holding down the tongue against the floor of the mouth to allow examination of the back of the throat.

## Tongue-tie

A minor defect of the mouth, also called ankyloglossia, in which the frenulum (band of tissue attaching the underside of the tongue to the floor of the mouth) is too short and extends forward to the tip of the tongue. There are usually no symptoms other than limited movement of the tongue. In rare cases, the condition causes a speech defect, in which case a minor operation is required to divide the frenulum.

## Tonic

One of a diverse group of remedies intended to relieve symptoms such as malaise, lethargy, and loss of appetite. Most tonics contain herbal extracts, vitamins, and minerals. Medical evidence suggests that tonics mainly have a *placebo* effect.

## Tonometry

The procedure for measuring the pressure of the fluid within the eye. A rise in intraocular pressure is one of the signs of *glaucoma*. Tonometry is usually performed by an *ophthalmologist* during an eye examination.

### HOW IT IS DONE

One method of measuring the pressure in the eye is called applanation tonometry. The ophthalmologist applies a drop of quick-acting anesthetic and a trace of *fluorescein* to each cornea; he or she then measures the pressure within the eye by means of a tonometer (measuring device) mounted on a *slit lamp* (light source with a magnifying viewer). The head of the tonometer is illuminated and touched gently against the anesthetized cornea. A visible circle of fluorescein-stained tear film is formed, which the ophthalmologist views through the slit-lamp microscope. The force with which the tonometer head is pressed against the cornea is gradually increased until the area of the circle reaches a fixed standard. The force needed to achieve this degree of corneal flattening, which is read off from a calibrated knob on the tonometer, is a measure of the pressure within the eye. (See also *Eye, examination of*.)

## Tonsil

A pair of oval masses at the back of the throat. The tonsils are made up of lymphatic tissue and form part of the *lymphatic system*, which is an important part of the body's defense against infection. Along with the adenoids at the base of the tongue, the tonsils protect against upper respiratory tract infections. The tonsils gradually enlarge from birth, reach their maximum size at about age 7, and then shrink substantially.

*Tonsillitis* (inflammation of the tonsils) is a common childhood infection. Rarely, *quinsy* (an abscess on the tonsil) may develop as a complication.

## Tonsillectomy

Surgical removal of the tonsils.

### WHY IT IS DONE

Tonsillectomy was once a common childhood operation; it is now performed only if a child suffers frequent recurrent attacks of severe *tonsillitis*. Less common problems that may necessitate the operation are *quinsy*

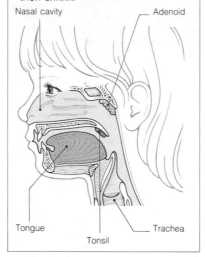

**LOCATION OF THE TONSILS**
The tonsils can be easily seen on either side of the back of the throat. They reach maximum size around the age of 7 years and then shrink.

Nasal cavity — Adenoid
Tongue — Tonsil — Trachea

(an abscess on the tonsil) or a single tonsil considered malignant because it is growing larger or is deeply ulcerated. In rare cases, removal of the tonsils may be advised for adolescents or young adults suffering from recurrent bouts of tonsillitis.

### HOW IT IS DONE

The operative technique is shown in the illustration at right.

### RECOVERY PERIOD

In the first 24 hours after the operation there may be bleeding from the throat; the patient must lie on his or her side to avoid choking. Postoperative pain in the throat and sometimes the ears is common and may require an analgesic (painkiller). Fluids and soft, easily digestible foods such as ice cream are usually given for a day or two until the patient can eat normally.

Sore throat, particularly at mealtimes, may persist for up to two weeks after the operation. Full recovery usually takes place within three weeks. In some people, late bleeding occurs, requiring examination.

## Tonsillitis

Inflammation of the tonsils due to infection. Tonsillitis mainly occurs in childhood, with most children suffering at least one attack.

### CAUSES AND INCIDENCE

The function of the tonsils is to help protect the upper respiratory tract against infection. However, some-

times the tonsils themselves become repeatedly infected by the microorganisms they fight. Tonsillitis is most common in children under 9; it infrequently occurs in adolescents and young adults.

### SYMPTOMS AND SIGNS

The main symptoms are a sore throat and difficulty swallowing (very young children may refuse to eat). The throat is visibly inflamed. Other common symptoms are fever, headache, earache, enlarged and tender glands in the neck, and unpleasant-smelling breath. Occasionally, the illness causes temporary deafness or *quinsy* (an abscess on the tonsil). If symptoms persist for more than 24 hours or if pus can be seen on the tonsils, a physician should be consulted.

### TREATMENT

The illness is treated with bed rest, plenty of fluids, and an *analgesic drug* (painkiller), such as acetaminophen. In some cases, *antibiotic drugs* may also be prescribed.

## Tooth abscess

See *Abscess, dental*.

## Toothache

Pain coming from one tooth, or from the teeth and gums generally. The pain may be felt either as a dull throb or a sharp twinge.

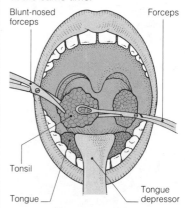

**PROCEDURE FOR TONSILLECTOMY**
Tonsillectomy is most commonly carried out around the age of 6 or 7. The adenoids may be removed at the same time.

Blunt-nosed forceps — Forceps
Tonsil
Tongue — Tongue depressor

**Standard technique**
With the patient under a general anesthetic, the tongue is depressed and the tonsils pried from the back of the throat and then cut away.

## CAUSES

Early dental *caries* (decay) may cause mild toothache when eating sweet or very hot or cold food. More advanced decay or, less commonly, a fracture in a tooth (see *Fracture, dental*) or a deep, unlined filling (see *Filling, dental*) may result in inflammation of the pulp. This usually causes sharp, stabbing pain, which is often worse when lying down. It is often difficult for the sufferer to locate the painful tooth.

If the inflammation spreads, periapical *periodontitis* (inflammation of supporting tissues around the root tip) may develop, causing localized pain that is brought on mainly by biting and chewing. A dental abscess (see *Abscess, dental*) may also occur. In this case, pain is severe and often continuous, the gum surrounding the affected tooth is tender and swollen, and there may be swelling of the face and neck accompanied by fever.

Chronic periodontitis (inflammation of all the supporting tissues), which causes the gums to recede, results in aching around exposed tooth roots when hot, cold, or sweet food is eaten. Gums around the affected teeth are tender and swollen.

A filling that is not quite level or a blow to a tooth may also result in inflammation of supporting tissues, causing pain when biting.

Sometimes toothache is not caused by a disorder of the teeth or gums. For example, in *sinusitis* (inflammation of the mucous membrane lining the facial air cavities) pain may be referred to the upper molar and premolar teeth (see *Referred pain*).

## TREATMENT

*Analgesic drugs* (painkillers) may provide temporary relief until a visit to the dentist can be arranged. An emergency appointment should be made if the symptoms suggest there is an abscess. The treatment carried out by the dentist depends on the underlying cause.

## Toothbrushing

Cleaning of the teeth with a special type of brush to remove plaque and food particles from tooth surfaces. Toothbrushing should be carried out at least once a day using a fluoride *dentifrice* (usually toothpaste); children should brush their teeth after every meal and at bedtime. For complete *oral hygiene*, flossing (see *Floss, dental*) should be performed daily.

A safe and effective toothbrush for general use has an easily gripped handle and soft, round-ended or

### BASIC TOOTHBRUSHING

Efficient toothbrushing is essential for the preservation of the teeth and the health of the gums. The enemy is plaque, a mixture of food debris, dried saliva, and bacteria, which develops at the gum margins and leads to caries (tooth decay) and gum disease.

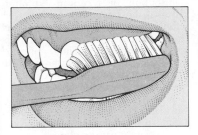

**1** With the bristle tips set at 45 degrees to the plane of the teeth, scrub gently along the gum line using ¼-inch strokes. The bristle tips should do the work.

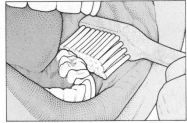

**2** Keep the bristles angled against the line of the gums and work over the outer and inner surfaces of the upper and lower teeth. Keep the strokes short.

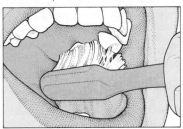

**3** Don't forget to scrub over the chewing surfaces of all four sets of premolar and molar teeth. Move slowly over the surfaces, cleaning each tooth in turn.

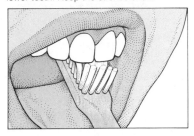

**4** Remember to brush the inside surfaces of the front teeth. Hold the brush almost vertical and scrub with an up-and-down movement.

polished bristles. The size and shape must allow every tooth to be reached; children need a smaller toothbrush than adults. Toothbrushes should be rinsed after each use and replaced when the bristles become frayed or bent. Interspace brushes, which have small, round heads, may be useful for cleaning around *bridges* and fixed *orthodontic appliances*. Electric toothbrushes are also available and may make brushing easier for people with some physical disabilities.

## Tooth decay
See *Caries, dental*.

## Tooth extraction
See *Extraction, dental*.

## Toothpaste
See *Dentifrice*.

## Tophus
A collection of *uric acid* crystals deposited in the tissues, especially around joints (such as the elbow) but occasionally in other places (such as the ear). A tophus is a sign of *hyperuricemia*, which accompanies *gout*. Tophi may occasionally ulcerate and discharge chalky white material.

## Topical
A term describing a *drug* that is applied to the surface of the body, as opposed to being swallowed or injected. Topical refers not only to drugs applied to the skin, but also to those administered into the ear canal, onto the surface of the eye, or as suppositories into the vagina or rectum.

## Torsion
A term that means twisting. Almost any structure that is relatively free to move in the body may become twisted, such as the intestine (see *Volvulus*), the spermatic cord from the testis (see *Testis, torsion of*), or a cyst on a stalk. One of the principal dangers of torsion is obstruction of the blood supply to the affected part; if this occurs, pain is usually the first symptom. If the torsion is not corrected, tissue death may develop.

**T**

## Torticollis

Twisting of the neck, causing the head to be rotated and tilted into an abnormal position. Also known as wry neck, torticollis is often accompanied by pain and stiffness in the neck.

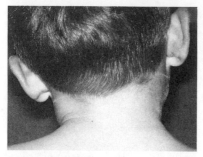

**Child with torticollis**
The muscles on one side of the neck have gone into spasm, pulling the head over to that side and causing pain.

#### CAUSES

The condition usually results from a minor neck injury that causes irritation of cervical nerves and consequent spasm of neck muscles. Torticollis may also result from muscle spasm caused by sleeping in an awkward position or by anxiety. Injury to a neck muscle at birth can also cause torticollis, as can a burn or other injury that has resulted in heavy scarring and shrinkage of the skin.

#### TREATMENT

Treatment for torticollis due to muscle spasm may include wearing an orthopedic *collar, heat treatment, ultrasound treatment,* or *physical therapy.* When the cause is birth injury, the muscle is gently stretched several times each day; occasionally, an operation is required to cut the lower end of the muscle. Skin contracture may be treated by *Z-plasty,* which relieves tension in the scar tissue.

## Touch

The sense by which certain characteristics of objects, such as their size, shape, temperature, and surface texture, can be ascertained through physical contact.

Many types of touch receptors are present in the skin. In hairy skin areas, some of the receptors consist of webs of sensory nerve cell endings wrapped around the hair bulbs. They are triggered if the hairs are moved. Other receptors are more common in nonhairy areas, such as lips and fingertips, and consist of nerve cell endings that may be free (i.e., naked) or surrounded by bulblike structures.

Signals from touch receptors pass, via sensory nerves, to the spinal cord, from there to the thalamus in the brain, and on to the *sensory cortex,* where touch sensations are perceived.

According to the number and distribution of receptors, different parts of the body vary in their sensitivity to painful stimuli and in touch discrimination (the ability to distinguish between a single pinprick and two pinpricks placed slightly apart). For example, the cornea is several hundred times more sensitive to painful stimuli than are the soles of the feet. The fingertips are good at touch discrimination but relatively insensitive to painful stimuli.

Touch sense becomes much more developed in people deprived of other senses, particularly blind people; it is this capacity for touch development that is used by systems such as braille. (See also *Sensation.*)

## Tourette's syndrome

See *Gilles de la Tourette's syndrome.*

## Tourniquet

A device placed around a limb to compress blood vessels. A tourniquet may be used to help locate a vein for an intravenous injection or withdrawal of blood. By preventing blood from flowing back to the heart, a tourniquet causes veins in the limb below it to swell and become more prominent.

An inflatable tourniquet, called *Esmarch's bandage,* is used to control blood flow in some limb operations. An inflatable tourniquet also forms part of a *sphygmomanometer,* an instrument for measuring *blood pressure.*

Tourniquets have caused more problems than they have solved. In the past, they were used as a first-aid measure to stop severe bleeding. This use is now discouraged because leaving a tourniquet in place for too long can cause *gangrene* (tissue death). First-aid courses now teach the control of bleeding by pressure over the bleeding site (see *Pressure points*). It is usually effective and safer.

## Toxemia

The presence in the bloodstream of toxins (poisons) produced by bacteria. Toxemia may be a feature of *septicemia* (the spread and multiplication of bacteria within the bloodstream from a localized site of infection), but it can also occur without any evidence of bacteria in the blood. Toxemia with or without septicemia is sometimes called blood poisoning.

Toxemia may cause symptoms such as a fever and headache and other symptoms specific to the particular toxin (e.g., muscle spasms caused by the toxin released by *tetanus* bacteria). Toxemia can lead to the highly dangerous condition of *septic shock,* in which there is widespread tissue damage and a drop in blood pressure.

Treatment of toxemia is as for septicemia and septic shock—*antibiotic drugs,* removal of a localized site of infection if one can be found, and measures to treat shock, including *intravenous infusions.* For some types of toxemia, an *antitoxin* may be given.

Toxemia of pregnancy, or *preeclampsia,* has some features common to other forms of toxemia, but no toxin has ever been identified. (See also *Toxic shock syndrome.*)

## Toxemia of pregnancy

A disorder of pregnant women characterized by raised blood pressure, tissue swelling, and leakage of protein from the kidneys into the urine (see *Preeclampsia*). If severe, toxemia of pregnancy may progress to seizures and coma (see *Eclampsia*).

## Toxicity

The property of being poisonous. The term is also used to refer to the severity of adverse effects or illness produced by a *toxin* (a poisonous protein produced by certain bacteria, animals, or plants), by a *poison,* or by a drug overdose (see *Drug poisoning*).

## Toxicology

The study of *poisons,* including their chemical composition, preparation, identification, effects on the body, and antidotes. (See also *Poisoning.*)

## Toxic shock syndrome

An uncommon condition linked with the use of certain brands of highly absorbent tampons. Toxic shock syndrome was first recognized in the late 1970s and many cases were diagnosed in young women in the early 1980s. About 70 percent of cases occur in women who are using tampons at the time of onset.

#### CAUSE

Toxic shock syndrome is caused by a *toxin* produced by the bacterium STAPHYLOCOCCUS AUREUS. Overgrowth of this bacterium in the vagina and increased production of the toxin have been associated with prolonged use of certain brands of highly absorbent tampons (now taken off the market).

# THE SENSE OF TOUCH

The skin contains many thousands of specialized cells that respond to external stimuli, such as touch, heat, cold, and pressure. These cells (receptors) are divided into two types. One type of receptor consists only of a thin nerve fiber, which may wrap around an individual hair and respond to its movement. The other type has a specialized structure, known as an end organ, surrounding the nerve ending. Some skin receptors consist of several layers of cells attached to one nerve fiber. Others contain several nerve fibers arranged in a loop or coil. Probably several varieties of receptors play a part in each touch modality.

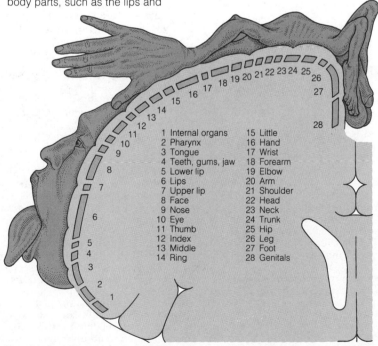

Merkel's disk

Meissner's corpuscle

Dermis

Free nerve endings

Epidermis

Organ of Ruffini

Pacinian corpuscle

## Skin receptors

These receptors vary from free nerve endings to corpuscular or bulblike structures. Individual receptors do not seem to be associated exclusively with any one sensation (e.g., cold or pain).

### Delicate touch
The ability to detect light contact between an object and the skin. Areas with more receptors are more sensitive.

### Pain
Pain warns the brain about possible injury from an external stimulus and can trigger a reflex withdrawal.

### Heat
Some free nerve endings respond specifically to heat. The skin of the wrist is good for testing temperature.

### Cold
Cold on the skin is detected by specialized end organs. Extreme cold also stimulates pain receptors.

### Pressure
A change in pressure on the skin is detected by specialized end organs called pacinian corpuscles.

## TOUCH PERCEPTION

General sensations from various parts of the body are perceived at specific points within the brain's cerebral cortex. Highly sensitive body parts, such as the lips and hands, are represented by correspondingly large regions within the cortex.

1 Internal organs
2 Pharynx
3 Tongue
4 Teeth, gums, jaw
5 Lower lip
6 Lips
7 Upper lip
8 Face
9 Nose
10 Eye
11 Thumb
12 Index
13 Middle
14 Ring

15 Little
16 Hand
17 Wrist
18 Forearm
19 Elbow
20 Arm
21 Shoulder
22 Head
23 Neck
24 Trunk
25 Hip
26 Leg
27 Foot
28 Genitals

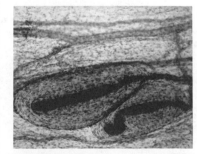

## Pacinian corpuscle
These receptors are 1 mm to 4 mm long and occur in nonhairy areas of skin, especially the fingers.

T

Of the cases that do not occur in association with menstruation, some have been linked to use of a contraceptive cap, diaphragm, or sponge. Other cases arise from skin wounds or infections caused by *s. AUREUS* elsewhere in the body.

### SYMPTOMS
The onset of toxic shock syndrome is sudden, with high fever, vomiting, diarrhea, headache, muscular aches and pains, dizziness, and disorientation. A skin rash resembling sunburn develops on the palms and soles, and peels within one or two weeks. The blood pressure may fall dangerously low, and *shock* may develop. Other serious complications include *renal failure* and *liver failure*. The mortality is about 3 percent, usually due to a prolonged fall in blood pressure or to lung complications.

### TREATMENT
Treatment is with *antibiotic drugs*. *Intravenous infusion* may be necessary to treat shock, and more treatment may be needed for complications.

Recurrence is common; women who have had toxic shock syndrome are advised not to use tampons, caps, diaphragms, or sponges.

## Toxin
A poisonous protein produced by pathogenic (disease-causing) bacteria, such as *CLOSTRIDIUM TETANI*, which causes *tetanus*; various animals, notably venomous snakes (see *Snakebites*); or certain plants, such as the death cap mushroom *AMANITA PHALLOIDES* (see *Mushroom poisoning*).

Bacterial toxins are sometimes subdivided into *endotoxins*, which are released only from the inside of dead bacteria; *exotoxins*, which are released from the surface of live bacteria; and *enterotoxins*, which inflame the intestine. (See also *Poison; Poisoning*.)

## Toxocariasis

An infestation of humans, usually children, with the larvae of *TOXOCARA CANIS*, a small, threadlike worm that lives in the intestines of dogs. The disease is also known as visceral larva migrans.

### CAUSES AND INCIDENCE
The causes and course of an infestation are shown in the illustrated box above right.

### PREVENTION
Dogs that live with children should be dewormed—monthly if they are less than 6 months old, when infestation is more likely.

### ORIGINS OF TOXOCARIASIS

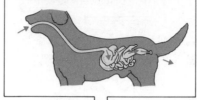

**1** A dog (often a puppy) harboring the small roundworm *TOXOCARA CANIS* in its digestive tract passes large numbers of worm eggs in its feces, which may contaminate soil.

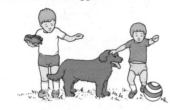

**2** Children who play with an infested dog, or with soil contaminated with dog feces, and who then put their fingers in their mouths, may swallow some of the worm eggs.

**3** The swallowed eggs hatch in the intestines to liberate larvae, which migrate through the tissues to organs such as the liver, lungs, brain, and eyes. They provoke allergic phenomena such as asthma and may have serious effects, such as loss of vision.

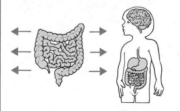

### SYMPTOMS AND SIGNS
Usually, infestation causes only mild fever and malaise, which soon clears up. However, following some cases of heavy infestation, *pneumonia* and *seizures* may develop. Another possible complication is loss of vision caused by a larva entering the eye and dying there.

### DIAGNOSIS AND TREATMENT
Toxocariasis is diagnosed from sputum (phlegm) analysis, and by a *liver biopsy* (removal of a small sample of the organ for analysis).

Severe cases of toxocariasis require treatment in the hospital, where the patient may be given the *antihelmintic drug* thiabendazole (to control the infestation) and an *anticonvulsant drug* (to control seizures).

## Toxoid
An inactivated bacterial *toxin* (poisonous protein). Inactivation, usually by heat or chemicals, removes the toxicity of the toxin but preserves its property of stimulating antibody production by the *immune system*. Certain toxoids are used to immunize against specific diseases, such as *diphtheria* or *tetanus*.

## Toxoplasmosis

An infection of mammals, birds, and reptiles that is also common in humans. Toxoplasmosis usually produces no ill effects except when transmitted by a woman to her unborn child or in people with an immunodeficiency disorder.

### CAUSES AND INCIDENCE
The infection is caused by the protozoan (single-celled microorganism) *TOXOPLASMA GONDII*. Humans are most commonly infected by eating undercooked meat from infected animals. An estimated 25 percent of pork and 10 percent of lamb eaten by humans contains toxoplasma organisms. In addition, the protozoa multiply in the intestines of cats, and about 1 percent of cats excrete cysts containing toxoplasma eggs in the feces. Infection in humans can occur through failure to wash the hands after handling the cat or its feces.

Toxoplasmosis contracted by a woman during pregnancy is transmitted to the child in about one third of cases, often with severe effects.

Infection is extremely common worldwide. In some areas of the US, *blood tests* show that about half the population have been infected.

### SYMPTOMS AND SIGNS
In most cases, the body's *immune system* provides adequate protection against the protozoa, so that the infection produces no symptoms. In some people with a normal immune system, however, the infection causes a feverish illness resembling infectious *mononucleosis*. It may also cause retinitis (inflammation of the retina) and *choroiditis* (inflammation of the blood vessels behind the retina).

Infection of an unborn child during early pregnancy may result in miscarriage or stillbirth. Infants may have

T

enlargement of the liver and spleen, *hydrocephalus*, blindness, mental retardation, and may die during infancy. Infection in late pregnancy usually has no ill effects.

Toxoplasmosis may also take a severe course in people with an immune system deficiency (such as *AIDS*), causing lung and heart damage and severe *encephalitis* (brain inflammation).

**DIAGNOSIS AND TREATMENT**

The diagnosis is made from blood tests. Treatment is necessary only in pregnant women, in children born with severe symptoms, in people with an immune system deficiency, and in cases of retinitis or choroiditis. Treatment is usually with the antimalarial drug *pyrimethamine* combined with a *sulfonamide drug*.

## TPA

The abbreviation for *tissue-plasminogen activator*.

## Trabeculectomy

A surgical procedure performed to reduce pressure in the eye. Trabeculectomy is used to control *glaucoma* when medication cannot keep the intraocular pressure within safe limits or when, despite medical treatment, visual field loss and optic nerve damage are progressing.

The procedure provides an alternative outlet route from the eye for aqueous humor (eye fluid) so that a better balance is achieved between the rate of secretion of aqueous humor and its rate of outflow. In this way, the pressure can be kept within normal limits and further damage to the optic nerve fibers prevented.

**HOW IT IS DONE**

The *conjunctiva* (mucous membrane covering the front of the eyeball) above the upper edge of the *cornea* is opened and a half-thickness flap of *sclera* (white part of the eye) is cut and folded forward. A small block is removed from the inner half near the scleral-corneal junction so that a connection is made into the front chamber of the eye. The outer flap is replaced and secured with a few delicate stitches and the conjunctiva is closed over it.

## Trace elements

A group of minerals that is required only in minute amounts in the diet to maintain health. The principal trace elements include *chromium*, *copper*, *selenium*, *sulfur*, and *zinc*. Although tiny amounts of these substances are needed, they are vital to numerous chemical processes in the body. (See also *Nutrition*.)

## Tracer

A radioactive substance introduced into the body so that its distribution, processing, and elimination from the body can be followed (by using a radiation detector). Radioactive iodine may be used as a tracer to study the functioning of the thyroid gland.

## Trachea

The anatomical name for the windpipe. The trachea begins immediately below the larynx (voice box) and runs down the center of the front of the neck to end behind the upper part of the sternum (breastbone), where it divides to form the two main bronchi.

The trachea consists of fibrous and elastic tissue and smooth muscle. It also contains about 20 rings of cartilage, which help keep the trachea open even during extremes of neck movement. The lining of the trachea includes cells that secrete mucus (called goblet cells) and other cells that bear minute, hairlike cilia. The mucus helps trap tiny particles in inhaled air; the beating of the cilia moves the mucus upward and out of the respiratory tract, thereby helping to keep the lungs and airways free.

**DISORDERS**

One of the most common disorders is *tracheitis* (inflammation of the lining of the trachea), which is usually caused by an infection (often by a virus) and is frequently associated with *bronchitis* or *laryngitis*. The principal symptoms are difficult, painful breathing and a harsh cough.

Obstruction of the trachea by an inhaled foreign object is rare because the narrowest part of the upper respiratory tract is the larynx, and any objects that pass through it usually continue through the trachea into a bronchus. However, the trachea may become obstructed by a tumor or narrowed as a result of scarring caused by the prolonged presence of a *tracheostomy* tube inserted to create an artificial airway through the front of the neck. Tracheal obstruction produces breathlessness and a loud, harsh, vibrating sound during breathing.

Rarely, a congenital malformation occurs in which a channel forms between the trachea and the esophagus, situated immediately behind it (a condition called a *tracheoesophageal fistula*).

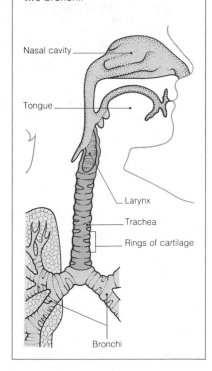

**LOCATION OF THE TRACHEA**
The trachea extends down from the larynx for 4.5 inches to the point where it divides into the two bronchi.

Nasal cavity

Tongue

Larynx

Trachea

Rings of cartilage

Bronchi

The trachea is sometimes injured by a direct blow or by strangulation. The seriousness of such an injury depends on the extent to which the airway is obstructed. In extreme cases, the trachea may collapse completely, which may be rapidly fatal unless an emergency tracheostomy is performed to reestablish an airway.

## Tracheitis

Inflammation of the *trachea* (the windpipe). Tracheitis is usually caused by viral infection and aggravated by inhaled fumes, especially tobacco smoke. It often occurs with *laryngitis* and *bronchitis*, a condition known as laryngotracheobronchitis, which is the most common cause of *croup* in young children.

Typical symptoms of tracheitis include dry cough and hoarseness. In most cases, the condition is short-lived and requires no treatment.

## Tracheoesophageal fistula

A rare *birth defect* in which there is an abnormal passage that connects the trachea (windpipe) and the

**T**

esophagus. About three babies per 10,000 are born with a tracheoesophageal fistula. In the most common form, the lower end of the esophagus connects with the trachea; the upper end is underdeveloped, forming a blind-ending pouch.

### SYMPTOMS AND SIGNS
The affected baby cannot swallow saliva, and thus drools constantly. During feeding, food is regurgitated and enters the lungs, causing the baby to choke, cough, and sometimes turn blue because of lack of oxygen. The abdomen becomes distended because inhaled air passes into the stomach through the fistula. The acidic fluid in the stomach passes up into the lungs through the fistula, causing *pneumonia* and *atelectasis* (lung collapse).

### DIAGNOSIS AND TREATMENT
In most cases the condition is discovered soon after birth. Milder forms of tracheoesophageal fistula may not be detected until childhood or even adult life, usually after recurrent attacks of pneumonia. The diagnosis is confirmed by *chest X ray*.

Treatment consists of an operation to close the fistula and connect the trachea and esophagus correctly. Before the 1940s, the condition was untreatable; today the survival rate is about 90 percent.

## Tracheostomy
An operation in which an opening is made in the trachea (windpipe) and a tube is inserted to maintain an effective airway.

### WHY IT IS DONE
Tracheostomy may be performed to treat an emergency or as a planned procedure. Today, acute airway problems are usually handled by an *endotracheal tube* passed via the mouth or nose. However, when the problem (such as a tumor or foreign body) involves the larynx, a tracheostomy is preferable in an emergency.

A planned tracheostomy is most frequently carried out on a person who has lost the ability to breathe naturally and is undergoing long-term *ventilation* (the pumping of air into the lungs by a machine) or who has lost the ability to keep oral and pharyngeal secretions out of the windpipe because of coma or a specific swallowing problem. For this purpose, tracheostomy is performed after passing an endotracheal tube through the nose or mouth and into the trachea. Permanent tracheostomy is necessary after *laryngectomy* (removal of the larynx).

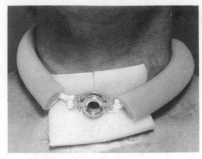

**Tracheostomy tube**
The tube readily becomes blocked by bronchial secretions; it has a metal inner lining removable for cleaning.

### HOW IT IS DONE
The operation is carried out using a local or a general anesthetic.

An incision is made in the skin overlying the trachea, between the Adam's apple and the clavicles (collarbones), the neck muscles are pulled apart, and the thyroid gland, which surrounds the trachea, is usually severed. A small vertical incision (called a "window") is made in the trachea and, in the case of laryngectomy, the cut edges of the trachea are brought forward and stitched to the edges of the skin wound. A metal or plastic tube is then inserted. If the patient cannot breathe unaided, the tube is connected to a ventilator.

### RECOVERY PERIOD
For patients able to breathe unaided, the air in the room is humidified to reduce drying of mucus in the airway. Air from a ventilator is humidified before it passes into the tube. Any excessive mucus that accumulates in the airway is sucked away through a catheter inserted into the tube.

While the tube is in place, the patient is usually unable to speak; he or she is provided with a bell or buzzer and pen and paper for communication. After laryngectomy, the tube is removed after several days; a permanent opening remains. In other cases, the tube is removed when the patient has recovered from the condition that necessitated the operation, and the opening soon closes and heals.

## Tracheotomy
Cutting of an airway into the trachea. (See also *Tracheostomy*.)

## Trachoma
A persistent infectious disease of the *conjunctiva* and *cornea*. Trachoma is caused by an organism, CHLAMYDIA TRACHOMATIS, that is spread by direct contact and possibly by flies (see *Chlamydial infections*). Untreated trachoma leads to complications that may cause blindness.

### SYMPTOMS AND SIGNS
Infection by C. TRACHOMATIS causes acute *conjunctivitis*, with pain, *photophobia*, and watering of the eyes. The eyes become red and inflamed and the conjunctiva that lines the lids becomes thickened and roughened with scar tissue and is studded with small lumps called follicles. Damage to the mucus-secreting cells of the conjunctiva and to the lacrimal (tear-producing) glands may lead to *keratoconjunctivitis sicca* (dry eye).

An abnormal growth of blood vessels can extend down from the conjunctiva into the upper part of the cornea, leading to opacity (loss of transparency) and loss of vision. More severe damage to the cornea occurs later when fibrous scarring of the inside of the upper lid causes it to be rolled inward so that the lashes rub against the cornea, causing ulceration and encouraging secondary bacterial infection. The secondary bacterial infection may lead to extensive ulceration, scarring, and even perforation, with spread of infection into the eye and permanent loss of vision.

### TREATMENT
Trachoma is treated in the early stages to attempt to eradicate the causative organism, which is sensitive to various *antibiotic drugs* applied to the eye. Antibiotic drugs taken by mouth are also used. Established trachoma with scarring is much more difficult to manage; treatment may involve surgical correction of lid deformities and corneal grafting to restore transparency and vision.

## Tract
A group of organs that forms a common pathway to perform a particular function. For example, the urinary tract comprises the kidneys, ureters, bladder, and urethra, which together form a series of connected structures for the removal of waste products from the body.

The term tract also refers specifically to a bundle of nerve fibers that have a common function, as in the pyramidal tract, which carries nerve impulses from the brain to the muscles.

## Traction
A procedure in which part of the body is placed under tension to correct the alignment of two adjoining structures or to hold them in position.

T

## TRACTION FOR FEMORAL FRACTURE

Because of the power of the thigh muscles and their tendency to go into spasm, fractures of the femur (thigh bone) tend to override.

Without traction to prevent this, the bone would heal with overlapping ends and the leg would be permanently shortened.

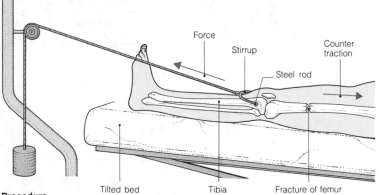

Force
Stirrup
Counter traction
Steel rod
Tilted bed
Tibia
Fracture of femur

**Procedure**
Traction is usually performed by means of a narrow steel rod through the upper end of the tibia (shin), to which a steel stirrup is attached so that a cord and weight can be used to apply the force. The other end of the femur must usually be immobilized, or countertraction applied, to keep the fractured bone ends aligned.

### WHY IT IS DONE
The most common use of traction is in the treatment of a *fracture* in which muscles around the bone ends are pulling the bones out of alignment. Fractures of the shaft of the *femur* (thigh bone) are most likely to be treated in this way. Traction is also used to align and immobilize unstable fractures of the cervical spine (the neck) when any movement of the vertebrae might injure the spinal cord (see *Spinal injury*).

### HOW IT IS DONE
To apply traction to a lower limb fracture, the person lies on a bed with the injured limb supported by attachments from an overhead frame. The upper end of the fractured bone is held immobilized while the lower end is pulled in a straight line away from it by a system of weights and pulleys. The traction grip is obtained by a pin inserted through the tibia (shin) or through a plaster cast applied to the limb. For spinal fractures, the patient lies flat on a firm surface and weights are attached to tongs inserted into holes drilled on either side of the skull. Both limb and spinal fractures are maintained in continuous traction until healing has occurred.

## Training
A program of *exercises* to prepare for a particular sport and improve technique. Training may be concentrated on improving skills (e.g., a golfer may practice putting) or on improving physical *fitness*.

Fitness training should include both *aerobic* and anaerobic exercises, which together build strength, flexibility, and endurance (the capacity to exercise for long periods).

Interval training is a type of fitness program in which a particular exercise, such as running a set distance at a timed pace, is repeated several times with a rest period between. Circuit training consists of performing a set number of different exercises, such as push-ups, sit-ups, and step-ups, one after the other.

The selection of an appropriate training program requires specialized assessment and advice. Self-imposed training schedules may be damaging to health; for example, bone and muscle disorders may develop in runners if their training is unsupervised.

## Trait
Any characteristic or condition determined by a *gene* or genes (i.e., inherited). Blue or brown eye color, dark or light skin, body proportions, and nose shape are all traits, reflecting the genetic variation among people.

The majority of common traits (such as eye color) have no obvious effect on health; others may have marginally advantageous effects in particular environments (such as dark skin in a sunny climate) or mildly disabling effects (such as color-vision deficiency). Severely handicapping traits, such as *cystic fibrosis* or *osteogenesis imperfecta*, are individually rare, but the fact that there are many different types means that they are collectively quite common (see *Genetic disorders*).

The term trait is also sometimes used in a more restricted sense to describe a mild form of a recessive genetic disorder. For example, a person who inherits the sickle cell gene in a single dose is said to have sickle cell trait. A double dose of the same gene causes the much more serious *sickle cell anemia*.

## Trance
A sleeplike state in which consciousness is reduced, voluntary actions are lessened or absent, and bodily functions are diminished. A trance usually results from separation of a group of mental processes from the rest of the mind rather than from any physical brain disturbance.

Trances are claimed to be induced by *hypnosis* and have been reported as part of a group experience, particularly in a religious context. Trances are sometimes a feature of *catalepsy*, *automatism*, and some forms of petitmal *epilepsy*.

## Tranquilizer drugs
Drugs with a sedative effect, subdivided into major tranquilizers (see *Antipsychotic drugs*) and minor tranquilizers (see *Antianxiety drugs*).

## Transcutaneous electrical nerve stimulation
A method of pain relief achieved by the application of minute electrical impulses to nerve endings that lie beneath the skin. Transcutaneous electrical nerve stimulation (TENS) seems to work by blocking pain messages to the brain by providing an alternative stimulus. TENS is carried out to relieve severe and persistent pain when it is not satisfactorily controlled by *analgesic drugs*.

### HOW IT IS DONE
A TENS unit provides electrical impulses to electrodes that are placed on the skin or sometimes surgically implanted. Adjustments of the unit can be made by the patient to achieve maximal relief.

### RISKS
TENS must not be used by anyone with a cardiac pacemaker; the electrical impulses from the transmitter may interfere with the pacemaker's action.

T

### OUTLOOK

TENS is beneficial in about 60 percent of the patients who use it. Pain relief in some people lasts only during stimulation; in others, pain relief persists after treatment.

## Transference

The unconscious displacement of emotions from important childhood figures, such as parents or siblings, to people in adult life. Transference is particularly important in *psychoanalysis*, in which the feelings the patient has toward the analyst are explored to show how such projected feelings affect other relationships.

## Transfusion

See *Blood transfusion*.

## Transfusion, autologous

The use of a person's own blood, donated on an earlier occasion, for *blood transfusion* during surgery. Autologous transfusion is used to avoid the risk that blood from another donor may transmit infection.

Autologous transfusions were first performed on a large scale in the early 1960s for certain major operations, and services continued to develop to some extent during the 1970s. Fear of *AIDS* during the 1980s created a demand for much greater availability and use of this technique.

### WHY IT IS DONE

Autologous transfusion eliminates the slight but serious risk of infecting a recipient with HIV (the AIDS virus) or *hepatitis* virus from contaminated blood. It also eliminates the risk of transmitting *cytomegalovirus*, *malaria*, and *syphilis*.

Another advantage of autologous transfusion is the reduced risk of a transfusion reaction occurring as a result of incompatibility between donor and recipient blood.

Autologous transfusion has been used illegally by people associated with professional sports. Carried out just before a sporting event, "blood doping" increases the oxygen-carrying capacity of the circulation and thus improves stamina.

### HOW IT IS DONE

Blood can be withdrawn (in the same way as for *blood donation*) in several sessions at least four days apart and up to three days before surgery is planned. A total of up to 8 pints of blood can be removed and stored until required. Iron tablets are prescribed to ensure that the bone marrow produces replacement blood cells.

## EFFECT OF CHROMOSOMAL TRANSLOCATION

A translocation is a rearrangement of the chromosomes in body cells. A person carrying a translocation may show no abnormality but there is a risk of his or her child having a *chromosomal disorder*.

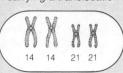

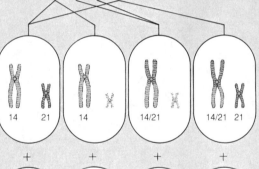

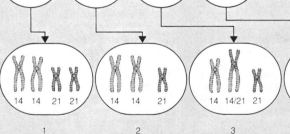

**Normal cell**
A body cell normally contains 22 paired chromosomes (called autosomes) plus two sex chromosomes (XX in women and XY in men). Just two pairs of autosomes—numbers 21 and 14—are shown here.

**Example of translocation**
In a typical translocation, a large part of one chromosome is joined to a large part of another. Here, most of a chromosome number 21 and a chromosome number 14 have joined.

**Balanced translocation (parent)**
The remaining bits of chromosomes 21 and 14 disappear. If, as here, the translocation is balanced—that is, the total chromosome complement is normal or near normal—no outward abnormality is seen.

**Eggs or sperm produced**
A parent with the example translocation makes four types of egg or sperm. They are (from left)—normal, missing a chromosome 21, carrying joined chromosomes 14 and 21, and the same with an extra chromosome 21.

**Normal egg or sperm**
An egg or sperm from the parent with the translocation combines with one from the other parent, which has one number 21 and one number 14 chromosome. Any of the four outcomes below may result.

**Child**
The child may have (1) normal chromosomes, (2) a missing chromosome 21 (incompatible with life), (3) a balanced translocation (like the parent), and (4) effectively, an extra chromosome 21, leading to Down's syndrome. In the latter case, the parents may benefit from genetic counseling.

## Transient ischemic attack

A brief interruption of the blood supply to part of the brain that results in temporary impairment of vision, speech, sensation, or movement. Typically, the episode lasts for several minutes or, at the most, for a few hours. Any attack that lasts for more than 24 hours is called a *stroke*. Transient ischemic attacks (TIAs) may be the prelude to a full-scale stroke.

### CAUSES

Some TIAs occur when an artery supplying the brain becomes temporarily blocked by a flake of clotted blood carried from elsewhere in the bloodstream (see *Embolism*). Other attacks are caused by narrowing of an artery due to *atherosclerosis*.

### SYMPTOMS AND SIGNS

Symptoms occur suddenly, and vary widely, according to the site and duration of the interruption to blood flow. They include weakness or numbness in an arm or leg, *aphasia* (disturbance of language functions), dizziness, or partial blindness. An attack is always followed by full recovery.

### DIAGNOSIS AND TREATMENT

Diagnostic testing usually includes *CT scanning* to rule out the possibility of a brain tumor or subdural *hematoma* (a swelling containing blood), which sometimes produces TIA-like symptoms. Blood tests to look for blood-clotting abnormalities are also used. Other tests, including *ultrasound scanning*, digital subtraction *angiography*, or conventional angiography, may be used to look at the vessels for evidence of atherosclerosis. In some instances, heart studies are performed to check the heart as a possible source of blood clots.

Treatment is aimed at preventing a major stroke, which occurs within five years in from one fourth to one third of the patients with TIA. Therapeutic options include *endarterectomy*, *anticoagulant drugs*, or aspirin (an antiplatelet drug). Thus far, only aspirin has been proven effective.

## Transillumination

A procedure carried out during physical examination of a lump or swelling. Light from a small flashlight is shined against one side of the lump; if light can be seen on the other side, the physician knows the lump contains clear fluid because fat or other tissue would block the light. For example, a *hydrocele* (fluid-containing swelling in the scrotum) allows light to pass, whereas a *varicocele* (mass of enlarged veins) in the scrotum does not.

## Translocation

A rearrangement of the *chromosomes* inside a person's cells. Translocation is a type of *mutation* (change in the genetic material). Sections of chromosomes may be exchanged, or the main parts of two chromosomes may be joined. A translocation may be inherited or acquired as the result of a new mutation.

Often, because there has been no net loss or gain of chromosomal material within the person's cells, a translocation has no outward effect, and causes no abnormality. However, the translocation can mean that some of the person's egg or sperm cells carry too much or too little chromosomal material, which leads to a risk of a *chromosomal abnormality* (such as *Down's syndrome*) in the person's children (see diagram on opposite page).

When a chromosomal abnormality occurs, the child's and the parents' chromosomes are checked to see whether a translocation is the cause (see *Chromosome analysis*). *Genetic counseling* can help determine the risk of another child being affected.

## Transmissible

A term meaning capable of being passed from one person to another or from one organism to another of the same or a different species (as in the transmission of disease from an insect to a human). The term is applied to *infectious diseases* and to *genetic disorders*.

## Transplant surgery

The replacement of a diseased organ or tissue with a healthy, living substitute. The organ is usually taken from a person who has just died. However, in the US, about one third of transplanted kidneys are taken from living relatives of the patient (see *Organ donation*).

Around the world about 100,000 major organs have been transplanted, mostly in the past 10 to 15 years. About 80 percent of patients are alive and well one year after the transplantation of a major organ (such as the heart or liver) and most survive at least five years.

The earliest successful transplant operation was *corneal grafting*, carried out early this century. The cornea is not affected by the rejection process (the automatic attempt by the body's *immune system* to destroy foreign cells) because it has no blood supply, and therefore no white blood cells and antibodies to bring about rejection after a transplant.

Kidney transplantation was shown to be technically possible in the 1950s, but early transplant operations ended in failure because of rejection. In the 1960s, however, *corticosteroid drugs* and cytotoxic agents (see *Anticancer drugs*) were found to suppress the rejection response, making transplantation practicable. The discovery in the 1970s and introduction in the early 1980s of *cyclosporine*, a more effective *immunosuppressant drug*, substantially improved the success rates for transplant surgery.

Every patient who undergoes an organ transplant operation must take immunosuppressant drugs indefinitely; this damping down of the body's natural defenses exposes him or her to a greater risk of infection, especially with fungi (see *Fungal infections*) and protozoal *parasites*. Patients

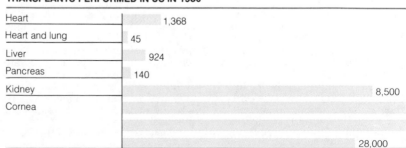

**TRANSPLANTS PERFORMED IN US IN 1986**

| | |
|---|---|
| Heart | 1,368 |
| Heart and lung | 45 |
| Liver | 924 |
| Pancreas | 140 |
| Kidney | 8,500 |
| Cornea | 28,000 |

**Factors affecting transplantation**
The number of specific transplant operations performed depends partly on demand (how many people would benefit) and partly on availability. For corneal transplants, there is a high demand and ready availability. But for some other types of transplantation, strict selection is necessary, due to shortages of suitable donor organs or because only a small number of specialist centers can offer the procedure.

undergoing long-term immunosuppressant treatment are also at increased risk of certain types of cancer, especially *lymphomas*.

A second important factor in improving the results of transplant surgery has been the steady improvement in techniques for matching the donors and recipients. Organ transplantation proceeds most smoothly when the donor and recipient share most of the same tissue types (see *Histocompatibility antigens; Tissue-typing*).

A third factor that has contributed to higher success rates is the development of techniques for organ preservation. After removal from the donor, the organ is washed with an oxygenated fluid and cooled; this reduces the risk of damage due to lack of blood. Nevertheless, it is still important to keep to a minimum the time the organ is deprived of a normal blood supply. In most cases of heart or liver transplantation, the organs are removed from the donor while the heart is still functioning, but after *brain death* has been certified. (See also *Heart transplant; Heart-lung transplant; Liver transplant; Kidney transplant.*)

## Transposition of the great vessels

A form of congenital *heart disease* in which the two major vessels that carry blood away from the heart—the aorta and the pulmonary artery—are in each other's normal position. This means that, unless the baby also has a septal defect (hole in the heart) through which blood can flow, insufficient oxygenated blood is supplied to the body's tissues. Transposition of the great vessels occurs in about 40 babies per 100,000 born.

### SYMPTOMS, DIAGNOSIS, AND TREATMENT
*Cyanosis* (blueness of the skin) usually develops and the baby becomes increasingly short of breath, and feeds poorly. Symptoms vary in severity according to the amount of oxygenated blood passing through the septal opening.

A firm diagnosis can be made only after a *chest X ray*, an *ECG* (electrocardiogram), an echocardiogram (see *Echocardiography*), and cardiac *catheterization*, in which a catheter is introduced into the heart.

Once the diagnosis is made, emergency surgical treatment is carried out to create or enlarge a hole in the septum. This allows enough oxygenated blood through to keep the child alive. Later, reconstructive *open*

*heart surgery* is performed to create normal circulation. The surgery usually allows the child to live a full and normal life.

## Transsexualism

A rare psychiatric disorder in which a person feels persistently uncomfortable about his or her anatomical sex.

Usually developing in early adulthood, transsexualism is much more common in men. The condition is often associated with a disturbed child-parent relationship and may follow a period of cross-dressing.

Unlike effeminate homosexual men or masculine lesbians who have no desire to change their anatomical gender, transsexuals wish to live as members of the opposite sex. Frequently, they obsessively seek surgical or hormonal treatment to bring about a physical *sex change*. A careful psychiatric evaluation is used by the physician to rule out a psychotic delusional system, which would make hormonal or surgical treatment extremely risky. Associated features include *personality disorder*, alcohol or drug excess, anxiety, depression, and work problems. Sexual drive is often quite low, although some transsexuals are actively homosexual.

Transsexualism should be distinguished from the delusion (false belief not responding to reasoned argument) of belonging to the other sex, which sometimes occurs in *schizophrenia*. Rare cases of physical intersex (see *Hermaphroditism*), in which there are congenital abnormalities of the sexual structures, are ruled out by the physician during a general and genital examination and by endocrine tests if necessary.

## Transvestism

A persistent desire by a man to dress in women's clothing; it is also called cross-dressing. Transvestism most often starts in childhood, usually with the boy dressing in the underwear of a female relative. It is done in private while masturbating. Transvestism should be differentiated from charades or female impersonation, which do not involve the component of sexual arousal.

Transvestism varies from the occasional wearing of female underclothes to constant, public dressing in women's clothes and extensive involvement in transvestite subculture. For some people, cross-dressing serves to relieve anxiety; for others it provides sexual excitement. No

biological factors have been established. Occasionally, transvestism develops into *transsexualism*.

Most transvestites are heterosexual and have a sexual relationship with a female partner who knows and can accept the cross-dressing as a special need. Transvestites rarely seek medical or psychiatric treatment.

An emergency may be created in a couple or family upon accidental revelation of the behavior. Crisis intervention consists of educating the partner and kin that the behavior does not break the law or indicate that the person is dangerous. The situation of the patient (child, teen, or adult) is evaluated carefully to determine why private sexual behavior has become public and therefore a problem.

## Tranylcypromine

A monoamine-oxidase inhibitor *antidepressant drug*.

## Trapezius muscle

A large, diamond-shaped muscle that extends from the back of the skull to the lower part of the thoracic spine (the part of the spine in the chest) and, at its broadest point, across the width of the shoulders. At the shoulders, the

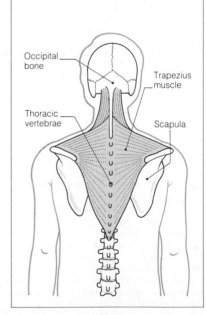

**LOCATION OF THE TRAPEZIUS MUSCLE**
This extensive, diamond-shaped muscle in the back provides power for activities such as swimming and lifting.

Occipital bone

Trapezius muscle

Thoracic vertebrae

Scapula

trapezius is attached to the top and back of the scapula (shoulder blade) and to the outermost part of the clavicle (collarbone). Along its midline, the trapezius is also attached by ligaments to the vertebrae.

The trapezius muscle helps support the neck and spine. It is also involved in movements of the arm. When an arm is raised, the trapezius on that side contracts, thereby causing the scapula to rotate.

## Trapped nerve
See *Nerve, trapped.*

## Trauma
A physical injury or a severe emotional shock. The psychological condition that can result from physical or emotional trauma is known as *post-traumatic stress disorder.*

## Trauma surgery
See *Traumatology.*

## Traumatology
Emergency treatment of patients suffering from acute trauma (physical injury), commonly as the result of traffic accidents, industrial accidents, domestic accidents, shootings, or stabbings. In the US, trauma is the most common cause of death in people up to age 30 and the fourth most common cause of death in the population as a whole, accounting for more than 100,000 deaths annually. In addition, more than 1 million more cases of trauma require hospitalization every year.

In cases of life-threatening trauma, the priorities of the trauma surgeon are to maintain a clear airway in the patient and so prevent asphyxia, to arrest bleeding, to treat shock, and to deal with major chest wounds affecting the heart or lungs. If there are abdominal injuries, an exploratory operation called a *laparotomy* or, in the case of head injuries, a *craniotomy*, may be required. Multiple injuries require coordinated treatment by members of many specialities.

Once the patient's condition is stable, other injuries, such as fractures and superficial cuts, are treated.

## Travelers' diarrhea
An affliction of people visiting foreign countries. Episodes of diarrhea range in severity from inconvenient to debilitating. Known by a variety of colorful names, such as Montezuma's revenge and the Tokyo trots, all are forms of *gastroenteritis.*

## Travel immunization
Any person planning to travel outside of the US, Canada, Europe, Australia, and New Zealand may need immunizations before departure. Few immunizations are now compulsory for international travel. Nevertheless, some immunizations are advisable for the traveler's own protection.

A prospective traveler should consult his or her physician about individual requirements. If necessary, the physician can check with state or local departments of health for the latest immunization recommendations for particular destinations.

The physician needs information on the countries to be visited, the duration and nature of the visit, and the individual's previous immunization history. Most US citizens have received childhood immunization against certain diseases, such as diphtheria, pertussis, tetanus, and polio, so may not need further protection (see *Immunization*). However, in

**GUIDELINES FOR TRAVEL IMMUNIZATION**

| Immunization | Reason for immunization | Effectiveness |
|---|---|---|
| Yellow fever | Compulsory for entry to some countries and advisable for visits to others within yellow fever zones in Africa and South America. May also be needed when traveling from yellow fever zones to neighboring states or to some Asian countries. | Near 100 percent protection for at least 10 years. Certificate provided. |
| Cholera | Occasionally compulsory for entry to some countries in Asia and Africa. Also advisable when traveling to many other Asian and African countries. | Gives moderate protection for six months. Other precautions against cholera needed in epidemic areas. |
| Typhoid | Recommended when traveling anywhere outside of the US, Canada, Europe, Australia, and New Zealand for anyone who has not received immunization or a booster within the past five years. | Gives moderate protection for about five years, after which a booster is needed. |
| Tetanus | Advisable for anyone who has not received childhood immunization or a booster within the past 10 years. | Highly effective, with booster needed every 10 years. |
| Polio | Advisable for anyone who has not received childhood immunization or a booster within the past 10 years. | Highly effective with booster needed every 10 years. |
| Immune serum globulin | Recommended when traveling to any country where hygiene and sanitary standards are low to protect against viral hepatitis, type A. | Moderate protection for up to three months. |
| Measles | Advisable for anyone who did not receive childhood immunization and who has not had measles. | Highly effective, lifelong protection. |
| Diphtheria | Advisable for anyone who did not receive childhood immunization and is shown by a test to be nonimmune. | Highly effective. |
| Hepatitis B Rabies Meningitis | Recommended only for individuals or groups at special risk through occupation, nature of visit abroad, and so on. | All highly effective. |
| Smallpox | No longer necessary, as the disease has been eradicated. | |

T

some cases, booster doses against tetanus and polio are advisable.

With knowledge of the individual's medical history, the physician can decide if there are grounds for not administering a particular vaccine. Infants younger than 1 year are not usually given certain travel vaccines, notably yellow fever, cholera, and typhoid injections. In general, infants should receive their scheduled immunizations before travel abroad.

After discussion, the physician establishes an appropriate schedule of injections. Some vaccines must be given in two or three doses several weeks apart, so it is wise to consult your physician at least two to three months before departure.

Antimalarial drugs (see *Malaria*) may also be needed for people planning to visit certain destinations.

## Trazodone

An *antidepressant drug*. Trazodone has a strong sedative effect and is particularly useful in the treatment of *depression* accompanied by *anxiety* or *insomnia*. Possible adverse effects include drowsiness, constipation, dry mouth, dizziness, and, rarely, *priapism* (painful, persistent erection).

## Treatment

Any measure taken to prevent or cure a disease or disorder or to relieve symptoms. Examples include *drug treatment, radiation therapy, surgery*, and bed rest.

## Trematode

The scientific names for any *fluke* or *schistosome* (flattened worms that may parasitize humans).

## Trembling

See *Tremor*.

## Tremor

An involuntary, rhythmic, oscillating movement in the muscles of part of the body, most commonly the hands, feet, jaw, tongue, or head. Tremor is caused by rapidly alternating contraction and relaxation of the muscles.

Occasional temporary tremors are experienced by almost everyone, usually at times of fear, excitement, or other heightened emotion; they are due to increased production of the hormone *epinephrine*.

A slight persistent tremor unrelated to any disease is common in elderly people. Another type of persistent tremor not associated with disease is essential tremor, a fine-to-moderate

tremor (six to 10 movements per second) that runs in families and may be temporarily relieved by a small amount of alcohol or by taking *beta-blocker drugs*. Both these tremors increase with movement of the affected part of the body.

Some types of persistent tremor indicate an underlying disorder. Coarse tremor (four to five muscle movements a second) present at rest but reduced during movement is often a sign of *Parkinson's disease*. Intention tremor (tremor that is worse on movement of the affected part) is a sign of disease of the *cerebellum*. Other disorders marked by tremor include *multiple sclerosis, Wilson's disease, mercury poisoning, thyrotoxicosis*, and hepatic *encephalopathy*.

Tremor may also be caused by drugs, among them *amphetamine drugs, antidepressant drugs, caffeine*, and *lithium*. It may also be a symptom of drug withdrawal. A tremor can occur in people taking *antipsychotic drugs* for certain psychiatric disorders.

Tremor is also a feature of alcohol withdrawal and, as such, may indicate *alcohol dependence*. The so-called morning shakes occur as blood alcohol levels fall and are relieved by the first drink of the day.

## Trench fever

An infectious illness that was common among troops in the trenches during World War I and World War II, but is now rare or unknown in most parts of the world. Like epidemic *typhus*, which it resembles, the disease is caused by rickettsiae (microorganisms similar to bacteria) spread by body lice. The symptoms include headache and muscle pains as well as fever, which may occur in bouts. It is treated with *antibiotic drugs*.

## Trench foot

See *Immersion foot*.

## Trench mouth

See *Vincent's disease*.

## Trephine

A hollow, cylindrical instrument with a saw-toothed edge used for cutting a circular hole, usually in bone. Trephines are most often used to bore holes in the skull to form a removable flap before performing operations on the brain.

Perforating the skull to relieve excess pressure is a recent innovation and is part of conventional surgery. Ancient peoples used trephines on the

skull (as evidenced by the skulls found by paleontologists) but the reason they did so is unknown; most likely it was done by witch doctors to encourage the release of evil spirits.

## Tretinoin

A drug chemically related to *vitamin A*, used topically to treat *acne* and certain skin disorders characterized by scaling and thickening, such as *ichthyosis*. Tretinoin may aggravate acne in the first few weeks of treatment but usually improves the condition within three to four months.

Tretinoin may cause skin irritation and peeling. Excessive exposure to sunlight may aggravate any irritation and lead to *sunburn*. In rare cases, it may bleach or darken the skin.

## Trial, clinical

A test on human volunteers of the effectiveness and safety of a drug, or a systematic comparison of alternative forms of medical or surgical treatment for a particular disorder. Clinical trials are also used to test the usefulness of new medical or surgical appliances, dressings, or equipment.

In the development of new drugs, clinical trials follow animal tests that mainly evaluate toxic effects (see *Animal experimentation*); clinical trials are usually undertaken at a late stage before the manufacturer proceeds to commercial production. The purpose of clinical trials is to demonstrate that the new drug is effective, safe, and superior to, or at least as good as, existing drugs. Such trials are also useful in revealing effects that may not have been suspected from results of the animal tests.

Careful precautions are necessary to ensure that the results of clinical trials are not misleading. Trials that fail to eliminate the effects of personal bias or the *placebo* effect may be of little value. For these reasons, most clinical trials are carried out in the form of randomized, *controlled trials*.

## Triamcinolone

| CORTICOSTEROID | | | | |
|---|---|---|---|---|

Tablet Liquid Injection Cream Ointment Inhaler Dental paste

Prescription needed

Available as generic

A *corticosteroid drug* used to treat inflammation of the mouth, gums, skin, and joints. Triamcinolone is also used to treat *asthma* and certain blood disorders, such as *thrombocytopenia* and *leukemia*.

## Triamterene

A potassium-sparing *diuretic drug*. Triamterene is used with thiazide or loop diuretics to treat *hypertension* (high blood pressure) and *edema* (fluid retention). Possible adverse effects include nausea, vomiting, lethargy, muscle weakness, and rash.

## Triazolam

A *benzodiazepine drug* used in the short-term treatment of *insomnia*.

## Triceps muscle

The name (meaning "three heads") of the muscle at the back of the upper arm. At the upper end of the muscle, one of its three heads is attached to the outer edge of the scapula (shoulder blade); the other two heads are attached to either side of the upper part of the humerus (the upper arm bone).

The lower part of the triceps is attached by a large tendon to the olecranon process of the ulna (the bony prominence at the back of the elbow). Contraction of the triceps muscle straightens the arm. (See also *Biceps muscle*.)

---

**LOCATION OF THE TRICEPS MUSCLE**
This muscle at the back of the arm functions to straighten the elbow joint, thus opposing the action of the biceps at the front of the arm.

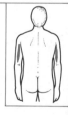

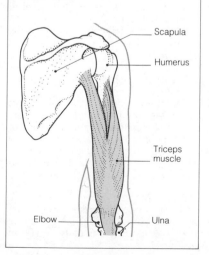

Scapula

Humerus

Triceps muscle

Elbow — Ulna

---

## Trichiasis

An alteration in the direction of growth of the eyelashes in which the lashes grow inward toward the eyeball. The abnormally directed lashes can rub against the eye, causing severe discomfort and sometimes damage to the *cornea*. Trichiasis can result from inflammation and scarring that occurs in *trachoma*. Severe scarring may lead to *entropion* (turning in of the lid margin).

Temporary treatment involves the manual removal of the offending lashes, but the lashes regrow and may again cause pain and damage. Permanent treatment involves destruction of the growth follicles of the offending eyelashes using *electrolysis*.

## Trichinosis

 An infestation with the larvae of a tiny worm, *TRICHINELLA SPIRALIS*, usually acquired by eating undercooked pork or pork products, such as ham or sausages.

### CAUSES AND INCIDENCE

Worm larvae are present as cysts in the muscles of infested animals, such as rats, dogs, bears, and pigs. If a person eats the raw or undercooked meat of an infested animal, the larvae are released from the cysts and develop into adults in the person's intestines. The adult worms discharge fresh larvae, which travel in the bloodstream to various tissues and organs, including the heart and brain, and to the muscles, where they form cysts.

Infestation of humans is practically confined to pork-eating populations, mainly in North America and Europe. Up to 5 percent of people in the US have had a trichiniferous infestation, but usually without symptoms. The principal preventive measure is thorough cooking of pork and pork products. Freezing to a temperature below 0°F (-18°C) for 24 hours also kills the larvae.

### SYMPTOMS AND COMPLICATIONS

Infestation with only a few worms usually causes no symptoms. A heavy infestation may cause diarrhea and vomiting within a day or two of eating infested meat, followed, a week or so later, by more symptoms as new larvae circulate through the body. The symptoms may include fever, swelling around the eyelids, and severe muscle pains, which may last for several weeks. Very rarely, the person becomes seriously ill and may die. In other people, the symptoms subside and gradually disappear.

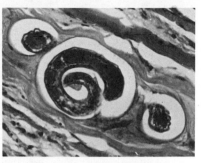

**Biopsy specimen showing trichinosis**
This photomicrograph of a section of a patient's muscle shows a cyst formed by a *TRICHINELLA SPIRALIS* larva.

### DIAGNOSIS AND TREATMENT

Trichinosis may be suspected by a physician from the symptoms; it is confirmed by *blood tests*, which detect antibodies to the larvae, or by a muscle *biopsy* (sample of tissue), which shows the larvae themselves.

The disease is treated with an *antihelmintic drug* (usually thiabendazole) that kills adult worms in the intestines and attacks larvae in the tissues. *Corticosteroid drugs* are given to reduce inflammation. This treatment generally leads to recovery within a few days to weeks.

## Trichomoniasis

 An infection of the vagina, often sexually transmitted, caused by the protozoan (single-celled microorganism) *TRICHOMONAS VAGINALIS*. In addition to being transmitted during sexual intercourse, trichomoniasis is occasionally contracted from an infected washcloth or towel or transmitted by a woman to her baby during childbirth. The infection may also occur in men, affecting the urethra, but usually does not cause any symptoms.

Trichomoniasis is not in itself a serious condition. It is estimated that 3 million people are infected every year in the US.

### SYMPTOMS AND SIGNS

The causative organism may inhabit the vagina for years without causing symptoms. If symptoms do occur, they include painful inflammation and itching of the vagina and vulva, and a profuse, yellow, frothy, offensive discharge. Sexual intercourse is usually painful. Men usually have no symptoms but some suffer from urethral discomfort, inflammation of the glans (head) of the penis, and signs of *nonspecific urethritis*.

T

### DIAGNOSIS AND TREATMENT

The diagnosis is made from a laboratory examination of a sample of the vaginal discharge or of swabs taken from the urethra. Diagnosis is usually difficult in men.

Treatment is with *metronidazole*, which usually clears up the condition. An infected person's sexual partner or partners should be treated at the same time to prevent reinfection and further spread of infection.

## Trichotillomania

The habit of constantly pulling out one's own hair. Trichotillomania is often associated with severe mental subnormality or with a psychotic illness, such as schizophrenia. It may also occur in psychologically disturbed children as an expression of anxiety and frustration.

The sufferer typically pulls, twists, and breaks off chunks of hair from the scalp, leaving bald patches; occasionally, pubic hair is pulled out. Children sometimes eat the removed hair, which may cause a trichobezoar, or hairball (see *Bezoar*).

Treatment may consist of *psychotherapy* and/or *antipsychotic drugs*.

## Tricuspid insufficiency

Failure of the tricuspid valve of the heart to close properly, allowing blood to leak back into the right atrium (upper chamber) during contractions of the right ventricle (lower chamber). This lowers the pumping efficiency of the heart.

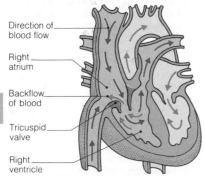

**Defect in tricuspid insufficiency**
The tricuspid valve lies between the atrium and ventricle in the right side of the heart. Insufficiency means that when the right ventricle contracts, some blood escapes back into the right atrium.

Direction of blood flow
Right atrium
Backflow of blood
Tricuspid valve
Right ventricle

### CAUSES AND INCIDENCE

The disorder is usually due to an increased work load on the right side of the heart as a result of *pulmonary* *hypertension* (high pressure in the blood. supply to the lungs). This causes the right ventricle to distend and leads to widening of the opening in which the tricuspid valve is situated. In rare cases, tricuspid insufficiency occurs as a result of *rheumatic fever* or, in intravenous drug abusers, as a result of a bacterial infection of the heart; it is then usually accompanied by other heart valve disorders.

### SYMPTOMS, DIAGNOSIS, AND TREATMENT

The tricuspid insufficiency causes symptoms of right-sided *heart failure*, notably *edema* (fluid collection and swelling) affecting the ankles and abdomen. The liver is congested with blood and is swollen and tender. Veins in the neck are distended.

The condition is diagnosed from the patient's symptoms, from a characteristic *murmur* heard through a stethoscope, and by tests that may include an *ECG*, *chest X rays*, *echocardiography*, and cardiac *catheterization*.

Treatment for heart failure, with *diuretic drugs* and *ACE inhibitor drugs*, often clears up the symptoms. If symptoms persist, *heart valve surgery* may be performed to repair or replace the malfunctioning valve.

## Tricuspid stenosis

Narrowing of the opening of the tricuspid valve in the heart between the right atrium (upper chamber) and right ventricle (lower chamber). Tricuspid stenosis is an uncommon heart valve disorder that occurs mainly in people who have had *rheumatic fever*. It may also occur in intravenous drug abusers as a result of bacterial infection of the heart. It is usually accompanied by other heart valve disorders, such as *mitral stenosis*.

The right atrium must work harder to pump blood through the narrowed valve, causing it to enlarge. The symptoms are very similar to those of *tricuspid insufficiency*; the condition is diagnosed by the same procedures.

Drug treatment is given with *diuretic drugs* to reduce edema and sometimes a *digitalis drug* to increase the force of the heart's contractions. If symptoms persist, *heart valve surgery* may be carried out to repair or replace the valve.

## Trifluoperazine

An *antipsychotic drug* used principally in the treatment of *schizophrenia*.

## Trifluridine

An *antiviral drug* used to treat and sometimes prevent eye infections caused by the same virus that causes *herpes simplex*. Adverse effects include dryness, stinging, itching, or redness of the eyes, and swollen eyelids.

## Trigeminal nerve

The fifth *cranial nerve*. The trigeminal nerve arises from the pons (part of the *brain stem*) and divides into three main branches, which then subdivide into a complex network of nerves. These nerves supply sensation to the face, scalp, nose, teeth, lining of the mouth, upper eyelid, sinuses, and front two thirds of the tongue; control the production of saliva by the salivary glands and of tears by the lacrimal glands; and stimulate contraction of the jaw muscles responsible for chewing.

Damage to, or disease in, one area supplied by a branch of the trigeminal nerve may cause *referred pain* in another area supplied by a different branch of the nerve. For example, sinusitis (infection of the sinuses) may cause toothache.

## Trigeminal neuralgia

A disorder of the trigeminal nerve (fifth cranial nerve) in which episodes of severe, stabbing pain affect the cheek, lips, gums, or chin on one side of the face. The pain is very brief (lasting only a few seconds to minutes) but is often so intense that the sufferer is unable to do anything for the duration of the attack. The pain often causes wincing and for this reason is commonly called tic douloureux (literally, "painful twitch").

Trigeminal neuralgia is unusual under the age of 50. When it does occur in younger people, it may be associated with *multiple sclerosis*. Attacks occur in bouts that may last for weeks at a time. Pain-free intervals between attacks tend to become shorter with time.

The cause of trigeminal neuralgia is uncertain. The pain nearly always starts from one trigger point on the face and can be brought on by touching the face, washing, shaving, eating, drinking, or even talking.

Treatment is difficult. *Carbamazepine* suppresses the pain in most sufferers, but resistance to the drug develops in some people or they are unable to tolerate a high enough dosage to relieve the pain. If drug treatment fails, surgical options are available.

## Trigger finger

Locking of one or several fingers in a bent position. Forcible straightening of an affected finger usually causes an audible click.

T

## LOCATION OF THE TRIGEMINAL NERVE

The trigeminal nerve splits into three main parts. The ophthalmic nerve supplies most of the scalp, the upper eyelid, tear gland, and cornea; the maxillary nerve supplies the upper jaw; and the mandibular nerve supplies the tongue, lower jaw, and jaw muscles.

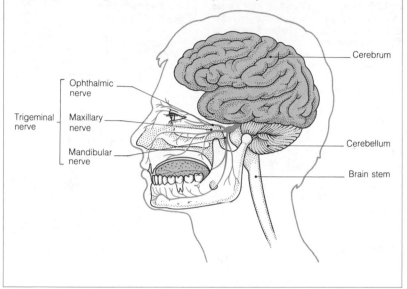

Trigger finger is caused by inflammation of the fibrous sheath that encloses the tendon of the affected finger and is accompanied by localized swelling of the tendon. When the finger is bent, the enlarged tendon is forced out of the narrowed mouth of the sheath and is then unable to reenter it. There is usually tenderness at the base of the affected finger. In addition, a small swelling may be felt over the tendon.

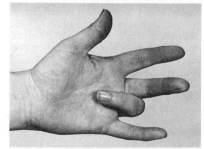

**Appearance of trigger finger**
The disorder is caused by inflammation of one of the tendons involved in controlling the finger's movements.

Treatment of trigger finger involves either the injection of a *corticosteroid drug* into the sheath to reduce inflammation or a surgical procedure to widen the opening.

## Trihexyphenidyl

An *anticholinergic drug* often used in conjunction with other drugs that relieve rigidity and tremor in *Parkinson's disease*. Trihexyphenidyl is also occasionally used to relieve the symptoms of *parkinsonism* caused by *antipsychotic drugs*.

## Trimeprazine

An *antihistamine drug* used mainly to relieve itching in allergic conditions, such as *urticaria* (hives) and atopic *eczema*. Since trimeprazine has a sedative effect, it is useful in the relief of itching that usually prevents sleep. Trimeprazine is also used as a *premedication* to sedate children before surgery or other medical procedures are performed.

The adverse effects of trimeprazine are typical of other antihistamines, although trimeprazine is more likely to cause drowsiness than some other drugs in this group.

## Trimethobenzamide

An *antiemetic drug* promoted for the treatment of nausea and vomiting caused by anesthetics, *radiation therapy*, or *anticancer drugs*. Trimethobenzamide may cause adverse effects such as drowsiness and, rarely, blurred vision, muscle cramps, diarrhea, tremor, rash, and jaundice.

## Trimethoprim

An *antibacterial drug* prescribed for a wide variety of infections. Trimethoprim is used to treat *urinary tract infection, prostatitis*, and some types of *gastroenteritis*. Combined with another antibacterial drug, *sulfamethoxazole*, trimethoprim is used to treat infections of the urinary tract, ear, and respiratory tract (including *pneumocystis pneumonia*) and *gonorrhea*.

Possible adverse effects include rash, itching, nausea, vomiting, diarrhea, and sore tongue.

## Trimipramine

A tricyclic *antidepressant drug*. Trimipramine has a strong sedative effect and is used to treat *depression* accompanied by *anxiety* or *insomnia*.

Possible adverse effects include dry mouth, blurred vision, dizziness, constipation, and nausea.

## Triprolidine

An *antihistamine drug* used to treat allergies, such as allergic *rhinitis* (hay fever) and *urticaria* (hives). Triprolidine is also a common ingredient of *cough remedies* and *cold remedies*. It is occasionally given to treat or prevent allergic reactions to *blood transfusions* or certain foods.

Possible adverse effects include dry mouth, dizziness, difficulty passing urine and, in children, *hyperactivity*.

## Trismus

Involuntary contraction of the jaw muscles, resulting in the mouth becoming tightly closed, a condition commonly known as lockjaw.

Trismus may occur as a symptom of *tetanus, tonsillitis, quinsy, mumps, Vincent's disease*, an abscess around a back tooth, nasopharyngeal cancer (see *Nasopharynx, cancer of*), or *Parkinson's disease*. Occasionally trismus is hysterical in origin (it sometimes occurs in *anorexia nervosa*). Treatment of trismus is directed toward the underlying cause.

## Trisomy

The presence, within the cells of a person, of an extra chromosome so that there are three *chromosomes* of a particular number, instead of the usual two. The result can range from the death and spontaneous abortion of an affected embryo to a range of abnormalities in a live-born child.

**CAUSES AND INCIDENCE**

A trisomy may result from a fault during the formation of an egg or sperm cell by which an extra chromosome

T

gets into the cell. If an affected egg or sperm takes part in fertilization, the resulting embryo also has an extra chromosome, causing trisomy. Trisomy can also result from a *translocation* (a rearrangement of the chromosomes) inherited from one of the parents. Most types of trisomy are more common in older mothers.

Certain trisomies (such as three number 11 chromosomes) have never been observed in live-born babies; if they do occur, such trisomies probably lead to early abortion or stillbirth. By far the most common trisomy in live-born infants is trisomy 21, also called *Down's syndrome*, in which there are three number 21 chromosomes. Much less common are trisomy 18 (Edwards' syndrome) and trisomy 13 (Patau's syndrome). Some others— such as trisomy 8 and trisomy 22—are extremely rare. Partial trisomies, in which only part of a chromosome is in triplicate, have also been found.

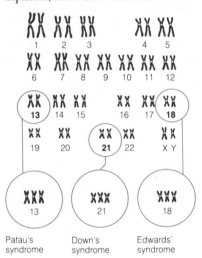

**Types of trisomy**
In all trisomies a child has three, instead of the usual two, chromosomes of a particular number. Down's syndrome is by far the most common trisomy.

**SYMPTOMS, DIAGNOSIS, AND TREATMENT**
All full trisomies cause multiple abnormalities, such as skeletal and heart defects, facial anomalies, and mental deficiency. The effect of a partial trisomy is variable, depending on how much extra chromosomal material is present. The conditions are diagnosed by *chromosome analysis*.

There is no specific treatment for these conditions. Many children with Down's syndrome survive into adulthood, but babies with other full trisomies usually die early in infancy.

Parents of an affected baby should obtain *genetic counseling* to assess the risk of a future child being affected.

## Trisomy 21 syndrome
A set of abnormalities caused when a child has three, instead of the usual two, number 21 chromosomes in each of his or her cells. It is better known as *Down's syndrome*.

## Trochlear nerve
The fourth *cranial nerve*. It arises from the midbrain (part of the *brain stem*) and passes through the skull to enter the eye socket through a gap in the skull bones. The trochlear nerve supplies only one muscle of each eye (the superior oblique muscle), the contraction of which rotates the eye outward.

Damage to the trochlear nerve (as a result of a skull fracture, for example) may lead to double vision when trying to look outward.

## Trophoblastic tumor
A growth arising from the tissues that develop into the placenta. The most common type of trophoblastic tumor is a benign growth called a *hydatidiform mole*. A malignant trophoblastic tumor that has spread outside the uterus is called a *choriocarcinoma*.

## Tropical diseases
Most diseases of temperate areas are also prevalent in the tropics. Many other diseases are virtually confined to tropical areas. In most cases, this is not due primarily to tropical geographic factors (such as temperature, humidity, or disease-carrying insects), but to the fact that large populations in many tropical countries live in poverty.

**DISEASES OF POVERTY**
*Malnutrition* is one of the major causes of illness in the tropics. Apart from causing nutritional deficiency disorders, a poor diet weakens the body's ability to fight infectious diseases such as *measles* and *diphtheria*. Overcrowded living conditions are a cause of such diseases as *tuberculosis*.

Low standards of public health administration, food inspection and handling, and a lack of sanitary facilities, which encourage water and soil contamination with human excrement, are the cause of a vast number of diseases including *typhoid fever*, *shigellosis*, *cholera*, *amebiasis*, and *tapeworm infestation*. Most of these diseases were common in temperate zones before improvements in public

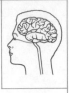

**LOCATION OF THE TROCHLEAR NERVE**
This nerve emerges from the brain and supplies a muscle that rotates the eye down and outward.

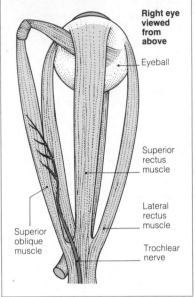

Right eye viewed from above

Eyeball

Superior rectus muscle

Lateral rectus muscle

Trochlear nerve

Superior oblique muscle

health and sanitation. Only some diseases, such as *hookworm infestation* and *schistosomiasis*, appear to be related to temperature or soil conditions found only in the tropics in addition to the lack of community sanitation and walking barefoot.

**DISEASES SPREAD BY INSECTS**
Some tropical diseases depend on the coincidence of a parasite and a specific insect *vector* (agent responsible for spread) such as a mosquito. These diseases include *malaria*, *yellow fever*, *sleeping sickness*, and *leishmaniasis*. It is worth noting, however, that at least some of the relevant insect vectors can survive in temperate zones; malaria was once common in parts of the US.

**LIGHT AND HEAT**
Certain conditions arise as a result of exposure to tropical sunlight. The most common is skin damage from ultraviolet light, leading to wrinkling, loss of elasticity, and an increased tendency to *skin cancer*, especially in white people with fair coloring. Ultraviolet light also damages the outer tissues of the eye (the conjunctiva and the cornea) and may lead to the development of *pinguecula* and *pterygium*. Overexertion in the tropics, with inadequate water intake

and salt replacement, may lead to *heat exhaustion*; prolonged exposure to high temperatures may lead to *heat stroke* in people who are not acclimated to the heat.

## Tropical ulcer

An area of persistent skin and tissue loss caused by infection and occurring predominantly in tropical regions. The ulcers are most common in people who are malnourished.

The classic form of tropical ulcer results from contamination of a cut or abrasion (usually on a foot or leg) by a mixture of various types of bacteria. Infections spread beneath the skin, and the affected tissue dies and is shed, leaving the ulcer in place.

Treatment consists of thorough cleaning of the ulcer, which is then dressed; the patient also needs antibiotic drugs and a nourishing, protein-rich diet. With this treatment, the ulcer usually heals, although it may leave some scarring and deformity.

Similar types of ulcer can occur as a result of more specific infections, such as *diphtheria* of the skin, cutaneous *leishmaniasis*, and *yaws*. Treatment is as described above, except that drug therapy may vary.

To avoid tropical ulcers, it is particularly important to wash any cuts, sores, or abrasions thoroughly and cover them with a sterile dressing.

## Tropicamide

A drug used to dilate the pupil before an eye examination and, occasionally, before eye surgery. Rare adverse effects include blurred vision, increased sensitivity to light, stinging, dry mouth, flushing, and *glaucoma*.

## Trunk

The central part of the body, comprising the chest and abdomen, to which the head and limbs are attached. The term trunk also refers to a large blood vessel or nerve from which smaller vessels or nerves branch off.

## Truss

An elastic, canvas, or padded metal appliance used to hold an abdominal *hernia* (protrusion of intestine through a weakened area in the abdominal wall) in place. A truss may be used to treat a hernia that is causing discomfort or is unsightly in people who are waiting for an operation or who are unfit for surgery. The hernia is pushed back through the abdominal wall before the truss is put on, usually while the person lies down.

## Trypanosomiasis

A tropical disease caused by protozoan (single-celled) parasites known as trypanosomes. In Africa, trypanosomes spread by tsetse flies are the cause of *sleeping sickness*. In South America, other trypanosomes, spread by beetlelike insects, are the cause of *Chagas' disease*.

## Tsetse fly bites

 Tsetse flies are found in Africa, where they spread the parasitic disease *sleeping sickness*. They are brown, about the size of houseflies, and each has a proboscis (biting and feeding apparatus) projecting forward at the front. Their bites can be painful. Measures to minimize the risk of bites include use of insecticide sprays and protective clothing impregnated with insect repellent.

## T-tube cholangiography

An X-ray procedure, also called operative or postoperative choledochography, performed to exclude the presence of residual gallstones in the common bile duct after removing the gallbladder and exploring the common bile duct (see *Cholecystectomy*).

The procedure is performed in the operating room following removal of the gallbladder eight to ten days after surgery. Contrast medium is injected into the T-tube (a T-shaped rubber tube placed, during surgery, in the common bile duct and brought out through a small abdominal skin incision) and X rays are taken. If there are no residual gallstones on the eighth day, the T-tube is removed. Otherwise, the tube is left until a decision is made concerning treatment to remove the stones.

## Tubal ligation

See *Sterilization, female*.

## Tubal pregnancy

See *Ectopic pregnancy*.

## Tubercle

Any of several small, nodular masses apparent in tissues that have been infected by the *tuberculosis* bacterium. The masses are gray in color and semitransparent.

The term tubercle (or tuberculum or tuberosity) also refers to any small, rounded protrusion on the surface of a bone. For example, the tibial tubercle is a bump at the top of the tibia (main bone of the lower leg), immediately below the knee.

## Tuberculin tests

Skin tests used to determine whether or not a person has been previously infected with *tuberculosis*. Tuberculin tests are performed in the diagnosis of suspected *tuberculosis* and are also carried out before *BCG vaccination*.

### HOW THEY ARE DONE

The skin of the forearm is first cleansed with alcohol. A small dose of tuberculin (a purified protein extract of tuberculosis bacilli) is then introduced into the skin by one of various techniques. In the Mantoux test, tuberculin is injected into the skin with a needle. In the Sterneedle test, a drop of tuberculin is put on the forearm and a spring-loaded device with a circle of sharp prongs is used to force the tuberculin through punctures in the skin.

### RESULTS

The forearm is examined after a few days and the skin reaction at the test site noted. If there is no change in the skin, the reaction is said to be negative. This indicates that the person has never been exposed to and has no immunity against tuberculosis. If a dime-sized area of the skin becomes red, hard, and raised, the reaction is positive. A positive reaction indicates previous exposure to tuberculosis, either through BCG vaccination or through actual infection.

## Tuberculosis

An infectious disease, commonly called TB, caused in humans by the bacterium *MYCOBACTERIUM TUBERCULOSIS*. Tuberculosis was once common worldwide and was a major killer in childhood and early adult life. In Europe, it was responsible for about one quarter of the deaths in the middle 19th century. Its incidence has fallen and continues to fall in developed

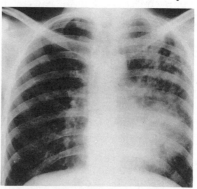

**Chest X ray showing tuberculosis**
The right lung appears normal, but the left shows dense opacities (white areas) adjoining the heart shadow.

T

countries, but tuberculosis remains a major problem in poorer countries.

**CAUSES**

Infection is passed from person to person in airborne droplets (produced by coughing or sneezing). The bacteria breathed into the lungs then multiply to form an infected "focus." In a high proportion of cases, the body's *immune system* then checks the infection and healing occurs, leaving a scar.

In about 5 percent of cases, however, the primary infection does not resolve. Spread occurs via the vessels of the lymphatic system to the lymph nodes. Sometimes at this stage bacteria enter the bloodstream and spread to other parts of the body; this is called miliary tuberculosis and may occasionally be fatal. In some people, the bacteria go into a dormant state in the lungs and other organs, only to become reactivated many years later. Progressive damage may then occur (e.g., cavities in the lungs).

In some cases, tuberculosis does not primarily affect the lung but may involve the lymph nodes (particularly of the neck), or the intestines, bones, or other organs. Such infections were especially common in bovine tuberculosis, acquired from contaminated cows' milk; this method of transmission has virtually disappeared from developed countries.

**INCIDENCE**

The incidence of tuberculosis in the US is about eight to 10 new cases per 100,000 population annually and is falling. However, this still represents more than 20,000 new cases in the US per year. The incidence is much higher in certain racial or social groups, such as Hispanics, Haitians, and immigrants from Southeast Asia. The disease is also more common in deprived city areas, in the elderly, in patients with *immunodeficiency disorders*, in diabetics, alcoholics, and in people who are in close contact with a person with tuberculosis.

Worldwide, there are 30 million people with active tuberculosis; about 3 million die of the disease annually. Tuberculosis is most prevalent where resistance has been lowered by malnutrition and other diseases.

**PREVENTION**

In the US, two types of preventive measures are used against tuberculosis. First is the use of *BCG vaccination* in high-risk groups. Second is *contact tracing*. Relatives and close friends of a tuberculosis victim are examined, X-rayed, and given a skin test so that tuberculosis is detected at an early stage and the risk of spread to other people is reduced. Any person—especially a child—who has contact in a household with someone who has active tuberculosis is given an antituberculosis antibiotic drug as a preventive measure.

**SYMPTOMS AND COMPLICATIONS**

Because tuberculosis usually affects the lungs, the main symptoms include coughing (sometimes bringing up blood), chest pain, shortness of breath, fever and sweating (especially at night), poor appetite, and weight loss. The main complications of tuberculosis of the lungs are *pleural effusion* (collection of fluid between the lung and chest wall), *pneumothorax* (air between the lungs and chest wall), and, in some cases, progression of the disease to death.

**DIAGNOSIS**

The diagnosis is made from the patient's symptoms and signs, and from a *chest X ray* and tests on the sputum and skin. The chest X ray is almost always abnormal. The upper parts of the lung are most commonly affected and may show cavities. Old healed areas of tuberculosis often remain as persistent shadows.

The sputum is examined for tuberculosis organisms. Attempts are also made to grow the bacteria from the sputum or other body fluids, although this procedure can take as long as six weeks. A skin test, called a *tuberculin test*, may be carried out. A positive test result indicates that the person has either been immunized against tuberculosis or has been infected. A strongly positive test result may indicate an active infection. Occasionally, *bronchoscopy* or the removal and examination of a piece of tissue (e.g., from a lymph node) may be necessary to make a firm diagnosis.

**TREATMENT AND OUTLOOK**

Modern drugs are very effective against tuberculosis, although at least two different antibiotic drugs must be taken to avoid bacterial *resistance* to the drugs. In the US, a common treatment is daily therapy for nine to 12 months with isoniazid and rifampin; other drugs, and sometimes a shorter course of treatment, may also be given. An adverse drug reaction (usually a rash or fever) develops in about 5 percent of patients, who then require a modified course of treatment. Blood tests are performed regularly during treatment to ensure that the drugs are not causing toxic effects on the liver.

Provided the full course of treatment is taken, the majority of patients are fully restored to health and suffer no recurrences.

## Tuberosity

A prominent area on a bone to which tendons are attached. The gluteal tuberosity is a ridge on the upper back part of the shaft of the femur (thigh bone) to which tendons of part of the gluteus maximus muscle are attached. Other bones with tuberosities include the ischium (one of the three fused bones that form the pelvis), humerus (upper arm bone), and radius and ulna (lower arm bones).

## Tuberous sclerosis

An inherited disorder affecting the skin and nervous system. The most typical skin feature of tuberous sclerosis is adenoma sebaceum (an acnelike condition on the face) but a variety of other skin conditions may also occur. Affected people characteristically suffer from epilepsy and mental retardation, although intelligence may be normal in mild cases. Other associated problems include the development of noncancerous tumors, especially of the brain, kidney, retina, and heart.

There is no cure for tuberous sclerosis. Treatment is aimed at relieving troublesome symptoms, including treatment of epilepsy and removal of tumors. Seriously affected people may not live beyond age 30. *Genetic counseling* is recommended for affected families who are considering children. The gene for tuberous sclerosis can now be detected at an early stage in pregnancy.

## Tuboplasty

An operation in which a damaged fallopian tube is repaired to treat infertility. Tuboplasty is performed if a tube has become scarred and blocked, usually following *salpingitis* (tubal infection) or *pelvic inflammatory disease*.

In performing tuboplasty, the gynecologist usually uses *microsurgery* techniques to unblock the delicate tubes. Recently, the use of balloon tuboplasty has been introduced.

The fertility rate following tuboplasty varies from 5 to 50 percent, depending on how badly the tube was damaged to start with and whether other causes of infertility exist. *Ectopic pregnancy* is more common in women who have had diseased tubes or tuboplasty than in those with healthy fallopian tubes.

T

## PROCEDURE FOR BALLOON TUBOPLASTY

A blocked fallopian tube may be treated by inserting a balloon catheter into the damaged tube and inflating the balloon. The balloon is then deflated and the catheter withdrawn.

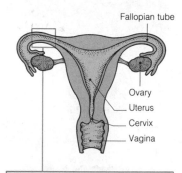

Fallopian tube
Ovary
Uterus
Cervix
Vagina

Blocked fallopian tube    Guide wire

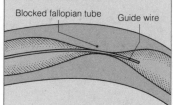

**1** A thin guide wire is maneuvered along the fallopian tube to the blockage and the tip of the wire is forced through the constricted area.

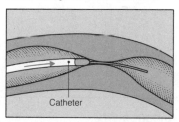

Catheter

**2** A balloon-tipped catheter is threaded over the guide wire until the balloon strikes the blockage; the balloon is then inflated.

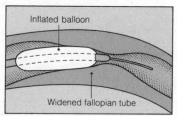

Inflated balloon

Widened fallopian tube

**3** The inflated balloon is pushed against the obstructed part. Gradually the blockage widens until the balloon can be pushed through.

## Tularemia

An infectious disease of wild animals, such as rabbits, squirrels, and muskrats. Tularemia is occasionally transmitted to humans.

### CAUSES AND INCIDENCE

Humans may be infected through direct contact with an infected animal or its carcass, in which case the causative bacteria enter the body via a cut or abrasion in the skin. Tularemia can also be acquired through a bite from an infected tick, flea, fly, or louse or, in rare cases, by eating infected meat.

Tularemia occurs only in North America and some parts of Europe and Asia. A few hundred cases are reported annually in the US. A vaccine is available for people at highest risk, such as hunters, trappers, game wardens, and laboratory workers.

### SYMPTOMS, DIAGNOSIS, AND TREATMENT

In most cases, a red spot develops on the skin at the site of infection, grows larger, and forms an ulcer. The lymph nodes in the armpits or groin enlarge and become tender, and there is a fever and often a headache, muscle pains, and malaise. The illness may continue for several weeks. In other cases, the eyes, throat, digestive tract, or lungs are affected.

Tularemia is diagnosed by a blood test that detects antibodies formed against the bacteria. Treatment is with *antibiotic drugs*, sucn as streptomycin. Without treatment, tularemia is fatal in about 5 percent of cases; with treatment, the fatality rate is less than 1 percent. One attack protects against future disease.

## Tumbu fly bites

A cause of *myiasis* (skin infestation with fly larvae) in Africa.

## Tumor

By strict definition, any swelling. Also known as a neoplasm, a tumor is an abnormal mass of tissue that forms when cells in a specific area reproduce at an increased rate.

Tumors may be *malignant* or *benign*. Malignant tumors invade surrounding tissues and may also spread via the bloodstream or lymphatic system to form a secondary growth (called a *metastasis*) elsewhere in the body. *Cancer* is the general term used to refer to all types of malignant tumors. A malignant tumor that arises from epithelial tissues (such as skin) is termed a *carcinoma*; one that arises from deep body tissues (such as muscle, bone, or fibrous tissue) is called a *sarcoma*.

Benign tumors usually grow slowly and do not metastasize, although they may sometimes be multiple. They tend to remain confined within a fibrous capsule, making surgical removal relatively straightforward. However, benign tumors may grow large enough to cause damage by pressing on nearby structures, which can be particularly dangerous in confined spaces, such as inside the skull.

At the microscopic level, one essential difference between benign and malignant tumors is that the former retain many of the features of the tissue from which they arose. In contrast, malignant tumors tend to comprise small, rapidly growing cells that form masses of tissue with less recognizable features of the tissue from which they originated.

## Tumor-specific antigen

A substance secreted by a specific type of tumor (or class of tumors) that is detectable in the blood. Tumor-specific antigens cannot be used accurately to screen for malignant tumors because most can also be produced in nonmalignant conditions.

Two tumor-specific antigens are carcinoembryonic antigen and *alpha-fetoprotein*. Carcinoembryonic antigen is produced in abnormal amounts by about half of the tumors of the colon, stomach, breast, lungs, and pancreas. Alpha-fetoprotein levels in blood serum are raised in 70 percent of the people who have hepatoma (a primary *liver cancer*) and in most people with teratoma, a type of testicular cancer (see *Testis, cancer of*).

## Tunnel vision

Constriction of the *visual field*; only objects straight ahead can be seen.

### CAUSES

The most common cause of tunnel vision is chronic *glaucoma*, in which raised pressure within the eye results in destruction of *optic nerve* fibers. Peripheral vision is gradually lost until the visual field is reduced to only a few degrees across.

Tunnel vision may also be caused by a tumor or other brain disorder that interferes with the fibers that connect the *optic nerve* to the brain. Pituitary tumors, for instance, can press on the point where the optic nerves come together, causing loss of the right half of the right eye's field of vision and the left half of the left eye's vision. *Retinitis pigmentosa* (retinal degeneration) may cause the loss of peripheral vision and result in tunnel vision.

## Turner's syndrome

A disorder caused by a *chromosomal abnormality* that affects only females.

### INCIDENCE AND CAUSES

Approximately one in 3,000 live-born girls is born with Turner's syndrome. The chromosomal abnormality may arise in one of three ways. Most affected females have only 45 chromosomes compared with the normal complement of 46, the missing chromosome being one of the X chromosomes. Sometimes, both X chromosomes are present but one is defective. Occasionally, the condition arises as a type of *mosaicism*, in which some cells are missing one X chromosome, some have extra chromosomes, and others have their normal number of chromosomes.

### SIGNS

The main features of the syndrome are shortness of stature, webbing of the skin of the neck, absence or very retarded development of secondary sexual characteristics (see *Sexual characteristics, secondary*), absence of menstruation, coarctation (narrowing) of the aorta, abnormalities of the eyes and bones, and a degree of mental retardation. The average adult height is 4 feet 6 inches (135 cm).

### TREATMENT

Coarctation of the aorta is treated by surgery at an early age. Menstruation may be induced by *estrogen drugs* but sufferers continue to be infertile.

## Twins

Two infants resulting from one pregnancy. Twins may develop from a single ovum (egg) or from two ova.

Monozygotic or monovular (identical) twins develop when a single, fertilized ovum divides completely and equally at an early stage of development; if this division is incomplete it results in *Siamese twins*. Monozygotic twins share the same placenta. Although one is often much bigger than the other at birth, they are always of the same sex and look remarkably alike, hence their common name of identical twins.

Twins from two ova are called dizygotic or binovular twins. The ova from which they develop may be released by the same or different ovaries; fertilization of the two ova occurs simultaneously. Each dizygotic twin has its own placenta. The twins may be of the same or different sexes, and may look quite different.

Twins occur in about one in 90 pregnancies. Dizygotic twins are more likely to occur in older women, in women who have had many previous pregnancies, and in women who have a history of twins in the family; they are also more common in Africa and Asia. These factors do not have any bearing on the incidence of monozygotic twins.

Twins face greater difficulties from the start. Deaths are more frequent before, during, or just after birth. When rearing twins, especially monozygotic twins, it is important to reinforce their importance as separate people. (See also *Pregnancy, multiple*.)

## Twins, conjoined

Another name for *Siamese twins*.

## Twitch

See *Fasciculation; Tic*.

---

## TWO TYPES OF TWINS

During each menstrual cycle, either one ovum or a small number of ova may be released. If one ovum is fertilized and the two cells formed from its first division develop independently, the result is identical twins. If two ova are fertilized and mature normally, nonidentical twins result.

### IDENTICAL TWINS

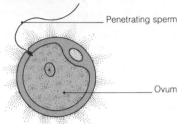

Penetrating sperm

Ovum

Identical twins come from a single fertilized ovum. When the ovum splits, the two cells formed develop independently.

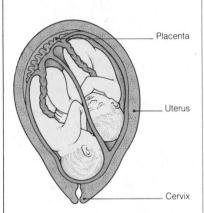

Placenta

Uterus

Cervix

The result is a pair of genetically identical twins sharing the same placenta. They are called monovular or monozygotic.

### NONIDENTICAL TWINS

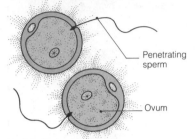

Penetrating sperm

Ovum

Nonidentical twins come from two separate ova that have been fertilized by two separate spermatozoa.

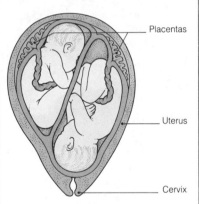

Placentas

Uterus

Cervix

The resulting individuals are genetically distinct and have separate placentas. They are dizygotic, or binovular, twins.

---

## Tympanometry

A type of *hearing test*, also called impedance audiometry.

## Tympanoplasty

An operation to repair a hole in the eardrum and/or ossicles (the tiny bones in the middle ear) to treat hearing loss.

### WHY IT IS DONE

In a healthy ear, sound waves are conducted from the eardrum to the oval window of the inner ear by a chain of three bones called ossicles (see *Ear*). Chronic *otitis media* (middle-ear infection) can fuse these bones in position or erode them, in either case interfering with sound conduction and thus causing some degree of conductive hearing loss. In such cases tym-

T

panoplasty offers the only chance of restoring some of the lost hearing.

**HOW IT IS DONE**

An incision is made adjacent to the eardrum (using general anesthesia) to provide access to the middle ear. Viewing the ear through an operating microscope, the surgeon then repositions or repairs the chain of ossicles. This may involve reshaping and transposing one of the bones, replacing an ossicle with a plastic substitute, grafting an ossicle taken from a donor, or fashioning an ossicle from cartilage. The bones are reset in their natural order and the eardrum is repaired.

**RESULTS**

The operation often improves hearing considerably, but there is no guarantee of success, especially in cases where poor eustachian tube function causes the eardrum to adhere to the ossicles. (See also *Myringoplasty; Stapedectomy.*)

## Tympanum

Part of the *ear*, comprising the middle-ear cavity (tympanic cavity) and eardrum (tympanic membrane).

## Typhoid fever

An infectious disease contracted by eating food or drinking water that has been contaminated with the bacterium *SALMONELLA TYPHOSA*. An almost identical disease, known as *paratyphoid fever*, is caused by a related bacterium.

**CAUSES AND INCIDENCE**

The source of infection is the feces of a person who has the disease or is a symptomless carrier of the causative bacteria. In areas of poor sanitation, typhoid is commonly spread by contamination of drinking water with sewage, or by flies carrying the bacteria from infected feces to food. Elsewhere, infection is usually due to handling of food by typhoid carriers. Shellfish that have been contaminated by sewage are an occasional source of typhoid outbreaks.

During the development of the disease, the bacteria pass from the intestines into the blood, and then to the spleen and liver, where they multiply. The organisms are excreted from the liver, accumulate in the gallbladder, and are released in enormous numbers into the intestine. Carriers, after recovering from typhoid fever, may continue to harbor typhoid bacilli in the gallbladder and shed them in the feces for many years.

Typhoid is uncommon in developed countries but epidemics occur regularly in developing countries. There are fewer than 600 cases per year in the US.

**PREVENTION**

Typhoid is a reportable disease and known cases should be isolated. Immunization against typhoid is recommended for travel anywhere outside of the US and Canada, northern Europe, Australia, and New Zealand. The vaccine is given in two doses, often causing some swelling and pain at the site of injection for one to two days. A booster dose is needed after two to three years. The vaccine does not provide complete protection; travelers at risk should drink only boiled water or bottled drinks and eat well-cooked food.

**SYMPTOMS AND SIGNS**

Typhoid has an incubation period of seven to 14 days. The course of the infection varies from a mild upset to a major life-threatening illness. The first symptom is usually severe headache, followed by fever, loss of appetite, malaise, abdominal tenderness, constipation, and often delirium. Constipation soon gives way to diarrhea. During the second week of the illness, small, raised pink spots appear on the chest and abdomen for several days; there is also enlargement of the liver and spleen at this time.

The illness usually clears up within four weeks. However, if treatment is delayed, severe, sometimes fatal, complications may develop, including intestinal bleeding, *urinary tract infection, renal failure,* or perforation of the intestine leading to *peritonitis.*

**DIAGNOSIS AND TREATMENT**

The diagnosis is confirmed by obtaining a *culture* of typhoid bacteria from a sample of blood, feces, or urine, or by a *blood test* that reveals the presence of antibodies against typhoid bacteria.

The *antibiotic drugs* chloramphenicol or ampicillin usually bring the disease under control within a few days; severely ill patients may require brief supplementary treatment with *corticosteroid drugs.*

The complication of intestinal perforation is the principal risk, but can be avoided by adequate control with antibiotics. An operation may be needed if widespread peritonitis or severe bleeding develops.

Given early diagnosis and proper treatment, the outlook is usually excellent. Permanent immunity most often follows an attack of typhoid, although relapses are common if the disease is not fully eradicated by thorough antibiotic treatment.

## Typhus

Any of a group of infectious diseases, with similar symptoms, caused by rickettsiae (microorganisms similar to bacteria) and spread by insects or similar animals.

**TYPES, CAUSES, AND INCIDENCE**

Historically, the most important type was epidemic typhus, spread by body lice. It once occurred in epidemics that killed hundreds of thousands during war, famine, or other natural disasters. Today it is rare except in some highland areas of tropical Africa and South America. Lice ingest the causative organism, *RICKETTSIA PROWAZEKI*, from the blood of infected people and deposit feces containing the microorganisms onto the skin of other hosts, where they enter the blood as the result of scratching.

Endemic, or murine, typhus is a disease of rats that may be spread to humans by fleas. About 50 cases occur in the US each year. Scrub typhus is spread by mites and occurs in India and Southeast Asia. *Rocky Mountain spotted fever* is a disease similar to typhus.

**PREVENTION**

In crowded conditions following natural disasters, epidemic typhus is prevented through control of human louse infestation with insecticides. A vaccine also exists against the disease.

Other types of typhus are avoided through measures to discourage bites by fleas, mites, or ticks (e.g., the use of protective clothing).

**SYMPTOMS AND SIGNS**

In epidemic typhus, severe headache, back and limb pain, coughing, and constipation develop suddenly and are followed by high fever, confusion, a rash similar to that of measles, prostration, a weak heart beat, and, often, delirium. Without treatment, death may occur from *septicemia, heart failure, renal failure,* or *pneumonia.*

Other types of typhus have similar symptoms and complications, although endemic typhus is milder.

**DIAGNOSIS AND TREATMENT**

Particular types of typhus fever are diagnosed by tests that can detect blood products formed in reaction to the rickettsial organisms. Typhus fevers are treated with *antibiotic drugs*. Other measures may be required to relieve severe symptoms and treat complications. Convalescence is often slow, particularly in the elderly.

## Typing

See *Tissue-typing.*

T

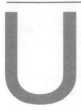

# U

## Ulcer

An open sore on the skin or on a mucous membrane that results from the destruction of surface tissue. An ulcer may be shallow or deep and crater-shaped and is usually inflamed and painful.

Skin ulcers most commonly occur on the leg (see *Leg ulcer*), usually as the result of inadequate blood supply to or drainage from the limb. Among the rarer forms of skin ulcers are those that develop in *basal cell carcinomas*, which are a form of skin cancer.

Ulcers on mucous membranes most commonly develop within the digestive tract, occurring in the mouth (see *Mouth ulcer*), in the stomach or the duodenum (see *Peptic ulcer*), or in the small or large intestine (see *Ulcerative colitis*).

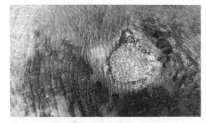

**Ulcer on forehead**
An ulcer in this skin area is often due to a basal cell carcinoma—a type of skin cancer that is easily treated.

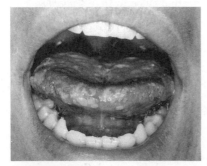

**Ulcers in mouth**
Aphthous ulcers (canker sores) are common, painful, and are usually precipitated by stress. Most heal well without scarring.

The skin or mucous membranes of the genitalia may also be affected by ulcers (see *Genital ulceration*). Most are caused by sexually transmitted disease. Examples of this type of ulcer are hard and soft chancres (see *Chancre, hard; Chancroid*).

Ulcers may also develop on the cornea, the transparent covering at the front of the eyeball (see *Corneal ulcer*).

## Ulceration

The formation of one or more *ulcers*.

## Ulcerative colitis

Chronic inflammation and ulceration of the lining of the colon and rectum. The disease sometimes begins by affecting the rectum only.

**CAUSES AND INCIDENCE**

The cause of ulcerative colitis is unknown. In the US, the disease affects between 40 and 50 people per 100,000. It is most common in young and middle-aged adults.

**SYMPTOMS AND SIGNS**

The main symptom is bloody diarrhea; the feces may also contain pus and mucus. In severe cases, diarrhea and bleeding are extensive and there may be abdominal pain and tenderness, fever, and general malaise. The incidence of attacks varies considerably from person to person. Most commonly, attacks occur at intervals of a few months; however, in some cases, symptoms are either continuous or occur infrequently.

One of the principal dangers of severe ulcerative colitis is *anemia*, caused by loss of blood. Other complications include a toxic form of *megacolon* (a grossly distended colon), which may be life-threatening; rashes; mouth ulcers; *arthritis*; and inflammation of the eye in the form of *conjunctivitis* or *uveitis*. In addition, people whose entire colon has been inflamed for more than 10 years are at increased risk of cancer of the colon (see *Intestine, cancer of*).

**DIAGNOSIS**

The diagnosis is based on examination of the rectum and lower colon with a viewing instrument (see *Sigmoidoscopy*) or of the entire colon by *colonoscopy* or by a barium enema (see *Barium X-ray examinations*). During sigmoidoscopy or colonoscopy, a *biopsy* (removal of a small sample of tissue for analysis) may be performed. Samples of feces may also be taken for analysis to exclude the possibility of infection (by bacteria or parasites) as a cause of the symptoms. *Blood tests* may be required.

People who have had ulcerative colitis for many years require periodic colonoscopy and biopsy to check for the development of cancer.

**TREATMENT**

In most cases, medical treatment effectively controls the disease. Treatment usually consists of *corticosteroid drugs* (to control symptoms by reducing inflammation) and the *sulfonamide drug* sulfasalazine (to maintain long-term freedom from symptoms). Newer drug treatments using salicylate derivatives of sulfasalazine have recently become available.

*Colectomy* (surgical removal of the colon) may be required if inflammation is extensive, severe, and uncontrollable; colectomy is required by most patients who have toxic megacolon. This operation usually produces a dramatic improvement in the patient's health.

## Ulcer-healing drugs

| COMMON DRUGS |
|---|
| Histamine-2 receptor antagonists |
| *Cimetidine Famotidine Ranitidine* |
| |
| Others |
| *Sucralfate* |
| *Antacids* |

A group of drugs used to treat and prevent *peptic ulcer*.

**HOW THEY WORK**

Ulcer-healing drugs work in one of two ways.

*Histamine-2 receptor antagonists* work by blocking the effects of histamine, an action that reduces the secretion of acid in the stomach and thus promotes the healing of ulcers.

Other ulcer-healing drugs, such as sucralfate, are believed to form a protective barrier over the ulcer, thereby allowing the underlying tissues time to heal. *Antacid drugs* taken regularly are also effective.

Ulcer-healing drugs usually relieve symptoms within one to two weeks; in most cases, the ulcer heals within eight weeks. Once healed, a maintenance dose may be prescribed. Without continuing treatment, the chance of an ulcer recurring is between 60 and 70 percent.

**POSSIBLE ADVERSE EFFECTS**

Adverse effects may include confusion, headaches, and dizziness. Ulcer-healing drugs may mask the symptoms of *stomach cancer*. These drugs are therefore not usually prescribed for periods longer than two months unless the possibility of cancer has been ruled out.

## Ulna

The longer of the two bones of the forearm; the other is the *radius*. With the palm facing forward, the ulna is the inner bone (i.e., the bone nearer the trunk) running down the forearm parallel to the radius.

---

**LOCATION OF THE ULNA**
The ulna hinges at the elbow on the inner side of the lower end of the humerus (upper arm bone). It is less mobile than the radius.

Right arm

Humerus

Radius

Ulna

Carpals

Thumb

---

The upper end of the ulna articulates with the radius and extends into a rounded projection (called the olecranon process) that fits around the lower end of the humerus (upper arm bone) to form part of the *elbow* joint. The lower end of the ulna is rounded and articulates with the carpals (*wrist* bones) and lower part of the radius.

## Ulna, fracture of

Fractures of the *ulna* typically occur across the shaft or at the olecranon process (tip of the elbow).

A shaft fracture is usually caused by a blow to the forearm or a fall onto the hand. In some cases, the radius is fractured at the same time (see *Radius, fracture of*). An operation is usually needed to reposition the broken bone ends and fix them together, using either a plate and screws or a long nail down the center of the bone. The arm is then immobilized in a plaster cast, with the elbow at a right angle, until the fracture heals.

A fracture of the olecranon process is usually caused by a fall onto the elbow. If the bone ends are not displaced, the arm is immobilized in a plaster cast with the elbow at a right-angle. Otherwise, an operation is

needed before immobilization. If the bone ends are displaced, they are fitted together and fixed with a metal screw; if the bone is broken into several pieces, the bone fragments are removed and the triceps muscle reattached to the broken end of the ulna.

## Ulnar nerve

One of the principal nerves of the arm, running down its full length into the hand. A branch of the *brachial plexus*, the ulnar nerve controls muscles that move the thumb and fingers. It also conveys sensation from the fifth and part of the fourth fingers, and from the palm at the base of these digits.

**DISORDERS**
A blow to the *olecranon* process (the bony prominence at the tip of the elbow), over which the ulnar nerve passes, causes a pins and needles sensation and pain in the forearm and fourth and fifth fingers.

Persistent numbness and muscle weakness in the areas controlled by the nerve may be caused by pressure from an abnormal bony outgrowth from the humerus (upper arm bone). Such a growth may be due to *osteoarthritis* or to a fracture of the humerus. If an operation is not performed to relieve the pressure on the nerve, the hand muscles controlled by the nerve may become permanently damaged, resulting in a *clawhand*.

## Ultrasound

Sound with a frequency greater than the human ear's upper limit of perception—that is, with a frequency higher than 20,000 hertz (cycles per second). Ultrasound used in medicine for diagnosis or treatment is typically in the frequency range of 1 million to 15 million hertz (see *Ultrasound scanning*; *Ultrasound treatment*).

## Ultrasound scanning

A diagnostic technique in which very high frequency sound waves (inaudible to the human ear) are passed into the body; the reflected echoes are detected and analyzed to build a picture of the internal organs or of a fetus in the uterus. The procedure is considered painless and safe.

Also called sonography, ultrasound scanning was originally a spin-off from naval sonar (used to detect submarines in World War II) and was first used medically in the 1950s. The original ultrasound scanners produced still images; most modern scanners produce moving pictures, which are easier to interpret.

**HOW IT WORKS**
The illustrated box (next page) explains how ultrasound scanners work and are operated.

**WHY IT IS DONE**
Ultrasound waves pass readily through soft tissues and fluids, making this procedure particularly useful for examining fluid-filled organs (such as the uterus in pregnancy and the gallbladder) and soft organs (such as the liver). Ultrasound waves cannot, however, pass through bone or gas. They are thus of limited use for examining regions that are surrounded by bone (such as the brain) or that contain gas (such as the lungs or intestines). Nevertheless, ultrasound has been used to examine most parts of the anatomy.

**OBSTETRIC USES** One of the most common uses of ultrasound is to view the uterus and fetus in pregnancy.

Ultrasound scanning is often performed about 16 to 18 weeks into the pregnancy. If the date of conception is known, the scan shows whether the fetus is of the expected size; fetal size can also help establish the accurate date of conception. The scan also reveals whether there is a multiple pregnancy (see *Pregnancy, multiple*). It is also possible to identify certain gross abnormalities, such as *anencephaly* or *spina bifida*. Congenital *heart disease* can sometimes be detected, enabling the baby to be delivered in a hospital that specializes in correcting such defects. The scan also shows the position of the placenta. If the placenta is in a position that could obstruct normal childbirth (*placenta previa*), delivery by *cesarean section* may be necessary.

Scans earlier in pregnancy may be performed to establish viability (whether the fetus is alive) if the physician suspects an *ectopic pregnancy* (presence of an embryo outside the uterus), *hydatidiform mole* (abnormal tumor in the uterus), impending *miscarriage*, or early fetal death.

Ultrasound is also vital for the procedure of *amniocentesis* (removal of amniotic fluid via a needle for analysis) and is used during *chorionic villus sampling* (removal of tissue from the placenta for analysis). A scan shows the position of the fetus and placenta before the procedure and also helps the physician guide the needle into the uterus.

Later in pregnancy, a scan may be carried out if the growth rate of the fetus seems slow, if fetal movements cease or are excessive, or if the mother experiences vaginal bleeding. For

U

## HOW ULTRASOUND SCANNING WORKS

Ultrasound waves are emitted by a device called a transducer, which is placed on the skin over the part of the body to be viewed. The transducer contains a crystal that converts an electrical current into sound waves. The waves used have frequencies in the range of 2.5 to 10 million hertz. At these high frequencies, the waves can be focused into a fine parallel beam, which passes through a "slice" of the body if the transducer crystal is made to oscillate back and forth. Some of the waves are reflected at tissue boundaries, so a series of echoes is returned. The transducer also acts as a receiver, converting these echoes into electrical signals, which are processed and displayed on a screen to give a two-dimensional image of the scanned body slice. By moving the transducer, different slices through the body can be seen.

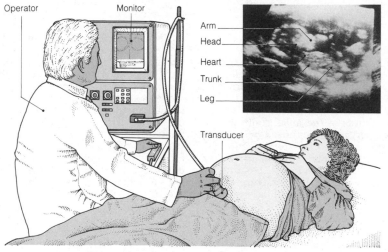

Operator    Monitor

Arm
Head
Heart
Trunk
Leg

Transducer

Ultrasound has wide applications in medicine and is especially useful in obstetrics. It offers no known risk to the baby. By moving the transducer across the outer wall of the abdomen, views of the growing fetus are obtained from various angles, so it is possible to screen for abnormalities.

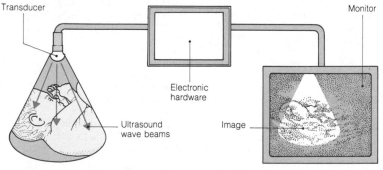

Transducer

Monitor

Electronic hardware

Ultrasound wave beams

Image

**Parts of an ultrasound scanner**
The transducer emits a beam of high frequency waves, which are passed through a slice of the body; the echoes are picked up by the transducer and converted by the electronic hardware into an image displayed on the cathode-ray tube viewing monitor.

*Echocardiography* is a type of ultrasound technique used to look at the heart; it is particularly useful for investigating congenital heart disease and disorders of the heart valves.

The liver can be clearly viewed by ultrasound, which can be used to diagnose *cirrhosis* and liver cysts, abscesses, or tumors. *Gallstones* in the gallbladder or bile ducts are visible; in a patient with *jaundice*, a scan can help establish whether the jaundice is due to obstruction of the bile ducts or liver disease. The pancreas can be scanned for cysts, tumors, or pancreatitis, and the kidneys for congenital defects, cysts, tumors, and *hydronephrosis* (swelling due to obstruction to the outflow of urine). Other organs that may be scanned by ultrasound for diagnostic purposes (primarily to look for cysts, solid tumors, or foreign bodies) include the thyroid gland, breasts, bladder, testes, ovaries, spleen, and eyes.

Doppler ultrasound is a modified version of ordinary ultrasound that is used for looking at moving objects, such as blood coursing through the blood vessels and the fetal heart beat in pregnancy (see *Doppler effect*).

Ultrasound scanning is also being used more frequently in conjunction with fine needle *biopsy* (inserting a very thin hollow needle into an organ to remove cells, tissue, or fluid for examination) to help guide the needle accurately to a specific spot.

**HOW IT IS DONE**
For a scan in early pregnancy, the woman is usually asked not to pass urine for a few hours beforehand; a full bladder helps improve the view of the uterus by displacing nearby loops of intestine. For a liver or gallbladder scan, the patient is usually asked to fast for several hours beforehand.

Clothing over the area to be scanned is removed and oil or jelly is smeared over the skin to achieve good contact as the transducer is passed back and forth over the skin. During the scan, which takes about 15 minutes, the patient can usually lie back and watch the images appearing on the screen.

The ultrasonic waves produce no detectable sensation. When a scan is performed in conjunction with a technique involving insertion of a needle, a local anesthetic is used and there is usually little or no discomfort.

## Ultrasound treatment

The use of high-frequency sound waves to treat injuries to soft tissues, such as ligaments, muscles, and ten-

high-risk or overdue pregnancies, a predelivery scan may be carried out to check on fetal size, development, and position in the uterus, the amount of amniotic fluid, and to recheck the position of the placenta.

**NONOBSTETRIC USES** In the newborn child, ultrasound can be used to scan the brain, via a gap (the anterior fontanelle) in the skull, to investigate *hydrocephalus*, or to diagnose a *brain tumor* or brain hemorrhage.

U

dons. The treatment reduces inflammation and speeds up healing. It is thought to work by improving blood flow through tissues under the skin.

During treatment, there may be a feeling of warmth and a slight tingling sensation. Occasionally, severe pain occurs if the sound waves are pointed at a bone surface just under the skin.

## Ultraviolet light

Invisible light from the part of the electromagnetic spectrum immediately beyond the violet end of the visible light spectrum (that is, between visible light and X rays). Long wavelength ultraviolet light (that nearest visible light) is often termed UVA; intermediate wavelength ultraviolet light is designated UVB; and short wavelength ultraviolet light (that nearest X rays) is called UVC.

### ELECTROMAGNETIC SPECTRUM

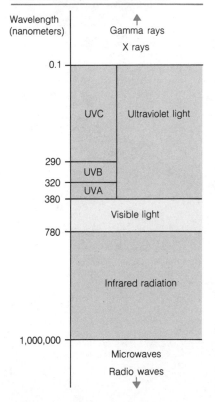

**Ultraviolet light in the spectrum**
Different types of electromagnetic radiation are defined according to their wavelengths. The diagram shows the different types within the electromagnetic spectrum, together with their wavelength limits (in nanometers, or billionths of a meter). Ultraviolet light falls in the band between visible light and extreme short wavelength radiation, such as X rays.

Ultraviolet light occurs naturally in sunlight, but most of it—including all UVC and much UVB (both of which are potentially harmful)—is absorbed by the *ozone* layer of the atmosphere. The ultraviolet light that reaches the earth's surface, mainly UVA, is responsible for the tanning and burning effects of sunlight and for the production of vitamin D in the skin. However, it is the ultraviolet component of sunlight, particularly the relatively small proportion of UVB, that can cause cataracts and, especially in fair-skinned people, skin cancer (see *Sunlight, adverse effects of*).

Suntanning lamps, which produce ultraviolet light artificially, are designed to emit only UVA rays, although, in practice, they also give off a small amount of UVB light.

A mercury-vapor lamp (Wood's light) can also be used to produce ultraviolet light artificially. This light is used to diagnose certain skin conditions, such as *tinea*, because it causes the infected area to fluoresce.

Ultraviolet light may also be used in *phototherapy* to treat certain skin conditions, including *psoriasis, vitiligo,* and *jaundice* of the newborn.

## Umbilical cord

The ropelike structure connecting the fetus to the *placenta* that supplies oxygen and nutrients from the mother's circulation. The umbilical cord is usually 16 to 24 inches (40 to 60 cm) long and consists of a jellylike substance in which two arteries and a vein are embedded.

Several minutes after delivery, the umbilical cord is clamped and then cut about an inch from the baby's abdominal wall. The stump falls off within a couple of weeks, leaving a scar called the *umbilicus* (navel).

### DISORDERS

In rare cases, the umbilical cord prolapses (protrudes down) through the mother's cervix during labor. This is a dangerous condition because the baby's oxygen supply can be cut off. Prompt delivery of the infant, either by *cesarean section* or a *forceps delivery*, is necessary. Sometimes the cord pulls tightly around the baby's neck during delivery; it can usually be freed easily by slipping it over the baby's head.

Rarely, there is only one artery in the umbilical cord. This condition may be associated with birth defects.

The newborn baby's umbilical stump sometimes becomes infected and may ooze pus. This condition, called omphalitis, generally begins

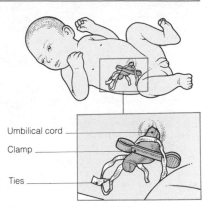

**Umbilical cord after birth**
The cord ceases to function after birth and is clamped and cut; the baby now obtains oxygen through his or her own lungs.

during the first week of life. Treatment involves gently wiping the umbilicus with sterile cotton and water. Treatment with antibiotics may be necessary to prevent serious infection.

Quite commonly, a fleshy protuberance called a *granuloma* grows on the umbilical stump, sometimes as a result of chronic infection. Umbilical granulomas may be removed by local application of *silver nitrate*. Umbilical polyps, also known as umbilical adenomas, are shiny, bright red, raspberrylike growths that also appear in the newborn period. They may require surgical removal.

## Umbilicus

The scar on the abdomen that marks the site of attachment of the *umbilical cord* to the fetus. The umbilicus is commonly called the navel.

### DISORDERS

An umbilical *hernia* is a soft swelling at the umbilicus caused by protrusion of the abdominal contents through a weak area of the abdominal wall.

Umbilical hernias are quite common in newborns, occurring twice as often in boys. When the baby cries, the

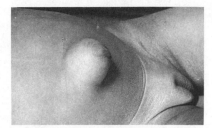

**Umbilical hernia**
This condition, present from birth, is due to a local weakness in the abdominal wall. Recovery without treatment is usual.

U

swelling increases in size and may cause discomfort. Umbilical hernias usually disappear without treatment by about age 2. They are unlikely to disappear without treatment after about age 4.

Occasionally, umbilical hernias develop in adults, especially in women following childbirth. Surgery may be necessary for large, persistent, or disfiguring hernias.

In rare cases, there may be a discharge from the umbilicus. It can be caused by an infection or by an abnormal connection between the umbilicus and the urinary, biliary, or intestinal tract. The abnormal connection may be due to a birth defect, to cancer, or to tuberculosis. Surgery is used to correct this condition.

Occasionally, benign or malignant tumors develop at the umbilicus. These tumors may be secondary to cancers in the breast, colon, ovary, or stomach. In women, *endometriosis* may in rare cases develop in the umbilicus, which bleeds at periodic intervals. The treatment is surgical excision.

## Unconscious

A specific part of the mind in which ideas, memories, perceptions, or feelings that a person is not currently aware of are stored and actively processed. The contents of the unconscious mind are not easily retrievable, in contrast to those of the *subconscious*. *Freudian theory* stresses the importance of the unconscious in determining behavior and causing neurotic symptoms. *Jungian theory* describes a collective unconscious, inherited by every person and derived from experiences in our distant past.

## Unconsciousness

Abnormal loss of awareness of self and of the surroundings resulting from a reduced level of activity of the reticular formation in the *brain stem.* Sleep is a normal state of altered consciousness from which a person can be roused easily; an unconscious person can be roused only with difficulty or not at all. Unconsciousness may be brief and light, as in *fainting*, or deeper and more prolonged (see *Coma*). The term *concussion* refers to a brief transient state of unconsciousness following a head injury.

## Underbite

A term that describes a type of *malocclusion* in which the lower jaw is set abnormally forward, which causes the lower incisors to overlap the upper incisors.

## Unsaturated fats

See *Fats and oils.*

## Uranium

A radioactive metallic element that does not occur naturally in its pure form but is widely distributed as various compounds in ores such as pitchblende, carnotite, and uraninite.

Natural radioactive decay of uranium yields a series of radioactive products, including *radium* and *radon*, and progresses ultimately to lead. During the various decay stages, *radiation* is emitted as alpha and beta particles and gamma rays. In addition to its *radiation hazards*, uranium is chemically poisonous in the body, where it damages the urinary system.

## Urea

A waste product of the breakdown of proteins and the main nitrogenous (nitrogen-containing) constituent of urine. Proteins in food are digested in the intestine to form *amino acids*, which are absorbed into the bloodstream and transported to the liver. In the liver, amino acids in excess of the body's requirements are converted into urea, which is transported by the bloodstream to the kidneys and excreted in the urine.

The kidneys are usually highly efficient at eliminating urea from the body. A high-protein diet increases the amount of urea produced. Healthy kidneys are able to cope with increased urea production, but *renal failure* impairs the kidneys' ability to eliminate urea and leads to uremia (abnormally high blood levels of urea). For this reason, measuring

---

### FIRST AID: UNCONSCIOUSNESS

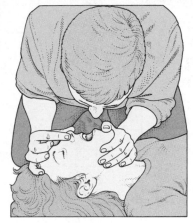

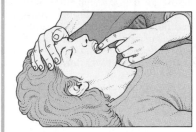

**DO NOT**
- leave an unconscious person alone
- give anyone who is, or has been, unconscious anything to eat or drink

**1** Make sure the victim is breathing. If breathing sounds difficult, check the airways and quickly clear the mouth.

**2** If the victim is not breathing, start *artificial respiration*. Loosen any tight clothing he or she is wearing.

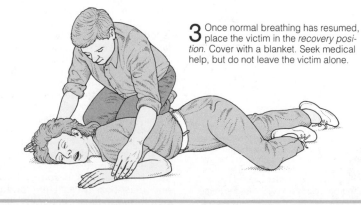

**3** Once normal breathing has resumed, place the victim in the *recovery position*. Cover with a blanket. Seek medical help, but do not leave the victim alone.

blood levels of urea is one of the routine kidney function tests.

Urea is also formed in the body from the breakdown of cell proteins. If there is a large increase in urea from this source (e.g., due to severe tissue damage from injury or surgery), the kidneys are sometimes unable to cope and uremia results.

Certain conditions (such as liver damage) may lead to a decrease in the blood level of urea. Blood levels of urea also fall during pregnancy, when the blood is more dilute than usual.

### MEDICAL USES

Urea is used in various creams and ointments to moisturize and soften the skin in the treatment of disorders such as *psoriasis*, atopic *dermatitis*, *ichthyosis*, and other conditions in which the skin is dry and scaly. Occasionally, urea is used as an osmotic *diuretic drug*, primarily to reduce pressure in the skull due to cerebral *edema* or pressure in the eye caused by *glaucoma*.

## Uremia

The presence of excess urea and other chemical waste products in the blood. Uremia develops as a result of kidney failure (see *Renal failure*).

## Ureter

Either of the two tubes that carry urine from the kidneys to the bladder. Each is about 10 to 12 inches (25 to 30 cm) long. The walls of each ureter have three layers—a fibrous outer layer, a muscular middle layer, and an inner membrane. Each ureter is supplied by blood vessels and nerves.

Urine flows down the ureters partly by gravity but mainly by peristalsis, a pumping action as waves of contraction pass several times per minute through the muscle layers in the ureteral walls. Each ureter enters the bladder via a tunnel in the bladder wall, which is angled to prevent reflux of urine back into the ureter when the bladder muscle contracts.

### DISORDERS

Some people are born with two ureters on one or both sides. A double ureter is usually accompanied by partial duplication of the kidney on that side. The two ureters may join farther down (to form a Y shape) or may be completely distinct. In many cases, a duplicated ureter causes no problems. However, when the ureters enter the bladder separately, there may be a tendency for urine to reflux up one of the tubes; when a ureter enters the urethra or vagina instead of the blad-

---

### ANATOMY OF THE URETER

The ureters are tubes that carry urine from the kidneys to the bladder. They enter the back of the bladder at an angle.

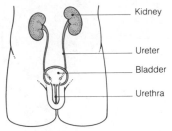

- Kidney
- Ureter
- Bladder
- Urethra

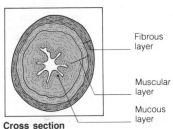

- Fibrous layer
- Muscular layer
- Mucous layer

**Cross section**

Each ureter has three layers—an outer, fibrous layer, a thick, muscular middle layer, and an inner, mucous membrane.

---

der at its lower end, it can cause *incontinence* or infection. These problems can be corrected surgically.

If a urinary tract *calculus* (stone) passes down or becomes stuck in a ureter, it can lead to spasms of the muscles in the ureteral walls, an extremely painful condition known as *renal colic*.

Ureteritis is an inflammatory condition of a ureter that may be caused by blockage with a stone or by infection spreading up from the bladder.

## Ureteral colic

See *Renal colic*.

## Ureterolithotomy

The surgical removal of a urinary tract *calculus* (stone) stuck in a ureter (tube that carries urine from a kidney to the bladder). The stone is removed if it is causing recurrent attacks of *renal colic* (severe pain in the loin area) or obstruction to urine flow from a kidney, which can rapidly lead to kidney damage.

Before the operation, intravenous *pyelography* is carried out to locate the stone. An incision is made in the patient's abdomen with the use of a general anesthetic, and the surgeon feels the ureter for the stone. The ure-

---

ter is then opened with a longitudinal cut, the stone is removed with forceps, and a check is made for more stones. The ureter and abdomen are then sewn up, leaving a tube inserted into the abdomen to drain any urine that leaks from the ureter. This tube is removed four or five days later and the patient can then leave the hospital.

Ureterolithotomy is not the only method of dealing with ureteral stones. Stones at the lower end of the ureter can sometimes be removed, after crushing, by means of *cystoscopy* (passage of a viewing tube into the bladder via the urethra). Stones at the top end may be dealt with by shock-wave *lithotripsy* (shattering of stones).

## Urethra

The tube by which urine is excreted from the bladder. In females, the urethra is short and opens to the outside just in front of the vagina between the labia minora. In males, the urethra is much longer. It is surrounded by the prostate gland at its upper end and then forms a channel through the length of the penis. The location and relative length of the male and female urethras are shown in the illustrated box (overleaf).

### DISORDERS

Although urethral infections, scarring, and congenital abnormalities occur in both sexes, these disorders are much more common and serious in males than in females.

In male infants, a urethral valve is sometimes present. The valve flap arises from the lining of the urethra and impedes the flow of urine. The resulting bottleneck causes back pressure on the kidneys as urine fills the bladder, ureters, and collecting ducts of the kidneys. Permanent and severe damage to the kidneys can occur if the urethral valve is not removed surgically.

*Urethritis* (inflammation of the urethra) may be due to infection, irritation, or minor injury. Inflammation may be followed by scarring and formation of a *urethral stricture* (a narrowed section of the urethra).

The male urethra is easily damaged in accidents involving pelvic injury and may require surgical repair, again with a risk of a urethral stricture.

## Urethral dilatation

Widening of a *urethral stricture* (narrowed urethra) in a male by means of a slim, round-tipped instrument inserted through the opening of the urethra at the tip of the penis.

U

## LOCATION OF THE URETHRA

The urethra is the tube through which urine is passed from the bladder. There is no voluntary muscle in the urethra. The flow of urine is controlled by muscles in the bladder wall and outlet.

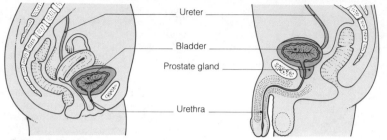

Ureter
Bladder
Prostate gland
Urethra

**Urethra in a woman**
The female urethra is short—about an inch and a half (4 cm) long—and runs down to open to the exterior just in front of the vagina.

**Urethra in a man**
The male urethra is about 9 inches (23 cm) long and passes through the prostate gland and along the full length of the penis.

## Urethral discharge

A fluid that flows from the urethra in some cases of *urethritis* caused by infection. In gonorrhea, the discharge is yellow and purulent (contains pus); in other types of infection the discharged fluid is clear.

## Urethral stricture

An uncommon condition in which the male urethra becomes narrowed and sometimes shortened along part of its length as a result of shrinkage of scar tissue within its walls.

### CAUSES AND SYMPTOMS

Scar tissue may form after injury to the urethra or after persistent *urethritis* (inflammation). Urethritis was once most commonly due to *gonorrhea*, but modern antibiotic treatment has made strictures from this cause uncommon.

A stricture can make it difficult or painful to pass urine or to ejaculate and may cause some deformation of the penis when erect. It can also cause damage to the kidneys by back pressure (buildup of fluid) and may encourage the development of a *urinary tract infection*.

### TREATMENT

A stricture may be treated by urethral dilatation, in which an attempt is made to stretch and widen the tube by means of an instrument passed into it via the opening at the tip of the penis. This procedure is performed using either local or general anesthesia and may need to be repeated. If dilatation fails, an instrument called a urethrotome may be inserted to cut through the scar tissue. Alternatively, it may be possible to remove the stricture altogether and reconstruct the urethra with plastic surgery.

## Urethral syndrome, acute

A set of symptoms of uncertain cause experienced by some women and, very rarely, by some men. The symptoms consist of pain and discomfort in the lower abdomen, a frequent urge to pass urine, and, in women, pain around the vulval region. Middle-aged women are the most commonly affected.

Usually, the physician cannot discover any causative infection, and the patient's kidney function and urinary tract anatomy are normal. Emotional and psychological factors may contribute. In women who have gone through the menopause, the symptoms may be due to inflammation of the vulva associated with thinning of tissues (see *Vulvitis*).

There is usually no effective treatment. Cases due to vulvitis may be relieved by use of *estrogen drugs* or *corticosteroid drugs* in cream form. Antiseptic creams and strong soaps should be avoided as they may cause irritation or an allergic reaction that worsens the symptoms. Scrupulous personal hygiene and a high fluid intake are usually recommended.

## Urethritis

Inflammation of the urethra, usually due to an infection but sometimes with other causes.

### CAUSES

Urethritis may be caused by a variety of infectious organisms, the best known of which is the bacterium that causes *gonorrhea*. Nonspecific urethritis may be caused by any of a large number of different types of microorganisms, including bacteria, yeasts, and *chlamydial infection*. Bacteria from the skin or rectum sometimes spread to infect the urethra.

Other causes of urethritis include trauma from an accident or from a surgically introduced catheter or cystoscope (viewing tube for examining the bladder). Irritant chemicals, such as antiseptics and some spermicidal preparations, are other possible causes of urethritis.

### SYMPTOMS AND COMPLICATIONS

Urethritis causes a burning sensation and pain when passing urine. The pain can be severe and is sometimes likened to passing small fragments of broken glass. The urine may be blood-stained and, particularly when gonorrhea is the cause, there is often a yellow, pus-filled, discharge.

Urethritis may be followed by scarring and the formation of a *urethral stricture* (narrowing of a section of the urethra), which can make passing urine difficult.

### TREATMENT

Gonorrhea is usually cured by penicillin or other *antibiotic drugs*. Treatment of nonspecific urethritis varies according to the causative organism, if it can be identified. Antibiotic treatment may be needed if bacterial infection follows urethritis due to a noninfective cause.

Urethral strictures are treated by the technique of *urethral dilatation*.

## Urethrocele

An anatomical abnormality caused by a weakness in the tissues in the front wall of the vagina. This weakness causes the overlying urethra to bulge backward and downward into the vagina. A urethrocele may be congenital (present from birth), may develop after childbirth, or may be associated with obesity.

A urethrocele may cause difficulty emptying the bladder and pain during sexual intercourse (see *Intercourse, painful*). It also increases susceptibility to *urinary tract infection*.

The usual treatment of a urethrocele is a surgical operation to tighten the tissues at the front of the vagina, thus giving the urethra better support (see *Vaginal repair*).

## -uria

A suffix relating to urine, as in *proteinuria*, the term for the presence of protein in the urine.

## Uric acid

A waste product of the breakdown of *nucleic acids* in body cells. A small amount of uric acid is also produced by the digestion of foods rich in nucleic acids, such as liver, kidneys, sweetbreads, and, to a lesser extent, fish and poultry.

Most uric acid produced in the body passes, via the bloodstream, to the kidneys, which remove the acid from the blood and excrete it in the urine. However, some uric acid passes into the intestine, where it is broken down by bacteria into chemicals that are excreted in the feces.

The kidneys of a healthy person maintain blood levels of uric acid within acceptable limits. When uric acid excretion is disrupted, it may result in *hyperuricemia* (abnormally high levels of uric acid in the blood), which, in turn, may lead to *gout* or kidney stones (see *Calculi, urinary tract*). Causes of hyperuricemia include kidney disease, *leukemia*, hemolytic *anemia*, genetic disorders in which an enzyme involved in uric acid excretion is lacking, and certain drugs, including some diuretic drugs and anticancer drugs.

## Urinal

A container for urine, useful for bedridden men (women use a *bedpan*). Also known as a urinal is an appliance for men suffering from urinary *incontinence*; it consists of a thick rubber tube with a hole in the end, connected by a plastic tube to a drainage bag strapped on the leg.

## Urinalysis

A battery of tests on a patient's urine, including measurements of the urine's physical characteristics (such as color, concentration, and cloudiness), microscopic examination, and chemical testing. Urinalysis can help check normal kidney function or detect and diagnose urinary tract and other disorders.

Microscopic examination may reveal the presence of red blood cells in the urine, indicating damage to the glomeruli (filtering units) of the kidneys or a disorder of the remaining kidney and upper and lower urinary tract. Microscopic examination of urine may also reveal fragments of protein and kidney cells, called casts, in any of various types of kidney disease; pus or bacteria when there is a *urinary tract infection*; crystals, indicating the possibility of an inborn error of metabolism (see *Metabolism,*

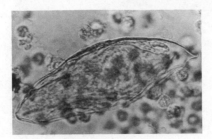

**Schistosome egg in urine**
The tropical disease schistosomiasis may be diagnosed by the finding of schistosome (fluke) eggs on urinalysis.

*inborn errors of*) or susceptibility to urinary tract *calculi* (stones); and worm eggs caused by the parasitic disease *schistosomiasis*.

If a single drop of fresh urine is spread thinly on the surface of a nutrient gel and incubated, any bacteria present will multiply and produce colonies. The appearance of these colonies under microscopic examination allows the microbiologist to identify the organism causing a urinary tract infection.

A wide variety of simple stick tests is available to measure substances such as glucose in the urine (a high level usually means that the patient has *diabetes mellitus*). Other substances or properties tested for include blood, protein, bile, the acidity of urine, and its concentration (ratio of dissolved substances to water). These tests rely on a simple color change in a test patch of the stick or strip when it is dipped into the urine.

Detection of human chorionic gonadotropin in the urine is the basis of many *pregnancy tests*. (See also *Kidney function tests*.)

## Urinary diversion

Any surgical procedure performed to allow passage of urine when the normal outlet channel, via the bladder and urethra, is obstructed or cannot be used, or when the bladder has been surgically removed.

#### TEMPORARY DIVERSION

Temporary urinary diversion is commonly required (if an indwelling catheter is not feasible) when passage of urine is blocked by enlargement of the *prostate gland* or by *urethral stricture*. In this case, a small opening is made through the abdominal wall just above the pubic bone and a tube is passed directly into the bladder (see *Catheterization, urinary*). Temporary diversion is also required after some operations on the urinary tract; a small

tube is introduced into the kidney and brought to the abdominal surface, bypassing the ureters and allowing healing to take place.

#### PERMANENT DIVERSION

Permanent urinary diversion is needed when the bladder has been removed, usually to treat advanced bladder cancer, or when neurological control of the bladder is severely disturbed, such as after severe spinal injury. Permanent diversion may also be required if there is an irreparable *fistula* (opening) between the bladder or urethra and the vagina.

Permanent diversion is usually achieved by creating what is known as an ileal conduit (see illustrated box, overleaf). A section of the ileum is removed to create a substitute bladder. The ureters are implanted into one end of this bladder; the other end is brought out through an incision in the abdominal wall, as in an *ileostomy*. The patient wears a bag attached to the skin to collect urine.

A variant of this method permits the patient to use a catheter to periodically empty the ileal conduit, thereby providing the person with a degree of continence.

## Urinary system

See *Urinary tract* and illustrated box on *Urine* formation and excretion.

## Urinary tract

The part of the body concerned with the formation and excretion of urine. The urinary tract consists of the *kidneys* (with their blood and nerve supplies), the renal pelves (funnel-shaped ducts that channel urine from the kidneys into the ureters), the *ureters, bladder,* and *urethra*.

The kidneys make urine by filtering blood. The urine collects in the renal pelves and then passes down the ureters into the bladder by gravity and by peristalsis (wavelike contractions of the ureteric walls). Urine is then stored in the bladder until a sufficient amount is present to stimulate micturition (passage of urine). When the bladder contracts, the urine is expelled from the body via the urethra.

## Urinary tract infection

An infection anywhere in the urinary tract. *Urethritis* (inflammation of the urethra) may be caused by mechanisms other than infection, but *cystitis* (inflammation of the bladder) and *pyelonephritis* (inflammation of the kidneys) are nearly always caused by bacterial infection.

U

## URINARY DIVERSION USING ILEAL CONDUIT

This is a standard operation performed when the bladder has been removed or is seriously malfunctioning and beyond hope of repair. A midline incision in the abdomen is used; before making it, the surgeon creates an opening through the abdominal wall in a good position for attaching the future collecting bag.

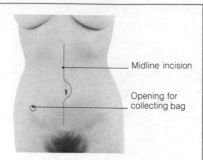

Midline incision

Opening for collecting bag

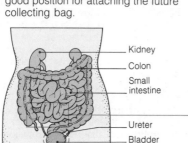

Kidney
Colon
Small intestine
Ureter
Bladder

**1** A short length is cut out of the ileum (the lower part of the small intestine), retaining the mesentery (supporting folds of tissue) and the essential blood vessels that supply the freed section.

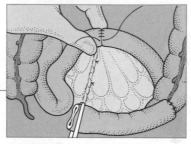

**2** The cut ends of the intestine are stitched together to reestablish continuity. One end of the freed length of intestine is closed and the other end is temporarily clamped.

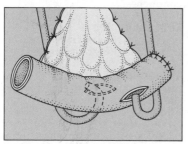

**3** The ureters are now implanted into the isolated length of ileum. The open end of this segment is brought through the abdominal wall and stitched in place.

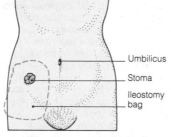

Umbilicus
Stoma
Ileostomy bag

**4** A collecting bag for the reception of the patient's urine is fixed with adhesive around the new stoma (mouth) in the wall of the abdomen.

### CAUSES

When urethritis is due to infection, the cause is usually a sexually transmitted disease, such as *gonorrhea* or nonspecific urethritis, often caused by chlamydia organisms. Otherwise, urinary tract infection is usually caused by organisms that have spread from the rectum, via the urethra, to the bladder or kidneys. Infections can also be bloodborne.

Because of the shortness of the urethra in women, infections above the urethra are more common in women than in men. In many women, they occur without any identifiable underlying cause. In most men and some women, however, there is an identifiable cause, usually some factor that impairs the drainage of urine. In men, this may be an enlarged prostate gland (see *Prostate, enlarged*) or a *urethral stricture*.

In either sex, urinary tract infection may be caused by a urinary tract *calculus* (stone), a *bladder tumor*, or a congenital abnormality of the urinary tract, such as a double kidney on one side. Defective bladder emptying as a result of *spina bifida* or spinal cord injury (see *Spinal injury*) leads almost inevitably to urinary tract infection. Urinary tract infection is also more common during pregnancy.

The risks of a urinary tract infection can be reduced by careful personal hygiene, drinking plenty of fluids, and regular emptying of the bladder.

### SYMPTOMS AND COMPLICATIONS

Urethritis causes a burning sensation when passing urine. Cystitis causes a frequent urge to pass urine, lower abdominal pain, *hematuria* (blood in the urine), and often general malaise with a mild fever. An infection in the kidneys leads to pain in the loins and high fever.

Urethritis can lead to scarring of the urethra and formation of a urethral stricture. Cystitis, provided there is no upward spread to the kidneys, does not usually produce complications. Without proper treatment, kidney infection can lead to permanent kidney damage, *septicemia* (spread of infective organisms to the blood), and *septic shock*. If a calculus in a kidney is the underlying cause of infection, it may grow rapidly during the course of the infection.

### DIAGNOSIS AND TREATMENT

Infection is diagnosed by a *culture* of a few drops of urine. The urine specimen is taken midstream to avoid contamination of the specimen by organisms that normally live in the last part of the urethra.

Further investigation is usually needed for men who have any urinary tract infection or for women suffering from recurrent cystitis or an infection above the level of the bladder. Such investigation is performed by *pyelography* (introduction of a radiopaque dye into the urinary tract, followed by X rays) or by *ultrasound scanning*.

Most urinary tract infections are treated with *antibiotic drugs*; the drug depends on the type of infection.

## Urination, excessive

The production of more than about 5 pints (2.5 liters) of urine per day. Excessive urination is known medically as polyuria. It is usually a sign of illness.

### CAUSES

Illnesses that cause excessive urination fall into several groups. First, certain psychiatric illnesses can cause a person to drink compulsively. This is called polydipsia and leads inevitably to a high urine output.

Second, a disorder of the pituitary gland that leads to reduced production of *ADH* (antidiuretic hormone) can cause a marked increase in urine volume (ADH acts on the kidneys to concentrate the urine). This is known as central *diabetes insipidus*. Alternatively, normal amounts of ADH may be produced, but the kidneys fail

U

to respond. This is called nephrogenic diabetes insipidus and can result from various diseases or damage to the kidneys.

Third, various diseases may cause abnormal amounts of certain substances to be excreted in the urine; these substances draw water with them, increasing the urine volume. The most important disease in this group is *diabetes mellitus*, in which excess glucose in the blood spills into the urine. Certain kidney diseases, known as salt-losing states, lead to too much salt being lost in the urine, with an accompanying increase in volume.

**DIAGNOSIS AND TREATMENT**

Any person who passes large quantities of urine should consult a physician, who may use a variety of tests to establish the cause. If the patient's water intake is restricted, urine volume soon drops in the compulsive drinker; however, this does not happen in diabetes insipidus. Central diabetes insipidus improves after administration of synthetic ADH, but nephrogenic diabetes insipidus does not. In patients with diabetes mellitus, the glucose level in the blood and urine is high; in salt-losing patients, excessive sodium is detectable in the urine.

Treatment of excessive urination depends on the underlying cause. (See also *Urination, frequent.*)

## Urination, frequent

Passing urine more frequently than usual, also called simply "frequency." Most people pass urine an average of four to six times daily and only occasionally need to urinate at night. A marked increase in this rate constitutes frequency.

In some cases, frequency is the inevitable result of excessive production of urine (see *Urination, excessive*). In other cases, the total volume of urine produced is not high or may even be lower than usual.

Often the cause is *cystitis* (bladder inflammation) due to infection. A common response to this is to drink less. However, the result is a more concentrated (and thus more irritant) urine, which increases urinary frequency. Sufferers from cystitis should drink more than usual, not less.

Anxiety is a common cause of increased frequency. Other causes include *calculi* (stones) in the bladder, an enlarged prostate gland (see *Prostate, enlarged*) in men, and, in rare cases, a *bladder tumor*. Some people with *renal failure* also notice that they

pass urine more frequently, particularly at night. Treatment is always of the underlying cause.

## Urination, painful

Pain or discomfort when passing urine, also known medically as dysuria. The pain is often described as having a burning or scalding quality. Sometimes it is preceded by difficulty in starting the flow. Pain after the flow has ceased, with a strong desire to continue, is called strangury.

The most common cause of dysuria is *cystitis* (inflammation of the bladder), especially in women. Dysuria may also be caused by a *bladder tumor* or *calculus* (stone), especially if blood clots or small stones or crystals are passed in the urine. Strangury is usually due to spasm of an inflamed bladder wall; it may also be caused by bladder stones.

Other possible causes of dysuria include *urethritis* (inflammation of the urethra), often due to gonorrhea; in men, *prostatitis* (inflammation of the prostate gland) or *balanitis* (inflammation of the glans of the penis); and in women, vaginal *candidiasis* (thrush) or an allergy to vaginal deodorants.

Mild discomfort when passing urine may be due to highly concentrated urine, which may occur during a fever or after heavy sweating.

Dysuria may be investigated by physical examination, *urinalysis*, and, sometimes, *pyelography*, or *cystoscopy*.

## Urine

The pale yellow fluid produced by the kidneys and excreted from the body via the ureters, bladder, and urethra. Urine carries waste products, and excessive water or chemical substances, from the body.

**URINE PRODUCTION**

Urine is produced by the filtration of blood through the kidneys. The filtering units of the kidneys remove about 230 pints (110 liters) of watery fluid from the blood every day. Nearly all of this fluid is then reabsorbed into the blood; the remainder is passed from the body as urine.

A healthy adult may produce between about 1 and 4 pints (0.5 to 2 liters) of urine per day. The minimum volume of urine needed to remove all waste products is about 1 pint; any volume produced above this level consists of excess water. A high fluid intake increases the amount of urine produced, while a high fluid loss from sweating, vomiting, or diarrhea leads to reduced production.

**COMPOSITION OF URINE** (g/liter)

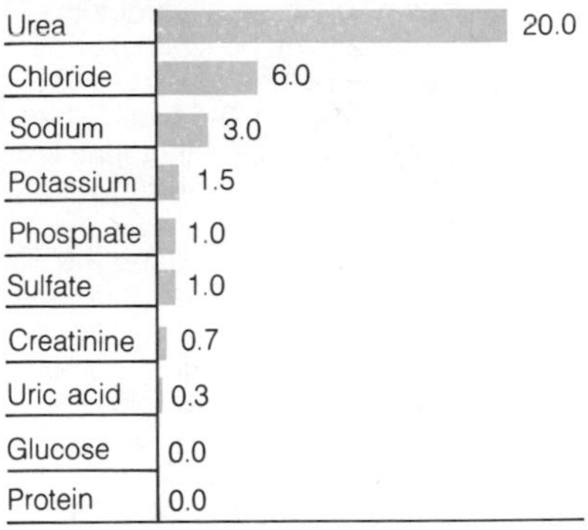

| | |
|---|---|
| Urea | 20.0 |
| Chloride | 6.0 |
| Sodium | 3.0 |
| Potassium | 1.5 |
| Phosphate | 1.0 |
| Sulfate | 1.0 |
| Creatinine | 0.7 |
| Uric acid | 0.3 |
| Glucose | 0.0 |
| Protein | 0.0 |

**Composition of urine**
The chart shows normal, average contents of urine, other than water. The main waste products excreted are urea, creatinine, and uric acid. Variable amounts of sodium, chloride, hydrogen, and other ions are excreted to adjust the body's water, salt, and acid-base balance.

**COMPOSITION**

The average composition of urine excreted by a healthy person is shown in the chart (above).

The volume, acidity, and salt concentration of the urine are carefully regulated by hormones such as *ADH* (antidiuretic hormone), *atrial natriuretic peptide*, and *aldosterone*. These hormones act on the kidneys to ensure that the body's water, salt, and acid-base balance (acidity or alkalinity of the blood and tissue fluids) is kept within narrow limits.

Measurements of the composition of urine are useful in the diagnosis of a wide variety of conditions, from kidney disease and diabetes to pregnancy (see *Urinalysis*).

Urine is normally sterile when passed and has only a faint odor. The unpleasant smell of stale urine is due to the action of bacteria, which causes the release of ammonia. A substance called urochrome, of unknown source, gives urine its yellow color.

## Urine, abnormal

Urine may be produced in abnormal amounts or may have an abnormal appearance or composition.

**ABNORMAL VOLUME**

Production by an adult of more than about 5 pints (2.5 liters) of urine per day is unusual unless he or she is drinking excessively or has a disease (see *Urination, excessive*).

Abnormally low urine production (*oliguria*) of less than about 0.8 pint (0.4 liters) per day may occur in severe

## THE URINARY SYSTEM

Also known as the urinary tract, the system consists of the kidneys, in which urine is formed to carry away waste materials from the blood; the ureters, which transport the urine from the kidneys; the bladder, where the urine is stored until it can be conveniently disposed of; and the urethra, through which the bladder is emptied to the outside.

The kidneys require a large blood supply and are connected close to the body's main artery, the aorta. More than 2 pints of blood pass through the kidneys every minute.

**X ray showing urinary tract**
The X ray at left, taken by the technique of intravenous *pyelography*, shows (as lighter areas) the calyces and pelvis of each kidney, the ureters and bladder, as well as the bones of the lower spine and pelvic girdle.

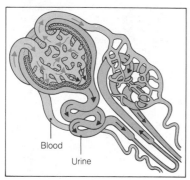

**The filtering units**
Each kidney has about 1 million of these units, which form dilute urine by filtering the blood.

Blood

Urine

**COMPOSITION OF URINE**
Urine consists mainly of water, with small amounts of urea (the main waste product), other waste products, and salt.

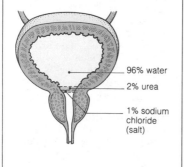

96% water

2% urea

1% sodium chloride (salt)

**Interior of bladder**
The two ureteral openings and the urethral orifice form a triangle on the base of the bladder. In males, the urethra runs through the body of the prostate gland situated below the bladder.

**Collecting system**
From the tubules that lead from the filtering units, much of the water and some other substances are reabsorbed into the blood. The remaining, more concentrated, urine runs into collecting ducts and then into the pyramid-shaped calyces of the kidney and the kidney pelvis. From there the urine passes into the ureter.

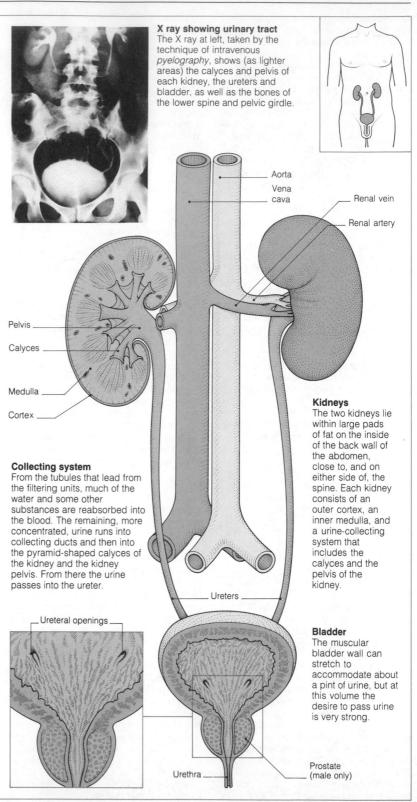

Aorta

Vena cava

Renal vein

Renal artery

Pelvis

Calyces

Medulla

Cortex

**Kidneys**
The two kidneys lie within large pads of fat on the inside of the back wall of the abdomen, close to, and on either side of, the spine. Each kidney consists of an outer cortex, an inner medulla, and a urine-collecting system that includes the calyces and the pelvis of the kidney.

Ureters

Ureteral openings

**Bladder**
The muscular bladder wall can stretch to accommodate about a pint of urine, but at this volume the desire to pass urine is very strong.

Urethra

Prostate (male only)

U

*dehydration* and in cases of acute *renal failure*. It also occurs when the kidneys are not receiving their normal blood supply due, for example, to *heart failure, shock,* or advanced liver disease.

No production of urine by the kidneys (*anuria*) may occur in extreme cases of kidney damage. However, lack of the passage of urine from the bladder is more commonly caused by obstruction in the lower part of the urinary tract as a result of a *bladder tumor, calculus* (stone), or an enlarged prostate gland (see *Prostate, enlarged*).

**ABNORMAL APPEARANCE**

Cloudy urine may be due to a *urinary tract infection,* in which case it may have an offensive smell. Urinary tract *calculi* (stones) can also produce cloudy urine, which is not necessarily infected. Cloudy urine may be caused by the presence of certain salts, such as phosphates. In rare instances, lymph fluid enters the urine and gives it a milky appearance.

Slight *hematuria* (blood in the urine) produces a smoky appearance. Larger amounts of blood produce easily recognizable red urine, which may contain clots. Red urine is not always due to blood, however. Some dyes used in candy may be excreted in the urine, and a wide variety of drugs can discolor it (rifampin turns urine orange). In some patients with *porphyria,* the urine turns red if it is left to stand; in some patients with *jaundice,* the urine is orange or brown. Frothy urine, particularly if the froth persists after shaking, may contain an excess of protein.

**ABNORMAL COMPOSITION**

In *diabetes mellitus,* the excess glucose present in the blood spills into the urine, causing *glycosuria.* In *glomerulonephritis* (inflammation of the filtering units of the kidneys) and in the *nephrotic syndrome,* excess protein may be present in the urine (*proteinuria*). In *renal failure,* the total amount of waste products, such as urea, is reduced.

Other kidney disorders, such as *Fanconi's syndrome* and *renal tubular acidosis,* may make the urine too acid or too alkaline, or may cause it to contain excess amino acids, phosphates, salt, or water.

## Urine retention

Inability to empty the bladder or difficulty doing so. Urinary retention may be complete, in which case urine cannot voluntarily be passed at all (although some may leak out) or incomplete, in which case some urine may be passed, but the bladder fails to empty completely.

**CAUSES**

Retention may be due to an obstruction to the flow of urine. This problem predominantly affects males. Causes include phimosis (tight foreskin), a *urethral stricture, calculus* (stone) in the bladder, *prostatitis* (inflammation of the prostate), or enlargement or a tumor of the prostate (see *Prostate, enlarged; Prostate, cancer of*). In women, urinary retention may result from pressure on the urethra from uterine *fibroids.* In either sex it may be due to a *bladder tumor.*

Alternatively, retention may be due to defective functioning of the nerve pathways concerned with sensing bladder enlargement and triggering bladder emptying. Defective nerve function may be induced by a surgical operation, by a general or spinal anesthetic, by the use of drugs that act on the bladder or the urinary sphincters, or it may be the result of a disease of the spinal cord or damage to the nerve pathways through injury.

**SYMPTOMS AND COMPLICATIONS**

Except when nerve pathways are defective, complete urinary retention causes discomfort and pain in the lower abdomen, which can be severe. The filled bladder may be felt on examination as a swelling above the pubic bone. Chronic or partial retention, by contrast, may not cause any serious symptoms and the sufferer may be unaware of it.

There is a risk that retention will lead to kidney damage from back pressure up the urinary tract. Incomplete emptying often leads to a *urinary tract infection.*

**TREATMENT**

Urinary retention is treated by inserting a drainage tube into the bladder, usually via the urethra (see *Catheterization, urinary*). The cause of the retention is then investigated if it is not already known. When obstruction is the cause, it can usually be treated; if nerve damage is the cause, the prospects are less hopeful. Permanent or intermittent catheterization is sometimes necessary.

## Urine tests

See *Urinalysis.*

## Urography

Imaging of the urinary tract (kidney, ureters, and bladder) by X rays after the introduction of a radiopaque dye. (See *Pyelography.*)

## Urokinase

A *thrombolytic drug* prepared from human urine or from a tissue culture of human kidney. Urokinase is given to dissolve blood clots in people who have had a recent *myocardial infarction* (heart attack) or *pulmonary embolism.* Given by injection in the early stages of a myocardial infarction, urokinase may limit the damage caused to the heart muscle.

Treatment with urokinase is strictly supervised due to a risk of excessive bleeding. Urokinase sometimes produces an allergic reaction that causes rash or fever.

## Urologist

A specialist in *urology.* A urologist is concerned with the investigation and treatment of such varied disorders or symptoms as *incontinence, cystitis, urine retention, urinary tract infection, calculi* (stones), and *bladder tumors.* In men, the urologist investigates and treats disorders of the prostate gland, testes, and penis.

In addition to a physical examination to establish a diagnosis, the urologist may employ the investigative techniques of *pyelography, cystoscopy, ultrasound scanning, cystometry,* and *urinalysis.* Because many urological problems are treated by surgical operation, most specialists in urology are qualified surgeons.

## Urology

A branch of medicine concerned with the structure, functioning, and disorders of the urinary tract in both males and females and of the reproductive tract in males.

Urology is thus concerned with the study of the kidneys, ureters, bladder, and urethra in members of both sexes, and with the testes, epididymis, prostate gland, seminal vesicles, and penis in males.

## Ursodeoxycholic acid

A drug under investigation for treating *gallstones* that is prepared from *chenodiol,* a natural acid in bile. Ursodeoxycholic acid seems to be effective in the treatment of small gallstones that do not contain calcium but are largely made up of cholesterol.

Ursodeoxycholic acid works by reducing the amount of cholesterol released by the liver into the bile; it also helps dissolve cholesterol from the surface of gallstones.

Possible adverse effects of ursodeoxycholic acid are diarrhea and temporary impairment of liver function.

**U**

## Urticaria

A skin condition, commonly known as hives, characterized by the development of itchy wheals (raised white lumps surrounded by an area of red inflammation). Wheals vary considerably in size and large ones may merge to form irregular, raised patches. The rash is most common on the limbs and trunk but may appear anywhere on the body. The wheals usually last for no longer than several hours.

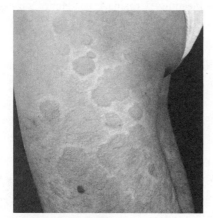

**Appearance of urticaria**
Possible causes are food or drug allergy, contact with certain plants, insect stings or bites, and desensitizing injections.

*Dermatographia* is a less common form of urticaria in which wheals form after stroking the skin. *Angioedema* is a more severe condition (which sometimes occurs with urticaria) in which the airways become closed.

### CAUSES

The cause of urticaria is often unknown. The most common known mechanism is an allergic reaction (see *Allergy*) in which the chemical *histamine* is released from skin cells, causing fluid to leak from capillaries into the skin tissues. Urticaria often results from an allergic reaction to a particular kind of food (such as milk, eggs, shellfish, strawberries, or nuts), food additive (such as some food dyes), or drug (such as penicillin or aspirin).

Less commonly, urticaria occurs in response to sweating brought on by heat or exercise, or to exposure to cold or sunlight.

### TREATMENT AND PREVENTION

Itching can be relieved by applying calamine lotion or by taking *antihistamine drugs*. More severe cases may require *corticosteroid drugs*. Identifying and avoiding known trigger factors can help prevent future allergic reactions. Even if the cause cannot be identified, a tendency to urticaria often disappears in time without any treatment.

## Uterus

The hollow, muscular organ of the female *reproductive system* in which the fertilized ovum (egg) normally becomes embedded and in which the developing embryo and fetus is nourished and grows.

The uterus is situated in the pelvic cavity behind the bladder and in front of the bowel.

### STRUCTURE

The uterus of a nonpregnant woman measures 3 to 4 inches (7.5 to 10 cm) in length and weighs about 2 to 3 ounces (60 to 90 grams). In shape, it resembles an upside down pear. The lower, narrow part of the uterus opens into the vagina at the *cervix* (neck of the uterus); the upper part opens into the *fallopian tubes*.

In most women the uterus is anteverted (tilts forward) at an angle of 90 degrees to the vagina. In about 20 percent of women the uterus is retroverted (tilts backward; see *Uterus, tipped*).

### ANATOMY OF THE UTERUS

The nonpregnant uterus lies deep in the pelvis immediately behind and above the urinary bladder and in front of the rectum. It is usually turned forward, at an angle to the vagina, and is curved downward slightly. When the bladder is full, the uterus is pushed up and back.

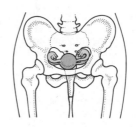
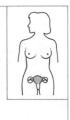
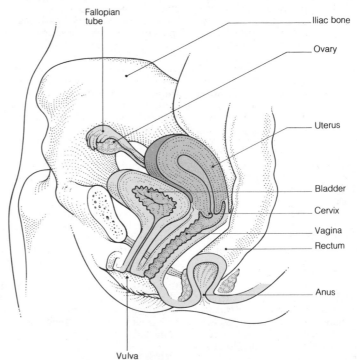

Fallopian tube

Iliac bone

Ovary

Uterus

Bladder

Cervix

Vagina

Rectum

Anus

Vulva

The uterus is a thick-walled organ that consists mainly of muscle. The fallopian tubes enter on both sides of the uterus just below its uppermost point. The small uterine cavity is lined with a mucous membrane called the endometrium, which undergoes changes during the different phases of the menstrual cycle. The cervix is lined with a flatter mucous membrane identical to that of the vagina.

U

## DISORDERS OF THE UTERUS
Conditions that affect the uterus include congenital disorders, infection, benign or malignant growths, and hormonal imbalances that may affect menstrual flow.

### CONGENITAL DISORDERS
In embryonic life, the uterus develops in two halves, which fuse along the midline. One percent of women have a congenital malformation of the uterus, usually resulting from a fusion error. Malformation is not usually serious, but may predispose a woman to preterm labor, *breech* presentation, or retention of the placenta after childbirth. Less commonly, the uterus may be absent, or there may be separate right and left halves, each with its own cervix and vagina. If a congenital malformation makes it difficult or impossible for a woman to conceive or to carry a pregnancy to term, surgical correction may be necessary.

### INFECTION AND INFLAMMATION
Endometritis (infection and inflammation of the lining of the uterus) may originate in the uterus or be caused by infection spreading from elsewhere in the reproductive tract, such as the cervix or fallopian tubes. *Endometritis* may also develop if placental fragments are retained after childbirth or a *miscarriage*.

### TUMORS
Benign tumors of the uterus include *polyps* and *fibroids*. Malignant tumors include cancer of the endometrium (see *Uterus, cancer of*).

**Endometriosis** The lining of the uterus may grow in abnormal places.

**Polyps** Polyps may arise from the cervix or endometrium. If they bleed they require investigation.

**Cancer of endometrium** This is the third most common cancer in women and causes abnormal bleeding.

**Fibroids** These may cause excessive menstrual bleeding.

**Endometritis** This infection of the uterus may be part of a wider infection.

Tumors may also affect placental tissue. Such tumors include *hydatidiform mole*, which is usually benign, and *choriocarcinoma*, which is malignant.

### HORMONAL DISORDERS
Excessive production of *prostaglandins* by the uterus may lead to *dysmenorrhea* (painful periods) or *menorrhagia* (heavy periods).

Hormonal disorders affecting the *ovary* or other organs may disrupt the normal buildup of endometrium during the menstrual cycle, causing menstrual disorders (see *Menstruation, disorders of*), especially *amenorrhea* (absence of periods) or irregular, heavy bleeding.

### INJURY
Injury to the uterus is rare, except following surgery, particularly an *abortion*. In rare cases, the uterus may be perforated by an *IUD*.

### OTHER DISORDERS
The uterus may move from its normal position (see *Uterus, prolapse of*).

Adenomyosis (invasion of the uterine muscle by endometrium) may lead to dysmenorrhea, menorrhagia, and pain during intercourse.

*Endometriosis* (the presence of endometrium outside the uterus) may be symptomless or may be associated with dysmenorrhea, menorrhagia, painful intercourse, and *infertility*.

### INVESTIGATION
A physical examination may be followed by *blood tests*, a *biopsy* (removal of a sample of tissue for microscopic analysis), imaging of the uterus by *hysterosalpingography* or *ultrasound scanning*, or *laparoscopy* (examination of the abdominal cavity through a viewing tube).

The uterus is lined with *endometrium*, which is a specialized tissue that undergoes changes during the menstrual cycle. The endometrium builds up under the influence of hormones from the *ovary*. When hormonal support is withdrawn at the end of each menstrual cycle, the blood supply to the endometrium is cut off and the tissue is shed (see *Menstruation*).

During pregnancy, the uterus expands in size to accommodate the growing baby. Muscle bulk also increases dramatically. At full-term, the uterus weighs about 2 pounds (1 kg), and the powerful uterine muscles expel the baby through the birth canal with great force.

After the *menopause* there is loss of muscle and connective tissue, and the endometrium atrophies (thins). Uterine fibroids almost always shrink after the menopause.

## Uterus, cancer of
Malignant growth in the tissues of the uterus. Cancer of the uterus affects two main sites—the cervix (see *Cervix, cancer of*) and the *endometrium* (lining of the uterus). The term uterine cancer usually refers to cancer of the endometrium.

### INCIDENCE AND CAUSES
In the US in 1987, there were 35,000 new cases of endometrial cancer (compared to 12,800 new cases of cervical cancer).

Endometrial cancer occurs more commonly in women who have had an excess of estrogen in their systems. Risk factors that raise the estrogen level include obesity, a history of failure to ovulate, or long-term use of estrogen hormones if not balanced by *progesterone hormones*. Excess estrogen is common in women with high blood levels of *estrogen hormones*, particularly if progesterone hormone levels are low.

Unlike cervical cancer, endometrial cancer may occur in women who have not had sexual intercourse; it is more common in women who have had few or no children. Use of the birth-control pill lowers the risk of this cancer.

### SYMPTOMS AND SIGNS

The first symptom of endometrial cancer in a woman after the menopause is usually a blood-stained vaginal discharge. In a younger woman, the first symptom may be *menorrhagia* (heavy periods), bleeding between periods, or bleeding after sexual intercourse. A variety of other conditions can also cause such bleeding.

### DIAGNOSIS

Diagnosis must be made by collecting a sample of uterine lining either by biopsy or dilatation and curettage (*D and C*). A *cervical smear test* (Pap), which screens for cervical cancer, is not an effective screening test for uterine cancer.

### TREATMENT

Treatment for very early endometrial cancer is most commonly simple *hysterectomy* and removal of tubes and ovaries. Many surgeons recommend removal of lymph nodes in the pelvis and abdomen to be certain that the cancer has not spread. If the cancer has spread, *radiation therapy* may be recommended. *Chemotherapy* may also be used.

With early treatment, the five-year survival rate is over 80 percent.

## Uterus, prolapse of

A condition in which the uterus descends from its normal position down into the vagina. The degree of prolapse varies from only slight displacement to a condition called procidentia, in which the uterus can be seen outside the vulva.

Related conditions include *cystocele* and *urethrocele* (in which the bladder and/or urethra bulge along the front wall of the vagina) as well as *rectocele* (in which the rectal wall bulges into the back wall of the vagina). A general term for these conditions is pelvic relaxation. Prolapse of the uterus always occurs with some degree of vaginal relaxation, but vaginal relaxation may occur without any prolapse of the uterus.

### CAUSES AND INCIDENCE

Normally, the uterus is kept in position by support ligaments. Stretching of these ligaments (such as during childbirth) is the most common cause of uterine prolapse. In addition, prolapse is more likely if the uterus is retroverted (see *Uterus, tipped*).

Prolapse occurs most commonly in middle-aged women who have had children, although it can occur in childless women. It was far more common earlier this century when women

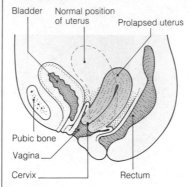

**PROLAPSE OF THE UTERUS**
This condition is caused by weakening of the various ligaments and muscles that help keep the uterus in position in the lower abdomen.

Bladder — Normal position of uterus — Prolapsed uterus — Pubic bone — Vagina — Cervix — Rectum

**First-degree prolapse**
In this least severe degree of prolapse, strain causes the cervix (neck) of the uterus to move farther down in the vagina; however, it remains well within the vagina.

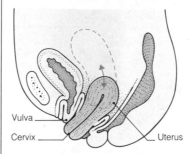

Vulva — Cervix — Uterus

**Second-degree prolapse**
The cervix projects beyond the vulva during straining, but retracts on relaxation. (In third-degree prolapse, the entire uterus projects permanently.)

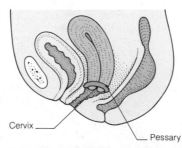

Cervix — Pessary

**Treatment of prolapse**
The uterus may be held in position by a plastic pessary inserted into the vagina; other patients are treated by hysterectomy or vaginal repair.

had more pregnancies and were in poorer general health. Obesity aggravates prolapse.

### SYMPTOMS

There are often no symptoms or the woman may complain of a dragging feeling in the pelvis or a sensation that something is being displaced downward. In severe cases, the uterus is visible from the outside. Other symptoms, such as leakage of urine or difficulty passing urine or feces, may result from an accompanying cystocele, urethrocele, or rectocele.

### DIAGNOSIS, PREVENTION, AND TREATMENT

Prolapse of the uterus is diagnosed by physical examination. In some cases, it is discovered during a routine pelvic examination. Evaluation of the urinary system may be necessary if the bladder is also prolapsed.

*Pelvic floor exercises* strengthen the muscles of the vagina and thus reduce the risk of a prolapse occurring, especially after childbirth.

In severe cases, a vaginal *hysterectomy* (removal of the uterus through the vagina), along with tightening of the support ligaments and, in some cases, *vaginal repair* may be recommended. For women who do not want surgery, or who are not fit enough to undergo general anesthesia, a plastic *pessary* may be inserted into the vagina to hold the uterus in position. The pessary requires periodic changing.

## Uterus, retroverted

See *Uterus, tipped*.

## Uterus, tipped

A condition in which the uterus inclines backward rather than forward. A tipped, or retroverted, uterus was once believed to be the cause of various gynecological symptoms. It is now generally considered to be a harmless variation of the normal.

### CAUSES AND INCIDENCE

About 20 percent of women have a retroverted uterus. Retroversion occurs in some women because the uterus has stayed in the retroverted position usual in infancy rather than becoming anteverted (tilted forward) as it matures. In others, the position of the uterus changes after childbirth—either becoming retroverted when it was previously anteverted, or vice versa. Less commonly, retroversion is caused by a disease, such as a tumor, scarring from *endometriosis*, or *pelvic inflammatory disease*.

### SYMPTOMS

Retroversion usually causes no symptoms, but an underlying disease

U

## TIPPED UTERUS

In about 80 percent of women, the uterus is anteverted (turned forward) In addition, the body of the

organ is anteflexed (bent forward). In retroversion, the organ is turned back, but not bent back. A

retroverted uterus may also be retroflexed. Retroversion may or may not be a cause of symptoms.

**ANTEFLEXION**

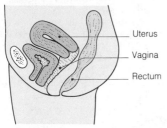

**RETROVERSION**

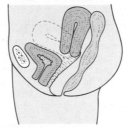

**RETROFLEXION**

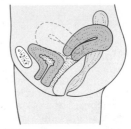

### Anteflexion
The illustration shows the usual position of the uterus, lying bent and turned forward, at right angles to the vagina.

### Retroversion
A retroverted uterus that can easily be anteverted by manipulation seldom causes trouble and requires no treatment.

### Retroflexion
If the retroversion and retroflexion are the result of disease, there are usually symptoms. Intercourse may be painful.

may produce painful periods, painful intercourse, and *infertility*.

**DIAGNOSIS AND TREATMENT**

A retroverted uterus is diagnosed by physical examination of the pelvis. Treatment is unnecessary if there are no symptoms. In rare cases when there are symptoms, the gynecologist may manipulate the uterus into a forward position and then insert a plastic vaginal pessary to hold the uterus in place. If this relieves the symptoms, surgery may be performed to change the position of the uterus permanently. If underlying gynecological disease is suspected, *laparoscopy* may be suggested.

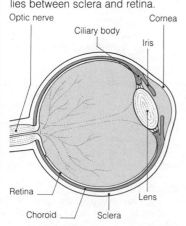

### LOCATION OF THE UVEA
The uvea consists of the iris, ciliary body, and choroid, which lies between sclera and retina.

## Uvea

The colored part of the *eye* and the middle, blood vessel-containing layer of the eye. The uvea is a pigmented structure consisting of the *iris* (the diaphragm of the pupil), the ciliary body and its muscle, which focuses the lens, and the *choroid* (the coat of the eye lying just under the retina).

The uvea contains many blood vessels that, in the iris, supply the active muscles that control the opening and closing of the pupil; in the choroid, the blood vessels assist with the nutrition of the retina. The pigment cells of the uvea are concentrated at the back of the iris; in the choroid they are scattered throughout. These pigment cells confer color on the eye and improve its optical efficiency. (See also *Uveitis*.)

## Uveitis

Inflammation of the *uvea*, which may seriously affect vision. Uveitis may affect any part of the uvea, including the iris (when it is called iritis), the ciliary body (when it is known as cyclitis), or the choroid (when it is called choroiditis).

The cause of uveitis is most commonly an *autoimmune disorder* rather than an infection.

Treatment involves monitoring the inflammation with a *slit lamp*. *Corticosteroid drugs* in the form of eye drops (or, occasionally, orally or by injection) are given; eye drops containing a substance related to *atropine* are given to block nerve impulses to the muscles of the iris and ciliary body, thus dilating the pupil. Other

medications may be given in the rarer cases of uveitis due to an infection.

## Uvula

The small, conical, fleshy protuberance that hangs from the middle of the lower edge of the soft *palate* (part of the roof of the mouth). The uvula is composed of muscle and connective tissue, with a covering of mucous membrane.

Some people are born with a bifid (forked) uvula. This is of little significance, but may be associated with *cleft lip and palate*.

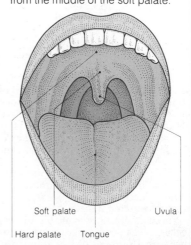

### LOCATION OF THE UVULA
This conical fold of loose, wet, mucous membrane hangs down from the middle of the soft palate.

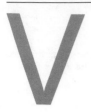

## Vaccination

One of the main types of *immunization* (a procedure to stimulate or bolster the body's *immune system*). Vaccination is another term for active immunization, in which killed or weakened microorganisms are introduced into the body, usually by injection. These microorganisms sensitize the immune system; if disease-causing organisms of the same type later enter the body, they are quickly destroyed through the action of *antibodies* produced by the immune system or by other immune mechanisms.

Vaccination does not encompass the other main type of immunization procedure—passive immunization—in which ready-made antibodies are given by injection to provide short-term immunity.

## Vaccine

A preparation given to induce *immunity* against an infectious disease. A vaccine works by sensitizing the body's *immune system* to a particular disease-causing bacterial toxin, virus, or bacterium. If the particular infectious agent invades the body at a later time, the sensitized immune system quickly produces *antibodies* that help destroy either the agent itself or the toxin it produces.

Most vaccines are preparations containing the very organisms (or parts of the organisms) against which protection is sought. So that these organisms themselves do not cause disease, they are killed or weakened. The term "live attenuated organisms" describes strains of organisms that have been rendered harmless either by artificial alteration of their genes or by successively infecting laboratory animals; this leads to changes in the organisms that considerably reduce their ability to cause disease without reducing their ability to induce immunity. Other vaccines contain chemically modified bacterial *toxins*.

Vaccines are now available to protect against a wide variety of infectious diseases. Examples of live attenuated vaccines are those given to protect against *measles*, *mumps*, and *rubella* (now often combined), *yellow fever*, and Sabin's oral *polio* vaccine. *Diphtheria* and *tetanus* vaccines contain inactivated bacterial toxins. *Cholera*, *typhoid fever*, *pertussis*, *rabies*, viral *hepatitis B*, *influenza*, and Salk injected polio vaccines contain killed organisms or, in the case of hepatitis B, only a part of the hepatitis B virus.

Vaccines are usually given by injection into the upper arm. Oral polio vaccine is given on a sugar lump or by drops on the tongue. Some vaccines require several doses, spaced some weeks apart; others require only one dose. The effectiveness of vaccines varies from near total protection in most cases, to only partial or weak protection (for typhoid or cholera). The duration of effectiveness also varies from a few months to lifelong. (See also *Immunization*.)

## Vacuum extraction

An obstetric procedure to facilitate delivery of a baby. Vacuum extraction was introduced in the 1950s as an alternative to *forceps delivery*. It may be used if the second stage of labor (see *Childbirth*) is prolonged, if the mother becomes exhausted, or if the baby shows signs of *fetal distress*. (Vacuum extraction is also one method used to perform an elective abortion; see *Abortion, elective*.)

### HOW IT IS DONE

The procedure is performed using an instrument called a ventouse, or vacuum extractor, consisting of a suction cup connected to a vacuum bottle. The cup is placed on the baby's head in the birth canal and the vacuum machine is turned on; this sucks the

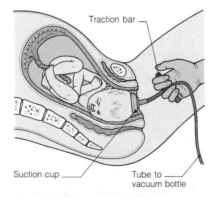

Traction bar

Suction cup

Tube to vacuum bottle

**Technique of vacuum extraction**
Once the suction cup is attached to the baby's head, the obstetrician pulls on the traction bar during each contraction, and the baby is drawn from the vagina.

baby's scalp firmly into the cup. The obstetrician draws the baby out of the mother's vagina by gently pulling on the cup with each uterine contraction.

Delivery by vacuum extraction is generally slower than with forceps, but there is less risk of damage to the woman's genital tract. The baby is born with a swelling on the scalp, but it is harmless and disappears without treatment within several days. *Cephalhematoma* (localized swelling of the scalp caused by bleeding over a skull bone), which may take two or three weeks to disappear, may develop in some babies.

## Vagina

The muscular passage, forming part of the female *reproductive system*, that connects the cervix (neck of the uterus) with the external genitalia.

### STRUCTURE

The vagina is 2.5 to 4 inches (7 to 10 cm) in length, the back wall being slightly longer than the front. The vagina is H-shaped in cross section. The muscular walls have a ridged inner surface and are richly supplied with blood vessels. The walls are usually in contact with each other, except during sexual arousal and intercourse when they become engorged with blood.

### FUNCTION

The vagina has three functions. It is a receptacle for the penis during *sexual intercourse*, bringing sperm closer to the ova for fertilization; it provides an outlet for blood shed at *menstruation*; and, during *childbirth*, it stretches to allow the baby to pass through.

### DISORDERS

*Vaginal discharge* and *vaginal itching* are very common symptoms; they may indicate a disorder in the vagina, vulva, or cervix.

Congenital abnormalities include vaginal atresia (partial or complete absence of the vagina) and blocking of the external opening of the vagina by an imperforate *hymen*.

Infections (see *Vaginitis*) and prolapse of the vagina (see *Urethrocele*; *Rectocele*) are the most common disorders. Cancer of the vagina occurs very rarely.

In *vaginismus*, sexual intercourse and pelvic examination are rendered impossible by abnormal spasm of the muscles around the vaginal entrance.

## Vaginal bleeding

Bleeding via the vagina that may come from the uterus, the cervix, or from the vagina itself.

## STRUCTURE OF THE VAGINA

The vagina has muscular walls, which are highly elastic to allow intercourse and childbirth; it has a ribbed inner lining that secretes a lubricating fluid during sexual excitation and intercourse.

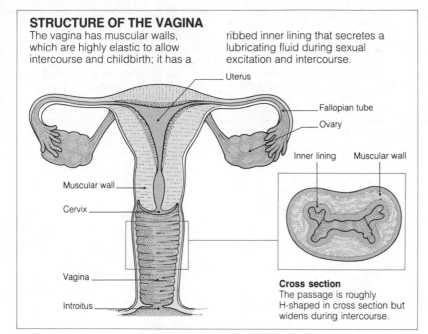

**Cross section**
The passage is roughly H-shaped in cross section but widens during intercourse.

The most common source of bleeding is the uterus and the most likely reason for it is *menstruation*. From puberty to the menopause, menstrual bleeding usually occurs at regular intervals. However, problems may occur either with the character or timing of the bleeding (see *Menstruation, disorders of*).

Possible causes of nonmenstrual bleeding from the uterus include *endometritis* (infection of the lining of the uterus) and endometrial cancer (see *Uterus, cancer of*). These conditions can also occur after the menopause. In addition, use of hormones (such as use of oral birth-control pills) can result in spotting, usually requiring dosage adjustment. Bleeding from the uterus may occur during pregnancy. In the early months, bleeding may be a sign of threatened *miscarriage*. Later in pregnancy, it may indicate serious fetal or maternal problems.

Bleeding from the cervix may be due to *cervical erosion*, in which case it may occur after sexual intercourse. *Cervicitis* (infection of the cervix) and *polyps* may also cause bleeding. More seriously, bleeding from the cervix may be a sign of cervical cancer (see *Cervix, cancer of*).

Vaginal bleeding, originating from the walls of the vagina, is less common than bleeding from the uterus or the cervix. The most likely cause is injury during intercourse, especially after the menopause, when the walls of the vagina become thinner and more fragile. In extreme cases, bleeding may occur without any apparent precipitating cause. Occasionally, severe *vaginitis* causes vaginal bleeding. In rare cases, vaginal bleeding is caused by cancer of the vagina.

Any bleeding not caused by menstruation should be investigated to exclude a serious cause. Infections can be treated with *antibiotic drugs*; fragile vaginal walls can be helped by use of a cream containing *estrogen drugs*. Growths, such as polyps, *fibroids*, or cancer of the uterus or cervix, may need surgical treatment.

## Vaginal discharge

Some mucous secretion from the walls of the vagina and neck of the cervix is normal in a woman of reproductive years. The amount and nature of the discharge varies considerably among women and at different times in the menstrual cycle. The birth-control pill can increase or decrease the discharge, and secretions are usually greater during pregnancy. Sexual stimulation, with or without intercourse, also produces increased vaginal discharge.

Discharge may be abnormal if it is excessive, offensive smelling, yellow or green, or if it causes itching. Abnormal vaginal discharge often occurs in *vaginitis*. Infection with the fungus *CANDIDA ALBICANS* causes a thick, white discharge (see *Candidiasis*); the protozoan parasite *TRICHOMONAS VAGINALIS* causes a profuse green-yellow discharge (see *Trichomoniasis*). A retained pessary or forgotten tampon may cause a profuse and highly offensive secretion. Very rarely, a vaginal discharge may occur in childhood before the beginning of menstruation; this is usually the result of infection or a foreign body. Abnormal vaginal discharge is often accompanied by itching of the vagina and the vulva.

Treatment depends on the cause. Infections are treated with an *antibiotic drug* or *antifungal drug*. Foreign bodies are removed.

## Vaginal itching

Intense irritation and tickling in the vagina and external genital area, also known as pruritus vulvae. Most commonly, vaginal itching is due to an allergic reaction to chemicals that are present in deodorants, spermicides, creams, and douches.

Also very common is itching after the *menopause* due to low estrogen levels. Vaginal infections may also cause itching (see *Vaginitis*). A group of vaginal skin changes, collectively called vulvar dystrophies, can make the skin itch. One form of vulvar dystrophy causes the skin to appear pale and white. Alternatively, the skin may be thickened and scarred.

Treatment for vaginal itching may be in the form of *antibiotic drugs* or hormones, sometimes taken orally and sometimes applied in cream form.

## Vaginal repair

An operation, also known as colporrhaphy, to correct prolapse (displacement) of the vaginal wall.

**TYPES**

There are two different forms of vaginal repair operations—anterior colporrhaphy and posterior colpoperineorrhaphy. Either type may be accompanied by a vaginal *hysterectomy* if the uterus is also prolapsed (see *Uterus, prolapse of*).

**ANTERIOR COLPORRHAPHY** This operation is performed for prolapse affecting the front wall of the vagina. The repair is performed through the vagina.

A triangle of vaginal skin is removed, with its base lying upward toward the uterus. Supporting stitches are inserted through the skin at one side of the triangle, across the gap, and through the skin at the other side. The tissues are then drawn together, narrowing the vagina.

V

After the operation, a catheter may be inserted into the bladder to drain urine for about 24 hours.

**POSTERIOR COLPOPERINEORRHAPHY** This procedure is performed for prolapse of the back wall of the vagina (see *Rectocele*). The repair is performed through the vagina using general anesthesia.

Triangles of skin are removed from the vagina and from the perineum (the area between the genitals and the anus), with the bases of the triangles at the vaginal opening. The perineal muscles are stitched tightly together and the skin on each side of the triangles is brought together and stitched, narrowing the vagina.

## Vaginismus

Painful, involuntary spasm of the muscles that surround the vaginal entrance, interfering with sexual intercourse. When penetration is attempted, the woman's pelvic floor muscles tighten and virtually close the vaginal entrance, making penetration very painful; her legs may straighten and come together. This spasm usually also occurs when a physician attempts a vaginal examination, which may require anesthesia.

**CAUSES**
Vaginismus usually occurs in women who fear that penetration will be painful. Often they have been previously unable to insert a tampon or a finger into the vagina. Any traumatic experience with painful penetration, such as rape or a history of sexual molestation as a child, may predispose a woman to vaginismus. Chronic *vaginitis* may result in painful intercourse and lead to vaginismus. Sufferers may also be particularly sensitive to the stretching sensation that occurs during penetration, which may trigger a spasm when intercourse is first attempted. A vicious circle of anxiety and spasm is then established.

In some women, a contributing factor may be underlying guilt or fear associated with the sexual act due to a restrictive upbringing or an inadequate sex education.

**DIAGNOSIS AND TREATMENT**
The physician first examines the woman to exclude any anatomical abnormalities of the *vagina* that might be causing pain, leading to spasm. Common causes of vaginal pain are infections such as *candidiasis* and atrophy (thinning of the vaginal lining) due to low hormone levels.

Medical problems, such as infection, are corrected; treatment is then by use of a series of graded dilators, which the woman introduces into her vagina. Starting with the smallest size, she practices inserting and removing the instrument, also learning to relax and tighten her vaginal muscles with the dilator in place. Over the course of several treatment sessions, the size of the dilator is gradually increased until the woman is comfortable with the largest size (about the size of the average erect penis). Intercourse can then be attempted.

Results of treatment are usually excellent, with the woman experiencing no discomfort during penetration. (See also *Intercourse, painful*.)

## Vaginitis

Inflammation of the vagina. Vaginitis may be caused by infection, allergic reaction, hormone deficiency associated with aging, or a foreign body, such as a forgotten tampon.

Vaginal infection is commonly caused by the fungus CANDIDA ALBICANS (see *Candidiasis*) and the protozoan parasite TRICHOMONAS VAGINALIS (see *Trichomoniasis*), both of which cause irritation and *vaginal discharge*. Vaginitis is also commonly caused by bacteria that are normal inhabitants of the vagina but which, for unknown reasons (possibly stress or a change of sexual partner), multiply and cause an offensive, fishy-smelling discharge; this is called nonspecific vaginitis.

Vaginitis may also be caused by a reaction to spermicidal creams used with barrier contraceptives, to chemicals in vaginal douches, or to soaps, bath oils, or bath salts.

After the menopause, the lining of the vagina becomes thin and dry and prone to inflammation. Such inflammation, known as atrophic vaginitis, is due to a reduction in the production of *estrogen hormones*.

**TREATMENT**
Infections are treated with *antibiotic drugs* or *antifungal drugs*, as appropriate. In cases of allergy, irritant agents should be avoided. Any foreign body should be removed and any secondary infection treated with drugs. Atrophic vaginitis is treated by giving *estrogen drugs*. (See also *Vulvitis*; *Vulvovaginitis*.)

## Vagotomy

An operation in which the *vagus nerve*, which controls production of digestive acid by the stomach lining, is cut to treat a *peptic ulcer*. Excessive production of digestive acid is a major factor in the development of a peptic ulcer. If a peptic ulcer is associated with obstruction of the outlet of the stomach, hemorrhage, or perforation, a vagotomy may be performed to cut the vagus nerve, thus reducing acid production at its source.

**HOW IT IS DONE**
An incision is made in the upper abdomen, with the use of a general anesthetic, and the two branches of the vagus nerve, which lie in front of and behind the lower esophagus, are exposed. All the nerve fibers are then cut (truncal vagotomy) or, less commonly, some of them are cut (selective vagotomy and highly selective vagotomy).

Since truncal and selective vagotomy cause the stomach to lose its ability to empty itself because muscles of the pylorus (the outlet from the stomach) fail to relax, the operation is usually accompanied by a *pyloroplasty* (surgical widening of the pylorus) or a *gastrojejunostomy* (a surgically created connection between the stomach and jejunum) to allow emptying of the stomach contents.

**RECOVERY PERIOD**
After the operation the patient is given fluids intravenously (by infusion into a vein) until the gastrointestinal tract can accept swallowed fluids.

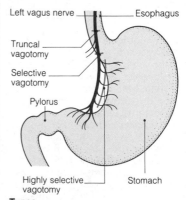

**TECHNIQUE OF VAGOTOMY**
One branch of the vagus nerve acts to increase the secretion of acid and pepsin into the stomach. Vagotomy reduces this secretion and helps to heal peptic ulcers.

Left vagus nerve — Esophagus

Truncal vagotomy

Selective vagotomy

Pylorus

Highly selective — Stomach
vagotomy

**Types**
The simplest operation is truncal vagotomy, in which the trunk of the nerve is cut. Selective vagotomy involves cutting only the twigs that supply the stomach.

V

## OUTLOOK
The operation cures peptic ulcers in about 90 percent of cases, but occasionally there are troublesome side effects, including diarrhea and *dumping syndrome* (premature passing of food from the stomach into the intestine, causing a feeling of weakness and distention after meals).

## Vagus nerve
The tenth *cranial nerve* and the principal component of the parasympathetic division of the *autonomic nervous system*. The vagus nerve is the longest of the cranial nerves, and it branches most widely. It emerges from the medulla oblongata (part of the *brain stem*), passes through the neck and chest to the abdomen, and has branches to most of the major organs in the body, including the larynx, pharynx (throat), trachea (windpipe), lungs, heart, and much of the digestive system.

The vagus nerve exerts its effects on target organs by releasing the chemical *acetylcholine*. This causes narrowing of the bronchi and slowing of the heart rate. It also stimulates the production of stomach acid and pancreatic juice; stimulates the activity of the gallbladder; and increases *peristalsis* (the rhythmic, muscular contractions that move food through the digestive tract).

The vagus nerve branches to the larynx and trachea supply the muscles of these structures, thus involving the vagus nerve in swallowing, coughing, sneezing, and speech quality.

### DISORDERS
Overactivity of the vagus nerve increases the production of stomach acid, which is a factor in the development of a *peptic ulcer*. Some cases of this type of ulcer may be successfully treated by a *vagotomy* (an operation to cut part of the vagus nerve).

The vagus nerve may be damaged by infection (such as *meningitis*), tumor, or *stroke*. In most such cases, the glossopharyngeal nerve (the ninth cranial nerve) and the spinal accessory nerve (the eleventh cranial nerve) are also affected. Possible effects of such damage include impairment or complete loss of the gag reflex, difficulty swallowing, and hoarseness. In severe cases, death may result.

## Valgus
The medical term for outward displacement of a part of the body. For example, in genu valgum (*knock-knee*), the lower leg is displaced outward.

**COURSE OF THE VAGUS NERVE**
There are two vagus nerves, right and left. The right vagus nerve supplies the rear portion of the stomach; the left vagus nerve supplies the front portion of the stomach.

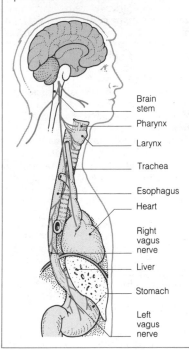

Brain stem
Pharynx
Larynx
Trachea
Esophagus
Heart
Right vagus nerve
Liver
Stomach
Left vagus nerve

## Valproic acid
An *anticonvulsant drug* used to treat *epilepsy*. Although valproic acid has less of a sedative effect than many other anticonvulsant drugs, it occasionally causes drowsiness. Other possible side effects include abdominal discomfort, temporary hair loss, weight gain, and rash. Since prolonged treatment may in rare cases cause liver damage, regular blood tests are usually performed to monitor liver function.

## Valsalva's maneuver
A forcible attempt to breathe out when the airway is closed. Valsalva's maneuver may be performed under certain circumstances without conscious effort or it may be carried out as a deliberate action.

Valsalva's maneuver occurs naturally when an attempt is made to breathe out while holding the vocal cords tightly together. This happens when lifting a heavy object, straining on the toilet, and at the beginning of a sneeze.

When performed deliberately by pinching the nose and holding the mouth closed, Valsalva's maneuver is useful in the prevention of pressure damage to the eardrums as it forces air through the ducts leading to the middle-ear cavities (see *Barotrauma*).

## Valve
A structure that allows fluid or semifluid material to flow in one direction through a tube or passageway but closes to prevent reflux in the opposite direction. The most important valves in the body are at the exits from the heart chambers and in the veins. By ensuring that blood flows in one direction only, these valves are vital to the circulatory system; without them, the heart would be ineffective as a pump and blood circulation could not occur.

There are also small valves in the vessels of the lymphatic system. The muscular rings at the junction of the stomach and duodenum and between the small and large intestines are also sometimes called valves. In fact, these structures are flow-regulating devices and do not prevent reverse direction flow.

Defects of the *heart valves* include stenosis (narrowing) and/or insufficiency (inability to prevent reflux). Either defect can lead to *heart failure*. Insufficiency of the valves in the veins—most commonly in the legs—causes *varicose veins*.

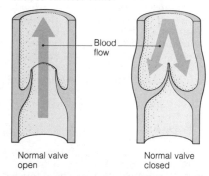

Blood flow

Normal valve open

Normal valve closed

**Valves in the circulatory system**
The valves are flaps that open to allow blood to flow in one direction but close to prevent counterflow in the other direction.

## Valve replacement
A surgical operation to replace a defective or diseased heart valve. (See *Heart valve surgery*.)

## Valvotomy
An operation performed to correct a stenosed (narrowed) *heart valve*. Cuts are made, or pressure applied, to separate the flaps of the valve where

V

they have joined and thus reduce the degree of narrowing.

In the past, valvotomy operations were usually performed, with the heart still beating, by means of a dilating instrument or even a finger introduced into the heart via an incision. Today, valvotomy is usually performed with the heart opened up (see *Heart valve surgery*). Balloon *valvuloplasty* is a newer technique for treating a narrowed valve without the need to open the chest.

## Valvular heart disease

A defect of one or more of the valves in the heart. (See *Heart valve.*)

## Valvuloplasty

A reconstructive or repair operation on a defective heart valve (see *Heart valve surgery*). Valvuloplasty can be performed as an open-heart operation (with the patient connected to a *heart-lung machine* and the heart opened up). However, the newer technique of balloon valvuloplasty makes it possible to treat a stenosed (narrowed) valve without opening the chest. A catheter containing a balloon at its tip is passed through the skin into a blood vessel and from there to the heart. Inflation of the balloon via the catheter may then help separate the flaps of a narrowed valve.

## Vancomycin

An *antibiotic drug* used in the treatment of a variety of infections. Vancomycin is usually given to treat infections caused by staphylococci bacteria (see *Staphylococcal infections*) resistant to other antibiotics. It is given by injection to treat *endocarditis*, *osteomyelitis*, *pneumonia*, and *meningitis* and by mouth to treat a rare form of infective *colitis*.

Possible adverse effects include tenderness at the injection site, fever, chills, itching, and rash. Taken over a long period in high doses, it may in rare cases cause deafness by damaging the *vestibulocochlear nerve*.

## V Vaporizer

A device for converting a drug or water into an aerosol so that medication can be taken by inhalation or so that inhaled air can be made more moist. A common example is an *inhaler*, used to administer *bronchodilator drugs* and *corticosteroid drugs* in the treatment of asthma and other respiratory disorders. Vaporizers are also used to moisten air breathed by children with croup.

## Varicella

Another name for *chickenpox.*

## Varices

Enlarged, tortuous, or twisted sections of vessels, usually veins. Varices is the plural of varix. A vein affected by varices is called a *varicose vein.* Although varicose veins can occur anywhere in the body, they most commonly occur in the legs. *Esophageal varices* are enlarged veins in the lower end of the esophagus.

## Varicocele

*Varicose veins* (abnormally distended veins) that surround the *testis.* Varicocele is a very common condition that affects about 10 to 15 percent of men. It more commonly involves the left testis.

The usual cause of varicocele is failure of the testicular valves. The condition is usually harmless, though there may be an aching discomfort in the scrotum.

Diagnosis is confirmed by examination of the scrotum. The condition may be relieved by wearing an athletic supporter or tight underpants. Further treatment is not usually required. However, an operation to divide and tie off the swollen veins is sometimes performed.

## Varicose veins

Twisted, distended superficial veins (just beneath the skin). Varicose veins in the legs are the best known type. Varicosities in other parts of the body include *hemorrhoids* (dilated veins in the anus), *esophageal varices* (in the esophagus), and *varicocele* (collections of varicose veins in the scrotum).

### CAUSES

There are two principal systems of veins in the legs—the deep veins, which lie among the muscles and carry about 90 percent of the blood, and the surface veins, which are often visible just under the skin and are less well supported. Once circulating blood has oxygenated the tissues of the legs, it is collected by the veins and, pumped upward by contractions of the leg muscles, it passes, via connecting veins, to veins in the abdomen, which return the blood to the heart.

Valves in the veins prevent blood from draining back down the leg under the force of gravity. However, these valves must support a high column of blood and, in many people, they become defective, causing pooling of blood in the superficial veins,

which become swollen and distorted. Factors that may contribute to the development of varicose veins include obesity, hormonal changes during pregnancy or at the menopause, pressure on pelvic veins when pregnant, and standing for long periods.

*Thrombophlebitis* (inflammation and clotting of blood in veins) or deep vein *thrombosis* (clotting in the deeper veins) may be associated with varicosities.

### INCIDENCE

Varicose veins are extremely common. In the US about 15 percent of adults are affected, women more often than men. The disorder tends to run in families.

### SYMPTOMS AND SIGNS

The most common sites for varicose veins are the back of the calf and anywhere on the inside of the leg. The veins are blue, prominent, swollen, and kinked. In some people they cause no symptoms, but others experience a severe ache in the affected area (which is made worse by prolonged standing), swelling of the feet and ankles, and persistent itching of the skin. These symptoms become progressively worse during the day and can be relieved only by sitting with the legs raised. In women, symptoms are often most troublesome just before menstruation.

If backflow of blood is severe enough to cause tissues to become starved of oxygen and nourishment, the skin becomes thin, hard, dry, scaly, and discolored, and *ulcers* may form. They should be treated by cleansing and dressing and facilitating the return of blood to the heart by elevating the legs.

Bumping a large varicose vein may cause severe bleeding. It can be stopped by keeping the affected leg raised and by tying a clean handkerchief around the leg to apply moderate pressure. A physician should then be consulted.

### DIAGNOSIS AND TREATMENT

Varicose veins in the legs are diagnosed from a physical examination done while the patient is standing.

In many cases, the only treatment needed is the wearing of elastic support stockings, regular walking, as little standing as possible, and sitting with the feet up.

In more severe cases, *sclerotherapy* may be carried out. An irritant solution is injected into the varicose veins. The consequent scarring and blockage of the vein causes its work to be taken over by other, healthy veins.

## VARICOSE VEINS

When valves in the veins work correctly, the weight of the blood column is well distributed. When valves fail, some veins become overfilled with blood and swell.

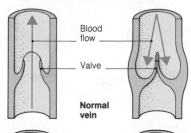

Blood flow

Valve

**Normal vein**

Blood flow

Valve failure

**Varicose vein**

**How varicosities are caused**

In a normal vein, valves stop blood from draining down due to gravity. If valves fail, blood is able to pool downward.

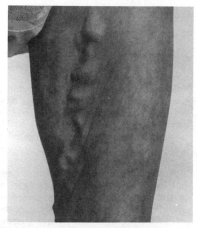

**Appearance of varicose vein**

This varicosity of the saphenous vein on the inside of the thigh shows the typical tortuous, swollen appearance.

### STRIPPING A VEIN

Vein stripping is performed only in severe cases when the valves in the main surface veins are shown to be malfunctioning (and there are symptoms) or the skin is ulcerated. Visible varicosities usually occur in the branches of the vein and these may have to be treated separately.

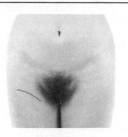

**Site of incision**

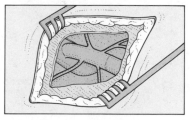

1 Here the greater saphenous vein and its four main upper branches are exposed through an incision in the groin.

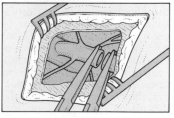

2 The vein is clamped and cut and both free ends tied off. The four branches are also securely tied off and cut. If branches remain, the operation may fail.

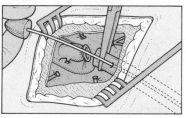

3 A small hole is made in the top of the vein and a flexible wire passed down the vein to the calf or ankle and brought out through a small incision.

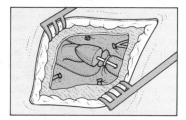

4 The upper end of the wire has a specially shaped metal head, and the vein is tied firmly to the wire just below it.

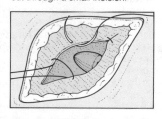

5 The upper incision is closed and the vein is then removed by pulling the wire out through the lower incision. The

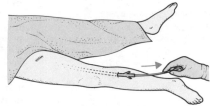

vein bunches up on the stripper and its branches tear off as it does so. Bleeding is not usually severe.

---

If varicose veins are very painful, ulcerated, or prone to bleed, they may require removal by an operation known as stripping (see box). The operation usually takes about half an hour. The patient must keep the leg bandaged for several weeks.

Both sclerotherapy and surgery are usually successful, but varicose veins may later develop elsewhere.

## Variola

Another name for *smallpox*. The term variolation was once used to describe smallpox vaccination.

## Varus

The medical term for an inward deformity of part of the body. For example, in genu varum (*bowleg*), the lower leg is displaced inward.

## Vasculitis

Inflammation of blood vessels. Vasculitis usually leads to damage to the lining of vessels, with narrowing or blockage, so that the blood flow is restricted or stopped. As a result, the tissues supplied by the affected vessels are also damaged, or destroyed, by *ischemia* (lack of blood supply and, therefore, oxygen).

V

Vasculitis is thought to be caused, in most cases, by bodies in the circulating blood known as immune complexes. Immune complexes consist of *antigens* (foreign materials, such as components of microorganisms) bound to *antibodies* that have been formed in response to the antigens. Normally, the immune complexes are destroyed by *phagocytes* (types of white blood cell), but sometimes they settle in the walls of the blood vessels, where they cause severe inflammation. In at least some cases, the causative antigens are known to be viruses.

Vasculitis is the basic disease process in a number of conditions, including *periarteritis nodosa*, *erythema nodosum*, *Schönlein-Henoch purpura*, *serum sickness*, *temporal arteritis*, and *Buerger's disease*.

## Vas deferens

A narrow tube that carries and stores *sperm* released from the *testis* and *epididymis*.

At the base of the bladder, the vas deferens connects to a tube from the seminal vesicles to form the ejaculatory duct. The duct passes into the prostate gland and connects to the urethra. Sperm and seminal fluid are passed through this duct into the urethra during *ejaculation*.

The vas deferens is about 2 feet (60 cm) long. *Vasectomy* involves blocking each vas deferens to prevent the passage of sperm.

### LOCATION OF THE VAS DEFERENS

The vas passes from the epididymis at the back of the testis, up and around the bladder, before entering the prostate.

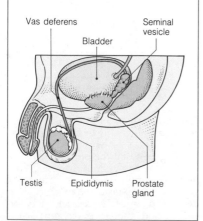

Vas deferens  Seminal vesicle
Bladder
Testis  Epididymis  Prostate gland

### HOW VASECTOMY IS PERFORMED

This operation blocks the passage of sperm from the testes but does not prevent the prostate and other glands from secreting the fluids that form most of the semen. Hence it has little effect on the volume of the ejaculate and no effect on orgasm.

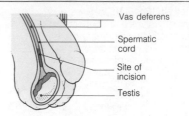

Vas deferens
Spermatic cord
Site of incision
Testis

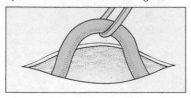

**1** Incisions are made on both sides near the root of the penis; the vas deferens is cut free of the spermatic cord. Blood vessels are avoided.

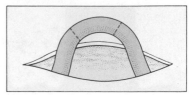

**2** A loop of the vas deferens is freed and brought out through the incision. There are now several possibilities; usually, a length of the vas is cut out.

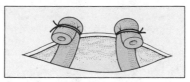

**3** To prevent the cut ends from rejoining, they are often bent back and tightly closed with ligatures. They are then pushed back into the cord.

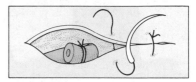

**4** The skin incision is now closed with three or four sutures. When the local anesthetic wears off, there is usually a mild, dull, aching pain for a few days.

## Vasectomy

The operation of male sterilization. Vasectomy is a minor surgical procedure that consists of cutting the two vas deferens, the ducts that carry sperm from the testes to the seminal vesicles. The man continues to ejaculate as usual, but the semen no longer carries sperm, which are reabsorbed within the testes.

**WHY IT IS DONE**

Male sterilization provides a method of birth control that is safe and virtually 100 percent effective; the risk of problems or complications is lower than for female sterilization. However, vasectomy is often irreversible, and the decision to have it performed should be carefully considered by the man and his partner.

**HOW IT IS DONE**

The operation is performed on an outpatient basis using a local anesthetic. The basic steps are shown in the illustrated box (above). The procedure takes 15 to 20 minutes.

**RECOVERY PERIOD**

The patient should rest in bed for 24 hours. There may be slight bruising of the scrotum and/or bleeding from the external wound for a few days. To relieve any pain, acetaminophen should be taken rather than aspirin, which can prolong bleeding.

Most men return to work within a few days, and sexual relations can be resumed as soon as the man is able, often within a week. For four to six weeks, tight-fitting underpants or a jockstrap should be worn to support the scrotum.

After a vasectomy, a man remains fertile until the sperm already present in the vas deferens are ejaculated or die. Between two and four months after the operation, the man returns to the hospital at least twice with specimens of semen for analysis. It is only when two consecutive specimens are found to be sperm-free that he is considered sterile. Until that time, either he or his partner needs to use some form of contraception.

**OUTLOOK**

In rare cases, a vasectomy fails because the severed parts of a vas deferens reunite. If this occurs, the man can safely undergo another vasectomy operation.

Although most men who have a vasectomy experience no sexual problems as a result, the operation occa-

V

sionally causes psychological problems that affect sexual performance. If counseling or psychotherapy fails to clear up these problems (or if a man strongly regrets that he has been sterilized) it may be possible to have the operation reversed. About half of reversal operations are successful in restoring fertility.

## Vasoconstriction
Narrowing of blood vessels, causing reduced blood flow to a part of the body. Vasoconstriction under the skin occurs in response to cold and reduces heat loss from the body. It also occurs due to a fall in blood pressure in physiological *shock*. Vasoconstriction is also caused by *decongestant drugs*, which relieve nasal congestion by reducing blood flow to the lining of the nose.

## Vasodilatation
Widening of blood vessels, causing increased blood flow to a part of the body. Vasodilatation under the skin occurs in response to hot weather and increases heat loss from the body. It also occurs as a response to *vasodilator drugs* and *alcohol*.

## Vasodilator drugs
A group of drugs that widens blood vessels. Vasodilator drugs include *ACE inhibitor drugs*, *calcium channel blockers*, *nitrate drugs*, and *sympatholytic drugs*.
### WHY THEY ARE USED
Vasodilator drugs are used to treat disorders in which abnormal narrowing of blood vessels reduces blood flow through tissues, impairing the supply of oxygen. Such disorders include *angina pectoris* (chest pain caused by inadequate blood supply to heart muscle) and *peripheral vascular disease*.

Vasodilator drugs are also used to treat *hypertension* (high blood pressure) and *heart failure* (reduced pumping efficiency). Drugs of the vasodilator group are also occasionally prescribed in the treatment of senile *dementia*, although they rarely improve symptoms.
### HOW THEY WORK
Vasodilator drugs widen blood vessels by relaxing surrounding muscles within the walls of the vessels; calcium channel blockers and nitrate drugs have a direct action on these muscles; sympatholytic drugs block the nerve signals that stimulate muscular contraction; and ACE inhibitors interfere with enzyme activity in

the blood—an action that reduces the production of angiotensin II (a chemical that narrows blood vessels).
### POSSIBLE ADVERSE EFFECTS
All vasodilator drugs may cause flushing, headaches, dizziness, fainting, and swollen ankles.

## Vasopressin
An alternative name for *ADH* (antidiuretic hormone).

## Vasovagal attack
Temporary loss of consciousness due to sudden slowing of the heart beat. A vasovagal attack, which is a common cause of *fainting* in healthy people, is a result of overstimulation of the *vagus nerve*, which helps to control breathing and blood circulation. A vasovagal attack is usually brought on by severe pain, stress, shock, or fear. The loss of consciousness is commonly preceded by sweating, nausea, dizziness, ringing in the ears, dimmed vision, and weakness. A person experiencing these symptoms can sometimes avoid fainting by putting his or her head between the knees.

This cause of fainting is often attributed to instances where no other cause can be found.

## VD
The abbreviation for venereal disease, another name for *sexually transmitted disease*.

## Vector
An animal that transmits a particular infectious disease. A vector picks up disease organisms from a source of infection (such as an infected person's or animal's blood or feces), carries them within or on its body, and later deposits them where they infect a new host, directly or indirectly.

Mosquitoes, fleas, lice, ticks, and flies are the most important vectors of disease to humans. When an organism develops or completes part of its life cycle inside a vector, this vector is called a biological vector. For example, mosquitoes are biological vectors for malarial parasites, which develop and multiply inside the insect and are injected into the blood of a new host by the mosquito's bite.

V

---

### TYPES OF VASODILATOR DRUGS
The different types of vasodilator drugs work in various ways to prevent or reduce the contraction of muscle cells in blood vessel walls, thus helping to widen the blood vessels.

Constricted          Dilated

**Action**
A blood vessel is shown contracted and dilated (above). Vasodilators widen vessels, improving blood flow (below).

Nerve fiber ending

Synaptic cleft

Drug

Muscle cell

**Sympatholytic drugs**
Muscles in blood vessel walls are made to contract by the action of neurotransmitters. Sympatholytic drugs block the sites where neurotransmitters act.

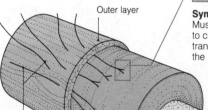

Outer layer

Nerve fibers

Muscle layer

Inner layer

**Calcium channel blockers and nitrates**
These drugs act directly on the contracted muscle cells in blood vessel walls, causing them to relax.

**ACE inhibitors**
These drugs work by blocking the activity of a particular enzyme in the blood—an action that reduces the production of angiotensin II, a chemical that acts to narrow blood vessels.

When a vector is not essential to the life cycle of a disease organism, it is called a mechanical vector. For example, flies may act as mechanical vectors of *shigellosis* (bacterial dysentery) by carrying the bacteria on their legs from infected feces to food.

## Vegetarianism

Eating a diet (see *Nutrition*) that excludes meat and fish, and sometimes all other animal products. A large proportion of the world's total population is vegetarian or primarily vegetarian. Humans do not need to eat meat or animal products to maintain health as long as the various nutrients supplied by plant foods provide a balanced diet.

### TYPES

Vegetarian diets can be classified into four types according to the foods that are eaten or are excluded (see chart, below).

### EATING A BALANCED DIET

All vegetarians, but especially vegans, must ensure that they eat a sufficient amount of *protein*. It is also necessary to eat different types of protein-containing foods. Whereas animal proteins are complete (containing all the essential *amino acids* needed for good health), individual plant proteins are incomplete (lacking a variety of essential amino acids). Plant proteins must therefore be eaten in combination if they are to provide all the body's amino acid requirements. A balanced vegetarian diet should consist of a wide selection of grains, dried beans and peas, nuts, and seeds. Rice and beans contain different essential amino acids; when eaten together they form a complete protein.

Vitamin $B_{12}$ is plentiful in all animal products. Vegetarians other than vegans are unlikely to suffer deficiency, but vegans should ensure that they are obtaining the vitamin from fortified food sources (such as soy milk or breakfast cereals) or from a vitamin $B_{12}$ supplement, often given by injections since vitamin $B_{12}$ is absorbed poorly when it is taken by mouth in tablet form.

Vegetarians should also receive adequate amounts of vitamin C, which helps the absorption of iron from plant foods.

Milk and milk products are rich in calcium. Lactovegetarians therefore receive a plentiful supply, but vegans must rely on grains, legumes, nuts, seeds, and dark green, leafy vegetables for this mineral. Vitamin D is important for calcium absorption from food in the intestinal tract. It is manufactured by our bodies from the action of sunlight on the skin or may be supplied by a supplement.

### ADVANTAGES OF A VEGETARIAN DIET

Vegetarians tend to eat a high-fiber diet. This may help protect them from certain intestinal diseases, such as cancer of the intestines and diverticular disease. Provided they do not eat a lot of high-fat dairy products, vegetarians have a reduced risk of coronary artery disease, high blood pressure, obesity, and non-insulin-dependent diabetes compared to nonvegetarians. Women who are vegetarians have been found to suffer less from *osteoporosis* (brittle bones).

## Vegetative state

A term sometimes used to describe a type of indefinite deep *coma*. Although the eyes may be open and occasional random movements of the head and limbs may occur, there are no other signs of consciousness and no responsiveness to stimuli. Only the basic body functions, such as breathing, heart beat, and body temperature, are maintained.

## Vein

A vessel that returns blood toward the heart from the various organs and tissues of the body.

The majority of veins carry deoxygenated (blue) blood. This blood collects in small vessels called venules in the tissues. The venules join to form veins, which deliver the blood to the two largest veins in the body, the venae cavae. The venae cavae then carry the deoxygenated blood to the right side of the heart to be pumped to the lungs.

The main exceptions to this design are the pulmonary veins in the chest, which carry oxygenated blood from the lungs to the left side of the heart. Another special vein is the portal vein, which carries nutrient-rich blood from the intestines to the liver.

The walls of veins, like those of arteries, consist of a smooth inner lining, a muscular middle layer, and a fibrous outer covering. However, blood pressure in veins is much lower than it is in arteries. Correspondingly, the walls of veins are thinner, less elastic, less muscular, and weaker. Veins collapse when empty, while arteries remain extended.

V

**TYPES OF VEGETARIANISM**

**Semivegetarian**

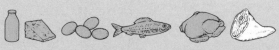

This diet includes milk, eggs, milk products such as cheese, cream, and yogurt, and allows occasional fish and poultry but no red meat.

**Lacto-ovovegetarian**

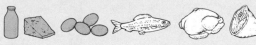

This diet allows milk, eggs, and milk products such as cheese, but excludes all types of fish and poultry as well as red meat.

**Lactovegetarian**

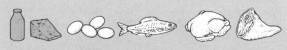

This is similar to the lacto-ovovegetarian diet except that eggs are excluded in addition to fish and meat. Milk and milk products are allowed.

**Vegan**

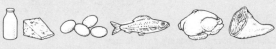

This is the most rigid form of vegetarianism; it excludes all foods of animal origin. Vegans must obtain all the nutrients they need from plant sources.

The inner linings of many veins contain folds, which act as valves, ensuring that blood can flow only toward the heart. The blood is helped on its way through the veins by pressure on the vessel walls from the contraction of surrounding muscles.

## Veins, disorders of

The most common vein disorder is a *varicose vein*—swelling, distortion, and twisting of a vein. Varicose veins occur most commonly in the legs, where they are caused by failure of the valves farther up the vein. *Esophageal varices* are varicose veins in the lower part of the esophagus; they commonly result from back pressure through the circulation from *cirrhosis* of the liver. *Hemorrhoids* are varicose veins in the anus.

Inflammation of a vein is called phlebitis. It is almost always associated with a tendency to blood clotting in the affected vein, in which case it is called *thrombophlebitis*. Clot formation in the small veins near the surface is not significant, although clots may cause swelling and tenderness. However, if clots form in deeper, larger

## LOCATION OF THE VENAE CAVAE

All the circulating blood, after being pumped to the body, returns to the heart via the venae cavae. The superior vena cava collects blood from the whole of the upper trunk, head, neck, and limbs. The inferior drains blood from all parts of the body below the chest.

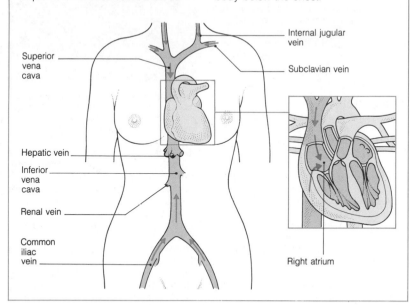

## STRUCTURE OF A VEIN AND AN ARTERY

Like arteries, the walls of veins have a smooth, inner layer, a muscular, middle layer, and a fibrous, outer layer. However, the walls are thinner and less muscular than those of arteries.

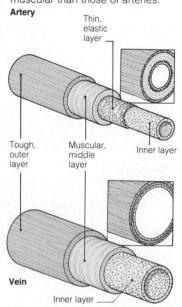

veins—a condition called deep vein thrombosis (see *Thrombosis, deep vein*)—they may become widespread and there is a risk that part of the clot will break off and cause blockage of the pulmonary artery.

The blood pressure in veins is much lower than in arteries; an injured vein will thus bleed much more slowly than an artery of the same size. Light pressure on an injured vein is usually sufficient to stop bleeding. Raising an injured part above the level of the heart will also stop bleeding from veins, though not from arteries.

## Vena cava

Either of two very large veins into which all the circulating venous (deoxygenated) blood drains. The venae cavae deliver this blood to the right atrium (one of the upper chambers of the heart) for pumping to the lungs. The veins are each nearly an inch in diameter and are situated deep within the chest and abdomen.

The superior vena cava starts at the top of the chest, behind the lower edge of the right first rib and close to the breastbone. It travels some 3 inches (7.5 cm) downward, passing through the pericardium (outer lining of the heart) before connecting to the right atrium. It is formed from the

right and left brachiocephalic veins, which themselves are formed from union of the subclavian veins (draining blood from the arms), the jugular veins (draining blood from the head), and several minor veins. The superior vena cava also receives blood from the azygos vein, which drains much of the chest. The superior vena cava thus collects blood from the whole of a person's upper trunk, head, neck, and limbs.

The inferior vena cava starts in the lower abdomen, in front of the fifth lumbar vertebra, and travels some 10 inches (25 cm) upward in front of the spine, behind the liver, and through the diaphragm before joining to the right atrium. It is formed from the union of the two common iliac veins, which receive blood from the legs and pelvic organs. The inferior vena cava also receives blood from the hepatic vein and from the renal veins, which drain the liver and the kidneys, respectively.

## Venereal diseases

See *Sexually transmitted diseases*.

## Venereology

The medical discipline concerned with the study and treatment of *sexually transmitted diseases*.

V

## Venesection

The process of withdrawing blood from a vein, also called phlebotomy, for *blood donation* or for therapeutic bloodletting. Regular bloodletting is used in the treatment of *polycythemia* (a disorder in which the blood is too thick); in *hemochromatosis* (a disorder of body iron chemistry) to reduce the amount of iron in the body; and very occasionally in some types of *heart failure* to reduce the blood volume and ease the heart's work load.

## Venipuncture

A common procedure in which a vein is pierced with a needle to withdraw blood or inject fluid. It is usually performed on a vein in the forearm.

### HOW IT IS DONE

A tourniquet is applied to the upper arm, causing the veins to become distended. A suitable vein, usually a large one that can be easily felt through the skin, is selected. The overlying skin is cleansed with a swab soaked in alcohol, and a sterile needle is inserted into the vein. For taking blood or injecting medication, a syringe is attached to the needle. For *intravenous infusion*, a cannula (hollow tube) is inserted into the vein via the needle; the needle is then withdrawn, and tubing for the fluid to flow through is attached to the cannula.

After the required amount of fluid has been injected or withdrawn, the needle or cannula is removed. The area is then covered with a piece of cotton and firm pressure applied for a minute or two until bleeding stops.

The procedure is not usually painful but it may cause some discomfort. Slight bruising may appear at the site of the venipuncture, although such bruising usually subsides within a few days.

## Venography

A diagnostic procedure, also known as phlebography, that enables veins to be seen on an X-ray film after they have been injected with a substance opaque to X rays.

### WHY IT IS DONE

Venography is used to detect anatomical abnormalities or diseases of the veins themselves—such as narrowing or blockage from *thrombosis* (abnormal clot) or tumor—as well as disease or injury in organs that are supplied by the veins. It is also used to evaluate the extent of disease so that treatment can be planned.

The veins most frequently studied are those in the leg, usually because of

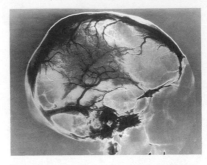

**Venogram showing veins within the skull**
This X-ray image of a skull shows both the veins and the venous sinuses (dark areas), which are wide blood drainage channels.

suspected deep vein thrombosis (see *Thrombosis, deep vein*). Other commonly studied veins include the axillary veins in the arm, the superior and inferior venae cavae (the main veins leading to the heart), and the renal veins (leading from the kidney).

### HOW IT IS DONE

Contrast medium is injected either through a needle directly into the veins to be examined or, if the veins are not readily accessible, through a catheter that has been guided, under X-ray control, along the venous system to the required vein. A sequence of X-ray pictures is taken so that blood flow along the veins can be studied. Leg venography takes about 20 minutes to perform; other types may take longer.

The newer technique of digital subtraction *angiography* adds to the information obtained through use of computer analysis to process images and remove unwanted shadowing.

## Venomous bites and stings

Many animals carry poison, or venom, which they can inject into other animals or humans via their mouthparts (bites) or by some other injecting apparatus (stings). Often, these venoms are carried for purely defensive purposes (to discourage predators). Sometimes they are used to kill or immobilize prey. It is rare for a venomous animal to attack a person unless cornered, provoked, stepped on, or otherwise disturbed.

Specific *antivenins* are available to treat many, though not all, animal venoms. In cases of serious poisoning, administration of antivenin can sometimes be lifesaving.

### TYPES OF VENOMOUS ANIMAL

For the better known types of venomous bites and stings, see *Snakebites, Spider bites, Insect stings, Scorpion*

*stings,* and *Jellyfish stings.* Other venomous animals include certain species of lizards, centipedes, millipedes, and fish.

**LIZARD BITES** Two types of biting lizard are found in the southwestern US and Mexico. A bite causes severe local pain, shock, and other symptoms such as vomiting. Some fatal bites have been reported. Treatment is with powerful *analgesic drugs* (painkillers).

**CENTIPEDES AND MILLIPEDES** Centipede bites can cause severe pain and local swelling but are not a danger to life. Certain millipedes secrete, and sometimes squirt out, an irritating liquid that may be dangerous if it enters the eyes. First aid is by thorough irrigation with water.

**FISH STINGS** Venomous fish inflict stings via certain fins or specialized spines on their bodies. These fish include stingrays (found in many parts of the world, including the coast of California), weeverfish (European waters), and scorpion fish, lionfish, and stonefish (throughout the Indian and Pacific oceans). They are a danger to swimmers, waders, snorkelers, and scuba divers.

The effects of a fish sting may include excruciating pain, shock, vomiting, sweating, and cardiac *arrhythmias.* Occasional fatalities occur. Stinging spines should be removed from the wound, which should be thoroughly washed. A useful first-aid procedure is to immerse the stung body part in hot water; the heat inactivates some of the components of the venom and relieves the intense pain. Alternatively, a physician may inject a local anesthetic. In some cases, *cardiopulmonary resuscitation* and life-support procedures are necessary.

## Ventilation

The use of a machine called a *ventilator* to take over respiration (and thus maintain life) in a person who has lost or who lacks the ability to breathe naturally.

### WHY IT IS DONE

Arrested or severe impairment of breathing may be caused by damage to the respiratory center in the brain stem due to head injury, brain disease, or an overdose of narcotic drugs. Breathing difficulties may also be due to damage to or malfunctioning of the breathing mechanism as a result of chest injury, respiratory disease, a nerve or muscle disorder, or major chest or abdominal surgery. Occasionally, difficulties arise as a result of

**V**

## TECHNIQUE OF ARTIFICIAL VENTILATION

Machine-assisted breathing may be needed when a person has lost the ability to breathe naturally—often following a severe head injury, narcotic overdose, or in various other emergency situations. It may also be needed when a muscle relaxant has been given during an operation as part of a general anesthetic.

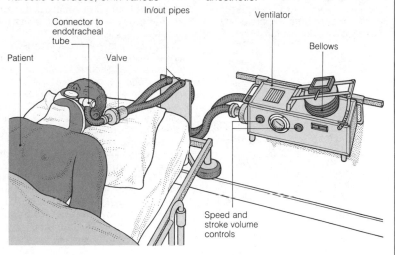

Patient · Connector to endotracheal tube · Valve · In/out pipes · Ventilator · Bellows · Speed and stroke volume controls

### Procedure
The air is delivered to the patient's lungs via a tube inserted into the windpipe. After each inflation, the air is expelled by the natural elasticity of the lungs. Fluids and drugs must be given to the patient by intravenous infusion.

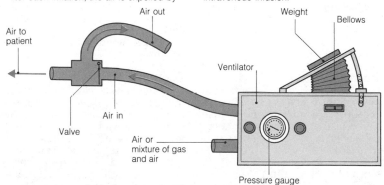

Air to patient · Air out · Valve · Air in · Air or mixture of gas and air · Ventilator · Weight · Bellows · Pressure gauge

### Ventilator components
The pump part of the ventilator consists of a bellows, which is expanded by an electric motor and compressed by a weight. The air (or other gas mixture) is driven through a humidifier and delivered via a hose and valve to the patient. The stroke volume, stroke rate, and oxygen content of the gas mixture can be varied according to the needs of the individual patient.

During ventilation the amount of oxygen and other gases in the patient's blood is checked by analyzing blood samples. X rays are taken to assess the state of the lungs; the pulse, blood pressure, heart rhythm, and temperature are monitored.

The patient is unable to eat or drink when connected to the ventilator. Fluids are therefore given by *intravenous infusion*. Drugs may need to be given in the same way.

The patient's inability to cough may cause secretions to accumulate in the lungs. They are removed by suction apparatus, and intensive *respiratory therapy* is given to prevent the secretions from building up again.

When the patient begins to recover, he or she is disconnected from the ventilator and allowed to breathe naturally for increasingly longer and more frequent periods. After the blood gases have returned to a normal level during spontaneous breathing, the patient is taken off the ventilator permanently.

## Ventilator
A device, also known as a life-support machine or respirator, used to take over respiration (and thus maintain life) in a patient who lacks or has lost the ability to breathe naturally.

A ventilator is an electrical pump connected to an air supply that works like bellows. The pump can be adjusted to vary the proportion of oxygen in the pumped air and to regulate the amount of air delivered. The air is first pumped through a humidifier, which adds sterile water vapor to prevent the lungs from drying out; the air is then directed through a tube that has been passed down the patient's trachea (see *Ventilation*). After the lungs have been inflated, the air is expelled by the natural elasticity of the lungs and rib cage. A valve on the ventilator prevents the expelled air from reentering the lungs.

Artificial ventilation is usually carried out in an *intensive-care* unit.

## Ventouse
See *Vacuum extraction*.

## Ventral
Relating to the front of the body, or describing the lowermost part of a body structure when a person is lying facedown. In human anatomy, the term ventral means the same as anterior. The opposite of ventral is dorsal (or posterior).

problems during anesthesia. Severely premature babies with *respiratory distress syndrome* may also need ventilation for a period until their lungs develop sufficiently to cope with breathing unaided.

**HOW IT IS DONE**
The patient is connected to the ventilator by means of an *endotracheal tube* passed through the nose or mouth into the trachea (windpipe); if prolonged ventilation is likely to be required, a tube is inserted into an opening made in the trachea, an operation called a *tracheostomy*. Conscious patients, and those nearing the end of anesthesia, are usually given muscle-relaxant and sedative drugs to prevent them from resisting the insertion and irritant presence of the tube.

V

## LOCATION OF VENTRICLES

The location of the ventricles in the brain (seen from above) and in the heart are shown below. Of the heart ventricles, the right ventricle pumps blood to the lungs, the left pumps blood to the rest of the body.

### VENTRICLES IN THE BRAIN

Together, these irregularly shaped cavities contain about a glassful of cerebrospinal fluid.

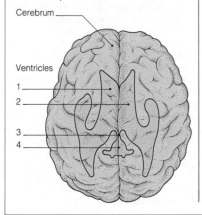

### VENTRICLES IN THE HEART

The ventricles of the heart are the large, lower chambers, separated by a muscular wall, the septum.

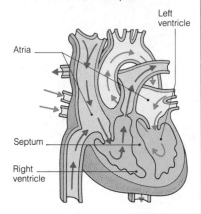

## Ventricle

A cavity or chamber. Both the *heart* and *brain* have anatomical parts known as ventricles.

There are four ventricles in the brain—one in each of the two cerebral hemispheres (which make up the cerebrum, or main mass of the brain), a third at the center of the brain, above the brain stem, and a fourth situated between the brain stem and the cerebellum. These cavities are filled with cerebrospinal fluid and are linked by ducts so that the fluid can circulate through them. The cavities are lined in part with tuftlike clusters of blood vessels called the choroid plexus, which secrete the cerebrospinal fluid.

In the heart, there are two ventricles. They are the lower, pumping chambers, which receive blood from the atria (upper heart chambers) and pump it to the lungs and to the rest of the body.

## Ventricular ectopic beat

An abnormal heart beat that has been initiated from electrical impulses in the ventricles (lower heart chambers) rather than the sinoatrial node in the right atrium (upper heart chamber). Many people, especially older people, have occasional ventricular ectopic beats that do not cause symptoms. Ventricular ectopic beats may also be caused by a *myocardial infarction* (heart attack) or *digitalis drugs*.

Occasionally, a ventricular ectopic beat causes the sensation that the heart has stopped for a second and then restarts with a thump.

Ventricular ectopic beats may be detected on an *ECG* (measurement of electrical activity of the heart) as a broad, bizarre-looking wave (see illustrated box, opposite).

If a person has frequent ventricular ectopic beats that cause symptoms or beats that arise from more than one site in the ventricles, treatment with an *antiarrhythmic drug* may be required.

## Ventricular fibrillation

Rapid, ineffective, uncoordinated contractions of the heart. Ventricular fibrillation is caused by abnormal heart beats initiated by electrical activity in the ventricles (lower heart chambers). It is a common complication of *myocardial infarction* (heart attack) and may also be caused by electrocution or drowning. The heart ceases to pump blood effectively and the condition is fatal unless the normal heart rhythm is quickly restored. Diagnosis is confirmed by *ECG* (measurement of electrical activity of the heart), which shows broad, irregular waves (see illustrated box, opposite).

Treatment is with *cardioversion* (administration of an electric shock to the heart) and *antiarrhythmic drugs*.

## Ventricular tachycardia

A serious cardiac *arrhythmia* (abnormal heart beat) in which each heart beat is initiated from electrical activity in the ventricles (lower heart chambers) rather than the sinoatrial node in the right atrium (upper heart chamber). The result is an abnormally fast heart rate of between 140 and 220 beats per minute.

Ventricular tachycardia is caused by serious heart disease, such as a *myocardial infarction* (heart attack) or *cardiomyopathy*. It may last for a few seconds or several days. Diagnosis is confirmed by *ECG* (recording of the electrical activity of the heart), which shows broad, regular abnormal waves (see box, opposite).

Emergency treatment is with *cardioversion* (administration of an electric shock to the heart) or by injection of an *antiarrhythmic drug*, such as lidocaine. Use of the drug is usually continued by mouth for several months. Untreated ventricular tachycardia may cause heart failure and death.

## Ventriculography

An outdated procedure that enables the ventricular cavities within the brain to be seen on X-ray film after the introduction of air or a contrast medium (a substance opaque to X rays). Ventriculography is performed very infrequently; *CT scanning* and *MRI* have largely taken its place.

## Verapamil

A *calcium channel blocker drug* used in the treatment of *hypertension* (high blood pressure), *angina pectoris* (chest pain due to inadequate blood supply to heart muscle), and certain types of *arrhythmia* (irregular heart rhythm).

Possible adverse effects include headache, facial flushing, dizziness, ankle swelling, and constipation.

## Vernix

The pale, greasy, cheeselike substance that covers the skin of a newborn baby. Vernix consists of fatty secretions and dead cells. It is thought to protect the baby's skin and insulate against heat loss before birth.

## Verruca

The medical term for a *wart*.

## Version

A change in the direction in which a fetus lies so that a *malpresentation* (abnormal presentation), most often *breech* (bottom down), becomes the normal cephalic (head down) presen-

V

## TYPES OF VENTRICULAR ARRHYTHMIA

The ventricles (lower chambers) of the heart usually beat regularly in response to excitatory waves spread from the upper chambers. If rhythm disturbances (which may be associated with heart disease) occur, they are visible on an electrocardiograph (ECG) recording.

Normal heart beat

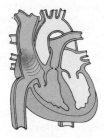

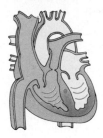

Ventricular ectopic beat

Ventricular tachycardia

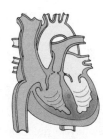

Ventricular fibrillation

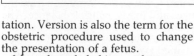

### Normal heart beat
This is the normal ECG appearance of the heart beat. The regular spikes coincide with beats of the ventricles (lower heart chambers). The small rises before each spike coincide with contractions of the atria (upper chambers).

### Ventricular ectopic beat
Here there is an abnormal beat, which has a broad, bizarre-looking wave form on the ECG; it occurs just before the expected normal beat. To the patient, the heart may seem to stop at time A and restart with a thump at time B.

### Ventricular tachycardia
Here there is a rapid succession of abnormal beats, caused by an abnormal focus of electrical activity in a ventricle. It usually indicates serious underlying heart disease. The rate of beating may be very high—up to 220 beats per minute.

### Ventricular fibrillation
This pattern is seen only when the heart is in a state of virtual arrest, usually after a heart attack, with the ventricles twitching in a rapid and totally irregular manner. Unless a normal rhythm can be restored, the condition is quickly fatal.

baby's buttocks, the obstetrician very gently attempts to rotate the baby, bringing its head down into the mother's pelvis. External version is performed between the 34th and 37th week of pregnancy and can be done with or without general anesthesia. Drugs may be used to relax the uterus.

Though effective if properly performed, external version carries small risks of inducing premature labor or rupture of membranes, antepartum hemorrhage, or knotting of the umbilical cord. The risks of external version must be weighed against the risks of vaginal breech delivery and the risks of *cesarean section*.

Internal version is the turning of a fetus by an obstetrician by reaching inside the uterus. Internal version is rarely done except in the case of a second twin who is malposed (not in the normal position) after delivery of the first twin.

## Vertebra
Any of the 33 approximately cylindrical bones that form the *spine*, or vertebral column. There are seven vertebrae in the cervical spine in the neck; 12 vertebrae in the thoracic spine in the chest; five vertebrae in the lumbar spine in the lower back; five fused vertebrae in the *sacrum*; and four fused vertebrae in the *coccyx* (see box, overleaf). Between each pair of separate vertebrae is an intervertebral disk (see *Disk, intervertebral*).

## Vertebrobasilar insufficiency
Intermittent episodes of dizziness, double vision, weakness, and difficulty speaking caused by reduced blood flow to the brain stem and cerebellum in the brain.

The obstruction to blood flow is usually caused by *atherosclerosis* (narrowing of arteries with deposits of fat) involving the basilar and vertebral arteries and other arteries in the base of the brain.

## Vertigo
An illusion that one's surroundings or self are spinning, either horizontally or vertically. Vertigo is a common complaint, but only rarely is it a sign of an underlying disorder. The term is sometimes used erroneously to describe *dizziness* or faintness.

### CAUSES
Vertigo results from a disturbance of the semicircular canals in the inner ear or the nerve tracts leading from them. It can occur in healthy people when sailing, on amusement park rides, or

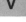

tation. Version is also the term for the obstetric procedure used to change the presentation of a fetus.

Many breech babies undergo version spontaneously, especially before the 34th week of pregnancy. If this does not occur, the obstetrician may be able to manipulate the fetus into the cephalic position by a procedure called external version. With one hand on the mother's abdomen over the baby's head and the other over the

## LOCATION AND STRUCTURE OF THE VERTEBRAE

The 33 vertebrae are arranged as shown. Apart from the top two, they all have a similar structure. The topmost cervical vertebra (the atlas) has no body. The second (the axis) forms a pivot on which the atlas can rotate, allowing the head to be turned in all directions.

**The spine**

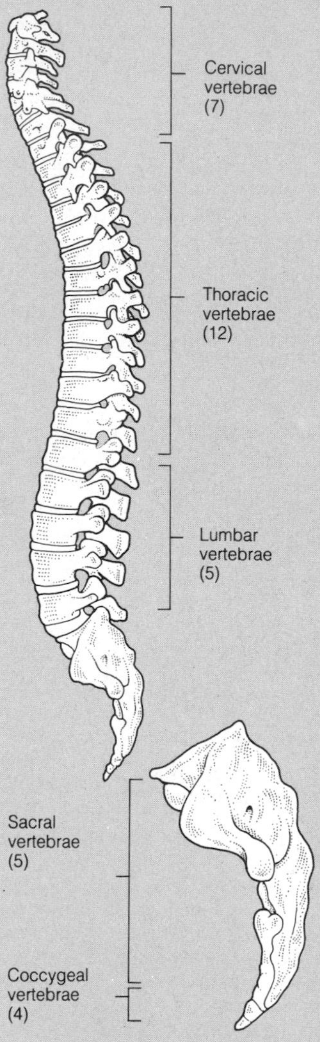

Cervical vertebrae (7)

Thoracic vertebrae (12)

Lumbar vertebrae (5)

Sacral vertebrae (5)

Coccygeal vertebrae (4)

**Cervical vertebrae**

Transverse process

Spinous process

Foramen

Body

**Thoracic vertebrae**

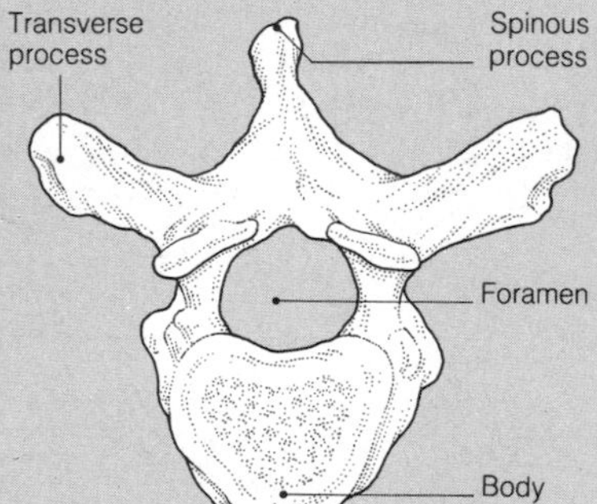

Transverse process

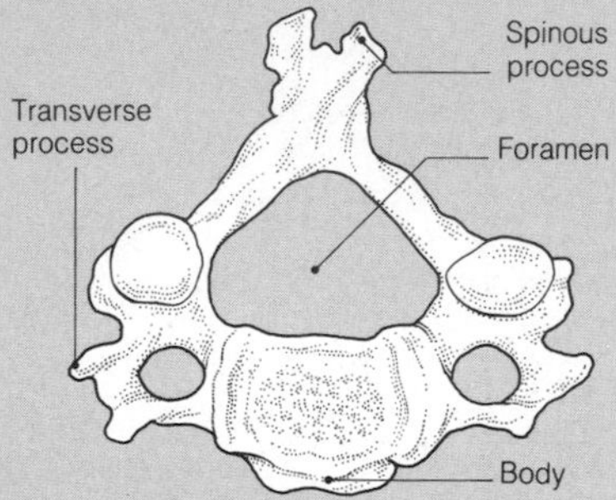

Spinous process

Foramen

Body

**Lumbar vertebrae**

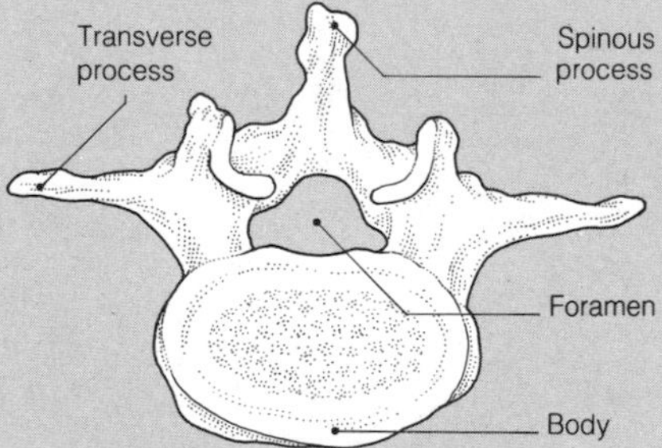

Transverse process

Spinous process

Foramen

Body

**Arrangement**
The vertebrae fall into five groups—cervical, thoracic, lumbar, sacral, and coccygeal. The top 24 are separated by disks of cartilage.

**Structure**
Three typical vertebrae are shown above. The foramen in each is the channel through which the spinal cord runs. The processes serve as muscle attachments.

even when watching a movie. Astronauts in zero gravity experience vertigo when moving their heads.

Severe vertigo, usually accompanied by other symptoms, may indicate a number of diseases. *Labyrinthitis* (inflammation of the semicircular canals) causes sudden vertigo accompanied by vomiting and unsteadiness. It often occurs in conjunction with an infection such as influenza or *otitis media* and usually clears up as the infection subsides. *Meniere's disease* is a more serious condition charac-

terized by attacks of vertigo that are sometimes severe enough to cause the sufferer to fall to the ground. The attacks of vertigo are accompanied by severe vomiting, *tinnitus* (ringing in the ears), *nystagmus* (jerky eye movements), and unsteadiness.

Elderly people with *atherosclerosis* often suffer from vertigo upon sudden movement of the head. Vertigo is less commonly caused by a tumor of the brain stem or by *multiple sclerosis*. Vertigo may also be psychological in origin, in which case it is usually associated with *agoraphobia* (fear of open spaces).

**INVESTIGATION AND TREATMENT**
If disease is the suspected cause of vertigo, the physician performs an examination of the ears, eyes, and nervous system, sometimes including *CT scanning* of the brain.

**TREATMENT**
Vertigo that comes on suddenly is usually assumed to be due to labyrinthitis and is treated with bed rest and *antihistamine drugs* or *anticholinergic drugs*. If vertigo persists for more than a few days, the sufferer should walk as much as possible to allow the body to develop compensatory measures. Antihistamine drugs may be prescribed to prevent recurrent attacks.

## Vesicle
A small skin blister, usually filled with clear fluid, that forms at the site of skin damage. Vesicle also refers to any small saclike structure in the body; the seminal vesicles are small sacs in which seminal fluid is stored.

## Vestibulocochlear nerve
The eighth *cranial nerve* concerned with *balance* and *hearing*. It carries sensory impulses from the inner *ear* to the brain, which it enters between the pons and the medulla oblongata (parts of the *brain stem*).

The vestibulocochlear nerve consists of two parts—the vestibular nerve and the cochlear nerve (also sometimes known as the acoustic, or auditory, nerve). The vestibular nerve carries sensory impulses from the semicircular canals in the inner ear to the cerebellum in the brain, which, in conjunction with information from the eyes and joints, controls balance. The cochlear nerve carries sensory impulses from the cochlea (the snail-shaped part of the inner ear responsible for detecting sound) to the hearing center in the brain, where the impulses are interpreted as sounds.

V

## DISORDERS

A tumor of the cells that surround the vestibulocochlear nerve (see *Acoustic neuroma*) may cause loss of balance, *tinnitus* (noises in the ear), and *deafness*. Damage to the vestibulocochlear nerve (e.g., due to an infection such as *meningitis* or *encephalitis*) or an adverse reaction to a drug (such as streptomycin) may also cause deafness.

## Viability

The capability of independent survival and development. It is widely accepted that a normal human fetus is viable from 28 weeks' gestation onward. However, today, fetuses born as early as the 23rd to 24th week can often survive after care in a neonatal intensive-care unit.

## Vibrator

A mechanical device applied to the body to tone or relax muscles and to massage the skin.

Vibrators may also be used as an aid to sexual stimulation or as an alternative to sexual intercourse for inducing orgasm. They are sometimes used as an aid in *sex therapy*. (See also *Orgasm, lack of*; *Ejaculation, disorders of*.)

---

### LOCATION OF THE VESTIBULOCOCHLEAR NERVE

The nerve conducts sensory impulses concerned with hearing and balance from different parts of the inner ear to the brain.

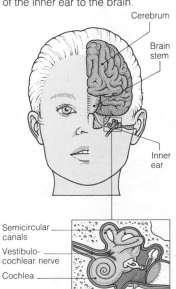

Cerebrum

Brain stem

Inner ear

Semicircular canals

Vestibulo-cochlear nerve

Cochlea

---

## Villus

One of the countless millions of minute fingerlike projections that occur on the mucous lining of the small intestine. Although villi are present in all three sections of the small intestine, they are largest and most numerous in the duodenum and jejunum (the first and second parts), where most of the absorption of food occurs.

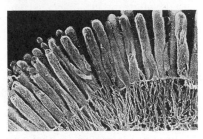

**Microvilli in the intestine**
This scanning electron micrograph shows numerous villi projecting from a single cell in the lining of the small intestine.

### STRUCTURE

Each villus contains a small lymph vessel and a network of capillaries. The outer surface of each villus is covered with hundreds of hairlike structures (microvilli) that increase the surface area of the small intestine to an area approximately equal to that of a tennis court.

### FUNCTION

The function of the villi is to provide a large intestinal surface area for the absorption of food molecules into the blood and lymphatic systems. Food particles that are broken down into small molecules by digestive enzymes reach the bloodstream via the capillaries of the villi.

## Vincent's disease

Painful bacterial infection and ulceration of the gums, also known as acute necrotizing ulcerative gingivitis, trench mouth, or Vincent's stomatitis.

### CAUSES AND INCIDENCE

The condition is caused by abnormal growth of microorganisms that usually exist harmlessly in small amounts in gum crevices. Predisposing factors include poor *oral hygiene*, smoking, throat infections, and emotional stress. In many cases Vincent's disease is preceded by *gingivitis* or by *periodontitis*. The condition is relatively rare, primarily affecting young adults aged 15 to 35.

### SYMPTOMS

The symptoms appear over the course of a day or two. The gums become sore and inflamed and bleed at the slightest pressure. Craterlike ulcers, which bleed spontaneously, develop on the gum tips between teeth, and there is a foul taste in the mouth, bad breath, and sometimes swollen lymph nodes. As the disease advances, ulcers spread along the gum margins and into deeper tissues. Occasionally, the infection spreads to the lips and the lining of the cheeks, resulting in destruction of tissues (see *Noma*).

### TREATMENT

The dentist usually prescribes a mouthwash containing hydrogen peroxide to relieve pain and inflammation. After a few days, when the gums are less tender, scaling (see *Scaling, dental*) is performed to remove calculus (a hard mineral deposit) and plaque from the teeth. In severe cases, the antibacterial drug *metronidazole* may be prescribed to control infection.

Regular follow-up visits to the dentist may be necessary. Counseling may focus on maintaining oral hygiene, giving up smoking, or learning to cope with stress.

## Viremia

The presence of virus particles in the blood. Viremia can occur at certain stages in a variety of viral infections.

Some viruses, such as those responsible for viral hepatitis, yellow fever, and poliomyelitis, may simply be carried in the bloodstream, which is used solely as a means of spreading. Symptoms arise when virus particles enter and start multiplying in target tissues rather than from the viremia.

Other viruses, such as the rubella virus and HIV (the AIDS virus), exist within lymphocytes (types of white blood cell), which they use as a place to multiply as well as for spreading.

If viremia is a feature of a viral infection, there is a risk that the infection may be transmissible in blood or blood products (as is the case with the AIDS virus) or by blood-feeding insects (as is the case with yellow fever).

## Virginity

The physical state of not having experienced *sexual intercourse*.

## Virilism

Masculine characteristics that affect the physical appearance of a woman. Virilism is caused by excessive levels of androgens. Androgens are male sex hormones that, in women, are normally secreted in small amounts by the adrenal glands and ovaries. Raised levels of these hormones induce

V

various changes in women, including *hirsutism* (excessive hair growth); a male-pattern hairline with balding at the temples; disruption or cessation of menstruation; enlargement of the clitoris; loss of normal fat deposits around the hips; development of the arm and shoulder muscles; and deepening of the voice as a result of enlargement of the larynx. (See also *Virilization*.)

## Virility

A term used to describe the quality of maleness, especially sexual characteristics and performance.

## Virilization

The process by which *virilism* occurs in women due to overproduction of androgens (male sex hormones) by the adrenal glands and/or ovaries. This process, in turn, may be caused by various underlying conditions, such as certain tumors of the adrenal glands (see *Adrenal glands* disorders box); some types of ovarian cysts (see *Polycystic ovary*); or congenital *adrenal hyperplasia*, a rare genetic disorder.

## Virion

A single, complete, virus particle. (See *Viruses*.)

## Virology

The study of *viruses* and the *epidemiology* and treatment of diseases caused by viruses. In a more restricted sense, virology also means the isolation and identification of viruses to diagnose specific viral infections. To achieve this, a tissue or fluid sample (such as a specimen of feces, sputum, blister fluid, blood, urine, cerebrospinal fluid, or even brain biopsy specimen, depending on the suspected virus) is needed.

Unlike bacteria, viruses cannot be grown in a suitable culture medium; they can multiply only within living cells. Therefore, viruses must be grown in cultures of cells, which can be any of many types of animal or human cell that are easily made to multiply in test tubes. The culture is exposed to the specimen or fluid containing the virus, and the cells are then observed for distinctive changes that occur when they are infected with certain viruses.

Alternatively, virus particles or components of viruses can sometimes be detected directly in specimens by the use of staining techniques or an electron microscope. Sometimes, the virus particles must first be made to

clump together by adding an *antiserum* (antibodies obtained from the blood of someone who has had the viral infection, and which will bind to the virus particles). *Immunoassay* techniques, in which "labeled" antibodies are added to the specimens and detected if they have bound to virus cell components, are another possibility.

Another method of diagnosing viral infections is to look for antibodies produced by the immune system to combat the viruses. A rapidly rising level of antibodies to a particular virus can provide good evidence of infection. Antibodies can be detected by types of immunoassay and other laboratory techniques (see *Serology*).

## Virulence

The ability of a microorganism to cause disease. Virulence can be assessed by measuring what proportion of the population exposed to the microorganism develops symptoms of disease, how rapidly the infection spreads through body tissues, or by the mortality from the infection.

## Viruses

The smallest known types of infectious agent. Viruses are about one half to one hundredth the size of the smallest bacteria, from which they differ in having a much simpler structure and method of multiplication. Viral infections range from the trivial and harmless, such as *warts*, the common cold (see *Cold, common*), and other minor respiratory tract infections, to extremely serious diseases, such as *rabies*, *AIDS*, and probably some types of *cancer*.

### NATURE OF VIRUSES

It is debatable whether viruses are truly living organisms or just collections of large molecules capable of self-replication under very specific favorable conditions. Their sole activity is to invade the cells of other organisms, which they take over to make copies of themselves. Outside living cells, viruses are wholly inert. They are incapable of activities typical of life, such as metabolism (internal processing of nutrients).

The number of different kinds of virus probably exceeds the number of types of all other organisms. They parasitize all recognized life-forms—mammals, birds, reptiles, insects, plants, algae, even bacteria. Not all viruses cause disease, but many do.

### STRUCTURE AND REPLICATION OF VIRUSES

A single virus particle (virion) consists simply of an inner core of *nucleic acid*

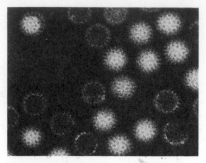

**Rotavirus particles**
This particular virus is a common cause of stomach upsets and diarrhea in infants. Each white sphere is a virus particle.

surrounded by one or two protective shells (capsids) made of protein. These capsids are built from a number of identical protein subunits arranged in a highly symmetrical form, usually either as a 20-faced solid (an icosahedron) or as a spiral tube. Surrounding the outer capsid may be another layer called the viral envelope. This layer also consists primarily of protein. In many cases, the viral envelope is lost when the virus invades a cell.

The nucleic acid at the core is called the genome; it consists of a string of *genes* that contain coded instructions for making copies of the virus. Depending on the type of virus, the nucleic acid may be either DNA, in which there are two complementary, intertwined strands of nucleic acid (the double helix), or RNA, consisting of a single strand.

The basic process by which a virus replicates is shown in the illustrated box (right). Different viruses employ different strategies, some highly complex, to make copies of themselves once they have invaded a host cell. During replication of the viral nucleic acid, the viral genes may first have to code the manufacture of special enzymes called polymerases or transcriptases to assist in replication, or may borrow these enzymes from the host cell. Sometimes the viral genome must invade the nucleus of the host cell and incorporate itself into the cell's chromosomes before it can replicate.

Sometimes, if the viral genome invades the nucleus of the host cell, it may not at first replicate but may "hide" there, sometimes becoming reactivated months or years later. It may also interact with the cell's chromosomes—a process that may convert the cell into a tumor cell.

V

## VIRUSES AND DISEASE

All viruses have the same basic structure (right), but they come in various shapes and sizes. Examples from the main families are shown below (some in cross section). All are tiny (from about one millionth to one hundred thousandths of an inch in diameter) and most cannot be seen even with a powerful light microscope. All types of viruses can multiply only after invading the cells of their human or other host (far right).

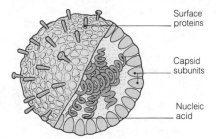

**Structure of a typical virus particle**
Nucleic acid in the center is surrounded by one or more capsids made of protein subunits.

### TYPES OF VIRUS

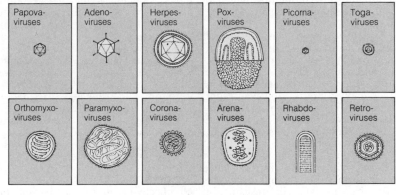

| Family | Examples of conditions or diseases |
|---|---|
| Papovaviruses | Warts |
| Adenoviruses | Respiratory and eye infections |
| Herpesviruses | Cold sores, genital herpes, chickenpox, herpes zoster (shingles), glandular fever, congenital abnormalities (cytomegalovirus) |
| Poxviruses | Cowpox, smallpox (eradicated), molluscum contagiosum |
| Picornaviruses | Poliomyelitis, viral hepatitis types A and B, respiratory infections, myocarditis |
| Togaviruses | Yellow fever, dengue, encephalitis |
| Orthomyxoviruses | Influenza |
| Paramyxoviruses | Mumps, measles, rubella |
| Coronaviruses | Common cold |
| Arenaviruses | Lassa fever |
| Rhabdoviruses | Rabies |
| Retroviruses | AIDS, degenerative brain diseases, and (possibly) various kinds of cancer |

## VIRAL REPLICATION

The sequence below shows how a virus multiplies. The signs and symptoms of viral infection are caused by the virus interfering with or destroying the host's cells.

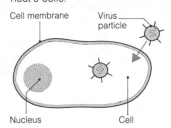

**1** The virus particle first attaches itself to and then injects itself into the host cell.

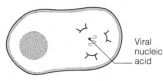

**2** The viral capsid breaks down and the viral nucleic acid (DNA or RNA) contained inside is released.

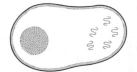

**3** The viral nucleic acid replicates itself; the new copies are made from raw materials within the host cell.

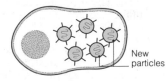

**4** Each of the new copies of the viral nucleic acid now directs the manufacture of a capsid for itself.

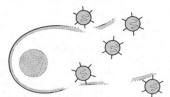

**5** The newly formed viral particles are released in large numbers, and the host cell may be destroyed.

V

## TYPES

Viruses that cause human disease are grouped into more than 20 large families; the most important are shown in the table (previous page).

In recent years, special attention has been paid to the family of retroviruses, which include *HIV* (human immunodeficiency virus), the agent responsible for AIDS. HIV is an RNA virus and, after invading a cell, first manufactures an enzyme called reverse transcriptase, which it needs to make copies of itself. Research into this enzyme may reveal a means of attacking HIV.

## HOW VIRUSES CAUSE DISEASE

Viruses gain access to the body by all possible entry routes. They are inhaled in droplets; swallowed in food and fluids; and passed through the punctured skin in the saliva of feeding insects or rabid dogs or accidentally on the needles of tattooists, those who pierce ears, or even physicians. Viruses are accepted directly by the mucous membranes of the genital tract during sexual intercourse and by the conjunctiva of the eye after accidental contamination.

Many viruses begin to invade cells and multiply near their site of entry. Some enter the lymphatic vessels and may spread to the lymph nodes, where many are engulfed by white blood cells. Some, such as HIV, invade and then multiply within *lymphocytes* (a type of white cell). Many pass from the lymphatics to the blood and within a few minutes are spread to every part of the body. They may then invade and start multiplying within specific target organs such as the skin, brain, liver, or lungs. Other viruses travel along nerve fibers to their target organs.

Viruses cause disease in a variety of ways. First, they may destroy or severely disrupt the activities of the cells they invade, possibly causing serious disease if vital organs are affected. Second, the response of the body's *immune system* to viral infection may lead to symptoms, such as fever and fatigue, or to a disease process. In particular, antibodies produced by the immune system may attach to viral particles and circulate as immune complexes in the bloodstream. The antibodies may then be deposited in various parts of the body and cause inflammation and severe tissue damage. Third, by interacting with the chromosomes of their host cells, viruses may cause cancer. Fourth, a virus may cause disease by weakening the cell-mediated arm of the immune system (i.e., the activity of T-*lymphocytes*). This is how HIV works, invading and disrupting one type of T-lymphocyte so that the normal defenses to a wide range of infections are lost.

## VIRUSES AND CANCER

The chromosomes in all normal body cells contain 50 or more genes (known as oncogenes) that are necessary for the growth or *differentiation* of the cells. Certain retroviruses contain almost identical oncogenes. In the process of replication, these viruses may modify the chromosomes of the host cell. A small mutation in these can "switch on" the oncogenes inappropriately, thus prompting the cell to begin unrestrained division, leading to cancer.

To date, this process has been found to cause many cancers in animals but only one type of cancer in humans. The virus responsible is similar to the AIDS virus and can cause leukemia in the person it infects. However, other viruses are known to be at least potentially cancer-producing in humans; this is a major area of research.

## RESISTANCE TO VIRUSES

The immune system deals fairly rapidly with most viruses. Each mechanism of the immune system may be involved in resisting a viral attack—including white cells (macrophages) that engulf the viral particles, and lymphocytes that produce antibodies against the virus or attack virally infected cells. This leads to recovery from most viral infections within a few days to weeks. Furthermore, the immune system is often sufficiently sensitized by the infection to make a second illness from the same virus rare (as is the case with measles).

With some viruses, however, the speed of the attack is such that serious damage or even death may occur before the immune system can adequately respond (as is the case with rabies and some cases of poliomyelitis). In other cases, a virus is able to dodge or hide from the immune system, so the infection becomes chronic or recurrent. This is common with many herpes virus infections (such as genital herpes and shingles) and with viral hepatitis B. Finally, the AIDS virus, by weakening the immune system, leaves the body open to many *opportunistic infections*.

## FIGHTING VIRAL DISEASE

Viruses are more difficult than bacteria to combat with drugs because it is difficult to design drugs that will kill viruses without also killing the cells they parasitize. Nevertheless, there has been remarkable progress in the development of antiviral agents, especially against the herpes group of viruses (see *Antiviral drugs*). Such drugs may work by helping to prevent viruses from entering cells or by interfering with their replication in cells.

*Interferon* refers to a group of natural substances, produced by virus-infected cells, that protects uninfected cells. Some interferons can now be produced artificially and have been tried in the treatment of various viral infections, including the common cold and viral hepatitis B.

Otherwise, treatment of viral infections depends largely on alleviating the patient's symptoms and trusting the body's immune defenses to bring about a cure.

A much more fruitful area in the fight against viruses is *immunization*. One viral disease, smallpox, has already been eradicated worldwide through a coordinated vaccination program. Highly effective vaccines are also now available to prevent many others, including poliomyelitis, measles, mumps, rubella, hepatitis B, yellow fever, and rabies.

## Viscera

A collective term used to describe the internal organs.

## Viscosity

The resistance to flow of a liquid or gas; the "stickiness" of a fluid. The viscosity of the blood affects its ability to flow through small blood vessels. An increase in the viscosity of the blood—caused by an increase in the proportion of red blood cells—increases the risk of *thrombosis* (abnormal clot formation).

## Vision

The faculty of sight. Vision involves two main components—the *eye* and the *brain*.

When light rays reach the eye, most of the focusing is done by the *cornea*. However, the eye also has an automatic fine-focusing facility, called *accommodation*, that operates by altering the curvature of the crystalline *lens*. Together, these two systems provide sufficient optical power to form an image on the *retina*. The light-sensitive rods and cones in the retina convert the elements of this image into nerve impulses that, after preliminary processing in the retina, pass into the brain via the *optic nerves*. The rods,

**V**

# THE SENSE OF VISION

Vision starts in the retina, the membrane at the back of the eye that contains the light-sensitive rod and cone cells. Much of the rest of the eye is concerned with focusing light, in the right quantities, onto the retina. Huge amounts of data are sent from the retina via the optic nerves to the brain for analysis.

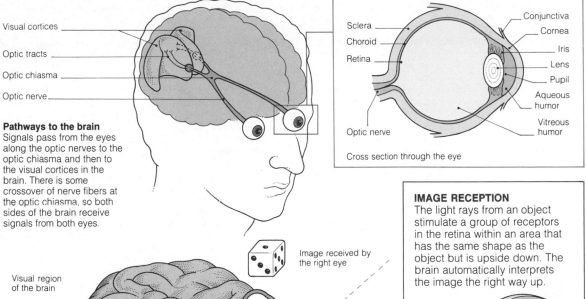

Visual cortices

Optic tracts

Optic chiasma

Optic nerve

Sclera
Choroid
Retina
Optic nerve

Conjunctiva
Cornea
Iris
Lens
Pupil
Aqueous humor
Vitreous humor

Cross section through the eye

## Pathways to the brain

Signals pass from the eyes along the optic nerves to the optic chiasma and then to the visual cortices in the brain. There is some crossover of nerve fibers at the optic chiasma, so both sides of the brain receive signals from both eyes.

Visual region of the brain

Combined 3-D image

Image received by the right eye

Image received by the left eye

## Stereoscopic vision

The two eyes receive slightly different views of all but the most distant objects; information from the two images is compared and processed in the brain to give a single 3-D interpretation of the object.

## IMAGE RECEPTION

The light rays from an object stimulate a group of receptors in the retina within an area that has the same shape as the object but is upside down. The brain automatically interprets the image the right way up.

Lens

Object

Cornea

Image on retina

## EYEBALL MOVEMENTS

To maintain the image of any moving object on the center of the retina, precise eyeball movements, achieved by the six muscles shown below, are necessary. The muscles act to swivel the eyeball in the directions indicated (the right eye is shown). The muscles always act in groups.

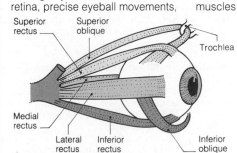

Superior rectus
Superior oblique
Trochlea
Medial rectus
Lateral rectus
Inferior rectus
Inferior oblique

**Inferior oblique**
Upward, outward, and anticlockwise rotation

**Lateral rectus**
Outward

**Superior oblique**
Downward, outward, and clockwise rotation

**Superior rectus**
Upward, inward, and clockwise rotation

**Medial rectus**
Inward

**Inferior rectus**
Downward, inward, and anticlockwise rotation

V

which are proportionately more concentrated at the periphery of the retina, are highly sensitive to light but not to color. The color-sensitive cones are concentrated more at the center of the retina (see *Color vision*).

Accurate alignment of the two eyes is achieved by coordination of the motor nerve impulses to the six tiny muscles that move each eye. This coordination is achieved in the brain, which correlates information from several sources, taking into account the brain's perception of the images, the position of the head, the position of the eyes relative to the head, and the position of the two eyes relative to each other.

Accurate alignment of the two eyes allows the brain to fuse the images from each eye, but because each eye has a slightly different view of a given object, the brain can interpret solidity or depth. This stereoscopic vision is important in judging distance.

## Vision, disorders of

The most common visual disorders are due to simple errors of *refraction*, such as *myopia*, *hyperopia*, and *astigmatism*. The blurring of vision from refractive errors can almost always be corrected by *glasses*. Defects of vision that cannot be eliminated in this way may have any of a wide variety of causes, including loss of binocular fusion (which can cause *double vision* or *amblyopia*), disorders of the eye or optic nerve, disorders of the nerve pathways that connect the optic nerves to the brain, and disorders of the brain itself.

### VISUAL DEFECT FROM EYE AND OPTIC NERVE DISORDERS

Eye or optic nerve disease often affects vision only on the side involved; it can affect one or both sides, often to different degrees. Any interference with the transparency of the eye affects vision. Loss of transparency may result from corneal opacities (opaqueness of the cornea) following infection, ulceration, or injury; from *cataract* (opacification of the crystalline lens); or from *vitreous hemorrhage* (bleeding into the gel of the eye behind the lens).

Defects near the center of the retina cause loss of the corresponding parts of the *visual field* of the affected eye. This is especially serious if the central part of the retina (where sharp *visual acuity* exists) is involved (see *Macular degeneration*). Peripheral retinal damage, which occurs in the early stages of chronic simple *glaucoma* or *retinitis pigmentosa*, may not cause noticeable visual disturbance if sharp central vision is unaffected.

*Floaters* (freely moving shadows perceived in the field of vision) are usually of no significance, but necessitate an eye examination. Floaters may signify a retinal tear or a hemorrhage. Floaters may herald a *retinal detachment*, especially if accompanied by bright flashing lights at the periphery of the field of vision.

A defect in the optic nerve in front of the optic nerve crossing causes visual disturbance in one eye only. It often takes the form of a central *scotoma* (a blind spot in the center of the field of vision). This condition can be due to *optic neuritis*, which is sometimes a sign of *multiple sclerosis*.

### VISUAL DEFECT FROM NERVE PATHWAY DISORDER

Disorders of one of the nerve pathways behind the optic nerve crossing always affect both eyes. This is because half of the fibers from each optic nerve—those from the inner half of each retina—cross over before they run back to the back of the brain. Each pathway thus has contributions from both eyes and any interruption thus causes loss of part of the visual field of each eye.

### VISUAL DEFECT FROM BRAIN DISORDER

Severe damage to one side of the visual area of the brain, such as from loss of blood supply (stroke), causes loss of the inner half of the field of vision of the eye on the same side and of the outer half of the field of the other eye. This is called *hemianopia*, in which the sufferer has only half of the field of vision.

Visual disturbance may also arise from involvement of the areas of the brain concerned with the psychological and associational aspects of vision. Disorders of these functions may cause visual *agnosia* (failure to recognize objects), visual perseveration (in which a scene continues to be perceived after the direction of gaze has shifted), and visual hallucinations.

## Vision, loss of

An inability to see, which may develop slowly or suddenly. Vision loss may affect one or both eyes. It can cause complete blindness, or may affect only peripheral vision or only central vision. Loss of vision may be temporary or permanent, depending on the cause.

### SLOW VISION LOSS

A progressive loss of visual clarity is common with advancing age as a result of loss of transparency of the crystalline lenses of the eyes (see *Cataract*). Other common causes of gradual loss of vision are *macular degeneration*, *diabetes mellitus*, and *glaucoma*. Gradual visual loss may also be due to progressive opacity of the cornea from *keratopathy* (disease of the cornea) of any kind, or to progressive distortion from *keratoconus* (a conical deformity of the cornea). *Retinitis pigmentosa* causes a variable degree of visual loss in both eyes.

### SUDDEN VISION LOSS

Sudden loss of vision may be caused by optical or neurological disorders. *Hyphema* (bleeding into the aqueous humor) usually results from injury; the blood can block the normal passage of the light to the retina. Severe *uveitis* (inflammation of the uvea) may cause serious reduction in vision. *Vitreous hemorrhage* (bleeding into the gel of the eye) and retinal disorders, such as *retinal detachment* and *retinal hemorrhage*, may also reduce vision suddenly.

*Optic neuritis* (inflammation of the optic nerve) can severely reduce vision in one eye. Any damage to the nerve connections between the eyes and the brain, or to the visual area of the brain itself, can cause loss of peripheral vision. Damage to the visual nerve pathways may sometimes be a result of *ischemia* (inadequate blood supply), tumor, injury, or inflammation.

## Vision tests

The part of an *eye examination* that determines if there is any reduction in the ability to see. Most vision tests are tests of *visual acuity* (sharpness of central vision). *Visual field* (side vision) tests may also be performed to assess disorders of the eye and the nervous system. Refraction tests are done to discover whether the patient has a refractive error (that is, an error that can be corrected with glasses), such as *hyperopia*, *myopia*, or *astigmatism*. Refraction tests also show whether there is a deficiency in the power of *accommodation* (see *Presbyopia*).

### VISUAL ACUITY TESTS

Visual acuity is tested, one eye at a time, using *Snellen's chart*. An attempt is made to read letters of standard sizes from a standard distance, classically 20 feet (6 meters).

### REFRACTION TESTS

These tests may be done in several ways. In one technique (retinoscopy) a narrow beam of light is projected into the eye, from a distance of about

V

## TYPES OF VISION TESTS

These tests are performed to measure a number of variables—the acuity of a patient's distance vision and the power of the lenses he or she may need (visual acuity and refraction tests), the extent of peripheral vision (visual field tests), and the ability to focus on objects close up (accommodation tests).

### VISUAL ACUITY TESTS

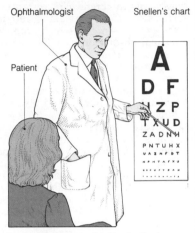

These tests use the familiar Snellen's chart. Visual acuity is measured according to how far down the chart the patient can read accurately.

### ACCOMMODATION TESTS

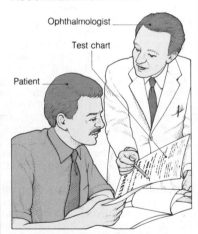

After any distance-focusing ability has been corrected, the ability to read small print close up is measured to test the patient's accommodation.

### REFRACTION TESTS

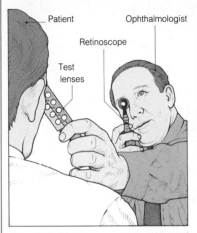

The effect of lenses on movements of light reflected from the eye (as the light source is moved) is observed to help calculate the corrective glasses needed.

### VISUAL FIELD TESTS

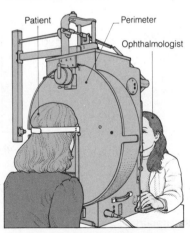

One eye is fixed straight ahead, the other covered, and lights are shined onto a white bowl or screen in front of the patient to find the field of vision of each eye.

### ACCOMMODATION TESTS

The power of accommodation (ability to focus on near objects) may be measured by correcting any refractive error with *glasses*, and then determining the nearest distance at which very small print can be read. Most people at age 45, unless nearsighted, need some assistance (e.g., glasses) with accommodation to read small print up close.

### VISUAL FIELD TESTS

Visual field tests can indicate disorders of the peripheral parts of the retinas, of the optic nerves, or of the optical pathways that convey nerve impulses from the eyes to the back of the brain. Most visual field tests involve the use of large black screens or white hollow bowls. The patient's head is secured, one eye is covered, and the other is directed to a point at the center of the inside of the bowl. Small spots of light are projected onto the inner surface of the bowl; the spots appear for brief periods in various places or are moved inward from the periphery. The person being tested responds when he or she sees the spot.

## Visual acuity

Sharpness of vision. Visual acuity is not concerned with the extent or clarity of the peripheral vision but with sharpness (discrimination) of central vision (see *Visual field*). A person's visual acuity is measured during a *vision test*.

Refractive errors (errors that can be corrected with glasses) are the most common cause of poor visual acuity. They include *myopia, hyperopia*, and *astigmatism*. Poor visual acuity for near objects occurs in *presbyopia*.

## Visual field

The total area in which visual perception is possible while looking straight ahead. The visual fields normally extend outward over an angle of about 90 degrees on either side of the midline of the face, but are more restricted above and below, especially if the eyes are deep-set or the eyebrows are prominent. The visual fields of the two eyes overlap to a large extent so that a defect in the field of one eye may be concealed if both eyes are open (see box, overleaf).

The level of *visual acuity* (sharpness of vision) in the visual field is much lower in areas remote from the point at which one is looking directly. For instance, it is impossible to read fine print as little as 5 degrees to one side of the fixation point. This is especially

**V**

26 inches (65 cm), by an instrument that allows the tester to observe the light reflected back through the pupil from the retina. Small movements of the light are made in various directions. The appropriate correction can be determined from the power and type of lenses needed to neutralize the movement of the light. Refinements of the refraction (correction with glasses) can be achieved by determining the person's subjective response to changes made in his or her vision by slight changes in the lenses.

## THE VISUAL FIELDS

The field of vision of each eye (with the head and eyes immobile) extends through an angle of about 130 degrees and is divided into an area that overlaps with the visual field of the other eye (binocular vision) and an area that can be seen with only the one eye.

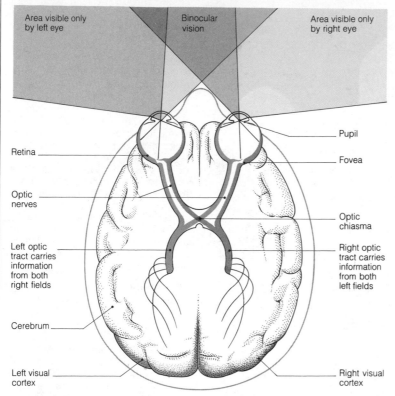

Area visible only by left eye

Binocular vision

Area visible only by right eye

Pupil

Retina

Fovea

Optic nerves

Optic chiasma

Left optic tract carries information from both right fields

Right optic tract carries information from both left fields

Cerebrum

Left visual cortex

Right visual cortex

**Route of visual signals**
Note that all light from the fields left of center of both eyes (gray) falls on the right sides of the two retinas; and information about these fields goes to the right visual cortex. Information about the right fields of vision (pink) goes to the left cortex. Data about the area of binocular vision go to both cortices.

apparent to people with *macular degeneration*, who have no central vision and must use other parts of the visual field.

Partial loss of visual field is less obvious than loss of central vision; even people with extensive visual field loss, as from *glaucoma* or *stroke*, may be unaware of it if they retain sharp central visual acuity. (See also *Vision, disorders of*; *Vision tests*.)

### Vital sign

An indication that a person is still alive. Vital signs include chest movements caused by breathing, the presence of a pulse (which indicates that the heart is beating) at the neck or wrist, and the constriction of the pupil of the eye when it is exposed to a bright light. A physician certifies *death* on the basis of the absence of all these signs. Additional tests, such as measurement of brain activity, may also be required in certain circumstances, notably if the patient is on a life-support system.

### Vitamin

Any of a group of complex chemicals that are essential for the normal functioning of the body. With few exceptions (notably vitamin D), the body cannot manufacture these substances itself, making it necessary to obtain them from the diet. There are 13 major vitamins—A, C, D, E, K, $B_{12}$, and the seven B-complex vitamins. Most are required only in extremely small amounts, and each vitamin is present in many different foods. Vitamin D is also produced in the skin when it is exposed to sunlight.

A balanced diet that includes a variety of different types of foods is likely to contain adequate amounts of all the vitamins, and supplements are not usually necessary. However, a physician may recommend *vitamin supplements* in certain circumstances, such as for a person taking certain *lipid-lowering drugs* (which reduce intestinal absorption of vitamins) or for some women who are pregnant or breast-feeding.

**TYPES**
Vitamins can be categorized into fat-soluble vitamins and water-soluble vitamins.

**FAT-SOLUBLE VITAMINS** The fat-soluble vitamins (A, D, E, and K) are absorbed with fats from the intestine into the blood and then stored in fatty tissue (mainly the liver). They are not normally excreted in the urine.

Body reserves of some of these vitamins may last for several years and a daily intake is thus not usually essential; in fact, an excessive intake of a fat-soluble vitamin may cause harmful levels to accumulate in the body. For most people, a balanced diet ensures a sufficient supply.

Deficiency of a fat-soluble vitamin is usually due to a disorder in which intestinal absorption of fats is impaired (see *Malabsorption*) or to a prolonged poor or restricted diet.

**WATER-SOLUBLE VITAMINS** The water-soluble vitamins are C, $B_{12}$, and the members of the B complex. Most of these vitamins are stored in the body for only a short period and are rapidly excreted in the urine if taken in greater amounts than the body requires. Vitamin $B_{12}$ is an exception, in that it is stored in the liver. It may take five or six years for deficiency symptoms to appear.

Deficiencies of the water-soluble vitamins are more likely to occur than fat-soluble vitamin deficiencies. Foods that contain water-soluble vitamins should therefore be eaten daily; moreover, prolonged cooking, preserving, and processing tend to destroy these vitamins, so fresh or lightly cooked foods are the best sources. Plain, frozen fruits and vegetables can also be a good source of water-soluble vitamins. Taking very large amounts of water-soluble vitamins does not usually cause toxic effects; adverse reactions to very large doses of vitamin C and vitamin $B_6$ (pyridoxine) have been reported.

V

## FUNCTION

The role of vitamins in the body is not fully understood; most knowledge about them is based on evidence provided by symptoms that occur as a result of deficiency. Most vitamins have been found to have several important actions on one or more body systems or functions; many are involved in the activities of *enzymes* (substances that promote chemical reactions in the body). See also articles on individual vitamins.

# Vitamin A

A *vitamin* essential for normal growth and for the formation of strong bones and teeth in children, for normal vision and cell structure, for protecting the linings of the respiratory, digestive, and urinary tracts against infection, and for healthy skin.

Many foods contain vitamin A. Particularly rich sources of this vitamin include liver, fish-liver oils, egg yolk, milk and other dairy products, margarine, and various vegetables and fruits, such as carrots, winter squashes, kale, broccoli, spinach, apricots, and peaches.

## DEFICIENCY

Vitamin A deficiency is rare in developed countries. In most cases, it is due to failure of the intestine to absorb enough of the vitamin, which may occur as a result of *cystic fibrosis*, *bile duct obstruction*, or long-term treatment with certain *lipid-lowering drugs*. Dietary deficiency occurs only in people who have an exceptionally poor diet; it is most common in some developing countries.

The effects of vitamin A deficiency include poor night vision; dry, inflamed eyes; dry, rough skin; loss of appetite; diarrhea; and lowered resistance to infection. Severe deficiency may cause weak bones and teeth, corneal ulcers, and, in extreme cases, *keratomalacia* (an eye disorder in which there is severe corneal damage that can lead to blindness if untreated).

## EXCESS

Prolonged, excessive intake of vitamin A can result in a condition called hypervitaminosis A, the symptoms of which include headache, tiredness, nausea, loss of appetite, diarrhea, dry and itchy skin, hair loss, and, in women, irregular menstruation. In extreme cases, there may also be bone pain and enlargement of the liver and spleen. Excessive intake during pregnancy may cause birth defects.

Contrary to popular belief, excessive intake of carotene (e.g., through eating huge amounts of carrots) does not cause hypervitaminosis A, but produces carotenemia (high blood levels of carotene), the most noticeable feature of which is a deep yellow coloration of the skin.

## RETINOIDS

Synthetic, vitamin A-like compounds called retinoids have been reported to reverse some of the skin wrinkling, roughness, and mottled pigmentation caused by chronic sun exposure.

Clinical testing of retinoids, which are applied directly to the skin, was begun in 1987.

# Vitamin B

See *Vitamin B₁₂*; *Vitamin B complex*.

## VITAMINS AND THEIR SOURCES IN THE DIET

| Fat-soluble | Good sources |
| --- | --- |
| Vitamin A | Liver, fish-liver oils, egg yolk, milk and dairy products, margarine, various fruits and vegetables (such as carrots and apricots) |
| Vitamin D | Fortified milk, oily fish (such as sardines, herring, salmon, and tuna), liver, dairy products, egg yolk |
| Vitamin E | Vegetable oils (such as corn, soy bean, olive, and sunflower oils), nuts, meat, green leafy vegetables, cereals, wheat germ, egg yolk |
| Vitamin K | Green leafy vegetables (especially cabbage, broccoli, and turnip greens), vegetable oils, egg yolk, cheese, pork, liver |
| **Water-soluble** | |
| Thiamine (vitamin B₁) | Wheat germ, bran, whole-grain or enriched cereals and breads, brown rice, pasta, liver, kidney, pork, fish, beans, nuts |
| Riboflavin (vitamin B₂) | Liver, milk, cheese, eggs, green leafy vegetables, whole grains, enriched breads and cereals, brewer's yeast |
| Niacin (nicotinic acid) | Liver, lean meat, poultry, fish, whole grains, enriched breads and cereals, peanuts, dried beans |
| Pantothenic acid | Liver, heart, kidney, fish, egg yolk, skimmed milk, brewer's yeast, wheat germ, most vegetables |
| Pyridoxine (vitamin B₆) | Liver, chicken, pork, fish, whole grains, wheat germ, bananas, potatoes, dried beans, peanuts |
| Biotin | Liver, kidney, peanuts, dried beans, egg yolk, mushrooms, cauliflower, bananas, grapefruit, watermelons |
| Folic acid | Green leafy vegetables (such as spinach and broccoli), mushrooms, liver, nuts, dried beans, peas, egg yolk, whole-wheat bread |
| Vitamin B₁₂ (cyanocobalamin) | Liver, kidney, chicken, beef, pork, fish, eggs, cheese, butter, yogurt, other dairy products |
| Vitamin C | Citrus fruits, tomatoes, potatoes, green leafy vegetables, green peppers, strawberries, cantaloupe |

**Vitamin needs**
A varied diet usually provides all vitamin needs. For vegans (who eat no animal products), vitamins B₁₂ and D may be lacking; these vitamins can be obtained from supplements or, in the case of vitamin D, through adequate exposure to sunlight.

V

# Vitamin B$_{12}$

Also known as cyanocobalamin, a *vitamin* that plays a vital role in the activities of several *enzymes* (substances that promote chemical reactions in the body). Vitamin B$_{12}$ is important in the production of the genetic material of cells (and thus in growth and development), in the production of red blood cells in bone marrow, in the utilization of folic acid (a constituent of the *vitamin B complex*) and carbohydrates in the diet, and in the functioning of the nervous system.

Foods rich in vitamin B$_{12}$ include liver, kidney, chicken, beef, pork, fish, eggs, and dairy products.

### DEFICIENCY AND EXCESS

A balanced diet contains sufficient amounts of vitamin B$_{12}$ for the body's needs. Deficiency of vitamin B$_{12}$ is almost always due to an inability of the intestine to absorb the vitamin, most commonly as a result of pernicious anemia (see *Anemia, megaloblastic*). In rare cases, deficiency of vitamin B$_{12}$ may result from following a vegan diet (one that excludes all kinds of animal products).

The principal effects of vitamin B$_{12}$ deficiency are megaloblastic anemia, a sore mouth and tongue, and symptoms caused by damage to the spinal cord, such as numbness and tingling in the limbs. There may also be depression and loss of memory.

No harmful effects are known to occur as a result of a high intake of vitamin B$_{12}$.

# Vitamin B complex

A group of *vitamins* that consists of thiamine (also known as vitamin B$_1$), riboflavin (vitamin B$_2$), niacin (nicotinic acid), pantothenic acid, pyridoxine (vitamin B$_6$), biotin, and folic acid. *Vitamin B$_{12}$* is not usually included in this group.

### THIAMINE

This vitamin plays a vital role in the activities of various *enzymes* (substances that promote chemical reactions in the body) involved in the breakdown and utilization of carbohydrates and in the functioning of the nerves, muscles, and heart.

Thiamine is present in most unrefined foods. Particularly good sources of thiamine include wheat germ, bran, whole-grain or enriched cereals and breads, brown rice, pasta, liver, kidney, pork, fish, beans, nuts, and eggs.

A balanced diet usually provides adequate amounts of thiamine. Those

susceptible to deficiency include elderly people on a poor diet, people with very high energy requirements (such as manual workers or people involved in high-level endurance activities), or those suffering from *hyperthyroidism* (overactivity of the thyroid gland), those with *malabsorption* disorders, and those with severe *alcohol dependence*. Deficiency may also occur as a result of severe illness, surgery, or serious injury.

Mild thiamine deficiency may cause tiredness, irritability, loss of appetite, and sleep disturbances. Severe deficiency may produce *beriberi*, abdominal pain, constipation, depression, memory impairment, and, in people who are severely dependent on alcohol, *Wernicke-Korsakoff syndrome*.

Excessive intake of thiamine is not known to cause harmful effects.

### RIBOFLAVIN

Riboflavin is essential for the activities of various enzymes involved in the breakdown and utilization of carbohydrates, fats, and proteins, the production of energy in cells, the utilization of other B vitamins, and the production of hormones by the adrenal glands.

Riboflavin is found in a wide range of foods. Particularly good sources of riboflavin are liver, milk, cheese, eggs, green leafy vegetables, whole grains, enriched breads and cereals, and brewer's yeast.

A balanced diet usually provides adequate amounts of riboflavin. People susceptible to deficiency include people taking phenothiazine *antipsychotic drugs*, tricyclic *antidepressant drugs*, or estrogen-containing *oral contraceptives*; those with *malabsorption* disorders; or those with severe *alcohol dependence*. Deficiency may also occur as a result of serious illness, surgery, or severe injury.

Prolonged deficiency of riboflavin may cause chapped lips, soreness of the tongue and corners of the mouth, and certain eye disorders, such as nutritional *amblyopia* (poor visual acuity) and *photophobia* (abnormal sensitivity to light).

Excessive dietary intake of riboflavin is not known to produce any harmful effects.

### NIACIN

This vitamin plays an essential role in the activities of various enzymes involved in the metabolism of carbohydrates and fats, the functioning of the nervous and digestive systems, the manufacture of sex hormones, and the maintenance of healthy skin.

The principal dietary sources of niacin include liver, lean meat, poultry, fish, whole grains, nuts, and dried beans.

A balanced diet usually provides adequate amounts of niacin. Most cases of deficiency are due to *malabsorption* disorders or to severe *alcohol dependence*. Prolonged niacin deficiency causes *pellagra*, the principal symptoms of which include soreness and cracking of the skin, inflammation of the mouth and tongue, and mental disturbances.

Excessive intake of niacin is not known to cause harmful effects.

### PANTOTHENIC ACID

Pantothenic acid is essential for the activities of various enzymes involved in the metabolism of carbohydrates and fats, the manufacture of corticosteroids and sex hormones, the utilization of other vitamins, the functioning of the nervous system and adrenal glands, and normal growth and development.

Pantothenic acid is present in almost all vegetables, cereals, and animal foods. Particularly rich sources of this vitamin include liver, heart, kidney, fish, egg yolks, brewer's yeast, and wheat germ.

A balanced diet generally provides adequate amounts of this vitamin. Deficiency usually occurs as a result of *malabsorption* disorders or severe *alcohol dependence*. Deficiency may also sometimes occur as a result of severe illness, surgery, or serious injury. The principal effects of deficiency include fatigue, headaches, nausea, abdominal pain, numbness and tingling, muscle cramps, and susceptibility to respiratory infections. In severe cases, a *peptic ulcer* may also result.

Excessive intake of pantothenic acid is not known to have harmful effects.

### PYRIDOXINE

This vitamin plays a vital role in the activities of various enzymes and hormones involved in the breakdown and utilization of carbohydrates, fats, and proteins, in the manufacture of red blood cells and antibodies, in the functioning of the digestive and nervous systems, and in the maintenance of healthy skin.

Good dietary sources of pyridoxine include liver, chicken, pork, fish, whole grains, wheat germ, bananas, potatoes, and dried beans.

A balanced diet contains adequate amounts of pyridoxine; it is also manufactured in small amounts by intestinal bacteria. Those susceptible to deficiency include some breast-fed

V

infants, elderly people on a poor diet, those with a *malabsorption* disorder, people with severe *alcohol dependence*, people being treated with certain drugs (including *penicillamine* and *hydralazine*), and women taking estrogen-containing *oral contraceptives*.

Deficiency of pyridoxine may cause weakness, irritability, depression, skin disorders, inflammation of the mouth and tongue, cracked lips, anemia, and, in infants, seizures.

Excessive intake—100 times or more above the normal daily intake—has been reported to cause *neuritis*.

### BIOTIN
Biotin is essential for the activities of various enzymes involved in the breakdown of fatty acids and carbohydrates and for the excretion of the waste products of protein breakdown.

Biotin is present in many foods. Particularly rich sources of this vitamin include liver, peanuts, dried beans, egg yolks, mushrooms, bananas, grapefruit, and watermelon.

A balanced diet provides enough biotin for the body's needs; biotin is also manufactured by intestinal bacteria. Deficiency may occur during long-term treatment with *antibiotic drugs* or *sulfonamide drugs*. Raw egg whites contain a substance that interferes with the intestinal absorption of biotin, and prolonged, high consumption has resulted in deficiency in several cases. The principal symptoms of biotin deficiency include weakness, tiredness, poor appetite, hair loss, depression, inflammation of the tongue, and eczema.

Excessive intake of biotin is not known to have harmful effects.

### FOLIC ACID
This vitamin plays a vital role in the activities of various enzymes involved in the manufacture of nucleic acids (the genetic material of cells) and therefore in growth and reproduction, in the production of red blood cells, and in the healthy functioning of the nervous system.

The principal dietary sources of folic acid include green, leafy vegetables, broccoli, spinach, mushrooms, liver, nuts, dried beans, peas, egg yolk, and whole-wheat bread.

A varied diet that includes fresh vegetables and fruit generally provides enough folic acid for the body's needs. Mild deficiency is relatively common, but can usually be corrected by increasing the daily consumption of foods containing folic acid. More severe deficiency may occur during pregnancy or breast-feeding, in pre-

mature or low birth weight infants, in people undergoing *dialysis*, with certain blood disorders, with *psoriasis*, with *malabsorption* disorders, with severe *alcohol dependence*, and in people taking certain drugs, including *anticonvulsant drugs*, antimalarial drugs, estrogen-containing *oral contraceptives*, and some *analgesic drugs* (painkillers), *corticosteroid drugs*, and *sulfonamide drugs*.

The principal effects of folic acid deficiency include anemia, sores around the mouth, a sore tongue, and, in children, poor growth.

Excessive intake of folic acid is not known to have harmful effects.

## Vitamin C
Also known by its chemical name, ascorbic acid, a vitamin that plays an essential role in the activities of various *enzymes* (substances that promote chemical reactions in the body). It is important for the growth and maintenance of healthy bones, teeth, gums, ligaments, and blood vessels; in the production of certain *neurotransmitters* (chemicals responsible for the transmission of nerve impulses between nerve cells) and of adrenal gland hormones; in the immune response to infection; in wound healing; and in the absorption of iron from the digestive tract.

The principal dietary sources of vitamin C are fresh fruits and vegetables. Citrus fruits, tomatoes, green leafy vegetables, potatoes, green peppers, strawberries, and cantaloupe are particularly rich sources.

### DEFICIENCY
A balanced diet usually provides enough vitamin C for the body's requirements. However, slight deficiency may occur as a result of a serious injury or burn, major surgery, use of *oral contraceptives*, fever, or continual inhalation of carbon monoxide (a constituent of tobacco smoke and traffic fumes). More pronounced deficiency is usually caused by a poor diet.

Mild deficiency may cause weakness, general aches and pains, swollen gums, and *nosebleeds*. Severe deficiency leads to *scurvy* and *anemia*.

### EXCESS
Large doses of vitamin C are taken by some people in the belief that they prevent colds, but there is no convincing evidence to support this. Excessive intake of vitamin C is not usually harmful unless the daily dose is more than about 1 gram, when it may cause nausea, stomach cramps, diarrhea, and, occasionally, kidney stones.

## Vitamin D
The collective term for a group of related substances—including calciferol (also known as ergocalciferol or vitamin $D_2$) and cholecalciferol (vitamin $D_3$)—that play several vital roles in the body. The vitamin helps regulate the balance of calcium and phosphate, aids the absorption of calcium from the intestine, and is essential for strong bones and teeth.

The richest dietary source of vitamin D is fortified milk. Other good sources include oily fish, such as sardines, herring, salmon, and tuna; liver; dairy products; and egg yolks. Vitamin D is also formed by the action of ultraviolet rays in sunlight on chemicals in the skin.

### DEFICIENCY
The body requires only small amounts of vitamin D, which are provided by a balanced diet and normal exposure to sunlight. Deficiency may occur in people on a poor diet or on a vegan diet (one that excludes animal products); in premature infants; in those deprived of sunlight, such as night workers; and in dark-skinned people, particularly those living in foggy urban areas, who do not absorb enough ultraviolet rays.

Deficiency also occurs in certain disorders, most commonly those in which intestinal absorption of the vitamin is impaired (see *Malabsorption*). Other causes include liver disorders, kidney disorders, and some genetic defects. Prolonged use of certain drugs, such as the *anticonvulsant drug* phenytoin, may also result in vitamin D deficiency.

Long-term deficiency of vitamin D leads to low blood levels of calcium and phosphate, which results in softening of the bones. This condition is known as *rickets* in children and as *osteomalacia* in adults.

### EXCESS
Excessive intake of vitamin D may cause weakness, abnormal thirst, increased urination, gastrointestinal disturbances, and depression. Over a long period, too much vitamin D disrupts the balance of calcium and phosphate in the body, which may lead to abnormal calcium deposits in the soft tissues, kidneys, and blood vessel walls, and sometimes retarded growth in children.

## Vitamin E
The collective term for a group of substances—of which alpha-tocopherol is the most important—that play several vital roles in the body.

V

Vitamin E is essential for normal cell structure, for maintaining the activities of certain enzymes, and for the formation of red blood cells. It also protects the lungs and other tissues from damage by pollutants and helps prevent red blood cells from being destroyed by poisons in the blood. In addition, vitamin E is believed to slow aging of cells.

The principal dietary sources of vitamin E are vegetable oils, nuts, meat, green leafy vegetables, cereals, wheat germ, and egg yolks.

### DEFICIENCY

A balanced diet provides adequate amounts of the vitamin. Deficiency usually occurs only in disorders that impair intestinal absorption (see *Malabsorption*), in certain liver disorders, and in premature infants.

Vitamin E deficiency leads to the destruction of red blood cells, which eventually results in *anemia*. In infants, deficiency causes irritability and edema (accumulation of fluid in body tissues).

### EXCESS

Prolonged, excessive intake of vitamin E may cause abdominal pain, nausea and vomiting, and diarrhea. It may also reduce intestinal absorption of vitamins A, D, and K, which, in severe cases, may produce symptoms of deficiency of these vitamins.

## Vitamin K

A *vitamin* that is essential for the formation in the liver of substances that promote blood clotting.

The principal dietary sources of vitamin K are green leafy vegetables (especially cabbage, broccoli, and turnip greens), vegetable oils, egg yolks, cheese, pork, and liver. Vitamin K is also manufactured by bacteria that normally live in the intestine.

### DEFICIENCY AND EXCESS

The combination of a balanced diet and the activity of intestinal bacteria usually provides enough vitamin K for the body's needs. Deficiency may develop as a result of prolonged treatment with antibiotics (which destroy intestinal bacteria), disorders in which intestinal absorption is impaired (see *Malabsorption*), certain liver disorders, and chronic diarrhea. Newborn infants lack the intestinal bacteria that produce vitamin K and are therefore given supplements to prevent deficiency.

Deficiency of vitamin K reduces the ability of the blood to clot. This may cause nosebleeds, seeping of blood from wounds, and bleeding from the gums, intestine, and urinary tract. In rare, very severe cases, brain hemorrhage may result.

Excessive intake of vitamin K has no known harmful effects.

## Vitamin supplements

A group of preparations containing one or more *vitamins*.

Most people who eat a balanced diet (see *Nutrition*) do not usually need vitamin supplements. Eating a variety of foods provides adequate amounts of all vitamins. Excessive amounts of some vitamins (especially A and D) may actually be harmful, and supplements should be taken only on the advice of a physician. Some multivitamin preparations contain up to five times the recommended daily intake of certain vitamins.

### MEDICAL USES

Vitamin supplements are used to treat diagnosed vitamin deficiency, to prevent vitamin deficiency in susceptible people, and to treat certain medical disorders.

In developed countries, deficiency most commonly occurs in people on a poor diet, such as those with severe *alcohol dependence* or *drug dependence*, those on a low income, and elderly people who do not eat properly. A vegan diet (one that excludes not only meat and fish, but also all other animal products, such as eggs and dairy foods) may sometimes result in vitamin deficiency. Deficiency may also result from *malabsorption* (a disorder in which intestinal absorption of nutrients is impaired), *liver disorders*, and *kidney disorders*.

Supplements are used to prevent deficiency during periods of increased requirements, such as pregnancy, breast-feeding, and infancy. They are also given to people who are taking certain drugs (such as *lipid-lowering drugs* and *sucralfate*) that may impair the absorption of vitamins, to those suffering from serious illness or injury, or to people who have had major surgery. People who are being fed intravenously or via a tube (see *Feeding, artificial*) are also likely to need vitamin supplements. In most cases, the vitamin dosage used to prevent deficiency is lower than that needed to treat a deficiency.

Certain vitamins are used to treat some conditions that are not specific deficiency disorders. Vitamin D, for example, is used in the treatment of *osteoporosis* and vitamin A derivatives (retinoids) are now prescribed for severe *acne*.

Although vitamin $B_6$ is given to treat *premenstrual syndrome* and it has been claimed that high doses of vitamin C help cure the common cold and that vitamin E improves well-being, such claims have not been clearly substantiated by medical evidence.

## Vitiligo

A common disorder of skin pigmentation in which patches of skin lose their color. Depigmented white patches are particularly obvious in dark-skinned people, occurring most commonly on the face, hands, armpits, and groin. Affected skin is particularly sensitive to sunlight.

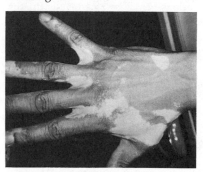

**Vitiligo affecting right hand**
Loss of pigment is the only skin change that occurs. The usual remedy is to mask the white patches with makeup.

Vitiligo is thought to be an *autoimmune disorder* that causes an absence of melanocytes, the specialized cells responsible for secreting the skin pigment *melanin*. The condition may occur at any age but usually develops in early adulthood. It affects about one in 200 people. Spontaneous repigmentation occurs in about 30 percent of cases.

### TREATMENT

Makeup may be used to disguise areas of vitiligo; in mild cases, no further treatment may be necessary. *Phototherapy* using *PUVA* induces significant repigmentation in more than 50 percent of cases, but many treatments are required. Creams containing *corticosteroid drugs* may also help. If areas of vitiligo are extensive, chemicals may be used to remove pigment from remaining areas of normal skin.

## Vitreous hemorrhage

Bleeding into the *vitreous humor*, the gellike substance that fills the main cavity of the eye between the crystalline lens and the retina. A common cause of vitreous hemorrhage is

V

diabetic *retinopathy*, in which new, fragile blood capillaries that bleed readily form on the retina.

Any bleeding into the vitreous humor is likely to affect vision; a major hemorrhage into the center of the gel causes very poor vision for as long as the blood remains. Blood released into the periphery of the vitreous humor may be absorbed and the transparency of the gel stored, but a large hemorrhage is likely to persist for weeks or months or may never clear.

## Vitreous humor

The transparent, gellike body that fills the large rear compartment of the eye between the crystalline *lens* and the *retina*. The vitreous humor consists almost entirely of water. Under certain conditions, it can exert sufficient pull on the retina to cause *retinal tears* and *retinal detachment*.

The vitreous humor tends to shrink with age; in most people over 65, it has separated from the retina, leaving a water-filled space. This separation is usually harmless but often causes numerous annoying *floaters* to be seen in the field of vision. The floaters usually disperse with time but at their onset should be evaluated by an ophthalmologist.

## Vivisection

Strictly, the performance of a surgical operation on a live animal, particularly for research purposes. However,

---

### LOCATION OF THE VITREOUS HUMOR

The vitreous humor occupies the large rear chamber of the eye, bounded by the back of the crystalline lens and the inner surface of the retina.

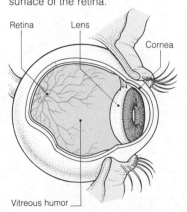

---

## LOCATION OF THE VOCAL CORDS

The vocal cords are located at the top of the larynx (voice box). Their top edges stretch between the thyroid cartilage at the front and the arytenoid cartilages at the back. If brought close together, the cords vibrate and emit sounds as air passes between them.

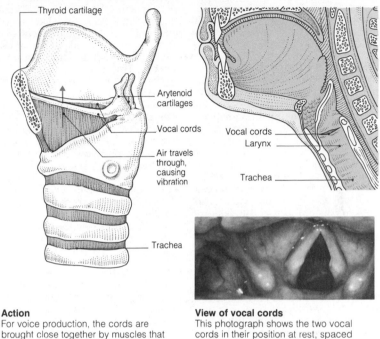

**Action**
For voice production, the cords are brought close together by muscles that act on the arytenoid cartilages.

**View of vocal cords**
This photograph shows the two vocal cords in their position at rest, spaced apart to give a V shape.

---

the term vivisection is often popularly used to refer to *animal experimentation* of any kind, even when surgery is not involved.

## Vocal cords

Two fibrous sheets of tissue in the *larynx* (voice box) that are responsible for voice production. The cords are attached at the front to the inner surface of the thyroid cartilage (Adam's apple) and at the rear to the arytenoid cartilages.

The so-called true vocal cords are the cords that vibrate and make sound; the false vocal cords are folds in the larynx that have nothing to do with sound production.

Most of the time the vocal cords lie apart, forming a V-shaped opening called the glottis through which air is breathed. Vocal sounds are produced when the cords tighten, close, and vibrate as air expelled from the lungs passes between them. Alterations in the tension of the cords produce sounds of different pitch, which are modified by the tongue, palate, and lips to produce *speech*. (For disorders that affect the vocal cords, see *Larynx, disorders of*.)

## Voice box

See *Larynx*.

## Voice, loss of

Partial loss of voice, also known as dysphonia, is fairly common and may be caused by any condition that interferes with the normal working of the vocal cords.

Temporary loss of voice frequently results from straining the muscles of the *larynx* (which control the vocal cords) through overuse of the voice. Temporary dysphonia also often results from inflammation of the vocal cords in *laryngitis*.

Persistent or recurrent dysphonia may be due to *polyps* (benign growths) on the vocal cords, thickening of the vocal cords due to *hypothyroidism*, or, less commonly, to interference with the nerve supply to the muscles of the larynx as a result of cancer of the larynx (see *Larynx, cancer of*), thyroid

V

gland (see *Thyroid cancer*), or esophagus (see *Esophagus, cancer of*). In rare cases, nerves or the vocal cords themselves may be accidentally damaged during surgery performed to treat thyroid cancer, resulting in permanent dysphonia.

Total loss of voice, known as *aphonia*, is rare and usually of psychological origin. (See also *Hoarseness; Larynx, disorders of*.)

## Volkmann's contracture

A disorder in which the wrist and fingers become permanently fixed in a bent position. It occurs as a result of ischemia (inadequate blood supply) in the forearm muscles that control them.

### CAUSES

Ischemia in the forearm muscles may be caused by damage to the brachial artery that results from a displaced fracture of the humerus (upper arm bone) or dislocation of the elbow. Ischemia may also follow any forearm injury that leads to *edema* (retention of fluid within tissues), with consequent swelling of tissues and compression of blood vessels.

### SYMPTOMS

Initially, the fingers become cold, numb, and white or blue. Finger movements are weak and painful, and no pulse can be felt at the wrist. Unless treatment is started within a few hours, the characteristic wrist and finger deformity develops.

### TREATMENT

Any displaced bones are first manipulated back into position, using a general anesthetic. If blood flow to the hand fails to improve, an operation is performed in which the tissues in the forearm are cut open to relieve pressure on the underlying muscles. Blockage of the artery may be relieved by injecting a *vasodilator drug* or

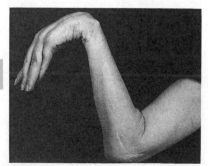

**Appearance of Volkmann's contracture**
The wrist is permanently bent due to formation of scar tissue and tautness affecting the forearm muscles.

by cutting open the artery and removing part of the lining. Occasionally, a section of damaged artery is cut out and replaced by a graft taken from a vein.

If there is permanent deformity, *physical therapy* may restore function to an acceptable level. In severe cases, surgery may be required to shorten the bones in the forearm, cut away damaged muscle, and transplant healthy muscle from another part of the forearm. This procedure is sometimes accompanied by *arthrodesis* (fusion) of the wrist joint.

## Volvulus

Twisting of a loop of intestine or, in rare cases, of the stomach. Volvulus is a serious condition that causes obstruction of the passage of intestinal contents (see *Intestine, obstruction of*) and a risk of *strangulation*. Symptoms of volvulus are severe *colic* followed by vomiting.

Volvulus may be present from birth or may be a result of *adhesions* (bands

of scar tissue). It is more common in Africa and Asia than in the US or Europe, possibly because of an association with an exceedingly high-fiber diet.

Surgical correction is usually necessary to treat the condition.

## Vomiting

Involuntary forcible expulsion of stomach contents through the mouth. Vomiting is usually preceded by nausea, pallor, sweating, excessive salivation, and a reduction in the heart rate.

### MECHANISM

Vomiting occurs when the vomiting center in the brain stem is activated. Activation of the vomiting center may occur as the result of information passing directly to it from the frontal lobes of the brain, the digestive tract, or the balancing mechanism in the inner ear when these mechanisms are either damaged or disturbed. The center may also be activated by the chemoreceptor trigger zone, also in

---

### THE VOMITING REFLEX

Many situations can provoke vomiting—including the presence of irritants in the stomach, high levels of certain substances in the blood, pressure within the skull, or disturbances of balance.

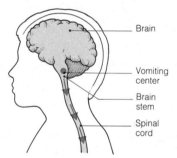

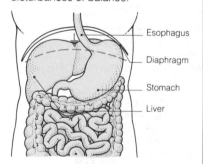

**1** In each case, a vomiting center in the brain stem is activated, causing nerve messages to pass toward the abdomen.

**2** The messages cause the diaphragm to press down on the stomach and the abdominal wall muscles to contract.

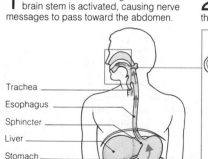

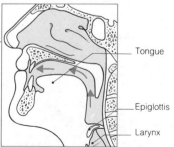

**3** The sphincter between the stomach and the esophagus relaxes and the stomach contents are propelled upward

via this sphincter toward the mouth. The epiglottis closes over the larynx to prevent vomit from entering the trachea.

V

**VOMITING** Forceful expulsion of stomach contents that usually has a simple explanation, such as irritation of the stomach by infection or overindulgence in food or alcohol. However, it may be a sign of a more serious disorder, particularly if there are accompanying symptoms. Vomiting may or may not be preceded by nausea.

Have you had severe abdominal pain that has not been relieved by the vomiting?

YES

☎ **EMERGENCY! GET MEDICAL HELP NOW!** A serious abdominal condition, such as appendicitis or a perforated duodenal ulcer, may cause such symptoms.

See • *Appendicitis*

NO

Have you vomited red blood, or black or dark brown matter that resembles coffee grounds?

YES

**Treatment for vomiting**
If you have been vomiting, provided you suspect no serious cause, try the following self-help measures:
• Eat no solid food until your nausea and vomiting subside.
• Drink plenty of clear (nonalcoholic) fluids in small sips even if you cannot keep anything down for long.
• Do not smoke.
• Do not take aspirin.

If you vomit repeatedly for more than 24 hours, or if more symptoms develop, consult your physician.

☎ **EMERGENCY! GET MEDICAL HELP NOW!** This could be caused by bleeding somewhere in the digestive tract.

NO

Do you have diarrhea OR is your temperature 100°F (38°C) or above?

YES

This may be caused by an infection of the digestive tract. If symptoms persist, consult your physician.

See • *Gastroenteritis*

NO

In the past few hours, have you done any of the following?
• overeaten
• eaten large amounts of rich, creamy, or spicy food
• consumed a large amount of alcohol

YES

Inflammation of the stomach lining often occurs as the result of overindulgence. Consult your physician if you have recurrent attacks.

See • *Gastritis*

NO

Have you eaten anything that may have gone bad or to which you may be allergic?

YES

Poisoning by food contaminated by bacteria or by poisonous chemicals or by food to which you are allergic may be responsible for the vomiting.

See • *Food poisoning*

NO

Continued on next page

V

Do you have a headache?

**YES** → Have you had a head injury within the past 24 hours?

**YES** → ☎ **EMERGENCY!**
**GET MEDICAL HELP NOW!**
You may have a brain injury.

**NO** ↓

Do you have one or more of the following symptoms?
- pain when you bend your head forward
- dislike of bright light
- drowsiness or confusion

**YES** → ☎ **EMERGENCY!**
**GET MEDICAL HELP NOW!**
These symptoms suggest the possibility of a serious brain disorder.

See • *Meningitis*
• *Subarachnoid hemorrhage*

**NO** ↓

Was your headache preceded by visual distortion, weakness of an extremity, and/or nausea AND is the headache one-sided (sometimes with blurred vision and nasal stuffiness)?

**YES** → The symptoms are probably due to a migraine attack. Consult your physician.

See • *Migraine*

**NO**

**NO** ↓

Do you have severe pain in or around one eye AND is your vision blurred?

**YES** → ☎
**Consult your physician without delay!**
These symptoms suggest the possibility of acute glaucoma, in which excess fluid causes increased pressure in the eye.

See • *Glaucoma*

**NO** ↓

Before you vomited, did everything around you seem to spin?

**YES** → Disorders of the inner ear cause vomiting and dizzy spells. Consult your physician.

See • *Labyrinthitis*
• *Meniere's disease*

**NO** ↓

**Vomiting and the Pill**
If you are taking the birth-control pill and suffer from an attack of vomiting, your protection against conception may be reduced. Continue to take your pills as usual, but use an extra form of contraception until you start a new packet of pills.

V

Continued on next page

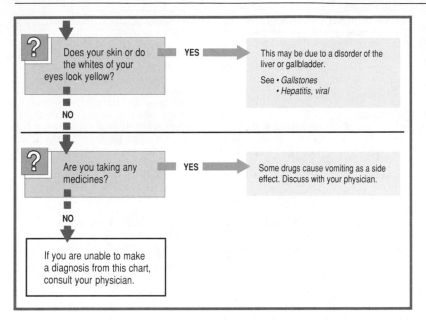

the brain stem, which is itself stimulated by the presence in the blood of poisons or other substances.

Once activated, the vomiting center sends messages to the diaphragm (the sheet of muscle separating the chest from the abdomen), which presses sharply downward on the stomach, and to the wall of the abdomen, which presses inward. Simultaneously, the pyloric sphincter between the base of the stomach and the intestine closes and the region between the top of the stomach and the esophagus relaxes. As a result, the stomach contents are expelled upward through the esophagus. As this happens, the larynx (voice box) is tightly closed by the epiglottis (the flap of cartilage at its entrance) to prevent vomit from entering the trachea (windpipe) and causing choking.

**CAUSES**

Vomiting commonly happens after overindulgence in food or alcohol. It is also a common adverse effect of many drugs and often follows general anesthesia (see *Anesthesia, general*).

Vomiting may also result from disorders of the stomach or intestine that result in inflammation, irritation, or distention of either organ. Such disorders include *peptic ulcer*, acute *appendicitis*, *gastroenteritis*, and *food poisoning*. Less commonly, vomiting is a symptom of intestinal obstruction due to *pyloric stenosis*, *intussusception*, or a tumor (see *Intestine, cancer of*).

Vomiting may also be caused by inflammation of organs associated with the digestive tract, such as the liver (see *Hepatitis*), pancreas (see *Pancreatitis*), and gallbladder (see *Cholecystitis*).

Another possible cause of vomiting is raised pressure within the skull, which may be due to *encephalitis, hydrocephalus*, a *brain tumor*, or a *head injury*. When the rise is rapid, it causes sudden, extremely forceful vomiting, often without any prior nausea. Vomiting is a common feature of *migraine* as well.

Vomiting is also a common feature of disorders affecting the balancing mechanism within the inner ear, such as *Meniere's disease* and acute *labyrinthitis*, or of disturbance of the mechanism by unusual movement, such as that experienced on a boat (see *Motion sickness*).

Disorders of the *endocrine system*, such as *Addison's disease*, may cause vomiting, as do disturbances of hormone production in early pregnancy (see *Vomiting in pregnancy*).

Vomiting is sometimes a symptom of a metabolic disorder, such as ketoacidosis (excessive production of ketones and acids), which may be due to poorly controlled *diabetes mellitus*.

Internal bleeding from the esophagus, stomach, or duodenum, or swallowing blood from a nosebleed, can also result in vomiting (see *Vomiting blood*).

Vomiting sometimes occurs as a reaction of disgust to a situation or food. It may also be a symptom of a psychological or emotional problem or be part of the psychiatric disorders *anorexia nervosa* or *bulimia*.

**INVESTIGATION AND TREATMENT**

Persistent vomiting requires investigation by a physician. Treatment depends on the underlying cause. Do not eat or drink or take any unnecessary medication during the active phase of vomiting. *Antiemetic drugs* may be prescribed.

## Vomiting blood

Known medically as hematemesis, vomiting blood is a symptom of bleeding from within the digestive tract. It usually occurs as a result of a serious disorder of the esophagus, stomach, or duodenum.

Vomiting blood may be caused by a tear at the lower end of the esophagus (see *Mallory-Weiss syndrome*), bleeding from *esophageal varices* (widened veins in the esophagus and upper stomach), severe erosive *gastritis* (inflammation of the stomach lining), *peptic ulcer*, or, in rare cases, a malignant stomach tumor (see *Stomach cancer*). Blood can also be vomited if it is swallowed from a nosebleed.

Vomited blood may be dark red, brown, black, or resemble coffee grounds (as a result of the action of stomach acid). Depending on the extent of internal bleeding and the quantity of stomach contents, the blood may either streak the vomit or constitute a major part of it. Vomiting blood is often accompanied by melena (black, tarry feces).

The underlying cause of vomiting blood is investigated by *endoscopy* (passing a viewing tube into the esophagus and stomach) or by *barium X-ray examinations*. If the loss of blood is severe, blood transfusion may be necessary and surgery may be required to stop the bleeding.

## Vomiting in pregnancy

Nausea and vomiting in early pregnancy are extremely common. It is experienced by about half of all pregnant women.

The vomiting usually starts before the sixth week of pregnancy and continues until about the 12th week; in some cases it occurs throughout pregnancy. The probable cause is activation of the vomiting center in the brain due to changed hormone levels during pregnancy.

The vomiting occurs most frequently in the morning, often after waking (hence its common name, morning sickness), but can occur at any time. It is sometimes precipitated by emotional stress, traveling, or food. Sufferers may find it helpful to eat small, regular meals.

In rare cases, the vomiting becomes severe and prolonged, a condition known as hyperemesis gravidarum. This can cause dehydration, nutritional deficiency, alteration in blood acidity, liver damage, and weight loss. Immediate hospital admission is required to replace lost fluids and chemicals by *intravenous infusion*, to rule out any serious underlying disorder, and to control the vomiting.

## Von Recklinghausen's disease
Another name for *neurofibromatosis*.

## Von Willebrand's disease
An inherited lifelong *bleeding disorder* with similarities to *hemophilia*.
### CAUSES AND INCIDENCE
Von Willebrand's disease is caused by a defective *gene* and is usually inherited in an autosomal dominant pattern (see *Genetic disorders*). A person needs to inherit only one copy of the defective gene to suffer from the disease. As many as one person in 1,000 is believed to have the gene but its effects are variable. Unlike hemophilia, the disease affects equal numbers of men and women.

The gene defect leads to a reduced concentration in the blood of a substance called von Willebrand factor. This factor plays a dual role in the arrest of bleeding. It helps platelets in the blood to plug injured blood vessel walls, and it forms part of the substance *factor VIII*, which is vital to blood coagulation. In the absence of von Willebrand factor, neither blood coagulation nor platelet plug formation can proceed normally, so there is a bleeding tendency.
### SYMPTOMS
The symptoms may include excessive bleeding from the gums and from cuts, nosebleeds, and, in women, *menorrhagia* (excessive menstrual bleeding). In the most severe forms, deep bleeding into joints and muscles may be a problem.
### DIAGNOSIS
The disease is diagnosed by *blood-clotting tests*, which show a long bleeding time, and by measurements that reveal reduced levels of von Willebrand factor in the blood.
### TREATMENT
There are various treatments available for the disease. One is to administer desmopressin (an *ADH*-like substance), which raises the body's natural production of von Willebrand

factor. Another treatment is to give cryoprecipitate (a preparation obtained from normal blood plasma), which is a rich source of von Willebrand factor. These treatments are generally successful in preventing bleeding episodes.

## Voyeurism
The repeated observation of unsuspecting people who are naked, in the act of undressing, or engaging in sexual activity. Commonly called Peeping Toms, voyeurs become sexually aroused through the act of looking and have no wish to engage in sexual activity. Voyeurs achieve orgasm (usually by masturbation) while watching or remembering the witnessed events. In its severe form, voyeurism is the only way in which orgasm is achieved.

## Vulva
The external, visible part of the female genitalia. The vulva comprises the *clitoris* and two pairs of skin folds called *labia*.

The most common symptom of a disorder affecting the vulva is itching, known medically as pruritus vulvae. Itching of the vulva often occurs with *vaginal itching*.

Various skin disorders, such as *dermatitis*, commonly affect the vulva and

---

**ANATOMY OF THE VULVA**
The outer skin folds (labia majora) are usually in contact. If parted, they reveal the clitoris and inner folds (labia minora), which enclose the urethral and vaginal openings.

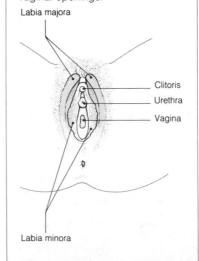

Labia majora

Clitoris
Urethra
Vagina

Labia minora

---

are usually easily relieved. More serious conditions include genital warts (see *Warts, genital*), *vulvitis*, *vulvovaginitis*, and cancer (see *Vulva, cancer of*).

## Vulva, cancer of
A rare disorder that most commonly affects postmenopausal women. It may be preceded by vulval itching but often no preliminary symptoms occur before the appearance of a lump or painful ulcer on the vulva.

Diagnosis is made by a biopsy (removal of a small sample of tissue for laboratory analysis).

Treatment of vulval cancer is by surgical removal of the affected area. The outlook depends on how soon the cancer is diagnosed and treated.

## Vulvitis
Inflammation of the *vulva* with a variety of different causes.

Infections causing vulvitis include *candidiasis*, genital herpes (see *Herpes, genital*), and warts (see *Warts, genital*). Infestations with *pubic lice* or *scabies* are other possible causes.

Vulvitis may occur as a result of changes in the vulval skin. These changes tend to affect women after the menopause, although there is no apparent cause. They may take the form of red or white patches and/or thickened or thinned areas that may be inflamed. Formerly called a variety of names, such as kraurosis vulvae and lichen sclerosus et atrophicus, the condition is now generally known as vulval dystrophy.

Other possible causes of vulvitis are allergic reactions to soap, cream, or detergent, excessive vaginal discharge, or urinary incontinence (see *Incontinence, urinary*).
### TREATMENT
Treatment depends on the cause; a combination of creams applied to the vulva along with good hygiene is the usual remedy. In some cases of vulval dystrophy, a *biopsy* (removal of a small sample of tissue for laboratory analysis) may be carried out to exclude the possibility of cancer. (See also *Vulvovaginitis*; *Vaginitis*.)

## Vulvovaginitis
Inflammation of the vulva and vagina. Vulvovaginitis is usually due to the infections *candidiasis* or *trichomoniasis*, which cause a profuse infected vaginal discharge that also affects the vulva.

Treatment of vulvovaginitis is with an *antifungal drug* or an *antibiotic drug*. (See also *Vaginitis*; *Vulvitis*.)

V

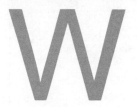

# Walking

Movement of the body in one direction by lifting the feet alternately and bringing one foot into contact with the ground before the other starts to leave it. The manner in which a person walks, known as gait, is determined by body shape, size, and posture; it often reflects the individual's personality. A normal pattern of walking is shown in the illustrated box below.

Walking is controlled by nerve signals from the motor cortex (part of the *cerebrum* of the brain) and by signals from the *basal ganglia* and the *cerebellum*, located at the back of the brain. The signals are sent via the spinal cord to nerve cells and from there are carried by nerve fibers to the muscles. In response to changes in position, the cerebellum also receives information from the muscles, joints, eyes, and the balance organ in the inner ear. This information is used to adjust new signals sent to the muscles by the brain centers to ensure balance and coordinated movement.

Some of the nerves that control walking are located in a very primitive part of the brain. This may account for the walking reflex that occurs in newborn babies in which the legs move automatically in a walking motion when the child is held upright (see *Reflex, primitive*). The age at which children walk varies enormously.

## DISORDERS

Abnormal gait may be caused by muscle weakness, by abnormalities of the skeleton, or by joint stiffness, causing immobility in the lower limbs or spinal column. Abnormal gait may also be the result of neurological disorders that affect the central control of locomotion and the balance and input of information to the nervous system from muscles and joints.

The different causes affect walking in a variety of ways; the physician can often gain clues to the underlying cause of a disorder by observing the way in which a person walks.

**MUSCULAR CAUSES** Any condition that causes wasting or loss of any of the muscles connected to the legs or feet may cause abnormal walking. In *muscular dystrophy*, the legs are held wide apart and the person waddles because of weakness of the buttock muscles. In *poliomyelitis* or after severe muscle injury, weakness of individual groups of muscles may cause limping because of unbalanced muscle action.

**SKELETAL CAUSES** Congenital deformities of the foot, such as *talipes* (clubfoot), may prevent normal walking. In talipes equinovarus, for example, the heel cannot be brought to the ground and a characteristic limping gait results. Congenital dislocation of the hip (see *Hip, congenital dislocation of*) that has not been detected in infancy may be noticed only when the child starts to walk—the foot on the affected side is placed flat on the ground while the opposite knee is flexed. *Scoliosis* (deformity of the spine) can also result in abnormal gait.

During a stage in their growth, *knock-knee* or *bowleg* often develops in children. These conditions may produce a strange walk, but both disappear within several years.

*Synovitis* of the hip is a common cause of limping in children, most often boys aged 2 to 12 years. The limp, which is accompanied by pain of varying severity, starts suddenly and lasts for only a few days or weeks. Another common cause of limping in boys, usually between the ages of 5 and 10, is *Perthes' disease*. The limp may or may not be painful. A painful

---

## THE MECHANICS OF WALKING

Many different muscles take part in the walking process. They contract in a complex, rhythmic sequence in response to programs of signals sent from the motor cortex in the brain. Feedback of information from the muscles and joints to the brain helps to ensure that the gait is smooth, steady, and coordinated.

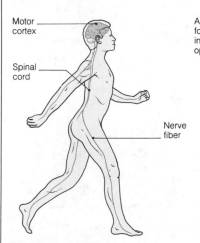

Motor cortex

Spinal cord

Nerve fiber

**Route of the signals**
The signals for walking originate in the motor cortex and are carried via the spinal cord and nerve fibers to muscles.

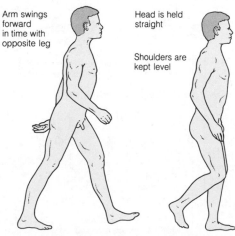

Arm swings forward in time with opposite leg

**1** As the left foot contacts the ground, the right arm swings forward and the right foot shifts onto tiptoe.

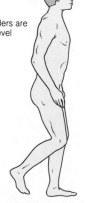

Head is held straight

Shoulders are kept level

**2** Once the left foot is fully planted on the ground and supporting the body, the right foot is raised.

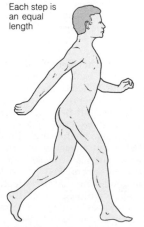

Each step is an equal length

**3** A sequence of muscle contractions advances the right leg, and the left arm swings forward.

limp may develop in young adolescents as a result of a slipped epiphysis (see *Femoral epiphysis, slipped*).

Other causes of limp include a painful *bone tumor* and *arthritis*.

Bone shortening may follow fracture or disease of one of the long bones of the leg; this condition always causes an abnormal gait, usually with a dip of the body to the shortened side.

NEUROLOGICAL CAUSES Among the most common of the neurological causes is *stroke*, which frequently results in *hemiplegia* (paralysis or weakness of one side of the body). Because the affected leg is held stiffly extended, it must be swung outward and forward in walking. When both legs are affected by weakness (a condition known as paraparesis), they are held extended and pressed together at the thighs so that only short steps are possible and the toes scrape along the ground. In some people with paraparesis, the legs cross with each step, which produces a characteristic scissors movement.

In *parkinsonism* there is difficulty starting to walk; the body is bent forward at the waist and hips, with bending at the knees and ankles. The steps are short and shuffling with the feet barely clearing the ground. As progress continues, the steps become more and more rapid, and the person may eventually fall unless assisted.

Other disorders, including severe peripheral *neuritis*, *multiple sclerosis*, tertiary *syphilis*, and various forms of *myelitis*, may damage the sensory nerves or the spinal cord. The damage causes loss of information to the brain about the position of the joints, resulting in an easily recognized gait. The body is bent forward and the eyes are fixed on the ground, the legs are held wide apart, and the feet are carried much higher than normal and thrown forward with sudden movements. People affected in this way are critically dependent on vision for walking; the gait becomes even worse if vision is defective.

Disease of the cerebellum or of the balancing mechanisms in the inner ears, such as *Meniere's disease*, may cause severe loss of balance and instability so that the affected person walks cautiously, with the legs apart, sometimes lurching to one side as though intoxicated (see *Ataxia*). In *chorea*, the gait may be bizarre and dancelike, with sudden thrusting movements of the hips and twisting of the trunk and limbs. The steps are irregular and of varying length.

W

## WALKING AIDS
Various types of walking aids are available for different forms and degrees of disability. The choice depends on factors such as whether the person is usually healthy or chronically disabled and whether the disability affects one or both of the person's legs.

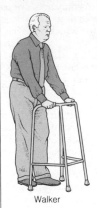 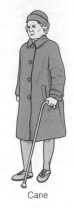 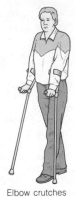 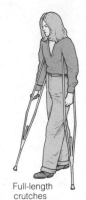

Walker          Cane          Elbow crutches          Full-length crutches

**Walkers and canes**
Walkers are useful for people affected by weakness on both sides, canes for those who have one-sided weakness or pain.

**Elbow and full-length crutches**
Elbow crutches are often useful for people recovering from strokes, full-length crutches for those with leg injuries.

## HOW TO USE CRUTCHES
Crutches are suitable only for people who are able to support their weight on at least one leg. There are various ways of using crutches, as shown in the illustrations below.

### FOUR-POINT WALKING

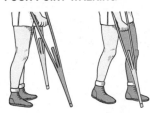 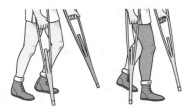

The feet and crutch tips are well separated, and one point is moved at a time. There are two possible sequences— right crutch, left foot, left crutch, right foot (above) or right then left crutch, right then left foot.

### THREE-POINT WALKING

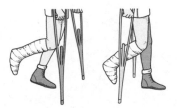

The crutches are advanced together while the person balances on one or both feet; the weight is then borne by the crutches while the feet are moved.

### TWO-POINT WALKING

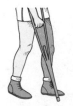 

In two-point walking with crutches, the person moves the left foot and right crutch forward together, followed by the left foot and right crutch.

## Walking aids

Equipment for increasing the mobility of people who have a disorder that affects *walking*. Support from a walking aid may be required by people with *arthritis* or other diseases affecting mobility, by those recovering from an injury (such as a *fracture* or *sprain*), or by those who are waiting to be fitted with a prosthesis after an amputation.

### WALKERS

Walkers provide a very stable form of support and may be useful for people with severe balancing problems or for those who are affected by weakness, pain, or stiffness on both sides. However, walkers tend to get in the way of the feet, allowing only slow progress.

Walkers are usually made of a light, strong alloy and have rubber-tipped legs to prevent sliding. They can be supplied with wheels on the front legs to make maneuvering easier.

### CRUTCHES

Crutches provide greater mobility than a walker, but they are suitable only for people who are able to support their own weight. Crutches are often used by people who need to avoid placing weight on an injured leg or foot while healing takes place.

Body weight may be borne by the hands with full-length crutches or by the elbows with elbow crutches. Full-length crutches are usually used by otherwise healthy people who have suffered a fracture or a severe strain or sprain of a bone, joint, or ligament or tendon of a lower extremity.

Elbow crutches are particularly useful for people recovering from *stroke* because they allow gradual progression from a high degree of support to almost natural walking. People with arthritis in their upper limbs should not use elbow crutches because the additional strain on the joints may make the arthritis worse.

Like walkers, crutches are usually made of a light alloy and are rubber-tipped. There are various ways of using crutches (see the illustrated box opposite).

### CANES

Canes are most commonly used by people who have weakness, pain, or stiffness on one side. They are usually made of wood and have various types of handles to suit different grips. For extra stability, canes can be supplied with three or four small feet on the end of the shaft.

It is important for a cane to be of the correct length; an upright posture should be achieved with the elbow slightly bent. It is generally best to walk with the cane on the strong side so that the cane is forward when the foot on the weak side comes forward. However, if one side is very weak, the cane may be held on the weak side, close to the leg, and moved with it, acting as a type of splint.

### ELECTROMUSCULAR STIMULATION

Computer-controlled electromuscular stimulation of the leg muscles to facilitate walking in quadriplegics and paraplegics was, as of 1988, an investigational procedure.

## Walking, delayed

Ninety percent of normal children walk by 14 or 15 months of age. Delayed walking may be suspected if the child is unable to walk alone by 18 months. (See *Developmental delay*.)

## Walleye

A form of *strabismus* in which the affected eye turns outward.

## Warfarin

> **WARNING**
> Always check with your physician before taking any other drug with warfarin since many drugs interfere with its anticlotting effect.

An *anticoagulant drug* used to treat and prevent abnormal blood clotting. Warfarin is used to treat *thrombosis* and to prevent *stroke* or treat *transient ischemic attack*. It is also prescribed to prevent blood clotting after heart valve replacement (see *Heart valve surgery*), in some *heart valve disorders*, or in chronic *atrial fibrillation*. Because warfarin is fully effective only after several days, a faster-acting anticoagulant, such as *heparin*, is usually also prescribed during this period.

### POSSIBLE ADVERSE EFFECTS

Warfarin may cause abnormal bleeding in different parts of the body; regular blood-clotting (prothrombin time) tests are therefore carried out to monitor treatment. Warfarin may also cause nausea, loss of appetite, abdominal pain, and rash.

## Wart

A contagious, harmless growth on skin or mucous membranes. Warts are caused by the papillomavirus, of which there are 30 types.

Warts infect only the topmost layer of skin. They do not have roots, seeds, or branches. The black dots that are sometimes evident are capillaries that have become clotted due to the rapid skin growth caused by the wart virus.

### TYPES

All warts are essentially the same but their appearance may be modified according to their position on the body. They are usually symptomless.

**COMMON WARTS** These are firm, sharply defined, round or irregular, flesh-colored to brown growths, up to about one quarter inch (6 mm) in diameter. They often have a rough surface. Common warts usually appear on sites subject to injury (e.g., the hands, face, knees, and scalp), particularly in young children.

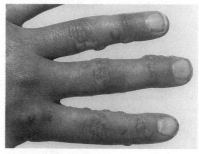

**Common warts on hand**
Warts often grow in crops. In time, they disappear spontaneously but can be removed by freezing.

**FLAT WARTS** Flat-topped, flesh-colored papules that occur mainly on the wrists, the backs of the hands, and the face; they may itch.

**DIGITATE WARTS** Dark-colored growths with fingerlike projections.

**FILIFORM WARTS** Long, slender growths that occur on the eyelids, armpits, or neck usually in overweight, middle-aged people.

**PLANTAR WARTS** These are warts on the sole of the foot (see *Plantar warts*). They are flattened simply because of the pressure placed on them; otherwise, they are just like other warts.

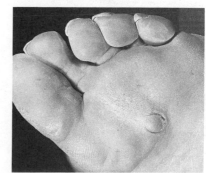

**Typical plantar wart**
This type of wart may need treatment—a physician may pare it down with a scalpel and apply a corrosive paint.

W

**GENITAL WARTS** These extensive, pink, cauliflowerlike areas may occur on the genitals of men or women (see *Warts, genital*). Genital warts need prompt treatment. There is some evidence that warts infecting a woman's cervix may predispose her to cervical cancer. It is important that both sexual partners be checked and rechecked since the infection can travel back and forth between them. Condoms can prevent the transfer of warts. Warts present around the genitals of young children may be a sign of sexual abuse.

**TREATMENT**
About 50 percent of warts disappear in six to 12 months without any treatment. With the exception of disabling plantar warts and genital warts, removal can be delayed. Common, flat, and plantar warts can be cured with several different treatments. Most commonly, liquid nitrogen is used to freeze the wart solid. As it thaws, a blister forms, lifting the wart off. Sometimes a blister-producing liquid (cantharidin) or corroding acid liquids or plasters are used. Several treatments may be needed and sometimes the wart returns. Surgical removal with a scalpel, electric needle, or laser may also be used.

## Warts, genital
Soft warts that grow in and around the entrance of the vagina and the anus and on the penis. Genital warts are transmitted by sexual contact and are caused by a papillomavirus. There may be an interval of up to 18 months between infection and the appearance of the warts.

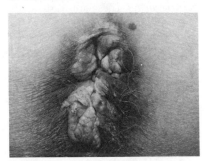

**Genital warts around the anus**
These growths are painless but need treatment—usually by application of podophyllin or surgical removal.

W

Genital warts have been linked with cases of cervical cancer (see *Cervix, cancer of*). A woman who has had genital warts—or whose partner has had genital warts—should have frequent *cervical smear tests*.

Genital warts may be removed by surgery or by the application of *podophyllin*. There is a tendency for the warts to recur.

## Wasp stings
See *Insect stings*.

## Water
Although only a simple chemical (consisting of two atoms of hydrogen bonded to one of oxygen—$H_2O$), water is essential to all forms of life. Some simple life-forms, such as certain microorganisms, can survive in a state of suspended animation for years or decades without water. However, even they require water to carry out functions such as growth and reproduction.

Water is the most common chemical in the human body (and also one of the most abundant substances on earth). About 99 percent of the molecules in the body are water, although it makes up a smaller proportion of body weight (about 60 percent in an average man). Thus, a man weighing 155 pounds (70 kg) contains about 87.5 pints (42 liters) of water, of which about 58 pints (28 liters) are within the body cells themselves; 29 pints (14 liters) are extracellular. Of the extracellular water, about 6.25 to 8.3 pints (3 to 4 liters) are in the blood plasma, lymph, and cerebrospinal fluid; the remaining 21 to 23 pints (10 to 11 liters) are in *tissue fluid*.

**ROLE IN THE BODY**
Water is essential to life because it provides the medium in which all metabolic reactions take place. It also provides the medium for the transportation of chemical substances dissolved in it, such as *ions*. The blood plasma carries water to all body tissues; it also carries excess water from tissues for elimination from the body by the liver, kidneys, lungs, and skin. The interchange of water between the blood and tissue cells occurs via the tissue fluid, which bathes all the individual cells. The passage of water in the tissue fluid into and out of cells takes place by a process called *osmosis*.

**WATER BALANCE**
Water is taken into the body not only by drinking, but also in food; in addition, a small amount is actually formed within the body by the metabolism of food.

Water is lost from the body in *urine*, sweat, *feces*, and as water vapor breathed out. However, the amount lost as sweat depends on physical

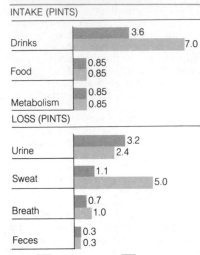

| INTAKE (PINTS) | | |
|---|---|---|
| Drinks | 3.6 | 7.0 |
| Food | 0.85 | 0.85 |
| Metabolism | 0.85 | 0.85 |

| LOSS (PINTS) | | |
|---|---|---|
| Urine | 3.2 | 2.4 |
| Sweat | 1.1 | 5.0 |
| Breath | 0.7 | 1.0 |
| Feces | 0.3 | 0.3 |

Key ▇ Cold climate ▇ Hot climate

**Water intakes and losses**
The charts show average intakes of water from various sources and losses in urine, sweat, and so on. In cool climates, people tend to drink more than the amount required to satisfy thirst; the excess water is lost in urine. In hot climates, large amounts of water are lost in sweat, and an increase in fluid intake is essential to avoid dehydration.

activity and the external temperature; the amount passed out of the body in the urine depends largely on the amount of fluid drunk (see chart above).

The amount of water in the body must remain within relatively narrow limits for the proper functioning of metabolic processes; this balance is achieved by the activities of the kidneys, which control the balance between fluid intake and output by regulating the amount of water excreted from the body in the urine. The minimum daily urinary output necessary to remove waste products is about 1 pint (0.5 liters), although most healthy adults usually produce about 3.1 pints (1.5 liters) of urine a day. The amount produced in excess of the minimum is controlled mainly by *ADH* (antidiuretic hormone), which is produced by the posterior portion of the pituitary gland and acts on the kidneys to reduce water excretion.

The body's water balance is also regulated in another way. If there is an excessive amount of any substance (such as sugar or salt) dissolved in the blood that must be excreted by the kidneys, extra water is needed to accomplish this function. This may lead to *dehydration* despite increased production of ADH, but is usually compensated for by increased water intake as a response to *thirst*.

In some disorders, such as *renal failure* or *heart failure*, insufficient water is excreted in the urine, resulting in *edema* (abnormal accumulation of water in body tissues).

## Waterborne infection

Water can be a source of infection if it contains infective or parasitic organisms and is drunk, contaminates food, or is played in.

### DRINKING WATER

Throughout the world, contamination of water used for drinking is an important means of spread of diseases, including viral *hepatitis A*, many viral and bacterial causes of *diarrhea*, *typhoid fever*, *cholera*, *amebiasis*, and some types of *worm infestation*.

Contamination results from the discharge of human or animal excretory products containing infective organisms into rivers, lakes, reservoirs, or wells used as a source of water supply. The discharge may be direct or in the form of untreated sewage. It can also occur through leakage between sewage and water supply systems. This could happen, for example, in a city affected by a major earthquake.

In developed countries such as the US, the risks of waterborne infection are minimized through measures such as adequate sanitary facilities, sewage treatment and disposal, and the sterilization and testing of water before it is supplied to homes. Tap water is therefore usually safe (unless there is a specific warning not to drink it).

In developing countries, sanitary facilities, sewage disposal, and water treatment may be inadequate. As a consequence, members of the population are more likely to carry the types of disease organisms spread by water. It is therefore best not to drink tap water in poorer countries and always to regard with suspicion any water taken directly from rivers, lakes, and wells.

**AVOIDANCE OF INFECTION** The accompanying table summarizes safe and suspect sources of drinking water in developed and developing countries. If safe tap water is unavailable, bottled or canned water or drinks of well-known brand names are usually safe; do not put ice made from suspect water into drinks. Rainwater is usually free of infective organisms provided it is not allowed to stand for a long period before drinking.

### SAFETY OF WATER AND OTHER DRINKS FOR CONSUMPTION

| | Developed countries | Developing countries |
|---|---|---|
| Usually safe | Tap water from public supply; rainwater; canned or bottled drinks; springwater | Canned or bottled drinks of well-known brands; rainwater |
| Suspect | Water direct from rivers, streams, lakes, ponds, canals, wells | Tap water (cities); springwater |
| Very suspect | Obviously polluted water, i.e., cloudy in appearance or with an unpleasant smell | Tap water (rural areas); water direct from rivers, streams, lakes, ponds, canals |

**Safe and suspect water**
Any source of water that falls into the suspect or very suspect categories should be sterilized. Techniques include boiling, filtering, and chemical treatment.

Water that may be infected should be sterilized before drinking. The most reliable method is to boil the water for five minutes. Boiling kills any infective organisms present. If boiling is impractical, the alternative is to filter the water and then to sterilize it chemically. Filtering is necessary to remove suspended particles, which can harbor disease organisms and interfere with sterilization. Various types of filters are available; some remove bacteria and other infective organisms as well as inanimate particles. The manufacturer's instructions should be followed carefully. For chemical sterilization, purifying tablets that contain chlorine or iodine are used. Water should be left for 20 to 30 minutes following treatment before it is used.

Vegetables or other food that have been washed in suspect water should not be eaten unless they have been thoroughly cooked.

### IMMERSION IN WATER

Swimming in polluted water is liable to cause an ear infection (see *Otitis externa*). The risk can be minimized by shaking the head to the left and the right after swimming to clear water out of the outer-ear canals.

Most swimmers inadvertently swallow some water. If it is contaminated, there is a risk of contracting any of the diseases transmitted in polluted drinking water. It is therefore advisable to avoid swimming in rivers possibly polluted with sewage (e.g., downstream of towns) or in the ocean near large coastal resorts.

*Leptospirosis* is caused by contact with water contaminated by rat's urine; sewage and canal workers are most at risk.

In tropical countries, swimming or wading in rivers, lakes, and ponds is highly inadvisable due to the risk of *schistosomiasis* (bilharziasis), a serious disease caused by a fluke that can burrow through the swimmer's skin. Swimmers' itch is caused by a similar type of fluke, which burrows into the skin and causes an itchy rash. Outbreaks of swimmers' itch have occurred in the US.

### OTHER MECHANISMS OF WATERBORNE INFECTION

Fish (particularly shellfish) that live in polluted water may collect infective organisms in their bodies. They must be expertly cleaned and prepared and then promptly and thoroughly cooked to avoid possible hepatitis, choleralike illnesses, *food poisoning*, or a *tapeworm infestation*.

*Legionnaires' disease* is caused by a bacterium that can contaminate the water systems of large buildings. It is not apparently contracted from actually drinking contaminated water; the route of infection seems to occur via inhalation from showers or air-conditioning systems. (See also *Food-borne infection*.)

## Waterhouse-Friderichsen syndrome

A serious, but very rare, condition caused by infection of the bloodstream by bacteria of the meningococcus group. Thus, meningitis is often associated with this syndrome. The main feature is bleeding into the adrenal glands, which leads to acute *adrenal failure* and *shock*.

The onset of Waterhouse-Friderichsen syndrome is abrupt; the victim collapses within several hours and sinks into a coma. Rapidly enlarging purple spots appear on the skin. The condition is almost invariably fatal unless it is immediately treated in a hospital.

## Watering eye

An increase in the volume of the tear film, usually producing epiphora (overflow of *tears*). Watering may be caused by excess tear production due to emotion or to conjunctival or corneal irritation. It may also be caused by an obstruction to the channel that drains tears from the eye.

## Water intoxication

A condition caused by excessive water retention in the brain. The principal symptoms are headaches, dizziness, nausea, confusion, and, in severe cases, seizures and unconsciousness.

Various disorders can disrupt the body's water balance, leading to accumulation of water in body tissues, including the brain. Such disorders include *renal failure*, liver *cirrhosis*, severe *heart failure*, diseases of the adrenal glands, and certain lung or ovarian tumors that produce a substance with a similar action to antidiuretic hormone (*ADH*).

There is also a risk of water intoxication for about 48 hours after surgery, because the stress of an operation leads to increased ADH production. Water intoxication may also occur during induction of labor with *oxytocin*.

## Water-on-the-brain

A nonmedical term for *hydrocephalus*.

## Water-on-the-knee

A popular term for accumulation of fluid within or around the knee joint. The most common cause is *bursitis* (inflammation of a bursa, one of the fluid-filled sacs that covers and cushions pressure points in the body). Another cause is fluid within the knee joint (see *Effusion, joint*).

## Water tablets

See *Diuretic drugs*.

## Wax bath

A type of *heat treatment* in which hot, liquid wax is applied to part of the body to relieve pain and stiffness in inflamed or injured joints. Wax baths are most frequently used to treat sufferers from *rheumatoid arthritis*.

A wax bath is given by dipping the body part, usually a hand or foot, into wax kept at a temperature of 120 to 130°F. The limb is held in the wax for a few seconds and then withdrawn; the wax solidifies, forming a thin layer. The wax may be broken off and the limb redipped or the procedure may be repeated until the wax coating is about half an inch thick. The treated area is then wrapped in a plastic sheet and blanket to retain the heat. After 20 minutes, the wax is peeled off and exercises are performed to encourage movement in the treated joints.

## Wax, ear

See *Earwax*.

## Weakness

A term used to describe a general lack of vigor or strength, which is a common symptom of a wide range of conditions, including *anemia*, *emotional problems*, and various disorders affecting the heart, nervous system, bones, joints, and muscles. When associated with emotional disorders (such as depression), weakness may represent a lack of desire or ambition rather than a lack of muscle strength.

More specifically, the term weakness is used to describe loss of power in certain muscle groups, which may or may not be accompanied by muscle wasting and loss of sensation. (See also *Paralysis*.)

## Weaning

The gradual substitution of solid foods for milk or formula in an infant's diet (see *Feeding, infant*).

## Webbing

A flap of skin between adjacent fingers or toes. Webbing is a common congenital abnormality that may affect two or more digits. Although mild webbing is completely harmless, surgical correction may be performed for cosmetic reasons. In severe cases, adjacent digits may be completely fused (see *Syndactyly*).

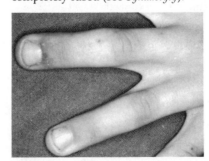

**Webbing of the fingers**
This curious feature is often an inherited trait, appearing in each of several generations of a family.

## Wegener's granulomatosis

A rare disorder in which *granulomas* (nodular aggregations of abnormal cells) associated with areas of chronic tissue inflammation due to *vasculitis* (inflammation of blood vessels) develop in the nasal passages, lungs, and kidneys.

### CAUSES AND SYMPTOMS

The cause of the condition is unknown, but it is thought to be an *autoimmune disorder* (a disorder in which the body's natural defenses attack its own tissues).

The principal symptoms include a bloody discharge from the nose, coughing (sometimes with the production of bloodstained sputum), breathing difficulty, chest pain, and blood in the urine. There may also be loss of appetite, weight loss, weakness, fatigue, and joint pains.

### DIAGNOSIS AND TREATMENT

A diagnosis usually requires the microscopic examination of a *biopsy* sample of abnormal tissue, which may be taken from inside the nose, from a lung, or from a kidney.

Treatment is with a combination of *immunosuppressant drugs*, such as cyclophosphamide or azathioprine, and *corticosteroid drugs* to alleviate the symptoms and in some instances to aid in the induction of a remission in the disease process.

### OUTLOOK

With prompt treatment, most people recover completely within about a year, although *renal failure* develops in some sufferers.

Without treatment, various complications may occur, including perforation of the nasal septum, causing deformity of the nose; inflammation of the eyes; a rash, nodules, or ulcers on the skin; and damage to the heart muscle, which may be fatal.

## Weight

The heaviness of a person or object, usually measured in pounds or kilograms. Weight is a routine physical measurement of *growth* in children. Accurate scales should be used; ideally, a person should be weighed before breakfast naked or wearing the same amount of clothing each day.

Weight can be compared to charts standardized for an individual's height, age, and sex. If weight is below 80 percent of the standard weight for height, the individual's *nutrition* is probably inadequate as a result of poor diet or disease.

In healthy adults, weight remains more or less stable because calorie intake from the diet matches calorie expenditure used to fuel all body activities (see *Metabolism*). *Weight loss* or weight gain occurs if the net balance is disturbed.

W

## WEIGHT TABLE: MEN

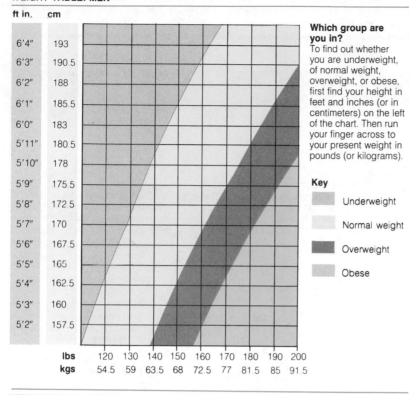

| ft in. | cm |
|---|---|
| 6'4" | 193 |
| 6'3" | 190.5 |
| 6'2" | 188 |
| 6'1" | 185.5 |
| 6'0" | 183 |
| 5'11" | 180.5 |
| 5'10" | 178 |
| 5'9" | 175.5 |
| 5'8" | 172.5 |
| 5'7" | 170 |
| 5'6" | 167.5 |
| 5'5" | 165 |
| 5'4" | 162.5 |
| 5'3" | 160 |
| 5'2" | 157.5 |

| lbs | 120 | 130 | 140 | 150 | 160 | 170 | 180 | 190 | 200 |
|---|---|---|---|---|---|---|---|---|---|
| kgs | 54.5 | 59 | 63.5 | 68 | 72.5 | 77 | 81.5 | 85 | 91.5 |

**Which group are you in?**
To find out whether you are underweight, of normal weight, overweight, or obese, first find your height in feet and inches (or in centimeters) on the left of the chart. Then run your finger across to your present weight in pounds (or kilograms).

**Key**

Underweight

Normal weight

Overweight

Obese

## WEIGHT TABLE: WOMEN

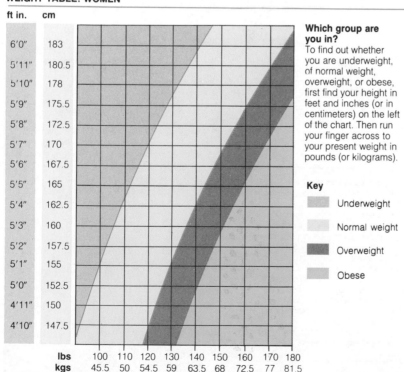

| ft in. | cm |
|---|---|
| 6'0" | 183 |
| 5'11" | 180.5 |
| 5'10" | 178 |
| 5'9" | 175.5 |
| 5'8" | 172.5 |
| 5'7" | 170 |
| 5'6" | 167.5 |
| 5'5" | 165 |
| 5'4" | 162.5 |
| 5'3" | 160 |
| 5'2" | 157.5 |
| 5'1" | 155 |
| 5'0" | 152.5 |
| 4'11" | 150 |
| 4'10" | 147.5 |

| lbs | 100 | 110 | 120 | 130 | 140 | 150 | 160 | 170 | 180 |
|---|---|---|---|---|---|---|---|---|---|
| kgs | 45.5 | 50 | 54.5 | 59 | 63.5 | 68 | 72.5 | 77 | 81.5 |

**Which group are you in?**
To find out whether you are underweight, of normal weight, overweight, or obese, first find your height in feet and inches (or in centimeters) on the left of the chart. Then run your finger across to your present weight in pounds (or kilograms).

**Key**

Underweight

Normal weight

Overweight

Obese

*Obesity* can be most easily assessed in terms of weight for height. A person is considered to be obese if his or her weight is 20 percent more than that given in a standard weight-for-height table. An alternative method of assessment is to use the body mass index, which is obtained by dividing weight in kilograms by the square of height in meters; a body mass index above 26 for a woman or 28 for a man constitutes obesity.

## Weight loss

Loss of body weight occurs any time there is a decrease in the net balance of calorie intake related to calorie expenditure. This decrease may be due to deliberate *weight reduction*, a change in diet, or change in level of activity; weight loss is also a symptom of a wide range of disorders.

**CAUSES**

Many diseases disrupt the appetite and may lead to weight loss by reducing the intake of calories. *Depression* reduces the motivation to eat, *peptic ulcer* causes pain and may lead to food avoidance, and *kidney* disorders cause loss of appetite due to the effect of uremia (raised levels of urea in the blood). In *anorexia nervosa* and *bulimia*, complex psychological factors affect the individual's eating pattern.

Calorie intake may also be affected by digestive disorders. Persistent *vomiting* due to *gastroenteritis*, for example, leads to weight loss. Cancer of the esophagus (see *Esophagus, cancer of*) or *stomach cancer* causes loss of weight, as does the *malabsorption* of nutrients that occurs in certain disorders of the intestine or pancreas.

Disorders that increase the rate of metabolic activity in cells cause weight loss by increasing the expenditure of calories. These disorders include any type of *cancer*, chronic infection such as *tuberculosis*, and *hyperthyroidism* (overactivity of the thyroid gland). Untreated *diabetes mellitus* also causes weight loss, initially due to a greater fluid loss from the increase in urine output and as a result of loss of calories from glycosuria (glucose in the urine); eventually, a wasting of tissue mass causes weight loss as fat stores are broken down.

Unexplained weight loss may be a sign of disease and should always be investigated by a physician. A working diagnosis may be established by means of a careful patient history and a physical examination. In some cases, appropriate tests can confirm a specific cause.

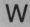

**WEIGHT LOSS** Minor fluctuations in weight as a result of temporary changes in the level of exercise taken or the amount of food eaten are normal. More drastic, unintentional weight loss, especially when combined with other symptoms such as loss of appetite, usually requires medical attention.

**? Is your appetite as good as ever?**

**YES →**

Have you noticed two or more of the following symptoms?
- excessive sweating
- weakness or trembling
- unexplained tiredness
- bulging eyes

**YES →**

An overactive thyroid gland is a possibility, especially if you are a woman. Consult your physician.

See • *Graves' disease*
 • *Hyperthyroidism*

**NO ↓**

**NO ↓**

Have you noticed one or more of the following symptoms?
- unusually frequent or abundant urination
- increased thirst
- unexplained tiredness
- genital itching
- absence of periods

**YES →**

This may be due to diabetes mellitus, a hormonal disorder in which insufficient insulin is produced by the pancreas.

See • *Diabetes mellitus*

**CANCER WATCH**
There is a possibility of cancer if weight loss and loss of appetite are combined with abdominal pain OR a change in bowel habits. **Consult your physician without delay!**

**NO ■ ■ ■ ■ ■ →**

If you feel well, there is probably no serious cause for your weight loss. However, if your weight continues to drop, discuss this with your physician to exclude the slight possibility of a serious underlying disorder.

**? Have you noticed one or more of the following symptoms?**
- recurrent bouts of diarrhea
- recurrent constipation
- recurrent abdominal pain
- blood in the feces

**YES →**

☎
**Consult your physician without delay!**
A disorder of the digestive tract may be responsible.

See • *Crohn's disease*
 • *Intestine, cancer of*
 • *Irritable bowel syndrome*
 • *Malabsorption*
 • *Peptic ulcer*
 • *Stomach cancer*

**NO ↓**

**Signs of weight loss**
If you lose weight without deliberately attempting to slim down, you should always take the matter seriously, especially if other symptoms suggest the possibility of illness. If you do not weigh yourself regularly, the following signs may indicate that you have lost weight:
- people remark on your changed appearance
- your cheeks become sunken
- your pants or skirts become loose around the waist
- your collars fit more loosely
- you need a smaller bra

Continued on next page

W

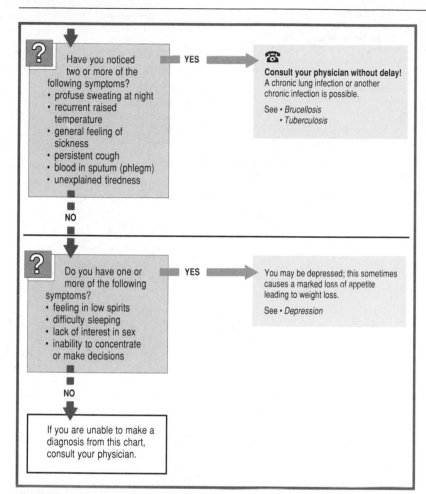

?
Have you noticed two or more of the following symptoms?
• profuse sweating at night
• recurrent raised temperature
• general feeling of sickness
• persistent cough
• blood in sputum (phlegm)
• unexplained tiredness

**YES** →

☎
**Consult your physician without delay!**
A chronic lung infection or another chronic infection is possible.

See • *Brucellosis*
    • *Tuberculosis*

**NO**

?
Do you have one or more of the following symptoms?
• feeling in low spirits
• difficulty sleeping
• lack of interest in sex
• inability to concentrate or make decisions

**YES** →

You may be depressed; this sometimes causes a marked loss of appetite leading to weight loss.

See • *Depression*

**NO**

If you are unable to make a diagnosis from this chart, consult your physician.

## RULES FOR WEIGHT REDUCTION

| | |
|---|---|
| Cut down drastically on all visible fats, such as butter, margarine, cream, and cooking oils, and also on the invisible fats | present in pastries, cookies, and cakes. Choose low-fat milk, cheeses, and yogurts. |
| Choose lean cuts of meat and avoid processed meat, such as salami. Broil or roast meat without adding fat instead of | frying. Choose fresh fish in preference to the smoked variety. |
| Eat more boiled legumes (e.g., lentils, peas, and beans); they provide plenty of | protein and are filling but contain very little fat. |
| Avoid refined carbohydrates such as sugar (dextrose) and cane syrup | (sucrose) as well as refined grain products such as white flour or white rice. |
| Increase your consumption of unrefined carbohydrates. Eat whole-wheat bread, whole-grain breakfast cereals (without | added sugar), unrefined rice, fresh fruit, and plenty of vegetables. |
| Reduce intake of alcoholic drinks, which | are high in calories. |

**Dietary recommendations for weight loss**
Careful choice of the right types of food—and, in particular, the avoidance of items with a high calorie content per unit of weight (mainly fats)—makes it easier to achieve a low-calorie diet without necessarily having to reduce the bulk of food you eat.

## Weight reduction

The process of losing excess body fat. Weight reduction is usually undertaken by people who are overweight (see *Obesity*) to improve their health or appearance. A person who is severely overweight is more at risk of suffering from various illnesses, such as *diabetes mellitus, hypertension* (high blood pressure), and heart disease.

### HOW IT IS DONE

The most efficient way to lose weight is to eat less. To lose weight, people should eat 500 to 1,000 calories a day less than their energy requirements. This should result in a weight loss of approximately 1.5 pounds per week until a desirable weight is achieved. The rate of weight loss may be faster at the beginning of a weight reduction diet, when the body's glycogen and fat stores, which contain water, are being depleted.

*Exercise* forms an important part of a reducing regime, burning excess calories and improving muscle tone. Some people believe that *aerobics* speed up the metabolism for a short period after exercising and thus make the body more efficient at using energy.

### FAD DIETS

Many people who are trying to lose weight want to do so quickly; they may follow fad diets that provide severely restricted calorie intakes. Though there may be a rapid weight loss in the beginning, most of these diets do not work in the long term and the lost weight usually returns.

A number of liquid diets providing about 330 calories per day have been developed. Some physicians are concerned about the effects of these liquid diets. Any diet providing less than 1,000 calories per day should be undertaken only with medical supervision and only briefly or intermittently for short periods.

## Weil's disease

Another name for *leptospirosis*.

## Welders' eye

Acute *conjunctivitis* and *keratopathy* (corneal damage) that is caused by the intense ultraviolet light radiation emitted by the electric welding arc. Welders' eye is a result of failure to wear adequate eye protection while welding.

## Werdnig-Hoffmann disease

A very rare inherited disorder of the nervous system that affects infants. Also known as infantile spinal muscular atrophy, Werdnig-Hoffmann

W

disease is a type of *motor neuron disease*. Werdnig-Hoffmann disease affects the nerve cells in the spinal cord that control muscle movement. Its underlying cause is unknown.

Marked floppiness and paralysis occur during the first few months. Affected babies move less than normal babies and sometimes the mother recalls being aware of reduced fetal movements before the baby was born. Severely affected infants tend to lie still in a froglike position with the knees bent up and turned out. The muscles of the face are unaffected, so the child has an alert expression that is in sharp contrast to his or her physical helplessness. The baby becomes increasingly floppy and deformed over the following few months. The muscles that control breathing and feeding are also affected, which usually causes death before the child is 3 years old.

There is no cure for Werdnig-Hoffmann disease. Treatment aims to keep the affected infant as comfortable as possible.

## Wernicke-Korsakoff syndrome

An uncommon brain disorder almost always due to the malnutrition that occurs in chronic *alcohol dependence* or, occasionally, in other conditions, such as cancer with malnutrition.

### CAUSES
The factor responsible is deficiency of thiamine (vitamin $B_1$, see *Vitamin B complex*), which affects the brain and nervous system. The thiamine deficiency is probably caused by the combined effects of poor eating habits and an inherited defect in thiamine metabolism.

### SYMPTOMS
The disease consists of two stages— Wernicke's encephalopathy and Korsakoff's psychosis—each characterized by particular symptoms.

Wernicke's encephalopathy usually develops suddenly and produces various abnormal eye movements, *ataxia* (difficulty coordinating body movements, especially walking), slowness, and confusion. Sufferers also usually have signs of *neuropathy*, such as loss of sensation, pins and needles sensation, or impaired reflexes. The level of consciousness progressively falls and may lead to coma and death without treatment.

Korsakoff's psychosis may follow Wernicke's encephalopathy if treatment is not instituted soon enough. Symptoms consist of severe *amnesia* (memory loss), apathy, and disorien-

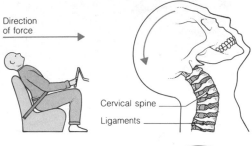

### CAUSE OF WHIPLASH INJURY
This injury to the neck section of the spine may occur when a car is subjected to a sudden violent force and the occupant's body is restrained in the seat but his or her head is not restrained.

**Sudden acceleration**
Here, there is a sudden force from behind (usually due to another vehicle striking the rear of the car). As the body accelerates forward, the head jerks violently backward relative to the body, stretching and bending the neck; the head then rebounds forward.

Direction of force

Cervical spine
Ligaments

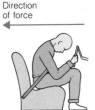

**Sudden deceleration**
Here, there is a sudden violent force from the front toward the back of the vehicle, due, for example, to a collision with a tree. The seat belt restrains the body, but the head continues to move forward, stretching the neck; the head then rebounds backward.

Direction of force

Cervical spine
Ligaments

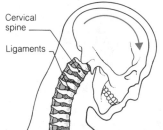

tation. Recent memory is affected more than distant memory, sufferers often not being able to remember what they did even a few minutes previously. Confabulation (invention of stories) may occur to make up for gaps in memory.

### TREATMENT AND OUTLOOK
Wernicke's encephalopathy is a medical emergency. If the diagnosis is even suspected, high doses of intravenous thiamine are given immediately. This treatment reverses most of the symptoms, often within a few hours.

In the absence of prompt treatment, Korsakoff's psychosis is usually irreversible, leaving the sufferer permanently handicapped by memory loss and in need of continual supervision.

## Wernicke's encephalopathy
See *Wernicke-Korsakoff syndrome*.

## Wheelchair
A chair mounted on wheels used to provide mobility for a person unable to walk. The simplest type of wheelchair is pushed by an attendant or hand-propelled by the disabled person. Manual wheelchairs have small wheels with casters at the front and large, narrow wheels at the back; these wheelchairs are designed to have metal handles that can be easily gripped.

Powered wheelchairs are battery-operated and controlled electronically by finger pressure or, if necessary, by chin pressure or breath control. The battery provides power for six to eight hours and is recharged overnight by connection to an electrical outlet. Wheels are usually small with wide, low-pressure tires. Several different types of powered chairs are available. Those suitable for outdoor use are capable of negotiating raised obstructions but are usually too wide and long for convenient use indoors; indoor models are lighter and more compact but cannot mount sidewalk curbs.

Wheelchairs may be made of light-weight metal (such as titanium or an alloy) and are often foldable for easy storage in the trunk of a car.

## Wheeze
A high-pitched, whistling sound produced in the chest during breathing; it is caused by narrowing of the airways. A wheeze may be loud enough to be heard by those in the room with the sufferer or just audible with a stethoscope. Wheeze is a feature of *asthma* and also occurs in *bronchitis*, *bronchiolitis*, and pulmonary edema (fluid in the lungs). Inhalation of a foreign body, such as a peanut, into the airways may also cause a wheeze. (See also *Breathing difficulty*.)

W

## Whiplash injury

An injury to the soft tissues, *ligaments*, and joints of the cervical spine (neck portion) caused by the neck being bent forcibly and violently forward and then backward or vice versa. Whiplash injury most commonly results from sudden acceleration or deceleration, as in a car collision. However, some degree of whiplash to the neck occurs in all forms of head injury.

Damage to the spine usually involves minor *sprain* of a neck ligament or *subluxation* (partial dislocation) of a cervical joint. Occasionally, a ligament may rupture or there may be a fracture of a cervical vertebra (see *Spinal injury*).

Characteristically, pain and stiffness in the neck are much worse 24 hours after the injury.

Treatment may include immobilization in an orthopedic *collar, analgesic drugs* (painkillers), *muscle-relaxant drugs*, and *physical therapy*. Recovery is usually complete but it can take several weeks before full pain-free neck movement is possible.

## Whipple's disease

A rare disorder that may affect many organs. Also called intestinal lipodystrophy, Whipple's disease causes a variety of symptoms and findings. The most common are malabsorption (impaired absorption of nutrients by the small intestine), diarrhea, pain in the abdomen, progressive weight loss, joint pains, swollen lymph nodes, abnormal skin pigmentation, anemia, and fever. The condition most commonly occurs in middle-aged men.

The precise cause of Whipple's disease remains unknown but it is probably due to an unidentified bacterial infection. Diagnosis is by jejunal biopsy (removal of a small sample of tissue from the jejunum for microscopic analysis). Affected tissues are found to contain macrophages (a type of cell) containing rod-shaped bacteria.

Treatment is with *antibiotic drugs* for at least one year. Attempts to correct nutritional deficiencies that have arisen from malabsorption are made with dietary supplements.

## Whipple's operation

A type of *pancreatectomy* in which the head of the pancreas and loop of the duodenum are surgically removed. It is named for the US surgeon Allen Whipple (1881-1963).

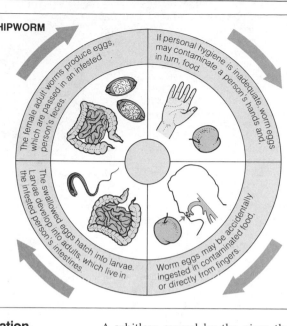

**LIFE CYCLE OF WHIPWORM**
Whipworm infestation occurs worldwide and is particularly common in the tropics. An estimated 2 million people in the US are affected at any given time—mainly children and residents of mental institutions. Adult worms are 1 to 2 inches in length, with long, whiplike tails; they may live in a person's intestines for up to 20 years. Most infestations do not cause symptoms.

The female adult worms produce eggs, which are passed in an infested person's feces.

If personal hygiene is inadequate, worm eggs may contaminate a person's hands and, in turn, food.

Worm eggs may be accidentally ingested in contaminated food or directly from fingers.

The swallowed eggs hatch into larvae. Larvae develop into adults, which live in the infested person's intestines.

## Whipworm infestation

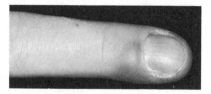

The whipworm is a small, cylindrical worm, 1 or 2 inches (2.5 to 5 cm) long, with a whiplike tail, that can live in human intestines. The life cycle and transmission of infection are shown above.

A light infestation causes no symptoms; a heavy infestation can cause abdominal pain, diarrhea, and sometimes *anemia*, because the worms consume a small amount of the host's blood every day. The condition is diagnosed by finding worm eggs during an examination of feces.

Treatment is with *antihelmintic drugs*, such as mebendazole, which usually bring about a satisfactory cure; heavy infestations may require more than one course of treatment.

## Whitehead

A very common type of skin blemish (see *Milia*).

## Whitlow

An abscess on the fingertip or, rarely, on the toe. A whitlow causes the finger to swell and become extremely painful and sensitive to pressure and touch. It may be caused by the virus that causes *herpes simplex* or by a bacterium, which usually enters the body through a cut.

A whitlow caused by bacterial infection may be treated with *antibiotic drugs* or, if the infection is severe, by incision and drainage in a minor surgical procedure using local anesthesia.

A whitlow caused by the virus that causes herpes simplex is treated by application of an *antiviral drug*; such whitlows should not be incised and drained because of the high risk of spreading the infection.

A very rare complication of untreated whitlow is *osteomyelitis*, a serious bacterial infection of bone and bone marrow.

**Herpetic whitlow**
This extremely painful finger infection, caused by the herpes simplex virus, may be helped by applying an antiviral ointment.

## Whooping cough

See *Pertussis*.

## Wife beating

See *Spouse abuse*.

## Will, living

A written declaration, signed by an adult person of sound mind, that instructs his or her physicians to withhold or withdraw life-sustaining treatment if the person suffers from an incurable and terminal condition.

The written declaration must be signed with the same type of formality as a regular will, hence the description of the document as a "living will."

**W**

In 1987, 38 states and the District of Columbia had enacted laws giving legal effect to living wills. Although the terms and provisions of the laws vary from state to state, in general they require the physician and the hospital to honor the patient's living will or to transfer the care of the patient to another physician who will honor the living will.

The law also provides legal immunity from liability for the physician and the hospital honoring the patient's wishes as expressed in his or her living will.

## Wilms' tumor
A type of *kidney cancer*, also called nephroblastoma, that occurs mainly in children.

## Wilson's disease
A rare, inherited disorder in which copper accumulates in the liver and is slowly released into other parts of the body. Eventually, Wilson's disease causes severe damage to both the liver and the brain.

### SYMPTOMS AND SIGNS
Symptoms vary in severity from person to person; they usually first appear in adolescence but sometimes occur as early as 5 or as late as 50. The toxic effects of copper on the liver can cause various disorders, progressing from *hepatitis* to *cirrhosis*. Accumulation of copper in the brain causes progressive problems ranging from mild intellectual impairment to crippling rigidity, tremor, and dementia.

### DIAGNOSIS AND TREATMENT
The diagnosis is based on analysis of blood and urine and a liver *biopsy* (removal of a small amount of tissue for microscopic analysis) to discover the amount of copper in the body.

Wilson's disease requires lifelong treatment with penicillamine, a drug that binds with copper and thus enables it to be excreted. If started soon after the onset of symptoms, penicillamine can sometimes improve liver and brain function. If the disease is discovered before toxic effects produce symptoms, the drug may be able to prevent symptoms from developing.

## Windpipe
A common name for the *trachea*.

## Wiring of the jaws
Immobilization of the jaws by means of metal wires to allow a fracture of the jaw to heal or as part of a treatment for *obesity*.

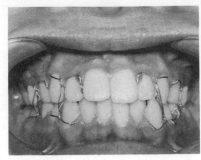

**Wired jaws**
A total of eight pairs of teeth have been wired together to immobilize the jaw while a fracture heals.

In the most commonly used method, thin, hairpin-shaped wires with a central eyelet (closed loop) are wound around pairs of adjacent teeth; about six wires are fixed to teeth in the upper and lower jawbones. Wires are then threaded through opposing pairs of upper and lower eyelets and twisted together to hold the jaws in a rigid position.

When a fracture of the jaw is being treated, the jaws are kept wired in a fixed position for about six weeks. As a means of achieving weight loss, the jaws are wired for as long as a year. In both cases, the person can take only a liquid or semiliquid diet, which for weight loss is calorie controlled. This form of diet treatment, though effective while the jaws are wired, usually fails when the overweight person resumes his or her previous eating habits.

## Wisdom tooth
One of the four rearmost *teeth*, also known as third molars. In most people, the wisdom teeth erupt between the ages of 17 and 21. However, in some people, one or more may neither develop nor erupt. In many cases, wisdom teeth are unable to emerge fully from the gum as a result of overcrowding (see *Impaction, dental*).

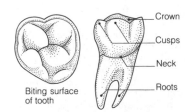

Crown
Cusps
Neck
Roots
Biting surface of tooth

**Structure of wisdom tooth**
Like other molars, each wisdom tooth has strong roots and a bulky crown with many cusps and an extensive grinding surface.

## Witches' milk
A thin, white discharge from the nipple of a newborn infant. Witches' milk occurs quite commonly and is usually accompanied by enlargement of one or both of the baby's breasts. The discharge is caused by maternal hormones that entered the fetus's circulation through the placenta. Witches' milk is a harmless sign that usually disappears within a few weeks.

## Withdrawal
The process of retreating from society and from relationships with others. Withdrawal is usually indicated by aloofness, lack of interest in social activities, preoccupation with one's own concerns, and difficulty communicating with others.

Withdrawal is also a term applied to the psychological and physical symptoms that develop upon discontinuation of a substance to which a person had become addicted (see *Withdrawal syndrome*).

## Withdrawal bleeding
Vaginal blood loss that occurs when the body's level of *progesterone* or *estrogen hormones* drops suddenly. *Menstruation* (sloughing of the uterine lining, which takes place each month that fertilization and implantation of an ovum do not occur) is a form of withdrawal bleeding because it is preceded by the withdrawal of both estrogen and progesterone in the menstrual cycle. The withdrawal bleeding that occurs at the end of each cycle of combined *oral contraceptive* pills mimics menstruation, but is usually shorter and lighter. Discontinuation of an estrogen-only preparation also produces bleeding, which may differ from normal menstruation in amount and duration.

## Withdrawal method
See *Coitus interruptus*.

## Withdrawal syndrome
A set of unpleasant mental and physical symptoms experienced when a person stops using a drug on which he or she is physically dependent (see *Drug dependence*).

In general, any drug that causes euphoria or that relieves pain or anxiety can cause dependence and withdrawal symptoms of varying degrees. Withdrawal syndromes most commonly result from *alcohol dependence*, *narcotic drug* dependence, *tobacco smoking*, or regular use of *tranquilizer drugs*. Other drugs that may

W

## FIRST AID: WOUNDS

> **DO NOT**
> - attempt to remove the object from the wound.

### FOREIGN BODY

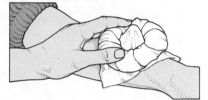

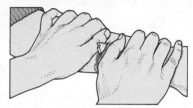

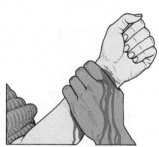

**1** Apply direct pressure above and below the object. Lay the victim down and raise and support the limb.

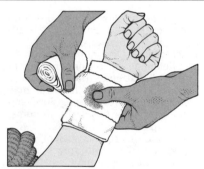

**2** Lightly drape a piece of gauze over object and wound and place a ring pad over it. Or use a roll of cotton to build up a pad around the wound. It should be high enough to prevent pressure on the object.

#### Ring pad

**1** Place a narrow bandage across one hand. Wind one end once or twice around your fingers to make a loop.

**2** Bring the other end through the loop, wind it repeatedly around the loop, pulling it tight each time.

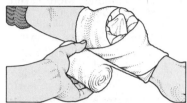

**3** Secure with a roller bandage. Make two straight turns, overlapping the pad, on either side. Then continue with diagonal turns until the pad is held firmly. Take the victim to the hospital.

### DEEPER WOUNDS

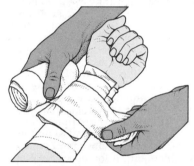

**1** Examine the wound for foreign bodies; if there are none, apply direct pressure to control bleeding by pressing on the wound with the fingers or palm. Lay the victim down and raise the injured part higher than the chest and heart.

**2** Put a sterile, unmedicated dressing over the wound so that it extends well beyond its edges. Secure it firmly with a bandage.

**3** If the blood seeps through, do not remove the bandage, but put more dressing and another bandage on top. Watch for *shock* and seek medical aid.

### CUTS AND SCRAPES

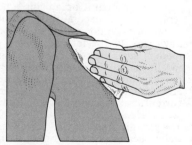

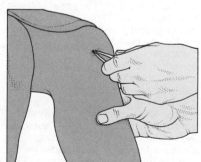

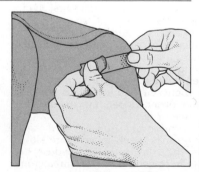

**1** Rinse the wound under cold, running water. Then, using a roll of cotton, gauze, or antiseptic wipes, clean around the wound. Work outward, using a clean pad for each stroke.

**2** Remove any loose foreign bodies, such as metal, glass, or gravel, with the gauze, cotton, or tweezers.

**3** Dry the surrounding area and dress the wound. If it is small, use an adhesive bandage. Otherwise, make a dressing with a piece of gauze and a piece of cotton. Secure with a bandage.

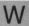

W

lead to withdrawal symptoms include *amphetamine drugs, cocaine, marijuana,* and *caffeine.*

## TYPES

**ALCOHOL** Withdrawal symptoms start six to eight hours after the last drink and may last four to seven days. Common symptoms include trembling of the hands and tongue, sweating, nausea, anxiety, and sometimes cramps and vomiting. More severe symptoms include seizures (see *Delirium tremens*), confusion, and hallucinations. Withdrawal symptoms may be frightening and frequently result in a resumption of drinking. Many alcohol-dependent people need a drink in the morning to ward off the withdrawal syndrome.

**NARCOTIC DRUGS** *Heroin* or *morphine* withdrawal syndrome starts eight to 12 hours after the last dose and may last for seven to 10 days. At first, a craving for the drug is the most prominent feature, accompanied by restlessness, sweating, runny eyes and nose, and yawning. As the syndrome progresses, a variety of other symptoms appear, including diarrhea, vomiting, abdominal cramps, dilated pupils, loss of appetite, gooseflesh (the origin of the term "cold turkey"), irritability, tremor, weakness, and depression.

Other narcotic drugs, such as *codeine* and some prescription analgesics, cause withdrawal symptoms similar to those produced by heroin or morphine, but, if the doses have not been too high, these withdrawal symptoms may be less intense and may develop more slowly.

**TRANQUILIZERS** Withdrawal syndrome from *barbiturate drugs* and *meprobamate* begins from 12 to 24 hours after the last dose and has many similarities to alcohol withdrawal. The first symptoms are usually tremor, anxiety, restlessness, and weakness sometimes followed by delirium, hallucinations, and, in some cases, seizures. A period of prolonged sleep occurs just before the symptoms clear up, which is between three and eight days after onset, depending on the individual drug.

Withdrawal from *benzodiazepine drugs* may begin much more slowly (up to 14 days after the last dose) and can in some cases be life-threatening.

**TOBACCO SMOKING** Withdrawal symptoms from *nicotine* (the substance in tobacco responsible for dependence) develops gradually over 24 to 48 hours. In addition to a desperate desire to smoke, the most common

### DRUGS USED TO TREAT WORM INFESTATIONS

| Infestation | Drugs |
|---|---|
| Pinworm | Mebendazole, pyrantel |
| Common roundworm (ascariasis) | Mebendazole, pyrantel, piperazine |
| Whipworm | Mebendazole |
| Hookworm | Mebendazole |
| Strongyloidiasis | Thiabendazole |
| Toxocariasis | Mebendazole, thiabendazole |
| Tapeworms | Niclosamide, praziquantel |
| Filariasis | Diethylcarbamazine |
| Schistosomiasis | Praziquantel |

**Antihelmintic drugs**
Drugs such as those listed above are the main treatment for worm infestations. Usually just one or two doses are required but

symptoms are irritability, difficulty concentrating, frustration, headaches, and restless anxiety.

**OTHER DRUGS** Discontinuation of an amphetamine or cocaine results in lethargy, extreme tiredness, and dizziness. Cocaine withdrawal may also lead to severe depression, and sometimes other physical symptoms, such as tremor and sweating.

Chronic marijuana users have reported various withdrawal symptoms, including tremor, sweating, nausea, vomiting, diarrhea, irritability, and sleep disturbances.

Symptoms of caffeine withdrawal, consisting of tiredness, headaches, and irritability, may occur in people accustomed to drinking large quantities of tea, coffee, or caffeine-containing soft drinks. The onset of these symptoms usually occurs several hours after the last drink of caffeine-containing liquid.

## TREATMENT
Severe withdrawal syndromes require medical treatment. Symptoms may be suppressed by giving the patient small quantities of the drug he or she was using. More commonly, however, a substitute drug is given, such as *methadone* for narcotic drugs or *diazepam* for alcohol. The dose of the drug is then gradually reduced. This substitution process requires careful adjustment and can be safely managed only in a medical setting.

## Womb
See *Uterus.*

sometimes longer treatment is needed. Laxatives may also be given to aid expulsion of worms living in the intestines.

## Word blindness
See *Alexia; Dyslexia.*

## World Health Organization
The World Health Organization (WHO) was established in 1948 as an agency of the United Nations with responsibilities for international health matters and public health. Its headquarters is in Geneva, Switzerland; there are also regional offices for Europe, Africa, North America, South America, Southeast Asia, the Eastern Mediterranean, and the Western Pacific (including Australia).

The WHO has campaigned effectively against certain infectious diseases, notably smallpox (which was officially declared as eradicated throughout the world in 1980), tuberculosis, and malaria. Its other functions include sponsoring medical research programs, organizing a network of collaborating national laboratories, and providing expert advice to its 160 member states on matters such as health service organizations, family health, the use of medicinal drugs, the abuse of drugs, and mental health. The organization's current strategy is described in its campaign "Health for all by the year 2000." The plan gives specific targets for basic public health measures, such as the provision of piped water supplies and other basic sanitation, the universal provision of immunization of children against infectious diseases, and reductions in the use of tobacco and alcohol.

## Worm infestation

Several types of worm, or their larvae, can exist as parasites of humans. They range in size from the microscopic to many feet in length and may live in the intestines, blood, lymphatic system, bile ducts, or organs such as the liver. Worms are more common than is realized; in many cases, they cause few or no symptoms, and a person may have an infestation for many years without realizing it. Other worms can cause chronic, sometimes severe and debilitating, illness.

There are two main classes of worm—the *roundworms*, which have long, cylindrical bodies, and the platyhelminths, which have flattened bodies. The platyhelminths are further subdivided into the cestodes (tapeworms) and trematodes (flukes).

Worm diseases found in developed countries, such as the US, include *pinworm infestation, ascariasis, whipworm infestation, toxocariasis*, and *trichinosis* (all caused by different types of roundworm), *liver fluke*, and some types of *tapeworm infestation*. Important types in tropical regions include *hookworm infestation, filariasis*, and *guinea worm disease* (caused by roundworms), and *schistosomiasis* (caused by a type of fluke).

Worms may be acquired by eating undercooked, infected meat, by contact with soil or water containing worm larvae, by accidental ingestion of worm eggs (via fingers or food), from soil contaminated by infected feces, or in day-care centers where hygiene may be compromised.

The diagnosis of a worm infestation may be alarming but most types can be easily eradicated with *antihelmintic drugs* (see box opposite).

## Wound

Any damage to the skin and/or underlying tissues caused by an accident, act of violence, or surgery. Wounds in which the skin or mucous membrane are broken are called open; those in which they remain intact are termed closed.

### TYPES

Wounds can be divided into the following broad categories—an incised wound (an injury in which the skin is cleanly cut, or a surgical *incision*); an abrasion (a graze in which surface tissue is scraped away); a *laceration* (a wound in which the skin is torn, such as an animal or human *bite*); a penetrating wound (such as a stab or gunshot wound); and a contusion (a wound in which the underlying

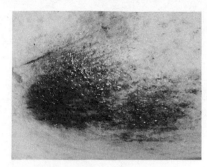

**Abrasion on arm**
Abrasions usually result from sliding falls and may contain dirt. They should be carefully cleaned and dressed.

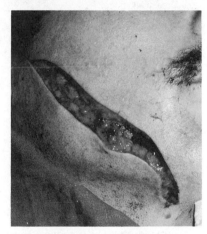

**Knife wound down side of face**
This is a deep, incised wound, cleanly cut, and likely to heal with minimal scarring once the edges have been sutured.

tissues are damaged by a blunt instrument). This type of soft tissue injury may include damage to subcutaneous tissue, muscle, bone, blood vessels, and/or nerves. When the wound lies over the thorax or abdomen, internal organs may also be bruised or more severely damaged. Considerable bleeding can occur with little outward evidence.

Many penetrating wounds and some contused wounds are deceptive in appearance, showing little external sign of damage but involving serious internal injury. Low-velocity gunshot injuries cause tissue damage all along the path of the projectile. High-velocity gunshot injuries may also damage distant structures as a result of shock waves traveling through tissues. In stab wounds, vital organs may be perforated or major blood vessels severed. In contusions, the liver, spleen, or kidney may be ruptured and cause internal bleeding.

### TREATMENT

Many minor wounds can be treated by first-aid measures (see *Bleeding, treatment of; Dressings*; and first-aid box on previous page). More extensive or deeper wounds require professional treatment.

If the wound contains any foreign material or dead tissue, it is removed; the wound is then cleansed with an antiseptic solution to decrease the risk of *wound infection*.

Clean, incised wounds may be closed by *suturing* if the wounds are fresh; they usually heal with minimal scarring. Lacerations may need to have the jagged skin edges cut away before they are stitched. Contaminated wounds are usually not closed.

Wounds in which there is extensive tissue damage and/or a high risk of infection are usually filled with layers of sterile gauze and covered with a bandage for four or five days. If, after this time, there is no sign of infection and the skin edges can be brought together without tension, the wound may be stitched. Otherwise, the wound may be left open and allowed to heal on its own.

Penetrating wounds or contusions may require an exploratory operation of the abdominal cavity (see *Laparotomy*) or the chest cavity (see *Thoracotomy*). Damage to blood vessels, nerves, or bones often necessitates repair by specialized surgical techniques, such as *microsurgery*. *Skin grafting* may also be required. (See also *Healing*.)

## Wound infection

Any type of wound is susceptible to the entry of bacteria; the resultant infection can delay healing, result in disability, or cause death. Complications of wound infection may result in local spread of the infection to adjacent organs or tissue or distant spread via the blood.

### SURGICAL WOUNDS

About 5 to 10 percent of surgical wounds become infected. Primary infection—occurring during the operation itself or while dressing the wound afterward—is a common occurrence despite routine *aseptic technique* (the creation of a germ-free environment). *Antibiotic drugs* are therefore administered as a preventive measure for 24 hours after surgery. Infection is more likely to develop in obese patients and in patients with reduced natural defenses against infection, such as the elderly and those suffering from cancer.

W

For surgery in which there is a higher-than-average risk of infection (such as an intestinal operation) or in which infection would have particularly serious consequences (such as a joint replacement operation), the patient is given antibiotic drugs as a preventive measure.

**NONSURGICAL WOUNDS**

Nonsurgical wounds most likely to become infected are wounds sustained in an agricultural accident or by soldiers in battle. There is a risk of the soilborne bacterium *CLOSTRIDIUM TETANI* causing the serious, sometimes fatal, infection *tetanus* or of related bacteria, such as *CLOSTRIDIUM PERFRINGENS*, causing gas *gangrene*.

In dealing with any serious nonsurgical wound, the physician attempts to prevent infection by removing any foreign material or dead tissue from the wound, thoroughly cleaning it with an antiseptic solution, and giving antibiotics. In addition, if there is a risk of the wound being contaminated with soil, an antitetanus injection is given unless the patient has received one within the previous five years.

**SIGNS AND TREATMENT**

The signs of infection in a wound are redness, swelling, warmth, pain, and sometimes the presence of pus. Pus is usually accompanied by an exquisitely tender dark swelling (an *abscess*) that either is draining pus or must be incised to permit drainage.

Once infection is discovered, a sample of blood or pus is taken and the patient is given an antibiotic drug. When a *culture* of the causative bacteria has been grown, treatment may need to be switched to a more appropriate antibiotic. Any abscess should be drained surgically.

## Wrinkle

A furrow in the skin. Wrinkling is a natural feature of aging caused by a reduction in collagen production and consequent loss of skin elasticity. Wrinkles are most obvious on the face and other exposed parts of the body but occur all over the skin. Premature deep wrinkling is usually caused by overexposure to sunlight.

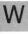

Despite the claims made for various "rejuvenating" skin preparations, treatments do not permanently restore skin elasticity. A *face-lift* smoothes out wrinkles by stretching the skin, but the effects last only about five years. *Vitamin A* derivatives are currently being evaluated as a means of reducing wrinkling.

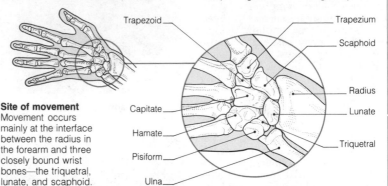

## STRUCTURE OF THE WRIST

The wrist is a complex joint that allows the hand to be bent forward and backward relative to the arm (through an angle of almost 180 degrees) and also moved side to side (through about 70 degrees).

Trapezoid — Trapezium — Scaphoid — Capitate — Hamate — Pisiform — Ulna — Radius — Lunate — Triquetral

**Site of movement**
Movement occurs mainly at the interface between the radius in the forearm and three closely bound wrist bones—the triquetral, lunate, and scaphoid.

## Wrist

The joint between the *hand* and the arm. The skeleton of the wrist consists of eight bones (known collectively as the carpus) arranged in two rows—the scaphoid, lunate, triquetral, and pisiform bones, which articulate with the radius and ulna (bones of the forearm); and the trapezium, trapezoid, capitate, and hamate, which are connected to the bones of the palm. The bones of the carpus articulate with each other.

Many tendons, which connect the forearm muscles to the fingers and thumb, run across the wrist. The extensor tendons, which straighten the fingers, are on the back of the wrist; the flexor tendons, which bend the fingers, are on the front. These tendons pass under ligaments to prevent them from springing away from the wrist. The gap between the ligaments and tendons at the front of the wrist is known as the carpal tunnel. Also passing across the wrist are the arteries and nerves supplying the muscles, bones, and skin of the hand and fingers.

**DISORDERS**

Wrist injuries may lead to serious disability by limiting hand movement. This is especially likely with fractures of the scaphoid bone, which often fail to heal, and with cutting injuries involving the tendons or nerves.

A common wrist injury in adults is *Colles' fracture*, in which the lower end of the radius is fractured and the wrist and hand are displaced backward. In young children, similar displacement results from a fracture through the epiphysis (growing end) of the radius.

*Sprain* of ligaments at the wrist joint can occur but is usually not severe.

Pressure on the median nerve as it passes through the carpal tunnel causes numbness, tingling, and pain in the thumb, index, and middle fingers (see *Carpal tunnel syndrome*). Damage to the radial nerve, which may be caused by fracture of the humerus (upper arm bone), results in *wristdrop* (inability to straighten the wrist).

Other conditions that may affect the wrist include *tenosynovitis* (inflammation of the inner lining of a tendon sheath) and *osteoarthritis*.

## Wristdrop

Inability to straighten the wrist, so that the back of the hand cannot be brought horizontal with the back of the forearm. This causes weakness of grip because the hand muscles can function efficiently only when the wrist is held straight.

Wristdrop is caused by damage to the *radial nerve*, usually at a point where it passes beneath the armpit or where it winds around the humerus (upper arm bone). The radial nerve may be damaged by prolonged pressure in the armpit (see *Crutch palsy*) or by a fracture of the humerus (see *Humerus, fracture of*).

Treatment involves holding the wrist straight. This may be achieved with a simple splint. However, if damage to the radial nerve is permanent, the usual treatment is *arthrodesis* (fusion) of the wrist bones.

## Wry neck

See *Torticollis*.

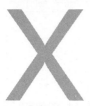

# X

## Xanthelasma

Yellowish deposits of fatty substance in the eyelids that are associated with a raised level of cholesterol in the blood. (See also *Xanthomatosis*.)

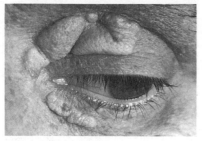

**Appearance of xanthelasma**
These fatty deposits around the eyes are common in elderly people but are usually of no more than cosmetic importance.

## Xanthoma

A yellow deposit of fatty material in the skin, often on the elbow or buttock. Xanthomas may indicate a lipid (fat) disorder. (See *Xanthomatosis*.)

## Xanthomatosis

A condition in which deposits of yellowish, fatty material occur in various parts of the body, particularly in the skin, internal organs, corneas, brain, and tendons. The deposits may occur in the eyelids only, a condition known as *xanthelasma*.

The most important feature of xanthomatosis is the tendency for cholesterol to be deposited in the linings of blood vessels, leading to generalized *atherosclerosis*.

Xanthomatosis is often associated with a range of disorders causing *hyperlipidemias* (raised levels of fats and cholesterol in the blood).

Treatment aims to lower the levels of fats and cholesterol in the blood. This is achieved by means of a diet that is low in cholesterol and high in polyunsaturated fat, and by drugs.

## Xeroderma pigmentosum

A rare, inherited skin disease. The skin is normal at birth, but extreme sensitivity to sunlight (see *Photosensitivity*) causes it to become dry, wrinkled, freckled, and prematurely aged by about the age of 5. Various types of benign and malignant skin tumors also develop. Xeroderma pigmentosum is often accompanied by conditions that involve the eye such as *photophobia* and *conjunctivitis*.

Treatment consists of preventing exposure to sunlight by wearing protective clothing and using *sunscreens*. Skin cancers are usually treated by surgical removal or with *anticancer drugs*.

## Xerophthalmia

An eye disorder in which vitamin A deficiency causes the conjunctiva and cornea to become abnormally dry. Without treatment, xerophthalmia may progress to *keratomalacia*, a condition in which there is severe damage to the cornea.

## Xerostomia

Abnormal dryness of the mouth (see *Mouth, dry*).

## Xiphisternum

An alternative name for the xiphoid process, the small, leaf-shaped projection that constitutes the lowest of the three parts of the *sternum* (breastbone).

## X-linked disorders

Sex-linked *genetic disorders* in which the abnormal gene or genes—the causative factors—are located on the X chromosome, and in which almost all those affected are males. *Color vision deficiency* and *hemophilia* are examples of this type of disorder. (See also *Fragile X syndrome*.)

## X rays

A form of invisible electromagnetic energy of short wavelength that is produced when high speed electrons strike a heavy metal. Discovered in 1896 by Wilhelm Conrad Roentgen, X rays are variably able to penetrate all substances. From the time of their discovery, X rays have been used to an increasingly important degree in medicine for both diagnosis and treatment.

**WHY THEY ARE USED**
X rays can be used to produce images of bones, organs, and internal tissues. Low doses of X rays are passed through the tissues and cast images—essentially shadows—onto film or a fluorescent screen. The X-ray image, also known as a radiograph or roentgenogram, shows structural changes in the area being examined.

X rays have the potential to damage living cells especially those that are dividing rapidly. Since cancer cells divide rapidly, high doses of radiation are used (along with other forms of radiant energy) for treating cancer (see *Radiation therapy*).

**HOW THEY WORK**
X rays are produced artificially by bombarding a small tungsten target with electrons in a device known as an X-ray tube (or cooling tube). The X rays that are emitted travel in straight lines and radiate outward from a point on the target in all directions. In an X-ray machine, the X-ray tube is surrounded by lead casing, except for a small aperture through which the X-ray beam emerges.

Each of the body's tissues absorbs X rays in a predictable way. Bones are dense and contain calcium; they absorb X rays well. Soft tissues—skin, fat, blood, and muscle—absorb X rays to a lesser extent. Thus, when an arm, for example, is placed in the path of an X-ray beam, the X rays pass readily through the soft tissues but penetrate the bones much less easily. The arm casts a shadow on film or a fluorescent screen, with the bone appearing white and the soft tissues dark gray.

**THE X-RAY EXAMINATION**
When a patient arrives for an X ray, the *X-ray technician* explains the procedure. The patient undresses to expose the area concerned; care is taken to remove any objects that might produce an image on the film, such as jewelry, hair clips, dentures, and wigs.

The position of the patient when the X ray is taken is carefully chosen to provide the clearest view of the part under examination, although this position may require modification if the patient is sick or in severe pain.

The X-ray film is usually contained in a flat cassette; the patient lies, sits, or stands with the region to be examined in contact with the cassette. Movement must be avoided while the X ray is taken since it results in a blurred image. Every effort is made to keep the patient comfortable and relaxed and to use the shortest possible exposure time—usually just a fraction of a second. If necessary, the region of interest can be supported or immobilized.

When the patient is in the correct position, the film is in place, and the X-ray tube is ready, the technician leaves the room for a few moments

## X-RAY EXAMINATION

Probably the best known of all imaging techniques, X rays are also one of the most useful, particularly for imaging the skeleton, the chest, and body conduits such as the blood vessels and digestive tract (after they have had a radiopaque material introduced into them).

Modern X-ray equipment is designed to produce high-quality images at the lowest possible radiation dose to the patient.

### Procedure
The technician makes sure the patient is correctly positioned, checks that the X-ray tube is ready, and then goes to a control panel behind a protective screen and presses a button to take the X ray. The technician can see and talk to the patient from behind the screen.

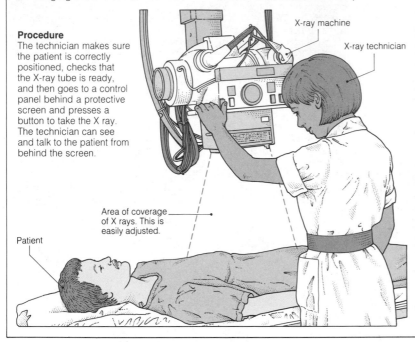

X-ray machine

X-ray technician

Area of coverage of X rays. This is easily adjusted.

Patient

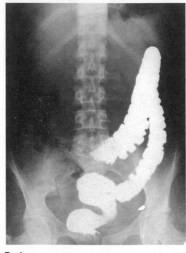

**Barium enema**
This X ray shows the lower part of the large intestine outlined by a radio-opaque contrast medium containing a barium compound.

and presses the exposure button on the control panel to take the X ray.

Once the X-ray film has been developed, it is interpreted by a *radiologist*. Some disorders, such as fractures, are immediately recognizable; others, such as some tumors, may take more time to assess.

### SPECIAL X-RAY TECHNIQUES
Hollow or fluid-filled parts of the body often do not show up well on X-ray film unless they first have a contrast medium introduced into them. Such contrast-medium techniques are used to look at the gallbladder (see *Cholecystography*), the bile ducts (see *Cholangiography*), the urinary tract (see *Pyelography*), the gastrointestinal tract (see *Barium X-ray examinations*), the blood vessels (see *Angiography*; *Venography*), the spinal cord (see *Myelography*), and the joint spaces (see *Arthrography*).

X rays can be used to obtain an image of a "slice" through an organ or part of the body by using a technique known as *tomography*. More detailed and accurate images of a body slice are produced by combining tomography with the capabilities of a computer (see *CT scanning*).

### X-RAY SAFETY
It is now understood that large doses of radiation can be extremely harmful (see *Radiation hazards*). Modern X-ray film, equipment, and techniques are designed specifically to produce high-quality images at the lowest possible radiation dose (exposure) to the patient. The possible hazard of genetic damage can be minimized by using a lead shield to protect the patient's reproductive organs from the X-ray beam. X-ray examinations are also generally avoided if there is any possibility of pregnancy.

X-ray technicians and radiologists wear a *film badge* to monitor their exposure to radiation. (See also *Imaging techniques*.)

## X rays, dental
See *Dental X rays*.

## X-ray technician
A person who prepares patients for *X-ray* examinations, takes and develops X-ray pictures, and assists with other imaging techniques.

The X-ray technician gives the patient any special instructions that he or she must follow during the X-ray examination. Once the examination begins, the technician is responsible for positioning the patient to provide the best possible picture of the part being studied.

X-ray technicians also assist *radiologists* in performing specialized X-ray examinations (such as contrast-medium studies) and carrying out other imaging procedures, such as *radionuclide scanning, ultrasound scanning,* and *MRI*. The sources of energy that produce the images for these last procedures are beta particles or gamma rays from radionuclides, high-frequency sound waves, and electromagnetic waves generated by extremely powerful magnets.

## Xylometazoline
A *decongestant drug* used to relieve nasal congestion caused by a common *cold, sinusitis,* or hay fever (see *Rhinitis, allergic*). Available in nose drops or nasal sprays, xylometazoline works by narrowing the small blood vessels in the lining of the nose.

Excessive use of xylometazoline may cause headache, palpitations, or drowsiness. Long-term use may cause congestion to become worse.

X

## USING X RAYS TO LOOK AT THE BODY

X rays are perhaps the most widely used method of imaging the body. When passed through body tissues onto photographic film, X rays cast images of internal structures, allowing alterations in silhouette to be seen. Soft tissues do not show up as well as bone on X rays, but, by using a contrast medium, they too can be visualized. New computer techniques produce even clearer, more detailed images.

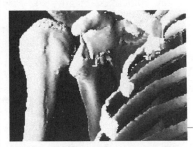

**3-D CT scan**
A computer can transform X-ray images of body slices into a three-dimensional image of part of the body. This scan shows a badly damaged shoulder blade.

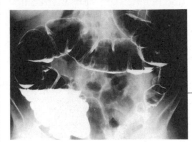

**Barium X ray**
Introducing barium, which is opaque to X rays, into the large intestine allows it to be visualized.

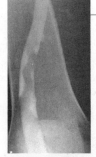

**Venography**
This technique for examining veins involves injecting them with a contrast medium before they are X rayed. The femoral vein shown here (in the foreground) is partially blocked by blood clots.

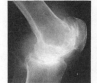

**X rays of knee joint**
The X ray at left shows erosion of bone and cartilage. The parts of an artificial knee are seen in the X ray at right.

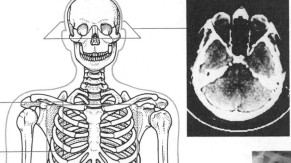

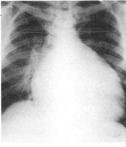

**CT scan**
Combined use of a computer and X rays produces cross-sectional images. In this brain scan, the eyes and nose are seen at the top; the central light area represents the brain stem.

**Chest X ray**
This heart appears enlarged due to excess fluid around it.

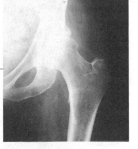

**X ray of hip joint**
This X ray of an osteo-arthritic hip shows almost complete degener-ation of the cartilage.

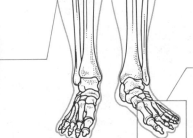

**X ray of foot**
All the bones can be clearly seen in this X ray of a 4-year-old's foot.

X

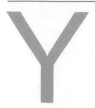

## Yawning

An involuntary act, usually associated with drowsiness or boredom, in which the mouth is opened wide and a slow, deep breath taken through it. Yawning is accompanied by a momentary increase in the heart rate, slight constriction of some blood capillaries, and, in many cases, watering of the eyes (possibly because of pressure on the tear glands as a result of the facial movements).

The purpose of yawning is unknown, but one theory suggests it is triggered by raised levels of carbon dioxide in the blood; thus, its purpose may be to reduce the blood carbon dioxide level and increase the blood oxygen level.

## Yaws

A disease found throughout poorer subtropical and tropical areas of the world that is caused by a spirochete (spiral-shaped bacterium) very similar to that which causes syphilis. Yaws is not, however, a sexually transmitted disease. The infection is almost always acquired in childhood.

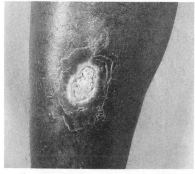

**Yaws ulcer on leg**
Yaws is an infection that mainly affects the skin and bones. Ulceration and tissue destruction may occur in advanced cases.

Three or four weeks after infection, a single, highly infectious, itchy, raspberrylike growth appears at the site of infection. Scratching spreads the infection and leads to the develop-

ment of more growths elsewhere on the skin. Without treatment, the growths heal slowly over the course of about six months. Recurrence of the growths is common.

Yaws can be cured by a single large dose of a penicillin. In about 10 percent of untreated cases, widespread tissue loss eventually occurs. This may lead to gross destruction of the skin, bones, and joints of the legs, nose, palate, and upper jaw.

## Yeasts

Types of *fungi*. Certain yeasts can cause infections of the skin or mucous membranes. The most important disease-causing yeast is CANDIDA ALBICANS, which causes *candidiasis*.

## Yellow fever

 An infectious disease of short duration and variable severity caused by a virus transmitted by mosquitoes. In severe cases, the skin of the sufferer becomes yellow from jaundice—hence the name yellow fever.

**CAUSES**
Today, yellow fever can be contracted only in Central America, parts of South America, and a large area of Africa. In forest areas, various species of mosquitoes may spread the infection from monkeys to humans. In urban areas, the disease is transmitted between humans by AEDES AEGYPTI mosquitoes.

**PREVENTION**
Eradication of the causative mosquito from populated areas has greatly reduced the incidence of yellow fever. Vaccination confers long-lasting immunity and should always be obtained before travel to or through affected areas. A vaccination certificate is required for entry to many countries, including parts of Asia as well as other countries where the disease is prevalent.

A single injection of the vaccine gives protection for at least 10 years. Children under 1 year of age should not be vaccinated. Reactions to the vaccine are rare and usually trivial.

**SYMPTOMS AND SIGNS**
Three to six days after infection, there is sudden onset of fever and headache, often with nausea and nose bleeding. Characteristically, despite the high fever, the heart rate is very slow. In many cases, the patient recovers in three days.

In more serious cases, the fever is higher and there is severe headache and pain in the neck, back, and legs.

Damage may occur rapidly to the liver and kidneys, causing jaundice and *renal failure*. This may be followed by a stage of severe agitation and delirium, leading to coma and death.

**DIAGNOSIS AND TREATMENT**
During epidemics, diagnosis is easy. Doubt is resolved by isolating the virus from the blood or by the demonstration of *antibodies* to the virus by a type of *immunoassay*.

No drug is effective against the yellow fever virus; treatment is directed at maintaining the blood volume. Transfusion of fluids is often necessary. In mild and moderate cases, the outlook is excellent and complications are few. Relapses do not occur and one attack confers lifelong immunity. Overall, however, about 10 percent of victims die.

## Yin and yang

Fundamental concepts in traditional *Chinese medicine* and philosophy. Yang embodies positive, active, "male" qualities and thus complements yin, which embodies negative, passive, "female" qualities. The concepts of yin and yang are also central to the theoretical basis of *macrobiotics*.

## Yoga

A system of Hindu philosophy and physical discipline. The main form of yoga practiced in the West is hatha-yoga, in which the follower adopts a series of poses, known as asanas, and uses a special breathing technique. This maintains flexibility of the body, teaches physical and mental control, and is a useful aid to *relaxation*.

If attempted by people in poor health or practiced incorrectly, yoga may pose health hazards, such as back disorders, *hypertension* (high blood pressure), and *glaucoma* (increased pressure in the eye).

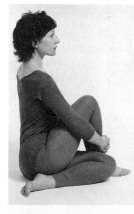

**Yoga pose**
This photograph shows a stage of the full twist asana, which is excellent for promoting flexibility.

# Z

## Zidovudine

An *antiviral drug* formerly known as azidothymidine (AZT). Zidovudine was approved for use in the treatment of *AIDS* in April 1987.

### WHY IT IS USED

Zidovudine is used to reduce the severity of AIDS-related conditions, such as *pneumocystis pneumonia* and infections of the brain and nervous system caused by the AIDS virus. Zidovudine does not cure these conditions but may improve symptoms or prolong remission. For example, it may reduce lymph gland swelling and promote weight gain. Although zidovudine slows the progress of AIDS, relapse commonly occurs after several months of treatment.

### HOW IT WORKS

Zidovudine blocks the action of the enzyme that stimulates the AIDS virus to grow and multiply. Clinical trials have shown that the resultant reduction in virus activity leads to an increase in the production and number of T-helper lymphocytes (a type of white blood cell). This in turn improves the efficiency of the immune system, making the occurrence of *opportunistic infections*, such as candidiasis (thrush), less likely. Zidovudine does not appear to stop the growth of other viruses.

### POSSIBLE ADVERSE EFFECTS

By reducing the number of red blood cells produced, zidovudine often causes severe *anemia*, requiring blood transfusion. For this reason, regular blood tests are performed and the drug is withdrawn if the blood count is dangerously low. Too high a dose of zidovudine may cause restlessness, insomnia, and fever.

Zidovudine also impairs the absorption and thus the effectiveness of *trimethoprim* and *sulfamethoxazole*, the antibiotic drugs used to treat pneumonia in people who have AIDS.

## Zinc

A *trace element* that is essential for normal growth, development of the reproductive organs, normal functioning of the prostate gland, healing of wounds, and the manufacture of proteins and nucleic acids (the genetic material of cells). Zinc also controls the activities of more than 100 enzymes and is involved in the functioning of the hormone insulin.

Small amounts of the element are present in a wide variety of foods; particularly rich sources include lean meat, whole-grain breads and cereals, dried beans, and seafood.

### DEFICIENCY

A balanced diet that contains natural, unprocessed foods provides sufficient zinc for the body's needs, so deficiency is rare; it most often occurs in people who are generally malnourished. Zinc deficiency may also be caused by a disorder that impairs intestinal absorption of the mineral (see *Malabsorption*; *Acrodermatitis enteropathica*) or by increased zinc requirements due to cell damage (e.g., as a result of a burn or in *sickle cell anemia*). Symptoms of deficiency include impairment of taste and loss of appetite; in severe cases, there may also be hair loss and inflammation of the skin, mouth, tongue, and eyelids. In children, zinc deficiency may impair physical growth and delay sexual development.

### EXCESS

Prolonged, excessive intake of zinc (usually through supplements) may interfere with the intestinal absorption of iron and copper, leading to a deficiency of these minerals and resultant symptoms of nausea, vomiting, fever, headache, tiredness, and abdominal pain.

### MEDICAL USES

Zinc compounds, such as *zinc oxide*, are included in many preparations for treating skin and scalp disorders.

## Zinc oxide

An ingredient of many skin preparations that has a mild *astringent* (drying) action and a soothing effect. Zinc oxide is used to treat painful, itchy, or

### A SELECTION OF ZOONOSES (DISEASES CAUGHT FROM ANIMALS)

| Animal | Disease | Animal | Disease |
|--------|---------|--------|---------|
| Bat | Histoplasmosis<br>Rabies | Parrot | Psittacosis |
| Cat | Toxoplasmosis<br>Cat-scratch fever<br>Fungal infections | Pig | Trichinosis<br>Pork tapeworm<br>Brucellosis |
| Cow | Brucellosis<br>Beef tapeworm<br>Q fever<br>Cowpox | Rabbit | Tularemia |
| Dog | Rabies<br>Toxocariasis<br>Mite infestations<br>Fungal infections | Rat | Leptospirosis<br>Plague<br>Rat-bite fever |
| Horse | Glanders<br>Equine encephalitis | Sheep | Liver fluke<br>Anthrax |
| Monkey | Yellow fever | Turtle | Salmonella infection |

**Relative importance**
With the exception of fungal infections and mites caught from pets, all the above are rare in the US. Some are confined to the tropics—such as yellow fever, which is not caught from monkeys directly, but can be transmitted from monkeys to humans by mosquitoes. Apart from the animals listed, bites from various other species (e.g., skunks, foxes, and mongeese) may transmit rabies to humans in different parts of the world.

moist skin conditions (such as eczema, bedsores, and diaper rash) and to ease the pain caused by hemorrhoids and insect bites or stings. It also blocks the ultraviolet rays of the sun.

Zinc oxide is also used to thicken lotions and creams, making them easier to apply.

## Zollinger-Ellison syndrome

A rare condition characterized by severe and recurrent *peptic ulcers* in the stomach, duodenum, and upper small intestine.

Zollinger-Ellison syndrome is caused by a tumor, usually found in the pancreas, that secretes the hormone gastrin; the hormone stimulates the stomach and duodenum to produce large quantities of acid, which leads to ulceration. The high levels of acid in the digestive tract also cause diarrhea and steatorrhea (fat in the feces) in almost half the sufferers.

The condition often goes unrecognized until the surgery for the peptic ulcers is rapidly followed by a recurrence of the ulceration. Once suspicion is aroused, the physician performs blood tests; high levels of gastrin are usually sufficient to confirm the diagnosis.

The tumor (or, more frequently, tumors) is most often cancerous, although of a slow-growing type. If possible, the tumor or tumors are removed surgically; otherwise, total *gastrectomy* (surgical removal of the stomach) is necessary.

## Zoonosis

Any infectious or parasitic disease of animals that can be transmitted to humans. Many disease organisms can infect only humans or particular animals, but zoonotic organisms are more flexible and can adapt themselves to many different species.

Zoonoses are usually caught from animals closely associated with humans, either as pets (such as dogs, cats, or parrots), food sources (such as pigs or cattle), or scavenging parasites (such as rats). Examples include *toxocariasis* (from dogs), *cat-scratch fever* and some *fungal infections* (from cats), *psittacosis* (from parrots or other birds), *brucellosis* (from cows, goats, or swine), *trichinosis* (from pigs), and *leptospirosis* (from rats). *Rabies* can infect virtually any mammal, but dog bites are a common cause of human infection worldwide.

Other zoonoses are transmitted from animals less obviously associated with humans, usually by insect

### TECHNIQUE OF Z-PLASTY
This relatively simple plastic surgery technique is carried out to revise unsightly scars or to relieve skin tension caused by scar contracture.

It can be particularly useful for dealing with facial scars or ones that cross natural skin creases.

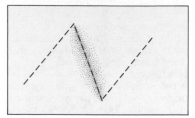

**1** Three incisions are made, forming a Z. The central incision is made lengthwise through the scar.

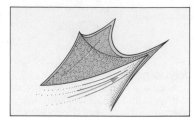

**2** Two triangular flaps are developed by cutting skin away from underlying tissue, and the flaps are then transposed.

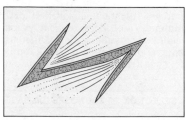

**3** This maneuver creates a new Z, of which the central arm is at right angles to the original direction of the scar.

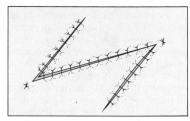

**4** The flaps are sutured in place. With careful planning, the suture lines can be hidden in natural skin creases.

*vectors*. For example, some cases of *yellow fever* are transmitted from forest monkeys to humans via the bites of mosquitoes. (See also *Dogs, diseases from; Cats, diseases from; Rats, diseases from; Insects and disease*.)

## Z-plasty

A technique used in *plastic surgery* to change the direction of a scar so that it can be hidden in natural skin creases or to relieve skin tension caused by scar *contracture*. Z-plasty is especially useful for revising unsightly scars on the face and for releasing scarring across joints, such as on the fingers or in the armpits, that may restrict movement or cause deformity.

A Z-shaped incision is made with the central arm of the Z along the scar. Two V-shaped flaps are created by cutting the skin away from underlying tissue. The flaps are then transposed and stitched. The procedure has the effect of redistributing tension perpendicular to the original defect.

## Zygote

The cell produced when a *sperm* fertilizes an *ovum*. A zygote contains all the genetic (hereditary) material for a new person—half coming from sperm and

half from the ovum. Measuring about 4 thousandths of an inch (0.1 mm) in diameter, a zygote is much larger than other body cells. It travels down one of the woman's fallopian tubes toward the uterus, dividing as it does so, but without growing larger. After about a week, the mass of cells (now called a blastocyst) implants into the lining of the uterus, and the next stage of embryological growth begins.

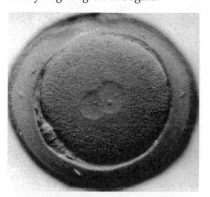

**Appearance of zygote**
The photograph shows a human egg just after fertilization by a sperm. The two circular areas at center are the nuclei of the sperm and egg merging.

Z

# SELF-HELP
# ORGANIZATIONS,
# DRUG GLOSSARY,
# AND INDEX

# SELF-HELP ORGANIZATIONS

The following list gives the names and telephone numbers of various organizations and support groups that exist to help people with particular health problems. Even if no specific support group is mentioned for your particular problem, it may be worth contacting one of the more broadly based groups for a referral.

Some numbers offer recorded information, others provide personalized counseling or referrals. In general, diagnoses and recommendations for treatment are not offered.

Portions of this information were derived from the *Healthfinder* booklet published by the US Department of Health and Human Services.

## ABORTION AND BIRTH CONTROL

**Planned Parenthood Hotline**
(800) 223-3303

Provides referrals to local clinics that offer abortion, birth control, pregnancy testing, and obstetrical/gynecological services, and screening for sexually transmitted diseases.

## ACQUIRED IMMUNODEFICIENCY SYNDROME (AIDS)

**AIDS Information Hotline Public Health Service**
(800) 342-AIDS

Provides information to the public on the prevention and spread of AIDS.

**National Gay Task Force Crisisline**
(800) 221-7044
(212) 529-1604 in NY, AK, and HI

Offers basic information on AIDS, including symptoms, possible causes, and preventive measures. Provides referrals.

## ALCOHOLISM

**Al-Anon Family Group Headquarters**
(800) 356-9996
(212) 245-3151 in NY and Canada

Provides printed materials on alcoholism specifically aimed at helping families.

**Alcoholism and Drug Addiction Treatment Center**
(800) 382-4357

Refers adolescents and adults to local facilities for help.

**National Council on Alcoholism**
(800) NCA-CALL

Refers to local affiliates and provides written information on alcoholism.

## ALZHEIMER'S DISEASE

**Alzheimer's Disease and Related Disorders Association**
(800) 621-0379
(800) 572-6037 in IL

Offers information on publications available from the association. Refers callers to local chapters and support groups.

## CANCER

**AMC Cancer Information**
(800) 525-3777

Provides information on causes of cancer, prevention, methods of detection and diagnosis, treatment and treatment facilities, rehabilitation, and counseling services. A service of AMC Cancer Research Center, Denver.

**Cancer Information Service (CIS)**
(800) 4-CANCER
(808) 524-1234 in Oahu (neighbor islands call collect)
(800) 638-6070 in AK

Answers cancer-related questions from the public, cancer patients and families, and health professionals. No diagnosis made or treatment recommended. Spanish-speaking staff available to callers from the following areas: CA, FL, GA, IL, northern NJ, New York City, and TX. A service of the National Cancer Institute.

## CHILD ABUSE

**National Child Abuse Hotline**
(800) 422-4453

Provides information and professional counseling on child abuse. Gives referrals to local social service groups offering counseling on child abuse.

**Parents Anonymous Hotline**
(800) 421-0353
(800) 352-0386 in CA

Provides information on self-help groups for parents involved in child abuse.

## CHILDREN

**National Child Safety Council Childwatch**
(800) 222-1464

Answers questions from callers and distributes literature on safety, including drug abuse, household dangers, and electricity. Provides safety information to local police departments.

**National Hotline for Missing Children**
(800) 843-5678
(202) 644-9836 in DC

Operates a hotline for reporting missing children and sightings of missing children. Offers assistance to law enforcement agents. A service of the National Center for Missing and Exploited Children.

**National Runaway Switchboard**
(800) 621-4000

Provides counseling and traveler's assistance to runaways. Gives referrals to shelters nationwide. Also relays messages to, or sets up conference calls with, parents at the request of the child.

## COOLEY'S ANEMIA

**Cooley's Anemia Foundation**
(800) 221-3571
(212) 598-0911 in New York City

Provides information on patient care, research, fund-raising, patient-support groups, and research grants. Makes referrals to local chapters.

## CYSTIC FIBROSIS

**Cystic Fibrosis Foundation**
(800) 344-4823
(301) 951-4422 in MD

Responds to patient and family questions and offers literature. Provides referrals to local clinics.

## DIABETES

**American Diabetes Association**
(800) 232-3472
(703) 549-1500 in VA and DC metro area

Provides free literature, newsletter, and information on health education and support group assistance.

**Juvenile Diabetes Foundation International Hotline**
(800) 223-1138
(212) 889-7575 in NY

Answers questions and provides brochures on juvenile diabetes. Gives referrals to physicians and clinics.

## DOWN'S SYNDROME

**National Down Syndrome Congress**
(800) 232-6372
(309) 452-3264 in IL

Answers questions from parents for assistance with health concerns. Refers to local organizations.

**National Down Syndrome Society Hotline**
(800) 221-4602
(212) 460-9330 in NY

Offers information on Down's syndrome and gives referrals to local programs for the newborn. Provides free information packet upon request.

## DRUG ABUSE

**"Just Say No" Kids Club**
(800) 258-2766

Responds to questions on how to start a club for 7 to 14 year olds.

**National Cocaine Hotline**
(800) COCAINE

Answers questions on the health risks of cocaine and provides counseling to cocaine users and their friends and families. Provides referrals. A service of Fair Oaks Hospital, Summit, NJ.

**National Federation of Parents for Drug-Free Youth**
(800) 554-KIDS
(301) 585-5437 in MD

Provides referrals to parent-support groups for parents of children with drug and alcohol problems. Sends educational materials.

**National Parents' Resource Institute for Drug Education (PRIDE)**
(800) 241-7946
(404) 658-2548 in GA

Provides a broad range of materials on drug-related issues, including alcohol and legal questions. Refers callers to related organizations for further information.

**NIDA Helpline**
(800) 662-HELP

Provides general information on drug abuse and on AIDS as it relates to intravenous drug users. Referrals offered. A service of the National Institute on Drug Abuse.

**Office of Substance Abuse Prevention**
(800) 638-2045
(301) 443-6500 in MD

Offers information and technical assistance to schools, parent groups, business and industry, and national organizations in developing drug abuse prevention activities. Does not provide crisis counseling, intervention treatment referral, or information on the pharmacology or criminal aspects of drugs.

## EATING DISORDERS

**Anorexia Bulimia Treatment and Education Center**
(800) 33-ABTEC
(301) 332-9800 in MD

Answers questions and provides literature on the disorders. A service of Mercy Hospital, Baltimore.

**Bulimia Anorexia Self-Help**
(800) 227-4785
(800) 762-3334 for 24-hour crisis information

Provides information on bulimia, anorexia, depression, anxiety, and phobias. Refers to local resources.

## FITNESS

**Aerobics and Fitness Foundation**
(800) BE FIT 86

Answers questions from the public regarding safe and effective exercise programs and practices.

## GENERAL HEALTH

**American Medical Radio News**
(800) 621-8094

Offers prerecorded messages that highlight daily health news and feature stories. A service of the American Medical Association.

**ODPHP National Health Information Center**
(800) 336-4797
(202) 429-9091 in DC

Provides a central source of information for health educators, health professionals, and the general public. No diagnosis made or treatment recommended. Spanish-speaking staff available. A service of the Office of Disease Prevention and Health Promotion, US Department of Health and Human Services.

## HANDICAPS
### (See also HEARING AND SPEECH and VISION)

**HEATH Resource Center**
(800) 544-3284
(202) 939-9320 in DC

Provides information on secondary education for the handicapped and on learning disabilities.

**Job Accommodation Network**
(800) 526-7234
(800) 526-4698 in WV

Offers ideas for accommodating handicapped persons in the workplace and information on obtaining aids and procedures.

**Library of Congress National Library Services for the Blind and Physically Handicapped**
(800) 424-8567
(202) 287-5100 in DC

Provides both audio and Braille formats for the blind and physically handicapped, or anyone who is unable to read print for any reason, through a network of state libraries.

## National Information System for Health Related Services (NIS)
(800) 922-9234
(800) 922-1107 in SC

Makes referrals to specialized services that emphasize diagnosis, treatment, and support for developmentally disabled and chronically ill children.

## National Rehabilitation Center
(800) 34-NARIC
(202) 635-5822 in DC

Provides rehabilitation information on assistive devices and disseminates other rehabilitation-related information.

### HEADACHE

## National Headache Foundation
(800) 843-2256
(800) 523-8858 in IL

Offers membership information and sends literature on headaches and their treatment.

### HEARING AND SPEECH

## American Cleft Palate Association
(800) 24-CLEFT
(800) 23-CLEFT in PA

Offers basic information to parents and health professionals on cleft palate syndrome. Makes referrals to local support groups and sends information, including lists of plastic surgeons, dentists, and speech pathologists for patients' review. The association does not refer individuals to specific physicians.

## Dial a Hearing Test
(800) 222-EARS
(800) 345-EARS in PA

Answers questions on hearing problems and makes referrals to local numbers for a two-minute hearing test, as well as referrals to ear, nose, and throat specialists. Also makes referrals to organizations that have information on ear-related problems, including questions on broken hearing aids.

## Grapevine
(800) 352-8888
(800) 346-8888 in CA

Offers information on deafness, including answers for raising and educating a deaf child. Refers callers to parents, professionals, and other resources in their own communities nationwide.

## Hearing Helpline
(800) 424-8576
(703) 642-0580 in VA

Provides information on better hearing and preventing deafness. Materials are mailed to callers on request. A service of the Better Hearing Institute.

## National Association for Hearing and Speech Action Line
(800) 638-8255
(301) 897-0039 in HI, AK, and MD call collect

Offers information and distributes materials on pathologists and audiologists certified by the American Speech-Language-Hearing Association for hearing and speech problems and hearing aids.

## National Hearing Aid Helpline
(800) 521-5247
(313) 478-2610 in MI

Provides information and distributes a directory of hearing aid specialists certified by the National Hearing Aid Society.

### HEART DISEASE

## Heartlife
(800) 241-6993
(404) 523-0826 in GA

Answers questions on heart diseases and pacemakers and distributes a quarterly periodical entitled *Pulse*.

### HOSPITAL CARE

## Hill-Burton Hospital Free Care
(800) 638-0742
(800) 492-0359 in MD

Provides a recording on hospitals and other health facilities participating in the Hill-Burton Hospital Free Care Program. A service of the Bureau of Resources Development, US Department of Health and Human Services.

## Shriners Hospital Referral Line
(800) 237-5055
(800) 282-9161 in FL

Gives information on free hospital care available to children under 18 who need orthopedic care or burn treatment. Sends application forms to those who meet eligibility requirements for treatment provided by 22 Shriners Hospitals in the US, Mexico, and Canada.

### HOSPICE CARE

## Hospice Education Institute Hospicelink
(800) 331-1620
(203) 767-1620 in CT

Offers general information about hospice care and makes referrals to local programs. Does not offer medical advice or counseling.

### HUNTINGTON'S CHOREA

## Huntington's Disease Society of America
(800) 345-4372
(212) 242-1968 in NY

Gives information on the disease and provides referrals to physicians and support groups. Answers questions on presymptomatic testing.

### IMPOTENCE

## Recovery of Male Potency
(800) 835-7667
(313) 966-3219 in MI

Provides referrals to self-help support groups and other agencies. Distributes an information packet. A service of Grace Hospital, Detroit, and affiliated with 23 hospitals nationwide.

### KIDNEY DISEASES

## American Kidney Fund
(800) 638-8299
(800) 492-8361 in MD

Grants financial assistance to kidney patients who are unable to pay treatment-related costs. Also provides information on the donation of organs and on kidney-related diseases.

### LEARNING DISORDERS
(See also HANDICAPS)

## The Orton Dyslexia Society
(800) ABCD-123

Answers questions about dyslexia and about how to become a

member of this society and makes referrals to other members of the society. Written materials are also available.

## LEPROSY (HANSEN'S DISEASE)

**American Leprosy Missions**
(800) 543-3131
(201) 794-8650 in NJ

Answers questions and distributes materials on the disease.

## LIVER DISEASES

**American Liver Foundation**
(800) 223-0179
(201) 857-2626 in NJ

Provides callers with information, including fact sheets. The foundation also makes physician referrals.

## LUNG DISEASE

**Lung Line**
**National Asthma Center**
(800) 222-5864
(303) 355-LUNG in Denver

Answers questions about asthma, emphysema, chronic bronchitis, allergies, juvenile rheumatoid arthritis, smoking, and other respiratory and immune system disorders. Callers' questions are answered by registered nurses or other health professionals. A service of the National Jewish Center for Immunology and Respiratory Medicine.

## LUPUS

**Lupus Foundation of America**
(800) 558-0121
(202) 328-4550 in DC

Answers basic questions about the disease and provides health professionals and patients and their families with information and literature. Refers callers to local affiliates.

## MENTAL HEALTH

**American Mental Health Fund**
(800) 433-5959
(800) 826-2336 in IL

Makes available via recorded message the AMHF pamphlet that includes general information about the organization, mental health, and warning signs of mental illness.

**National Alliance for the Mentally Ill**
(703) 524-7600

Self-help advocacy organization for families of people with mental illness. Refers callers to its more than 600 state and local affiliates.

## NEUROFIBROMATOSIS

**National Neurofibromatosis Foundation**
(800) 323-7938
(212) 460-8980 in NY

Responds to inquiries from health professionals and from patients and their families. Makes referrals to physicians on the clinical advisory board.

## ORGANS
## (See also KIDNEY DISEASES and RETINITIS PIGMENTOSA)

**The Living Bank**
(800) 528-2971
(713) 528-2971 in TX

Operates a registry and referral service for people wanting to commit their tissues, bones, or vital organs to transplantation or research. Offers information to the public about organ donation and transplantation.

**Organ Donor Hotline**
(800) 24-DONOR
(800) 552-2138 in VA

Offers information and referrals for organ donation and transplantation. Answers callers' requests for organ donor cards.

## PARALYSIS AND SPINAL CORD INJURY
## (See also HANDICAPS)

**American Paralysis Association**
(800) 225-0292
(201) 379-2690 in NJ

Answers questions about research on head and spinal injuries. Raises money to fund research to find a cure for paralysis caused by spinal and head injuries or stroke.

**National Spinal Cord Injury Association**
(800) 962-9629
(617) 964-0521 in MA

Provides peer counseling to those suffering from spinal cord injuries and makes referrals to local chapters and other organizations. Produces the *National Resource Directory*, which deals with topics that are helpful to people who have handicaps.

**Spinal Cord Injury Hotline**
(800) 526-3456
(800) 638-1733 in MD

Offers literature on spinal cord injuries, including a quarterly newsletter, and makes referrals to a variety of organizations and support groups. This hotline is a service of the Maryland Institute for Emergency Medical Services Systems.

## PARKINSON'S DISEASE

**National Parkinson Foundation**
(800) 327-4545
(800) 433-7022 in FL
(305) 547-6666 in Miami

Questions about the disease answered by nurses. Also makes physician referrals and provides written materials.

**Parkinson's Education Program**
(800) 344-7872
(714) 640-0218 in CA

Provides materials such as newsletters, glossary of definitions, and publications catalog, and offers patient-support group information and physician referrals.

## PESTICIDES

**National Pesticide Telecommunications Network**
(800) 858-7378
(806) 743-3091 in TX

Responds to nonemergency questions concerning the effects of pesticides, toxicology and symptoms, environmental effects, waste disposal and cleanup, and safe use of pesticides. The National Pesticide Telecommunications Network is a service of the Environmental Protection Agency and Texas Tech University.

## PLASTIC SURGERY

**American Society of Plastic and Reconstructive Surgeons**
(800) 635-0635

Provides referrals to board-certified plastic surgeons nationwide and from Canada. Offers pamphlets describing plastic and reconstructive procedures and realistic results of some operations.

## PREGNANCY

**ASPO/Lamaze (American Society for Psychoprophylaxis in Obstetrics)**
(800) 368-4404
(703) 524-7802 in VA

Provides list of local certified childbirth educators for people who are interested in this type of birth method. The Virginia number gives information on local Lamaze classes and on becoming a certified Lamaze educator.

**Bethany Lifeline**
(800) 238-4269

Provides callers with referrals to professional counseling services, adoption services, shepherding home care, and limited group home placement.

**The Edna Gladney Home**
(800) 433-2922
(800) 772-2740 in TX
(817) 926-3304 (call collect for 24-hour service)

Provides a residential program for unwed, pregnant women in addition to counseling, schooling, and adoption services.

**National Pregnancy Hotline**
(800) 852-5683
(800) 831-5881 in CA
(213) 380-8750 in Los Angeles

Provides pregnant women with a full range of information, counseling services, and referrals.

**Pregnancy Crisis Center**
(800) 368-3336
(804) 847-6828 in VA only

Provides a residential program for unwed mothers as well as shepherding homes for those over 18. The center is run by Family Life Services and is also an adoption agency.

## RARE DISEASES

**National Information Center for Orphan Drugs and Rare Diseases**
(800) 336-4797
(202) 429-9091 in DC

Gathers and disseminates information to patients, health professionals, and the public.

## RETINITIS PIGMENTOSA

**National Retinitis Pigmentosa Foundation**
(800) 638-2300
(301) 225-9400 in MD

Covers genetics, current research, and retina donor programs. Responds to questions and makes available an information packet on the disease.

## REYE'S SYNDROME

**National Reye's Syndrome Foundation**
(800) 233-7393
(800) 231-7393 in OH

Provides callers with general information and referrals to families for peer counseling.

## SAFETY

**Consumer Product Safety Commission**
(800) 638-CPSC
(800) 638-8270
(800) 492-8104 in MD

Answers questions and provides material on consumer product safety, including product hazards and product defects and injuries sustained in using products. Covers only products used in and around the home, excluding automobiles, foods, drugs, cosmetics, boats, and firearms.

**National Child Safety Council (See CHILDREN)**

**National Highway Traffic Safety Administration**
(800) 424-9393
(202) 366-0123 in DC

Provides information and referral on the effectiveness of occupant protection, such as safety belt use and child safety seats, and auto recalls. Staffed by experts who investigate consumer complaints and provide assistance to resolve problems. Gives referrals to other government agencies for consumer questions on warranties, service, and auto safety regulations.

**National Safety Council**
(800) 621-7619 for placing orders
(312) 527-4800 in IL

Provides posters, brochures, and booklets on safety and the prevention of accidents.

## SICKLE CELL DISEASE

**National Association for Sickle Cell Disease**
(800) 421-8453
(213) 936-7205 in CA

Offers genetic counseling and an information packet.

## SPINA BIFIDA

**Spina Bifida Information and Referral**
(800) 621-3141
(301) 770-7222 in MD

Provides information to consumers and health professionals and makes referrals to its local chapters. A service of the Spina Bifida Association of America.

## SUDDEN INFANT DEATH SYNDROME

**National SIDS Foundation**
(800) 221-SIDS
(301) 459-3388 or 3389 in MD

Provides literature on medical information and referrals, as well as information on support groups.

## SURGERY

**National Second Surgical Opinion Program Hotline**
(800) 638-6833
(800) 492-6603 in MD

Helps consumers locate a specialist near them for a second opinion in nonemergency surgery. A service of the Health Care Financing Administration, US Department of Health and Human Services.

## TOXIC SUBSTANCES
### (See also PESTICIDES)

### Asbestos Hotline
(800) 334-8571

Answers questions and maintains a list of laboratories that test consumers' homes for asbestos. Also handles and maintains the US Environmental Protection Agency's bulk sampling analysis program.

## TRAUMA

### American Trauma Society (ATS)
(800) 556-7890
(301) 328-6304 in MD

Offers information to health professionals and the public on ATS activities. Answers questions about trauma and medical emergencies.

## TUBEROUS SCLEROSIS

### National Tuberous Sclerosis Association
(800) 225-6872
(312) 668-0787 in IL

Answers questions about the disease and makes parent-to-parent contact referrals. Literature is provided.

## URINARY INCONTINENCE

### Simon Foundation
(800) 23-SIMON

Provides a recorded message on incontinence and gives ordering information for a quarterly newsletter and other publications.

## VENEREAL DISEASES

### VD Hotline
### (Operation Venus)
(800) 227-8922

Provides information on sexually transmitted diseases and confidential referrals for diagnosis and treatment. The hotline is a service of the American Social Health Association and the United Way.

## VISION
### (See also HANDICAPS)

### American Council of the Blind
(800) 424-8666
(202) 393-3666 in DC

Offers information on blindness. Provides referrals to clinics, rehabilitation organizations, research centers, and local chapters. Also publishes resource lists.

### American Foundation for the Blind (AFB)
(800) 232-5463
(212) 620-2147

Gives callers information on visual impairments and blindness and on AFB services, products, and publications.

### National Eye Care Project Helpline
(800) 222-EYES

Offers information on free eye examinations. To qualify for this program, people must be financially disadvantaged, at least 65 years old, US citizens, and must not have seen an ophthalmologist in three years.

## WOMEN

### HERS Foundation
(215) 667-7757

Offers information to women who are considering having, or who have already had, a hysterectomy.

### PMS Access
(800) 222-4767
(608) 833-4767 in WI

Provides information, literature, and counseling on premenstrual syndrome (PMS). Gives referrals to physicians and clinics in the caller's locale. A service of Madison Pharmacy Associates, Inc.

### Women's Sports Foundation
(800) 227-3988
(212) 972-9170 in AK, HI, and New York City metro area

Provides information on women's sports, physical fitness, and sports medicine.

# DRUG GLOSSARY

The drug glossary includes all the most important generic drugs, a broad range of brand-name drugs, and the various vitamins, minerals, and other substances that may be used as drugs. The generic names are the official names for drugs, as approved by the USAN (US Adopted Name) Council. The brand names for drugs are chosen by individual drug manufacturers.

If a generic drug has a separate entry within the encyclopedia, the page number of this entry is given directly after the drug's name. If a drug belongs to a group of drugs that has its own encyclopedia entry, this information is given in the glossary together with the relevant page number. If a generic drug belongs to a drug group that does not have an encyclopedia entry, the glossary tells you the dis-order or disorders for which the drug you are looking up is most commonly used and gives appropriate page references.

In the case of brand-name drugs, glossary entries give the equivalent generic drug names and appropriate page references to entries within the main part of the encyclopedia. If a brand-name drug contains several generic drugs or if its ingredients do not have separate encyclopedia entries, the glossary will direct you to appropriate drug group or disorder entries.

This selection of drugs is designed to reflect the wide diversity of products available for the treatment or prevention of disease. Inclusion of any drug does not imply AMA endorsement, nor does exclusion indicate AMA disapproval.

## A

**Accubron** a brand name for theophylline 977

**Accutane** a brand name for isotretinoin 608

**Acebutolol** 61, a generic beta-blocker drug 165

**Acecainide** a generic antiarrhythmic drug 114

**Aceclidine** a generic drug used to treat glaucoma 488

**Acetaminophen** 61, a generic analgesic drug 97

**Acetazolamide** 62, a generic diuretic drug 366, used to treat glaucoma 488

**Acetic acid** 62, an ingredient of antiseptics 119

**Acetohexamide** 62, a generic hypoglycemic drug 560

**Acetophenazine** a generic antipsychotic drug 119

**Acetylcysteine** 62, a generic mucolytic drug 700

**Achromycin** a brand-name tetracycline drug 976

**Acrisorcin** a generic antifungal drug 117

**Acrivastine** a generic antihistamine drug 118

**ACTH** 65, the abbreviation for adrenocorticotropic hormone

**Acthar** a brand name for corticotropin 313

**Acticort** a brand name for hydrocortisone 550

**Actidil** a brand-name antihistamine drug 118

**Actifed** a brand-name decongestant drug 336

**Activase** a brand name for tissue-plasminogen activator 989

**Acyclovir** 67, a generic antiviral drug 120

**Adalat** a brand name for nifedipine 727

**Adapettes** a brand-name artificial tear preparation 966

**Adapin** a brand name for doxepin 372

**Adeflor** a brand-name multivitamin 702 containing fluoride 460

**Adipex-P** a brand name for phentermine 790

**Adriamycin** a brand name for doxorubicin 372

**Adrucil** a brand name for fluorouracil 460

**Adsorbocarpine** a brand name for pilocarpine 795

**Advil** a brand name for ibuprofen 566

**AeroBid** a brand-name corticosteroid drug 312

**Aerolate** a brand name for theophylline 977

**Aerolone** a brand name for isoproterenol 608

**Aeroseb-Dex** a brand name for dexamethasone 348

**Aerosporin** a brand-name antibiotic drug 114

**Afrin** a brand name for oxymetazoline 761

**Afrinol** a brand name for pseudoephedrine 829

**Agoral** a brand-name laxative drug 630

**Akarpine** a brand name for pilocarpine 795

**AK-Cide** a brand-name drug containing prednisolone 813 and sulfacetamide 954

**AK-Dilate** a brand name for phenylephrine 791

**Akne-Mycin** a brand name for erythromycin 418

**AK-Neo-Cort** a brand-name drug containing hydrocortisone 550 and neomycin 717

**AK-Pred** a brand name for prednisolone 813

**AK-Sulf** a brand name for sulfacetamide 954

**AK-Tate** a brand name for prednisolone 813

**AK-Tracin** a brand name for bacitracin 150

**AK-Trol** a brand name for dexamethasone 348

**AK-Zol** a brand name for acetazolamide 62

**Alatone** a brand name for spironolactone 932

**Albalon-A** a brand-name decongestant drug 336

**Albalon Liquifilm** a brand name for naphazoline 714

**Albuterol** 81, a generic bronchodilator drug 215

**Alcohol, rubbing** 85, a type of antiseptic 119

**Alconefrin** a brand name for phenylephrine 791

**Aldactazide** a brand-name drug containing hydrochlorothiazide 550 and spironolactone 932

**Aldactone** a brand name for spironolactone 932

**Aldoclor** a brand-name drug containing chlorothiazide 271 and methyldopa 684

**Aldomet** a brand name for methyldopa 684

**Aldoril** a brand-name drug containing hydrochloro-thiazide 550 and methyldopa 684

**Alfacalcidol** another name for vitamin D 1059

**Algicon** a brand-name antacid drug 113

**Alka-Seltzer** a brand-name analgesic drug 97 containing aspirin 137 and sodium bicarbonate 922

**Alkeran** a brand name for melphalan 674

**Allbee C-800** a brand-name multivitamin 702

**Allbee with C** a brand-name multivitamin 702

**Aller-Chlor** a brand name for chlorpheniramine 271

**Allerest** a brand-name decongestant drug 336

**Allerfrin** a brand name for triprolidine 1011

**Allergen Ear Drops** a brand-name analgesic drug 97

**Allersone** a brand-name preparation containing hydrocortisone 550

**Allopurinol** 88, a generic drug used to treat gout 495

**Alphaderm** a brand name for hydrocortisone 550

**AlphaRedisol** a brand name for hydroxocobalamin 551

**Alpha-tocopherol** 89, a constituent of vitamin E 1059

**Alphatrex** a brand name for betamethasone 166

**Alphosyl** a brand name for coal tar 285

**Alprazolam** 89, a generic antianxiety drug 114

**Alprostadil** 89, a generic prostaglandin drug 824 used to treat congenital heart disease 518

**Alseroxylon** a generic antihypertensive drug 118

**ALternaGEL** a brand-name antacid drug 113

**Alu-Cap** a brand-name antacid drug 113

**Aluminum acetate** a generic astringent 139

**Aluminum carbonate**  a generic antacid drug 113

**Aluminum chloride**  a generic antiperspirant 118

**Aluminum hydroxide**  a generic antacid drug 113

**Alupent**  a brand name for metaproterenol 683

**Alurate**  a brand-name barbiturate drug 157

**Alu-Tab**  a brand-name antacid drug 113

**Amantadine**  92, a generic antiviral drug 120 now used to treat Parkinson's disease 772

**Ambenonium**  a generic drug used to treat myasthenia gravis 708

**Ambenyl**  a brand-name cough remedy 316

**Amcill**  a brand name for ampicillin 96

**Amcinonide**  a generic corticosteroid drug 312

**Amdinocillin**  a generic penicillin drug 779, a type of antibiotic drug 114

**Amen**  a brand name for medroxyprogesterone 671

**Americaine**  a brand-name local anesthetic 106

**Amikacin**  a generic antibiotic drug 114

**Amikin**  a brand-name antibiotic drug 114

**Amiloride**  94, a generic potassium-sparing diuretic drug 366

**Aminoglutethimide**  94, a generic anticancer drug 115

**Aminophylline**  94, a generic bronchodilator drug 215

**Aminosalicylate**  another name for aminosalicylic acid 94

**Aminosalicylic acid**  94, a generic drug used to treat tuberculosis 1013

**Amiodarone**  a generic antiarrhythmic drug 114

**Amitril**  a brand name for amitriptyline 94

**Amitriptyline**  94, a generic antidepressant drug 116

**Amobarbital**  a generic barbiturate drug 157

**Amoxapine**  95, a generic antidepressant drug 116

**Amoxicillin**  95, a generic penicillin drug 779, a type of antibiotic drug 114

**Amoxil**  a brand name for amoxicillin 95

**Amphojel**  a brand-name antacid drug 113

**Amphotericin B**  96, a generic antifungal drug 117

**Ampicillin**  96, a generic penicillin drug 779, a type of antibiotic drug 114

**Amrinone**  a generic drug used to treat heart failure 519

**Amyl nitrite**  96, a generic vasodilator drug 1041, formerly used in the treatment of angina pectoris 108, now considered a drug of abuse

**Amytal**  a brand-name barbiturate drug 157

**Anacin**  a brand-name analgesic drug 97 containing aspirin 137 and caffeine 222

**Anacin-3**  a brand name for acetaminophen 61

**Anadrol**  a brand-name anabolic steroid drug 940

**Anamine**  a brand-name decongestant drug 336

**Anaprox**  a brand name for naproxen 714

**Anaspaz**  a brand-name antispasmodic drug 120

**Anatuss**  a brand-name cough remedy 316

**Anavar**  a brand name for oxandrolone 761

**Anbesol**  a brand-name local anesthetic 106

**Ancef**  a brand-name cephalosporin 248, a type of antibiotic drug 114

**Android**  a brand name for testosterone 974

**Anectine**  a brand-name muscle-relaxant drug 706 used in general anesthesia 104

**Anergan**  a brand name for promethazine 823

**Anestacon**  a brand name for lidocaine 639

**Anexsia-D**  a brand-name analgesic drug 97

**Anhydron**  a brand-name diuretic drug 366

**Anisindione**  a generic anticoagulant drug 116

**Anisotropine**  a generic antispasmodic drug 120 used to treat irritable bowel syndrome 607

**Anorex**  a brand-name appetite suppressant drug 128

**Anspor**  a brand-name cephalosporin 248, a type of antibiotic drug 114

**Antabuse**  a brand name for disulfiram 366

**Anthra-Derm**  a brand name for anthralin 113

**Anthralin**  113, a generic antimitotic drug used to treat psoriasis 830

**Antiminth**  a brand name for pyrantel 841

**Antipyrine**  a generic analgesic drug 97 used in ear drops

**Antispas**  a brand name for dicyclomine 357

**Antivert**  a brand name for meclizine 669

**Anturane**  a brand name for sulfinpyrazone 954

**Anuject**  a brand-name local anesthetic 106

**Anusol-HC**  a brand-name preparation used to relieve anal itching 608

**Apap**  a brand name for acetaminophen 61

**A.P.L.**  a brand-name gonadotropin drug 494

**Apresazide**  a brand-name drug containing hydralazine 549 and hydrochlorothiazide 550

**Apresoline**  a brand name for hydralazine 549

**Apresoline with Esidrix**  a brand-name drug containing hydralazine 549 and hydrochlorothiazide 550

**Aprobarbital**  a generic barbiturate drug 157

**Aquamethyton**  a brand name for phytonadione 794

**Aquasol A**  a brand name for vitamin A 1057

**Aquatag**  a brand-name thiazide diuretic drug 366

**Aquatar**  a brand-name for coal tar 285

**Aquatensen**  a brand name for methyclothiazide 684

**Arachis oil**  a generic preparation used to treat scaly skin 910

**Aralen**  a brand name for chloroquine 270

**Aristocort**  a brand name for triamcinolone 1008

**Aristospan**  a brand name for triamcinolone 1008

**Armour Thyroid**  a brand name for a thyroid hormone preparation 985

**Arnica**  a generic herbal preparation used to treat bruising 217

**Artane**  a brand name for trihexyphenidyl 1011

**Arthropan**  a brand-name analgesic drug 97

**A.S.A.**  a brand name for aspirin 137

**Asbron G**  a brand-name bronchodilator drug 215

**Ascorbic acid**  136, another name for vitamin C 1059

**Ascriptin**  a brand-name analgesic drug 97

**Asendin**  a brand name for amoxapine 95

**Asparaginase**  a generic anticancer drug 115

**Aspergum**  a brand-name drug containing aspirin 137

**Aspirin**  137, a generic analgesic drug 97

**Astemizole**  a generic antihistamine drug 118

**Atabrine**  a brand name for quinacrine 842

**Atarax**  a brand name for hydroxyzine 551

**Atenolol**  140, a generic beta-blocker drug 165

**Ativan**  a brand name for lorazepam 649

**Atracurium**  a generic muscle-relaxant drug 706 used in general anesthesia 104

**Atromid-S**  a brand name for clofibrate 284

**Atropine**  143, a generic anticholinergic drug 115

**A/T/S**  a brand name for erythromycin 418

**Attenuvax**  a brand-name measles vaccine 668

**Augmentin**  a brand-name antibiotic drug 114

**Auralgan**  a brand-name analgesic drug 97 in ear-drop form

**Auranofin**  144, a generic antirheumatic drug 119

**Aureomycin**  a brand-name antibiotic drug 114

**Aurothioglucose**  a generic drug containing gold 494

**Aventyl**  a brand name for nortriptyline 731

**Axotal**  a brand-name analgesic drug 97

**Aygestin**  a brand name for norethindrone 731

**Azacitidine**  a brand-name anticancer drug 115

**Azatadine**  149, a generic antihistamine drug 118

**Azidothymidine**  another name for zidovudine 1087

**Azlocillin**  a generic penicillin drug 779, a type of antibiotic drug 114

**Azmacort**  a brand name for triamcinolone 1008

**Azo Gantanol**  a brand-name drug containing an analgesic drug 97 and an antibiotic drug 114, used to treat cystitis 328

**Azo Gantrisin**  a brand-name drug containing an analgesic drug 97 and an antibiotic drug 114, used to treat cystitis 328

**Azolid**  a brand name for phenylbutazone 790

**Azo-Sulfisoxazole**  a brand-name drug containing an analgesic drug 97 and an antibiotic drug 114, used to treat cystitis 328

**AZT**  149, an abbreviation of the former name for zidovudine 1087

**Azulfidine**  a brand name for sulfasalazine 954

**Azulfidine EN-tabs**  a brand name for sulfasalazine 954

# B

**Bacampicillin**  150, a generic penicillin drug 779, a type of antibiotic drug 114

**Bacarate** a brand-name appetite suppressant drug 128

**Baciguent** a brand name for bacitracin 150

**Bacitracin** 150, a generic antibacterial drug 114

**Baclofen** 153, a generic muscle-relaxant drug 706

**Bactine** a brand-name skin antiseptic 119 containing lidocaine 639

**Bactocill** a brand name for oxacillin 761

**Bactrim DS** a brand-name drug containing sulfamethoxazole 954 and trimethoprim 1011

**Balmex ointment** a brand-name preparation containing bismuth 174 and zinc oxide 1087

**Balneol** a cleansing lotion that relieves anal itching 608

**Balnetar** a brand name for coal tar 285

**Bancap HC** a brand-name analgesic drug 97

**Banflex** a brand name for orphenadrine 750

**Banthine** a brand-name antispasmodic drug 120

**Baratol** a brand-name antihypertensive drug 118

**Barbidonna** a brand-name antispasmodic drug 120

**Barbita** a brand name for phenobarbital 790

**Basaljel** a brand-name antacid drug 113

**Beclomethasone** 161, a generic corticosteroid drug 312

**Beclovent** a brand name for beclomethasone 161

**Beconase** a brand name for beclomethasone 161

**Beepen-VK** a brand-name penicillin drug 779, a type of antibiotic drug 114

**Belap** a brand-name antispasmodic drug 120

**Belganyl** a brand-name drug used to treat worm 1081 and protozoa infestations 827

**Belladenal** a brand-name antispasmodic drug 120

**Belladonna** 164, a generic anticholinergic drug 115

**Bellafoline** another name for belladonna 164

**Bellergal-S** a brand-name drug used to treat migraine 688

**Beminal-500** a brand-name multivitamin 702

**Benacen** a brand name for probenecid 822

**Benactyzine** a generic antianxiety drug 114

**Benadryl** a brand name for diphenhydramine 361

**Bendroflumethiazide** 164, a generic diuretic drug 366

**Bendylate** a brand name for diphenhydramine 361

**Benemid** a brand name for probenecid 822

**Ben Gay** a brand-name analgesic drug 97

**Benisone** a brand name for betamethasone 166

**Benoquin** a brand-name drug used to treat vitiligo 1060

**Benoxinate** a generic local anesthetic 106

**Benoxyl** a brand name for benzoyl peroxide 164

**Bentyl** a brand name for dicyclomine 357

**Benylin** a brand-name cough remedy 316

**Benzac W** a brand name for benzoyl peroxide 164

**Benzagel** a brand name for benzoyl peroxide 164

**Benzalkonium chloride** a generic skin antiseptic 119

**Benzamycin** a brand-name drug containing benzoyl peroxide 164 and erythromycin 418

**Benzathine penicillin G** a generic penicillin drug 779, a type of antibiotic drug 114

**Benzedrex** a brand-name decongestant drug 336

**Benznidazole** a generic drug used to treat trypanosomiasis 1013

**Benzocaine** a generic local anesthetic 106

**Benzoic acid** a generic antifungal drug 117

**Benzoin** an aromatic resin added to inhalations 589

**Benzonatate** a generic cough remedy 316

**Benzoyl peroxide** 164, a generic skin antiseptic 119 used to treat acne 63

**Benzphetamine** a generic appetite suppressant drug 128

**Benzquinamide** a generic antiemetic drug 117

**Benzthiazide** a generic thiazide diuretic drug 366

**Benztropine** a generic drug used to treat Parkinson's disease 772

**Benzyl alcohol** a generic local anesthetic 106

**Benzyl benzoate** a generic drug used to treat scabies 881

**Benzylpenicillin** a generic penicillin drug 779, a type of antibiotic drug 114

**Bephenium** a generic antihelmintic drug 118

**Berocca** a brand-name multivitamin 702

**Berubigen** a brand name for vitamin $B_{12}$ 1058

**Beta carotene** another name for vitamin A 1057

**Betadine** a brand-name skin antiseptic 119

**Betagan** a brand-name beta-blocker drug 165 used to treat glaucoma 488

**Betahistine** a generic drug used to treat Meniere's disease 674

**Betalin 12** a brand name for vitamin $B_{12}$ 1058

**Betalin S** a brand name for thiamine (vitamin B complex) 1058

**Betamethasone** 166, a generic corticosteroid drug 312

**Betapen-VK** a brand-name penicillin drug 779, a type of antibiotic drug 114

**Betatrex** a brand name for betamethasone 166

**Beta-Val** a brand name for betamethasone 166

**Betaxolol** a generic beta-blocker drug 165 used to treat glaucoma 488

**Bethanechol** a generic drug used to treat urine retention 1029

**Betoptic** a brand-name beta-blocker drug 165 used to treat glaucoma 488

**Bevantolol** a generic beta-blocker drug 165

**Bezafibrate** a generic lipid-lowering drug 642

**Bichloracetic acid** a generic drug used to treat warts 1069

**Bicillin** a brand-name penicillin drug 779, a type of antibiotic drug 114

**Bicitra** a brand-name antacid drug 113

**BiCNU** a brand-name anticancer drug 115

**Biltricide** a brand name for praziquantel 812

**Biopar Forte** a brand-name vitamin $B_{12}$ preparation 1058

**Biotin** part of the vitamin B complex 1058

**Biozyme C** a brand-name ointment used to treat skin ulcers 1018

**Biperiden** a generic drug used to treat Parkinson's disease 772

**Biphetamine** a brand-name amphetamine drug 95

**Bisacodyl** a generic stimulant laxative drug 630

**Bithin** a brand-name antihelmintic drug 118

**Bithionol** a generic antihelmintic drug 118

**Bitolterol** a generic bronchodilator drug 215

**Blenoxane** a brand-name anticancer drug 115

**Bleomycin** a generic anticancer drug 115

**Bleph-10** a brand-name drug used for eye infections 431

**Blephamide** a brand-name drug used to treat eye infections 431

**Blocadren** a brand name for timolol 988

**Bluboro** a brand-name astringent 139

**Bonine** a brand name for meclizine 669

**Bontril** a brand-name appetite suppressant drug 128

**Borofax** a brand-name ointment used to relieve skin irritation 608

**Brasivol** a brand-name drug used in the treatment of acne 63

**Breonesin** a brand-name cough remedy 316

**Brethaire** a brand name for terbutaline 971

**Brethine** a brand name for terbutaline 971

**Bretylium** a brand-name antiarrhythmic drug 114

**Bretylol** a brand-name antiarrhythmic drug 114

**Brevicon** a brand-name oral contraceptive 747

**Brevital** a brand-name barbiturate drug 157 used to induce general anesthesia 104

**Brexin** a brand-name cough remedy 316

**Bricanyl** a brand name for terbutaline 971

**Bromfed** a brand-name cold remedy 287

**Bromocriptine** 213, a generic drug used to treat Parkinson's disease 772

**Bromodiphenhydramine** a generic antihistamine drug 118

**Bromovinyldeoxyuridine** a generic antiviral drug 120

**Bromphen** a brand-name antihistamine drug 118

**Brompheniramine** a generic antihistamine drug 118

**Brondecon** a brand-name cough remedy 316 containing a bronchodilator drug 215

**Bronkaid Mist** a brand name for epinephrine 414

**Bronkodyl S-R** a brand name for theophylline 977

**Bronkolixir** a brand-name cough remedy 316 containing a bronchodilator drug 215

**Bronkometer** a brand-name bronchodilator drug 215

**Bronkosol** a brand-name bronchodilator drug 215

**Bronkotabs** a brand-name cough remedy 316 containing a bronchodilator drug 215

**Bucladin-S** a brand-name antiemetic drug 117

**Buclizine** a brand-name antiemetic drug 117

**Budesonide** a generic investigational corticosteroid drug 312

**Buff-A Comp** a brand-name analgesic drug 97 containing aspirin 137

**Bufferin** a brand name for aspirin 137

**Buf-Oxal 10** a brand name for benzoyl peroxide 164

**Bumetanide** a generic loop diuretic drug 366

**Bumex** a brand-name loop diuretic drug 366

**Bupivacaine** a generic local anesthetic 106

**Buprenex** a brand-name narcotic drug 715, a type of analgesic drug 97

**Buprenorphine** a generic narcotic drug 715, a type of analgesic drug 97

**Busulfan** a generic anticancer drug 115

**Butabarbital** a generic barbiturate drug 157, a type of sleeping drug 916

**Butalbital** a generic barbiturate drug 157, a type of sleeping drug 916

**Butamben** a generic drug used to relieve skin irritation 608

**Butazolidin** a brand name for phenylbutazone 790

**Butesin Picrate** a brand-name drug used to relieve skin irritation 608

**Butibel** a brand-name drug containing belladonna 164

**Butisol** a brand-name barbiturate drug 157, a type of sleeping drug 916

**Butoconazole** a generic antifungal drug 117

**Butorphanol** a generic narcotic drug 715, a type of analgesic drug 97

# C

**Cafergot** a brand-name drug used to treat migraine 688

**Caladryl** a brand-name drug containing diphenhydramine 361 and calamine 223

**Calan** a brand-name calcium channel blocker drug 224

**Calcet** a brand-name drug containing calcium 223 and vitamin D 1059

**Calcidrine** a brand-name cough remedy 316

**Calcifediol** another name for vitamin D 1059

**Calcimar** a brand name for calcitonin 223

**Calciparine** a brand name for heparin 531, an anticoagulant drug 116

**Calcitonin** 223, a generic drug used to treat bone disorders 194

**Calcitrel** a brand-name antacid drug 113

**Calcitriol** another name for vitamin D 1059

**Calcium carbonate** a generic antacid drug 113

**Calderol** a brand name for vitamin D 1059

**Caldesene** a brand-name preparation used to treat diaper rash 354

**Calel-D** a brand-name preparation containing calcium 223 and vitamin D 1059

**Calmol 4** brand-name rectal suppositories 955 used to relieve anal irritation 608

**Caltrate 600** a brand-name antacid drug 113

**Cama** a brand name for aspirin 137

**Camalox** a brand-name antacid drug 113

**Cambendazole** a generic antihelmintic drug 118

**Camphor** a generic drug used to relieve skin irritation 608

**Cannabis** 230, a generic central nervous system depressant

**Cantharidin** a generic drug used to treat warts 1069

**Cantharone** a brand-name drug used to treat warts 1069

**Cantil** a brand-name antispasmodic drug 120 used to treat irritable bowel syndrome 607

**Capreomycin** a generic antibacterial drug 114 used to treat tuberculosis 1013

**Captopril** 231, a generic ACE inhibitor drug 61

**Carafate** a brand-name ulcer-healing drug 1018

**Caramiphen** a generic cough remedy 316

**Carbachol** 231, a generic drug used to treat glaucoma 488

**Carbamazepine** 231, a generic anticonvulsant drug 116

**Carbamide peroxide** a generic preparation used to soften earwax 387

**Carbaryl** a generic drug used to treat lice 638

**Carbenicillin** a generic penicillin drug 779, a type of antibiotic drug 114

**Carbenoxolone** a generic ulcer-healing drug 1018

**Carbetapentane** a generic cough remedy 316

**Carbimide** a generic drug used to treat alcohol dependence 81

**Carbinoxamine** a generic antihistamine drug 118

**Carbocaine** a brand-name local anesthetic 106

**Carbocysteine** a generic decongestant drug 336

**Carboprost** a generic prostaglandin drug 824

**Carboxymethylcellulose** a generic laxative drug 630

**Cardec DM** a brand-name cough remedy 316

**Cardilate** a brand-name drug used to treat angina pectoris 108

**Cardioquin** a brand name for quinidine 842, an antiarrhythmic drug 114

**Cardizem** a brand name for diltiazem 361, a calcium channel blocker drug 224

**Cardovar** a brand-name antihypertensive drug 118

**Carisoprodol** 238, a generic muscle-relaxant drug 706

**Carmol** a brand-name drug used to treat dry skin 910

**Carmustine** a generic anticancer drug 115

**Carphenazine** a generic antipsychotic drug 119

**Casanthranol** a generic stimulant laxative drug 630

**Cascara** a generic stimulant laxative drug 630

**Castellani's Paint** a brand-name antifungal drug 117

**Castor oil** 239, a generic stimulant laxative drug 630

**Catapres** a brand-name antihypertensive drug 118

**Ceclor** a brand-name cephalosporin 248, a type of antibiotic drug 114

**Cefaclor** 245, a generic cephalosporin 248, a type of antibiotic drug 114

**Cefadroxil** a generic cephalosporin 248, a type of antibiotic drug 114

**Cefadyl** a brand-name cephalosporin 248, a type of antibiotic drug 114

**Cefamandole** a generic cephalosporin 248, a type of antibiotic drug 114

**Cefazolin** a generic cephalosporin 248, a type of antibiotic drug 114

**Cefizox** a brand-name cephalosporin 248, a type of antibiotic drug 114

**Cefobid** a brand-name cephalosporin 248, a type of antibiotic drug 114

**Cefol** a brand-name multivitamin 702

**Cefonicid** a generic cephalosporin 248, a type of antibiotic drug 114

**Cefoperazone** a generic cephalosporin 248, a type of antibiotic drug 114

**Ceforanide** a generic cephalosporin 248, a type of antibiotic drug 114

**Cefotaxime** a generic cephalosporin 248, a type of antibiotic drug 114

**Cefotetan** a generic cephalosporin 248, a type of antibiotic drug 114

**Cefoxitin** a generic cephalosporin 248, a type of antibiotic drug 114

**Ceftazidime** a generic cephalosporin 248, a type of antibiotic drug 114

**Ceftizoxime** a generic cephalosporin 248, a type of antibiotic drug 114

**Ceftriaxone** a generic cephalosporin 248, a type of antibiotic drug 114

**Cefuroxime** a generic cephalosporin 248, a type of antibiotic drug 114

**Celestone** a brand name for betamethasone 166, a corticosteroid drug 312

**Celontin** a brand-name anticonvulsant drug 116

**Cenocort** a brand-name corticosteroid drug 312

**Centrax** a brand-name antianxiety drug 114

**Centrum** a brand-name multivitamin 702

**Cephalothin** a generic cephalosporin 248, a type of antibiotic drug 114

**Cephapirin** a generic cephalosporin 248, a type of antibiotic drug 114

**Cephradine** a generic cephalosporin 248, a type of antibiotic drug 114

**Cephulac** a brand-name laxative drug 630

**Cerespan** a brand-name vasodilator drug 1041

**Cerose-DM Expectorant** a brand-name cough remedy 316

**Cesamet** a brand-name antiemetic drug 117

**Cetacaine** a brand-name local anesthetic 106

**Cetacort** a brand-name corticosteroid drug 312

**Cetamide** a brand name for sulfacetamide 954, an antibacterial drug 114

**Cetapred** a brand-name drug containing prednisolone 813 and sulfacetamide 954

**Cetrimide** a type of antiseptic 119

**Cevalin** a brand name for vitamin C 1059

**Chardonna-2** a brand-name drug containing belladonna 164

**Chealamide** a brand-name chelating agent 258

**Chenix** a brand name for chenodiol 258

**Chenodiol** 258, a generic drug used to treat gallstones 474

**Cheracol** a brand-name cough remedy 316

**Chloral hydrate** 270, a generic sleeping drug 916

**Chlorambucil** 270, a generic anticancer drug 115

**Chloramphenicol** 270, a generic antibiotic drug 114

**Chloraseptic** a brand-name drug used to treat sore mouth 697 or throat 789

**Chlordiazepoxide** 270, a generic antianxiety drug 114

**Chlorhexidine** a type of antiseptic 119

**Chlormezanone** a generic antianxiety drug 114

**Chlorofon-F** a brand-name muscle-relaxant drug 706

**Chloroform** 270, a generic general anesthetic 104

**Chloroguanide** a generic drug used to treat malaria 659

**Chloromycetin** a brand-name antibiotic drug 114

**Chlorophenothane** another name for DDT 333

**Chloroprocaine** a generic local anesthetic 106

**Chloroptic** a brand-name antibiotic drug 114

**Chloroquine** 270, a generic drug used to treat malaria 659

**Chlorothiazide** 271, a generic thiazide diuretic drug 366

**Chlorotrianisene** a generic anticancer drug 115

**Chloroxylenol** a type of antiseptic 119

**Chlorphenesin** a generic muscle-relaxant drug 706

**Chlorpheniramine** 271, a generic antihistamine drug 118

**Chlorphentermine** a generic appetite suppressant drug 128

**Chlorpromazine** 271, a generic antipsychotic drug 119

**Chlorpropamide** 271, a generic drug used to treat diabetes mellitus 349

**Chlorprothixene** a generic antipsychotic drug 119

**Chlortetracycline** a generic tetracycline drug 976, a type of antibiotic drug 114

**Chlorthalidone** 271, a generic thiazide diuretic drug 366

**Chlor-Trimeton** a brand name for chlorpheniramine 271

**Chlorzoxazone** 271, a generic muscle-relaxant drug 706

**Cholecalciferol** 272, another name for vitamin D 1059

**Choledyl** a brand-name bronchodilator drug 215

**Cholestyramine** 275, a generic lipid-lowering drug 642

**Choline magnesium trisalicylate** a generic drug used to treat arthritis 132

**Choline salicylate** a generic drug used to treat arthritis 132

**Choloxin** a brand-name lipid-lowering drug 642

**Chromagen capsules** a brand-name vitamin 1060 and mineral supplement 689

**Chronulac** a brand-name laxative drug 630

**Chymopapain** an enzyme for chemonucleolysis 258

**Chymoral** an enzyme used to reduce edema 390

**Chymotrypsin** an enzyme used in the treatment of cataracts 240

**Ciclopirox** a generic antifungal drug 117

**Cimetidine** 280, a generic ulcer-healing drug 1018

**Cinnamates** a generic sunscreen 955

**Cinnarizine** a generic antihistamine drug 118

**Cinoxacin** a generic antibacterial drug 114

**Ciprofibrate** a generic lipid-lowering drug 642

**Cisplatin** 283, a generic anticancer drug 115

**Citracal** a brand name for calcium 223

**Citra Forte** a brand-name cough remedy 316

**Citrocarbonate** a brand-name antacid drug 113

**Claforan** a brand-name cephalosporin 248, a type of antibiotic drug 114

**Clemastine** a generic antihistamine drug 118

**Cleocin** a brand name for clindamycin 284

**Clerz** a brand-name artificial tear preparation 966

**Clidinium bromide** a generic antispasmodic drug 120 used to treat irritable bowel syndrome 607

**Clindamycin** 284, a generic antibiotic drug 114

**Clinoril** a brand-name nonsteroidal anti-inflammatory drug 730

**Clioquinol** a generic antibacterial 114 and antifungal drug 117

**Clobetasol** a generic corticosteroid drug 312

**Clocortolone** a generic corticosteroid drug 312

**Cloderm** a brand-name corticosteroid drug 312

**Clofazimine** a generic drug used to treat leprosy 634

**Clofibrate** 284, a generic lipid-lowering drug 642

**Clomid** a brand-name drug used to treat infertility 586

**Clomiphene** 284, a generic drug used to treat infertility 586

**Clomipramine** a generic antidepressant drug 116

**Clonidine** 284, a generic antihypertensive drug 118

**Clonopin** a brand-name anticonvulsant drug 116

**Clorazepate** 284, a generic antianxiety drug 114

**Clotrimazole** 284, a generic antifungal drug 117

**Cloxacillin** 285, a generic penicillin drug 779, a type of antibiotic drug 114

**Cloxapen** a brand-name penicillin drug 779, a type of antibiotic drug 114

**Clozapine** a generic antipsychotic drug 119

**Clusivol** a brand-name multivitamin 702

**Clysodrast** a brand-name laxative drug 630

**Coactin** a brand-name penicillin drug 779, a type of antibiotic drug 114

**Coal tar** 285, a generic ingredient in preparations for skin disorders 910

**Cobalt edetate** a generic drug used to treat cyanide poisoning 326

**Cocaine** 285, a generic central nervous system stimulant 942

**Codeine** 286, a generic narcotic drug 715, a type of analgesic drug 97

**Codiclear** a brand-name cough remedy 316

**Codimal** a brand-name cough remedy 316

**Cod liver oil** 286, a dietary supplement containing vitamin A 1057 and vitamin D 1059

**Cogentin** a brand-name drug used to treat Parkinson's disease 772

**Co-Gesic** a brand-name analgesic drug 97

**Colace** a brand-name laxative drug 630

**ColBENEMID** a brand-name drug containing probenecid 822 and colchicine 287

**Colchicine** 287, a generic drug used to treat gout 495

**Colestid** a brand-name lipid-lowering drug 642

**Colestipol** a generic lipid-lowering drug 642

**Colistin** 289, a generic polymyxin 808, a type of antibiotic drug 114

**Collyrium** a brand-name preparation used to relieve eye irritation 431

**Cologel** a brand name for methylcellulose 684

**Colrex** a brand-name cold remedy 287 containing acetaminophen 61

**Coly-Mycin** a brand name for colistin 289

**Colyte** a brand-name laxative drug 630

**Combid** a brand-name drug containing prochlorperazine 822 and an antispasmodic drug 120

**Combipres** a brand-name antihypertensive drug 118

**Comhist LA** a brand-name cold remedy 287

**Compal** a brand-name analgesic drug 97

**Compazine** a brand name for prochlorperazine 822

**Compete** a brand-name multivitamin 702 containing iron 606 and zinc 1087

**Compound W** a brand-name preparation used to treat warts 1069

**Comtrex** a brand-name cold remedy 287 containing acetaminophen 61

**Conar A** a brand-name cough remedy 316

**Conex DA** a brand-name cold remedy 287

**Congespirin** a brand-name cough remedy 316

**Congess** a brand-name cough remedy 316

**Constant-T** a brand-name bronchodilator drug 215

**Contac** a brand-name cold remedy 287

**Cophene PL** a brand-name cold remedy 287

**Cordran** a brand-name corticosteroid drug 312

**Corgard** a brand-name beta-blocker drug 165

**Coricidin** a brand-name drug containing aspirin 137 and chlorpheniramine 271

**Corilin** a brand-name drug containing chlorpheniramine 271 and an analgesic drug 97 similar to aspirin 137

**Cortaid** a brand name for hydrocortisone 550

**Cort-Dome** a brand name for hydrocortisone 550

**Cortef** a brand name for hydrocortisone 550

**Cortenema** a brand name for hydrocortisone 550

**Corticaine** a brand-name preparation containing hydrocortisone 550 and a local anesthetic 106 used to treat anal discomfort

**Corticotropin** 313, another name for ACTH 65

**Cortifoam** a brand name for hydrocortisone 550

**Cortinal** a brand name for hydrocortisone 550

**Cortisol** 313, another name for hydrocortisone 550

**Cortisone** 313, a generic corticosteroid drug 312

**Cortisporin Cream** a brand-name preparation containing a corticosteroid drug 312 and an antibacterial drug 114

**Cortone** a brand name for cortisone 313

**Cortrophin Zinc** a brand name for corticotropin 313

**Coryban-D** a brand-name cough remedy 316

**Coryztime** a brand-name cold remedy 287

**Cosyntropin** a synthetic form of corticotropin 313

**Cotazym** a brand name for pancrelipase 767

**Cotrim** a brand-name drug containing sulfamethoxazole 954 and trimethoprim 1011

**CoTylenol** a brand-name cold remedy 287 containing acetaminophen 61

**Coumadin** a brand name for warfarin 1069

**Cromolyn sodium** 321, a generic drug used for the prevention of asthma 137

**Crotamiton** a generic drug used to treat scabies 881

**Crysticillin** a brand-name penicillin drug 779, a type of antibiotic drug 114

**Crystodigin** a brand name for digitoxin 361

**Cuprimine** a brand name for penicillamine 779

**Curare** 325, a generic muscle-relaxant drug 706

**Curretab** a brand name for medroxyprogesterone 671

**Cyanocobalamin** 326, another name for vitamin B$_{12}$ 1058

**Cyanoject** a brand name for vitamin B$_{12}$ 1058

**Cyclacillin** 326, a generic penicillin drug 779, a type of antibiotic drug 114

**Cyclandelate** a generic vasodilator drug 1041

**Cyclapen-W** a brand name for cyclacillin 326

**Cyclizine** a generic antiemetic drug 117

**Cyclobenzaprine** 326, a generic muscle-relaxant drug 706

**Cyclocort** a brand-name corticosteroid drug 312

**Cyclomethycaine** a generic local anesthetic 106

**Cyclopar** a brand-name tetracycline drug 976, a type of antibiotic drug 114

**Cyclopentamine** a brand-name decongestant drug 336

**Cyclophosphamide** 326, a generic anticancer drug 115

**Cycloserine** a generic antibiotic drug 114

**Cyclospasmol** a brand-name vasodilator drug 1041

**Cyclosporine** 326, a generic immunosuppressant drug 576

**Cyclothiazide** a generic thiazide diuretic drug 366

**Cylert** a brand name for pemoline 778

**Cyproheptadine** a generic appetite stimulant drug 128

**Cyronine** a brand-name synthetic thyroid hormone 985

**Cystospaz** a brand name for hyoscyamine 552

**Cytadren** a brand name for aminoglutethimide 94

**Cytarabine** a generic anticancer drug 115

**Cytomel** a brand-name synthetic thyroid hormone 985

**Cytosar-U** a brand-name anticancer drug 115

**Cytosine Arabinoside** a brand-name anticancer drug 115

**Cytoxan** a brand name for cyclophosphamide 326

# D

**Dacarbazine** a generic anticancer drug 115

**Dactinomycin** a generic anticancer drug 115

**Dalalone** a brand name for dexamethasone 348

**Dalicote** a brand name for dexamethasone 348

**Dalidyne** a brand name for dexamethasone 348

**Dallergy** a brand-name drug used to treat nasal congestion 715

**Dalmane** a brand name for flurazepam 460

**Damason-P** a brand-name cough remedy 316

**Danazol** 332, a generic drug used to treat endometriosis 404

**Danocrine** a brand name for danazol 332

**Danthron** a generic stimulant laxative drug 630

**Dantrium** a brand name for dantrolene 333

**Dantrolene** 333, a generic muscle-relaxant drug 706

**Daranide** a brand-name drug used to treat glaucoma 488

**Daraprim** a brand name for pyrimethamine 841

**Darbid** a brand-name antispasmodic drug 120 used to treat irritable bowel syndrome 607

**Daricon** a brand-name antispasmodic drug 120 used for irritable bowel syndrome 607

**Darvocet-N** a brand-name drug containing acetaminophen 61 and propoxyphene 824

**Darvon** a brand name for propoxyphene 824

**Darvon Compound 65** a brand-name analgesic drug 97 containing aspirin 137

**Daunorubicin** a generic anticancer drug 115

**Dazamide** a brand name for acetazolamide 62

**DDAVP** a brand-name drug used to treat diabetes insipidus 349

**Debrox** a brand-name preparation for softening earwax 387

**Decaderm** a brand name for dexamethasone 348

**Decadron** a brand name for dexamethasone 348

**Deca-Durabolin** a brand name for nandrolone 714

**Decaject** a brand name for dexamethasone 348

**Decapryn** a brand-name antihistamine 118 sleeping drug 916

**Decaspray** a brand name for dexamethasone 348

**Decholin** a brand-name laxative drug 630

**Declomycin** a brand-name antibiotic drug 114

**Deconade** a brand-name cold remedy 287

**Deconamine SR** a brand-name cold remedy 287

**Deconsal** a brand name for phenylephrine 791

**Deferoxamine** a generic drug used to treat iron poisoning 606

**Dehydrocholic acid** a generic laxative drug 630

**Dehydroemetine** a generic drug used for amebiasis 92

**Deladumone** a brand-name drug containing estradiol 421 and testosterone 974

**Delfen** a brand-name spermicide 927

**Delsym** a brand-name cough remedy 316

**Delta-Cortef** a brand name for prednisolone 813

**Deltasone** a brand name for prednisone 813

**Demazin** a brand-name cold remedy 287

**Demecarium** a generic drug used to treat glaucoma 488

**Demeclocycline** a generic tetracycline drug 976

**Demerol** a brand name for meperidine 680

**Demi-Regroton** a brand-name drug containing chlorthalidone 271 and reserpine 863

**Demulen** a brand-name oral contraceptive 747

**Depakene** a brand name for valproic acid 1037

**Depakote** a brand name for valproic acid 1037

**Depen** a brand name for penicillamine 779

**Depo-Estradiol** a brand name for estradiol 421

**Depo-Medrol** a brand name for methylprednisolone 684

**Depo-Provera** a brand name for medroxyprogesterone 671

**Depo-Testadiol** a brand-name drug containing estradiol 421 and testosterone 974

**Deprenyl** a generic drug used to treat Parkinson's disease 772

**Deprol** a brand-name antidepressant drug 116

**Dermacort** a brand name for hydrocortisone 550

**Dermolate** a brand name for hydrocortisone 550

**Dermoplast** a brand-name local anesthetic 106

**Desipramine** 347, a generic tricyclic antidepressant drug 116

**Desonide** a generic corticosteroid drug 312

**Desoximetasone** a generic corticosteroid drug 312

**Desoxycorticosterone** a generic corticosteroid drug 312

**Desoxyn** a brand name for a derivative of amphetamine 95

**Desquam-X** a brand name for benzoyl peroxide 164

**Desyrel** a brand name for trazodone 1008

**Dexamethasone** 348, a generic corticosteroid drug 312

**Dexatrim** a brand name for phenylpropanolamine 791

**Dexbrompheniramine** a generic antihistamine drug 118

**Dexchlorpheniramine** a generic antihistamine drug 118

**Dexone** a brand name for dexamethasone 348

**Dextroamphetamine** 348, a generic central nervous system stimulant 942

**Dextromethorphan** a generic cough remedy 316

**Dextrothyroxine** a generic lipid-lowering drug 642

**Dey-Dose Atropine Sulfate** a brand name for atropine 143

**DHE-45** a brand-name drug used to treat migraine 688

**DHS Zinc** a brand-name antifungal agent 117 used to treat dandruff 332

**DHT** a brand name for vitamin D 1059

**DiaBeta** a brand name for glyburide 493

**Diabinese** a brand name for chlorpropamide 271

**Diacetylmorphine** 351, another name for heroin 535

**Dia-Gesic** a brand-name narcotic cough remedy 316

**Dialose** a brand-name laxative drug 630

**Dialume** a brand-name antacid drug 113

**Diamidine** a generic drug used to treat leishmaniasis 633

**Diamox** a brand name for acetazolamide 62

**Diapid** a brand name for lypressin 657

**Diazepam** 357, a generic benzodiazepine antianxiety drug 114

**Diazoxide** a generic antihypertensive drug 118

**Dibenzyline** a brand-name vasodilator 1041 antihypertensive drug 118

**Dibucaine** a generic local anesthetic 106

**Dical-D** a brand-name preparation containing calcium 223 and vitamin D 1059

**Dichlorphenamide** a generic drug used to treat glaucoma 488

**Dicloxacillin** a generic penicillin drug 779, a type of antibiotic drug 114

**Dicumarol** 357, a generic anticoagulant drug 116

**Dicyclomine** 357, a generic antispasmodic drug 120 used to treat irritable bowel syndrome 607

**Dideoxycytidine** 357, a generic anticancer drug 115 that is being investigated as a treatment for AIDS 76

**Didronel** a brand-name drug used to treat Paget's disease 762

**Dienestrol** 357, a generic estrogen drug 421

**Diethylcarbamazine** a generic antihelmintic drug 118

**Diethylpropion** a generic appetite suppressant drug 128

**Diethylstilbestrol** 359, an estrogen drug 421

**Diflorasone** a generic corticosteroid drug 312

**Diflunisal** 359, a nonsteroidal anti-inflammatory drug 730

**Di-Gel** a brand name for simethicone 906

**Digitoxin** 361, a generic digitalis drug 361

**Digoxin** 361, a generic digitalis drug 361

**Dihydrocodeine** a generic narcotic drug 715, a type of analgesic drug 97

**Dihydroergotamine** a generic drug used to treat migraine 688

**Dihydrotachysterol** another name for vitamin D 1059

**Dihydroxyaluminum** a generic antacid drug 113

**Diiodohydroxyquin** a generic drug used to treat amebiasis 92

**Dilantin** a brand name for phenytoin 791

**Dilatrate-SR** a brand name for isosorbide dinitrate 608

**Dilaudid** a brand-name narcotic drug 715, a type of analgesic drug 97

**Dilor** a brand-name xanthine bronchodilator drug 215

**Diloxanide** a generic drug used to treat amebiasis 92

**Diltiazem** 361, a generic calcium channel blocker drug 224

**Dimacol** a brand-name cough remedy 316

**Dimenhydrinate** 361, a generic antihistamine drug 118

**Dimercaprol** a generic drug used to treat lead poisoning 631

**Dimercaptosuccinic acid** a generic drug used to treat lead poisoning 631

**Dimetane** a brand-name antihistamine drug 118

**Dimetapp** a brand-name cold remedy 287

**Dimethindene** a generic antihistamine drug 118

**Dimethisoquin** a generic local anesthetic 106

**Dimethyl sulfoxide** a generic drug used to treat cystitis 328

**Dimethyl tubocurarine** a generic muscle-relaxant drug 706 used in general anesthesia 104

**Dinoprost** a generic prostaglandin drug 824 used to stimulate uterine contractions in childbirth 263

**Dinoprostone** a generic prostaglandin drug 824 used to stimulate uterine contractions in childbirth 263

**Diphenatol** a brand-name drug containing diphenoxylate 361 and atropine 143

**Diphenhydramine** 361, a generic antihistamine drug 118

**Diphenidol** a generic antiemetic drug 117

**Diphenoxylate** 361, a generic antidiarrheal drug 117

**Diphenylpyraline** a generic antihistamine drug 118

**Dipivalyl epinephrine** another name for dipivefrin, a generic drug used to treat glaucoma 488

**Dipivefrin** a generic drug used to treat glaucoma 488

**Diprolene** a brand name for betamethasone 166

**Diprosone** a brand name for betamethasone 166

**Dipyridamole** 362, a generic drug used to treat abnormal blood clotting 184

**Disalcid** a brand-name nonsteroidal anti-inflammatory drug 730

**Disipal** a brand name for orphenadrine 750

**Disodium azodisalicyclic acid** a generic investigational drug used to treat inflammatory bowel disease 588

**Disophrol** a brand-name cold remedy 287

**Disopyramide** 365, a generic antiarrhythmic drug 114

**Disulfiram** 366, a generic drug used to treat alcohol dependence 81

**Ditropan** a brand-name anticholinergic drug 115 used to treat urinary incontinence 579

**Diucardin** a brand-name thiazide diuretic drug 366

**Diulo** a brand name for metolazone 684

**Diupres** a brand-name drug containing chlorothiazide 271 and reserpine 863

**Diuril** a brand name for chlorothiazide 271, a thiazide diuretic drug 366

**Diutensen-R** a brand-name drug containing methyclothiazide 684 and reserpine 863

**Dobutamine** a generic drug used to treat heart failure 519

**Docusate** a generic laxative drug 630

**Dolene** a brand-name narcotic drug 715, a type of analgesic drug 97

**Dolobid** a brand name for diflunisal 359

**Dolophine** a brand name for methadone 683

**Domperidone** a generic antiemetic drug 117

**Donatussin** a brand-name cough remedy 316

**Donnagel** a brand-name antidiarrheal drug 117

**Donnatal** a brand-name drug used to treat irritable bowel syndrome 607

**Donnazyme** a brand-name drug used to treat indigestion 580

**Dopamine** a natural neurotransmitter 725 used to treat heart failure 519

**Dopar** a brand name for levodopa 638

**Dopram** a brand-name drug used to stimulate respiration

**Dorcol** a brand-name cough remedy 316

**Doriden** a brand-name sleeping drug 916

**Dormalin** a brand-name benzodiazepine 164 sleeping drug 916

**Doryx** a brand name for doxycycline 372

**Doss** a brand-name laxative drug 630

**Dow-Isoniazid** a brand name for isoniazid 608

**Doxaphene** a brand name for propoxyphene 824

**Doxapram** a generic drug used to stimulate respiration

**Doxidan** a brand-name stimulant laxative drug 630

**Doxorubicin** 372, a generic anticancer drug 115

**Doxy-II** a brand name for doxycycline 372

**DOXY-CAPS** a brand name for doxycycline 372

**Doxycycline** 372, a generic tetracycline drug 976, a type of antibiotic drug 114

**Doxylamine** a generic antihistamine 118 sleeping drug 916

**Doxy-Lemmon** a brand name for doxycycline 372

**DOXY-TABS** a brand name for doxycycline 372

**Dramamine** a brand name for dimenhydrinate 361

**Drisdol** a brand name for ergocalciferol 415

**Dristan** a brand name for oxymetazoline 761

**Drithocreme** a brand name for anthralin 113

**Dritho-Scalp** a brand-name cream containing anthralin 113 and salicylic acid 879

**Drixoral** a brand-name antihistamine drug 118

**Dromostanolone** a generic androgen drug 100

**Dronabinol** a generic antiemetic drug 117 derived from marijuana 664

**Droperidol** a generic antiemetic drug 117

**Drysol** a brand-name antiperspirant 118

**Dulcolax** a brand-name stimulant laxative drug 630

**Duofilm** a brand name for salicylic acid 879

**Duolube** a brand-name drug used to relieve dry eyes 615

**Duo-Medihaler** a brand-name aerosol containing isoproterenol 608 and phenylephrine 791

**Duotrate** a brand-name nitrate drug 728 used in the treatment of angina pectoris 108

**Duphrene** a brand-name cold remedy 287

**Durabolin** a brand name for nandrolone 714

**Duracillin** a brand-name penicillin drug 779, a type of antibiotic drug 114

**Duramorph** a brand name for morphine 694

**Duraphyl** a brand name for theophylline 977

**Duraquin** a brand name for quinidine 842

**Duricef** a brand-name cephalosporin 248, a type of antibiotic drug 114

**Durrax** a brand-name antihistamine drug 118

**Duvoid** a brand-name drug used to treat urine retention 1029

**DV** a brand-name estrogen drug 421

**Dyazide** a brand-name drug containing hydrochloro-thiazide 550 and triam-terene 1009

**Dycill** a brand-name penicillin drug 779, a type of antibiotic drug 114

**Dyclonine** a generic local anesthetic 106

**Dymelor** a brand name for acetohexamide 62

**Dynapen** a brand-name penicillin drug 779, a type of antibiotic drug 114

**Dyphylline** a generic xanthine bronchodilator drug 215

**Dyrenium** a brand name for triamterene 1009

# E

**Easprin** a brand name for aspirin 137

**Echothiophate** a generic drug used to treat glau-coma 488

**Econazole** 388, a generic antifungal drug 117

**Econochlor** a brand name for chloramphenicol 270

**Econopred** a brand name for prednisolone 813

**Ecotrin** a brand name for aspirin 137

**Edecrin** a brand-name loop diuretic drug 366

**Edetate calcium disodium** a generic chelating agent 258 used to treat metal poisoning 805

**Edetate disodium** a generic chelating agent 258 used in the treatment of hypercalcemia 552

**EDTA** a generic chelating agent 258 used to treat hypercalcemia 552

**E.E.S.** a brand name for erythromycin 418

**Effersyllium** a brand name for psyllium 834

**Eflornithine** a generic investigational anticancer drug 115

**Efodine** a brand-name antiseptic 119

**Efudex** a brand name for fluorouracil 460

**E-Ionate PA** a brand name for estradiol 421

**Elavil** a brand name for amitriptyline 94

**Eldopaque** a brand-name preparation used to lighten the skin in disorders of pigmentation 794

**Eldoquin** a brand-name preparation used to lighten the skin in disorders of pigmentation 794

**Elixicon** a brand name for theophylline 977

**Elixophyllin** a brand name for theophylline 977

**Embolex** a brand name for heparin 531

**Emcyt** a brand-name anticancer drug 115

**Emete-con** a brand-name antiemetic drug 117

**Emetine** a generic drug used to treat amebiasis 92

**Emko** a brand-name spermicide 927

**Empirin** a brand-name drug containing aspirin 137 and codeine 286

**E-Mycin** a brand name for erythromycin 418

**Enalapril** 400, a generic ACE inhibitor drug 61

**Enarax** a brand-name drug containing hydroxyzine 551 used to treat irritable bowel syndrome 607

**Encainide** a generic antiarrhythmic drug 114

**Encaprin** a brand name for aspirin 137

**Encare** a brand-name spermicide 927

**Endep** a brand name for amitriptyline 94

**Enduron** a brand name for methyclothiazide 684

**Enduronyl** a brand-name antihypertensive drug 118

**Enflurane** a generic general anesthetic 104

**Enovid** a brand-name oral contraceptive 747

**Entex** a brand-name cough remedy 316

**Entozyme** a brand-name drug used to treat indigestion 580

**Entuss** a brand-name cough remedy 316

**Enuclene** a brand-name artificial tear preparation 966

**Ephedrine** 410, a generic bronchodilator 215 decongestant drug 336

**Epifrin** a brand name for epinephrine 414

**E-Pilo** a brand-name drug containing epinephrine 414 and pilocarpine 795

**Epinal** a brand-name epinephrinelike drug 414

**EpiPen** a brand name for epinephrine 414

**Epitrate** a brand name for epinephrine 414

**Eppy/N** a brand-name epinephrinelike drug 414

**Equagesic** a brand-name analgesic drug 97 containing aspirin 137

**Equanil** a brand name for meprobamate 680

**Ergocalciferol** 415, another name for vitamin D 1059

**Ergomar** a brand name for ergotamine 416

**Ergonovine** 416, a generic drug used to stop bleed-ing after childbirth 263

**Ergostat** a brand name for ergotamine 416

**Ergotamine** 416, a drug used to treat migraine 688

**Ergotrate maleate** a brand name for ergonovine 416

**ERYC** a brand name for erythromycin 418

**ERYC 125** a brand name for erythromycin 418

**Erycette** a brand name for erythromycin 418

**EryDerm** a brand name for erythromycin 418

**Erymax** a brand name for erythromycin 418

**Ery-Tab** a brand name for erythromycin 418

**Erythrityl tetranitrate** a generic nitrate drug 728 used to treat angina pectoris 108

**Erythrocin** a brand name for erythromycin 418

**Erythromycin** 418, a generic antibiotic drug 114

**Esgic** a brand-name analgesic drug 97 containing acetaminophen 61

**Esidrix** a brand name for hydrochlorothiazide 550

**Esimil** a brand name for hydrochlorothiazide 550

**Eskalith CR** a brand name for lithium 643

**Estar** a brand name for coal tar 285

**Estinyl** a brand name for ethinyl estradiol 422

**Estrace** a brand name for estradiol 421

**Estradiol** 421, a generic estrogen drug 421 used to treat symptoms of the menopause 676

**Estradurin** a brand-name estrogen drug 421 used to treat prostate cancer 824

**Estramustine** a generic anticancer drug 115

**Estratab** a brand-name estrogen drug 421

**Estratest** a brand-name drug containing an estrogen drug 421 and an androgen drug 100

**Estrone** 422, a generic estrogen drug 421 used to treat symptoms of the menopause 676

**Estropipate** a generic estrogen drug 421

**Estrovis** a brand name for quinestrol 842

**Ethacrynate sodium** a generic loop diuretic drug 366

**Ethacrynic acid** a generic loop diuretic drug 366

**Ethambutol** 422, a generic drug used to treat tuberculosis 1013

**Ethchlorvynol** a generic sleeping drug 916

**Ethinamate** a generic sleeping drug 916

**Ethinyl estradiol** 422, a generic estrogen drug 421 used in oral contraceptives 747

**Ethionamide** a generic drug used to treat tuberculosis 1013 and leprosy 634

**Ethopropazine** a generic phenothiazine drug 790 used to treat Parkinson's disease 772

**Ethosuximide** 423, a generic anticonvulsant drug 116

**Ethotoin** a generic anticonvulsant drug 116

**Ethrane** a brand-name general anesthetic 104

**Ethylestrenol** a generic anabolic steroid drug 940

**Ethynodiol** a generic progesterone drug 823

**Etidocaine** a generic local anesthestic 106

**Etidronate** a generic drug used for Paget's disease 762

**Etomidate** a generic general anesthetic 104

**Etoposide** a generic anti-cancer drug 115

**Etrafon** a brand-name drug containing amitriptyline 94 and perphenazine 786

**Etretinate** a generic drug used to treat psoriasis 830

**Eurax** a brand-name drug used to treat scabies 881

**Euthroid** a brand-name synthetic thyroid hor-mone 985

**Evac-Q-Kit** a brand-name stimulant laxative drug 630

**Excedrin** a brand-name analgesic drug 97

**Ex-Lax** a brand-name stimulant laxative drug 630

**Exsel** a brand-name preparation used to treat dandruff 332 and tinea versicolor 989

**Extend 12** a brand-name cough remedy 316

**Extendryl** a brand-name cold remedy 287

# F

**Famotidine** 440, a generic ulcer-healing drug 1018

**Fansidar** a brand-name drug used to treat malaria 659

**Fastin** a brand name for phentermine 790

**Fedahist** a brand-name cold remedy 287

**Fedrazil** a brand-name decongestant drug 336

**Feen-a-Mint** a brand-name stimulant laxative drug 630

**Feldene** a brand name for piroxicam 796

**Feminone** a brand name for ethinyl estradiol 422

**Femiron** a brand-name preparation containing iron 606

**Femstat** a brand-name vaginal cream containing an antifungal agent 117

**Fenfluramine** a generic appetite suppressant drug 128

**Fenofibrate** a generic lipid-lowering drug 642

**Fenoprofen** 445, a nonsteroidal anti-inflammatory drug 730

**Fentanyl** a generic analgesic drug 97 used in general anesthesia 104

**Feosol** a brand name for ferrous sulfate 445

**Feostat** a brand-name preparation containing iron 606

**F-E-P Creme** a brand-name preparation containing a corticosteroid drug 312 and a local anesthetic 106

**Ferancee** a brand-name preparation containing vitamin C 1059 and iron 606

**Fergon** a brand-name preparation containing iron 606

**Fer-In-Sol** a brand name for ferrous sulfate 445

**Fermalox** a brand-name drug containing iron 606 and an antacid drug 113

**Fero-Folic-500** a brand-name preparation containing iron 606

**Fero-Grad-500** a brand-name preparation containing iron 606

**Fero-Gradumet** a brand name for ferrous sulfate 445

**Ferralet Plus** a brand-name preparation containing iron 606

**Ferro-Sequels** a brand-name preparation containing iron 606

**Ferrous fumarate** an iron salt 606

**Ferrous gluconate** an iron salt 606

**Ferrous sulfate** 445, an iron salt 606

**Festal II** a brand name for pancrelipase 767

**Fiberall** a brand name for psyllium 834

**Fibrinolysin** a generic drug used to treat skin ulcers 1018

**Fiogesic** a brand-name cold remedy 287 containing aspirin 137

**Fiorinal** a brand-name analgesic drug 97 containing aspirin 137

**Flagyl** a brand name for metronidazole 684

**Flavoxate** 458, a generic antispasmodic drug 120 used to treat symptoms of urinary tract infections 1025

**Flecainide** a generic antiarrhythmic drug 114

**Fleet Bisacodyl** a brand-name stimulant laxative drug 630

**Fleet Relief** a brand-name local anesthetic 106

**Fletcher's Castoria for Children** a brand name for senna 891

**Flexeril** a brand name for cyclobenzaprine 326

**Flexoject** a brand name for orphenadrine 750

**Flintstones** a brand-name multivitamin 702

**Florinef** a brand-name corticosteroid drug 312

**Florone** a brand-name corticosteroid drug 312

**Floropryl** a brand-name drug used to treat glaucoma 488

**Florvite** a brand-name vitamin supplement 1060

**Floxuridine** a generic anticancer drug 115

**Flucytosine** a generic antifungal drug 117

**Fludarabine** a generic anticancer drug 115

**Fludrocortisone** a generic corticosteroid drug 312

**Fluidil** a brand-name diuretic drug 366

**Flunisolide** a generic corticosteroid drug 312

**Fluocinolone** 459, a generic corticosteroid drug 312

**Fluocinonide** a generic corticosteroid drug 312

**Fluonid** a brand name for fluocinolone 459

**Fluoritab** a brand name for fluoride 460

**Fluorometholone** a generic corticosteroid drug 312

**Fluoroplex** a brand name for fluorouracil 460

**Fluorouracil** 460, a generic anticancer drug 115

**Fluothane** a brand name for halothane 505

**Fluoxymesterone** a generic anticancer drug 115

**Fluphenazine** 460, a generic antipsychotic drug 119

**Flura** a brand name for fluoride 460

**Flurandrenolide** a generic corticosteroid drug 312

**Flurazepam** 460, a generic benzodiazepine 164 sleeping drug 916

**Flurbiprofen** a generic nonsteroidal anti-inflammatory drug 730

**Flurosyn** a brand name for fluocinolone 459

**FML** a brand-name corticosteroid drug 312

**Foille** a brand-name topical antibacterial drug 114

**Foldan** a brand name for thiabendazole 978

**Folex** a brand name for methotrexate 683

**Folic acid** 460, a vita-min 1056

**Folvite** a brand name for folic acid 460

**Formula 44** a brand-name cough remedy 316

**Fortaz** a brand-name cephalosporin 248, a type of antibiotic drug 114

**Fostex** a brand-name drug used to treat acne 63

**Fototar** a brand name for coal tar 285

**FUDR** a brand-name anticancer drug 115

**Fulvicin U/F** a brand name for griseofulvin 498

**Fungizone** a brand name for amphotericin 96

**Furacin** a brand-name antibacterial drug 114

**Furadantin** a brand name for nitrofurantoin 728

**Furazolidone** a generic drug used to treat giardiasis 486 and shigellosis 901

**Furosemide** 471, a generic loop diuretic drug 366

# G

**Gallamine** a generic muscle-relaxant drug 706

**Gamimune** a brand name for immune serum globulin 570

**Gamma benzene hexa-chloride** another name for lindane 641

**Gammacorten** a brand name for dexamethasone 348

**Gantanol** a brand name for sulfamethoxazole 954

**Gantrisin** a brand name for sulfisoxazole 954

**Garamycin** a brand name for gentamicin 485

**Gaviscon** a brand-name antacid drug 113

**Gelusil** a brand name for simethicone 906

**Gemfibrozil** 478, a generic lipid-lowering drug 642

**Gemnisyn** a brand-name drug containing acetaminophen 61 and aspirin 137

**Genoptic** a brand name for gentamicin 485

**Gentamicin** 485, a generic aminoglycoside, a type of antibiotic drug 114

**Geocillin** a brand-name antibacterial drug 114

**Geopen** a brand-name penicillin drug 779, a type of antibiotic drug 114

**Geravite** a brand-name multivitamin 702

**Gerimed** a brand-name multivitamin 702 and mineral supplement 689

**Geriplex** a brand-name multivitamin 702 containing iron 606

**Geritol** a brand-name multivitamin 702 containing iron 606

**Glaucon** a brand name for epinephrine 414

**Gliclazide** a generic hypoglycemic drug 560

**Glucamide** a brand name for chlorpropamide 271

**Glucotrol** a brand name for glipizide 490

**Glutaral** a type of anti-septic 119

**Glutethimide** a generic sleeping drug 916

**Glyburide** 493, a generic hypoglycemic drug 560

**Glycopyrrolate** a generic drug used to treat irritable bowel syndrome 607

**Glycotuss** a brand-name cough remedy 316

**Gold** 494, a generic drug used to treat rheumatoid arthritis 870

**Gold sodium thiomalate** a generic antirheumatic drug 119 containing gold 494

**Gramicidin** 497, a generic antibiotic drug 114

**Grisactin** a brand name for griseofulvin 498

**Griseofulvin** 498, a generic antifungal drug 117

**Gris-PEG** a brand name for griseofulvin 498

**Guaiacolsulfonate** a generic cough remedy 316

**Guaifed** a brand-name cough remedy 316

**Guaifenesin** a generic cough remedy 316

**Guanabenz** a generic antihypertensive drug 118

**Guanethidine** 501, a generic antihypertensive drug 118

**Gynecort** a brand name for hydrocortisone 550

**Gyne-Lotrimin** a brand name for clotrimazole 284

**Gynogen LA** a brand name for estradiol 421

**Gynol II** a brand-name spermicide 927

# H

**Halazepam** a generic benzodiazepine 164 antianxiety drug 114

**Halcinonide** a generic corticosteroid drug 312

**Halcion** a brand name for triazolam 1009

**Haldol** a brand name for haloperidol 505

**Haley's MO** a brand-name laxative drug 630

**Halofenate** a generic lipid-lowering drug 642

**Halog** a brand-name corticosteroid drug 312

**Haloperidol** 505, a generic antipsychotic drug 119

**Haloprogin** a generic antifungal drug 117

**Halotestin** a brand-name anticancer drug 115

**Halotex** a brand-name antifungal drug 117

**Halothane** 505, a generic general anesthetic 104

**Haponal** a brand-name drug used to treat irritable bowel syndrome 607

**Harmonyl** a brand-name antihypertensive drug 118

**HCG** an abbreviation for human chorionic gonadotropin 494

**Helmex** a brand name for pyrantel 841

**Helmizin** a brand name for piperazine 796

**Hemocyte** a brand-name preparation containing iron 606

**Hetacillin** a generic penicillin drug 779, a type of antibiotic drug 114

**Hexachlorophene** a type of antiseptic 119

**Hexadrol** a brand name for dexamethasone 348

**Hexocyclium** a generic antispasmodic drug 120 used to treat irritable bowel syndrome 607

**Hexylcaine** a generic local anesthetic 106

**Hexylresorcinol** a type of antiseptic 119

**H-H-R** a brand-name antihypertensive drug 118

**Hibiclens** a brand-name antiseptic 119

**Hibistat** a brand-name antiseptic 119

**Hiprex** a brand-name drug used to treat urinary tract infections 1025

**Hispril** a brand-name antihistamine drug 118

**Histabid** a brand-name cold remedy 287

**Histadyl** a brand-name cough remedy 316

**Histagesic** a brand-name cold remedy 287

**Histalet** a brand-name cold remedy 287

**Histamic** a brand-name cold remedy 287

**Histaspan** a brand name for chlorpheniramine 271

**Histex** a brand name for chlorpheniramine 271

**Historal** a brand-name cold remedy 287

**Histor-D** a brand-name cold remedy 287

**Histosal** a brand-name cold remedy 287

**HMS Liquifilm** a brand-name corticosteroid drug 312

**Homatropine** 544, a generic anticholinergic drug 115

**Homicebrin** a brand-name multivitamin 702

**Humorsol** a brand-name drug used to treat glaucoma 488

**Humulin** a brand name for insulin 594

**Hurricaine** a brand-name local anesthetic 106

**Hyaluronidase** an enzyme used topically to reduce bruising 217

**Hycanthone** a generic antihelmintic drug 118

**Hycodan** a brand-name cough remedy 316

**Hycodaphen** a brand-name cough remedy 316

**Hycomine** a brand-name cough remedy 316

**Hycotuss** a brand-name cough remedy 316

**Hydeltrasol** a brand name for prednisolone 813

**Hydeltra-T.B.A.** a brand name for prednisolone 813

**Hydoril** a brand name for hydrochlorothiazide 550

**Hydralazine** 549, a generic antihypertensive drug 118

**Hydrea** a brand-name anticancer drug 115

**Hydrocet** a brand-name analgesic drug 97

**Hydrochlorothiazide** 550, a generic thiazide diuretic drug 366

**Hydrocil** a brand name for psyllium 834

**Hydrocodone** a generic narcotic drug 715 used mainly in cough remedies 316

**Hydrocort** a brand name for hydrocortisone 550

**Hydrocortisone** 550, a generic corticosteroid drug 312

**Hydrocortone** a brand name for hydrocortisone 550

**HydroDIURIL** a brand name for hydrochlorothiazide 550

**Hydroflumethiazide** a generic thiazide diuretic drug 366

**Hydrogen peroxide** 550, a type of antiseptic 119

**Hydromal** a brand name for hydrochlorothiazide 550

**Hydromorphone** a generic narcotic drug 715, a type of analgesic drug 97

**Hydromox** a brand-name thiazide diuretic drug 366

**Hydropres** a brand-name drug containing hydrochlorothiazide 550 and reserpine 863

**Hydroprin** a brand-name drug containing hydrochlorothiazide 550 and reserpine 863

**Hydroquinone** a generic drug used to lighten the skin in disorders of pigmentation 794

**Hydroserpine** a brand-name drug containing hydrochlorothiazide 550 and reserpine 863

**Hydrotensin-50** a brand-name drug containing hydrochlorothiazide 550 and reserpine 863

**Hydroxocobalamin** 551, a synthetic form of vitamin B 1057

**Hydroxychloroquine** a generic derivative of chloroquine 270

**Hydroxyprogesterone** 551, a generic progesterone drug 823

**Hydroxyurea** a generic anticancer drug 115

**Hydroxyzine** 551, a generic antihistamine drug 118

**Hygroton** a brand name for chlorthalidone 271

**Hyoscyamine** 552, a generic anticholinergic drug 115

**Hyperetic** a brand name for hydrochlorothiazide 550

**Hyperstat** a brand-name antihypertensive drug 118

**Hytakerol** a brand name for vitamin D 1059

**Hytinic** a brand name for iron 606

**Hytone** a brand name for hydrocortisone 550

# I

**Iberet** a brand-name multivitamin 702 containing iron 606

**Iberol** a brand-name multivitamin 702 containing iron 606

**Ibuprofen** 566, a generic nonsteroidal anti-inflammatory drug 730

**Idoxuridine** 566, a generic antiviral drug 120

**Iletin** a brand name for insulin 594

**Ilosone** a brand name for erythromycin 418

**Ilotycin** a brand name for erythromycin 418

**Ilozyme** a brand name for pancrelipase 767

**Imferon** a brand name for iron 606

**Imipenem/cilastatin** a generic antibiotic drug 114

**Imipramine** 570, a generic antidepressant drug 116

**Imodium** a brand name for loperamide 649

**Imuran** a brand name for azathioprine 149

**Inapsine** a brand-name antiemetic drug 117

**Incremin with Iron** a brand-name multivitamin 702 containing iron 606

**Indapamide** a brand-name diuretic drug 366

**Inderal** a brand name for propranolol 824

**Inderal LA** a brand name for propranolol 824

**Inderide** a brand-name drug containing hydrochlorothiazide 550 and propranolol 824

**Indocin** a brand name for indomethacin 581

**Indomethacin** 581, a generic nonsteroidal anti-inflammatory drug 730

**Indoramin** a generic antihypertensive drug 118

**Inflamase** a brand name for prednisolone 813

**INH** a brand name for isoniazid 608

**Innovar** a brand-name drug containing an analgesic drug 97 and a tranquilizer drug 1003 used in general anesthesia 104

**Inocor** a brand-name drug used for heart failure 519

**Inosiplex** a generic investigational antiviral drug 120

**Intal** a brand name for cromolyn sodium 321

**Interferon** 598, a generic antiviral 120 and anticancer drug 115

**Intron A** a brand name for interferon 598

**Intropin** a natural neurotransmitter 725 used to treat heart failure 519 and shock 901

**Iodine** 605, an element

**Iodo** a brand-name antifungal 117 and antibacterial drug 114

**Iodochlorhydroxyquin** a brand-name antifungal 117 and antibacterial drug 114

**Iodoquinol** a generic drug used to treat amebiasis 92

**Ionamin** a brand name for phentermine 790

**Ionax** a type of antiseptic 119

**Ionil** a brand name for salicylic acid 879

**Iopanoic acid** a generic drug used to treat hyperthyroidism 557

**Ipecac** 606, a generic drug used to induce vomiting in the treatment of drug overdose and poisoning 379

**Ipodate** a generic drug used to treat hyperthyroidism 557

**Ipratropium** 606, a generic investigational anticholinergic drug 115 used as a bronchodilator drug 215

**Ipsatol** a brand-name cough remedy 316

**Iromin-G** a brand-name multivitamin 702 containing iron 606

**Iron** 606, an essential mineral

**Ismelin** a brand name for guanethidine 501

**Iso-Bid** a brand name for isosorbide dinitrate 608

**Isocarboxazid** 607, a generic antidepressant drug 116

**Isoclor** a brand-name drug containing chlorpheniramine 271 and pseudoephedrine 829

**Isoetharine** a generic bronchodilator drug 215

**Isofluorophate** a generic drug used to treat glaucoma 488

**Isoflurane** a generic general anesthetic 104

**Isoniazid** 608, a generic drug used to treat tuberculosis 1013

**Isopropamide** a generic antispasmodic drug 120 used to treat irritable bowel syndrome 607

**Isoproterenol** 608, a generic bronchodilator drug 215

**Isoptin** a brand name for verapamil 1046

**Isopto Carbachol** a brand name for carbachol 231

**Isopto Carpine** a brand name for pilocarpine 795

**Isopto Cetamide** a brand name for sulfacetamide 954

**Isopto P-ES** a brand-name drug used to treat glaucoma 488

**Isordil** a brand name for isosorbide dinitrate 608

**Isordil Sublingual** a brand name for isosorbide dinitrate 608

**Isordil Tembids** a brand name for isosorbide dinitrate 608

**Isosorbide dinitrate** 608, a generic vasodilator drug 1041

**Isotretinoin** 608, a generic drug derived from vitamin A 1057 used in the treatment of acne 63

**Isoxsuprine** 608, a generic vasodilator drug 1041

**Isuprel** a brand name for isoproterenol 608

## J

**Janimine** a brand name for imipramine 570

**Jenamicin** a brand name for gentamicin 485

## K

**Kabikinase** a brand name for streptokinase 945

**Kahlenberg solution** a brand-name preparation used to treat warts 1069

**Kanamycin** a generic antibiotic drug 114

**Kantrex** a generic antibiotic drug 114

**Kaochlor** a brand-name potassium supplement 812

**Kaolin** 614, a generic ingredient of some antidiarrheal drugs 117

**Kaon** a brand-name potassium supplement 812

**Kaopectate** a brand-name antidiarrheal drug 117

**Karaya gum** a generic bulk-forming laxative drug 630

**Kasof** a brand-name laxative drug 630

**Kato** a brand-name potassium supplement 812

**Kay Ciel** a brand-name potassium supplement 812

**Keflex** a brand name for cephalexin 247

**Keflin** a brand-name cephalosporin 248, a type of antibiotic drug 114

**Kefzol** a brand-name cephalosporin 248, a type of antibiotic drug 114

**Kemadrin** a brand name for procyclidine 822

**Kenacort** a brand-name corticosteroid drug 312

**Kenalog** a brand-name corticosteroid drug 312

**Keralyt** a brand name for salicylic acid 879

**Ketamine** a generic sedative drug 890 used as a general anesthetic 104

**Ketoconazole** 616, a generic antifungal drug 117

**Ketoprofen** 616, a generic nonsteroidal anti-inflammatory drug 730

**Ketrax** a brand-name antihelmintic drug 118

**Kie Syrup** a brand-name decongestant 336 cough remedy 316

**Kinesed** a brand-name antispasmodic drug 120 used in the treatment of irritable bowel syndrome 607

**Klebcil** a brand-name antibiotic drug 114

**Kleer compound** a brand-name cold remedy 287

**Klonopin** a brand-name anticonvulsant drug 116

**K-Lor** a brand-name potassium supplement 812

**Klor-con** a brand-name potassium supplement 812

**Klorvess** a brand-name potassium supplement 812

**Klotrix** a brand-name potassium supplement 812

**K-Lyte** a brand-name potassium supplement 812

**Kolantyl** a brand-name antacid drug 113

**Kolyum** a brand-name potassium supplement 812

**Komed** a brand-name preparation used to treat acne 63

**Konakion** a brand name for phytonadione 794

**Kondremul Plain** a brand name for mineral oil 689

**Konsyl** a brand name for psyllium 834

**Koromex** a brand-name spermicide 927

**K-Phos** a brand-name mineral supplement 689

**Kronofed** a brand-name drug containing chlorpheniramine 271 and pseudoephedrine 829

**Kronohist** a brand-name cold remedy 287

**K-Tab** a brand-name potassium supplement 812

**Kudrox** a brand-name antacid drug 113

**KU Zyme** a brand name for pancrelipase 767

**Kwell** a brand name for lindane 641

**Kwildane** a brand name for lindane 641

**KY Jelly** a brand-name vaginal lubricant 598

## L

**Labetalol** 624, a generic beta-blocker drug 165

**LaBID** a brand name for theophylline 977

**Lac-Hydrin** a brand-name preparation used to treat dry scaly skin 910

**Lacril** a brand-name artificial tear preparation 966

**Lacrisert** a brand-name artificial tear preparation 966

**Lactocal-F** a brand-name multivitamin 702

**Lactulose** 625 a generic laxative drug 630

**Lanacort** a brand name for hydrocortisone 550

**Laniazid** a brand name for isoniazid 608

**Lanolin** 626, a generic preparation used in the treatment of dry skin

**Lanorinal** a brand-name analgesic drug 97 containing aspirin 137

**Lanoxicaps** a brand name for digoxin 361

**Lanoxin** a brand name for digoxin 361

**Larobec** a brand-name multivitamin 702

**Larodopa** a brand name for levodopa 638

**Larotid** a brand name for amoxicillin 95

**Larylgan** a brand-name analgesic throat spray 97

**Lasan** a brand name for anthralin 113

**Lasix** a brand name for furosemide 471

**Laudanum** 630, a solution of opium 745

**Ledercillin VK** a brand-name penicillin drug 779, a type of antibiotic drug 114

**Lente** a brand name for insulin 594

**Leucovorin** a generic form of folic acid 460

**Leukeran** a brand name for chlorambucil 270

**Leuprolide** a generic anticancer drug 115

**Levamisole** a generic antihelmintic drug 118

**Levlen** a brand-name oral contraceptive 747

**Levobunolol** a generic beta-blocker drug 165 used to treat glaucoma 488

**Levodopa** 638, a generic drug used to treat Parkinson's disease 772

**Levo-Dromoran** a brand-name narcotic drug 715, a type of analgesic drug 97

**Levonorgestrel** 638, a generic progesterone drug 823 used in oral contraceptives 747

**Levophed**   a brand name for norepinephrine 730

**Levorphanol**   a generic narcotic drug 715, a type of analgesic drug 97

**Levothroid**   a brand name for levothyroxine 638

**Levothyroxine**   638, a generic thyroid hormone 985

**Levsin**   a brand name for hyoscyamine 552

**Levsinex**   a brand name for hyoscyamine 552

**Librax**   a brand-name antispasmodic drug 120 used for irritable bowel syndrome 607

**Libritabs**   a brand name for chlordiazepoxide 270

**Librium**   a brand name for chlordiazepoxide 270

**Lidex**   a brand-name corticosteroid drug 312

**Lidocaine**   639, a generic local anesthetic 106

**Lidoflazine**   a generic drug for angina pectoris 108

**Limbitrol**   a brand-name drug containing amitriptyline 94 and chlordiazepoxide 270

**Lincocin**   a brand name for lincomycin 641

**Lincomycin**   641, a generic antibiotic drug 114

**Lindane**   641, a generic drug used to treat scabies 881 and lice 638

**Lioresal**   a brand name for baclofen 153

**Liothyronine**   a generic synthetic thyroid hormone 985

**Liotrix**   a generic synthetic thyroid hormone 985

**Lipo-Hepin**   a brand name for heparin 531

**Lipotriad**   a brand-name multivitamin 702

**Liquaemin**   a brand name for heparin 531

**Liqui-Doss**   a brand-name laxative drug 630

**Liquid Pred**   a brand name for prednisone 813

**Liquifilm**   a brand-name artificial tear preparation 966

**Liquiprin**   a brand name for acetaminophen 61

**Lithane**   a brand name for lithium 643

**Lithium**   643, a generic drug used to treat manic-depressive illness 663

**Lithobid**   a brand name for lithium 643

**Lithonate**   a brand name for lithium 643

**Lithotabs**   a brand name for lithium 643

**Lomotil**   a brand-name drug containing diphenoxylate 361 and atropine 143

**Lomustine**   a generic anticancer drug 115

**Loniten**   a brand name for minoxidil 689

**Lo/Ovral**   a brand-name oral contraceptive 747

**Loperamide**   649, a generic antidiarrheal drug 117

**Lopid**   a brand name for gemfibrozil 478

**Lopressor**   a brand name for metoprolol 684

**Lopressor HCT**   a brand name for hydrochlorothiazide 550 and metoprolol 684

**Loprox**   a brand-name antifungal drug 117

**Lopurin**   a brand name for allopurinol 88

**Lorazepam**   649, a generic benzodiazepine 164 sleeping drug 916

**Lorcainide**   a generic antiarrhythmic drug 114

**Lorcet**   a brand-name analgesic drug 97

**Lorelco**   a brand name for probucol 822

**Loroxide-HC**   a brand name for benzoyl peroxide 164

**Lotrimin**   a brand name for clotrimazole 284

**Lotrisone**   a brand-name drug containing clotrimazole 284 and betamethasone 166

**Lotusate**   a brand-name barbiturate 157 sleeping drug 916

**Lovastatin**   650, a generic lipid-lowering drug 642

**Loxapine**   a generic antidepressant drug 116

**Loxitane**   a brand-name antidepressant drug 116

**Lozol**   a brand-name diuretic drug 366

**Lubrin**   a brand-name vaginal lubricant 596

**Ludiomil**   a brand name for maprotiline 664

**Lufyllin**   a brand-name bronchodilator drug 215

**Lugol's solution**   a brand-name preparation used to treat hyperthyroidism 557

**Lupron**   a brand-name anticancer drug 115

**Luride**   a brand-name fluoride supplement 460

**Lypressin**   657, a generic preparation of ADH 68

**Lysergic acid**   another name for LSD 650

**Lyteers**   a brand-name artificial tear preparation 966

---

# M

**Maalox**   a brand-name antacid drug 113

**Macrodantin**   a brand name for nitrofurantoin 728

**Mafenide**   a generic antibacterial drug 114

**Magan**   a brand-name antirheumatic drug 119

**Magnesium**   658, a mineral 689

**Magnesium citrate**   a generic laxative drug 630

**Magnesium gluconate**   a generic magnesium supplement 658

**Magnesium hydroxide**   a generic antacid drug 113

**Magnesium oxide**   a generic laxative drug 630

**Magnesium salicylate**   a generic antirheumatic drug 119

**Magnesium sulfate**   a generic magnesium supplement 658

**Magnesium trisilicate**   a generic antacid drug 113

**Magsal**   a brand-name magnesium supplement 658 and antihistamine drug 118

**Malathion**   a generic drug used to treat lice 638

**Mandelamine**   a brand-name drug used to treat urinary tract infections 1025

**Mandol**   a brand-name cephalosporin 248, a type of antibiotic drug 114

**Mannitol**   663, a generic osmotic diuretic drug 366

**Mantadil**   a brand-name drug used to treat skin irritation 608

**Maolate**   a brand-name muscle-relaxant drug 706

**Maprotiline**   664, a generic antidepressant drug 116

**Marax**   a brand-name drug used to treat asthma 137

**Marbaxin-750**   a brand name for methocarbamol 683

**Marcaine**   a brand-name epidural anesthetic 412

**Marezine**   a brand-name antiemetic drug 117

**Marflex**   a brand name for orphenadrine 750

**Marijuana**   664, a generic central nervous system depressant

**Marplan**   a brand name for isocarboxazid 607

**Materna**   a brand-name multivitamin 702

**Maxibolin**   a brand-name anabolic steroid drug 940

**Maxidex**   a brand name for dexamethasone 348

**Maxiflor**   a brand-name corticosteroid drug 312

**Maxitrol**   a brand name for dexamethasone 348

**Maxzide**   a brand-name drug containing hydrochlorothiazide 550 and triamterene 1009

**Mazanor**   a brand-name appetite suppressant drug 128

**Mazindol**   a generic appetite suppressant drug 128

**Measurin**   a brand name for aspirin 137

**Mebaral**   a brand-name anticonvulsant drug 116

**Mebendazole**   669, a generic antihelmintic drug 118

**Mecamylamine**   a rarely used generic antihypertensive drug 118

**Mechlorethamine**   a generic anticancer drug 115

**Meclan**   a brand-name drug used to treat acne 63

**Meclizine**   669, a generic antihistamine 118 and antiemetic drug 117

**Meclocycline**   a generic drug used to treat acne 63

**Meclofenamate**   669, a nonsteroidal anti-inflammatory drug 730

**Meclomen**   a brand name for meclofenamate 669

**Medicone**   a brand-name drug used to treat skin irritation 608

**Medigesic**   a brand-name analgesic drug 97

**Medihaler-Epi**   a brand name for epinephrine 414

**Medihaler-Ergotamine**   a brand name for ergotamine 416

**Medihaler-Iso**   a brand name for isoproterenol 608

**Mediplast**   a brand name for salicylic acid 879

**Mediquell**   a brand-name cough remedy 316

**Medrol**   a brand name for methylprednisolone 684

**Medrol Enpak**   a brand name for methylprednisolone 684

**Medrol Oral**   a brand name for methylprednisolone 684

**Medroxyprogesterone**   671, a generic progesterone drug 823

**Medrysone**   a generic corticosteroid drug 312 used to treat eye inflammation

**Mefenamic acid**   671, a generic nonsteroidal anti-inflammatory drug 730

**Mefoxin**   a brand-name antibiotic drug 114

**Megace**   a brand name for megestrol 672

**Megestrol**   672, a generic progesterone drug 823

**Melanex**   a brand-name preparation used to treat pigmentation disorders 794

**Melarsoprol**   a generic drug used to treat worm infestation 1081 and protozoa infestation 827

**Melfiat**   a brand-name appetite suppressant drug 128

**Mellaril**   a brand name for thioridazine 978

**Melphalan**   674, a generic anticancer drug 115

**Menadiol** another name for vitamin K 1060

**Menadione** another name for vitamin K 1060

**Menest** a brand-name estrogen drug 421

**Menogaril** a generic anticancer drug 115

**Menotropins** 677, a generic drug used to treat infertility 586

**Menthol** an extract from mint used in inhalations 589 and for skin irritation 608

**Mepenzolate** a generic antispasmodic drug 120 used to treat irritable bowel syndrome 607

**Mepergan** a brand-name drug containing meperidine 680 and promethazine 823

**Meperidine** 680, a generic narcotic drug 715, a type of analgesic drug 97

**Mephenytoin** a generic anticonvulsant drug 116

**Mephobarbital** a generic anticonvulsant drug 116

**Mephyton** a brand name for phytonadione 794

**Mepivacaine** a generic local anesthetic 106

**Meprobamate** 680, a generic antianxiety drug 114

**Meptazinol** a generic analgesic drug 97

**Mequitazine** a generic investigational antihistamine drug 118

**Mercaptopurine** 681, a generic anticancer drug 115

**Merthiolate** a brand-name antibacterial skin preparation 114

**Mesantoin** a brand-name anticonvulsant drug 116

**Mescaline** 681, a generic hallucinogenic drug 504

**Mesoridazine** a generic antipsychotic drug 119

**Mestinon** a brand name for pyridostigmine 841

**Mestranol** 681, a generic estrogen drug 421

**Metamucil** a brand name for psyllium 834

**Metandren** a brand-name androgen drug 100

**Metaprel** a brand name for metaproterenol 683

**Metaproterenol** 683, a generic bronchodilator drug 215

**Metaraminol** a generic drug used to treat shock 901

**Metatensin** a brand-name drug containing reserpine 863 and a diuretic drug 366

**Metaxalone** a generic muscle-relaxant drug 706

**Meted 2** a brand-name preparation containing salicylic acid 879 and sulfur 954

**Methacycline** a generic antibiotic drug 114

**Methadone** 683, a generic narcotic drug 715, a type of analgesic drug 97

**Methamphetamine** a generic amphetamine drug 95

**Methanol** 683, a type of alcohol

**Methantheline** a generic antispasmodic drug 120 used to treat irritable bowel syndrome 607

**Metharbital** a generic anticonvulsant drug 116

**Methazolamide** a generic drug used to treat glaucoma 488

**Methdilazine** a generic antihistamine drug 118

**Methenamine** a generic drug used to treat urinary tract infection 1025

**Methergine** a brand-name drug used to induce labor 263

**Methicillin** a generic penicillin drug 779, a type of antibiotic drug 114

**Methimazole** 683, a generic drug used to treat hyperthyroidism 557

**Methocarbamol** 683, a generic muscle-relaxant drug 706

**Methohexital** a generic sedative drug 890 used to induce general anesthesia 104

**Methotrexate** 683, a generic anticancer drug 115

**Methoxsalen** 683, a generic psoralen drug 829

**Methoxyflurane** a generic drug used to induce general anesthesia 104

**Methscopolamine** a generic antispasmodic drug 120

**Methsuximide** a generic anticonvulsant drug 116

**Methyclothiazide** 684, a generic diuretic drug 366

**Methylbenzethonium** a generic antiseptic preparation 119

**Methyl-CCNU** a brand-name anticancer drug 115

**Methylcellulose** 684, a generic bulk-forming laxative drug 630

**Methyldopa** 684, a generic antihypertensive drug 118

**Methylergonovine** a generic drug used to induce labor 263

**Methyl-glyoxalbisguanyl-hydrazone** a generic anticancer drug 115

**Methylphenidate** a generic central nervous system stimulant 942

**Methylprednisolone** 684, a generic corticosteroid drug 312

**Methyl salicylate** a generic analgesic drug 97 in cream form used for muscle and joint pain 132

**Methyltestosterone** a generic androgen drug 100

**Methyprylon** a generic sleeping drug 916

**Methysergide** 684, a generic drug used to prevent migraine 688

**Meticorten** a brand name for prednisone 813

**Metimyd** a brand-name drug containing prednisolone 813 and sulfacetamide 954

**Metoclopramide** 684, a generic antiemetic drug 117

**Metocurine** a generic muscle-relaxant drug 706 used during general anesthesia 104

**Metolazone** 684, a generic diuretic drug 366

**Metoprolol** 684, a generic beta-blocker drug 165

**Metreton** a brand name for prednisolone 813

**Metronid** a brand name for metronidazole 684

**Metronidazole** 684, a generic antibiotic drug 114

**Metryl** a brand name for metronidazole 684

**Metyrapone** a generic investigational drug for Cushing's syndrome 325

**Metyrosine** a generic antihypertensive drug 118

**Mevacor** a brand name for lovastatin 650

**Mexate** a brand name for methotrexate 683

**Mexiletine** 684, a generic antiarrhythmic drug 114

**Mezlocillin** a generic penicillin drug 779, a type of antibiotic drug 114

**Micatin** a brand name for miconazole 684

**Miconazole** 684, a generic antifungal drug 117

**Micrainin** a brand-name analgesic drug 97 containing aspirin 137

**Micro-K** a brand-name potassium supplement 812

**Micronase** a brand name for glyburide 493

**Micronefrin** a brand name for epinephrine 414

**Micronor** a brand-name oral contraceptive 747

**Midamor** a brand name for amiloride 94

**Midazolam** a generic benzodiazepine drug 164 used for premedication 818

**Midol 200** a brand name for ibuprofen 566

**Midrin** a brand-name drug containing an analgesic drug 97 and a sedative drug 890, used for migraine 688

**Milkinol** a brand-name laxative drug 630

**Milk of Magnesia** a brand-name antacid drug 113

**Milpath** a brand-name drug used to treat irritable bowel syndrome 607

**Milprem** a brand-name drug containing an estrogen 421 and an antianxiety drug 114

**Milrinone** a generic digitalis drug 361

**Miltown** a brand name for meprobamate 680

**Minipress** a brand name for prazosin 812

**Minocin** a brand name for minocycline 689

**Minocycline** 689, a generic tetracycline drug 976, a type of antibiotic drug 114

**Minoxidil** 689, a generic vasodilator drug 1041

**Mintezol** a brand name for thiabendazole 978

**Miochol** a brand name for acetylcholine 62

**Mitomycin** a generic anticancer drug 115

**Mitotane** a generic anticancer drug 115

**Mitrolan** a brand-name laxative drug 630

**Mity-Quin** a brand-name preparation containing hydrocortisone 550, an antifungal drug 117, and an antibacterial drug 114

**Mixtard** a brand name for insulin 594

**Moban** a brand-name antipsychotic drug 119

**Mobidin** a brand-name antirheumatic drug 119

**Mobigesic** a brand-name analgesic drug 97

**Modane** a brand-name laxative drug 630

**Modicon** a brand-name oral contraceptive 747

**Modrastane** a brand-name corticosteroid drug 312

**Moduretic** a brand-name drug containing amiloride 94 and hydrochlorothiazide 550

**Molindone** a generic antipsychotic drug 119

**Mol-Iron** a brand-name iron supplement 606

**Monistat** a brand name for miconazole 684

**Monobenzone** a generic drug for removal of normal skin pigmentation in severe vitiligo 1060

**Monocid** a brand-name antibiotic drug 114

**Mono-Gesic** a brand-name nonsteroidal anti-inflammatory drug 730

**Monosodium glutamate** 694, a food additive 461

**Monosulfiram** a generic drug used for scabies 881

**Motrin** a brand name for ibuprofen 566

**Moxalactam** a generic antibiotic drug 114

**MS Contin** a brand name for morphine 694

**Mucomyst** a brand name for acetylcysteine 62

**Murine Plus** a brand name for tetrahydrozoline 976

**Murocel** a brand name for methylcellulose 684

**Murocoll-2** a brand name for phenylephrine 791

**Muromonab CD3** a generic immunosuppressant drug 576

**Muro's Opcon-A** a brand-name preparation used to treat conjunctivitis 297

**Muro Tears** a brand-name artificial tear preparation 966

**Mutamycin** a brand-name anticancer drug 115

**Myadec** a brand-name multivitamin 702

**Myambutol** a brand name for ethambutol 422

**Mycelex** a brand name for clotrimazole 284

**Mycifradin** a brand name for neomycin 717

**Myciguent** a brand name for neomycin 717

**Mycitracin** a brand-name drug containing bacitracin 150 and neomycin 717

**Mycolog** a brand name for triamcinolone 1008

**Mycolog II Cream** a brand-name preparation containing nystatin 737 and triamcinolone 1008

**Mycostatin** a brand name for nystatin 737

**Myco-Triacet** a brand-name drug containing triamcinolone 1008 and nystatin 737

**Mydfrin** a brand name for phenylephrine 791

**Mydriacyl** a brand name for tropicamide 1013

**Myidil** a brand name for triprolidine 1011

**Myidone** a brand name for primidone 822

**Mykinac** a brand name for nystatin 737

**Mylanta** a brand-name antacid drug 113

**Myleran** a brand-name anticancer drug 115

**Mylicon** a brand name for simethicone 906

**Myobid** a brand name for papaverine 768

**Myochrysine** a brand-name drug containing gold 494

**Myoflex** a brand-name cream containing an analgesic drug 97

**Mysoline** a brand name for primidone 822

**Mysteclin-F** a brand-name drug containing amphotericin 96 and tetracycline 976

**Mysteclin-F Syrup** a brand-name syrup containing amphotericin 96 and tetracycline 976

**Mytrex** a brand name for triamcinolone 1008

## N

**Nabilone** a generic antiemetic drug 117

**Nadolol** 714, a generic beta-blocker drug 165

**Nafcillin** a generic penicillin drug 779, a type of antibiotic drug 114

**Nalbuphine** a generic analgesic drug 97

**Naldecon** a brand-name cough remedy 316

**Nalfon** a brand name for fenoprofen 445

**Nalidixic acid** 714, a generic antibiotic drug 114

**Naloxone** 714, a generic drug that blocks the action of narcotic drugs 715

**Naltrexone** 714, a generic drug that blocks the action of narcotic drugs 715

**Nandrolin** a brand name for nandrolone 714

**Nandrolone** 714, a generic anabolic steroid drug 940

**Naphazoline** 714, a generic decongestant drug 336

**Naphcon** a brand name for naphazoline 714

**Naprosyn** a brand name for naproxen 714

**Naproxen** 714, a generic nonsteroidal anti-inflammatory drug 730

**Naqua** a brand-name thiazide diuretic drug 366

**Naquival** a brand-name drug containing reserpine 863 and a thiazide diuretic drug 366

**Narcan** a brand name for naloxone 714

**Nardil** a brand name for phenelzine 790

**Nasahist** a brand-name cold remedy 287

**Nasalcrom** a brand name for cromolyn sodium 321

**Nasalide** a brand-name corticosteroid nasal spray 312

**Natabec** a brand-name multivitamin 702

**Natafort** a brand-name multivitamin 702

**Natalins** a brand-name multivitamin 702

**Natamycin** a generic antifungal drug 117

**Naturacil** a brand name for psyllium 834

**Nature's Remedy** a brand-name laxative drug 630

**Naturetin** a brand name for bendroflumethiazide 164

**Navane** a brand name for thiothixene 978

**ND-Stat** a brand-name antihistamine drug 118

**Nebcin** a brand name for tobramycin 993

**NegGram** a brand name for nalidixic acid 714

**Nembutal** a brand name for pentobarbital 780

**Neo-Calglucon** a brand-name calcium supplement 223

**Neo-Cortef** a brand-name drug containing hydrocortisone 550 and neomycin 717

**NeoDecadron** a brand name for dexamethasone 348

**Neomycin** 717, a generic antibiotic drug 114

**Neo-Polycin** a brand name for neomycin 717

**Neoquess** a brand name for dicyclomine 357

**Neosar** a brand name for cyclophosphamide 326

**Neosporin** a brand-name preparation containing antibacterial drugs 114

**Neostigmine** 718, a generic drug used to treat myasthenia gravis 708

**Neo-Synalar** a brand-name drug containing fluocinolone 459 and neomycin 717

**Neo-Synephrine 12 Hour** a brand name for oxymetazoline 761

**Neo-Tears** a brand-name artificial tear preparation 966

**Neotep** a brand-name cold remedy 287

**Neothylline** a brand-name bronchodilator drug 215

**Nephrocaps** a brand-name multivitamin 702

**Neptazane** a brand-name drug used to treat glaucoma 488

**Nestabs FA** a brand-name multivitamin 702

**Netilmicin** 720, a generic antibiotic drug 114

**Netromycin** a brand name for netilmicin 720

**Neutrogena** a brand-name soap containing coal tar 285

**Niacin** a member of the vitamin B complex 1058

**Niacinamide** a form of niacin, a member of the vitamin B complex 1058

**Niclocide** a brand name for niclosamide 727

**Niclosamide** 727, a generic antihelmintic drug 118

**Nico-400** a brand name for niacin, a member of the vitamin B complex 1058

**Nicobid** a brand name for niacin, a member of the vitamin B complex 1058

**Nicotine** 727, a stimulant drug found in tobacco 991

**Nico-vert** a brand name for dimenhydrinate 361

**Nifedipine** 727, a generic calcium channel blocker 224

**Niferex** a brand-name multivitamin 702

**Nifurtimox** a generic drug for trypanosomiasis 1013

**Nilstat** a brand name for nystatin 737

**Nimodipine** a generic calcium channel blocker 224

**Nitro-Bid** a brand name for nitroglycerin 729

**Nitrodisc** a brand name for nitroglycerin 729

**Nitro-Dur** a brand name for nitroglycerin 729

**Nitrofurantoin** 728, a generic antibacterial drug 114

**Nitrofurazone** a generic antibacterial drug 114

**Nitrogen mustard** a generic anticancer drug 115

**Nitroglycerin** 729, a generic vasodilator drug 1041

**Nitrol** a brand name for nitroglycerin 729

**Nitrolingual spray** a brand name for nitroglycerin 729

**Nitropress** a brand-name vasodilator drug 1041

**Nitrospan** a brand name for nitroglycerin 729

**Nitrostat** a brand name for nitroglycerin 729

**Nitrous oxide** 729, a gas used to induce general anesthesia 104

**Nizoral** a brand name for ketoconazole 616

**Noctec** a brand name for chloral hydrate 270

**Nolahist** a brand-name antihistamine drug 118

**Nolamine** a brand-name cold remedy 287

**Noludar** a brand-name sleeping drug 916

**Nolvadex** a brand name for tamoxifen 963

**Nonoxynol 9** a generic spermicide 927

**Norcet** a brand-name cough remedy 316

**Nordette** a brand-name oral contraceptive 747

**Norepinephrine** 730, a type of hormone 547

**Norethindrone** 731, a generic progesterone drug 823

**Norethynodrel** a generic progesterone drug 823 used in oral contraceptives 747

**Norflex** a brand name for orphenadrine 750

**Norgesic** a brand-name analgesic 97 containing aspirin 137

**Norgestrel** 731, a generic progesterone drug 823

**Norinyl** a brand-name oral contraceptive 747

**Norlestrin** a brand-name oral contraceptive 747

**Norlutate** a brand name for norethindrone 731

**Norlutin** a brand name for norethindrone 731

**Normodyne** a brand name for labetalol 624

**Norpace** a brand name for disopyramide 365

**Norpace CR** a brand name for disopyramide 365

**Norpramin** a brand name for desipramine 347

**Nor-Q-D** a brand name for norethindrone 731

**Nortriptyline** 731, a generic antidepressant drug 116

**Noscapine** a generic cough remedy 316

**Nostrilla** a brand name for oxymetazoline 761

**Notezine** a brand-name antihelmintic drug 118

**Novafed** a brand name for pseudoephedrine 829

**Novafed A** a brand-name cold remedy 287

**Novahistine DMX** a brand-name cough remedy 316

**Novocain** a brand name for procaine 822

**Novolin L, N, R** brand-name preparations of insulin 594

**NPH Insulin** a brand-name preparation of insulin 594

**Nubain** a brand-name narcotic drug 715, a type of analgesic drug 97

**Nucofed** a brand-name cough remedy 316

**Numorphan** a brand-name analgesic drug 97

**Nupercainal** a brand-name local anesthetic 106

**Nuprin** a brand name for ibuprofen 566

**Nutracort** a brand name for hydrocortisone 550

**Nutraplus** a brand name for urea 1022

**Nydrazid** a brand name for isoniazid 608

**Nylidrin** a generic vasodilator drug 1041

**Nystatin** 737, a generic antifungal drug 117

**Nystex** a brand name for nystatin 737

## O

**Obermine** a brand name for phentermine 790

**Obetrol** a brand-name appetite suppressant drug 128 containing amphetamine drugs 95

**Occlusal** a brand name for salicylic acid 879

**Octoxynol** a brand-name spermicide 927

**Ocusert PILO** a brand name for pilocarpine 795

**Ogen** a brand-name estrogen drug 421

**Olive oil** 742, a type of oil used to treat cradle cap 317

**Omeprazole** a generic investigational drug for peptic ulcers 780

**Omnipen** a brand name for ampicillin 96

**Omnipen-N** a brand name for ampicillin 96

**Oncovin** a brand-name anticancer drug 115

**Ophthaine** a brand-name local anesthetic 106 for eye surgery

**Ophthetic** a brand-name local anesthetic 106 for eye surgery

**Ophthochlor** a brand name for chloramphenicol 270

**Ophthocort** a brand-name preparation containing an antibiotic drug 114 and a corticosteroid drug 312 used to treat eye infections 431

**Opium** 745, a naturally occurring narcotic drug 715, a type of analgesic drug 97

**Opti-Clean** a brand-name contact lens cleaning solution 300

**Opticrom** a brand name for cromolyn sodium 321

**Optigene 3** a brand name for tetrahydrozoline 976

**Optilets-M-500** a brand-name multivitamin 702

**Optimine** a brand name for azatadine 149

**Optimyd** a brand-name drug containing prednisolone 813 and sulfacetamide 954

**Orabase HCA** a brand name for hydrocortisone 550

**Orajel** a brand-name local anesthetic 106 gel used to treat toothache 996 and mouth and lip irritation 697

**Oramide** a brand name for tolbutamide 994

**Orap** a brand name for pimozide 795

**Orasone** a brand name for prednisone 813

**Orazinc** a brand-name zinc supplement 1087

**Oretic** a brand name for hydrochlorothiazide 550

**Oreticyl** a brand-name drug containing hydrochlorothiazide 550 and reserpine 863

**Oreton Methyl** a brand-name androgen drug 100

**Orgatrax** a brand name for hydroxyzine 551

**Orinase** a brand name for tolbutamide 994

**Ornade** a brand-name cold remedy 287

**Ornex** a brand-name cold remedy 287 containing acetaminophen 61

**Orphenadrine** 750, a generic muscle-relaxant drug 706

**Ortho-Novum 1/35** a brand-name oral contraceptive 747

**Ortho-Novum 1/50** a brand-name oral contraceptive 747

**Ortho-Novum 7/7/7** a brand-name oral contraceptive 747

**Ortho-Novum 10/11** a brand-name oral contraceptive 747

**Orudis** a brand name for ketoprofen 616

**Os-Cal** a brand-name drug containing calcium 223 and vitamin D 1059

**Osmoglyn** a brand name for glycerin 493

**Otic-HC** a brand-name solution used to treat infections of the external ear 385

**Otobiotic** a brand-name drug containing hydrocortisone 550 and a polymyxin 808 antibiotic drug 114 used to treat infections of the external ear 385

**Otocort** a brand-name solution used to treat infections of the external ear 385

**Otrivin** a brand name for xylometazoline 1084

**Ouabain** a generic digitalis drug 361

**Ovcon** a brand-name oral contraceptive 747

**Ovral** a brand-name oral contraceptive 747

**Ovrette** a brand-name oral contraceptive 747

**O-V Statin** a brand name for nystatin 737

**Ovulen** a brand-name oral contraceptive 747

**Oxacillin** 761, a generic penicillin drug 779, a type of antibiotic drug 114

**Oxalid** a brand-name nonsteroidal anti-inflammatory drug 730

**Oxandrolone** 761, a generic anabolic steroid drug 940

**Oxazepam** 761, a generic benzodiazepine drug 164

**Oxprenolol** a generic beta-blocker drug 165

**Oxsoralen** a brand name for methoxsalen 683

**Oxtriphylline** 761, a generic bronchodilator drug 215

**Oxybenzone** a generic drug used in sunscreen preparations 955

**Oxybutynin** a generic anticholinergic drug 115 used to treat urinary incontinence 579

**Oxycodone** 761, a generic narcotic drug 715, a type of analgesic drug 97

**Oxymetazoline** 761, a generic decongestant drug 336

**Oxymetholone** a generic anabolic steroid drug 940

**Oxymorphone** a generic narcotic drug 715, a type of analgesic drug 97

**Oxyphenbutazone** a generic nonsteroidal anti-inflammatory drug 730

**Oxyphencyclimine** a generic antispasmodic drug 120 used to treat irritable bowel syndrome 607

**Oxyphenonium** a generic antispasmodic drug 120 used to treat irritable bowel syndrome 607

**Oxytetracycline** 761, a generic tetracycline drug 976, a type of antibiotic drug 114

**Oxytocin** 761, a type of hormone 547

## P

**P-200** a brand name for papaverine 768

**Pabalate** a brand-name analgesic drug 97

**Pamabrom** a brand-name diuretic drug 366 used to treat premenstrual syndrome 818

**Pamelor** a brand name for nortriptyline 731

**Pamine** a brand-name antispasmodic drug 120

**Pancrease** a brand name for pancrelipase 767

**Pancuronium** a generic muscle-relaxant drug 706

**Panmycin** a brand-name tetracycline drug 976, a type of antibiotic drug 114

**Panoxyl, Panoxyl AQ** brand-name preparations containing benzoyl peroxide 164

**Panthenol** a form of pantothenic acid, a member of the vitamin B complex 1058

**Pantopon** a brand-name narcotic drug 715 containing morphine 694, used as an analgesic 97

**Panwarfin** a brand name for warfarin 1069

**Papaverine** 768, a generic vasodilator drug 1041

**Para-aminobenzoic acid** 768, a generic drug used in many sunscreen preparations 955

**Paraflex** a brand name for chlorzoxazone 271

**Parafon Forte**   a brand-name drug containing acetaminophen 61 and chlorzoxazone 271

**Paraldehyde**   a generic anticonvulsant drug 116

**Paramethadione**   a generic anticonvulsant drug 116

**Paramethasone**   a generic corticosteroid drug 312

**Paregoric**   a generic narcotic 715 antidiarrheal drug 117

**Parlodel**   a brand name for bromocriptine 213

**Parmine**   a brand name for phentermine 790

**Parnate**   a brand name for tranylcypromine 1006

**Paromomycin**   a generic antihelmintic drug 118

**Parsidol**   a brand-name drug used to treat Parkinson's disease 772

**Pathibamate**   a brand name for meprobamate 680

**Pathocil**   a brand-name penicillin drug 779, a type of antibiotic drug 114

**Pavabid**   a brand name for papaverine 768

**Pavacen**   a brand name for papaverine 768

**Paveral**   a brand name for codeine 286

**Pavulon**   a brand-name muscle-relaxant drug 706

**Paxipam**   a brand-name antianxiety drug 114

**PBZ**   a brand-name antihistamine drug 118

**PCNU**   a generic investigational anticancer drug 115

**Pediacof**   a brand-name cough remedy 316

**Pediaflor**   a brand name for sodium fluoride 460

**Pediamycin**   a brand name for erythromycin 418

**Pediazole**   a brand-name drug containing erythromycin 418 and sulfisoxazole 954

**Peganone**   a brand-name anticonvulsant drug 116

**Pemoline**   778, a generic stimulant drug 942

**Penapar VK**   a brand-name penicillin drug 779, a type of antibiotic drug 114

**Penbutolol**   a generic beta-blocker drug 165

**Penecort**   a brand name for hydrocortisone 550

**Penfluridol**   a generic antipsychotic drug 119

**Penicillamine**   779, a generic antirheumatic drug 119 and chelating agent 258

**Penicillin V**   a generic penicillin drug 779, a type of antibiotic drug 114

**Penntuss**   a brand-name cough remedy 316

**Pentaerythritol**   a generic nitrate drug 728

**Pentamidine**   a generic drug used to treat trypanosomiasis 1013, leishmaniasis 633, and pneumocystis pneumonia 803

**Pentazocine**   780, a generic narcotic drug 715, a type of analgesic drug 97

**Pentids**   a brand-name penicillin drug 779, a type of antibiotic drug 114

**Pentobarbital**   780, a generic barbiturate drug 157

**Pentostatin**   a generic anticancer drug 115

**Pentothal**   a brand name for thiopental 978

**Pentoxifylline**   780, a generic drug used to treat peripheral vascular disease 784

**Pentrax**   a brand-name shampoo containing coal tar 285

**Pen-Vee K**   a brand-name penicillin drug 779, a type of antibiotic drug 114

**Pepcid**   a brand name for famotidine 440

**Peppermint oil**   780, used as a flavoring in some drug preparations

**Pepto Bismol**   a brand-name antidiarrheal drug 117

**Percocet**   a brand-name drug containing acetaminophen 61 and oxycodone 761

**Percodan**   a brand-name drug containing aspirin 137 and oxycodone 761

**Percogesic**   a brand-name analgesic drug 97

**Percorten**   a brand-name preparation of synthetic ACTH 65

**Perdiem**   a brand name for psyllium 834

**Pergolide**   a generic investigational drug used to treat Parkinson's disease 772

**Pergonal**   a brand name for menotropins 677

**Periactin**   a brand-name antihistamine drug 118

**Peri-Colace**   a brand-name laxative drug 630

**Peritrate**   a brand-name nitrate drug 728

**Permapen**   a brand-name penicillin drug 779, a type of antibiotic drug 114

**Permethrim**   a generic drug used to treat lice 638

**Permitil**   a brand name for fluphenazine 460

**Perphenazine**   786, a generic phenothiazine-type drug 790 used as an antipsychotic drug 119 and an antiemetic drug 117

**Persa-Gel**   a brand name for benzoyl peroxide 164

**Persantine**   a brand name for dipyridamole 362

**Pertofrane**   a brand name for desipramine 347

**Pertussin**   a brand-name cough remedy 316

**Peruvian balsam**   an ingredient of some preparations used to treat hemorrhoids 530

**Petrogalar**   a brand-name laxative drug 630

**Petrolatum**   another name for petroleum jelly 788

**Petroleum jelly**   788, a greasy substance used as an emollient 399

**Pfizerpen VK**   a brand-name penicillin drug 779, a type of antibiotic drug 114

**Phazyme**   a brand name for simethicone 906

**Phenacemide**   a generic anticonvulsant drug 116

**Phenaphen**   a brand name for acetaminophen 61

**Phenazine**   a brand-name appetite suppressant drug 128

**Phenazopyridine**   790, a generic analgesic drug 97

**Phenelzine**   790, a generic monoamine oxidase inhibitor antidepressant drug 116

**Phenergan**   a brand name for promethazine 823

**Phenergan-D**   a brand-name drug containing promethazine 823 and pseudoephedrine 829

**Phenformin**   a generic investigational drug used to treat diabetes mellitus 349

**Phenindamine**   a generic antihistamine drug 118

**Pheniramine**   a generic antihistamine drug 118

**Phenobarbital**   790, a generic barbiturate drug 157

**Phenol**   a type of antiseptic 119

**Phenolphthalein**   a generic laxative drug 630

**Phenoxybenzamine**   a generic antihypertensive drug 118

**Phenprocoumon**   a generic anticoagulant drug 116

**Phensuximide**   a generic anticonvulsant drug 116

**Phentermine**   790, a generic appetite suppressant drug 128

**Phentolamine**   a generic antihypertensive drug 118

**Phenurone**   a brand-name anticonvulsant drug 116

**Phenylbutazone**   790, a generic nonsteroidal anti-inflammatory drug 730

**Phenylephrine**   791, a generic decongestant drug 336

**Phenylpropanolamine**   791, a generic decongestant drug 336

**Phenyltoloxamine**   a generic antihistamine drug 118

**pHisoHex**   a brand-name antiseptic 119

**Phospholine Iodide**   a brand-name drug used to treat glaucoma 488

**Phrenilin**   a brand-name drug containing an analgesic 97 and a sedative drug 890

**Phyllocontin**   a brand name for aminophylline 94

**Physostigmine**   794, a generic drug used to treat glaucoma 488

**Pilocarpine**   795, a generic drug used to treat glaucoma 488

**Pilocel**   a brand name for pilocarpine 795

**Pilopine HS Gel**   a brand name for pilocarpine 795

**Pimozide**   795, a generic drug used to treat Gilles de la Tourette's syndrome 487

**Pindolol**   795, a generic beta-blocker drug 165

**Piperacillin**   a generic penicillin drug 779, a type of antibiotic drug 114

**Piperazine**   796, a generic antihelmintic drug 118

**Piperonyl butoxide**   a generic drug used to treat skin parasites 771

**Pipracil**   a brand-name penicillin drug 779, a type of antibiotic drug 114

**Pirenzepine**   a generic ulcer-healing drug 1018

**Pirmenol**   a generic antiarrhythmic drug 114

**Piroxicam**   796, a generic nonsteroidal anti-inflammatory drug 730

**Pitocin**   a brand name for oxytocin 761

**Pitressin**   a brand name for ADH 68

**Placidyl**   a brand-name sleeping drug 916

**Plaquenil**   a brand-name drug used to treat malaria 659

**Platinol**   a brand name for cisplatin 283

**Plegine**   a brand-name appetite suppressant drug 128

**Plicamycin**   a generic anticancer drug 115

**Podophyllin**   805, a generic drug used to treat genital warts 1070

**Polaramine**   a brand-name antihistamine drug 118

**Polycarbophil calcium**   a generic bulk-forming laxative drug 630

**Polycillin**   a brand name for ampicillin 96

**Polyestradiol**   a generic estrogen-containing anticancer drug 115

**Polyethylene glycol** an ingredient of some skin preparations and certain laxative drugs 630

**Poly-Histine CS** a brand-name cough remedy 316

**Poly-Histine D** a brand-name decongestant drug 336

**Poly-Histine DM** a brand-name cough remedy 316

**Polymox** a brand name for amoxicillin 95

**Poly-Pred** a brand name for prednisolone 813

**Polythiazide** a generic thiazide diuretic drug 366

**Poly-Vi-Flor** a brand-name multivitamin 702 containing fluoride 460 and iron 606

**Polyvinyl alcohol** an ingredient of artificial tear preparations 966

**Poly-Vi-Sol** a brand-name multivitamin 702 containing iron 606

**Pondimin** a brand-name appetite suppressant drug 128

**Ponstel** a brand name for mefenamic acid 671

**Pontocaine** a brand name for tetracaine 975

**Posture** a brand-name drug containing calcium 223 and vitamin D 1059

**Potassium** 812, a mineral 689

**Potassium chloride** a generic potassium supplement 812

**Potassium citrate** a generic antacid drug 113

**Potassium clavulanate** a generic drug used to enhance the activity of some penicillin drugs 779

**Potassium gluconate** a generic potassium supplement 812

**Potassium iodide** a generic antifungal drug 117, also used to treat hyperthyroidism 557

**Potassium permanganate** 812, a substance used as an antiseptic 119 and astringent 139

**Povan** a brand-name antihelmintic drug 118

**Povidone-iodine** a generic antiseptic 119

**Pragmatar** a brand-name preparation containing coal tar 285

**Pralidoxime** a generic drug used to treat poisoning with parathion 771 and certain other pesticides 788

**Pramet** a brand-name multivitamin 702

**Pramilet** a brand-name multivitamin 702

**Pramosone** a brand-name corticosteroid drug 312

**Pramoxine** a generic local anesthetic 106

**Prax** a brand-name local anesthetic 106

**Praziquantel** 812, a generic antihelmintic drug 118

**Prazosin** 812, a generic vasodilator drug 1041

**Precef** a brand-name cephalosporin 248, a type of antibiotic drug 114

**Pred Forte** a brand name for prednisolone 813

**Pred Mild** a brand name for prednisolone 813

**Prednisolone** 813, a generic corticosteroid drug 312

**Prednisone** 813, a generic corticosteroid drug 312

**Prefrin** a brand name for phenylephrine 791

**Pregnyl** a brand name for human chorionic gonadotropin 494

**Prelone** a brand name for prednisolone 813

**Prelu-2** a brand-name appetite suppressant drug 128

**Preludin** a brand-name appetite suppressant drug 128

**Premarin** a brand-name estrogen drug 421

**Prenalterol** a generic drug used for heart failure 519

**Prenate 90** a brand-name multivitamin 702

**Presalin** a brand-name analgesic drug 97 containing aspirin 137 and acetaminophen 61

**Prilocaine** a generic local anesthetic 106

**Primaquine** 821, a generic drug used to treat malaria 659

**Primatene Mist** a brand name for epinephrine 414

**Primaxin** a brand-name antibacterial drug 114

**Primidone** 822, a generic anticonvulsant drug 116

**Principen** a brand name for ampicillin 96

**Pro-Banthine** a brand name for propantheline 824

**Probenecid** 822, a generic drug used to treat gout 495

**Probucol** 822, a generic lipid-lowering drug 642

**Procainamide** 822, a generic antiarrhythmic drug 114

**Procaine** 822, a generic local anesthetic 106

**Procan SR** a brand name for procainamide 822

**Procarbazine** 822, a generic anticancer drug 115

**Procardia** a brand name for nifedipine 727

**Prochlor-Iso** a brand-name antiemetic drug 117

**Prochlorperazine** 822, a generic phenothiazine 790 and an antiemetic drug 117

**Proctocort** a brand name for hydrocortisone 550

**Proctofoam HC** a brand-name corticosteroid drug 312

**Procyclidine** 822, a generic anticholinergic drug 115

**Progens** a brand-name estrogen drug 421

**Progestasert** a brand-name progesterone drug 823

**Progestin** 823, another name for a progesterone drug 823 or hormone 823

**Proglycem** a brand-name antihypertensive drug 118

**Progynon** a brand name for estradiol 421

**Pro-Iso** a brand name for prochlorperazine 822

**Prolamine** a brand name for phenylpropanolamine 791

**Prolixin** a brand name for fluphenazine 460

**Proloprim** a brand name for trimethoprim 1011

**Promazine** 823, a generic phenothiazine 790, a type of antipsychotic drug 119

**Promethazine** 823, a generic antihistamine drug 118

**Promist** a brand-name cough remedy 316

**Prompt** a brand name for psyllium 834

**Pronestyl-SR** a brand name for procainamide 822

**Propacet 100** a brand-name drug containing acetaminophen 61 and propoxyphene 824

**Propafenone** a generic antiarrhythmic drug 114

**Propantheline** 824, a generic antispasmodic drug 120

**Prophene 65** a brand name for propoxyphene 824

**Propine** a brand-name drug used to treat glaucoma 488

**Propoxyphene** 824, a generic narcotic drug 715, a type of analgesic drug 97

**Propranolol** 824, a generic beta-blocker drug 165

**Propylene glycol** a substance used as an emollient 399

**Propylhexedrine** a generic decongestant drug 336

**Propylthiouracil** 824, a generic drug used to treat hyperthyroidism 557

**Prorex** a brand name for promethazine 823

**ProSobee** a brand-name multivitamin 702

**Prostaphlin** a brand name for oxacillin 761

**Prostigmin** a brand name for neostigmine 718

**Prostin/15M** a brand-name prostaglandin drug 824

**Prostin VR** a brand-name prostaglandin drug 824

**Protostat** a brand name for metronidazole 684

**Protriptyline** 828, a generic antidepressant drug 116

**Protropin** a brand name for growth hormone 501

**Proventil** a brand name for albuterol 81

**Provera** a brand name for medroxyprogesterone 671

**Pseudo Bid** a brand-name cough remedy 316

**Pseudoephedrine** 829, a generic decongestant drug 336

**Pseudohist** a brand-name cold remedy 287

**Psilocybin** 829, a hallucinogenic drug 504

**Psorigel** a brand-name preparation containing coal tar 285

**Psyllium** 834, a generic laxative drug 630

**Purinethol** a brand name for mercaptopurine 681

**Purodigin** a brand name for digitoxin 361

**P.V. Carpine** a brand name for pilocarpine 795

**P-V-Tussin** a brand-name cough remedy 316

**Pyocidin-Otic** a brand-name drug containing hydrocortisone 550 and a polymyxin 808

**Pyrantel** 841, a generic antihelmintic drug 118

**Pyrazinamide** 841, a generic drug used to treat tuberculosis 1013

**Pyrethrins** a generic drug used to treat skin parasites 771

**Pyridiate** a brand name for phenazopyridine 790

**Pyridium** a brand name for phenazopyridine 790

**Pyridium Plus** a brand-name analgesic drug 97 used for urinary tract infections 1025

**Pyridostigmine** 841, a generic drug used to treat myasthenia gravis 708

**Pyridoxine** 841, a member of the vitamin B complex 1058

**Pyrilamine** 841, a generic antihistamine drug 118

**Pyrimethamine** 841, a drug used to treat malaria 659 and toxoplasmosis 1000

**Pyrroxate** a brand-name cold remedy 287

**Pyrvinium** a generic antihelmintic drug 118

---

# Q

**Quadrinal** a brand-name drug used in the treatment of asthma 137

**Quazepam** a generic benzodiazepine 164 sleeping drug 916

**Quelidrine** a brand-name cough remedy 316

**Questran** a brand name for cholestyramine 275

**Quibron** a brand-name drug used to treat asthma 137

**Quibron-T/SR** a brand name for theophylline 977

**Quinacrine** 842, a generic drug used to treat giardiasis 486

**Quinaglute** a brand name for quinidine 842

**Quinamm** a brand name for quinine 842

**Quindan** a brand name for quinine 842

**Quinestrol** 842, a generic synthetic estrogen drug 421

**Quinethazone** a generic thiazide diuretic drug 366

**Quinidine** 842, a generic antiarrhythmic drug 114

**Quinine** 842, a generic drug used to treat malaria 659

**Quinora** a brand name for quinidine 842

**Quiphile** a brand name for quinine 842

---

# R

**R & C** a brand-name shampoo used to treat lice 638

**Racet** a brand-name drug containing hydrocortisone 550 and a drug that is both antibacterial 114 and antifungal 117

**Ranitidine** 849, a generic ulcer-healing drug 1018

**Raudixin** a brand-name antihypertensive drug 118

**Rauwiloid** a brand-name antihypertensive drug 118

**Rauwolfia serpentina** a generic antihypertensive drug 118

**Rauzide** a brand-name antihypertensive drug 118

**Redisol** a brand name for vitamin $B_{12}$ 1058

**Regitine** a brand-name antihypertensive drug 118

**Reglan** a brand name for metoclopramide 684

**Regonol** a brand name for pyridostigmine 841

**Regroton** a brand name for chlorthalidone 271

**Rela** a brand name for carisoprodol 238

**Remegel** a brand-name antacid drug 113

**Remsed** a brand name for promethazine 823

**Renese** a brand-name thiazide diuretic drug 366

**Rescinnamine** a generic antihypertensive drug 118

**Reserpine** 863, a generic antihypertensive drug 118

**Resorcinol** a generic preparation used to treat acne 63, dermatitis 345, and fungal infections 470

**Respbid** a brand name for theophylline 977

**Respinol-G** a brand-name cough remedy 316

**Restoril** a brand name for temazepam 968

**Retet** a brand-name tetracycline drug 976, a type of antibiotic drug 114

**Reticulogen** a brand-name drug used in the treatment of iron-deficiency anemia 102

**Retin-A** a brand name for tretinoin 1008

**Retinoic acid** a derivative of vitamin A 1057

**Retinol** 868, the principal form of vitamin A 1057

**Retrovir** a brand name for zidovudine 1087

**Rhindecon** a brand name for phenylpropanolamine 791

**Rhinolar** a brand-name cold remedy 287

**Rhinosyn** a brand-name cold remedy 287

**Ribavirin** a generic antiviral drug 120

**Riboflavin** 874, another name for vitamin $B_2$ 1058

**Rid** a brand-name preparation used to treat lice 638

**Ridaura** a brand name for auranofin 144

**Rifadin** a brand name for rifampin 874

**Rifamate** a brand-name drug containing isoniazid 608 and rifampin 874

**Rifampin** 874, a generic antibacterial drug 114

**Rimactane** a brand name for rifampin 874

**Rimactane INH** a brand-name drug containing isoniazid 608 and rifampin 874

**Ritalin** a brand-name central nervous system stimulant 942

**Ritodrine** 875, a generic drug used to delay premature labor 263

**Robaxin** a brand name for methocarbamol 683

**Robaxisal** a brand-name drug containing aspirin 137 and methocarbamol 683

**Robicillin VK** a brand-name penicillin drug 779, a type of antibiotic drug 114

**Robimycin** a brand name for erythromycin 418

**Robinul** a brand-name anticholinergic 115 and antispasmodic drug 120

**Robitet** a brand-name tetracycline drug 976, a type of antibiotic drug 114

**Robitussin** a brand-name cough remedy 316

**Rocaltrol** a brand-name drug used to treat low blood calcium 223

**Rocephin** a brand-name cephalosporin 248, a type of antibiotic drug 114

**Roferon-A** a brand name for interferon 598

**Rolaids** a brand-name antacid drug 113

**Ronase** a brand name for tolazamide 994

**Rondec** a brand-name cold remedy 287

**Rondomycin** a brand-name antibiotic drug 114

**Roxanol** a brand name for morphine 694

**RP-Mycin** a brand name for erythromycin 418

**Rubramin** a brand name for vitamin $B_{12}$ 1058

**Rufen** a brand name for ibuprofen 566

**Ru-Tuss** a brand-name cold remedy 287

**Ru-Vert-M** a brand name for meclizine 669

**Rynatan** a brand-name cold remedy 287

**Rynatuss** a brand-name cough remedy 316

---

# S

**Safeguard** a brand-name antibacterial soap 114

**SalAc** a brand-name preparation containing salicylic acid 879

**Salicylic acid** 879, a generic keratolytic drug 615

**Salicylsalicylic acid** a generic nonsteroidal anti-inflammatory drug 730

**Saligel** a brand-name preparation containing salicylic acid 879

**Salsalate** a generic nonsteroidal anti-inflammatory drug 730

**Saluron** a brand-name thiazide diuretic drug 366

**Salutensin** a brand-name drug containing a diuretic drug 366 and reserpine 863

**Sandimmune** a brand name for cyclosporine 326

**Sanorex** a brand-name appetite suppressant 128

**Sansert** a brand name for methysergide 684

**Sarna Lotion** a brand-name preparation used to treat skin irritation 608

**SAS 500** a brand name for sulfasalazine 954

**SAStid** a brand-name preparation containing salicylic acid 879 and sulfur 954

**Satric 500** a brand name for metronidazole 684

**Savacort-50** a brand name for prednisolone 813

**Scabene** a brand name for lindane 641

**Schamberg's Lotion** a brand-name preparation used to treat skin irritation 608

**Scopolamine** 887, a generic antispasmodic drug 120

**Scot-Tussin** a brand-name cough remedy 316

**Sebulex** a brand-name preparation containing salicylic acid 879 and sulfur 954

**Sebulon** a brand-name shampoo used to treat dandruff 332

**Secobarbital** 889, a generic barbiturate drug 157

**Seconal** a brand name for secobarbital 889

**Sectral** a brand name for acebutolol 61

**Sedapap-10** a brand-name analgesic drug 97 containing acetaminophen 61 and a barbiturate drug 157

**Seffin** a brand-name cephalosporin 248, a type of antibiotic drug 114

**Seldane** a brand name for terfenadine 971

**Selegiline** a generic investigational drug used to treat Parkinson's disease 772

**Selenium sulfide** an agent used to treat dandruff 332 and tinea versicolor 989

**Selsun** a brand-name preparation used to treat dandruff 332 and tinea versicolor 989

**Semets** a brand-name local anesthetic 106

**Semicid** a brand-name spermicide 927

**Semustine** a generic anticancer drug 115

**Senna** 891, a generic stimulant laxative drug 630

**Senokot** a brand-name stimulant laxative drug 630

**Septisol** a brand-name antiseptic 119

**Septra** a brand-name drug containing sulfamethoxazole 954 and trimethoprim 1011

**Ser-Ap-Es** a brand-name antihypertensive drug 118

**Serax** a brand name for oxazepam 761

**Serentil** a brand-name antipsychotic drug 119

**Serophene** a brand name for clomiphene 284

**Serpasil** a brand name for reserpine 863

**Serpasil-Apresoline** a brand-name drug containing hydralazine 549 and reserpine 863

**Serpate** a brand name for reserpine 863
**Sevin** a shampoo containing a generic drug used to treat lice 638
**Silain Gel** a brand-name antacid drug 113
**Silvadene** a brand name for silver sulfadiazine 906
**Silver nitrate** 906, an astringent 139
**Silver sulfadiazine** 906, a generic antibacterial drug 114
**Simeco** a brand name for simethicone 906
**Simethicone** 906, a generic drug used to relieve flatulence 458
**Simron** a brand-name iron preparation 606
**Sine-Aid** a brand-name drug containing acetaminophen 61 and pseudoephedrine 829
**Sinemet** a brand-name drug used to treat Parkinson's disease 772
**Sinequan** a brand name for doxepin 372
**Singlet** a brand-name cold remedy 287
**Sinubid** a brand-name cold remedy 287 containing acetaminophen 61
**Sinufed** a brand name for pseudoephedrine 829
**Sinulin** a brand-name cold remedy 287
**Sinutab** a brand-name cold remedy 287
**Skelaxin** a brand-name muscle-relaxant drug 706
**Slo-bid** a brand name for theophylline 977
**Slo-Phyllin** a brand name for theophylline 977
**Slo-Phyllin GG** a brand-name drug for asthma 137
**Slow FE** a brand name for ferrous sulfate 445
**Slow-K** a brand name for potassium 812
**Sodium bicarbonate** 922, a generic antacid drug 113
**Sodium citrate** a generic antacid drug 113
**Sodium fluoride** a type of fluoride 460
**Sodium iodide** a type of iodine 605 used to treat hyperthyroidism 557 and thyroid cancer 983
**Sodium nitrite** a generic drug used to treat cyanide poisoning 326
**Sodium salicylate** 922, a generic nonsteroidal anti-inflammatory drug 730
**Sodium thiosulfate** a generic drug used to treat acne 63, tinea versicolor 989, and cyanide poisoning 326
**Solatene** a brand name for vitamin A 1057

**Solfoton** a brand name for phenobarbital 790
**Solganal** a brand-name drug containing gold 494
**Solu-Cortef** a brand name for hydrocortisone 550
**Solu-Medrol** a brand name for methylprednisolone 684
**Soma** a brand name for carisoprodol 238
**Soma Compound** a brand-name drug containing aspirin 137 and carisoprodol 238
**Somophyllin** a brand name for aminophylline 94
**Somophyllin-CRT** a brand name for theophylline 977
**Somophyllin-T** a brand name for theophylline 977
**Soothe** a brand name for eye drops containing tetrahydrozoline 976
**Soprodol** a brand name for carisoprodol 238
**Sorbitrate** a brand name for isosorbide dinitrate 608
**Sotalol** a generic beta-blocker drug 165
**Sparine** a brand name for promazine 823
**Spectazole** a brand name for econazole 388
**Spectinomycin** a generic antibiotic drug 114
**Spectrobid** a brand name for bacampicillin 150
**Spectrocin** a brand-name drug containing gramicidin 497 and neomycin 717
**Spironolactone** 932, a potassium-sparing diuretic drug 366
**Spirozide** a brand name for spironolactone 932
**S-P-T** a brand name for thyroid hormone 985
**SSKI** a generic antifungal drug 117 also used to treat hyperthyroidism 557
**Stadol** a brand-name narcotic drug 715, a type of analgesic drug 97
**Stanozolol** 938, a generic anabolic steroid drug 940
**Staphcillin** a brand-name penicillin drug 779, a type of antibiotic drug 114
**Staticin** a brand name for erythromycin 418
**Statobex** a brand-name appetite suppressant 128
**Statrol** a brand-name antibacterial drug 114 used to treat eye infections 431
**Stelazine** a brand name for trifluoperazine 1010
**Sterane** a brand name for prednisolone 813
**Stibocaptate** a generic antihelmintic drug 118
**Stibogluconate** a generic drug used to treat leishmaniasis 633

**Stilphostrol** a brand name for diethylstilbestrol 359
**Stoxil** a brand name for idoxuridine 566
**Streptase** a brand name for streptokinase 945
**Streptokinase** 945, a generic thrombolytic drug 981
**Streptomycin** 945, a generic antibiotic drug 114
**Streptozocin** a generic anticancer drug 115
**Stuart Natal, Stuart Prenatal** brand-name multivitamin 702 and mineral 689 preparations
**Succinylcholine** a generic muscle-relaxant drug 706
**Sucralfate** 952, a drug used to treat peptic ulcer 780
**Sucrets Cold Decongestant Formula** a brand name for phenylpropanolamine 791
**Sudafed** a brand name for pseudoephedrine 829
**Sufentanil** a generic narcotic analgesic drug 97
**Sulamyd** a brand name for sulfacetamide 954
**Sulf-10** a brand name for sulfacetamide 954
**Sulfabenzamide** a generic antibacterial drug 114
**Sulfacetamide** 954, a generic antibacterial drug 114
**Sulfacet-R** a brand name for sulfacetamide 954
**Sulfacytine** a generic antifungal drug 117
**Sulfadiazine** a generic antifungal drug 117
**Sulfadoxine** a generic drug used to treat malaria 659
**Sulfamethizole** a generic sulfonamide 954, a type of antibacterial drug 114
**Sulfamethoxazole** 954, a generic antibacterial drug 114
**Sulfasalazine** 954, a generic anti-inflammatory drug 118
**Sulfinpyrazone** 954, a generic drug used to treat gout 495
**Sulfisoxazole** 954, a generic antibacterial drug 114
**Sulfoxyl** a brand-name drug containing benzoyl peroxide 164 and sulfur 954
**Sulfur** 954, a mineral 689
**Sulindac** 954, a generic nonsteroidal anti-inflammatory drug 730
**Sulphrin** a brand name for prednisolone 813
**Sulqui** a brand name for niclosamide 727
**Sultrin** a brand-name drug used to treat vaginitis 1036
**Sumox** a brand name for amoxicillin 95
**Sumycin** a brand-name tetracycline drug 976, a type of antibiotic drug 114

**Supen** a brand name for ampicillin 96
**Suramin** a generic drug used to treat sleeping sickness 916
**Surbex** a brand-name multivitamin 702
**Surmontil** a brand name for trimipramine 1011
**Sus-Phrine** a brand name for epinephrine 414
**Sustaire** a brand name for theophylline 977
**Sutilains** an enzyme used to treat infected burns 219 and skin ulcers 1018
**Syllact** a brand name for psyllium 834
**Symmetrel** a brand name for amantadine 92
**Synacort** a brand name for hydrocortisone 550
**Synalar** a brand name for fluocinolone 459
**Synalgos-DC** a brand-name analgesic drug 97 containing aspirin 137
**Synemol** a brand name for fluocinolone 459
**Synkayvite** a brand name for vitamin K 1060
**Synophylate** a brand name for theophylline 977
**Synthroid** a brand name for levothyroxine 638
**Syntocinon** a brand name for oxytocin 761

# T

**Tabloid** a brand-name anticancer drug 115
**Tabron** a brand-name multivitamin 702 and mineral 689 preparation
**Tacaryl** a brand-name antihistamine drug 118
**TACE** a brand-name anticancer drug 115
**Tagamet** a brand name for cimetidine 280
**Talacen** a brand-name analgesic drug 97 containing acetaminophen 61 and pentazocine 780
**Talbutal** a generic barbiturate 157 sleeping drug 916
**Talwin** a brand name for pentazocine 780
**Talwin Nx** a brand-name drug containing naloxone 714 and pentazocine 780
**Tambocor** a brand-name antiarrhythmic drug 114
**Tamoxifen** 963, a generic anticancer drug 115
**Tandearil** a brand-name nonsteroidal anti-inflammatory drug 730
**Tapar** a brand name for acetaminophen 61
**Tapazole** a brand name for methimazole 683

**Taractan** a brand-name antipsychotic drug 119

**Tavist** a brand-name antihistamine drug 118

**Tazicef** a brand-name cephalosporin 248, a type of antibiotic drug 114

**Tazidime** a brand-name cephalosporin 248, a type of antibiotic drug 114

**Tear-Efrin** a brand name for phenylephrine 791

**Tearisol** a brand-name artificial tear preparation 966

**Tears Naturale** a brand-name artificial tear preparation 966

**Tedral** a brand-name drug containing ephedrine 410 and theophylline 977

**Teebacin** a brand name for aminosalicylic acid 94

**Teebaconin** a brand name for isoniazid 608

**Tegafur** a generic anticancer drug 115

**Tegison** a brand-name drug used in the treatment of psoriasis 830

**Tegopen** a brand name for cloxacillin 285

**Tegretol** a brand name for carbamazepine 231

**Tegrin** a brand name for coal tar 285

**Teldrin** a brand name for chlorpheniramine 271

**Temaril** a brand name for trimeprazine 1011

**Temazepam** 968, a generic benzodiazepine drug 164

**Tempra** a brand name for acetaminophen 61

**Teniposide** a generic anticancer drug 115

**Tenoretic** a brand-name drug containing atenolol 140 and chlorthalidone 271

**Tenormin** a brand name for atenolol 140

**Tenuate** a brand-name appetite suppressant drug 128

**Tepanil** a brand-name appetite suppressant drug 128

**Teramine** a brand name for phentermine 790

**Terazosin** a generic antihypertensive drug 118

**Terbutaline** 971, a generic bronchodilator drug 215

**Terfenadine** 971, a generic antihistamine drug 118

**Terpin hydrate** a generic cough remedy 316

**Terra-Cortril** a brand-name drug containing hydrocortisone 550 and oxytetracycline 761

**Terramycin** a brand name for oxytetracycline 761

**Tessalon** a brand-name cough remedy 316

**Testolactone** a generic anticancer drug 115

**Testosterone** 974, an androgen hormone 100

**Testred** a brand name for testosterone 974

**Tetrabenazene** an investigational generic drug used to treat movement disorders 699

**Tetracaine** 975, a generic local anesthetic 106

**Tetrachloroethylene** a generic drug used to treat hookworm infestation 545

**Tetracyn** a brand-name tetracycline drug 976, a type of antibiotic drug 114

**Tetrahydroaminoacridine** 976, a generic investigational drug used to treat Alzheimer's disease 91

**Tetrahydrozoline** 976, a generic decongestant drug 336

**Tetrex** a brand-name tetracycline drug 976

**Texacort** a brand name for hydrocortisone 550

**T/Gel** a brand name for coal tar 285

**Thalidomide** 977, a generic sleeping drug 916

**Thalitone** a brand name for chlorthalidone 271

**Theo-24** a brand name for theophylline 977

**Theobid** a brand name for theophylline 977

**Theoclear** a brand name for theophylline 977

**Theo-Dur** a brand name for theophylline 977

**Theolair** a brand name for theophylline 977

**Theo-Organidin** a brand name for theophylline 977

**Theophyl** a brand name for theophylline 977

**Theophylline** 977, a generic bronchodilator drug 215

**Theospan** a brand name for theophylline 977

**Theostat** a brand name for theophylline 977

**Theovent** a brand name for theophylline 977

**Theozine** a brand name for hydroxyzine 551

**Theragran** a brand-name multivitamin 702 containing iron 606

**Thiabendazole** 978, a generic antihelmintic drug 118

**Thiamylal** a generic barbiturate drug 157 used in general anesthesia 104

**Thiethylperazine** a generic antiemetic drug 117

**Thimerosal** a mercury compound 681 used as an antiseptic 119 and as a disinfectant 364

**Thioguanine** a generic anticancer drug 115

**Thiopental** 978, a generic barbiturate drug 157

**Thioridazine** 978, a generic antipsychotic drug 119

**Thiosulfil** a brand name for sulfamethizole, a sulfonamide antibacterial drug 954

**Thiosulfil-A** a brand-name drug containing phenazopyridine 790 and sulfamethizole, a sulfonamide antibacterial drug 954

**Thiotepa** a generic anticancer drug 115

**Thiothixene** 978, a generic antipsychotic drug 119

**Thiuretic** a brand name for hydrochlorothiazide 550

**Thorazine** a brand name for chlorpromazine 271

**Thymoxamine** a generic drug used to treat glaucoma 488

**Thyrar** a brand name for thyroid hormone 985

**Thyroid Strong** a brand-name thyroid hormone 985

**Thyrolar** a brand-name thyroid hormone 985

**Ticarcillin** a generic penicillin drug 779, a type of antibiotic drug 114

**Ticlopidine** a generic drug used to prevent blood clotting 184

**Tigan** a brand name for trimethobenzamide 1011

**Timentin** a brand-name penicillin drug 779, a type of antibiotic drug 114

**Timolide** a brand-name drug containing hydrochlorothiazide 550 and timolol 988

**Timolol** 988, a generic beta-blocker drug 165

**Timoptic** a brand name for timolol 988

**Tinactin** a brand name for tolnaftate 994

**Tindal** a brand-name antipsychotic drug 119

**Tinidazole** a generic drug used to treat amebiasis 92

**Tinver** a brand-name drug used to treat tinea versicolor 989

**Tioconazole** an investigational generic antifungal drug 117

**T-Ionate P.A.** a brand name for testosterone 974

**Tiopronin** an investigational generic drug used to treat urinary tract calculi 224

**Tissue-plasminogen activator** 989, a generic thrombolytic drug 981

**Tixocortol** an investigational generic drug for inflammatory bowel disease 588

**Tobramycin** 993, a generic antibiotic drug 114

**Tobrex** a brand name for tobramycin 993

**Tocainide** 993, a generic antiarrhythmic drug 114

**Tocopheryl acetate** another name for vitamin E 1059

**Tofranil** a brand name for imipramine 570

**Tolazamide** 994, a generic hypoglycemic drug 560

**Tolazoline** a generic drug used to treat pulmonary hypertension in the newborn 836

**Tolbutamide** 994, a generic hypoglycemic drug 560

**Tolectin** a brand name for tolmetin 994

**Tolinase** a brand name for tolazamide 994

**Tolmetin** 994, a generic nonsteroidal anti-inflammatory drug 730

**Tolnaftate** 994, a generic antifungal drug 117

**Tonocard** a brand name for tocainide 993

**Topicort** a brand-name corticosteroid drug 312

**Topicycline** a brand-name tetracycline drug 976

**Topsyn** a brand-name corticosteroid drug 312

**Torecan** a brand-name antiemetic drug 117

**Tornalate** a brand-name bronchodilator drug 215

**Totacillin** a brand name for ampicillin 96

**TPA** the abbreviation for tissue-plasminogen activator 989

**Trancopal** a brand-name antianxiety drug 114

**Trandate** a brand name for labetalol 624

**Transderm-Nitro** a brand name for nitroglycerin 729

**Transderm-Scop** a brand name for scopolamine 887

**Tranxene** a brand-name benzodiazepine 164 antianxiety drug 114

**Tranylcypromine** 1006, a generic monoamine-oxidase inhibitor antidepressant drug 116

**Trasicor** a brand-name beta-blocker drug 165

**Travase** a brand-name enzyme-containing preparation used to treat infected burns 219 and skin ulcers 1018

**Trazodone** 1008, a generic antidepressant drug 116

**Trecator-SC** a brand-name drug used to treat tuberculosis 1013 and leprosy 634

**Tremin** a brand name for trihexyphenidyl 1011

**Trental**   a brand name for pentoxifylline 780

**Tretinoin**   1008, a generic drug used to treat acne 63

**Trexan**   a brand name for naltrexone 714

**Triacetin**   a generic antifungal drug 117 used to treat tinea 988

**Triad**   a brand-name analgesic drug 97

**Triafed-C**   a brand name for triprolidine 1011

**Triamcinolone**   1008, a generic corticosteroid drug 312

**Triaminic**   a brand name for phenylpropanolamine 791

**Triamterene**   1009, a generic potassium-sparing diuretic drug 366

**Triaprin**   a brand-name analgesic drug 97

**Triavil**   a brand-name drug containing amitriptyline 94 and perphenazine 786

**Triazolam**   1009, a generic benzodiazepine drug 164

**Trichlormethiazide**   a generic thiazide diuretic drug 366

**Trichloracetic acid**   a generic treatment for warts 1069

**Triclocarban**   a type of antiseptic 119

**Triclosan**   a type of antiseptic 119

**Tricodene**   a brand-name cold remedy 287

**Tridesilon**   a brand-name corticosteroid drug 312

**Tridihexethyl chloride**   a generic antispasmodic drug 120 for irritable bowel syndrome 607

**Tridil**   a brand name for nitroglycerin 729

**Tridione**   a brand-name anticonvulsant drug 116

**Trientine**   a generic chelating agent 258 used to treat Wilson's disease 1078

**Triethylenetetramine**   a generic chelating agent 258 used to treat Wilson's disease 1078

**Trifluoperazine**   1010, a generic antipsychotic drug 119

**Triflupromazine**   a generic antipsychotic 119 and antiemetic drug 117

**Trifluridine**   1010, a generic antiviral drug 120

**Trigesic**   a brand-name analgesic drug 97 containing aspirin 137

**Trihexane**   a brand name for trihexyphenidyl 1011

**Trihexyphenidyl**   1011, a generic anticholinergic drug 115

**Tri-Hydroserpine**   a brand-name vasodilator drug 1041

**Trilafon**   a brand name for perphenazine 786

**Tri-Levlen**   a brand-name oral contraceptive 747

**Trilisate**   a brand name for sodium salicylate 922

**Trilostane**   a generic synthetic corticosteroid drug 312 for Cushing's syndrome 325

**Trimazosin**   a generic antihypertensive drug 118

**Trimeprazine**   1011, a generic antihistamine drug 118

**Trimethadione**   a generic anticonvulsant drug 116

**Trimethaphan**   a generic antihypertensive drug 118

**Trimethobenzamide**   1011, a generic antiemetic drug 117

**Trimethoprim**   1011, a generic antibacterial drug 114

**Trimipramine**   1011, a generic tricyclic antidepressant drug 116

**Trimox**   a brand name for amoxicillin 95

**Trimpex**   a brand name for trimethoprim 1011

**Trinalin**   a brand-name drug containing azatadine 149 and pseudoephedrine 829

**Trind**   a brand-name cold remedy 287

**Tri-Norinyl**   a brand-name oral contraceptive 747

**Trinsicon**   a brand-name multivitamin 702 and mineral 689 preparation

**Trioxsalen**   a generic psoralen drug 829 used in PUVA treatment 839

**Tripelennamine**   a generic antihistamine drug 118

**Triphasil**   a brand-name oral contraceptive 747

**Triphed**   a brand name for triprolidine 1011

**Tri-Phen-Chlor**   a brand-name cold remedy 287

**Triple antibiotic**   a generic antibiotic drug 114

**Triple Sulfas**   a brand-name sulfonamide drug 954

**Triprolidine**   1011, a generic antihistamine drug 118

**Trisoralen**   a brand-name psoralen drug 829 used in PUVA treatment 839

**Tri-Vi-Flor**   a brand-name multivitamin 702 containing fluoride 460

**Tri-Vi-Sol**   a brand-name multivitamin 702

**Trobicin**   a brand-name antibiotic drug 114

**Trofan**   a brand-name nonbenzodiazepine, nonbarbiturate sleeping drug 916

**Trolamine**   a generic drug used as drops to remove earwax 387

**Troleandomycin**   a generic antibiotic drug 114

**Tromethamine**   a generic drug used to treat urinary tract calculi 224

**Tronolane**   a brand-name local anesthetic 106

**Tronothane**   a brand-name local anesthetic 106

**Tropicacyl**   a brand name for tropicamide 1013

**Tropicamide**   1013, a generic drug used to dilate the pupil

**Trymex**   a brand name for triamcinolone 1008

**Trypsin**   an intestinal enzyme used to treat indigestion 580

**Tryptophan**   a generic nonbenzodiazepine, nonbarbiturate sleeping drug 916

**Trysul**   a brand-name sulfonamide drug 954

**T-Stat**   a brand name for erythromycin 418

**Tubocurarine**   a generic muscle-relaxant drug 706 used in general anesthesia 104

**Tuinal**   a brand-name barbiturate 157 sleeping drug 916

**Tums**   a brand-name antacid drug 113

**Tussagesic**   a brand-name cough remedy 316

**Tussanil**   a brand-name cold remedy 287

**Tussar**   a brand-name cough remedy 316

**Tussend**   a brand-name cough remedy 316

**Tussionex**   a brand-name cough remedy 316

**Tussi-Organidin**   a brand-name cough remedy 316

**Tussi-Organidin DM**   a brand-name cough remedy 316

**Tussirex**   a brand-name cough remedy 316

**Tuss-Ornade**   a brand-name cold remedy 287

**Twin-K**   a brand-name cough remedy 316

**Tylenol**   a brand name for acetaminophen 61

**Tylox**   a brand-name drug containing acetaminophen 61 and oxycodone 761

**Tympagesic Otic Solution**   a brand-name analgesic drug 97 used to treat otitis externa 757

**Tyzine**   a brand name for tetrahydrozoline 976

---

## U

**Ultracef**   a brand-name cephalosporin 248, a type of antibiotic drug 114

**Undecylenic acid**   a generic antifungal drug 117 used to treat athlete's foot 141

**Unibase**   a brand-name emollient 399

**Unilax**   a brand-name laxative drug 630

**Unipen**   a brand-name penicillin drug 779, a type of antibiotic drug 114

**Uniphyl**   a brand name for theophylline 977

**Unipres**   a brand-name antihypertensive drug 118

**Unisom**   a brand-name antihistamine 118 sleeping drug 916

**Unproco**   a brand-name cough remedy 316

**Urecholine**   a brand-name drug used to treat urine retention 1029

**Urex**   a brand-name drug used to treat urinary tract infection 1025

**Urised**   a brand-name drug used to treat urinary tract infection 1025

**Urispas**   a brand-name antispasmodic drug 120

**Uritabs**   a brand-name drug used to treat urinary tract infection 1025

**Urobiotic-250**   a brand-name drug containing oxytetracycline 761 and phenazopyridine 790

**Urodine**   a brand name for phenazopyridine 790

**Urogesic**   a brand-name analgesic drug 97 used for urinary tract infection 1025

**Urokinase**   1029, a generic thrombolytic drug 981

**Uro-Phosphate**   a brand-name drug used to treat urinary tract infections 1025

**Ursodeoxycholic acid**   a generic drug used to treat gallstones 474

**Uticillin VK**   a brand-name penicillin drug 779, a type of antibiotic drug 114

**Uticort**   a brand name for betamethasone 166

**Utimox**   a brand name for amoxicillin 95

---

## V

**Vacon**   a brand name for phenylephrine 791

**Vaginex**   a brand-name cream containing an antihistamine drug 118 used to relieve genital irritation 608

**Vagitrol**   a brand-name vaginal cream containing a sulfonamide antibacterial drug 114

**Valdrene**   a brand name for diphenhydramine 361

**Valergen**   a brand name for estradiol 421

**Valertest** a brand-name drug containing estradiol 421 and testosterone 974

**Valisone** a brand name for betamethasone 166

**Valium** a brand name for diazepam 357

**Valmid** a brand-name sleeping drug 916

**Valpin 50** a brand-name antispasmodic drug 120 used to treat irritable bowel syndrome 607

**Valrelease** a brand name for diazepam 357

**Vancenase** a brand name for beclomethasone 161

**Vanceril** a brand name for beclomethasone 161

**Vanoxide-HC** a brand-name drug containing benzoyl peroxide 164 and hydrocortisone 550

**Vanseb** a brand name for salicylic acid 879

**Vaponefrin** a brand name for epinephrine 414

**Vaseline Petroleum Jelly** 788, a brand name for petroleum jelly 788

**Vasocidin** a brand-name drug containing prednisolone 813 and sulfacetamide 954

**VasoClear** a brand name for naphazoline 714

**Vasocon** a brand name for naphazoline 714

**Vasocon-A** a brand-name drug used to treat allergic conjunctivitis 297

**Vasodilan** a brand name for isoxsuprine 608

**Vasosulf** a brand name for sulfacetamide 954

**Vasotec** a brand name for enalapril 400

**Vatronol** a brand name for ephedrine 410

**V-Cillin K** a brand-name penicillin drug 779, a type of antibiotic drug 114

**Vecuronium** a generic muscle-relaxant drug 706

**Veetids** a brand-name penicillin drug 779, a type of antibiotic drug 114

**Velban** a brand-name anticancer drug 115

**Velosef** a brand-name cephalosporin 248, a type of antibiotic drug 114

**Velosulin** a brand name for pork insulin 594

**Velvachol** a brand-name preparation containing lanolin 626 and petroleum jelly 788

**Ventolin** a brand name for albuterol 81

**Vepesid** a brand-name anticancer drug 115

**Vermox** a brand name for mebendazole 669

**Verrex** a brand-name drug containing podophyllin 805 and salicylic acid 879

**Verrusol** a brand-name preparation used to treat warts 1069

**Vesprin** a brand-name antipsychotic 119 and antiemetic drug 117

**Vibramycin** a brand name for doxycycline 372

**Vibra-Tabs** a brand name for doxycycline 372

**Vicks** a brand-name cold remedy 287

**Vicodin** a brand-name analgesic drug 97

**Vicon-C** a brand-name multivitamin 702

**Vidarabine** a generic antiviral drug 120

**Vi-Daylin** a brand-name multivitamin 702

**Viloxazine** a generic central nervous system stimulant 942

**Vinblastine** a generic anticancer drug 115

**Vincristine** a generic anticancer drug 115

**Vindesine** a generic anticancer drug 115

**Vioform** a cream containing a generic antibacterial drug 114 and an antifungal drug 117

**Viokase** a brand name for pancrelipase 767

**Vira-A** a brand-name antiviral drug 120

**Viranol** a brand name for salicylic acid 879

**Virazole** a brand-name antiviral drug 120

**Viroptic** a brand name for trifluridine 1010

**Visine** a brand name for tetrahydrozoline 976

**Visken** a brand name for pindolol 795

**Vistaril** a brand name for hydroxyzine 551

**Vitron-C** a brand-name preparation containing iron 606 and vitamin C 1059

**Vivactil** a brand name for protriptyline 828

**Vivalin** a brand-name central nervous system stimulant 942

**Vontrol** a brand-name antiemetic drug 117

**Vosal** a brand name for acetic acid 62

**VoSol HC** a brand-name drug containing hydrocortisone 550 and acetic acid 62

**Voxsuprine** a brand name for isoxsuprine 608

**Vytone** a brand-name drug containing hydrocortisone 550 and an antibiotic drug 114

---

# W

**Wans** a brand-name drug containing pentobarbital 780 and pyrilamine 841

**Wart-Off** a brand-name preparation for warts 1069

**Wehless** a brand-name appetite suppressant 128

**Wellcovorin** a brand name for folic acid 460

**Westcort** a brand name for hydrocortisone 550

**Whitfield's Ointment** a brand-name preparation used to treat warts 1069

**Wigraine** a brand name for ergotamine 416

**Wigrettes** a brand name for ergotamine 416

**Wilpowr** a brand name for phentermine 790

**Winstrol** a brand name for stanozolol 938

**Witch hazel** a generic mild astringent 139

**Wyamycin S** a brand name for erythromycin 418

**Wyanoids** brand-name rectal suppositories used to relieve anal itching 608

**Wycillin** a brand-name penicillin drug 779

**Wydase** a brand-name enzyme used to reduce bruising 217

**Wygesic** a brand-name analgesic drug 97

**Wymox** a brand name for amoxicillin 95

**Wytensin** a brand-name antihypertensive drug 118

---

# X

**Xanax** a brand name for alprazolam 89

**Xerac** a brand-name antiperspirant 118

**Xerac BP** a brand name for benzoyl peroxide 164

**X-Otag** a brand name for orphenadrine 750

**X-Prep** a brand name for senna 891

**X seb** a brand name for salicylic acid 879

**Xylocaine** a brand name for lidocaine 639

**Xylometazoline** a generic decongestant drug 336

---

# Y

**Y-Itch** a brand name for tetracaine 975

**Yocon** a brand-name antihypertensive drug 118

**Yodoxin** a brand-name drug used to treat amebiasis 92

**Yohimbine** a generic antihypertensive drug 118

**Yohimex** a brand-name antihypertensive drug 118

**Yomesan** a brand name for niclosamide 727

**Yutopar** a brand name for ritodrine 875

---

# Z

**Zantac** a brand name for ranitidine 849

**Zarontin** a brand name for ethosuximide 423

**Zaroxolyn** a brand name for metolazone 684

**Z-Bec** a brand-name multivitamin 702

**Zeasorb-AF** a brand name for tolnaftate 994

**Zemo** a brand-name preparation used to relieve skin irritation 608

**Zenate** a brand-name multivitamin 702 and mineral 689 preparation

**Zentinic** a brand-name multivitamin 702 containing iron 606

**Zentron** a brand-name multivitamin 702 containing iron 606

**Zephiran Chloride** a brand-name antiseptic 119

**Zephrex** a brand-name cough remedy 316

**Zetar** a brand name for coal tar 285

**Zide** a brand name for hydrochlorothiazide 550

**Zidovudine** 1087, a generic antiviral drug 120

**Zinacef** a brand-name cephalosporin 248, a type of antibiotic drug 114

**Zincfrin** an astringent 139

**Zinc gluconate** a generic compound of zinc 1087

**Zincon** a brand-name antifungal drug 117 used to treat dandruff 332

**Zinc pyrithione** a generic antifungal drug 117 used to treat dandruff 332

**Zinc sulfate** an astringent 139

**Ziradryl** a brand name for diphenhydramine 361

**Zone-A** a brand-name corticosteroid drug 312

**Zorprin** a brand name for aspirin 137

**Zyloprim** a brand name for allopurinol 88

**Zymenol** a brand name for mineral oil 689

# INDEX

This index covers the three major sections of the encyclopedia: **Medicine Today**; the **A to Z of Medicine**; and the **Drug Glossary**. **Self-help Organizations** (see pages 1090-1095) are not included in the index.

Index entries begin with either a capital or a lower-case letter. Most index entries with an initial capital correspond to titles of entries in the **Medicine Today** or the **A to Z of Medicine** sections. Other index entries with an initial capital refer you to a **Drug Glossary** entry. With the exception of a few capitalized abbreviations or eponyms, all other index entries have a lower-case first letter.

Index entries that correspond to the titles of encyclopedia entries usually refer you to the page on which the encyclopedia entry starts. (In the case of encyclopedia entries that are simple cross-references to other encyclopedia entries, the index refers you directly to the cross-referenced entries or to major index entries.) Other index entries and all index subentries refer you to the title of an encyclopedia entry or to an illustration title, accompanied by a page number. This number refers to the page where the index topic appears.

Index entries, subentries, or page numbers in *italic* type refer you to illustrations.

## A

Abdomen 50
  fluid in: Ascites 136
  removal of fluid from:
    Paracentesis 768
  surgical opening of:
    Laparotomy, exploratory 626
Abdomen, acute 50
*abdominal incisions 579*
abdominal organs, reversed:
  and Dextrocardia 349
  medical term: Situs inversus 908
Abdominal pain 50
  *diagnosing abdominal pain 55*
  *symptom charts 51, 53*
Abdominal swelling 55
  *symptom chart 56*
Abdominal X ray 55
abdominoplasty:
  Body contour surgery 191
Abducent nerve 55
  *functions of cranial nerves 318*
Abduction 55
  and *joint movements 99*
Ablation 57
Abnormality 57
ABO blood classification:
  Blood groups 187
Abortifacient 57
Abortion 57
  spontaneous: Miscarriage 690
Abortion, elective 57
abrasion:
  type of Wound 1081
Abrasion, dental 58
Abreaction 58
Abscess 58
  and Pus 839
Abscess, dental 59
Absence 59
  feature of Epilepsy 413
absorption of nutrients:
  by Digestive system 359; Ileum 568
  *the digestive process 360*
Acanthosis nigricans 59

causing Pigmentation 795
Access to care 59
Accident-prone 59
Accidents 59
  *causes and incidence of accidental death 60*
  causing Eye injuries 432
  Falls in the elderly 438
  Health hazards 511
acclimation:
  and Environmental constraints 47; Heat disorders 525
Accommodation 61
  and Eye 428; Vision 1052
  loss of: Presbyopia 820
  testing of: *vision tests 1055*
Accreditation 61
Accubron 1096
Accutane 1096
Acebutolol 61
Acecainide 1096
Aceclidine 1096
ACE inhibitor drugs 61
  effect on Angiotensin 110;
    Renin 861
  examples of: Captopril 231;
    Enalapril 400
  group of Vasodilator drugs 1041
acetabulum:
  part of Hip 538; Pelvis 778
Acetaminophen 61
  an Analgesic drug 97
  causing Hepatitis 532; *disorders of the liver 646*
  overdose, treatment of:
    Acetylcysteine 62
Acetazolamide 62
Acetic acid 62
Acetohexamide 62
acetone:
  inhalation of: Solvent abuse 923
  excess: Ketosis 616
Acetophenazine 1096
Acetylcholine 61
  action of: Muscle 705; *how neurotransmitters work 726*
  type of Neurotransmitter 725
Acetylcysteine 62

Achalasia 62
  causing Swallowing difficulty 958
Achilles tendon 62
  Tendon 970
Achlorhydria 62
Achondroplasia 63
  and Short stature 902
Achromycin 1096
Acid 63
  causing Caries, dental 236;
    Decalcification, dental 335;
    Plaque, dental 800
  excess: Peptic ulcer 780;
    Zollinger-Ellison syndrome 1088
  in eye: *disorders of the cornea 308*
    and pH 788
Acid-base balance 63
  regulation of: Kidney 617
Acidosis 63
  causes of: Hypercapnia 553;
    Lactic acid 625
acid rain:
  Pollution 807
Acid reflux 63
  causes of: Hiatal hernia 538;
    Pregnancy 813
  causing Heartburn 516
acid regurgitation:
  see index entry Acid reflux
Acne 63
  and Sebaceous glands 889
  symptom of: Pimple 795
  treatment of: Isotretinoin 608;
    Tretinoin 1008; Vitamin supplements 1060
Acoustic nerve 64
  *functions of cranial nerves 318*
  part of Vestibulocochlear nerve 1048
  testing of: Hearing tests 513
Acoustic neuroma 64
acquired immune deficiency syndrome (AIDS):
  see index entry AIDS
Acrisorcin 1096
Acrivastine 1096
Acrocyanosis 64
Acrodermatitis enteropathica 64

Acromegaly 65
  cause of: Pituitary tumors 798
Acromioclavicular joint 65
  part of Shoulder 902
acromion:
  and Acromioclavicular joint 65;
    Shoulder 902
  part of Scapula 882
Acroparasthesia 65
ACTH 65
  abnormal production of:
    Addison's disease 67;
    Cushing's syndrome 325;
    *disorders of the adrenal glands 71; endocrine disorders 404*
  normal production of: *endocrine system 403; hormonal system 546;* Pituitary gland 797
Acthar 1096
Acticort 1096
Actidil 1096
Actifed 1096
Acting out 66
  to achieve Catharsis 241
  and Play therapy 801;
    Psychodrama 832; Role-playing 875
Actinic 66
Actinomycosis 66
  *a disorder of the lung 652*
Activase 1096
Acuity, visual:
  see index entry Visual acuity
Acupressure 66
Acupuncture 66
  and role of Endorphins 405
Acute 67
acute mountain sickness (AMS):
  Mountain sickness 696
Acyclovir 67
  in treatment of Cold sore 288;
    Herpes, genital 536; Herpes zoster 537
Adalat 1096
Adam's apple 67
  part of Larynx 628
  and Vocal cords 1061
Adapettes 1096
Adapin 1096
Addiction 67

and Alcohol dependence 81;
Drug dependence 378
Addison's disease 67
a *disorder of the adrenal glands 71;
endocrine disorder 404*
Adduction 67
and *joint movements 99*
Adeflor 1096
adenine:
as constituent of Nucleic acids
733
and *DNA and genetic disorders
40; what genes are and what
they do 480*
Adenitis 67
Adenocarcinoma 68
type of Lung cancer 651
Adenoidectomy 68
Adenoids 68
anatomy of: Nasopharynx 716
and Otitis media 757; Sleep
apnea 916
removal of: Adenoidectomy 68
Adenoma 68
adenoma sebaceum:
and Tuberous sclerosis 1014
Adenomatosis 68
adenosine diphosphate (ADP):
ADP 70
adenosine triphosphate (ATP):
see index entry ATP
adenovirus:
causing Pneumonia 803
*viruses and disease 1051*
ADH 68
deficiency of: Urination,
excessive 1026
excess: SIADH 904
function of: Urine 1027; Water
1070
production of: *endocrine system
403; hormonal system 546;*
Pituitary gland 797
Adhesion 68
causing Intestine, obstruction
of 602
following Peritonitis 786
type of Scar 882
adhesive bandages:
Dressings 374
Adie's pupil:
Pupil 838
Adie's syndrome:
and Mydriasis 709
Adipex-P 1096
Adipose tissue 69
Tissue 989
Adjuvant 69
Adlerian theory 69
Adolescence 69
ADP 70
Adrenal failure 70
Adrenal glands 70
and Corticosteroid drugs 312
disorders of: *disorders of the
adrenal glands 71; endocrine
disorders 404*
part of *endocrine system 403;
hormonal system 546*
Adrenal hyperplasia, congenital
72
causing Pseudohermaphro-
ditism 829
Adrenaline:

see index entry Epinephrine
Adrenal tumors 72
Adrenocorticotropic hormone
(ACTH):
see index entry ACTH
Adrenogenital syndrome:
see index entry Adrenal
hyperplasia, congenital
Adriamycin 1096
Adrucil 1096
Adsorbocarpine 1096
Advil 1096
Aerobic 72
and Oxygen 761
Aerobics 72
and Exercise 425; Fitness 457;
Training 1003
Aerobid 1096
Aerodontalgia 73
Aerolate 1096
Aerolone 1096
Aerophagia 73
causing Belching 164;
Flatulence 458
Aeroseb-Dex 1096
aerosols:
effects of: Ozone 761; Pollution
807
inhalation of: Solvent abuse 923
medical use of: Inhaler 589;
Vaporizer 1038
Aerosporin 1096
Affect 73
abnormal: Psychosis 833
Affective disorders 73
Affinity 73
Aflatoxin 73
and Fungi 471; Nutritional
disorders 737
Afrin 1096
Afrinol 1096
Afterbirth 73
medical term: Placenta 798
Afterpains 73
agammaglobulinemia:
type of Immunodeficiency
disorder 575
Agar 73
Age 73
see also index entry Aging
Agenesis 74
Agent 74
Agent orange 74
Age spots 74
Ageusia 74
common term: Taste, loss of
965
Aggregation 74
Aggression 74
and Inferiority complex 586
Aging 74
*practical effects of aging 75*
and Cancer 226; Osteoporosis
756
see also index entry Age
Agitation 75
Agnosia 76
Agoral 1096
Agoraphobia 76
and Panic attack 768; Vertigo
1048
type of Phobia 792
Agraphia 76
Ague 76

and Malaria 659
AIDS 44, 76
associated with Hemophilia 530
causes of: *causes and prevention
of AIDS 77;* HIV 541
and development of Fungal
infections 470; Kaposi's
sarcoma 614; Pneumocystis
pneumonia 803;
Toxoplasmosis 1001
effect on *the adaptive immune
system 573*
prevention of: *causes and
prevention of AIDS 77;* "Safe"
sex 879
transmission of: *how AIDS has
been contracted in the US 78;
no-risk activities 78;* Blood
transfusion 190
treatment of: Dideoxycytidine
357; Zidovudine (AZT) 1087
AIDS-related complex 79
see also index entry AIDS
Air 79
Air conditioning 79
and Legionnaires' disease 632;
Sick building syndrome 904
air conduction:
in Hearing 511
testing of: *types of hearing test
513*
Air embolism 80
type of Embolism 396
Air pollution:
Pollution 807
air pressure:
and Aviation medicine 148;
Eustachian tube 423
changes of: Barotrauma 159;
Mountain sickness 696
Air swallowing:
see index entry Aerophagia
air travel:
and Aviation medicine 147
causing Barotrauma 159
*conditions affecting suitability for
air travel 148*
Airway 80
Airway obstruction 80
Akarpine 1096
Akathisia 80
AK-Cide 1096
AK-Dilate 1096
Akinesia 80
akinetic seizure:
common term: Drop attack 375
Akne-Mycin 1096
AK-Neo-Cort 1096
AK-Pred 1096
AK-Sulf 1096
AK-Tate 1096
AK-Tracin 1096
AK-Trol 1096
AK-Zol 1096
Alatone 1096
Albalon-A 1096
Albalon Liquifilm 1096
Albinism 80
symptoms of: Nystagmus 737;
Pallor 765; Pigmentation 794
Albumin 81
production of: Liver 644
type of Plasma protein 801
Albuminuria 81

Albuterol 81
in treatment of Childbirth,
complications of 265
Alcohol 81
*alcohol and the body 82
alcohol and pregnancy 83
deaths from alcohol-related causes
in the US 83*
and Heat stroke 526; Nocturia
729; Sleep apnea 916
Smoking and drinking 20
see also index entries Alcohol
dependence; Alcohol
intoxication; Alcohol-related
disorders
Alcohol dependence 81
Alcoholics Anonymous 84
associated with Child abuse
263; Suicide 953; Suicide,
attempted 954
leading to Delirium tremens
338; Dementia 339; Wernicke-
Korsakoff syndrome 1076
see also index entries Alcohol;
Alcohol intoxication;
Alcohol-related disorders;
alcohol withdrawal
Alcoholics Anonymous 84
Alcohol intoxication 84
*alcohol and the body 82*
and Drowning 375; Hangover
506
see also index entries Alcohol;
Alcohol-related disorders
Alcoholism:
see index entry Alcohol
dependence
Alcohol-related disorders 84, 85
*alcohol and mortality 21
deaths from alcohol-related causes
in the US 83
effects of alcohol on the liver 21*
examples: Cardiomyopathy
235; Cirrhosis 282; Dementia
339; Encephalopathy 401;
Fetal alcohol syndrome 447;
Gastritis 476; *disorders of the
liver 646;* Liver disease,
alcoholic 647; Neuropathy
724; Pancreas, cancer of 766;
Pancreatitis 767; Wernicke-
Korsakoff syndrome 107
Smoking and drinking 20
see also index entries: Alcohol
dependence; Alcohol
intoxication
Alcohol, rubbing 85
alcohol withdrawal:
Alcoholics Anonymous 84
causing Delirium tremens 338;
Epilepsy 412; Withdrawal
syndrome 1080
see also index entry Alcohol
dependence
Alconefrin 1096
Aldactazide 1096
Aldactone 1096
Aldoclor 1096
Aldomet 1096
Aldoril 1096
Aldosterone 85
and Angiotensin 110; Renin
861; Urine 1027
effect on Kidney 617

Aldosterone (continued)
excess: Conn's syndrome 298
Aldosteronism 85
see also index entry
Aldosterone
Alexia 85
Alfacalcidol 1096
Algicon 1096
alginate:
use of: Antacid drugs 113;
Impression, dental 578
Alienation 85
Alignment, dental 86
Alimentary tract 86
see also index entry Digestive
system
Alka-Seltzer 1096
Alkali 86
in eye: *disorders of the cornea 308*
and pH 788
Alkaloids 86
Alkalosis 86
cause of: Hyperventilation 558
and pH 789
Alkeran 1096
Allbee C-800 1096
Allbee with C 1096
alleles:
and Gene 479; Inheritance 590
Aller-Chlor 1096
Allerest 1096
Allerfrin 1096
allergen:
*allergy and the body 87*
and Sensitization 893
see also index entry Allergy
Allergen Ear Drops 1096
allergic reaction:
see index entry Allergy
allergic rhinitis:
Rhinitis, allergic 872
Allergist 86
Allergy 86
*allergy and the body 87*
causing Anaphylactic shock 98;
Asthma 138; Conjunctivitis
297; Rhinitis, allergic 872;
Urticaria 1030
to Cephalosporins 248; Drug
378; Insect bites 591
Food allergy 461
and Hypersensitivity 555;
Immune system 571
treatment of: Antihistamine
drugs 118; Corticosteroid
drugs 312; Cromolyn sodium
321; Immunotherapy 576;
Triprolidine 1011
see also index entries allergen;
allergic alveolitis
Allersone 1096
allografting:
Grafting 496
Allopathy 88
Allopurinol 88
in treatment of Arthritis 132
Alopecia 88
treatment of: Minoxidil 689
alpha₁-antitrypsin:
and Emphysema 399
type of Globulin 490
alpha chains:
and Thalassemia 977
Alphaderm 1096

Alpha-fetoprotein 88
in diagnosis of Liver cancer
647; Spina bifida 928
measurement of:
Amniocentesis and chorionic
villus sampling 42
type of Tumor-specific antigen
1015
alpha particles:
type of Radiation 844
AlphaRedisol 1096
Alpha-tocopherol 89
constituent of Vitamin E 1059
*recommended daily dietary
allowances (RDAs) of selected
vitamins 19*
Alphatrex 1096
Alphosyl 1096
Alprazolam 89
Alprostadil 89
ALS (amyotrophic lateral
sclerosis):
type of Motor neuron disease
696
Alseroxylon 1096
ALternaGEL 1096
Alternative medicine 89
and Ethics, medical 422; Folk
medicine 460
Altitude sickness:
alternative term: Mountain
sickness 696
and Environmental constraints
46
Alu-Cap 1096
Aluminum 89
Aluminum acetate 1096
Aluminum carbonate 1097
Aluminum chloride 1097
Aluminum hydroxide 1097
Alupent 1097
Alurate 1097
Alu-Tab 1097
Alveolectomy:
Alveoloplasty 90
Alveolitis 90
Alveoloplasty 90
Alveolus, dental 90
Alveolus, pulmonary 90
damage to: Emphysema 399;
*the effects of emphysema on the
lungs 21*
part of Lung 651; Respiratory
system 865
Alzheimer's disease 91
causing Dementia 339
role of Neurotransmitter 725
treatment of:
Tetrahydroaminoacridine 976
AMA:
American Medical Association
93
Amalgam, dental 92
constituent of: Mercury 681
in treatment of Caries, dental
236
use of: Filling, dental 455
Amantadine 92
in treatment of Influenza 588
Amaurosis fugax 92
Amaurotic familial idiocy 92
alternative term: Tay-Sachs
disease 966
Ambenonium 1097

Ambenyl 1097
Ambidexterity 92
and Handedness 506
Amblyopia 92
causes of: Ptosis 834;
Strabismus 944; deficiency of
Vitamin B complex 1058
*a disorder of the eye 431*
treatment of: Occlusion 739
Ambulance 92
Ambulatory care 92
Ambulatory surgery 92
Amcill 1097
Amcinonide 1097
Amdinocillin 1097
ameba:
causing Colitis 289
see also index entry Amebiasis
Amebiasis 92
*the cycle of amebiasis 93*
cause of: Protozoa 827
causing Liver abscess 645;
Rectal bleeding 855
prevalence of: *areas of amebic
dysentery 382*
treatment of: Amebicides 93;
Metronidazole 684
type of Dysentery 382
Amebic dysentery:
see index entry Amebiasis
Amebicides 93
Amelogenesis imperfecta 93
effect on Calcification, dental
223
Amen 1097
Amenorrhea 93
*a disorder of menstruation 678*
treatment of: Norethindrone
731
Americaine 1097
American Medical Association 93
Ametropia 94
*a disorder of the eye 431*
Amikacin 1097
Amikin 1097
Amiloride 94
Amino acids 94
as constituent of Proteins 827
constituent of: Nitrogen 728
metabolism of: Liver 644
as source of Urea 1022
Aminoglutethimide 94
aminoglycoside antibiotics:
side effect of: Ototoxicity 759
types of Antibiotic drugs 114
Aminophylline 94
Aminosalicylate 1097
Aminosalicylic acid 94
Amiodarone 1097
Amitril 1097
Amitriptyline 94
Ammonia 94
from breakdown of Urine 1027
Amnesia 94
Amniocentesis 42, 95
in diagnosis of Genetic
disorders 484; Muscular
dystrophy 707; Rh
incompatibility 872
using Ultrasound scanning
1019
Amnion 95
Amnioscopy 95
Amniotic fluid 95

deficiency of: Oligohydramnios
742
amniotic sac:
and Embryo 397
Amniotomy 95
Amobarbital 1097
Amoxapine 95
Amoxicillin 95
Amoxil 1097
Amphetamine drugs 95
causing Schizophrenia 884
and Withdrawal syndrome
1080
Amphojel 1097
Amphotericin B 96
in treatment of Cryptococcosis
323; Sporotrichosis 935
Ampicillin 96
amplifier:
in Hearing aids 511
ampulla of Vater:
anatomy of: Biliary system 169;
Duodenum 380; Pancreas 765
Amputation 96
leading to Phantom limb 789
in treatment of Osteosarcoma
757; Peripheral vascular
disease 785
treatment of: Limb, artificial
640; *types of artificial limb 641*;
Prosthesis 827
Amputation, congenital 96
Amputation, traumatic 96
Amrinone 1097
AMS (acute mountain sickness):
Mountain sickness 696
amygdala:
part of Limbic system 641
Amyl nitrite 96
Amyloidosis 96
causing Nephrotic syndrome
719
as complication of Familial
Mediterranean fever 440;
Rheumatoid arthritis,
juvenile 871; Osteomyelitis
755
Amyotrophic lateral sclerosis:
type of Motor neuron disease
696
Amyotrophy 97
Amytal 1097
anabolic effect:
of Androgen hormones 100;
Steroids, anabolic 940
Anabolic steroids:
Steroids, anabolic 940
anabolism:
in Biochemistry 170;
Metabolism 681
Anacin 1097
Anacin-3 1097
Anadrol 1097
Anaerobic 97
anaerobic exercise:
in Training 1003
Anal dilatation 97
Anal discharge 97
anal disorders:
*disorders of the anus 121*
examples: Anal fissure 97; Anal
fistula 97; Anal stenosis 98;
Anus, cancer of 122; Anus,
imperforate 122; Crohn's

disease 320; Hemorrhoids 530;
Pinworm infestation 796
symptoms of: Itching 608;
Rectal bleeding 855
Analeptic drugs 97
Anal fissure 97
*a disorder of the anus 121*
symptom of: Rectal bleeding
855
Anal fistula 97
*a disorder of the anus 121*
symptom of: Rectal bleeding
855
Analgesia 97
see also index entry Analgesic
drugs
Analgesic drugs 97
*how analgesics work 98*
examples: Acetaminophen 61;
Aspirin 137; Codeine 286;
Heroin 536; Ibuprofen 566;
Meperidine 680; Methadone
683; Morphine 694; Narcotic
drug 715; Opium 745;
Oxycodone 761; Pentazocine
780; Phenazopyridine 790;
Propoxyphene 824; Sodium
salicylate 922
*landmarks in drug development 32*
anal itching:
*a disorder of the anus 121*
Itching 608
anal phase:
and Fixation 457;
Psychoanalytic theory 831
anal sphincter:
Sphincter 927
Anal stenosis 98
*a disorder of the anus 121*
Anal stricture:
see index entry Anal stenosis
anal tags:
type of Skin tag 913
Analysis, psychological:
Psychoanalysis 830
Analysis, scientific 98
Anamine 1097
Anaphylactic shock 98
and Allergy 86;
Hypersensitivity 555
cause of: Immunotherapy 576;
Insect stings 592
type of Shock 901
Anaprox 1097
anasarca:
alternative term: Edema 390
Anaspaz 1097
Anastomosis 99
Anatomy 99
Anatuss 1097
Anavar 1097
Anbesol 1097
Ancef 1097
Ancylostomiasis:
alternative term: Hookworm
infestation 545
Androgen drugs 100
Androgen hormones 100
Android 1097
Anectine 1097
Anemia 100
*types and causes of anemia 101*
causes of: Hookworm
infestation 545;

Spherocytosis, hereditary 927;
deficiency of Vitamin B
complex 1059; deficiency of
Vitamin C 1059; deficiency of
Vitamin E 1060
and Hypersplenism 557;
Rheumatoid arthritis 871
symptoms of: Glossitis 492;
Pallor 765
Anemia, aplastic 101
Anemia, hemolytic 102
see also index entry Hemolytic
disease of the newborn
Anemia, iron-deficiency 102
Anemia, megaloblastic 103
Anemia, pernicious 104
anemia, sickle cell:
Sickle cell anemia 905
Anencephaly 104
diagnosis of: Ultrasound
scanning 1019
and Neural tube defect 722
Anergan 1097
Anestacon 1097
Anesthesia 104
complications of: Sickle cell
anemia 905
see also index entries Epidural
anesthesia; Spinal anesthesia
Anesthesia, dental 104
Anesthesia, general 104
*techniques for general anesthesia
105*
*landmarks in surgery 33*
*operating room 744*
Anesthesia, local 106
see also index entries Epidural
anesthesia; Spinal anesthesia
Anesthesiologist 106
Anesthesia, general 104
Aneurysm 107
treatment of: Arterial
reconstructive surgery 130;
Neurosurgery 725
Anexsia-D 1097
Angel dust 108
Angiitis:
type of Vasculitis 1039
Angina 108
Angina pectoris 108
*a disorder of the heart 517;
disorder of muscle 705*
symptom of: Chest pain 259
treatment of: Amyl nitrite 96;
Calcium channel blockers
224; Isosorbide dinitrate 608;
Nadolol 714; Nifedipine 727;
Nitroglycerin 729; Pindolol
795; Propranolol 824;
Vasodilator drugs 1041
angiodynography:
Diagnostic ultrasound 30
Angioedema 108
associated with Urticaria 1030
treatment of:
Chlorpheniramine 271
angiogram:
see index entry Angiography
Angiography 109
in diagnosis of Periarteritis
nodosa 782; Subarachnoid
hemorrhage 950
example: *diet and atherosclerosis
20*

uses of: Neurology 723; Kidney
imaging 619
see also index entry Digital
subtraction angiography
Angioma 109
causing Subarachnoid
hemorrhage 950
Angioplasty, balloon 110
use of: Heart surgery 522
Angiotensin 110
and Kidney 617; Renin 861;
Vasodilator drugs 1041
angiotensin-converting enzyme
(ACE) inhibitors:
ACE inhibitors 61
Anhydron 1097
Animal experimentation 110
Animals, diseases from:
alternative term: Zoonoses 1088
anion:
and Acid 63
type of Ion 605
Anisindione 1097
Anisometropia 111
*a disorder of the eye 431*
Anisotropine 1097
Ankle joint 111
and Clonus 284
disorders of: Pott's fracture 812;
Sprain 936
ankyloglossia:
alternative term: Tongue-tie 995
Ankylosing spondylitis 111
treatment of: Indomethacin
581; Ketoprofen 616
and Sacroiliitis 878
*a disorder of the spine 933*
Ankylosis 112
Anodontia 112
Anomaly 112
Anorex 1097
Anorexia 112
alternative term: Appetite, loss
of 127
Anorexia nervosa 112
and Bulimia 218
symptoms of: Lanugo hair 626;
Weight loss 1073
Anorgasmia 113
common term: Frigidity 469
feature of Psychosexual
dysfunction 832
Anosmia 113
absence of Smell 918
anovulation:
causing Infertility 586
Anoxia 113
and Hypoxia 565
Anspor 1097
Antabuse 1097
Antacid drugs 113
examples: Simethicone 906;
Sodium bicarbonate 922
in treatment of Hiatal hernia
538
Antepartum hemorrhage 113
Anterior 113
alternative term: Ventral 1045
Anthracosis 113
Anthra-Derm 1097
Anthralin 113
Anthrax 114
Antianxiety drugs 114
examples: Alprazolam 89;

Chlordiazepoxide 270;
Clorazepate 284; Diazepam
357; Lorazepam 649;
Meprobamate 680
and Psychopharmacology 832
Antiarrhythmic drugs 114
examples: Disopyramide 365;
Mexiletine 684; Procainamide
822; Quinidine 842; Tocainide
993
Antibacterial drugs 36, 114
examples: Aminosalicylic acid
94; Nitrofurantoin 728;
Sulfonamide drugs 954;
Trimethoprim 1011
*landmarks in drug development 32*
see also index entry Antibiotic
drugs
Antibiotic drugs 36, 114
examples: Ampicillin 96;
Cefaclor 245; Cephalexin 247;
Chloramphenicol 270;
Clindamycin 284; Cloxacillin
285; Colistin 289; Cyclacillin
326; Doxycycline 372;
Erythromycin 418;
Gentamicin 485; Gramicidin
497; Lincomycin 641;
Metronidazole 684;
Minocycline 689; Nalidixic
acid 714; Oxacillin 761;
Oxytetracycline 761;
Penicillin drugs 779;
Polymyxins 808; Tetracycline
drugs 976; Tobramycin 993;
Vancomycin 1038
*landmarks in drug development 32*
see also index entry
Antibacterial drugs
Antibody 115
alternative term:
Immunoglobulin 575
as constituent of Serum 895
in diagnosis of Infectious
disease 585
function of: Immune response
570; Immune system 571; *the
adaptive immune system 573;
the innate immune system 572*
and Immunization 574;
Immunodeficiency disorders
575; Immunotherapy 576;
Plasmapheresis 800; Vaccine
1034
production of: Lymphocyte 657
use of: Gamma globulin 474;
Immunoassay 575;
Radioimmunoassay 847;
Serology 895
Antibody, monoclonal 115
*landmarks in diagnosis 25*
use of: Immunotherapy 576
Anticancer drugs 115
examples: Aminoglutethimide
94; Chlorambucil 270;
Cisplatin 283;
Cyclophosphamide 326;
Doxorubicin 372; Fluorouracil
460; Mercaptopurine 681;
Methotrexate 683;
Procarbazine 822
in treatment of Leukemia 637;
Lung cancer 651
Anticholinergic drugs 115

Anticholinergic drugs (continued)
*how anticholinergics work 116*
examples: Homatropine 544;
Hyoscyamine 552;
Trihexyphenidyl 1011
Anticoagulant drugs 116
examples: Dicumarol 357;
Heparin 531; Warfarin 1069
use of: Heart valve surgery 525;
Thrombectomy 980;
Thrombosis 981
Anticonvulsant drugs 116
examples: Ethosuximide 423;
Phenobarbital 790; Phenytoin
791; Primodone 822; Valproic
acid 1037
Antidepressant drugs 116
examples: Maprotiline 664;
Nortriptyline 731; Phenelzine
790; Protriptyline 828;
Tranylcypromine 1006;
Trazodone 1008;
Trimipramine 1011
and Psychopharmacology 832
Antidiarrheal drugs 117
examples: Kaolin 614;
Loperamide 649
Antidiuretic hormone (ADH):
see index entry ADH
Antidote 117
anti-D serum:
in prevention of Hemolytic
disease of the newborn 529
Antiemetic drugs 117
examples: Metoclopramide 684;
Prochlorperazine 822;
Trimethobenzamide 1011
antiestrogen drug:
example: Tamoxifen 963
Antifreeze poisoning 117
Antifungal drugs 117
examples: Clotrimazole 284;
Ketoconazole 616;
Miconazole 684; Nystatin
737; Tolnaftate 994
Antigen 118
and Immune response 570;
Immune system 571; *the*
*adaptive immune system 573;*
*the innate immune system 572;*
Immunoassay 575;
Immunoglobulins 575;
Serology 895; Tissue-typing
990
Antihelmintic drugs 118
examples: Mebendazole 669;
Niclosamide 727; Piperazine
796; Praziquantel 812;
Pyrantel 841; Thiabendazole
978
in treatment of Hookworm
infestation 545; Pinworm
infestation 796; Whipworm
infestation 1077
*drugs used to treat worm*
*infestations 1080*
Antihistamine drugs 118
examples: Azatadine 149;
Chlorpheniramine 271;
Dimenhydrinate 361;
Diphenhydramine 361;
Hydroxyzine 551; Meclizine
669; Promethazine 823;
Pyrilamine 841; Terfenadine

971; Trimeprazine 1011;
Triprolidine 1011
and Histamine 540
in treatment of Conjunctivitis
298; Rhinitis, allergic 873
Antihypertensive drugs 118
examples: Guanethidine 501;
Hydralazine 549; Methyldopa
684
Anti-inflammatory drugs 118
antimalarial drugs:
*drugs from plants 32*
examples: Chloroquine 270;
Quinine 842
*landmarks in drug development 32*
Malaria 659
and Travel immunization 1008
Antiminth 1097
Antiperspirant 118
constituent of: Aluminum 90
Antipsychotic drugs 119
examples: Chlorpromazine 271;
Fluphenazine 460;
Haloperidol 505;
Perphenazine 786;
Thioridazine 978;
Thiothixene 978;
Trifluoperazine 1010
and Psychopharmacology 832
Antipyretic drugs 119
Antipyrine 1097
Antirheumatic drugs 119
examples: Chloroquine 270;
Penicillamine 779
Antiseptics 119
examples: Boric acid 195;
Hydrogen peroxide 550;
Iodine 605; Potassium
permanganate 812
and *landmarks in surgery 33;*
Sterilization 939
Antiserum 119
antisocial behavior:
and Acting out 66
see also index entry Antisocial
personality disorder
Antisocial personality disorder
119
*diagnosis of antisocial personality*
*disorder 120*
and Somatization disorder 923;
Suicide 953
type of Personality disorder
786
Antispas 1097
Antispasmodic drugs 120
examples: Atropine 143;
Dicyclomine 357;
Propantheline 824
antithrombin:
and Blood clotting 185
Antitoxin 120
Antitussive drugs 120
alternative term: Cough
remedies 316
Antivenin 120
in treatment of Jellyfish stings
611; Scorpion stings 887;
Snakebites 921; Venomous
bites and stings 1044
Antivert 1097
Antiviral drugs 120
examples: Acyclovir 67;
Amantadine 92; Idoxuridine

566; Trifluridine 1010;
Zidovudine 1087
Antral irrigation 121
Anturane 1097
Anuject 1097
Anuria 121
feature of Renal failure 860
and Urine, abnormal 1029
Anus 121
and Rectum 856
see also index entry anal
disorders
Anus, cancer of 122
Anus, imperforate 122
*a disorder of the anus 121*
and Rectum 856
treatment of: Plastic surgery
801
Anusol-HC 1097
Anxiety 122
causing Chest pain 259;
Insomnia 593; Irritable bowel
syndrome 607; Night terror
738; Panic attack 768; Sleepwalking 917; Torticollis 998
treatment of: Relaxation
techniques 859
see also index entry
Antianxiety drugs
Anxiety disorders 122
Aorta 123
abnormalities of: *types of*
*congenital heart disorder 518;*
Marfan's syndrome 664
part of Circulatory system 280,
281
Aortic insufficiency 123
and *disorders of the heart 517*
Aortic stenosis 124
Aortitis 124
Aortography 124
Apap 1097
Aperient 124
type of Laxative drug 630
Apgar score 124
in assessment of Newborn 726
Aphakia 125
Aphasia 125
type of Speech disorder 926
Apheresis 125
and Blood donation 187
Aphonia 125
common term: Voice, loss of
1062
Aphrodisiacs 125
A.P.L. 1097
Aplasia 126
Aplastic anemia:
Anemia, aplastic 101
Apnea 126
Apocrine gland 126
type of Sweat gland 958
Aponeurosis 126
and Tendon 970
Apoplexy 126
common term: Stroke 947
Apothecary 126
common term: Pharmacist 789
Appendectomy 126
Appendicitis 127
causing Pelvic infection 777;
Peritonitis 785
treatment of: Appendectomy
126

Appendix 127
removal of: Appendectomy 126
see also index entry
Appendicitis
Appetite 127
and Hypothalamus 562
Appetite, loss of 127
and Anorexia nervosa 112
Appetite stimulants 128
Appetite suppressants 128
examples: Amphetamine drugs
95; Phentermine 790
Apraxia 128
Apresazide 1097
Apresoline 1097
Apresoline with Esidrex 1097
Aprobarbital 1097
aptitude testing:
part of Psychometry 832
APUD cell tumor 128
Aquamethyton 1097
Aquasol A 1097
Aquatag 1097
Aquatar 1097
Aquatensen 1097
aqueous humor:
part of Eye 429
arachidonic acid:
type of Fatty acid 442
Arachis oil 1097
Arachnodactyly 128
feature of Marfan's syndrome
664
Arachnoiditis 128
arachnoid tumor:
type of Meningioma 675
Aralen 1097
arboviruses:
and Insects and disease 592
ARC 128:
AIDS-related complex 79
arcus juvenilis:
and Arcus senilis 129
Arcus senilis 128
areola:
part of Breast 206; Nipple 728
Argyll Robertson pupil:
Pupil 839
Aristocort 1097
Aristospan 1097
arm:
bones of: Humerus 547; *location*
*of humerus 548*; Radius 849;
Ulna 1019
disorders of: Humerus, fracture
of 548; Radius, fracture of
849; Shoulder, dislocation of
903; Shoulder-hand
syndrome 903; Ulna, fracture
of 1019
joints of: Elbow 393; Shoulder
902; *structure of the shoulder*
*903*; Wrist 1082
and *movement 698*
muscles of: Biceps muscle 167;
Triceps muscle 1009
Armour Thyroid 1097
Arnica 1097
Aroma therapy 129
Arousal 129
Arrhenoblastoma 129
Arrhythmia, cardiac 129
*a disorder of the heart 517*
Arsenic 130

causing Squamous cell
carcinoma 937
and Occupational disease and
injury 739
Artane 1097
arterial blood sampling:
type of Blood test 189
arterial lining, removal of:
medical term: Endarterectomy
401
Arterial reconstructive surgery
130
in treatment of Subclavian steal
syndrome 951
Arteries, disorders of 130
leading to Stroke 947;
Subarachnoid hemorrhage
950; Thrombosis 981
see also index entry
Atherosclerosis
Arteriography 131
type of Angiography 109
Arteriole 131
part of Circulatory system 280
Arteriopathy 131
common term: Arteries,
disorders of 130
Arterioplasty 131
alternative term: Arterial
reconstructive surgery 130
Arteriosclerosis 131
see also index entry
Atherosclerosis
Arteriovenous fistula 131
type of Fistula 457
Arteritis 131
Artery 131
part of Circulatory system 280,
281
and Pulse 838
see also index entry Arteries,
disorders of
Arthralgia 131
Arthritis 132
causing Stiffness 941
as complication of Obesity 738
effect on Joints 613
and Paget's disease 763;
Reiter's syndrome 859
arthrocentesis:
in diagnosis of Synovitis 960
Arthrodesis 132
in treatment of Neuropathic
joint 723
Arthrography 133
Arthrogryposis:
Contracture 306
Arthropan 1097
Arthropathy 133
Arthroplasty 133
and Pseudarthrosis 828
Arthroscopy 133
in diagnosis of Loose bodies
649; Osteochondritis
dessicans 753
use of: Meniscectomy 676
artificial body part:
alternative term: Prosthesis 827
and Heart valve surgery 524;
Hip replacement 539; Knee
622; Limb, artificial 640; types
of artificial limb 641
see also index entry Implant
Artificial insemination 133

and Surrogacy 957
Artificial kidney 134
use of: Dialysis 352; procedure
for dialysis 353
Artificial respiration 134
Artificial sweeteners 135
artificial tears:
in treatment of
Keratoconjunctivitis sicca 615
A.S.A. 1097
asbestos:
as Carcinogen 233
causing Lung cancer 651;
Mesothelioma 681
see also index entry Asbestosis
Asbestosis 135
a disorder of the lung 652
type of Pneumoconiosis 802
Asbron G 1097
Ascariasis 135
life cycle of the ascariasis worm
136
cause of: Roundworms 876
ascending colon:
part of Intestine 601
Ascites 136
feature of Liver failure 647;
Pancreatitis 767; Portal
hypertension 809
Ascorbic acid 136
alternative term: Vitamin C
1059
Ascriptin 1097
Asendin 1097
Aseptic technique 136
in prevention of Wound
infection 1081
Asparaginase 1097
aspartame:
an Artificial sweetener 135
Aspergillosis 136
a Fungal infection 470; disorder
of the lung 652
Aspergum 1097
Aspermia 137
Asphyxia 137
Aspiration 137
for biopsy procedures 171; Bone
marrow biopsy 195
Aspirin 137
an Analgesic drug 97
associated with Reye's
syndrome 869
causing Gastritis 476; Occult
blood, fecal 739
landmarks in drug development 32
in treatment of Transient
ischemic attack 1005
Assay 137
assigned sex:
Sex change 896
Assignment 137
Astemizole 1097
Astereognosis 137
Asthenia 137
Asthenia, neurocirculatory:
alternative term: Cardiac
neurosis 234
Asthma 137
living with asthma 138
and Allergy 86; Rhinitis,
allergic 872
assessment of: Peak flow meter
775

Status asthmaticus 939
treatment of: Albuterol 81;
Aminophylline 94; Cromolyn
sodium 321; Hydrocortisone
550; Inhaler 589;
Isoproterenol 608; Nebulizer
716; Oxtriphylline 761;
Prednisolone 813
Asthma, cardiac 139
Astigmatism 139
a disorder of the eye 431
treatment of: Contact lenses
301; why glasses are used 489
Astringent 139
Astrocytoma 139
Asylum 139
alternative term: Mental
hospital 678
Asymptomatic 139
Asystole 139
causing Cardiac arrest 234
Atabrine 1097
Atarax 1097
Ataxia 139
Atelectasis 140
Atenolol 140
Atheroma 140
leading to Thrombosis 981
and Plaque 800
treatment of: Arterial
reconstructive surgery 130
Atherosclerosis 140
and Arteries, disorders of 130;
disorders of the heart 517;
hypertension 556; Plaque 800;
disorders of the retina 867
arterial degeneration in
atherosclerosis 141
diet and atherosclerosis 20
in Down's syndrome 372
leading to Ischemia 607;
Peripheral vascular disease
784; Raynaud's phenomenon
853; Stroke 947
treatment of: Arterial
reconstructive surgery 130;
Endarterectomy 401
Athetosis 141
resulting from Kernicterus 616
Athlete's foot 141, 142
cause of: Tinea 988
treatment of: Miconazole 684
Ativan 1097
atlas bone:
and Skull 914
location and structure of the
vertebrae 1048
atmospheric pressure:
see index entry air pressure
atomic bomb:
and Nuclear energy 733;
Radiation 845
atomic energy:
and Nuclear energy 732;
Radiation 844; Radiation and
disease 45
atomic radiation:
see index entry Radiation
Atony 142
atopic eczema:
and Skin allergy 911
type of Eczema 390
Atopy 142
ATP 142

and ADP 70; Energy 407
constituent of: Phosphates 792
Atracurium 1097
Atresia 142
causing Intestine, obstruction
of 602
Atrial fibrillation 142
causing Palpitation 765
type of Arrhythmia, cardiac 129
Atrial flutter 142
type of Arrhythmia, cardiac 129
Atrial natriuretic peptide 142
effect on Urine 1027
atrioventricular node:
anatomy of Heart 514; Vena
cava 1043
and cardiac arrhythmia 129; heart
cycle 515
Atrium 143
part of Heart 514
Atromid-S 1097
Atrophy 143
Atropine 143
drugs from plants 36
A/T/S 1097
Attachment 143
Attending physician 143
Attenuvax 1097
Audiogram 143
Audiologist 143
Audiology 143
Audiometry 143
types of hearing test 513
auditory evoked response:
Evoked responses 424
types of hearing test 513
Auditory nerve 143
and functions of cranial nerves
318
part of Vestibulocochlear nerve
1048
auditory ossicles:
parts of Ear 384
Augmentin 1097
Aura 143
feature of Epilepsy 412
Auralgan 1097
Auranofin 144
Aureomycin 1097
Auricle 144
alternative term: Pinna 795
part of Ear 384
Aurothioglucose 1097
Auscultation 144
use of: Examination, physical
424; types of physical
examination 425
Autism 145
feature of Rett's syndrome 869
Autoclave 145
use of: Sterilization 939
autograft:
Corneal graft 308
Grafting 496
Autoimmune disorders 145
and Immune system 571
examples: Addison's disease
67; Dermatomyositis 356;
Graves' disease 497;
Hashimoto's thyroiditis 507;
Hypothyroidism 563;
Diabetes mellitus 349;

autoimmune disorders
(continued
Lupus erythematosus 653;
Myasthenia gravis 709;
Pernicious anemia 786;
Polymyalgia rheumatica 808;
Polymyositis 808;
Rheumatoid arthritis 870;
Scleroderma 886; Temporal
arteritis 968; Vitiligo 1060
treatment of: Azathioprine 149;
Plasmapheresis 800
Automatism 147
feature of Epilepsy 413
Autonomic nervous system 147
*functions of the autonomic nervous
system 146*
divisions of: Parasympathetic
nervous system 771;
Sympathetic nervous system
959
part of Nervous system 720
Autopsy 147
autosomes:
and Chromosome abnormal-
ities 277; Genetic disorders
482; Inheritance 589
Autosuggestion 147
Aventyl 1097
Aversion therapy 147
and Behavior therapy 163
Aviation medicine 147
*conditions affecting passenger
suitability for air travel 148*
Avoidant personality disorder 148
type of Personality disorder 786
Avulsed tooth 149
Avulsion 149
Axilla 149
axillary nerve:
part of Brachial plexus 198
axis bone:
and Skull 914
*location and structure of the
vertebrae 1048*
axon:
part of Neuron 723; *structure of
a neuron 724*
Axotal 1097
Aygestin 1097
Ayurvedism 149
type of Indian medicine 580
Azacitidine 1097
Azatadine 149
Azathioprine 149
in treatment of Rheumatoid
arthritis 871; Wegener's
granulomatosis 1072
azidothymidine (AZT):
modern term: Zidovudine 1087
Azlocillin 1097
Azmacort 1097
Azo Gantanol 1097
Azo-Gantrisin 1097
Azolid 1097
Azo-Sulfisoxazole 1097
Azoospermia 149
diagnosis of: Semen analysis
891
feature of Klinefelter's
syndrome 621
AZT 149
new name: Zidovudine 1087
Azulfidine 1097

Azulfidine EN-tabs 1097
azygos veins:
anatomy of: Vena cava 1043

## B

Babesiosis 150
Babinski's sign 150
baby:
Birth weight 174
Bottle-feeding 197
Breast-feeding 207
Childbirth 263
Child development 267
*268-269*
Fetus 448
Infant 581
Newborn 726
Postmaturity 810
Pregnancy 813
Prematurity 817
Twins 1016
Baby blues 150
medical term: Postpartum
depression 810
Baby Doe case 150
Bacampicillin 150
type of Penicillin drug 779
Bacarate 1098
Baciguent 1098
bacillary dysentery:
alternative term: Shigellosis 901
Bacilli 150
types of Bacteria 154
Bacitracin 150
Back 150
*reducing strain on the back 153*
Spine 932
backache:
see index entry Back pain
backbone:
Spine 932
Back disorders 150
*disorders of the spine 933*
see also index entry Back pain
Back pain 150, 153
causes of: Disk prolapse 364;
Fibroid 453; Lumbrosacral
spasm 650; *disorders of the
spine 933*; Tension 971
*symptom chart 151*
Baclofen 153
Bacteremia 153
and Sepsis 894; Septicemia 894
Bacteria 153, *154*
causing *bacterial infections 584*;
Food poisoning 463; Infection
581; Infectious disease 582;
Staphylococcal infections 938,
Streptococcal infections 945
culturing of: Culture 324;
*culturing and testing bacteria
155*
examples: Bacilli 150;
Salmonella 880; Spirochete
932
producing Endotoxin 407;
Enterotoxin 408; Exotoxin
427; Toxin 1000
staining of: Gram's stain 497
study of: Bacteriology 155
type of Microorganism 685

Bactericidal 155
types of: Antibacterial drugs
114; Antibiotic drugs 114
Bacteriology 155
see also index entry Bacteria
Bacteriostatic 155
types of: Antibacterial drugs
114; Antibiotic drugs 114
Bacteriuria 155
Bactine 1098
Bactocill 1098
Bactrim DS 1098
Bad breath:
medical term: Halitosis 504
Bagassosis 155
causing Alveolitis 90
Baker's cyst 155
affecting Knee 621
and Rheumatoid arthritis 871
Balance 156
affected by Acoustic neuroma
64; *disorders of the ear 385*;
Streptomycin 946; Vertigo
1047
control of: Cerebellum 248; Ear
384; Vestibulocochlear nerve
1048
Balance billing:
Assignment 137
Balanitis 156
affecting Penis 780
Baldness:
medical term: Alopecia 88
ball-and-socket joint:
in Hip 538
*types of joints 612*
balloon angioplasty:
Angioplasty, balloon 110
Balloon catheter 156
in treatment of Pulmonary
stenosis 838
balloon tuboplasty:
type of Tuboplasty 1014
*procedure for balloon tuboplasty
1015*
balloon valvuloplasty:
type of Valvuloplasty 1038
Balm 156
Balmex ointment 1098
Balneol 1098
Balnetar 1098
Bancap HC 1098
Bandage 156
*first aid: applying bandages 157*
type of Dressing 374
Banflex 1098
Banthine 1098
Baratol 1098
barber's itch:
medical term: Sycosis vulgaris
959
Barbidonna 1098
Barbita 1098
Barbiturates 157
examples: Phenobarbital 790;
Thiopental 978
and Withdrawal syndrome
1080
Barium X-ray examinations 158
Barnard, Christiaan:
*landmarks in surgery 33*
Barotrauma 159
Barrett's esophagus:
complication of Esophagitis 420

barrier contraceptives:
see index entry Contraception,
barrier methods
Barrier cream 160
in prevention of Chapped skin
258
Barrier method 160
see also index entry
Contraception, barrier
methods
bartholinitis:
disorder of Bartholin's glands
160
Bartholin's cyst:
disorder of Bartholin's glands
160
Bartholin's glands 160
Bartonellosis 160
transmission of: Sand-fly bites
881
Basal cell carcinoma 160
cause of: Occupational disease
and injury 739
and Eyelid 433; *disorders of the
nose 732*
treatment of: Fluorouracil 460;
Radiation therapy 38, 846
type of Skin cancer 912; *disorder
of the skin 910*
Basal ganglia 160
and Huntington's chorea 548;
Parkinson's disease 773
Basaljel 1098
basal metabolic rate (BMR):
and Energy 407; Metabolism
682
base:
and Acid-base balance 63
alternative term: Alkali 86
constituent of Nucleic acids 733
Baseball elbow 160
Baseball finger 161
basophil cells:
and Allergy 86
basophil leukocyte:
type of Blood cell 183
Battered baby syndrome 161
Child abuse 262
B cell:
type of Lymphocyte 655
BCG vaccination 161
in prevention of Tuberculosis
1014
Beclomethasone 161
Beclovent 1098
Beconase 1098
Becquerel:
*a radiation unit 845*
Bed bath 161
Bedbug 161
Bedpan 161
Bed rest 161
Bedridden 161
Beds 161
Bedsores 162
and Nursing care 735
treatment of: Zinc oxide 1088
type of: Leg ulcer 633
Bed-wetting 162
medical term: Enuresis 408
Beepen-VK 1098
Bee stings:
Insect stings 592
Behavioral problems in children

162, *163*
and Conduct disorders 296;
Diet and disease 358
type of: Tantrum 964
Behaviorism 163
behavior modification:
by Behavior therapy 163;
Conditioning 296; Learning
631
Behavior therapy 163
method of: Conditioning 296
use of: Marital counseling 665
Behcet's syndrome 163
Belap 1098
Belching 164
and Indigestion 580
Belganyl 1098
Belladenal 1098
Belladonna 164
Bellafoline 1098
Bellergal-S 1098
Bell's palsy 164
alternative term: Facial palsy
434
Beminal-500 1098
Benacen 1098
Benactyzine 1098
Benadryl 1098
Bendroflumethiazide 164
Bends 164
cause of: Nitrogen 728
medical term: Decompression
sickness 335
and Scuba-diving medicine 888
Bendylate 1098
Benemid 1098
Ben Gay 1098
Benign 164
Benisone 1098
Benoquin 1098
Benoxaprofen 164
Benoxinate 1098
Benoxyl 1098
Bentyl 1098
Benylin 1098
Benzac W 1098
Benzagel 1098
Benzalkonium chloride 1098
Benzamycin 1098
Benzathine penicillin G 1098
Benzedrex 1098
Benznidazole 1098
Benzocaine 1098
Benzodiazepine drugs 164
causing Withdrawal syndrome
1080
examples: Chlordiazepoxide
270; Lorazepam 649;
Oxazepam 761; Triazolam
1009
*landmarks in drug development 32*
Benzoic acid 1098
Benzoin 1098
Benzonatate 1098
Benzoyl peroxide 164
in treatment of Acne 64
Benzphetamine 1098
Benzquinamide 1098
Benzthiazide 1098
Benztropine 1098
Benzyl alcohol 1098
Benzyl benzoate 1098
Benzylpenicillin 1098
Bephenium 1098

Bereavement 164
Berger's disease:
form of Glomerulonephritis 491
Beriberi 165
cause of: deficiency of Vitamin
B complex 1058
Berocca 1098
Berubigen 1098
Berylliosis 165
Beta-blocker drugs 165
abuse of: Sports, drugs and 935
*how beta-blockers work 166;*
examples: Acebutolol 61;
Atenolol 140; Labetolol 624;
Metoprolol 684; Nadolol 714;
Pindolol 795; Propranolol
824; Timolol 988
group of Sympatholytic drugs
959
*landmarks in drug development 32*
in treatment of Migraine 689
Beta carotene 1098
Betadine 1098
Betagan 1098
beta-globulins:
types of Globulin 490
Betahistine 1098
Betalin 12 1098
Betalin S 1098
Betamethasone 166
beta particles:
type of Radiation 844
Betapen-VK 1098
Betatrex 1098
Beta-Val 1098
Betaxolol 1098
beta-receptors:
and *how beta-blockers work 166*
types of Receptors 854
Betatrex 1098
Beta-Val 1098
Betaxolol 1098
Bethanechol 1098
Betoptic 1098
Bevantolol 1098
Bezafibrate 1098
Bezoar 166
Bi- 167
bicarbonate ion:
type of ion 605
Bicarbonate of soda:
Sodium bicarbonate 922
Biceps muscle 167
Bichloracetic acid 1098
Bicillin 1098
Bicitra 1098
BiCNU 1098
Bicuspid 167
Bifocal 167
type of Glasses 488
big toe:
medical term: Hallux 505
Bilateral 167
Bile 167
and Biliary system 169; *function
of the biliary system 168*
constituent of: Bilirubin 169
production of: Liver 644
storage of: Gallbladder 473
Bile duct 167
part of Biliary system 169
and *function of the biliary system
168;* Intestine 601
Bile duct cancer:
medical term:
Cholangiocarcinoma 272
Bile duct obstruction 167

cause of: Gallstones 474
causing Jaundice 610
Bilharziasis 167
alternative term:
Schistosomiasis 883
Biliary atresia 168
a *disorder of the liver 646*
Biliary cirrhosis 169
a *disorder of the liver 646*
Biliary colic 169
cause of: Gallstones 474
a *disorder of the gallbladder 473*
Biliary system 169
functions of: Bile 167; *function of
the biliary system 168*
parts of: Bile duct 167;
Gallbladder 473; Liver 644
Biliousness 169
Bilirubin 169
in Blood 182
causing Jaundice 610;
Kernicterus 616
as constituent of Bile 167
in diagnosis of Anemia 101
excess of: Hyperbilirubinemia
552
Billings' method 169
Billroth's operation 169
*types of gastrectomy 475*
Biltricide 1098
Binet's test 169
type of Intelligence test 595
binge eating:
feature of Binge-purge
syndrome 169; Bulimia 218
Binge-purge syndrome 169
binocular vision:
mechanism of: *the function of the
optic nerve 746; the sense of
vision 1053*
Bio- 169
Bioavailability 169
Biochemical analysis 30
Biochemistry 169
Biofeedback training 170
Relaxation techniques 859
Biological limits 46
Biomechanical engineering 170
Biopar Forte 1098
Biopsy 31, 170
*biopsy procedures 171*
in diagnosis of Breast, cancer of
206; Cancer 225; Esophagus,
cancer of 420; Lung cancer
651; Pharynx, cancer of 790;
Proctitis 822; Rectum, cancer
of 856; Stomach cancer 943;
Sprue, tropical 936
and Endoscopy 405; *endoscopes
406;* Sigmoidoscopy 906
types of: Bone marrow biopsy
195; *biopsy of the cervix 254;*
Liver biopsy 645; Renal
biopsy 860; Skin biopsy 912
Biorhythms 171
and Jet lag 611
biotin:
constituent of Vitamin B
complex 1059
Biozyme C 1098
Biperiden 1098
Biphetamine 1098
Bipolar disorder 172
example: Manic-depressive

illness 663
birds, diseases from:
examples: Alveolitis 90;
Histoplasmosis 541;
Psittacosis 829
Birth:
see index entry Childbirth
Birth canal 172
Birth control 172
methods of: Contraception 302;
Contraception, barrier
methods 304; Contraception,
hormonal methods 305;
*methods of contraception 303;*
Contraception, periodic
abstinence 305;
Contraception, postcoital
306; Family planning 440;
Sterilization, female 940;
Vasectomy 1040
birth-control pill:
Oral contraceptives 747
Birth defects 172, *173*
causes of: Chromosomal
abnormalities 277; Genetic
disorders 482; Pregnancy,
drugs in 815
and Embryo 397; Infant
mortality 581; Newborn 726
Birth injury 173
and Newborn 727
Birthmark 174
treatment of: Cryosurgery 323;
Laser treatment 629; *removing
skin blemishes 35*
types of: Hemangioma 526;
Nevus 726; Port-wine stain
810
birth rates:
Statistics, vital 939
Birth weight 174
and Prematurity 817; Sudden
infant death syndrome 952
Bisacodyl 1098
Bisexuality 174
and Sexuality 898
Bismuth 174
causing Melena 673
Bite (dentistry):
abnormality of: Malocclusion
966
affected by Thumb-sucking 893
medical term: Occlusion 739
Bites, animal 174
*first aid: insect stings and bites
593; snakebite 921*
types of: Insect bites 591;
Snakebites 920; Spider bites
928; Venomous bites and
stings 1044
Bites, human 175
Bithin 1098
Bithionol 1098
Bitolterol 1098
Black death 175
modern term: Plague 799
Black eye 175
Child abuse 263
black feces:
see index entry Feces,
abnormal
Blackhead 175
feature of Acne 64
Blackout 175

Blackout (continued)
Fainting 435
Black teeth:
Discolored teeth 363
Blackwater fever 175
Bladder 175
*anatomy of the bladder 176*
*disorders of the bladder 177*
and Catheterization, urinary 242
investigation of: Cystometry 329; Cystoscopy 330
part of Urinary tract 1025; *the urinary system 1028*
removal of: Cystectomy 327
stone in: Calculus, urinary tract 224
Bladder cancer:
Bladder tumors 175
bladder control:
in children: Developmental delay 348; Toilet-training 994
defective: Disk prolapse 365; Enuresis 408; Incontinence, urinary 579
Bladder tumors 175
causing Incontinence, urinary 580
Blastomycosis 176
type of Fungal infection 470
blastocyst:
development of: Zygote 1088
blastula:
development of: *the process of fertilization 446*
Bleaching, dental 177
bleaching, hair:
Hair 503
Bleb 177
Bleeder 177
Bleeding disorders 178
Bleeding 177
causing Hypotension 562; Hypovolemia 564; Renal failure 860; Shock 901
and Menstruation 677; Nosebleed 731; Placenta previa 799; Postpartum hemorrhage 811; Uterus, cancer of 1032; Varicose veins 1038
stopping: Bleeding, treatment of 179; Blood clotting 185; Hemostasis 531; Pressure points 820
see also index entry Bleeding disorders
Bleeding disorders 178
and Blood clotting 185; Platelets 801
diagnosis of: Blood clotting tests 185
treatment of: Blood products 189; Factor VIII 435; Hemostatic drugs 531; Phytonadione 794
types of: Christmas disease 277; Hemophilia 530; Thrombocytopenia 980; Von Willebrand's disease 1066
Bleeding gums:
Gingivitis 487
bleeding, rectal:
Rectal bleeding 855

bleeding time:
measurement of: Blood-clotting tests 185
Bleeding, treatment of 179
Pressure points 820
in Shock 901
Blenoxane 1098
Bleomycin 1098
Bleph-10 1098
Blephamide 1098
Blepharitis 179
causing Eyelashes, disorders of 433
treatment of: Sulfacetamide 954
Blepharoplasty 179
Blepharospasm 180
spasm of Eyelid 433
Blind loop syndrome 180
Blindness 180
causes of: Cataract 240; Cavernous sinus thrombosis 244; Chloroquine 271; Corneal abrasion 307; Filariasis 454; Glaucoma 488; Keratomalacia 615; Onchocerciasis 742; Tay-Sachs disease 966; Trachoma 1002
and *disorders of the cornea 308; disorders of the eye 431; disorders of the retina 867*
partial: Transient ischemic attack 1005
temporary: Migraine 688
types of: Color vision deficiency 292; Night blindness 727
Vision, loss of 1054
Blind spot 181
blinking, abnormal:
Tic 988
Blister 181
bloating:
Abdominal swelling 55
and Feces, abnormal 443; Hirschsprung's disease 540
Blocadren 1098
Blocked nose:
Nasal congestion 715
Nasal obstruction 715
Blocking 182
Blood 182
and Blood clotting 184; Circulatory system 280, *281*
constituents of: Blood cells 182; *constituents of blood 183*; Hemoglobin 528; Lymphocyte 655; Plasma 800; Plasma proteins 801; Platelet 801; Serum 895
disorders of: Bleeding disorders 178; *disorders of the blood 186*
blood alcohol levels:
*alcohol and the body 82*
blood calcium levels:
abnormally high: Hypercalcemia 552; Hyperparathyroidism 554, 555
abnormally low: Hypoparathyroidism 561
regulation of: Calcitonin 223; Calcium 224; Parathyroid glands 771; Vitamin D 1059

blood cancer:
medical term: Leukemia 635
Blood cells 182
*constituents of blood 183*
*disorders of the blood 186*
and Hemoglobin 528
types of: Lymphocyte 655; Platelet 801
blood cholesterol levels:
see index entry Blood lipid levels
blood clot:
causing Embolism 396; Thrombosis 981; Thrombosis, deep vein 981; *deep vein thrombosis 982*
medical term: Thrombus 982
removal of: Embolectomy 396; Thrombectomy 980
type of Embolus 397
see also index entry Blood clotting
Blood clotting 184
Blood-clotting tests 185
and Calcium 224; Factor VIII 435; Fibrinolysis 452; Vitamin K 1060
Coagulation, blood 285
disorders of: Bleeding disorders 178; *disorders of the blood 186*
prevention of: Anticoagulant drugs 116
see also index entry blood clot
Blood-clotting tests 185
in diagnosis of Purpura 839
blood coagulation:
see index entry Blood clotting
blood, coughing up:
see index entry Coughing up blood
Blood count 185
Blood culture:
Culture 324
Blood donation 187
and AIDS 79; Hemophilia 530; Transfusion, autologous 1004
blood fat levels:
see index entry Blood lipid levels
blood flow:
in Circulatory system 280, *281*
disorders of: Arteries, disorders of 130; Ischemia 607; Veins, disorders of 1043
investigation of: Diagnostic ultrasound 30; Plethysmography 801
and Resistance 863
Blood gases 187
blood glucose levels:
and Diabetes mellitus 349; *living with diabetes mellitus 350*; Glucose 492
effect on: Glucagon 492; Hypoglycemics, oral 560; Insulin 594
high: Hyperglycemia 553
low: Hunger 548; Hypoglycemia 560
Blood groups 187
in Blood transfusion 190; Forensic medicine 466
and Paternity testing 774; Prenatal treatment 43; Rh

incompatibility 871
*landmarks in surgery 33*
blood in feces:
see index entries Feces, abnormal; Rectal bleeding
blood in urine:
medical term: Hematuria 527
bloodletting:
medical term: Venesection 1044
blood lipid levels:
and Cholesterol 275; Coronary heart disease 311; Diet and disease 357; Oral contraceptives 748
high: Hyperlipidemias 553; *types of hyperlipidemia 554*
reduction of: Lipid-lowering drugs 642
Blood loss:
see index entry Bleeding
Blood poisoning 188
causing Toxemia 998
medical term: Septicemia 894
from Sepsis 894
Blood pressure 22, 188
high: Hypertension 556, 557
low: Hypotension 561; Shock 901
measurement of: Sphygmomanometer 927
regulation of: Angiotensin 110; Renin 861
and Sodium 922
Blood products 189
and AIDS 79; Hepatitis, viral 533
types of: Factor VIII 435; Immune serum globulin 570; Immunoglobulins 576
use of: Hemostatic drugs 531; Immunization 574
Blood smear 189
blood sugar levels:
see index entry blood glucose levels
Blood tests 189
for AIDS 79; Blood groups 187
types of: Blood-clotting tests 185; Blood count 185; Blood smear 189
Blood transfusion 190
leading to AIDS 78; Hepatitis, viral 533
type of: Transfusion, autologous 1004
uses of: Bleeding, treatment of 179; Hemolytic disease of the newborn 529; Hemophilia 530; Leukemia 637; Shock 902
blood urea levels:
measurement of: Kidney function tests 619
and Urea 1022
Blood vessels 190
and Circulatory system 280, *281*
disorders of: Arteries, disorders of 130; Bleeding disorders 178; Broken blood vessels 213; Veins, disorders of 1043
examples: Aorta 123; Vena cava 1043
investigation of: Angiography 109
joining: Anastomosis 99

narrowing of: Vasoconstriction 1041
types of: Arteriole 131; Artery 131; Capillary 231; Vein 1042
widening of: Vasodilation 1041
blood volume:
abnormally low: Hypovolemia 564; Shock 901
and Blood 182
blood, vomiting:
see index entry Vomiting blood
Bluboro 1098
Blue baby 190
cause of: Heart disease, congenital 518
and Cyanosis 326
Blue bloater 190
and Emphysema 400
Blue Cross/Blue Shield 190
blue skin:
medical term: Cyanosis 326
Blurred vision 190
causes of: Multiple sclerosis 701; Neuropathy 725; Polycythemia 807; Vision, disorders of 1054
tests for: Vision tests 1054; *types of vision tests 1055*
Blushing 191
B-lymphocyte:
part of Immune system 571
type of Lymphocyte 655
BMR:
see index entry Basal metabolic rate
Board certification 191
body chemistry:
medical term: Metabolism 681
study of: Biochemistry 169; Physiology 794
body "clock":
Biorhythms 171
Body contour surgery 191
body imaging:
see index entry Imaging techniques
Body odor 191
causes of: Hyperhidrosis 553; Metabolism, inborn errors of 682
and Sweat glands 958
treatment of: Antiperspirant 119; Deodorant 343
body temperature:
see index entry Temperature
Boil 191, *192*
compound: Carbuncle 233
multiple: Folliculitis 460
Bolus 192
and Swallowing 958
bolus feeding:
type of Feeding, artificial 443
Bonding 192
and Separation anxiety 893
Bonding, dental 192
Bone 192
*disorders of the bone 194*
growth of: Epiphysis 414; Vitamin A 1057; Vitamin C 1059; Vitamin D 1059
features of: Foramen 464; Periosteum 784; Sinus 907; Tuberosity 1014
formation of: Ossification 752

and Skeleton 909; *bones of the skeleton 908*
structure of: *the structure of bone 193;* Calcium 224; Phosphates 792
type of: Ossicle 752
Bone abscess 193
bone age:
Age 73
bone, broken:
see index entry Fracture
Bone cancer 193
diagnosis of: Bone imaging 195; *radionuclide bone scanning 27*
types of: Chondrosarcoma 275; Ewing's sarcoma 424; Fibrosarcoma 453; Multiple myeloma 701; Osteosarcoma 756
see also index entry Bone tumor
bone conduction:
and Deafness 333; Hearing 511
bone, cutting of:
Osteotomy 757
Bone cyst 194
bone density:
decrease of: Osteoporosis 756
increase of: Osteopetrosis 755; Osteosclerosis 757; Paget's disease 762
measurement of: Densitometry 340
bone, fracture of:
see index entry Fracture
Bone graft 194
in treatment of Osteomyelitis 755
type of Plastic surgery 801
Bone imaging 194
methods of: *radionuclide bone scanning 27;* Radionuclide scanning 848; X rays 26, 1083
type of: *three-dimensional bone imaging 27*
bone implant:
use of: Plastic surgery 801
bone, infection of:
causing Osteomyelitis 755
diagnosis of: Radionuclide scanning 848
leading to Sequestration 895
bone, inflammation of:
medical term: Osteitis 752
in Osteochondritis juvenilis 754; Osteomyelitis 755
Bone marrow 195
production of Blood cells 182
Bone marrow biopsy 195
Bone marrow transplant 34, 195
*performing a bone marrow transplant 196*
complication of: Graft-versus-host disease 497
in treatment of Anemia, aplastic 102; Leukemia 637; Lymphoma, non-Hodgkin's 657; Radiation sickness 846
bone pain:
feature of: Osteoid osteoma 754; Osteomalacia 755; Osteomyelitis 755; Paget's disease 763; Sickle cell anemia 905

bones, brittle:
see index entry Brittle bones
bone scanning:
see index entry Bone imaging
bones, deformed:
causes of: Fracture 468; Metabolism, inborn errors of 682; Osteochondritis juvenilis 754; Osteogenesis imperfecta 754; Osteomalacia 755; Paget's disease 762; Rickets 874
bones, hard:
feature of Osteopetrosis 755
bones, soft:
feature of Osteomalacia 755; Rickets 874; deficiency of Vitamin D 1059
bones, weak:
feature of Osteogenesis imperfecta 754; Osteomalacia 755; Osteoporosis 756; Paget's disease 762; Rickets 874
Bone tumor 195
cause of: Strontium 949
types of: Chondromatosis 275; Osteochondroma 754; Osteoma 754
see also index entry Bone cancer
Bonine 1098
Bontril 1098
Booster 195
Travel immunization 1008
Vaccine 1034
Borborygmi 195
Borderline personality disorder 195
Boric acid 195
Bornholm disease 195
alternative term: Pleurodynia 802
Borofax 1098
Bottle-feeding 197
and Feeding, infant 443
Botulism 197
type of Food poisoning 463
Bougie 198
Bowel 198
medical term: Intestine 601
opening into: Colostomy 293; Ileostomy 567
removal of: Colectomy 288
bowel control:
in children: Developmental delay 348; Toilet-training 994
defective: Disk prolapse 365; Incontinence, fecal 579
bowel habit, change of:
and Abdominal pain 54
causes of: Diverticular disease 367; Rectum, cancer of 856
investigation of: Barium X-ray examinations 158
Bowel movements, abnormal:
Feces, abnormal 442
Bowel sounds:
medical term: Borborygmi 195
Bowen's disease 198
type of Skin cancer 912
Bow leg 198
medical term: Varus 1039
resulting from Rickets 874

and Walking 1067
Brace, orthopedic 198
Braces, dental:
Orthodontic appliances 750
brachial artery:
damage to: Humerus, fracture of 548
Brachialgia 198
Brachial plexus 198
branches of: Radial nerve 844; Ulnar nerve 1019
damage to: Klumpke's syndrome 621; Thoracic outlet syndrome 979
brachytherapy:
type of Interstitial radiation therapy 599
Bradycardia 199
and Heart rate 520
type of Arrhythmia, cardiac 129
Braille 199
*aids for the blind 180*
Brain 199
anatomy of: Basal ganglia 160; Brain stem 203; *location of the brain stem 204; structure of the brain 200;* Cerebellum 248; Cerebrospinal fluid 249; Cerebrum 250; Cranial nerves 318; Hypothalamus 562; Limbic system 640; Meninges 675; *structure of a neuron 724;* Pineal gland 795; Pituitary gland 796; Thalamus 976; Ventricle 1046
*disorders of the brain 202*
part of Central nervous system 247; Nervous system 720, *721*
Brain abscess 201
causes of: Mastoiditis 667; Nocardiosis 729
treatment of: Neurosurgery 725
brain biopsy:
by Stereotactic surgery 939
Brain damage 201
causes of: DPT vaccination 373; Encephalitis 401; Head injury 507; Hypoglycemia 560; Kernicterus 616; Lead poisoning 631; Meningitis 675; Skull, fractured 914; Stroke 947
causing Cerebral palsy 248; Coma 294; Paralysis 769; Schizophrenia 884
and Concussion 295; Nerve damage 720
Brain death 203
and Organ donation 749
brain dysfunction:
in Alzheimer's disease 91; Dementia 339; Epilepsy 412; Liver failure 647; Temporal lobe epilepsy 969
and Brain damage 201; *disorders of the brain 202*
Minimal brain dysfunction 689
brain, electrical activity in:
and Concussion 295; Sleep 915
investigation of: EEG 391
Brain failure:
Brain syndrome, organic 204
Brain hemorrhage 203
causing Paralysis 769

Brain hemorrhage (continued)
  types of: Extradural
    hemorrhage 428;
    Intracerebral hemorrhage
    602; Subarachnoid
    hemorrhage 950; Subdural
    hemorrhage 951
Brain imaging 203
  methods of: CT scanning 323;
    MRI 28, 700; PET scanning
    29, 788; Ultrasound scanning
    1020
brain, impaired blood supply to:
    and Cerebrovascular disease
    250; Stokes-Adams syndrome
    942; Stroke 947; Transient
    ischemic attack 1005
brain, lack of:
    medical term: Anencephaly 104
Brain stem 203
  location of the brain stem 204
Brain syndrome, organic 204
Brain tumor 204
  causing Paralysis 769
  diagnosis of: PET scanning 29,
    788; Ultrasound scanning
    1020
  treatment of: Neurosurgery 725
  types of: Glioma 490;
    Medulloblastoma 671;
    Meningioma 675;
    Oligodendroglioma 742
Bran 205
  source of Fiber, dietary 452
  in treatment of Irritable bowel
    syndrome 607
Branchial disorders 205
Brash, water 205
Brasivol 1098
Braxton Hicks' contractions 205
  stages and features of pregnancy
    814
Breakbone fever 205
  medical term: Dengue 340
Breakthrough bleeding 205
Breast 205
  disorders of the breast 207
  Nipple 728
breast abscess:
  complication of Mastitis 667
Breastbone:
  medical term: Sternum 940
Breast cancer 206
  a disorder of the breast 207
  detection of: Breast self-
    examination 208; examining
    your breasts 209;
    Mammography 22, 662
  features of: Paget's disease of
    the nipple 763; Peau
    d'orange 775
  treatment of: Mastectomy 666;
    Megestrol 672; Radiation
    therapy 846; Tamoxifen 963
  see also index entry Breast
    reconstruction
breast engorgement:
  feature of Breast-feeding 207;
    Mastitis 667
Breast enlargement:
  medical term: Mammoplasty
    662
  procedure for mammoplasty 663
  see also index entries breast

growth (female); breast
    growth (male)
Breast-feeding 207
  causing Mastitis 667
  Feeding, infant 443
breast growth (female):
  and Puberty 834; changes of
    puberty 835
breast growth (male):
  associated with Cirrhosis 282;
    Klinefelter's syndrome 621
  causes of: Prolactinoma 823;
    Spironolactone 933
  medical term: Gynecomastia
    502
breast implant:
  use of: Mammoplasty 662
breast, inflammation of:
  medical term: Mastitis 667
Breast lump 208
  cause of: Mastitis 667
  detection of: Breast self-
    examination 208; examining
    your breasts 209
  see also index entry Breast
    cancer
Breast pump 208
breast quadrantectomy:
  type of Mastectomy 666
Breast reconstruction:
  type of Mammoplasty 662
  procedure for mammoplasty 663
Breast reduction:
  type of Mammoplasty 662
  procedure for mammoplasty 663
breast, removal of:
  medical term: Mastectomy 666
Breast, self-examination 208
  examining your breasts 209
Breast tenderness 208
  a disorder of the breast 207
Breath-holding attacks 209
  feature of Tantrum 964
Breathing 209
  abnormally deep: Anxiety 122;
    Hyperventilation 558
  abnormally rapid: Anxiety 122;
    Hyperventilation 558; Panic
    attack 768; Tachypnea 963
  abnormal rhythms: Apnea 126;
    Cheyne-Stokes respiration
    262; Sleep apnea 916; Sudden
    infant death syndrome 952
  noisy: Croup 321; Stridor 947;
    Wheeze 1076
  see also index entries Breathing
    difficulty; breathing stoppage
Breathing difficulty 210
  feature of Alveolitis 90; Asthma
    137; Atelectasis 140;
    Bronchitis 214; Choking 271;
    Diphtheria 362; Emphysema
    400; Epiglottiditis 412;
    Guillain-Barre syndrome 501;
    Heart block 516; Heart
    disease, congenital 518;
    disorders of the heart 517; Heart
    failure 519; Histoplasmosis
    541; Hyperventilation 558;
    Larynx, cancer of 628; Lung
    cancer 651; Mitral
    insufficiency 692; Myasthenia
    gravis 709; Panic attack 768;
    Pneumoconiosis 803;

Pneumonia 803; Pneumonitis
    804; Pneumothorax 805;
    Pulmonary embolism 836;
    Pulmonary fibrosis 836;
    Pulmonary stenosis 837;
    Respiratory distress
    syndrome 865; Septal defect
    894; Tobacco smoking 992;
    Transposition of the great
    vessels 1006
  symptom chart 211
Breathing exercises 210
breathing passages, infection of:
    Respiratory tract infection 866
breathing stoppage:
  causes of: Airway obstruction
    80; Choking 271
  feature of Apnea 126; Cheyne-
    Stokes respiration 262; Sleep
    apnea 916
  and Respiratory arrest 865
  treatment of: Artificial
    respiration 134
Breathlessness 212
  see also index entry Breathing
    difficulty
breech birth:
  see index entry Breech delivery
Breech delivery 212
  causing Birth injury 173
  and Malpresentation 661
Breonesin 1098
Brethaire 1098
Brethine 1098
Bretylium 1098
Bretylol 1098
Brevicon 1098
Brevital 1098
Brexin 1098
Bricanyl 1098
Bridge, dental 213
  Prosthodontics 827
Bright's disease 213
  alternative term:
    Glomerulonephritis 491
Brittle bones 213
  causes of: Osteogenesis
    imperfecta 754; Osteomalacia
    755; Osteoporosis 756
  following Menopause 676
brittle nails:
  and Koilonychia 623
Broca's area of brain:
  function of: Speech 925
Broken blood vessels 213
Broken tooth:
  Fracture, dental 468
Bromfed 1098
Bromides 213
Bromocriptine 213
  in treatment of Acromegaly 65;
    Pituitary tumors 798
Bromodiphenhydramine 1098
Bromovinyldeoxyuridine 1098
Bromphen 1098
Brompheniramine 1098
Bronchiectasis 214
  treatment of: Lobectomy, lung
    649
bronchiole:
  Bronchus 217
Bronchiolitis 214
  a disorder of the lung 652
Bronchitis 214

a disorder of the lung 652
  treatment of: Isoproterenol 608;
    Oxtriphylline 761
Bronchoconstrictor 215
Bronchodilator drugs 215
  how bronchodilators work 216
  examples: Albuterol 81;
    Isoproterenol 608;
    Metaproterenol 683;
    Oxtriphylline 761;
    Terbutaline 971;
    Theophylline 977
Bronchography 216
Bronchopneumonia 216
  type of Pneumonia 803, 804
Bronchoscopy 31, 216
  in diagnosis of Lung cancer 651
  in treatment of Choking 272
Bronchospasm 217
Bronchus 217
  part of Lung 651
  and Vagus nerve 1037
Bronchus, cancer of:
  Lung cancer 651
Brondecon 1098
Bronkaid Mist 1098
Bronkodyl S-R 1098
Bronkolixir 1098
Bronkometer 1098
Bronkosol 1098
Bronkotabs 1098
bronze diabetes:
  medical term:
    Hemochromatosis 528
Brown fat 217
Brucellosis 217
Bruise 217
  causes of: Bleeding disorders
    178; Purpura 839
Bruits 217
  detection of: Auscultation 144
Bruxism 217
Bubonic plague 217
  type of Plague 799
Buccal 217
Buck teeth 217
  treatment of: Orthodontic
    appliances 751
Bucladin-S 1098
Buclizine 1098
Budd-Chiari syndrome 218
  a disorder of the liver 646
Budesonide 1098
Buerger's disease 218
  causing Raynaud's
    phenomenon 853
Buff-A Comp 1098
Bufferin 1099
Buff-Oxal 10 1099
Bulimia 218
  causing Weight loss 1073
  feature of: Binge-purge
    syndrome 169
bulking agents:
  in treatment of Irritable bowel
    syndrome 607
  types of Antidiarrheal drugs
    117
Bulla 218
Bumetanide 1099
Bumex 1099
Bundle-branch block:
  Heart block 516
Bunion 218

cause of: Hallux valgus 505
Buphthalmos 219
Bupivacaine 1099
Buprenex 1099
Buprenorphine 1099
Burkitt's lymphoma 219
  type of Lymphoma, non-
    Hodgkin's 657
Burns 219
  causing Contracture 306;
    Hypotension 562;
    Hypovolemia 564; Renal
    failure 860; Shock 901
  first aid: treating burns 220
Burping 221
  alternative term: Belching 164
Burr hole 221
Bursa 221
Bursitis 221
  causing Water-on-the-knee
    1072
  feature of Rheumatoid arthritis
    870
  treatment of: Piroxicam 796
Busulfan 1099
Butabarbital 1099
Butalbital 1099
Butamben 1099
Butazolidin 1099
Butesin Picrate 1099
Butibel 1099
Butisol 1099
Butoconazole 1099
Butorphanol 1099
butter:
  Fats and oils 442
buttocks:
  Gluteus maximus 493
Bypass operations 221
  in treatment of Ischemia 607
  types of: Coronary artery
    bypass 309, 310; Shunt 904
Byssinosis 221

# C

Cachexia 222
Cadaver 222
  use in transplants: Corneal
    transplant 308; Heart-lung
    transplant 520; Heart
    transplant 522; Kidney
    transplant 619; Liver
    transplant 648; Organ
    donation 749; Transplant
    surgery 1005
Cadmium poisoning 222
  Occupational disease and
    injury 739
Café au lait spots 222
  type of Nevus 726
Cafergot 1099
Caffeine 222
  causing Palpitation 765;
    Tachycardia 963
  Withdrawal syndrome 1080
Caladryl 1099
Calamine 223
Calan 1099
Calcaneus 223
  part of Foot 463; Skeleton 909
Calcet 1099

Calcidrine 1099
Calcifediol 1099
Calciferol 223
  constituent of Vitamin D 1059
Calcification 223
Calcification, dental 223
Calcimar 1099
Calcinosis 223
Calciparine 1099
Calcitonin 223
Calcitrel 1099
Calcitriol 1099
Calcium 223
  abnormal blood levels of:
    Parathyroidectomy 771;
    Vitamin D 1059; Tetany 975
  deficiency of: Rickets 874;
    Osteoporosis 756
  deposition of: Nephrocalcinosis
    718
  in treatment of
    Hypoparathyroidism 561
  type of Ion 605
Calcium carbonate 1099
Calcium channel blockers 224
  action of: types of vasodilator
    drugs 1041
  examples: Diltiazem 361;
    Nifedipine 727; Verapamil
    1046
  in treatment of Migraine 689
Calculus 224
  alternative term: Stones 944
Calculus, dental 224
  causing Gingivitis 487;
    Periodontitis 783
  and Dental examination 342
  removal of: Periodontics 783;
    Preventive dentistry 820;
    Scaling, dental 881
  resulting from Plaque, dental
    800
Calculus, urinary tract 224
  urinary tract calculi 225
Calderol 1099
Caldesene 1099
Calel-D 1099
Calendar method 226
Calf muscles 226
Caliper splint 226
Callosity:
  Callus, skin 226
Callus, bony 226
Callus, skin 226
  treatment of: Keratolytic drugs
    615
Calmol 4 1099
Caloric test 226
Calorie 226
  Kilocalorie 621
  unit of Energy 407
Calorie requirements:
  Energy requirements 407
Calorimetry 227
Caltrate 600 1099
Cama 1099
Camalox 1099
Cambendazole 1099
Camphor 1099
campylobacter bacterium:
  causing Colitis 289
Cancer 227
  incidence of cancer 228
  causes of: Carcinogen 233;

Carcinogenesis 233;
  Metastasis 683
diagnosis of: Biopsy 170;
  Cancer screening 230; types of
  cancer test 229
examples: Bladder tumors 175;
  Bone cancer 193; Brain tumor
  204; Breast cancer 206;
  Cervix, cancer of 254;
  Esophagus, cancer of 420;
  Intestine, cancer of 601;
  Kidney cancer 617; Larynx,
  cancer of 638; Leukemia 635;
  Lip cancer 642; Liver cancer
  647; Lung cancer 651; Mouth
  cancer 607; Nasopharynx,
  cancer of 856; Ovary, cancer
  of 760; Penis, cancer 995;
  Uterus, concer of 1031;
  Vulva, cancer of 1066
and Obesity 738
study of: Oncology
treatment of: treatment of cancer
  229; Chemotherapy 258;
  Cytotoxic drugs 331;
  Immunotherapy 576;
  Radiation therapy 846, 847
  type of Neoplasm 718; Tumor
  1015
types of: Carcinoma 234;
  Sarcoma 881
Cancerphobia 230
Cancer screening 230
Cancrum oris 230
  alternative term: Noma 730
Candidiasis 230
  affecting Penis 780
  causing Itching 608; disorders of
    the lung 652; Vulvitis 1066
  example of Opportunistic
    infection 746
  as a Sexually transmitted
    disease 898; Superinfection
    956
  treatment of: Clotrimazole 284;
    Ketoconazole 616;
    Miconazole 684; Nystatin 737
  type of Fungal infection 470
Canine tooth:
  Teeth 966
Canker sore 230
  type of Mouth ulcer 699
Cannabis 230
  and Marijuana 664
Cannula 230
  use of: Intravenous infusion
    603; Venipuncture 1044
Cantharidin 1099
Cantharone 1099
Cantil 1099
Cap, contraceptive 231
Capgras' syndrome 231
Capillary 231
  part of Circulatory system 280
Capitation 231
Capping, dental:
  Crown, dental 321
Capreomycin 1099
Capsule 231
Capsulitis:
  Bursitis 221
Captopril 231
Caput 231
Carafate 1099

Caramiphen 1099
Carbachol 231
Carbamazepine 231
  in treatment of Trigeminal
    neuralgia 1010
Carbamide peroxide 1099
Carbaryl 1099
Carbenicillin 1099
Carbenoxolone 1099
Carbetapentane 1099
Carbimide 1099
Carbinoxamine 1099
Carbocaine 1099
Carbocysteine 1099
Carbohydrates 232
  in Nutrition 736
carbolic acid:
  use of: Skin peeling, chemical
    913
Carbon 232
Carbon dioxide 232
  carbon dioxide laser: use of a
    laser 630
  carbon dioxide "snow": Dry ice
    379
Carbon monoxide 233
  poisoning, effects of: Brain
    damage 201; Hypoxia 565
  poisoning, treatment of:
    Hyperbaric oxygen treatment
    552
  and Tobacco smoking 992
Carbon tetrachloride 233
carbonic acid:
  and Acidosis 63
Carboprost 1099
Carboxymethylcellulose 1099
Carbuncle 233
Carcinogen 233
  and Carcinogenesis 233
  see also index entry Cancer
Carcinogenesis 233
  and Carcinogen 233
  see also index entry Cancer
Carcinoid syndrome 234
carcinoid tumors:
  in Intestine, cancer of 601
Carcinoma 234
  type of Tumor 1015
Carcinomatosis 234
Cardec DM 1099
Cardiac arrest 234
  first aid: cardiopulmonary
    resuscitation 237
  and Myocarditis 712;
    Respiratory arrest 865;
    Shock, electric 902; Sick sinus
    syndrome 905
cardiac catheterization:
  in diagnosis of disorders of the
    heart 517
cardiac compression:
  in first aid: cardiopulmonary
    resuscitation 237
cardiac cycle:
  heart cycle 515
cardiac muscle:
  type of Muscle 706
Cardiac neurosis 234
Cardiac output 234
Cardiac stress test 234
Cardilate 1099
Cardiologist 235
Cardiology 235

Cardiomegaly 235
Cardiomyopathy 235
cardiopulmonary bypass:
  alternative term: Heart-lung
    machine 520
Cardiopulmonary resuscitation
  236
  and Cardiac arrest 234
  *first aid: cardiopulmonary*
    *resuscitation 237*
Cardioquin 1099
Cardiovascular 236
Cardiovascular disorders 236
Cardiovascular surgeon 236
Cardioversion 236
  alternative term: Defibrillation
    336
Carditis 236
Cardizem 1099
Cardovar 1099
Caries, dental 236
  associated with Nutritional
    disorders 737
  causes of: *causes of tooth decay*
    *238;* Plaque, dental 800
  causing Toothache 997
  and Decalcification, dental 335
Carisoprodol 238
Carmol 1099
Carmustine 1099
Carotene 238
  source of Vitamin A 1057
Carotid artery 238
carotid body:
  in Carotid artery 238
carotid sinus:
  in Carotid artery 238
carotenemia:
  and Vitamin A 1057
Carpal tunnel syndrome 238
carpals:
  part of *the skeletal structure of the*
    *hand 506;* Skeleton 909
Carphenazine 1099
carpus:
  alternative term: Wrist 1082
Carrier 239
Cartilage 239
  in Joints 613
  removal of: Meniscectomy 676
  tumors of: Dyschondroplasia
    382
Casanthranol 1099
Cascara 1099
Cast 239
Castellani's Paint 1099
Castor oil 239
Castration 239
  and Eunuch 423
catabolism:
  and Biochemistry 170
  in Metabolism 681
Catalepsy 239
Cataplexy 240
Catapres 1099
Cataract 240
  causes of: Galactosemia 472;
    Metabolism, inborn errors of
    682; Rubella 877
  a *disorder of the eye 431*
  and Radiation hazards 845
  treatment of: Cataract surgery
    240; Microsurgery 687
Cataract surgery 240

*procedure for cataract surgery 241*
  and Retinal detachment 867
Catastrophic insurance 241
Catatonia 241
  feature of Schizophrenia 884
Catharsis 241
Cathartic 242
Catheter 242
  type of: Balloon catheter 156
  uses of: Catheterization,
    cardiac 242; Catheterization,
    urinary 242
Catheterization, cardiac 242
  use of: Angiography 109
Catheterization, urinary 242
cation:
  and Acid 63
  type of Ion 605
CAT scanning 243
  alternative term: CT scanning
    323
Cat-scratch fever 243
Cats, diseases from 243
Cauda equina 244
  and Spinal nerves 931
Caudal 244
Caudal block 244
  type of Nerve block 719
Cauliflower ear 244
Causalgia 244
  treatment of: Sympathectomy
    959
Caustic 244
  and Alkali 86
Cauterization 244
Cavernous sinus thrombosis 244
  a *disorder of the nose 732*
Cavity, dental:
  see index entry Caries, dental
CDC:
  Centers for Disease Control 247
Ceclor 1099
Cecum 244
  *location of cecum 245*
Cefaclor 245
Cefadroxil 1099
Cefadyl 1099
Cefamandole 1099
Cefazolin 1099
Cefizox 1099
Cefobid 1099
Cefol 1099
Cefonicid 1099
Cefoperazone 1099
Ceforanide 1099
Cefotaxime 1099
Cefotetan 1099
Cefoxitin 1099
Ceftazidime 1099
Ceftizoxime 1099
Ceftriaxone 1099
Cefuroxime 1099
Celestone 1099
Celiac sprue 245
  causing Short stature 902
Cell 245
  abnormal changes in: Cervical
    smear test 252; Computer-
    aided diagnosis 295;
    Dysplasia 383; Oncogenes
    742
  *cell types 246*
  coded instructions in:
    Chromosomes 279; DNA 369;

Nucleic acids 733; RNA 875
cultures: Culture 324; Virology
  1050
replication of: Cell division 247
study of: Cytology 330; *cytology*
  *methods 331;* Staining 938
surface receptors: *types of*
  *receptor 854*
transformation of: Metaplasia
  683
Cell division 247
  and Chromosomes 279
Cellulitis 247
cellulose:
  in Carbohydrates 232; Fiber,
    dietary 452
Celontin 1099
Celsius scale 247
Cementum 247
Cenocort 1099
Centers for Disease Control 247
  and AIDS 76; Public health 835;
    Reportable diseases 861
Centigrade scale 247
  modern term: Celsius scale 247
Central nervous system 247
  part of Nervous system 720,
    721
central nervous system
  syndrome:
  and Radiation sickness 846
Centrax 1099
Centrifuge 247
Centrum 1099
Cephalexin 247
Cephalhematoma 247
  associated with Vacuum
    extraction 1034
  in Newborn 727
Cephalic 247
cephalic presentation:
  and Version 1046
Cephalosporins 248
Cephalothin 1099
Cephapirin 1099
Cephradine 1099
Cephulac 1099
Cerebellum 248
cerebral embolism:
  and stroke: *types and causes of*
    *stroke 948*
  type of Embolism 396
Cerebral hemorrhage 248
  and stroke: *types and causes of*
    *stroke 948*
Cerebral palsy 248
  associated with Spina bifida 928
  cause of: Kernicterus 616;
    Rubella 877
  causing Spasticity 924
  *types of cerebral palsy 249*
Cerebral thrombosis 249
  and stroke: *types and causes of*
    *stroke 948*
Cerebrospinal fluid 249
  excess of: Hydrocephalus 550
  sampling of: Lumbar puncture
    650
  and Spinal cord 929; Ventricle
    1046
Cerebrovascular accident 249
Cerebrovascular disease 249
Cerebrum 250
  disorders of: Brain damage 201;

*disorders of the brain 202;* Brain
  syndrome, organic 204;
  Cerebral palsy 248; Dementia
  339; Epilepsy 412
part of Brain 199; Central
  nervous system 247; Nervous
  system 720, 721
parts of: Basal ganglia 160;
  Gray matter 496; Meninges
  675; Ventricle 1046
Cerespan 1099
Cerose-DM Expectorant 1099
Certificate-of-need 251
Certification 251
Certification, board:
  Board certification 191
Cerumen 251
  common term: Earwax 387
Cervical 251
Cervical cancer:
  see index entry Cervix, cancer
  of
Cervical erosion 251
Cervical eversion:
  Cervical erosion 251
Cervical incompetence 252
  causing Miscarriage 690
cervical intraepithelial neoplasia
  (CIN) classification:
  in Cervical smear test 253
cervical mucus method 252
  and Contraception, periodic
    abstinence 305
Cervical osteoarthritis 252
  causing Paralysis 769
  and Neck 716
Cervical rib 252
  causing Thoracic outlet
    syndrome 979
  and Neck 716
Cervical smear test 252
  *procedure for a cervical (Pap)*
    *smear 253*
  and Colposcopy 293; Cytology
    330
  in diagnosis of Cervix, cancer
    of 254
cervical spine:
  injury to: Whiplash injury 1077
  part of Spine 932
Cervicitis 253
  resulting from Nonspecific
    urethritis 730
Cervix 254
  *disorders of the cervix 255*
  investigation: Cervical smear
    test 252
  part of Reproductive system,
    female 862
Cervix, cancer of 254
  associated with Herpes, genital
    536; Warts, genital 1070
  a *disorder of the cervix 255*
  diagnosis of: Cervical smear
    test 252; Colposcopy 293;
    Cone biopsy 296; Cytology
    330
  treatment of: Cryosurgery 323
Cesamet 1099
Cesarean section 256
  *procedure for a cesarean section*
    *257*
  in treatment of Childbirth,
    complications of 265; Fetal

distress 448; Malpresentation 661
Cestodes 256
  causing Tapeworm infestation 964
  type of Flatworm 458
Cetacaine 1099
Cetacort 1099
Cetamide 1099
Cetapred 1099
Cetrimide 1099
Cevalin 1099
Chagas' disease 256
  causing Myocarditis 712
  type of Trypanosomiasis 1013
Chain, Ernst:
  and *landmarks in drug development* 32
Chalazion 256
Chancre, hard 258
  feature of Syphilis 961
Chancroid 258
Chapped skin 258
Character disorders:
  Personality disorders 786
Charcoal 258
Charcot-Marie-Tooth disease 258
  alternative term: Peroneal muscular atrophy 786
Charcot's joint 258
Chardonna-2 1099
Chealamide 1099
Checkup:
  Examination, physical 424
Cheilitis 258
Chelating agents 258
  in treatment of Hemochromatosis 528; Lead poisoning 631; Mercury poisoning 681; Thalassemia 977
Chemonucleolysis 258
Chemotherapy 258
Chenix 1099
Chenodiol 258
Cheracol 1099
Chest 259
  medical term: Thorax 979
  removal of fluid from: Paracentesis 768
  surgical opening of: Thoracotomy 979
  X ray of: Chest X ray 259
Chest pain 259
  central: Myocardial infarction 712; Retrosternal pain 869
  feature of Tietze's syndrome 988
  and Palpitation 765
  *symptom chart 260*
Chest X ray 259
  X rays 26
Cheyne-Stokes respiration 262
"chi":
  in Chinese medicine 267
Chickenpox 262
  leading to Herpes zoster 537
Chigger bite 262
Chigoe 262
Chilblain:
  Pernio 786
Child abuse 262
  and Pedophilia 776
Childbed fever:

medical term: Puerperal sepsis 835
Childbirth 263
  anesthesia in: Epidural anesthesia 412; Nerve block 719; *pain relief in labor and delivery 265*; Pudendal block 835
  artificial initiation of: Induction of labor 581
  *stages of birth 264*
  complications of: Childbirth, complications of 265; Puerperal sepsis 835
  *first aid: emergency childbirth 266*
  and Postpartum depression 810
  preparation for: Prenatal care 818
Childbirth, complications of 265
  *maternal mortality 263*
Child development 267, 268-269
  assessment of: Developmental delay 348
Child guidance 267
child specialist:
  Pediatrician 776
Chill 267
  medical term: Rigor 875
Chinese medicine 267
Chinese restaurant syndrome 267
Chiropody:
  alternative term: Podiatry 805
Chiropractic 270
Chlamydial infections 270
  causing Lymphogranuloma venereum 657; Pelvic inflammatory disease 777; Pneumonia 803; Salpingitis 880; Urethritis 1024
  treatment of: Oxytetracycline 761
  types of Infectious disease 582; Sexually transmitted disease 898
Chloasma 270
  and abnormal Pigmentation 795
  associated with Pregnancy 813
Chloral hydrate 270
Chlorambucil 270
Chloramphenicol 270
  in treatment of Conjunctivitis 298
Chloraseptic 1100
Chlorate poisoning 270
Chlordiazepoxide 270
Chlorhexidine 1100
Chlormezanone 1100
Chlorofon-F 1100
Chloroform 270
Chloroguanide 1100
Chloromycetin 1100
Chlorophenothane 1100
Chloroprocaine 1100
Chloroptic 1100
Chloroquine 270
  causing *disorders of the retina 867*
Chlorosis 271
Chlorothiazide 271
Chlorotrianisene 1100
Chloroxylenol 1100
Chlorphenesin 1100
Chlorpheniramine 271
Chlorphentermine 1100
Chlorpromazine 271

in treatment of Anorexia nervosa 113
Chlorpropamide 271
Chlorprothixene 1100
Chlortetracycline 1100
Chlorthalidone 271
Chlor-Trimeton 1100
Chlorzoxazone 271
Choking 271
  *first aid: choking, infant and child 272*
  and Larynx 628
Cholangiocarcinoma 272
  type of Liver cancer 647
Cholangiography 272
cholangiopancreatography:
  type of Pancreatography 767
Cholangitis 272
  and *disorders of the liver 646*
Chole- 272
Cholecalciferol 272
  constituent of Vitamin D 1059
Cholecystectomy 272
  *procedure for cholecystectomy 273*
Cholecystitis 273
  causing Peritonitis 785
  a *disorder of the gallbladder 473*
Cholecystography 274
  in diagnosis of Gallstones 474
cholecystokinin:
  and function of Gallbladder 473
  a Gastrointestinal hormone 477
Choledyl 1100
Cholera 274
Cholestasis 274
Cholesteatoma 274
  causing Labyrinthitis 624
  following Otitis media 758
Cholesterol 275
  and Amaurosis fugax 92; Gallstones 474; Hyperlipidemias 553
  production of: Liver 644
  high blood levels of: Atherosclerosis 140; Coronary heart disease 311; Xanthomatosis 1083
Cholestyramine 275
Choline magnesium trisalicylate 1100
Choline salicylate 1100
Choloxin 1100
Chondritis 275
Chondro- 275
Chondromalacia patellae 275
  affecting Knee 621; Patella 774
chondromas:
  affecting Finger 456
  leading to Chondromatosis 275
Chondromatosis 275
Chondrosarcoma 275
Chordee 275
  associated with Hypospadias 561
Chorea 276
  causing Spasm 924
  affecting Walking 1068
Choreoathetosis 276
Choriocarcinoma 276
  and *disorders of the uterus 1031*
  resulting from Hydatidiform mole 549; Trophoblastic tumor 1012
chorion:

and development of Placenta 798
chorionic gonadotropin, human: Gonadotropin, human chorionic 494
Chorionic villus sampling 42, 276
  and Abortion, elective 57
  in diagnosis of Genetic disorders 484; Muscular dystrophy 707
Choroid 277
  part of Eye 429; Uvea 1033
Choroiditis 277
choroid plexus:
  in brain: Ventricle 1046
  part of Eye 429
Christian Science 277
Christmas disease 277
Chromagen capsules 1100
chromatin:
  in Chromosomes 279
Chromium 277
Chromosomal abnormalities 277
  and Abortion, elective 57
  causing Down's syndrome 372; Genetic disorders 482
  types of: Mosaicism 695; Trisomy 1011
  see also index entry Chromosome analysis
Chromosome analysis 278
  and Genetic analysis 31
Chromosomes 279
  in cell: Nucleus 735
  and Gene 479; *what genes are and what they do 480*; Inheritance 589
  replication of: Meiosis 673; *mechanism of meiosis 672*; Mitosis 691
  structure of: Nucleic acids 733
  translocation of: *effect of chromosomal translocation 1004*; Translocation 1005
  see also index entries Chromosomal abnormalities; Chromosome analysis
Chronic 280
Chronic obstructive lung disease: Lung disease, chronic obstructive 652
chronological age:
  and Age 73; Intelligence tests 595
Chronulac 1100
chylomicrons:
  in Hyperlipidemias 553
Chymopapain 1100
Chymoral 1100
Chymotrypsin 1100
Ciclopirox 1100
cilia:
  on Epithelium 415
  in Trachea 1001
ciliary body:
  part of Uvea 1033
ciliary muscle:
  part of Uvea 1033
Cimetidine 280
Cinnamates 1100
Cinnarizine 1100
Cinoxacin 1100
Ciprofibrate 1100
Circadian rhythm 280

Circadian rhythm (continued)
    and Jet lag 611; Pineal gland
        795
    type of Biorhythm 172
Circulation, disorders of 280
    Arteries, disorders of 130
    Capillary 231
    *disorders of the heart 517*
    Veins, disorders of 1043
Circulatory system 280, *281*
    and Blood 182; Respiration
        864
    parts of: Aorta 123; Arterioles
        131; Artery 131; Capillary
        231; Heart 514; *structure of a
        vein and an artery 1043*; Valve
        1037; Vein 1042; Vena cava
        1043
    see also index entry
        Circulation, disorders of
Circumcision 282
    complication of: Balanitis 156
    in treatment of Paraphimosis
        770; Phimosis 791
    see also index entry
        Circumcision, female
Circumcision, female 282
Cirrhosis 282
    associated with Liver disease,
        alcoholic 647
    causing Gynecomastia 502;
        Liver failure 647
    diagnosis of: Liver biopsy 645
    a *disorder of the liver 646*
    resulting from *effects of alcohol
        on the liver 21*
    treatment of:
        Hydrochlorothiazide 550;
        Metolazone 684
Cisplatin 283
Citracal 1100
Citra Forte 1100
Citrocarbonate 1100
Claforan 1100
Clap 283
    medical term: Gonorrhea 495
Claudication 283
    intermittent: Peripheral
        vascular disease 784
    a *disorder of muscle 705*
    treatment of: Pentoxifylline
        780
Claustrophobia 283
    type of Phobia 792
Clavicle 283
    part of Skeleton *908, 909*
    and Shoulder 902, *903*
Clawfoot 283
Clawhand 283
    and Ulnar nerve 1019
cleft lip:
    common term: Hare lip 507
    feature of Cleft lip and palate
        283
Cleft lip and palate 283
    treatment of: Plastic surgery
        801
cleft palate:
    associated with Hare lip 507
    cause of: Fetal alcohol
        syndrome 447
    feature of Cleft lip and palate
        283
Clemastine 1100

Cleocin 1100
Clergyman's knee 283
    type of Bursitis 221
Clerz 1100
Clidinium bromide 1100
Climacteric 284
    alternative term: Menopause
        676
Clindamycin 284
Clinoril 1100
Clioquinol 1100
Clitoridectomy 284
    Circumcision, female 282
Clitoris 284
    enlargement of:
        Pseudohermaphroditism 829;
        Sex determination 897;
        Virilism 1050
Clobetasol 1100
Clocortolone 1100
Cloderm 1100
Clofazimine 1100
Clofibrate 284
Clomid 1100
Clomiphene 284
Clomipramine 1100
Clone 284
Clonidine 284
Clonopin 1100
Clonus 284
Clorazepate 284
Closed panel:
    Health Maintenance
        Organization 511
clot:
    see index entries blood clot;
        Blood clotting
Clotrimazole 284
Clove oil 285
Cloxacillin 285
Cloxapen 1100
Clozapine 1100
Clubbing 285
    feature of Heart disease,
        congenital 518
    and Finger 455
Clubfoot 285
    medical term: Talipes 963
Clusivol 1100
Clysodrast 1100
CNS 285
    see also index entry Central
        nervous system
CNS stimulants 285
    group of Stimulant drugs 942
Coactin 1100
Coagulation, blood 285
    see also index entry Blood
        clotting
coal dust:
    and Occupational disease and
        injury 739
    causing Pneumoconiosis 802
Coal tar 285
Coarctation of the aorta 285
    a *type of congenital heart disorder
        518*
Cobalamin 285
    constituent of Vitamin B$_{12}$ 1058
Cobalt 285
    constituent of Vitamin B$_{12}$ 1058
    radioactive: Radiation therapy
        846
Cobalt edetate 1100

Cocaine 285
    and Withdrawal syndrome
        1080
cocci:
    types of Bacteria 154
Coccygodynia 285
Coccyx 285
    *anatomy of coccyx 286*
    part of Pelvis 778; *structure of
        the spine 932*
    and Sacrum 878
cochlea:
    function of: Hearing 512
    part of Ear 384
    and Vestibulocochlear nerve
        1048
Cochlear implant 286
Codeine 286
Codiclear 1100
Codimal 1100
Cod liver oil 286
coffee:
    causing Insomnia 593
    constituent of: Caffeine 222
Cogentin 1100
Co-Gesic 1100
Cognitive-behavioral therapy 286
Coil 287
    Contraception 302
    *methods of contraception 303*
    *effectiveness of contraceptives 304*
    IUD 609
Coinsurance 287
Coitus 287
    common term: Sexual
        intercourse 898, *899*
Coitus interruptus 287
Colace 1100
ColBENEMID 1100
Colchicine 287
    in treatment of Gout 495
cold agglutinin disorder:
    a *disorder of the blood 186*
Cold, common 287
    leading to Sinusitis 908
    treatment of: Cold remedies
        287
Cold injury 287
Cold remedies 287
Cold sore 287
    cause of: Herpes simplex 537
Colectomy 288
    in treatment of Intestine,
        cancer of 602: Polyposis
        familial 808; Ulcerative colitis
        1018
Colestid 1100
Colestipol 1100
Colic 288
Colic, infantile 288
Colistin 289
Colitis 289
Collagen 289
    constituent of: Sulfur 954
    in formation of Scar 882
    in Tendon 970
Collagen diseases 289
    associated with Scurvy 888
    example: Ehlers-Danlos
        syndrome 392
Collarbone 289
    medical term: Clavicle 283
Collar, orthopedic 289
Colles' fracture 289

Colloid 290
Collyrium 1100
Cologel 1100
Colon 290
    examination of: Colonoscopy
        290; Sigmoidoscopy 906
    inflammation of: Ulcerative
        colitis 1018
    opening into: Colostomy 293
    part of Intestine 601
    removal of: Colectomy 288;
        Hemicolectomy 528
Colon and rectal surgeon 290
Colon, cancer of:
    Intestine, cancer of 601
Colon, disorders of:
    *disorders of the intestine 290*
Colon, irritable:
    alternative term: Irritable bowel
        syndrome 607
Colonoscopy 290
    in diagnosis of Abdominal pain
        55; Peutz-Jeghers syndrome
        788
Colon, spastic:
    alternative term: Irritable bowel
        syndrome 607
Color blindness:
    Color vision deficiency 292
colorectal cancer:
    type of Intestine, cancer of 601
Colorex 1100
Color vision 291
Color vision deficiency 292
Colostomy 293
    in treatment of Hirschsprung's
        disease 540; Rectum, cancer
        of 856
Colostrum 293
    production of: Breast 206
Colposcopy 293
Coly-Mycin 1100
Colyte 1100
Coma 294
    causes of: Hypoglycemia 560;
        Shock 901
    type of Vegetative state 1042
Combid 1100
Combination drug 294
Combipres 1100
Comedo 294
    common term: Blackhead 175
Comhist LA 1100
Commensal 294
Commitment 294
Commode 294
Communicable disease 294
community dentistry:
    Public health dentistry 835
Compal 1100
Compartment syndrome 294
    causing Shin splints 901
    a *disorder of muscle 705*
    treatment of: Fasciotomy 441
Compazine 1100
Compensation neurosis 294
Compete 1100
complement:
    constituent of Blood 182
complement system:
    part of Immune system 571
Complex 294
complexion, florid:
    medical term: Plethora 801

Compliance 294
Complication 295
Compos mentis 295
Compound W 1100
Compress 295
  and Heat treatment 526
Compression syndrome 295
Compulsive behavior:
  Obsessive-compulsive behavior 738
compulsive personality:
  type of Personality disorder 786
Computer-aided diagnosis 295
computer imaging:
  Progress in medicine 16
Computerized tomography 295
  alternative term: CT scanning 323
Comtrex 1100
Conar A 1100
Conception 295
  failure of: Infertility 586
Concussion 295
conditioned reflex:
  and Conditioning 295
  type of Reflex 857
Conditioning 295
Condom 296
  how to use a condom 879
  Contraception, barrier methods 304
  in prevention of AIDS 79;
    Sexually transmitted diseases 898
  and "Safe" sex 879
Conduct disorders 296
conductive deafness:
  assessment of: Hearing tests 513
  resulting from Otosclerosis 759
  type of Deafness 333
Condyloma acuminatum:
  Warts, genital 296
Condyloma latum 296
Cone biopsy 296
  type of biopsy of the cervix 254
Conex DA 1100
Confabulation 296
  feature of Wernicke-Korsakoff syndrome 1076
Confidentiality 296
Confusion 296
  causes of: Dementia 339;
    Hypoxia 565; Subdural hemorrhage 951
congeners:
  causing Hangover 506
Congenital 297
congenital disorders:
  alternative term: Birth defects 172, 173
Congespirin 1100
Congess 1100
Congestion 297
Congestion, nasal 297
Congestive heart failure:
  Heart failure 519
Conjunctiva 297
  disorders of: Conjunctivitis 297;
    Pinguecula 795;
    Xerophthalmia 1083
  part of Eye 429
Conjunctivitis 297

causing Eye, painful, red 433
  a disorder of the eye 431
  and Reiter's syndrome 859;
    Rhinitis, allergic 872
Connective tissue 298
Connective tissue diseases:
  alternative term: Collagen diseases 289
Conn's syndrome 298
  alternative terms:
    Aldosteronism 85;
    Hyperaldosteronism 552
  cause of: Adrenal tumors 72
Consciousness 298
  loss of: Unconsciousness 1022;
    Vasovagal attack 1041
Consent 298
  and Ethics, medical 422
  Informed consent 588
Constant-T 1100
Constipation 298
  causes of: Codeine 286; Fibroid 453; Megacolon 671
  causing Fecal impaction 442
  and Feces, abnormal 442;
    Hirschsprung's disease 540;
    Soiling 922
  in Pregnancy 813
  symptom chart 299
  treatment of: Enema 407; Fiber, dietary 452; Lactulose 625;
    Laxative drugs 631;
    Methylcellulose 684; Psyllium 834
Contac 1100
contact dermatitis:
  Dermatitis 345
  and Skin allergy 911
Contact lenses 300
  care and insertion of contact lenses 301
Contact tracing 302
  and Gonorrhea 495; Sexually transmitted diseases 900
Contagious 302
continent ileostomy:
  and Sphincter, artificial 927
Contraception 302
  methods of contraception 303
  effectiveness of contraceptives 304
Contraception, barrier methods 304
  methods of contraception 303
  in prevention of AIDS 79;
    Sexually transmitted diseases 898
  and "Safe" sex 879
Contraception, hormonal methods 305
  methods of contraception 303
Contraception, postcoital 306
  effectiveness of contraceptives 304
  Oral contraceptives 747
Contraception, periodic abstinence 305
  methods of contraception 303
  effectiveness of contraceptives 304
Contraception, postcoital 306
Contraceptive 306
  Contraception 302
  methods of contraception 303
  effectiveness of contraceptives 304
contraceptive pill:
  Oral contraceptives 747

Contractions 306
  stimulation of: Prostaglandin 824
Contract practice:
  Corporate practice 312
Contracture 306
Contraindication 306
contrast media:
  uses of: Angiography 109;
    Imaging techniques 568;
    X rays 1084
Controlled trial 306
  type of: Double-blind 371
Contusion 306
  type of Wound 1081
Convalescence 306
Conversion disorder 307
Convulsion:
  Seizure 890
Convulsion, febrile:
  Seizure, febrile 890
Cooley's anemia 307
  type of Thalassemia 977
Cophene PL 1100
Copper 307
Cordotomy 307
Cordran 1100
Corgard 1100
Coricidin 1100
Corilin 1100
Corn 307
  associated with Hammer toe 505; Mallet toe 661
Cornea 307
  and Contact lenses 301
  disorders of: disorders of the cornea 308; disorders of the eye 431
  function of: Vision 1052; the sense of vision 1053
  part of Eye 429
  see also index entry Corneal graft
Corneal abrasion 307
Corneal graft 308
  by Microsurgery 687
  in treatment of Keratoconus 615; Trachoma 1002
  type of Transplant surgery 1005
corneal transplant:
  see index entry Corneal graft
Corneal ulcer 308
  associated with
    Keratoconjunctivitis sicca 615; Keratomalacia 615
  causes of: Herpes simplex 537;
    Herpes zoster 537
  causing Eye, painful, red 433
Coronary 309
  arteries: Heart 514
Coronary artery bypass 309, 310
  in treatment of Myocardial infarction 712
Coronary artery disease 309
Coronary care unit 309
Coronary heart disease 309
  associated with Obesity 738;
    Tobacco smoking 992
  cause of: Plaque 800
  causing Sick sinus syndrome 905; Sudden death 952
Coronary thrombosis 311
  Thrombosis 981
coronaviruses:

causing Cold, common 287
  viruses and diseases 1051
Coroner 312
  Medical examiner 670
corpora cavernosa:
  part of Penis 779
Corporate practice 312
Cor pulmonale 312
  cause of: Pneumoconiosis 802
  a disorder of the heart 517
corpus callosum:
  part of Cerebrum 250
Corpuscle 312
corpus luteum:
  anatomy of the ovary 759
corpus spongiosum:
  part of Penis 779
Corset 312
Cortaid 1100
Cort-Dome 1100
Cortef 1100
Cortenema 1100
cortex, cerebral:
  part of Cerebrum 250
Corticaine 1100
Corticosteroid drugs 312
  causing Cataract 240; Short stature 902
  and Cushing's syndrome 325
  examples: Dexamethasone 348;
    Fluocinolone 459;
    Hydrocortisone 550;
    Methylprednisolone 684;
    Prednisone 813;
    Triamcinolone 100
  in treatment of Crohn's disease 320; Rheumatoid arthritis 871; Rhinitis, allergic 873;
    Temporal arteritis 969;
    Uveitis 1033
Corticosteroid hormones 313
Corticotropin 313
  alternative term: ACTH 65
Cortifoam 1100
Cortinal 1100
Cortisol 313
  alternative term:
    Hydrocortisone 550
Cortisone 313
Cortisporin cream 1101
Cortone 1101
Cortrophin Zinc 1101
Coryban-D 1101
Coryza:
  Cold, common 287
Coryztime 1101
Cosmetic dentistry 313
Cosmetic surgery 313
  for Gynecomastia 502
  and Plastic surgery 801
  types of: Body contour surgery 191; Face-lift 434;
    Mammoplasty 662; Otoplasty 758
Costalgia 314
Cosyntropin 1101
Cotazym 1101
Cotrim 1101
CoTylenol 1101
Cough 314
  symptom chart 315
  treatment of: Cough remedies 316
Coughing up blood 314

Coughing up blood (continued)
  causes of: Bronchitis 215;
    Larynx, cancer of 628;
    Pneumonia 803; Tuberculosis
    1014
Cough remedies 316
Cough, smokers' 317
  and Tobacco smoking 992
Coumadin 1101
Counseling 317
  Psychotherapy 833
Cowpox 317
Coxa vara 317
  treatment of: Osteotomy 757
coxsackievirus:
  causing Hand-foot-and-mouth
    disease 506; Pneumonia 803
Crab lice:
  alternative term: Pubic lice 835
"crack":
  medical term: Cocaine 285
Cradle cap 317
Cramp 317
  cause of: Lactic acid 625
Cramp, writers' 318
Cranial nerves 318
  Nerve 719
Craniopharyngioma 318
Craniosynostosis 319
Craniotomy 319
  in treatment of Skull, fractured
    914
Cranium 319
  part of Skull 913
Creatinine clearance:
  type of Kidney function test
    619
Cremation 319
crepitations:
  detection of: Auscultation 144
Crepitus 319
Cretinism 319
  causes of: deficiency of Iodine
    605; disorders of the thyroid
    gland 986
Creutzfeldt-Jakob syndrome 319
Crib death:
  Sudden infant death syndrome
    952
Cri du chat syndrome 320
Crisis 320
Crisis intervention 320
Critical 320
Crohn's disease 320
  treatment of: Sulfasalazine
    954
Cromolyn sodium 321
  in treatment of Asthma 139;
    Rhinitis, allergic 873
Crosby capsule:
  use of: Jejunal biopsy 611
Crossbite 321
Cross-eye 321
  type of Strabismus 944
Cross matching 321
  and Blood groups 187; Blood
    transfusion 190
Crotamiton 1101
Croup 321
  associated with Stridor 947
  cause of: Tracheitis 1001
Crowding, dental 321
Crown, dental 321
  how crowns are fitted 322

Cruciate ligaments 321
  part of Knee 621
Crush syndrome 322
crutches:
  causing Crutch palsy 322
  how to use crutches 1068
  Walking aids 1069
Crutch palsy 322
Crying in infants 322
Cryo- 322
cryopexy:
  in treatment of Retinal
    detachment 868
Cryopreservation 322
Cryosurgery 323
Cryptococcosis 323
Cryptorchidism 323
  common term: Testis,
    undescended 973
  treatment of: Gonadotropin,
    human chorionic 495;
    Orchiopexy 749
Crysticillin 1101
Crystodigin 1101
CT scanning 26, 323
  performing a CT scan 324
  and Imaging techniques 568;
    imaging the body 569
  uses of: Heart imaging 520;
    Lung imaging 652
Culture 324
  of bacteria: Bacteriology 155
  of chromosomes:
    Amniocentesis 42, 95;
    Chorionic villus sampling 43,
    276; Chromosome analysis
    278
Cupping 325
Cuprimine 1101
Curare 325
Cure 325
  and Faith healing 438
Curet 325
Curettage 325
Curettage, dental 325
Curling's ulcer 325
Curretab 1101
Cushing's syndrome 325
  causes of: disorders of the adrenal
    glands 71; endocrine disorders
    404; Pituitary tumors 798
  causing Hyperlipidemias 553;
    Pigmentation 795; Stria 947
Cusp, dental 326
Cuspid 326
Cutaneous 326
Cutdown 326
cuts:
  first aid: wounds 1079
CVS:
  Chorionic villus sampling 276
Cyanide 326
Cyanocobalamin 326
  alternative term: Vitamin $B_{12}$
    1058
Cyanoject 1101
Cyanosis 326
  feature of Heart disease,
    congenital 518; Respiratory
    failure 865; Septic shock 895;
    Tetralogy of Fallot 976
Cyclacillin 326
Cyclandelate 1101
Cyclapen-W 1101

Cyclizine 1101
Cyclobenzaprine 326
Cyclocort 1101
Cyclomethycaine 1101
Cyclopar 1101
Cyclopentamine 1101
Cyclophosphamide 326
  in treatment of Wegener's
    granulomatosis 1072
Cycloplegia 326
cycloplegic drug:
  in treatment of Corneal
    abrasion 307
Cycloserine 1101
Cyclospasmol 1101
Cyclosporine 326
  use of: Transplant surgery 1005
Cyclothiazide 1101
Cyclothymia 326
Cylert 1101
Cyproheptadine 1101
Cyronine 1101
Cyst 327
Cyst-/cysto 327
Cystectomy 327
cystic duct:
  and Bile duct 167; Gallbladder
    473
Cysticerosis 328
  cause of: Tapeworm infestation
    964
Cystic fibrosis 328
  causing Short stature 902
  inheritance of: DNA and genetic
    disorders 40; Genetic
    disorders 484; unifactorial
    genetic disorders 483
  and disorders of the pancreas 766
cystic hygroma:
  type of Lymphangioma 654
Cystitis 328
  causing Abdominal pain 50;
    Intercourse, painful 598;
    Nocturia 729; Urination,
    frequent 1027; Urination,
    painful 1027
  avoiding cystitis 329
  leading to Nonspecific
    urethritis 730; Pyelonephritis
    840
  type of Urinary tract infection
    1025
Cystocele 329
  and Uterus, prolapse of 1032
Cystometry 329
cystosarcoma phylloides:
  type of Breast lump 208
Cystoscopy 330
  in diagnosis of Incontinence,
    urinary 580
Cystospaz 1101
Cystostomy 330
Cystourethrogram, voiding 330
Cytadren 1101
Cytarabine 1101
-cyte 330
Cyto- 330
Cytologist 330
Cytology 330
  cytology methods 331
  use of: types of cancer test 229
Cytomegalovirus 331
Cytomel 1101
Cytopathologist 331

cytoplasm:
  part of Cell 245
Cytosar-U 1101
cytosine:
  as constituent of Nucleic acids
    733
  and DNA and genetic disorders
    40; what genes are and what
    they do 480
Cytosine Arabinoside 1101
cytotoxic cells:
  part of Immune system 571
  types of Lymphocyte 657
Cytotoxic drugs 331
  types of Anticancer drugs 115
Cytoxan 1101

# D

Dacarbazine 1101
Dacryocystitis 332
Dactinomycin 1101
Dalalone 1101
Dalicote 1101
Dalidyne 1101
Dallergy 1101
Dalmane 1101
Damason-P 1101
Danazol 332
D and C 332
  and Abortion, elective 58
  in diagnosis of Menorrhagia
    677; Uterus, cancer of 1032
Dander 332
  allergy and the body 87
  causing Allergy 86; Asthma 138
Dandruff 332
  associated with Blepharitis 179
  cause of: Dermatitis 345
Danocrine 1101
Danthron 1101
Dantrium 1101
Dantrolene 333
Dapsone 333
Daranide 1101
Daraprim 1101
Darbid 1101
Daricon 1101
Darvocet-N 1101
Darvon 1101
Darvon Compound 65 1101
Daunorubicin 1101
Daydreaming 333
Dazamide 1101
DDAVP 1101
DDT 333
Deafness 333
  causes of: Acoustic neuroma
    64; Barotrauma 159; Birth
    defects 173; some possible
    causes of deafness 334; disorders
    of the ear 385; Earwax 387;
    Meniere's disease 674;
    Middle-ear effusion,
    persistent 688; Noise 729;
    Otitis media 758; Otosclerosis
    759; Ototoxicity 759; Paget's
    disease 763; Presbycusis 819;
    Rubella 877; Streptomycin
    946
  causing Developmental delay
    348

and Cleft lip and palate 283;
Labyrinthitis 624; Lipreading
642; Tinnitus 989;
Vestibulocochlear nerve 1049
diagnosis of: Hearing tests *513*
treatment of: Cochlear implant
286; Hearing aids 511, 513;
Myringotomy 713;
Stapedectomy 938;
Tympanoplasty 1016
Death 334
and Autopsy 147; Brain death
203; Coroner 312; Dying, care
of the 381; Forensic medicine
465; Life expectancy 639;
Pathologist 775; Pathology
775
causes of: *causes and incidence of
accidental death 60*; Accidents
59; *major causes of death in the
US in a representative year 694*;
Maternal mortality 668;
Occupational mortality 741
see also index entries Death
rates; Sudden death
death rates:
*causes and incidence of accidental
death 60*
*major causes of death in the US in
a representative year 694*
and Infant mortality 581;
Maternal mortality 263, 668;
Mortality 695; Occupational
mortality 741; Statistics, vital
939
death, sudden:
see index entry Sudden death
Debility 335
Debridement 335
Debrox 1101
Decaderm 1101
Decadron 1101
Deca-Durabolin 1101
Decaject 1101
Decalcification, dental 335
decapitation:
Neck 716
Decapryn 1101
Decaspray 1101
Decay, dental:
alternative term: Caries, dental
236
Decerebrate 335
Decholin 1101
Deciduous teeth:
alternative term: Primary teeth
822
Declomycin 1101
Decompression sickness 335
cause of: Nitrogen 728
common term: Bends 164
and Scuba-diving medicine 888
Decompression, spinal canal 335
Deconade 1101
Deconamine SR 1101
Decongestant drugs 336
examples: Ephedrine 410;
Naphazoline 714;
Oxymetazoline 761;
Phenylpropanolamine 791;
Pseudoephedrine 829;
Xylometazoline 1084
in treatment of Rhinitis, allergic
873

Deconsal 1101
decubitus ulcers:
common term: Bedsores 162
Deductible 336
deep vein thrombosis:
see index entry Thrombosis,
deep vein
Defecation 336
and Anus 121; Feces 442; Feces,
abnormal 442; Peristalsis 785;
Rectum 856
see also index entries
Constipation; Diarrhea
defense mechanisms (against
disease):
see index entry Immune
system
Defense mechanisms
(psychological) 336
in Bereavement 164
and Psychoanalysis 831
Defensive medicine 336
Deferoxamine 1101
Defibrillation 336
Defoliant poisoning 337
and Pollution 807
Deformity 337
Degeneration 337
Degenerative disorders 337
Deglutition 337
common term: Swallowing 958
Dehiscence 337
Dehydration 337
causes of: Cholera 274;
Delirium tremens 338;
Diarrhea 356; Fever 449;
Gastroenteritis 476;
Hangover 506; Heat
disorders 525
causing Thirst, excessive 979;
Urine, abnormal 1029
treatment of: Rehydration
therapy 858
and Water 1070
Dehydrocholic acid 1101
Dehydroemetine 1101
Déjà vu 338
in Seizure 890; Temporal lobe
epilepsy 969
Deladumone 1101
Delfen 1101
Delinquency 338
Behavioral problems in
children 162
Child guidance 267
Delirium 338
and Confusion 296
feature of Fever 449; Reye's
syndrome 869
see also index entry Delirium
tremens
Delirium tremens 338
and Alcohol dependence 83;
Withdrawal syndrome 1080
Delivery 338
and *stages of birth 264*;
Childbirth, complications of
265; Malpresentation 661
methods of: Breech delivery
212; Cesarean section 256;
*procedure for cesarean section
257*; Childbirth 263; Forceps
delivery 464; Vacuum
extraction 1034

*pain relief in labor and delivery
265*
Delsym 1101
Delta-Cortef 1101
Deltasone 1101
Deltoid 339
part of Shoulder 902
Delusion 339
in Dementia 339; Mania 663;
Megalomania 672; Paranoia
769; Psychosis 833;
Schizophrenia 884
Demazin 1101
Demeclocycline 1101
Demecarium 1101
Dementia 339
and *alcohol-related disorders 85*;
Parkinson's disease 773;
Pseudodementia 829;
Wilson's disease 1078
causes of: Alzheimer's disease
91; Brain syndrome, organic
204; Cerebrovascular disease
250; HIV 541
causing Delusion 339; Insomnia
593; Kleptomania 621
treatment of: Isoxsuprine 608
Dementia praecox 339
alternative term: Schizophrenia
884
Demerol 1101
Demi-Regroton 1101
De Morgan's spots 339
Demulen 1101
Demyelination 340
causing Retrobulbar neuritis
868
effect on Myelin 710
feature of Multiple sclerosis 701
Dendritic ulcer 340
Dengue 340
Densitometry 340
Density 340
relative density: Specific gravity
924
dental abscess:
see index entry Abscess, dental
Dental assistant 340
dental calculus:
see index entry Calculus,
dental
dental caries:
see index entry Caries, dental
dental crowns:
see index entry Crown, dental
Dental emergencies 340
Dental examination 341
dental floss:
see index entry Floss, dental
Dental hygienist:
Hygienist, dental 551
dental implants:
*fitting dental implants 992*
Titanium dental implants 991
dental impression:
see index entry Impression,
dental
dental plaque:
see index entry Plaque, dental
Dental X ray 342
Dentifrice 342
use of: Toothbrushing 997
Dentin 342
decay of: Caries, dental 237;

*causes of tooth decay 238
structure and arrangement of
teeth 967*
Dentist 342
Dentistry 342
Dentition 343
alternative term: Eruption of
teeth 416
and Permanent teeth 786;
Primary teeth 822; Teeth 966;
*structure and arrangement of
teeth 967*
Denture 343
and Impression, dental 578;
Prosthodontics 827
Deodorant 343
causing Itching 609; Vaginal
itching 1035
in prevention of Body odor 191
Deoxyribonucleic acid (DNA):
see index entry DNA
Depakene 1101
Depakote 1101
Depen 1101
Dependence 343
and Addiction 67
see also index entries Alcohol
dependence; Drug
dependence
dependent personality:
Personality disorders 786
Depersonalization 343
and Derealization 345
feature of Panic attack 768
Depilatory 344
and Hair removal 503
Depo-Estradiol 1101
Depo-Medrol 1101
Depo-Provera 1101
Depo-Testadiol 1101
Depot injection 344
Deprenyl 1101
Depression 344
causing Insomnia 593;
Pseudodementia 829; Sexual
desire, inhibited 898; Suicide
953; Suicide, attempted 954;
Weight loss 1073
in Influenza 588; Manic-
depressive illness 663;
Postpartum depression 810;
Post-traumatic stress
disorder 811; Pregnancy 814;
Premenstrual syndrome 818;
Psychosis 833
and Personality disorders 786;
Phobia 792
following Rape 850
treatment of: Antidepressant
drugs 116; Cognitive-
behavioral therapy 286; ECT
388; Exercise 425; Imipramine
570; Maprotiline 664;
Protriptyline 828
Deprol 1101
Derangement 345
Derealization 345
associated with
Depersonalization 343
feature of Panic attack 768
Dermabrasion 345
in treatment of Tattooing 966
Dermacort 1101
Dermatitis 345

Dermatitis (continued)
and *allergy and the body 87;*
Eczema 390; *disorders of the skin 910*
causes of: Allergy 86; Gold 494; Nickel 727; Skin allergy 911
diagnosis of: Skin tests 913
treatment of: Corticosteroid drugs 312; Hydrocortisone 550; Lanolin 626; Potassium permanganate 812
Dermatitis artefacta 345
Dermatitis herpetiformis 345
and Celiac sprue 245
Dermatographia 345
form of Urticaria 1030
Dermatologist 345
Dermatology 345
Dermatome 346
Dermatomyositis 346
type of Autoimmune disorder 145; *disorder of muscle 705;* Myositis 713; *disorder of the skin 910*
Dermatophyte infections 346
dermis:
part of Skin 909
Dermoid cyst 346
type of Ovarian cyst 759; Teratoma 971
Dermoid tumor:
Dermoid cyst 346
Dermolate 1101
Dermoplast 1101
DES 346
Diethylstilbestrol 359
descending colon:
part of Intestine 601
Desensitization, allergy:
type of Immunotherapy 576
Desensitization (psychological):
use of: Behavior therapy 163
Designer drugs 346
Desipramine 347
Desmoid tumor 347
Desonide 1101
Desoximetasone 1101
Desoxycorticosterone 1101
Desoxyn 1101
Desquam-X 1101
Desyrel 1101
Detergent poisoning 347
Developmental delay 347
and Child development 267, 268-269; Failure to thrive 435
resulting from Metabolism, inborn errors of 682
deviated septum:
Nasal septum 715
Deviation, sexual 348
Dexamethasone 348
Dexatrim 1101
Dexbrompheniramine 1101
Dexchlorpheniramine 1101
Dexone 1101
Dextroamphetamine 348
type of Amphetamine drug 95
Dextrocardia 349
Dextromethorphan 1101
Dextrose 349
Dextrothyroxine 1101
Dey-Dose Atropine Sulfate 1101
D factor:
causing Rh incompatibility 871

DHE-45 1101
DHS Zinc 1101
DHT 1101
DiaBeta 1102
Diabetes, bronze 349
alternative term: Hemochromatosis 528
Diabetes insipidus 349
and ADH 68
cause of: Pituitary tumors 798
causing Urination, excessive 1026
Diabetes mellitus 349
causes of: *disorders of the pancreas 766;* Pancreatectomy 767
causing Gangrene 474; Glycosuria 493; Impotence 578; Itching 608; Leg ulcer 633; Neuropathy 724; Nocturia 729; Paralysis 769; Peripheral vascular disease 784; *disorders of the retina 867;* Retinal hemorrhage 868; Strabismus 944; Thirst, excessive 979; Urination, excessive 1027; Weight loss 1073
*living with diabetes 350*
and Hyperglycemia 553; Hypoglycemia 560; Ketosis 616; Obesity 738
treatment of: Chlorpropamide 271; Glucagon 492; Guar gum 501; Hypoglycemics, oral 560; Insulin 594; Pump, insulin 838
diabetic neuropathy:
Neuropathy 724
Diabetic pregnancy 351
diabetic retinopathy:
causing Vitreous hemorrhage 1061
treatment of: Photocoagulation 793
type of Retinopathy 868
Diabinese 1102
Diacetylmorphine 351
common term: Heroin 535
Dia-Gesic 1102
Diagnosis 351
*diagnosing abdominal pain 55*
*diagnosing chest pain 259*
steps in diagnosing a condition 352
Diagnosing disease 24-31
*landmarks in diagnosis 25*
Examination, physical 424
*types of physical examination 425*
Imaging techniques 568
*imaging the body 569*
Diagnosis-related group 352
Dialose 1102
Dialume 1102
Dialysis 39, 352
*procedure for dialysis 353*
in treatment of Goodpasture's syndrome 495; Kidney, polycystic 619; poisoning with Paraquat 770; Renal failure 861
Diamidine 1102
Diamox 1102
Diaper rash 354
treatment of: Zinc oxide 1088

Diaphragm, contraceptive 354
associated with Toxic shock syndrome 1000
Contraception, barrier methods 304
Diaphragm muscle 354
and Breathing 209
nerve supply to: Phrenic nerve 793
part of Respiratory system 866
Diapid 1102
Diarrhea 356
causes of: Amebiasis 92; Cholera 274; Colitis 289; Crohn's disease 320; Dysentery 382; Food allergy 461; Food poisoning 463; Gastroenteritis 476; Diverticular disease 367; Intestine, cancer of 601; Irritable bowel syndrome 607; Polyposis coli 808; Shigellosis 901; Typhoid fever 1017; Ulcerative colitis 1018; deficiency of Vitamin A 1057
causing Dehydation 338; Incontinence, fecal 579
*symptom chart 355*
treatment of: Antidiarrheal drugs 117; Colectomy 288; Diphenoxylate 361; Kaolin 614; Rehydration therapy 859
Diastole 357
and Heart 515; Systole 962
diastolic blood pressure:
abnormally high: Hypertension 557
Blood pressure 188
Diathermy 357
uses of: Operating room 745; Physical therapy 793
Diathesis 357
Diazepam 357
Diazoxide 1102
Dibenzyline 1102
Dibucaine 1102
Dical-D 1102
Dichlorphenamide 1102
Dicloxacillin 1102
Dicumarol 357
Dicyclomine 357
Dideoxycytidine 357
Didronel 1102
Dienestrol 357
die, right to:
and Euthanasia 424; Will, living 1077
Diet:
constituents of: Artificial sweeteners 135; Calorie 226; Carbohydrates 232; Cholesterol 275; Fats and oils 441; Fiber, dietary 452; Food additives 461; *the four food groups and recommended daily servings 737;* Junk food 613; Minerals 689; *minerals and main food sources 690;* Mineral supplements 689; Nutrient 736; Nutrition 736; Proteins 827; Trace elements 1001; Vitamin 1056; *vitamins and their sources in the diet 1057;*

vitamins and minerals 19; Vitamin supplements 1060
Diet and exercise 18
*good dietary habits 358*
and Pregnancy 813
types of: Macrobiotics 658; Vegetarianism 1042
and weight: Fasting 441; Obesity 738; Weight 1072; Weight reduction 1075; *weight tables 1073*
see also index entries Alcohol; Diet and disease
Diet and disease 357
*infected animal products 462*
Atherosclerosis 141
Cholesterol 275
Coronary heart disease 311
*diet and atherosclerosis 20*
Diet and exercise 18
*world dietary habits and disease 358*
Food allergy 461
Food-borne infection 461
Food intolerance 462
Food poisoning 463
Nutritional disorders 737
Obesity 738
see also index entries Alcohol-related disorders; Diet
Dietetics 359
and Nutrition 736
Diethylcarbamazine 1102
Diethylpropion 1102
Diethylstilbestrol 359
Differentiation 359
Diffusion 359
Diflorasone 1102
Diflunisal 359
Di-Gel 1102
digestion:
see index entry Digestive system
Digestive system 359
disorders of: *disorders of the anus 121; disorders of the esophagus 421; disorders of the gallbladder 473; disorders of the intestine 600; disorders of the liver 646; disorders of the pancreas 766; disorders of the stomach 943*
functions of: Bile 167; *function of the biliary system 168; the digestive process 360;* Enzyme 410; liver structure and function 645; Peristalsis 785; Saliva 879
parts of: Anus 121; Appendix 127; Bile duct 167; Biliary system 169; Cecum 244; *location of cecum 245;* Colon 290; Duodenum 380; Esophagus 420; Gallbladder 473; Ileum 568; Intestine 601; Jejunum 611; Liver 644; Mouth 697; Pancreas 765; Pharynx 789; *location of the pharynx 790;* Rectum 856; Salivary glands 880; Stomach 942
Digitalis drugs 361
Digital subtraction angiography 26
type of Angiography 109

Digitoxin 361
Digoxin 361
Dihydrocodeine 1102
Dihydroergotamine 1102
Dihydrotachysterol 1102
Dihydroxyaluminum 1102
Diiodohydroxyquin 1102
Dilantin 1102
Dilatation 361
 of heart chambers:
  Cardiomegaly 235
Dilatation and curettage:
 see index entry D and C
dilation:
 see index entry Dilatation
Dilator 361
 in treatment of Vaginismus
  1036
Dilatrate-SR 1102
Dilaudid 1102
Dilor 1102
Diloxanide 1102
Diltiazem 361
Dimacol 1102
Dimenhydrinate 361
Dimercaprol:
 in treatment of Lead poisoning
  631
Dimercaptosuccinic acid 1102
Dimetane 1102
Dimetapp 1102
Dimethindene 1102
Dimethisoquin 1102
Dimethyl sulfoxide 1102
Dimethyl turbocurarine 1102
Dinoprost 1102
Dinoprostone 1102
Dioxin 361
 as constituent of Agent Orange
  74
 and Defoliant poisoning 337;
  Pollution 807
Diphenatol 1102
Diphenhydramine 361
Diphenidol 1102
Diphenoxylate 361
Diphenylpyraline 1102
Diphtheria 362
 causing Pharyngitis 789
 and Pertussis 787; Tropical
  ulcer 1013
 prevention of: DPT vaccination
  373; Vaccine 1034
Dipivalyl epinephrine 1102
Dipivefrin 1102
Diplopia 362
 common term: Double vision
  371
Diprolene 1102
Diprosone 1102
Dipsomania 362
Dipyridamole 362
Disability 362
 aids for the disabled 363
 Handicap 506
 Rehabilitation 858
 and Sexual problems 900
Disalcid 1102
Discharge 362
Disclosing agents 362
 and Oral hygiene 748
 revealing Plaque, dental 800
discoid lupus erythematosus
 (DLE):

see index entry Lupus
 erythematosus
Discolored teeth 363
disease:
 causes: of: Autoimmune
  disorders 145; Cancer 227;
  Carcinogen 233; Diet and
  disease 357; endocrine
  disorders 404; Genetic
  disorders 482; Iatrogenic 566;
  Infection 581; Infection,
  congenital 582; Infectious
  disease 582; Inheritance 589;
  Metabolism, inborn errors of
  682; Nutritional disorders
  737; Occupational disease
  and injury 739; Parasite 771;
  Pathogen 775; Pathogenesis
  775; Radiation hazards 845;
  Radiation sickness 846;
  Vector 1041; Zoonosis 1088
 diagnosis of: steps in diagnosing
  a condition 352; Diagnosing
  disease 24-31; Diagnosis 351;
  Pathognomonic 775; Sign
  906; Symptom 959
 and Illness 568
 nature of: Incubation period
  580; Morbidity 694; New
  diseases 44-45; Primary 821;
  Prognosis 823; Secondary
  889; Syndrome 960;
  Transmissible 1005
 occurrence of: Incidence 579;
  incidence of cancer 228;
  incidence of relatively short-lived
  conditions in the US 578;
  incidence of some reportable
  diseases in the US 862;
  Endemic 401; Epidemic 411;
  Pandemic 767; Prevalence
  820; prevalence of various
  chronic conditions in the US
  821; Reportable diseases 861;
  top 20 reportable diseases in the
  US in 1986 862; Statistics,
  medical 939; Statistics, vital
  939
 prevention of: Preventive
  medicine 22-23, 820;
  Immunization 571;
  Quarantine 842; Vaccination
  1034; Vaccine 1034
 study of: Environmental
  medicine 409; Epidemiology
  411; Etiology 423;
  Occupational medicine 740;
  Oncology 743 Pathologist
  775; Pathology 775;
  Pathology, cellular 775;
  Pathophysiology 775
 treatment of: Chemotherapy
  258; Drug 376; Radiation
  therapy 846, 847; Surgery
  956; Therapy 978; Treating
  disease 32-39; Treatment 1008
 see also index entries Birth
  defects; Immune system;
  Immunity; Mental illness
Disinfectants 364
 types of: Antiseptics 119
 use of: Sterilization 939
Disipal 1102
Disk, intervertebral 364

 part of Spine 932
Diskography 364
Disk prolapse 364
 cause of: Lordosis 650
 causing Back pain 150;
  Paralysis 769; Radiculopathy
  847; Sciatica 885
 diagnosis of: Diskography 364;
  Myelography 710
 symptoms and treatment of disk
  prolapse 365
 and Spinal nerves 931; disorders
  of the spine 933
 treatment of: Decompression,
  spinal canal 335
Dislocation, joint 364
 and Elbow 393; Hip 538; Hip,
  congenital dislocation of 538;
  Jaw, dislocated 610; Joint 613;
  Shoulder, dislocation of 903
 partial: Subluxation 951
Disodium azodisalicyclic acid
 1102
Disophrol 1102
Disopyramide 365
disorder:
 see index entry disease
Disorientation 365
 and Cerebrum 251
 in Reye's syndrome 869;
  Wernicke-Korsakoff
  syndrome 1076
displaced fracture:
 Fracture 466
displaced tooth:
 medical term: Luxated tooth
  653
Displacement activity 365
disseminated intravascular
 coagulation:
 type of Bleeding disorder 178
Dissociative disorders 366
Distal 366
Disulfiram 366
Ditropan 1102
Diucardin 1102
Diulo 1102
Diupres 1102
Diuretic drugs 366
 examples: Acetazolamide 62;
  Amiloride 94; Chlorothiazide
  271; Chlorthalidone 271;
  Furosemide 471;
  Hydrochlorothiazide 550;
  Mannitol 663;
  Methyclothiazide 684;
  Metolazone 684;
  Spironolactone 932;
  Triamterene 1009
 in treatment of Heart failure
  519
 and Sodium 922
Diuril 1102
Diutensen-R 1102
Diverticular disease 367
 causing Peritonitis 785
 treatment of: Psyllium 834
diverticulitis:
 and Diverticular disease 367
diverticulosis:
 and Diverticular disease 367
Diving medicine:
 Scuba-diving medicine 887
Dizziness 367

 causes of: Cervical
  osteoarthritis 252;
  Hypotension 561; Hypoxia
  565; Shock 901; Subclavian
  steal syndrome 950;
  Transient ischemic attack
  1005; Vertigo 1047
 symptom chart 368
Djerassi, Carl:
 landmarks in drug development 32
DLE (discoid lupus
 erythematosus):
 see index entry Lupus
  erythematosus
DNA 369
 constituent of Chromosomes
  279; Gene 478
 and disease: Carcinogenesis
  234; DNA and genetic disorders
  40; Radiation 845
 function of: what genes are and
  what they do 480; Genetic code
  481; Inheritance 589; Protein
  synthesis 827; steps in protein
  synthesis 828
 and RNA 875
 type of Nucleic acid 733
DNA fingerprinting:
 use of: Paternity testing 774;
  paternity testing using DNA
  fingerprints 775
Dobutamine 1102
doctor:
 Physician 793
Docusate 1102
Dogs, diseases from 369
 and Insect bites 591;
  Toxocariasis 1000
Dolene 1102
Dolobid 1102
Dolophine 1102
Domagk, Gerhard:
 landmarks in drug development 32
dominance (genetics):
 and Genes 481; Inheritance 590
Domperidone 1102
Don Juanism:
 and Nymphomania 737
Donatussin 1102
Donnagel 1102
Donnatal 1102
Donnazyme 1102
Donor 370
 and Artificial insemination 134;
  Blood donation 187; Organ
  donation 749; Tissue-typing
  990
Do not resuscitate 370
dopamine:
 deficiency of: Parkinson's
  disease 773
 excess of: Manic-depressive
  illness 663
 and Schizophrenia 884
 type of Neurotransmitter 725
Dopar 1102
Doppler effect 370
 in diagnosis of Aortic
  insufficiency 123; Peripheral
  vascular disease 785
 and Diagnostic ultrasound 30;
  Echocardiography 388;
  Ultrasound scanning 1020
Dopram 1102

Dorcol 1102
Doriden 1102
Dormalin 1102
Dorsal 371
Doryx 1102
Dose 371
Doss 1102
Double-blind 371
Double vision 371
  causes of: Exophthalmos 426;
    Head injury 507; Multiple
    sclerosis 701; Strabismus 944
  from nerve damage: Abducent
    nerve 55; Oculomotor nerve
    741; Trochlear nerve 1012
Douche 371
  in treatment of Vaginal itching
    1035
Dow-Isoniazid 1102
Down's syndrome 372
  causing Hypotonia in infants
    564; Short stature 902
  resulting from Translocation
    1005; Trisomy 1012
Doxaphene 1102
Doxapram 1102
Doxepin 372
Doxidan 1102
Doxorubicin 372
Doxy-II 1102
DOXY-CAPS 1102
Doxycycline 372
Doxylamine 1102
Doxy-Lemmon 1102
DOXY-TABS 1102
DPT vaccination 373
Drain, surgical 373
Dramamine 1102
Dream analysis 373
  in Psychoanalysis 831
Dreaming 373
  and Nightmare 727; Sleep 915
dream, wet:
  medical term: Nocturnal
    emission 729
Dressings 374
Dressler's syndrome 374
DRG 375
  Diagnosis-related group 352
Dribbling 375
  Incontinence, urinary 580
  see also index entry Drooling
drill, dental:
  use of: Filling, dental 455
drinking:
  see index entries Alcohol;
    Alcohol dependence; Alcohol
    intoxication; Alcohol-related
    disorders; Thirst; Thirst,
    excessive
Drip:
  medical term: Intravenous
    infusion 603
Drisdol 1102
Dristan 1102
Drithocreme 1102
Dritho-Scalp 1102
Drixoral 1102
Dromostanolone 1102
Dronabinol 1102
Drooling 375
  cause of: Teething 967
Drop attack 375
Droperidol 1102

Dropsy 375
  alternative term: Edema 390
Drowning 375
  drowning: rescue methods 376
Drowning, dry 376
  types of drowning 375
drowning, partial:
  and Respiratory distress
    syndrome 865
Drowsiness 376
Drug 376
  administration of: Compliance
    294; Contraindication 306;
    Depot injection 344; Dose
    371; methods of administering
    drugs 377; Injection 591;
    Intravenous infusion 603;
    Polypharmacy 808; Pump,
    infusion 838; Suppository
    956; Topical 997
  effects of: Drug poisoning 379;
    Pharmacokinetics 789; Side
    effect 905; Tolerance 994
  landmarks in drug development 32
  and Pregnancy, drugs in 815
  study of: Pharmacologist 789;
    Pharmacology 789;
    Psychopharmacology 832
  supply of: Druggist 378;
    Pharmacist 789; Pharmacy
    789
  types of: Generic drug 481;
    Pharmaceutical 789;
    Pharmacopeia 789;
    Proprietary 824
  uses of: Drug abuse 378; Drug
    treatment 36-37;
    Immunization and
    preventive drug treatment
    23; Treating disease 32
  see also index entry Drug
    dependence
Drug abuse 378
Drug addiction 378
  see also index entry Drug
    dependence
Drug dependence 378
  and Child abuse 263;
    Endocarditis 402; Sudden
    infant death syndrome 952;
    Tolerance 994; Withdrawal
    syndrome 1078
Druggist 378
drug interactions:
  and Compliance 294; Drug 377;
    Polypharmacy 808
Drug overdose 379
  see also index entry Drug
    poisoning
Drug poisoning 379
  and Suicide 953; Suicide,
    attempted 954
  treatment of: Antidote 117
drug tolerance:
  Tolerance 994
Drug treatment 36-37
drug trials:
  Double-blind 371
drug withdrawal:
  causing Withdrawal syndrome
    1078
  and Drug dependence 378;
    Epilepsy 412
dry drowning:

see index entry Drowning, dry
Dry eye:
  medical term:
    Keratoconjunctivitis sicca 615
Dry ice 379
Dry socket 379
Drysol 1102
DSM III 379
DTPA scan:
  type of kidney imaging 619
Dual personality:
  Multiple personality 701
Duchenne muscular dystrophy:
  type of Muscular dystrophy 706
Duct 379
ductus arteriosus:
  part of Fetal circulation 447
Dulcolax 1102
Dumbness:
  Mutism 708
Dumping syndrome 379
  following Vagotomy 1037
duodenal bypass:
  medical term:
    Gastrojejunostomy 477
Duodenal ulcer 380
  type of Peptic ulcer 780
Duodenitis 380
Duodenum 380
  part of Intestine 601
Duofilm 1102
Duolube 1102
Duo-Medihaler 1102
Duotrate 1103
Duphrene 1103
Dupuytren's contracture 380
Durabolin 1103
Duracillin 1103
Duramorph 1103
Duraphyl 1103
Duraquin 1103
Duricef 1103
Durrax 1103
Dust diseases 380
  examples: Asbestosis 135;
    Pneumoconiosis 802
  type of Occupational disease
    and injury 739
Duvoid 1103
DV 1103
Dwarfism:
  medical term: Short stature 902
Dyazide 1103
Dycill 1103
Dyclonine 1103
Dying, care of the 381
Dymelor 1103
dynamic psychotherapy:
  Psychotherapy 834
Dynapen 1103
Dyphylline 1103
Dyrenium 1103
Dys- 382
Dysarthria 382
  type of Speech disorder 926
Dyschondroplasia 382
Dysentery 382
  causing Diarrhea 356; Proctitis
    822
  types of: Amebiasis 92; the cycle
    of amebiasis 93; Shigellosis 901
Dyskinesia 382
Dyslexia 382
  type of Learning disability 632

Dysmenorrhea 383
  and Menstruation, disorders of
    678; disorders of the uterus 1031
dysosmia:
  defect of Smell 918
Dyspareunia 383
  common term: Intercourse,
    painful 596
Dyspepsia 383
  common term: Indigestion 580
Dysphagia 383
  common term: Swallowing
    difficulty 958
Dysphasia 383
  and Aphasia 125
Dysphonia 383
  and Voice, loss of 1061
Dysplasia 383
  detection of: Cervical smear
    test 252
  in diagnosis of Cervix, cancer
    of 254
Dyspnea 383
  common term: Breathing
    difficulty 210
Dysrhythmia, cardiac 383
Dystonia 383
Dystrophy 383
  type of Muscular dystrophy
    706
Dysuria 383
  common term: Urination,
    painful 1027

# E

Ear 384
  disorders of: Deafness 333;
    Earache 384; disorders of the
    ear 385; ear infections 758
  drainage tube: Ear tube 387
  noises in: Tinnitus 989
  surgery on: Otoplasty 758;
    Stapedectomy 938
  Syringing of ears 962
  see also index entries Balance;
    Hearing
Earache 384
  cause of: Otitis media 757
Ear, cauliflower:
  Cauliflower ear 244
Ear, discharge from 386
eardrum:
  damage to: Eardrum,
    perforated 386; Valsalva
    maneuver 1037
  inflammation of: Myringitis
    713; Middle ear effusion,
    persistent 688
  part of Ear 384
  surgery on: Myringotomy 713;
    Tympanoplasty 1016
Eardrum, perforated 386
  causes of: Otitis media 758;
    Syringing of ears 962
  treatment of: Myringoplasty
    713
Ear, examination of 386
Ear, foreign body in 386
ear, nose, and throat diseases:
  Otorhinolaryngology 759
Ear piercing 386

causing Hepatitis, viral 533
Ears, pinning back of:
   Otoplasty 758
ears, ringing in:
   causes of: Noise 730;
      Streptomycin 946
   medical term: Tinnitus 989
   and Vertigo 1048
Ear tube 387
Earwax 387
   treatment of: Syringing of ears
      962
Easprin 1102
eating, excessive:
   and Obesity 738
Ecchymosis:
   common term: Bruise 217
eccrine gland:
   type of Sweat gland 958
ECG 387
   and Coronary heart disease
      311; Heart rate 520
   *electrocardiography (ECG) 23*
Echocardiography 388
   in diagnosis of *disorders of the
      heart 517*; Pericarditis 783
   type of Diagnostic ultrasound
      30; Ultrasound scanning 1020
Echolalia 388
Echothiophate 1103
Eclampsia 388
   and Preeclampsia 813
Econazole 388
Econochlor 1103
Econopred 1103
Ecotrin 1103
ECT 388
   in treatment of Depression 344;
      Manic-depressive illness 663
   type of Shock therapy 902
Ectasia 389
ectomorphic body type:
   a Somatotype 923
-ectomy 389
Ectoparasite 389
Ectopic 389
Ectopic heart beat 389
Ectopic pregnancy 389
   causing Abdominal pain 50
   following Pelvic inflammatory
      disease 777
   and Oral contraceptives 748
Ectropion 390
Eczema 390
   of Nipple 728
   a *disorder of the skin 910*
   treatment of: Prednisolone 813;
      Promethazine 823; Zinc oxide
      1088
   type of: Pompholyx 808
eczema herpeticum:
   and Herpes simplex 537
Edecrin 1103
Edema 390
   causes of: Nephrotic syndrome
      719; Preeclampsia 813
   *chronic edema 391*
   treatment of: Furosemide 471
   type of: Angioedema 108
Edentulous 391
Edetate calcium disodium 1103
Edetate disodium 1103
EDTA 1103
Edwards' syndrome:

and Trisomy 1012
EEG 391
   *EEG changes during a seizure 890*
E.E.S. 1103
Effersyllium 1103
Effusion 392
   and Pericarditis 782
Effusion, joint 392
Eflornithine 1103
Efodine 1103
Efudex 1103
Egg:
   *egg and sperm cells 279*
   medical term: Ovum 761
Ego 392
   and Freudian theory 468;
      Psychoanalytic theory 831
Egomania 392
Ehlers-Danlos syndrome 392
*Ehrlich, Paul 32*
E-Ionate PA 1103
Eisenmenger complex 392
   type of Heart disease,
      congenital 518
ejaculate:
   and Artificial insemination 134
Ejaculation 392
   and Sexual intercourse 898
   during sleep: Nocturnal
      emission 729
Ejaculation, disorders of 393
ejaculatory ducts:
   and Vas deferens 1040
EKG:
   see index entry ECG
Elavil 1103
Elbow 393
Elderly, care of the 393
Eldopaque 1103
Eldoquin 1103
Elective 394
Elective surgery 394
Electra complex:
   and Oedipus complex 741
Electrical injury 394
   *first aid: electrical injury 395*
   causing Respiratory arrest 865
Electric shock treatment:
   ECT 388
electrocardiogram:
   see index entry ECG
Electrocardiography (ECG):
   see index entry ECG
Electrocautery:
   Electrocoagulation 395
Electrocoagulation 395
Electroconvulsive therapy:
   see index entry ECT
electrocution:
   Electrical injury 394
Electrodessication 395
Electroencephalography (EEG):
   EEG 391
Electrolysis 395
   method of Hair removal 503
Electrolyte 396
electromagnetic radiation:
   and Color vision 291; Radiation
      844
   *electromagnetic spectrum 1021*
electromuscular stimulation:
   Walking aids 1069
electromyogram:
   EMG 399

Electromyography (EMG):
   EMG 399
electron microscope:
   Microscope 685
Electronystagmography 396
Electrophoresis 396
Elephantiasis 396
   cause of: Filariasis 454
ELISA test 396
   and Serology 895
   type of Immunoassay 575
Elixicon 1103
Elixir 396
Elixophyllin 1103
Embolectomy 396
Embolex 1103
Embolism 396
   in Peripheral vascular disease
      784
   see also index entry Embolus
Embolism, therapeutic 397
embolization:
   Embolism, therapeutic 397
Embolus 397
   removal of: Embolectomy 396
   and Thrombosis 981
   see also index entry Embolism
Embryo 397
   abnormalities of: Teratogen 971
   *the developing embryo 398*
   *stages and features of pregnancy
      814*
   see also index entry Fetus
Embryology 399
Embryo, research on 399
Emcyt 1103
Emergence of new diseases 44
Emergency 399
Emergency physician 399
Emesis:
   see index entry Vomiting
Emete-con 1103
Emetic 399
Emetine 1103
EMG 399
   in diagnosis of *disorders of
      muscle 705*
Emko 1103
Emollient 399
emotion:
   abnormalities of: Personality
      disorders 786; Psychosis 833;
      Schizophrenia 884
   and Limbic system 640;
      Personality 786
Emotional deprivation 399
   causing Short stature 902
   and Child abuse 263
Emotional problems 399
Empathy 399
   in Psychotherapist 833
Emphysema 399
   causes of: Cadmium poisoning
      222; Pneumoconiosis 803;
      Pulmonary hypertension 837;
      *smoking and emphysema 21;*
      Tobacco smoking 992
   a *disorder of the lung 652*
   and Pink puffer 795
   treatment of: Isoproterenol 608
Emphysema, surgical 400
Empirical treatment 400
Empirin 1103
Empyema 400

E-Mycin 1103
Enalapril 400
Enamel, dental 400
   erosion of: Caries, dental 236
Enarax 1103
Encainide 1103
Encaprin 1103
Encare 1103
Encephalitis 400
   causes of: Herpes simplex 537;
      Measles 669; Smallpox 918
   causing Paralysis 769
   spread by Mosquito bites 695
Encephalitis lethargica 401
encephalocele:
   in Spina bifida 928
Encephalomyelitis 401
Encephalopathy 401
Encopresis 401
   common term: Soiling 922
Endarterectomy 401
Endemic 401
Endep 1103
Endocarditis 402
   affecting Heart valve 524
   cause of: Streptococcal
      infections 945
   following Mitral insufficiency
      692; Septal defect 894
   a *disorder of the heart 517*
   treatment of: Rifampin 874
endocardium:
   lining of Heart 514
Endocrine gland 402
   Gland 487
   see also index entry Endocrine
      system
Endocrine system 402, *403*
   *endocrine disorders 404*
   and Hormones 547
   part of *the hormonal system 546*
Endocrinologist 402
Endocrinology 402
Endodontics 402
Endodontist 404
Endogenous 404
Endometrial cancer:
   Uterus, cancer of 1031
Endometriosis 404
   causing Abdominal pain 50;
      Intercourse, painful 598
   treatment of: Danazol 332;
      Hysterectomy 565;
      Norethindrone 731
   a *disorder of the uterus 1031*
Endometritis 405
   a *disorder of the uterus 1031*
Endometrium 405
   buildup of: Menorrhagia 677
   cancer of: Uterus, cancer of
      1031
endomorphic body type:
   a Somatotype 924
endophthalmos:
   a *disorder of the eye 431*
Endorphins 405
   and Enkephalins 408
   type of Neurotransmitter 725;
      Peptide 782
Endoscope 405, *406*
   uses of: Endoscopic
      investigation 31; Endoscopic
      surgery 33, 35
   see also index entry Endoscopy

Endoscopic investigation 31
endoscopic retrograde
cholangiopancreatography:
ERCP 415
Endoscopic surgery 33, 35
Endoscopy 405
and Fiberoptics 452
types of: Arthroscopy 133;
Bronchoscopy 216;
Colonoscopy 290;
Cystoscopy 330; ERCP 415;
Gastroscopy 478;
Laparoscopy 626;
Laryngoscopy 627
see also index entry Endoscope
Endothelium 407
Endotoxin 407
causing Poisoning 805
fever-causing: Pyrogen 841
Endotracheal tube 407
in treatment of Respiratory
distress syndrome 865
and Ventilation 1045
endurance:
Fitness 457
Sports medicine 936
Enduron 1103
Enduronyl 1103
Enema 407
Energy 407
units of: Calorie 226; Joule 613
Energy requirements 407
Enflurane 1103
Engagement 407
engorgement, breast:
Expressing milk 428
Enkephalins 408
Enophthalmos 408
Enovid 1103
enteral nutrition:
common term: Feeding,
artificial 443
Enteric-coated tablet 408
Enteric fever:
alternative terms: Paratyphoid
fever 772; Typhoid fever 1017
Enteritis 408
Enteritis, regional:
alternative term: Crohn's
disease 320
Enterobiasis 408
type of Pinworm infestation
796
enteroglucagon:
type of Gastrointestinal
hormone 477
Enterostomy 408
Enterotoxin 408
causing Poisoning 805
Entex 1103
Entozyme 1103
Entropion 408
and Eyelid 433
ENT surgeon:
Otolaryngologist, head and
neck surgeon 758
Entuss 1103
Enuclene 1103
Enuresis 408
Environmental constraints 46
Environmental medicine 409
Environment and development
48
Environment Protection Agency:

Pesticides 788
Enzyme 410
abnormal functioning of:
Metabolism, inborn errors of
682
structure of: Proteins 827
synthesis of: Nucleic acids 733
enzyme-linked immunosorbent
assay (ELISA)
see index entry ELISA test
eosinophils:
types of Blood cells 183
Ependymoma 410
Ephedrine 410
Epicanthic fold 410
epicondyle:
part of Elbow 393; Humerus
547
Epicondylitis 410
inflammation of Elbow 393
Epidemic 410
Infectious disease 585
widespread: Pandemic 767
Epidemiology 411
epidermis:
part of Skin 910
structure of skin 909
Epidermolysis bullosa 411
Epididymal cyst 411
alternative term: Spermatocele
927
causing Testis, swollen 973
Epididymis 411
part of Reproductive system,
male 862; Testis 972
and Sperm 927
Epididymitis:
see index entry Epididymo-
orchitis
Epididymo-orchitis 411
cause of: Nonspecific urethritis
730
and Orchitis 749; inflammation
of Testis 972
Epidural anesthesia 412
and Spinal anesthesia 929
type of Nerve block 719
Epifrin 1103
Epiglottiditis 412
causing Stridor 947
a disorder of the larynx 629
Epiglottis 412
part of Larynx 628
Epilepsy 412
and brain activity: PET
scanning 29, 788
causes of: Head injury 510;
Spina bifida 928; Sturge-
Weber syndrome 949;
Tuberous sclerosis 1014
first aid: epileptic seizure 413
and Infantile spasms 581;
Seizure 890; Seizure, febrile
890
treatment of: Carbamazepine
231; Neurosurgery 725;
Phenobarbital 790; Phenytoin
791; Primidone 822
types of: Grand mal 497; Petit
mal 788; Status epilepticus
939
E-Pilo 1103
Epiloia:
Tuberous sclerosis 1014

Epinal 1103
Epinephrine 414
abnormal secretion of:
Pheochromocytoma 791
in treatment of Anaphylactic
shock 98; Insect stings 592
EpiPen 1103
Epiphora:
common term: Watering eye
1072
Epiphysis 414
inflammation of: Perthes'
disease 787
premature ossification of:
Achondroplasia 63
Epiphysis, slipped:
Femoral epiphysis, slipped 444
Episcleritis 414
Episiotomy 414
Epispadias 415
Epistaxis:
common term: Nosebleed 731
Epithelium 415
tumor of: Papilloma 768
Epitrate 1103
Eppy/N 1103
Epstein-Barr virus 415
as a Carcinogen 233
causing Burkitt's lymphoma
219; Mononucleosis,
infectious 693
and Lymphoma, non-
Hodgkin's 657
Equagesic 1103
Equanil 1103
equinovarus deformity:
type of Talipes 963
ERCP 415
Erection 415
Erection, disorders of 415
assessment of:
Plethysmography 802
examples: Chordee 275;
Impotence 578; Priapism 821
Ergocalciferol 415
constituent of Vitamin D 1059
Ergomar 1103
Ergometer 416
Ergonovine 416
Ergostat 1103
Ergot 416
causing Cataract 240
production of: Fungi 471
Ergotamine 416
Ergotrate maleate 1103
erogenous zones:
Eroticism 416
Erosion, dental 416
Eroticism 416
Eruption 416
Eruption of teeth 416, 417
ERYC 1103
ERYC 125 1103
Erycette 1103
EryDerm 1103
Erymax 1103
Erysipelas 416
cause of: Streptococcal infection
945
Ery-Tab 1103
Erythema 416
Erythema ab igne 417
Erythema infectiosum:
Fifth disease 454

Erythema multiforme 417
form of: Stevens-Johnson
syndrome 941
Erythema nodosum 417
Erythrityl tetranitrate 1103
Erythrocin 1103
Erythrocyte 418
see also index entries Blood;
Blood cells
erythrocyte sedimentation rate
(ESR):
ESR 421
Erythroderma:
alternative term: Exfoliative
dermatitis 425
Erythromycin 418
erythropoietin:
effect of: Bone marrow 195
excess: Polycythemia 807
production of: Kidney 617
Eschar 418
Esgic 1103
Esidrix 1103
Esimil 1103
Eskalith CR 1103
Esmarch's bandage 418
type of Tourniquet 998
Esophageal atresia 418
causing Swallowing difficulty
958
Esophageal dilatation 418
Esophageal diverticulum 418
location of esophageal diverticulum
419
Esophageal spasm 419
causing Swallowing difficulty
958
esophageal speech:
following Laryngectomy 627
Esophageal stricture 419
in Hiatal hernia 538
esophageal ulcer:
type of Peptic ulcer 780
Esophageal varices 419
treatment of: Sclerotherapy 886;
Shunt 904
Esophagitis 419
causing Heartburn 516;
Salivation, excessive 880;
Swallowing difficulty 958
resulting from Hiatal hernia 538
Esophagogastroscopy:
Gastroscopy 478
Esophagogram 420
Esophagoscopy 420
Esophagus 420
bleeding in: Melena 673
disorders of the esophagus 421
narrowing of: Swallowing
difficulty 958
Esophagus, cancer of 420
causing Swallowing difficulty
958; Weight loss 1073
Esotropia 421
ESP (extrasensory perception):
Parapsychology 770
ESR 421
Estar 1103
Estinyl 1103
Estrace 1103
Estradiol 1103
Estradurin 1103
Estramustine 1103
Estratab 1103

Estratest 1103
Estriol 421
Estrogen drugs 421
  examples: Dienestrol 357;
    Diethylstilbestrol 359;
    Mestranol 681; Quinestrol
    842
Estrogen hormones 422
  and Breast cancer 206
  excess: Gynecomastia 502;
    Uterus, cancer of 1031
  production of: Placenta 798
  in treatment of Osteoporosis
    756; Prostate, cancer of 825
  uses of: Hormone replacement
    therapy 545; Oral
    contraceptives 747
Estrone 422
Estropipate 1103
Estrovis 1103
ESWL 422
  lithotripsy procedures 643
  in treatment of Calculus,
    urinary tract 226
  type of Lithotripsy 39, 644
Ethacrynate sodium 1103
Ethacrynic acid 1103
Ethambutol 422
Ethanol 42
  see also index entry: Alcohol
Ethchlorvynol 1103
Ether 422
Ethical drug 422
Ethics, medical 422
Ethinamate 1103
Ethinyl estradiol 422
Ethionamide 1103
Ethopropazine 1103
Ethosuximide 423
Ethotoin 1103
Ethrane 1103
Ethyl alcohol 423
  see also index entry: Alcohol
Ethyl chloride 423
Ethylestrenol 1103
Ethynodiol 1103
Etidocaine 1103
Etidronate 1103
Etiology 423
Etomidate 1103
Etoposide 1103
Etrafon 1103
Etretinate 1103
Eunuch 423
Euphoria 423
  cause of: Cocaine 285
Eurax 1103
Eustachian tube 423
  blockage of: Middle-ear
    effusion, persistent 688;
    Otitis media 757
  and Ear 384; Nasopharynx 716
Euthanasia 424
  and Consent 298
Euthroid 1103
Euthyroid 424
Evac-Q-Kit 1103
Eversion 424
Evoked responses 424
Ewing's sarcoma 424
Examination, physical 424
  types of physical examination 425
Excedrin 1103
Excision 424

Excoriation 424
excrement:
  Feces 442
  and Food-borne infection 462
Excretion 424
Exenteration 425
Exercise 425
  Aerobics 72
  Diet and exercise 18
  the effects of exercise 426
  Physical therapy 793
  in Pregnancy 813
  and Weight reduction 1075
Exfoliation 425
Exfoliative dermatitis 425
exhaustion, nervous:
  alternative term: Neurasthenia
    722
Exhibitionism 425
Ex-Lax 1104
Exocrine gland 426
  Gland 487
Exomphalos 426
Exophthalmos 426
Exostosis 427
Exotoxin 427
  causing Poisoning 805
Exotropia 427
Expectorants 427
  types of Cough remedies 316
Expectoration 427
Expiration 427
Exploratory surgery 427
Explosive disorder 427
Exposure 427
Expressing milk 427
  Breast-feeding 207
Exstrophy of the bladder 428
Exsel 1104
Extend 12 1104
Extendryl 1104
extracorporeal shock wave
  lithotripsy (ESWL):
  see index entry ESWL
Extraction, dental 428
extradural hematoma:
  cause of: Extradural
    hemorrhage 428
  type of Hematoma 527
Extradural hemorrhage 428
Extrapyramidal system 428
extrasensory perception (ESP):
  Parapsychology 770
extrasystoles:
  causing Palpitation 765
extroversion-introversion:
  assessment of: Personality tests
    787
  and Extrovert 428; Introvert 603
Extrovert 428
  and Jungian theory 613
Exudation 428
Eye 428
  disorders of: Blindness 180;
    Color vision deficiency 292;
    disorders of the cornea 308;
    disorders of the eye 431;
    disorders of the retina 867;
    Vision, disorders of 1054;
    Vision, loss of 1054
  anatomy of the eye 429
  function of: Color vision 291;
    Vision 1052; the sense of vision
    1053; Visual acuity 1055;

  Visual field 1055, 1056
  study of: Ophthalmology 745
  see also index entries Eye,
    examination of; Eyelid; eye
    movements; eye muscles; eye
    socket
Eye, artificial 430
eyeball, protruding:
  medical term: Exophthalmos
    426
eyeball, sunken:
  medical term: Enophthalmos
    408
Eye drops 430
eye, dry:
  medical term:
    Keratoconjunctivitis sicca 615
Eye, examination of 430
  and Tonometry 996; Vision
    tests 1054; types of vision tests
    1055
Eye, foreign body in 432
Eye injuries 432
Eyelashes, disorders of 433
  Trichiasis 1009
Eye, lazy 433
Eyelid 433
  drooping: Ptosis 834
  glands, inflammation of:
    Meibomianitis 673
  sewing together: Tarsorrhaphy
    964
  surgery on: Blepharoplasty
    179
  swollen: Conjunctivitis 298
  turning inward: Entropion 408
  turning outward: Ectropion 390
Eyelid, drooping:
  medical term: Ptosis 834
Eyelid surgery:
  Blepharoplasty 179
eye movements:
  abnormal: Kernicterus 616;
    Nystagmus 737; Vertigo 1048
  control of: Abducent nerve 55;
    Oculomotor nerve 741;
    Trochlear nerve 1012
  normal: anatomy of the eye 429;
    the sense of vision 1053
  painful: Optic neuritis 746
  paralysis of: Ophthalmoplegia
    745
eye muscles:
  control of: Abducent nerve 55;
    Oculomotor nerve 741;
    Trochlear nerve 1012
  disorders of: Double vision 371;
    Myasthenia gravis 709
  and Eye 429; the sense of vision
    1053
Eye, painful red 433
eye socket:
  alternative term: Orbit 748
  component of: sphenoid
    bone 927
  location of orbit 749
Eyestrain 433
Eye teeth 433
  structure and arrangement of teeth
    967
eye tests:
  see index entry Eye,
    examination of
Eye tumors 433

F

face:
  appearance of: Facies 435
  bones of: structure of the skull
    913
  hair growth on: Androgen
    hormones 100
  nerve supply to: Facial nerve
    434; Trigeminal nerve 1010
  see also index entries Face-lift;
    Facial pain; Facial palsy;
    Facial spasm
face-downward position:
  Pronation 824
Face-lift 434
  removal of Wrinkle 1082
  type of Cosmetic sugery 313
facet joint:
  displacement of: Back pain 150
  in Spine 932
face-upward position:
  Supination 956
Facial nerve 434
Facial pain 434
  causes of: Nasopharynx, cancer
    of 716; Trigeminal neuralgia
    1010
Facial palsy 434
  cause of: tumor of Salivary
    glands 880
  causing Ectropion 390
Facial spasm 435
  and Tetany 975; Tic 988
Facies 435
Factitious disorders 435
Factor VIII 435
  deficiency of: Hemophilia 530
  in Von Willebrand's disease
    1066
factor IX:
  deficiency of: Christmas
    disease 277
  and Hemostatic drugs 531
Fahrenheit scale 435
Failure to thrive 435
  and Child abuse 263
Fainting 435
  causes of: Heart block 516;
    Hypotension 561;
    Neuropathy 725; Shock 901;
    Vasovagal attack 1041
  symptom chart 436
  and Unconsciousness 1022
Faith healing 436
Fallen arches 438
Fallopian tube 438
  damage to: Pelvic infection 777;
    Salpingitis 880
  and Ectopic pregnancy 389;
    Infertility 586; Sterilization,
    female 940
  examination of:
    Hysterosalpingography 565
  part of Reproductive system,
    female 862
  removal of: Salpingectomy 880;
    Salpingo-oophorectomy 880
  repair of: Microsurgery 687;
    Tuboplasty 1014
Fallot's tetralogy: Tetralogy of
  Fallot 976

Fallout:
Radiation hazards 845
Falls in the elderly 438
*preventing falls 439*
False teeth:
Denture 343
Familial 439
Familial Mediterranean fever 439
familial polyposis:
Polyposis, familial 808
Family planning 440
Family practitioner 440
Family therapy 440
Famotidine 440
Fanconi's anemia 440
Fanconi's syndome 440
causing Urine, abnormal 1029
Fansidar 1104
Fantasy 440
Farmers' lung 440
Farsightedness:
medical term: Hyperopia 554
treatment of: *why glasses are used 489*
Fascia 441
Fasciculation 441
cause of: Motor neuron disease 696
Fasciitis 441
fascioliasis:
infestation with Liver fluke 648
Fasciotomy 441
Fastin 1104
Fasting 441
causing Gallstones 474; Ketosis 616
fat:
embolism: Embolism 396
excess body: Obesity 738
tumor: Lipoma 642
see also index entry Fats and oils
Fatigue:
Tiredness 989
Fats and oils 441
Nutrition 736
excess intake of: Coronary heart disease 311; Diet and disease 357; Pancreas, cancer of 766
Fatty acids 442
fatty liver:
associated with Liver disease, alcoholic 647
Favism 442
cause of: G6PD deficiency 472
FDA:
Food and Drug Administration 461
Febrile 442
febrile seizure:
Seizure, febrile 890
Fecal impaction 442
causing Incontinence, fecal 579
Fecalith 442
Feces 442
color of: Bilirubin 169
formation of: Colon 290; Digestive system 359
leakage of: Crohn's disease 320; Fecal impaction 442; Incontinence, fecal 579
see also index entry Feces, abnormal

Feces, abnormal 442
black: Esophageal varices 419; Gastritis 476; Indigestion 581; Iron 606; Melena 673; Peptic ulcer 780; Portal hypertension 810
blood in: Colitis 289; Crohn's disease 320; Intestine, cancer of 601; Rectal bleeding 855; Shigellosis 901; Ulcerative colitis 1018
foul-smelling: Celiac sprue 245
greasy: Steatorrhea 939
hard: Fecal impaction 442; Fecalith 442
liquid: Diarrhea 356
Feces, blood in the:
see index entries Feces, abnormal; Rectal bleeding
Fedahist 1104
Fedrazil 1104
Feeding, artificial 443
by Nasogastric tube 715
type of: Intravenous infusion 603
Feeding, infant 443
Bottle-feeding 197
Breast-feeding 207
*introducing solids 444*
Fee for service 444
Feen-a-Mint 1104
Feldene 1104
female gender:
and Chromosome abnormalities 277; Inheritance 590; Sex determination 897; Sex hormones 897
Feminone 1104
Femiron 1104
Femoral epiphysis, slipped 444
Femoral nerve 444
Femstat 1104
Femur 445
part of Skeleton 909
Femur, fracture of 445
causing Leg, shortening of 633
Fenfluramine 1104
Fenofibrate 1104
Fenoprofen 445
Fentanyl 1104
Feosol 1104
Feostat 1104
F-E-P Creme 1104
Ferancee 1104
Fergon 1104
Fer-in-Sol 1104
Fermalox 1104
fermentation:
in bowel: Flatulence 458
Fero-Folic-500 1104
Fero-Grad-500 1104
Fero-Gradumet 1104
Ferralet Plus 1104
ferric oxide:
ingredient of Calamine 223
Ferro-Sequels 1104
Ferrous fumarate 1104
Ferrous gluconate 1104
Ferrous sulfate 445
form of Iron 606
fertile period:
*the process of fertilization 446*
Fertility 445

effect on: Gonorrhea 495; Oral contraceptives 748
Fertility drugs 447
causing Pregnancy, multiple 815
Fertilization 447
Conception 295
*the process of fertilization 446*
In vitro fertilization 605
Pregnancy 813
Reproduction, sexual 862
Festal II 1104
fetal abnormalities:
diagnosis of: Amniocentesis 95; Chorionic villus sampling 276; Fetoscopy 448; Prenatal care 818; *prenatal screening procedures 819*; Prenatal diagnosis 41-43; Ultrasound scanning 1019
drug-related: Drug 378; Teratogen 971
types of: Birth defects 172
see also index entries Fetus; fetus, death of
Fetal alcohol syndrome 447
fetal blood transfusion:
methods of: Fetoscopy 42; Prenatal treatment 43
fetal cell culture:
and Amniocentesis and chorionic villus sampling 42
Fetal circulation 447
Fetal distress 448
Fetal heart monitoring 448
fetal tissue transplant:
*landmarks in surgery 33*
Fetal ultrasonography 41
Fetishism 448
Fetoscopy 42, 448
Fetus 448
and drugs: Drug 378; Teratogen 971
examination of: Fetoscopy 42, 448
*development of the fetus 449*
genetic analysis of: Genetic analysis 31
poor growth of: Fetal alcohol syndrome 447; Intrauterine growth retardation 603
surgery on: Prenatal treatment 43
movements of: Quickening 842
sex determination of: Amniocentesis 95; Chorionic villus sampling 276
size determination of: Ultrasound scanning 1019
viability of: Ultrasound scanning 1019
see also index entries fetal abnormalities; fetus, death of
fetus, death of:
diagnosis of: Ultrasound scanning 1019
and Miscarriage 690; Stillbirth 941
FEV:
see index entry forced expiratory volume
Fever 449
cause of: Infectious disease 585; Pyrogen 841

*symptom chart 450*
Fever blister 449
fever-producing substance:
medical term: Pyrogen 841
Fiberall 1104
Fiber, dietary 452
Diet and disease 358
and Nutrition 736
in treatment of Constipation 300
Fiberoptics 452
use of: Endoscopy 405
Fibrillation 452
fibrin:
and Blood clotting 185; Coagulation, blood 285; Hemostasis 531
breakdown of: Fibrinolysis 452
fibrinogen:
component of Blood 182
in Fibrinolysis 452
type of Plasma protein 801
Fibrinolysin 1104
Fibrinolysis 452
Fibrinolytic drugs 452
alternative term: Thrombolytic drugs 981
Fibroadenoma 452
type of Breast lump 208
fibroadenosis:
causing Breast lump 208
Fibrocystic breast disease:
Breast lump 208
Fibrocystic disease 452
Fibroid 453
causing Intercourse, painful 598
treatment of: Hysterectomy 565
*a disorder of the uterus 1031*
Fibroma 453
Fibrosarcoma 453
Fibrosis 453
and *disorders of the lung 652*
Fibrositis 453
Fibula 453
*location of the fibula 454*
part of Skeleton 909
Fifth disease 454
Fight or flight response 454
mediated by Hypothalamus 562
Filariasis 454
causing Lymphedema 655
type of: Onchocerciasis 742
and Roundworms 876
Filling, dental 455
Restoration, dental 866
Film badge 455
Finger 455
bent: Dupuytren's contracture 380; Volkmann's contracture 1062
bones of: Phalanges 789
clubbing of: Tetralogy of Fallot 976
cold, white: Raynaud's disease 853; Volkmann's contracture 1062
extra: Polydactyly 808
*finger tendons 970*
joined: Syndactyly 960
movement of: Ulnar nerve 1019
Finger joint replacement 456
Fingerprint 456
Fiogesic 1104

Fiorinal 1104
First aid 456
  *arm sling* 918
  *artificial respiration* 134
  *applying bandages* 157
  *bleeding* 179
  *burns* 220
  *cardiopulmonary resuscitation* 237
  *choking (adult)* 271
  *choking (infant and child)* 272
  *dressings* 374
  *electrical injury* 395
  *emergency childbirth* 266
  *epileptic seizure* 413
  *fainting* 435
  *first-aid kit* 456
  *foreign body in ear* 386
  *foreign body in the eye* 432
  *frostbite* 469
  *heat exhaustion* 525
  *heat stroke* 526
  *hypothermia* 563
  *insect stings and bites* 593
  *nosebleed* 731
  *poisoning* 805
  *pressure points* 820
  *recovery position* 855
  *shock* 902
  *snakebite* 921
  *splints* 934
  *sprains* 937
  *strain* 945
  *suffocation* 953
  *unconsciousness* 1022
  *wounds* 1079
Fistula 457
  in Crohn's disease 320
Fitness 457
Fitness testing 457
  Sports medicine 936
Fixation 457
  in Psychoanalytic theory 831
Flagyl 1104
Flail chest 458
  cause of: Rib, fractured 873
flashbacks:
  cause of: LSD 650
  and Memory 674
Flatfoot 458
Flatulence 458
  and Flatus 458
  associated with Indigestion 580
  treatment of: Simethicone 906
Flatus 458
  and Flatulence 458
Flatworm 458
  alternative term: Platyhelminth
  801
Flavoxate 458
Flea bites:
  Insect bites 591
Flecainide 1104
Fleet Bisacodyl 1104
Fleet Relief 1104
Fleming, Alexander:
  *landmarks in drug development* 32
Fletcher's Castoria for Children
  1104
Flexeril 1104
Flexoject 1104
Flies:
  Insects and disease 592
Flintstones 1104
Floaters 458

as symptom of Retinal
  detachment 867
in Vitreous humor 1061
flooding technique:
  in Behavior therapy 163
Floppy infant syndrome 459
  medical term: Hypotonia in
  infants 564
Floppy valve syndrome:
  medical term: Mitral valve
  prolapse 692
Florey, Howard:
  *landmarks in drug development* 32
Florinef 1104
Florone 1104
Floropryl 1104
Florvite 1104
Floss, dental 459
  and Oral hygiene 748;
  Toothbrushing 997
  in treatment of Plaque, dental
  800
Flow cytometry 459
Floxuridine 1104
Flu:
  medical term: Influenza 588
Fluctuant 459
Flucytosine 1104
Fludarabine 1104
Fludrocortisone 1104
Fluidil 1104
fluid accumulation:
  in abdomen: Ascites 136
  associated with Nephrotic
  syndrome 719
  in tissues: Edema 390
  treatment of: Diuretic drugs
  366
Fluke 459
  causing Infectious disease 583;
  Worm infestation 1081
  infestation, treatment of:
  Praziquantel 812
  type of Parasite 771;
  Platyhelminth 801;
  Trematode 1008
Flunisolide 1104
Fluocinolone 459
Fluocinonide 1104
Fluonid 1104
Fluorescein 459
  in diagnosis of Corneal ulcer
  309; *disorders of the retina* 867
  use of: Eye, examination of 430
Fluoridation 459
  see also index entry Fluoride
Fluoride 460
  and Calcification, dental 223;
  Caries, dental 236; *fluoride
  and dental caries* 459;
  Toothbrushing 997
  recommended levels of:
  Fluoridation 460
Fluoritab 1104
Fluorometholone 1104
Fluoroplex 1104
Fluorosis 460
Fluorouracil 460
Fluothane 1104
Fluoxymesterone 1104
Fluphenazine 460
Flura 1104
Flurandrenolide 1104
Flurazepam 460

Flurbiprofen 1104
Flurosyn 1104
Flush:
  Blushing 191
  feature of Mitral stenosis 692;
  Rosacea 876
fly larvae infestation:
  medical term: Myiasis 710
FML 1104
Foam, contraceptive:
  Spermicides 927
Foille 1104
Foldan 1104
Folex 1104
Folic acid 460
  in treatment of Sickle cell
  anemia 905; Sprue, tropical
  936
  part of Vitamin B complex 1058
folie à deux:
  feature of Paranoia 769
Folk medicine 460
Follicle 460
Follicle-stimulating hormone 460
  causing Ovulation 760
  and contraception: *how oral
  contraceptives work* 747
  production of: Pituitary gland
  797
Folliculitis 460
Folvite 1104
Fomites 461
Fontanelle 461
Food additives 461
  and Nutrition 736
Food allergy 461
  causing Urticaria 1030
  Diet and disease 358
Food and Drug Administration
  461
  and Drug 377; Public health 835
Food-borne infection 461
  *infected animal products* 462
Food fad 462
Food intolerance 462
food irradiation:
  Radiation hazards 845
Food poisoning 463
  and Poisoning 805
  types of: Botulism 197;
  Salmonella 880;
  Staphylococcal infections 938
food preservatives:
  types of Food additives 461
Foot 463
  *skeleton of the foot* 464
  pain in: Metatarsalgia 683
Footdrop 464
Foramen 464
  in Skull 914
foramen ovale:
  and Fetal circulation 447
forced expiratory volume (FEV):
  measurement of: Spirometry
  932
forced vital capacity (FVC):
  measurement of: Spirometry
  932
Forceps 464
Forceps delivery 464
  assisted by Episiotomy 414
  causing Postpartum
  hemorrhage 811
  using Forceps, obstetric 464

Forceps, obstetric 464
  *obstetric forceps* 465
  use of: Forceps delivery 464
Foreign body 465
  on Cornea 307
  in ear: *first aid: foreign body in
  ear* 386
  in eye: *first aid: foreign body in
  the eye* 432
  in nose: *disorders of the nose* 732
  in wounds: *first aid: wounds*
  1079
Foreign medical graduate 465
Forensic medicine 465
Foreskin 466
  part of Penis 779
  removal of: Circumcision 282
  secretions of: Smegma 918
  tight: Paraphimosis 770;
  Phimosis 791
Forgetfulness:
  Memory 674
Formaldehyde 466
Formication 466
  type of Sensation, abnormal
  893
Formula 44 1104
Formula, chemical 466
Fortaz 1104
Fostex 1104
Fototar 1104
fovea:
  and Color vision 292
  of Retina 866
Fracture 466
  causes of: Falls in the elderly
  439; March fracture 664;
  Stress fracture 946
  causing Malalignment 659
  *fractures: types and treatment* 467
  susceptibility to: Osteogenesis
  imperfecta 754; Osteomalacia
  755; Osteoporosis 756
  treatment of: Cast 239; Traction
  1002
Fracture, dental 468
Fragile X syndrome 468
  causing Mental retardation 678
Freckle 468
  and Lentigo 634; Melanin 673
  type of Nevus 726
free association:
  in Psychoanalysis 831
Free-floating anxiety 468
  feature of Generalized anxiety
  disorder 481
Frequency:
  Urination, frequent 1027
Freudian slip 468
Freudian theory 468
Freud, Sigmund:
  and Freudian slip 468; Freudian
  theory 468: Psychoanalysis
  830; Psychoanalytic theory
  831
Friedreich's ataxia 468
  causing Paralysis 769
Frigidity 469
frontal lobe:
  of Cerebrum 250
Frostbite 469
Frottage 469
Frozen section 469
  type of Biopsy 170

Frozen shoulder 469
  cause of: Bursitis 221
  and Shoulder 903
fructose:
  type of Carbohydrate 232
Frustration 470
FSH 470
  see also index entry Follicle-
    stimulating hormone
FUDR 1104
Fugue 470
Fulminant 470
Fulvicin U/F 1104
Fumes:
  Pollution 807
Functional disorders 470
Fungal infections 470
  cause of: Fungi 471
  *fungal diseases 471*
  treatment of: Antifungal drugs
    117
Fungi 470
  type of Microorganism 685
  see also index entry Fungal
    infections
Fungicidal:
  Antifungal drugs 117
Fungizone 1104
Funny bone 471
  medical term: Olecranon 741
  part of Elbow 393
Furacin 1104
Furadantin 1104
Furazolidone 1104
Furosemide 471
Furuncle 471
FVC:
  see index entry forced vital
    capacity


# G

G6PD deficiency 472
GABA 472
Gait 472
  abnormal: Ataxia 139
  Walking 1067
galactocele:
  affecting Nipple 728
Galactorrhea 472
  from Nipple 728
  as symptom of Pituitary
    tumors 798; Prolactinoma
    23
galactose:
  abnormal metabolism of:
    Galactosemia 472
  type of Carbohydrate 232
Galactosemia 472
Galen:
  history of Medicine 670
Gallamine 1104
Gallbladder 473
  function of: Bile 167; *function of
    the biliary system 168*
  inflammation of: Cholecystitis
    273; Vomiting 1065
  part of Biliary system 169
  removal of: Cholecystectomy
    272; *procedure for
    cholecystectomy 273*
  role in Typhoid fever 1017

Gallbladder cancer 473
Gallium 473
Gallstones 474
  diagnosis of: T-tube
    cholangiography 1013
  *a disorder of the gallbladder 473*
  in *disorders of the pancreas 766;*
    Pancreatitis 767;
    Spherocytosis, hereditary 927
  susceptibility to: Lipid-lowering
    drugs 642
  treatment of: Ursodeoxycholic
    acid 1029
Gambling, pathological 474
Gamimune 1104
gamma-aminobutyric acid
  (GABA):
  GABA 472
Gamma benzene hexachloride
  1104
gamma camera:
  uses of: Nuclear medicine 733;
    Radionuclide scanning 27,
    848; Scanning techniques 882
Gammacorten 1104
Gamma globulin 474
  type of Immune serum globulin
    570; Globulin 490
gamma rays:
  type of Radiation 844
Ganglion (swelling) 474
Gangrene 474
  and Buerger's disease 218;
    *disorders of muscle 705;*
    Tobacco smoking 992
  causes of: Periarteritis nodosa
    782; Peripheral vascular
    disease 784; Raynaud's
    disease 853; Thrombus 893;
    Tourniquet 998
Ganser's syndrome 475
Gantanol 1104
Gantrisin 1104
Garamycin 1104
Gardnerella vaginalis 475
Gargle 475
gargoylism:
  in Hurler's syndrome 548
gas gangrene:
  form of Gangrene 475
  occurring in Wound infection
    1082
  treatment of: Hyperbaric
    oxygen treatment 552
gas, intestinal:
  causing Flatulence 458
gas in urine:
  medical term: Pneumaturia 802
Gastrectomy 475
Gastric bubble 476
gastric cancer:
  common term: Stomach cancer
    943
Gastric erosion 476
gastric lavage:
  Lavage, gastric 630
gastric tube:
  use of: Intubation 604
Gastric ulcer 476
  Peptic ulcer 780
gastrin:
  excess: Zollinger-Ellison
    syndrome 1088
  a Gastrointestinal hormone 477

Gastritis 476
Gastroenteritis 476
Gastroenterologist 477
Gastroenterology 477
Gastrointestinal hormones 477
Gastrointestinal tract 477
  part of Digestive system 359
Gastrojejunostomy 477
Gastroscopy 478
  in diagnosis of Abdominal pain
    55; Pyloric stenosis 841;
    Stomach cancer 944
Gastrostomy 478
Gauze 478
Gavage 478
Gaviscon 1104
Gay bowel syndrome 478
Gelusil 1104
Gemfibrozil 478
Gemnisyn 1104
gender:
  genetic basis of: Inheritance 590
Gender identity 478
Gene 478
  as constituent of Chromosomes
    279
  constituents of: Nucleic acids
    733
  *gene mapping 31*
  *what genes are and what they do
    480*
  *where do your genes come from?
    479*
  and Genetic code 481; Genetic
    probes 484; Genetics 485;
    Inheritance 589; Mutation
    708; Protein synthesis 827
  recessive: Sex-linked 897
  see also index entries DNA;
    Genetic analysis; Genetic
    counseling; genetic damage;
    Genetic disorders; Genetic
    engineering
*gene mapping 31*
general anesthesia:
  see index entry Anesthesia,
    general
Generalized anxiety disorder 481
General paralysis of the insane
  481
  feature of Neurosyphilis 725;
    Syphilis 961
Generic drug 481
  Drug 376
Genetically engineered drugs 37
Genetic analysis 31
  and Blood groups 188
  see also index entry
    Chromosome analysis
Genetic code 481
  determining Protein synthesis
    827
Genetic counseling 40, 481
  for Cystic fibrosis 328; Genetic
    disorders 484; Hemophilia
    530; Retinoblastoma 868;
    Sickle cell anemia 905; Spina
    bifida 929
genetic damage:
  and Mutation 708; Radiation
    hazards 846
Genetic disorders 482
  examples: Achondroplasia 63;
    Charcot-Marie-Tooth disease

258; Cystic fibrosis 328;
    Ehlers-Danlos syndrome 392;
    Familial Mediterranean fever
    439; Friedreich's ataxia 468;
    G6PD deficiency 472;
    Galactosemia 472; Gilbert's
    disease 487; Hemophilia 530;
    Homocystinuria 544;
    Huntington's chorea 548;
    Hurler's syndrome 548;
    Marfan's syndrome 664;
    McArdle's disease 668;
    Mucopolysaccharidosis 700;
    Muscular dystrophy 706;
    Neurofibromatosis 722;
    Osteogenesis imperfecta 754;
    Osteopetrosis 755; Peroneal
    muscular atrophy 786;
    Peutz-Jehger's syndrome 788;
    Phenylketonuria 791;
    Polyposis, familial 808;
    Porphyria 809; Sickle cell
    anemia; Spherocytosis,
    hereditary 927; Tay Sachs
    disease 966; Thalassemia 977;
    Tuberous sclerosis 1014;
    Wilson's disease 1078
  *unifactorial genetic disorders 483*
  see also index entry Genetic
    counseling
Genetic engineering 484
  Genetically engineered drugs
    37
genetic markers:
  determination of: Genetic
    probe 484
  in Paternity testing 774
Genetic modifications 48
Genetic probe 484
Genetics 485
  and Inheritance 589
Genital herpes:
  Herpes, genital 536
  and Sexually transmitted
    diseases 898
Genitalia 485
  ambiguous: Intersex 599
genital phase:
  in Psychoanalytic theory 831
genitals, exposing:
  Exhibitionism 425
  and Regression 858
Genital ulceration 485
Genital warts:
  Warts, genital 1070
Genoptic 1104
Gentamicin 485
Gentian violet 485
Genu valgum 485
  common term: Knock-knee
    622
  example of Valgus 1037
Genu varum 485
  common term: Bow leg 198
  example of Varus 1039
Geocillin 1104
Geopen 1104
Geravite 1104
Geriatrician 485
Geriatric medicine 485
Gerimed 1104
Geriplex 1104
Geritol 1104
Germ 486

medical term: Microorganism 685
German measles: Rubella 876
Germ cell tumor 486
Gerontology 486
Gestalt theory 486
Gestation 486
see also index entry Pregnancy
giant: Gigantism 487
giant cell arteritis:
alternative term: Temporal arteritis 968
Giardiasis 486
cause of: Protozoa 828
treatment of: Metronidazole 684; Quinacrine 842
Giddiness: Dizziness 367
Gigantism 487
cause of: Pituitary tumors 798
Gilbert's disease 487
Gilles de la Tourette's syndrome 487
treatment of: Haloperidol 505; Pimozide 795
type of Tic 988
Gingiva 487
alternative term: Gum 501
Gingivectomy 487
Gingivitis 487
cause of: Plaque, dental 800
and Oral hygiene 748; Periodontal disease 783
Gland 487
Glanders 488
Glands, swollen 488
Glandular fever:
medical term: Mononucleosis, infectious 693
glans: part of Penis 779
Glasses 488
why glasses are used 489
Glass eye: Eye, artificial 430
Glaucoma 488
acute closed-angle glaucoma 489
associated with raised Intraocular pressure 603; Lens dislocation 634; Retinal vein occlusion 868; Sturge-Weber syndrome 949
causing Tunnel vision 1015
diagnosis of: Eye, examination of 430; Tonometry 996
a disorder of the eye 431
treatment of: Acetazolamide 62; Carbachol 231; Physostigmine 794; Pilocarpine 795; Pindolol 795; Timolol 988; Trabeculectomy 1001; Urea 1023
Glaucon 1104
glia cells: in Cerebrum 250
Gliclazide 1104
Glioblastoma multiforme 490
Glioma 490
Glipizide 490
globin: constituent of Hemoglobin 528
production of: Liver 644

Globulin 490
and ESR 421
type of Plasma protein 801
Globus hystericus 490
Glomerulonephritis 491
a disorder of the kidney 618
following Scarlet fever 883
Glomerulosclerosis 491
glomerulus:
inflammation of: Glomerulonephritis 491
part of Nephron 718; Kidney 616
scarring of: Glomerulosclerosis 491
Glomus tumor 492
Glossectomy 492
Glossitis 492
inflammation of Tongue 995
Glossolalia 492
Glossopharyngeal nerve 492
a Cranial nerve 318
Glottis 492
and Vocal cords 1061
Glucagon 492
antagonist to Insulin 594
effect on Carbohydrates 232; Glucose 492; Glycogen 493
production of: Pancreas 766
in treatment of Hypoglycemia 560
Glucamide 1104
Glucocorticoids 492
Glucose 492
blood levels: Glucagon 492; living with diabetes mellitus 350; Insulin 594
as energy source: Carbohydrates 232
in urine: living with diabetes mellitus 350; Glycosuria 493
glucose-tolerance test: in diagnosis of Diabetes mellitus 350
Glucotrol 1104
Glue sniffing: Solvent abuse 923
Glutaral 1104
Gluten 493
allergy to: Dermatitis herpetiformis 345
causing Celiac sprue 245
Gluten enteropathy: Celiac sprue 245
Gluten intolerance: Celiac sprue 245
Glutethimide 1104
Gluteus maximus 493
Glyburide 493
Glycogen 493
metabolism of: Carbohydrate 232; Glucagon 492; Glucose 492; Insulin 594
production of: Liver 644
glycogen storage diseases: and Metabolism, inborn errors of 682
Glycopyrrolate 1104
Glycosuria 493
Glycotuss 1104
Gnat bites: Insect bites 591
Goiter 493
appearance of goiter 494

in Hypothyroidism 563
and deficiency of Iodine 605
causing Swallowing difficulty 958
treatment of: Thyroidectomy 984
Gold 494
preparation of: Auranofin 144
in treatment of Rheumatoid arthritis, juvenile 871
use of: Filling, dental 455
Gold sodium thiomalate 1104
Golfers' elbow 494
type of Overuse injury 760
Gonadotropin hormones 494
and Oral contraceptives 747
production of: Pituitary gland 797
types of: Follicle-stimulating hormone 460; Gonadotropin, human chorionic 494; Luteinizing hormone 653; Menotropins 677
Gonadotropin, human chorionic 494
Gonads 495
Ovary 759
Testis 972
underactivity of: Hypogonadism 560
Gonorrhea 495
affecting Penis 780
causing Pelvic inflammatory disease 777; Salpingitis 880; Urethral discharge 1024; Urethral stricture 1024; Urethritis 1024
incidence of gonorrhea in the US 900
type of Sexually transmitted disease 898
and Urinary tract infection 1026
Goodenough-Harris test: type of Intelligence test 595
Goodpasture's syndrome 495
treatment of: Plasmapheresis 800
Good Samaritan laws 495
Gout 495, 496
cause of: Uric acid 1025
causing Tophus 997
treatment of: Colchicine 287; Indomethacin 581; Piroxicam 796; Probenecid 822; Sulfinpyrazone 954
Grafting 496
graft rejection: and Graft-versus-host disease 497
following Transplant surgery 34
Graft-versus-host disease 497
Gramicidin 497
Gram's stain 497
in microscopy: Staining 938
Grand mal 497
type of Epilepsy 413; Seizure 890
Granulation tissue 497
granulocyte: type of Phagocyte 789
Granuloma 497
in Periodontitis 783
of Umbilical cord 1021
Granuloma annulare 497

Granuloma inguinale 497
Granuloma, lethal midline 497
grasp reflex:
type of Reflex 857; Reflex, primitive 857
Graves' disease 497
a disorder of the thyroid gland 986
Gravida 498
Gray 498
a Radiation unit 845
Gray matter 498
in Brain 199; Spinal cord 929
Grief 498
cause of: Bereavement 164
causing Sexual desire, inhibited 898
Grip 498
Grippe 498
Grisactin 1104
Griseofulvin 498
in treatment of Tinea 988
Gris-PEG 1104
Groin 498
Groin, lump in the 498
Groin strain 498
Ground substance 498
Group therapy 499
in Psychiatric treatment 39
Growing pains 499
Growth 499
Growth, childhood 499
growth charts 500
see also index entries Child development; Puberty; Short stature
Growth hormone 501
abuse of: Sports, drugs and 935
deficiency: Short stature 902
production of: Pituitary gland 797
growth, retarded:
Growth, childhood 499
Short stature 902
Grüntzig, Andreas:
landmarks in surgery 33
Guaiacolsulfonate 1104
Guaifed 1105
Guaifenesin 1105
Guanabenz 1105
Guanethidine 501
example of Sympatholytic drug 959
guanine:
as constituent of Nucleic acids 733
in genes: what genes are and what they do 480
Guar gum 501
Guillain-Barré syndrome 501
Guilt 501
and Dying, care of the 381; Post-traumatic stress disorder 811; Sudden infant death syndrome 952
Guinea worm disease 501
Gum 501
bleeding: Gingivitis 487; Scurvy 888; Vincent's disease 1049
health of: Vitamin C 1059
inflammation of: Gingivitis 487; Salivation, excessive 880; Vincent's disease 1049
receding: Dental examination 341

Gum (continued)
removal of: Gingivectomy 487
swelling of: Hyperplasia, gingival 555
gumboil:
cause of: Periodontitis 784
medical term: Abscess, dental 59
Gumma 502
feature of Syphilis 961
Gut 502
Intestine 601
Guthrie test 502
for the Newborn 726
Gynecologist 502
Obstetrician 739
Gynecology 502
Gynecomastia 502
cause of: Prolactinoma 823
in Klinefelter's syndrome 621
Gynecort 1105
Gyne-Lotrimin 1105
Gynogen LA 1105
Gynol II 1105
gyri:
of Brain 199; Cerebrum 250

# H

Habituation 503
Habsburg jaw 503
Hair 503
color of: Melanin 673
constituent of: Keratin 614
follicle: Acne 63; Pore 809
growth of: *hair growth 504*; Minoxidil 689
Hairball 503
hair cells:
damage to: Noise 730
part of Ear 384
Hairiness, excessive:
associated with Polycystic ovary 807; Virilism 1050
medical terms: Hirsutism 540; Hypertrichosis 558
see also index entry Hair removal
hair loss:
medical term: Alopecia 88
Hair removal 503
methods of: Depilatory 344; Electrolysis 395
Hair transplant 504
Halazepam 1105
Halcinonide 1105
Halcion 1105
Haldol 1105
Haley's MO 1105
Half-life 504
Halitosis 504
cause of: Ozena 761
treatment of: Mouthwash 699; Oral hygiene 748
Hallucination 504
feature of Confusion 297; Paranoia 769; Psychosis 833; Schizophrenia 884; Sleep deprivation 916; Temporal lobe epilepsy 969; Thought disorders 979
following Bereavement 164;

damage to Cerebrum 251
Hallucinogenic drug 504
alternative term: Psychedelic drug 830
examples: LSD 650; Marijuana 664; Mescaline 681; Peyote 788
Hallux 505
common term: big Toe 993
Hallux rigidus 505
Hallux valgus 505
affecting Toe 994
causing Bunion 218
Halofenate 1105
Halog 1105
Haloperidol 505
Haloprogin 1105
Halotestin 1105:
Halotex 1105
Halothane 505
Hamartoma 505
Hammer toe 505
Hamstring muscles 505
tearing: Running injuries 877
Hand 505
*the skeletal structure of the hand 506*
protection of: Eczema 390
and Shoulder-hand syndrome 903
spasms of:
Hypoparathyroidism 561
weakness of: Carpal tunnel syndrome 239
see also index entry Finger
Handedness 506
hand-eye coordination:
in old Age 74; Child development 267
and Developmental delay 348
Hand-foot-and-mouth disease 506
Handicap 506
Disability 362
handwashing:
causing Paronychia 773
continual: Obsessive-compulsive behavior 738
in prevention of Food poisoning 463; Shigellosis 901
Hangnail 506
Hangover 506
causes of: Alcohol 81; Sleeping drugs 916
causing Headache 507
Hansen's disease:
common term: Leprosy 634
Haponal 1105
haptoglobin:
type of Globulin 490
Hardening of the arteries 507
medical terms: Arteriosclerosis 131; Atherosclerosis 140
Hare lip 507
associated with Cleft lip and palate 283
Harmonyl 1105
Harvey, William:
history of Medicine 670
Hashimoto's thyroiditis 507
*a disorder of the thyroid gland 986*
symptom of: Goiter 494
hashish:
preparation of Marijuana 664
haversian canals:

part of Bone 193
Hay fever 507
alternative term: Rhinitis, allergic 872
HCG (human chorionic gonadotropin):
Gonadotropin, human chorionic 494
HDL:
see index entry high-density lipoprotein
head:
abnormally small: Microcephaly 685
flattening of: Rickets 874
parts of: Brain 199; Ear 384; Eye 428; Jaw 610; Mouth 697; Nose 731; Skull 913
see also index entries Headache; Head injury; Head lag
Headache 507
resulting from Brain hemorrhage 203; Cervical osteoarthritis 252; Hangover 506; Head injury 507; Pheochromocytoma 791; Polycythemia 807; Spinal anesthesia 929; Temporal arteritis 968; Yellow fever 1086
*symptom chart 508*
see also index entry Migraine
Head injury 507
causing Brain hemorrhage 203; Cerebral palsy 249; Respiratory arrest 865
treatment of: Ventilation 1044
Head lag 510
head louse:
Lice 638
Healing 510
acceleration of: Ultrasound treatment 1021
Health 511
Diet and disease 357
*good dietary habits 358*
Exercise 425
*the effects of exercise 426*
Fitness 457
Nutrition 736
Preventive medicine 820
Staying healthy 17-23
see also index entry Health hazards
Health food 511
Health hazards 511
Alcohol 81
Smoking and drinking 20-21
Tobacco smoking 991
Health Maintenance Organization 511
Hearing 511, *512*
and Cerebrum 251; Child development 267; Ear 384; Speech 926; Vestibulocochlear nerve 1048
impaired: Cerebral palsy 248; Developmental delay 347; *disorders of the ear 385*; Noise 729; Speech therapy 926
see also index entries Deafness; Hearing aids; Hearing tests
Hearing aids 511, *513*

in treatment of Presbycusis 820
see also index entry Deafness
Hearing loss:
Hearing tests 513
see index entries Deafness; Hearing; Hearing aids
Hearing tests 513
Heart 514
abnormal position of: Dextrocardia 349
*disorders of the heart 517*
*heart cycle 515*
see also index entries Heart beat; heart covering; heart muscle; Heart rate; Heart valve
Heart, artificial 516
Heart attack:
see index entry Myocardial infarction
Heart beat 516
abnormal: Stroke 947; Supraventricular tachycardia 956; Ventricular ectopic beat 1046
abnormal, treatment of: Calcium channel blockers 224; Phenytoin 791
awareness of: Palpitation 765
cessation of: Cardiac arrest 234
normal: Diastole 357; *heart cycle 515*; Systole 962
Heart block 516
Heartburn 516
causes of: Esophagitis 420; Hiatal hernia 538
in Pregnancy 813
heart compression:
medical term: Tamponade 963
heart covering:
inflammation of: Pericarditis 782
medical term: Pericardium 783
*heart cycle 515*
heart disease:
treatment of: Digitalis drugs 361; Weight reduction 1075
types of: *disorders of the heart 517*; Heart disease, congenital 518; Heart disease, ischemic 519
see also index entry Coronary heart disease
Heart disease, congenital 518
cause of: Rubella 877
Heart disease, ischemic 519
heart, enlargement of:
associated with Pulmonary hypertension 837; Pulmonary stenosis 837
medical term: Cardiomegaly 235
Heart failure 519
causes of: damaged Heart valve 524; Septal defect 894; Sleep apnea 916; Tricuspid insufficiency 1010
causing Nocturia 729
and Pulmonary hypertension 837
treatment of: Amiloride 94; Aminophylline 94; Digitoxin 361; Digoxin 361; Hydrochlorothiazide 550;

Isosorbide dinitrate 608;
  Metolazone 684; Prazosin 812;
  Venesection 1044
Heart imaging 519
heart lining, inflammation of:
  medical term: Endocarditis 402
Heart-lung machine 520
  use of: Open heart surgery 744
Heart-lung transplant 520, 521
heart murmur:
  causes of: Pulmonary
    insufficiency 837; Septal
    defect 894
  Heart sounds 522
  Murmur 703
heart muscle:
  death of: Coronary heart
    disease 311; Myocardial
    infarction 710
  disease of: Cardiomyopathy
    235
  inflammation of: Myocarditis
    712
  structure of: the body's muscles
    704; Muscle 706
Heart rate 520
  abnormally fast: Arrhythmia,
    cardiac 129; Sinus
    tachycardia 908; Tachycardia
    963; Ventricular tachycardia
    1046
  abnormally slow: Arrhythmia,
    cardiac 129; Bradycardia 199;
    Sick sinus syndrome 905;
    Sinus bradycardia 907
  normal: Fitness 457
  slowing of: Vagus nerve 1037
  see also index entry Heart beat
heart rhythm:
  abnormal: Arrhythmia, cardiac
    129
  see also index entries Heart
    beat; Heart rate
Heart sounds 520
  see also index entry heart
    murmur
heart stoppage:
  Cardiac arrest 234
Heart surgery 522
  types of: Angioplasty, balloon
    110; Coronary artery bypass
    309, 310; heart valve
    replacement 523; Heart valve
    surgery 524; Open heart
    surgery 744; Valvotomy 1037
Heart transplant 522
Heart valve 523
  Valve 1037
heart valve abnormalities:
  and Cardiomegaly 235;
    Pulmonary insufficiency 837
  diagnosis of: Echocardiography
    388
  causes of: Rheumatic fever 869;
    Streptococcal infections 945
  causing Murmur 703
heart valve, mechanical:
  in Heart valve surgery 524
Heart valve surgery 524
  types of: heart valve implants 34;
    heart valve replacement 523;
    Valvotomy 1037
Heat cramps 525
Heat disorders 525

Heat exhaustion 525
  and Sunlight, adverse effects of
    955
Heat stroke 525
  first aid: heat stroke 526
Heat treatment 526
  Physical therapy 793
Heel 526
Heimlich maneuver 526
  in treatment of Choking 271
Heliotherapy 526
Helmex 1105
Helminth infestation 526
  Worm infestation 1081
Helmizin 1105
helper cells:
  of Immune system 571
  types of Lymphocyte 657
Hem- 526
Hemangioblastoma 526
Hemangioma 526
  common term: Stork bite 944
  in Newborn 727; Sturge-Weber
    syndrome 949
  and disorders of the nose 732
  type of Kidney tumor 619; Skin
    tumor 913
Hemarthrosis 527
  of Knee 621
Hematemesis 527
  cause of: Esophageal varices
    419
  common term: Vomiting blood
    1065
Hematologist 527
Hematology 527
Hematoma 527
  of brain: Subdural hemorrhage
    951
  in muscle: disorders of muscle 705
  of Nasal septum 715;
    Quadriceps muscle 842
  and Tissue-plasminogen
    activator 990
Hematoma auris 527
  common term: Cauliflower ear
    244
hematoxylin-eosin:
  use of: Staining 938
Hematuria 527
  causes of: Bladder tumors 176;
    Cystitis 329; Kidney cancer
    617; Kidney, polycystic 619;
    Sickle cell anemia 905
  and Urine, abnormal 1029
heme:
  constituent of Hemoglobin 528
Hemianopia 527
Hemiballismus 528
Hemicolectomy 528
Hemiparesis 528
Hemiplegia 528
  form of Paralysis 769
  and types and causes of stroke 948
Hemochromatosis 528
  and disorders of the liver 646
  causing Pancreatitis 767;
    Pigmentation 795
  treatment of: Venesection 1044
Hemocyte 1105
Hemodialysis 528
  type of Dialysis 353
Hemoglobin 528
  abnormal: Sickle cell anemia

904; Thalassemia 977
  function of: Oxygen 761
  and Iron 606
Hemoglobinopathy 528
hemoglobin S:
  in Sickle cell anemia 904
Hemoglobinuria 529
Hemolysis 529
  causing Anemia, hemolytic 102;
    Hemoglobinuria 529
  example of Lysis 657
  in Spherocytosis, hereditary
    927
Hemolytic anemia:
  Anemia, hemolytic 102
Hemolytic disease of the
  newborn 43, 529
Hemolytic-uremic syndrome 529
Hemophilia 530
  and Factor VIII 435
  causing Hemarthrosis 527
  type of Bleeding disorder 178
hemophilia B:
  alternative term: Christmas
    disease 277
Hemoptysis 530
  common term: Coughing up
    blood 314
Hemorrhage 530
  common term: Bleeding 177
Hemorrhoidectomy 530
  removing hemorrhoids 531
Hemorrhoids 530
  causing Occult blood, fecal 739;
    Rectal bleeding 855
  and Pregnancy 813
  removal of: Hemorrhoidectomy
    531; removing hemorrhoids 531
  treatment of: Sclerotherapy 886;
    Suppository 956
Hemosiderosis 531
Hemospermia 531
  common term: Semen, blood in
    the 891
Hemostasis 531
Hemostatic drugs 531
Hemothorax 531
  and disorders of the lung 652
Heparin 531
  and Heart-lung machine 520
Hepatectomy, partial 532
Hepatectomy, total 532
Hepatic 532
hepatic encephalopathy:
  in Liver failure 647
  type of Encephalopathy 401
Hepatitis 532
  diagnosis of: Liver biopsy 645
  a disorder of the liver 646
  and Pancreatitis 767
  in Q fever 842
Hepatitis A:
  a disorder of the liver 646
  type of Hepatitis, viral 533
Hepatitis B:
  a disorder of the liver 646
  type of Hepatitis, viral 533
  and Liver cancer 647
Hepatitis, chronic active 532
hepatitis immunoglobulin:
  in treatment of Hepatitis, viral
    534
hepatitis non-A, non-B:
  type of hepatitis, viral 533

Hepatitis, viral 533
Hepatoma 534
  and Tumor-specific antigen
    1015
  type of Liver cancer 647
Hepatomegaly 534
herald patch:
  in Pityriasis rosea 798
Herbal medicine 534
Heredity 534
  and Inheritance 589
Heritability 534
Hermaphroditism 534
  and Sex determination 897
Hernia 534
  treatment of: Hernia repair 534,
    535; Truss 1013
  types of: main types of abdominal
    hernia 535; Hiatal hernia 537
Hernia repair 534, 535
Herniated disk:
  Disk prolapse 364
Herniorrhaphy 535
  alternative term: Hernia repair
    534
Heroin 535
  alternative term:
    Diacetylmorphine 351
  detoxification: Methadone 683
  Pregnancy, drugs in 815
Herpangina 536
Herpes 536
Herpes, genital 536
  causing Vulvitis 1066
Herpes gestationis 536
Herpes simplex 536
  causing Whitlow 1077
  and Infection, congenital 582
  as Opportunistic infection 746
  treatment of: Acyclovir 67;
    Idoxuridine 566; Trifluridine
    1010
Herpes zoster 537
  treatment of: Acyclovir 67
herpes zoster ophthalmicus:
  and Herpes zoster 537
herpetic whitlow 1077
  cause of: Herpes simplex 537
Hetacillin 1105
Heterosexuality 537
  Sexuality 898
Heterozygote 537
Hexachlorophene 1105
Hexadrol 1105
Hexocyclium 1105
hexosaminidase deficiency:
  causing Tay-Sachs disease 966
Hexylcaine 1105
Hexylresorcinol 1105
H-H-R 1105
Hiatal hernia 537
  causing Heartburn 516
  and Phrenic nerve 793
  treatment of: Plication 802
Hibiclens 1105
Hibistat 1105
Hiccup 538
  and Phrenic nerve 793
high blood pressure:
  medical term: Hypertension
    557
high-density lipoprotein (HDL):
  and Cholesterol 275; Fats and
    oils 442; Hyperlipidemias 553

Hip 538
and Pelvis 778
Hip, congenital dislocation of 538
treatment of: Osteotomy 757
and Walking 1067
hippocampus:
part of Limbic system 641
Hippocrates:
and Diagnosing disease 24;
Hippocratic oath 539;
Medicine 670
Hippocratic oath 539
in history of Medicine 670
Hip replacement 539
and Surgical implants 34
Hip, snapping 540
Hiprex 1105
Hirschsprung's disease 540
Hirsutism 540
Hispril 1105
Histabid 1105
Histadyl 1105
Histagesic 1105
Histalet 1105
Histamic 1105
Histamine 540
causing Allergy 86;
Inflammation 588; Rhinitis,
allergic 872; Urticaria 1030
production of: Mast cell 666
Histamine-2 receptor antagonists
540
histamine-blocking drugs:
types of: Antihistamine drugs
118; Histamine-2 receptor
antagonists 540; Ulcer-
healing drugs 1018
Histaspan 1105
Histex 1105
Histiocytosis X 540
Histocompatibility antigens 540
and Paternity testing 774
in Tissue-typing 990
Histologist 541
Histology 541
and Staining 938
using Microscope 686
Histopathology 541
and Pathology 775
using Microscope 686
Histoplasmosis 541
a Fungal infection 470
Historal 1105
Histor-D 1105
history, medical:
see index entry History-taking
History-taking 541
and Diagnosing disease 24;
Diagnosis 351; steps in
diagnosing a condition 352;
Examination, physical 424
Histosal 1105
HIV 541
causing AIDS 76; AIDS-related
complex 79; Encephalitis 401;
Infection, congenital 582
type of Virus 1052
Hives 541
medical term: Urticaria 1030
HLA-B27 tissue type:
and Reiter's syndrome 859
HLA:
see index entry human
leukocyte antigens

HMO:
Health Maintenance
Organization 511
HMS Liquifilm 1105
Hoarseness 543
causes of: Laryngitis 627;
Larynx, cancer of 628;
Thyroid cancer 984
symptom chart 542
Hodgkin's disease 543
type of Lymphoma 657
Hodgkin's lymphoma:
alternative term: Hodgkin's
disease 543
Hoffmann, Felix:
landmarks in drug development 32
Hole in the heart 544
medical term: Septal defect 894
Holistic medicine 544
Holter monitor 544
Homatropine 544
Homeopathy 544
Homeostasis 544
Homicebrin 1105
Homocystinuria 544
type of Metabolism, inborn
error of 682
homograft:
example: Corneal graft 308
use of: Grafting 496
Homosexuality, female:
Lesbianism 635
Homosexuality, male 544
Sexuality 898
Homozygote 545
and Genetic disorders 483
Homunculus 545
Hookworm infestation 545
and Roundworms 876
Hormonal disorders:
endocrine disorders 404
Hormonal methods of
contraception:
Contraception, hormonal
methods 305
hormonal system 546
see also index entry Endocrine
system
Hormone antagonist 545
Hormone replacement therapy
545
following Menopause 676
in Osteoporosis 756
using Medroxyprogesterone
671; Norethindrone 731;
Progesterone drugs 823
Hormones 547
abuse of: Sports, drugs and 935
constituent of: Peptide 782
measurement of: Immunoassay
575; Radioimmunoassay 847
and pregnancy: effects of
hormones during pregnancy 815
production of: Endocrine
system 402, 403; the hormonal
system 546
type of: Gastrointestinal
hormones 477
Horn, cutaneous 547
Horner's syndrome 547
in Klumpke's syndrome 621
Hornet sting:
Insect stings 592
Horseshoe kidney 547

a disorder of the kidney 618
Hospice 547
and Dying, care of the 381
Hospitals, types of 547
Hot flushes 547
and Menopause 676
Housemaid's knee 547
medical term: Bursitis 221
HPV16 (virus):
associated with Cervix, cancer
of 255
HSV1 (virus):
type of Herpes simplex 536
HSV2 (virus):
type of Herpes simplex 536
HTLV III (virus) 547
modern term: HIV 541
Human chorionic gonadotropin
(HCG):
Gonadotropin, human
chorionic 494
human growth hormone:
manufacture of: Genetically
engineered drugs 37
human immunodeficiency virus
(HIV):
see index entry HIV
human leukocyte antigens
(HLAs):
group of Histocompatibility
antigens 540
in Tissue-typing 990
Human potential 46-48
human T-cell lymphotropic virus,
strain III:
HTLV III 547
Humerus 547
location of the humerus 548
part of Skeleton 909
and Shoulder 902
Humerus, fracture of 548
humidifier:
use of: Croup 321; Ventilator
1045
Humors 548
Humorsal 1105
Hump back:
medical term: Kyphosis 623
Humulin 1105
Hunch back:
medical term: Kyphosis 623
Hunger 548
and Appetite 127
Hunter's syndrome:
type of Mucopolysaccharidosis
700
Huntington's chorea 548
and GABA 472
Hurler's syndrome 548
type of Metabolism, inborn
error of 682;
Mucopolysaccharidosis 700
Hurricane 1105
Hutchinson-Gilford syndrome:
form of Progeria 822
Hyaluronidase 1105
Hycanthone 1105
Hycodan 1105
Hycodaphen 1105
Hycomine 1105
Hycotuss 1105
Hydatid disease 548
hydatid disease cycle 549
treatment of: Mebendazole 669

Hydatidiform mole 549
form of Trophoblastic tumor
1012
leading to Choriocarcinoma 276
a disorder of the uterus 1031
Hydeltrasol 1105
Hydeltra-T.B.A. 1105
Hydoril 1105
Hydralazine 549
a Sympatholytic drug 959
Hydramnios 549
Hydrea 1105
Hydrocele 550
and Testis 972; Testis, swollen
973
Hydrocephalus 550
diagnosis of: Ultrasound
scanning 1020
and Spina bifida 928
treatment of: Neurosurgery 725
Hydrocet 1105
Hydrochloric acid 550
production of: Stomach 943
Hydrochlorothiazide 550
Hydrocil 1105
Hydrocodone 1105
Hydrocort 1105
Hydrocortisone 550
Hydrocortone 1105
HydroDIURIL 1105
Hydroflumethiazide 1105
hydrogen:
Ion 605
Hydrogen peroxide 550
in treatment of Vincent's
disease 1049
Hydromal 1105
Hydromorphone 1105
Hydromox 1105
Hydronephrosis 550
diagnosis of: Ultrasound
scanning 1020
and Kidney cancer 617
Hydrophobia 551
alternative term: Rabies 843
Hydropres 1105
Hydroprin 1105
Hydrops 551
Hydroquinone 1105
Hydroserpine 1105
Hydrotensin-50 1105
Hydrotherapy 551
in Physical therapy 793
Hydroxocobalamin 551
Hydroxychloroquine 1105
Hydroxyprogesterone 551
Hydroxyurea 1105
Hydroxyzine 551
Hygiene 551
and Infection 581
Hygiene, oral:
Oral hygiene 748
Hygienist, dental 551
Hygroma, cystic 551
type of Lymphangioma 654
Hygroton 1105
Hymen 551
imperforate: Vagina 1034
Hyoid 551
Hyoscyamine 552
Hyper- 552
Hyperacidity 552
Hyperactivity 552
and Food additives 461

treatment of: Pemoline 778;
Stimulant drugs 942
Hyperacusis 552
Hyperaldosteronism 552
alternative term: Aldosteronism 85
Hyperalimentation 552
Hyperbaric oxygen treatment 552
Oxygen 761
Hyperbilirubinemia 552
Hypercalcemia 552
abnormally high blood level of Calcium 224
and Rickets 874
Hypercapnia 553
Hyperemesis 553
excessive Vomiting 1062
hyperemesis gravidarum:
common term: Vomiting in pregnancy 1066
Hyperetic 1105
Hyperglycemia 553
abnormally high blood level of Glucose 492
symptom of Diabetes mellitus 349
treatment of: Insulin 594
Hypergonadism 553
Hyperhidrosis 553
hyperkalemia:
abnormally high blood level of Potassium 812
Hyperkeratosis 553
Hyperkinetic syndrome 553
alternative term: Hyperactivity 552
Hyperlipidemias 553
types of hyperlipidemia 554
treatment of: Lipid-lowering drugs 642
Hypermetropia:
Hyperopia 554
Hypernephroma 554
type of Kidney cancer 617
Hyperopia 554
treatment of: why glasses are used 489
Hyperparathyroidism 554, 555
cause of: Parathyroid tumor 771
Hyperplasia 555
Hyperplasia, gingival 555
Hyperpyrexia 555
Hypersensitivity 555
to Contact lenses 302
reactions: Immune system 571
Hypersplenism 557
Hyperstat 1105
Hypertension 556, 557
cause of: Pheochromocytoma 791
and disorders of the kidney 618;
Peripheral vascular disease 784; Polycythemia 807
treatment of: Amiloride 94;
Hydrochlorothiazide 550;
Labetolol 624; Methyldopa 684; Minoxidil 689; Nadolol 714;
Nephrectomy 718; Nifedipine 727; Pindolol 795; Propranolol 824; Prazosin 812; Relaxation techniques 859
hypertensive retinopathy:
a disorder of the retina 867

Hyperthermia 557
Hyperthermia, malignant 557
Hyperthyroidism 557
and Pituitary tumors 798;
disorders of the thyroid gland 986
symptoms and signs of hyperthyroidism 558
treatment of: Methimazole 683:
Nadolol 714; Propranolol 824;
Propylthiouracil 824
Hypertonia 558
Hypertrichosis 558
Hypertrophy 558
of heart muscle: Cardiomegaly 235
Hyperuricemia 558
abnormally high blood level of Uric acid 1025
Hyperventilation 558
causing Tetany 975
in Panic attack 768
treatment of: Relaxation techniques 859
hypervitaminosis A:
excess of Vitamin A 1057
Hyphema 559
cause of: Eye injuries 432
causing Vision, loss of 1054
Hypnosis 559
and Freudian theory 468;
Trance 1003
Hypnotic drugs 559
alternative term: Sleeping drugs 916
Hypo- 559
Hypoaldosteronism 559
hypocalcemia:
causing disorders of muscle 705
abnormally low blood level of Calcium 224
Hypochondriasis 559
hypodermic syringe:
Syringe 962
hypogammaglobulinemia:
and Immunodeficiency disorders 575
Hypoglossal nerve 560
functions of cranial neves 318
Hypoglycemia 560
abnormally low blood level of Glucose 492
cause of: Insulin 594
feature of Prematurity 817
Hypoglycemics, oral 560
examples: Tolazamide 994;
Tolbutamide 994
Hypogonadism 560
treatment of: Progesterone drugs 823
Hypohidrosis 560
hypokalemia:
abnormally low blood level of Potassium 812
causing disorders of muscle 705
Hypomania 560
form of Mania 663
Hypoparathyroidism 560
Hypophysectomy 561
Hypoplasia 561
Hypoplasia, enamel 561
Hypoplastic left heart syndrome 561
type of Heart disease,

congenital 519
Hypospadias 561
abnormality of Penis 780
treatment of: Plastic surgery 801
Hypotension 561
Hypothalamus 562
and Pituitary gland 796; control of Temperature 968; Thirst 979
Hypothermia 562
first aid: hypothermia 563
Hypothermia, surgical 563
use of: Open heart surgery 744
Hypothyroidism 563
causing Myxedema 713
and Hyperlipidemias 553;
Iodine 605; Pallor 765;
disorders of the thyroid gland 986
in the Newborn 726
Hypotonia 564
Hypotonia in infants 564
Hypovolemia 564
Hypoxia 564
Hysterectomy 565
performing a hysterectomy 564
and Oophorectomy 743
in treatment of Fibroid 453;
Hydatidiform mole 549;
Menorrhagia 677; Uterus, cancer of 1032
Hysteria 565
and Faith healing 438
hysterical amnesia:
and Dissociative disorders 366
Hysterosalpingography 565
in diagnosis of disorders of the uterus 1031
in investigating infertility 587
hysteroscope:
use of: Sterilization, female 940
Hysterotomy 565
Hytakerol 1105
Hytinic 1105
Hytone 1105

I

Iatrogenic 566
Iberet 1105
Iberol 1105
Ibuprofen 566
type of Nonsteroidal anti-inflammatory drug 730
Ice packs 566
in treatment of Sprain 936
Ichthyosis 566
Icterus 566
alternative term: Jaundice 610
Id 566
and Freudian theory 468;
Psychoanalytic theory 831
in relation to Ego 392; Superego 955
identical twins:
type of Twins 1016
Idiocy 566
Idiopathic 566
IDL:
see index entry intermediate-

density lipoprotein
Idoxuridine 566
ileal conduit:
use of: Urinary diversion 1025;
urinary diversion using ileal conduit 1026
Ileostomy 566
procedure for ileostomy 567
in treatment of Polyposis coli 808
Iletin 1096
Ileum 568
part of Intestine 601
surgical opening into:
Ileostomy 566
Ileus, paralytic 568
ilium:
part of Pelvis 778
Illness 568
Illusion 568
Ilosone 1105
Ilotycin 1105
Ilozyme 1105
Imaging techniques 568
imaging the body 569
and Modern diagnostic techniques 26-29
Scanning techniques 882
Imferon 1105
Imipenem/cilastatin 1105
Imipramine 570
Immersion foot 570
Immobility 570
causing Constipation 300;
Osteoporosis 756
leading to Pulmonary embolism 836; Thrombosis, deep vein 981
Immobilization 570
immune complexes:
causing Glomerulonephritis 491; Hypersensitivity 557;
Serum sickness 896;
Vasculitis 1040
formation of: Viruses 1052
removal of: Plasmapheresis 800
immune globulin:
alternative term: Immune serum globulin 570
Immune response 570
and Sensitization 893
Immune serum globulin 570
Immune system 571
function of Antibody 115;
Blood cells 183;
Immunoglobulins 575;
Interferon 598; Lymphocyte 655; Phagocyte 789; Thymus 893
parts of: the adaptive immune system 573; the innate immune system 572
Immunity 571
Immunization 23, 571
typical childhood immunization schedule 574
Travel immunization 1007
types of: types of immunization 574; Vaccination 1034
using Immune serum globulin 570; Vaccine 36, 1034
Immunoassay 575
and Serology 895

immunocomplexes:
see index entry immune complexes

Immunodeficiency disorders 575
leading to AIDS 76; Nocardiosis 729; Opportunistic infections 746

Immunoglobulins 575
alternative term: Antibodies 115
function of: Immune system 571; *the adaptive immune system 573*
production of: Lymphocyte 657
types of Plasma proteins 801

Immunologist 576
Immunology 576
Immunostimulant drugs 576
Immunosuppressant drugs 576
example: Cyclosporin 326
leading to Fungal infections 470; Opportunistic infections 746
in treatment of Autoimmune disorders 147; Cardiomyopathy 236
uses of: Heart transplant 523; Transplant surgery 1005

immunosuppression:
and Immune system 571
see also index entry Immunosuppressant drugs

Immunotherapy 576
Imodium 1105
Impaction, dental 576
and Eruption of teeth 416
*impacted wisdom teeth 577*

impedance audiometry:
*types of hearing test 513*

imperforate anus:
Anus, imperforate 122

imperforate hymen:
Hymen 551

Impetigo 577
*the appearance of impetigo 578*

Implant 578
*types of implants 577*

Implantation, egg 578
and *the developing embryo 398;* Pregnancy 813

Impotence 578
causes of: Cystectomy 327; Heroin 536; Neuropathy 725; Prolactinoma 823; Shy-Drager syndrome 904
causing Infertility 586
and Penis 780
treatment of: Penile implant 779; Sensate focus technique 892; Sex therapy 898
type of Psychosexual dysfunction 832

Impression, dental 578
use of: Denture 343

Impulse control disorders 578
Imuran 1105
Inapsine 1105
Incest 579
causing Sexual desire, inhibited 898
and Child abuse 263; Rape 849

Incidence 579
*incidence of relatively short-lived conditions in the US 578*

and Prevalence 820
Incision 579
Incisor 579
*structure and arrangement of teeth 967*

Incompetent cervix:
Cervical incompetence 252

Incontinence, fecal 579
cause of: Fecal impaction 442
treatment of: Sphincter, artificial 927
see also index entry Diarrhea

Incontinence, urinary 579
causes of: Irritable bladder 606; Multiple sclerosis 701; Neuropathy 725; Prostate, enlarged 825; abnormality of Ureter 1023
treatment of: Sphincter, artificial 927

Incoordination 580
feature of Ataxia 139

Incremin with Iron 1105
Incubation period 580
of *some important infectious diseases 583-585*

Incubator 39, 580
for the Newborn 726
in treatment of Prematurity 817

incus:
bone in Ear 384
example of Ossicle 752

Indapamide 1105
Inderal 1105
Inderal LA 1105
Inderide 1105
Indian medicine 580
Indigestion 580
Indocin 1105
Indomethacin 581
Indoramin 1105
Induction of labor 581
uses of: Childbirth, complications of 265; Postmaturity 810

Industrial diseases:
Occupational disease and injury 739

Infant 581
Newborn 726

Infantile spasms 581
Infant mortality 581
Infarction 581
example: Myocardial infarction 710

Infection 581
types of: Food-borne infection 461; Infection, congenital 582
see also index entry Infectious disease

Infection, congenital 582
Infectious disease 582
causes of: Bacteria 153; Fungi 470; Protozoa 827; Rickettsia 874; Viruses 1050; *viruses and disease 1051*
immunity against: Immunity 571
prevention of: Immunization 571; Quarantine 842; Vaccination 1034; Vaccine 1034
transmission of: Cats, diseases from 243; Dogs, diseases

from 369; Food-borne infection 461; *infected animal products 462;* Insects and disease 593; Rabies 843; Rats, diseases from 853; Transmissible 1005; Vector 1041; Zoonosis 1008
type of Health hazard 511; Occupational disease and injury 739
types of: Chlamydial infections 270; Fungal infections 470; Infection, congenital 582; *some important infectious diseases 583-585;* Reportable diseases 861; Sexually transmitted diseases 898

infectious hepatitis:
Hepatitis, viral 533

Infectious mononucleosis:
Mononucleosis, infectious 693

Inferiority complex 586
Infertility 586
causes of: Fibroid 453; Gonorrhea 495; Pelvic inflammatory disease 777; Prolactinoma 823; Puerperal sepsis 836; Testis, undescended 974
following Abortion, elective 58
*investigating infertility 587*
treatment of: Artificial insemination 133; Clomiphene 284; Gonadotropin, human chorionic 494; In vitro fertilization 604; Tamoxifen 963

Infestation 586
Infiltrate 586
Inflamase 1105
Inflammation 588
and *the innate immune system 572*

Inflammatory bowel disease 588
Influenza 588
Informed consent 588
Consent 298

Infrared 588
and Thermography 978

Infusion, intravenous:
Intravenous infusion 603

Ingestion 588
Ingrown toenail 589
Inguinal 589
INH 1105
Inhalation 589
Breathing 209
of medication: Inhaler 589; Vaporizer 1038

Inhaler 589
in treatment of Asthma 139

Inheritance 589
*inheritance of eye color 590*
and Intelligence 594
see also index entries Chromosomes; Gene

Inhibition 590
Injection 591
Injury 591
Ink blot test 591
type of: Rorschach test 876

Inlay, dental 591
and Restoration, dental 866

innominate bone:

part of Pelvis 778
Innovar 1105
Inocor 1105
Inoculation 591
Inoperable 591
Inorganic 591
Inosiplex 1105
Inpatient treatment 591
Insanity 591
former term: Lunacy 650

Insect bites 591
and *insect-borne diseases 592;* Insects and disease 591

insecticide:
type of Pesticide 788

Insects and disease 591
*insect-borne diseases 592*
and Tropical diseases 1012

Insect stings 592
*first aid: insect stings and bites 593*

Insecurity 592
insemination, artificial:
Artificial insemination 133

Insight 592
In situ 593
Insomnia 593
treatment of: Lorazepam 649; Pentobarbital 780; Sleeping drugs 916; Temazepam 968; Triazolam 1009

Instinct 593
Institutionalization 594
Insulin 594
administration of: Pump, insulin 838
production of: Genetically engineered drugs 37; Pancreas 766; Recombinant DNA 854
in treatment of Diabetes mellitus 349; Hypoglycemia 560

insulin coma therapy:
type of Shock therapy 902

insulin-dependent diabetes:
type of Diabetes mellitus 349

Insulinoma 594
treatment of: Pancreatectomy 767

insulin pump:
Pump, insulin 838

Intal 1105
Intelligence 594
assessment of: Intelligence tests 595
and Child development 267; Personality 786

intelligence quotient:
and Intelligence 594
measurement of: Intelligence tests 595

Intelligence tests 595
and Intelligence 594; Psychology 832
type of Psychometry 832

Intensive care 38, 595
of Newborn 726

Inter- 596
interactions, drug:
Drug 377

Intercostal 596
Intercourse, painful 596
leading to Orgasm, lack of 750

*symptom chart (men) 596*
*symptom chart (women) 597*
type of Psychosexual
dysfunction 832
Interferon 598
*how interferon fights viral
infections 599*
production of: Immune system
571; Viruses 1052
in treatment of Cold, common
287
intermediate-density lipoprotein
(IDL):
and Hyperlipidemias 553; *types
of hyperlipidemia 554*
intermittent claudication:
see index entry Claudication
Intern 599
interneuron:
*structure of a neuron 724*
in Spinal cord 929
type of Neuron 723
Internist 599
Intersex 599
and Transsexualism 1006
type of: Testicular feminization
syndrome 971
interstitial fluid:
alternative term: Tissue fluid
989
Interstitial pulmonary fibrosis 599
causing Pulmonary
hypertension 837
Interstitial radiation therapy 599
type of Radiation therapy 846
Intertrigo 601
Intestinal imaging:
Barium X-ray examinations 158
Intestinal lipodystrophy:
alternative term: Whipple's
disease 1077
Intestine 601
disorders of: Abdominal pain
50; *disorders of the anus 121;*
Colic, infantile 288;
Flatulence 458; Intestine,
cancer of 601; *disorders of the
intestine 600;* Intestine,
obstruction of 602; Intestine,
tumors of 602; Rectum,
cancer of 856
function of: *the digestive process
360;* Peristalsis 785
imaging of: Barium X-ray
examinations 158
part of Digestive system 359
parts of: Anus 121; Appendix
127; Cecum 244; *location of
cecum 245;* Colon 290;
Duodenum 380; Ileum 568;
Jejunum 611; Rectum 856
surgical joining of:
Anastomosis 99
Intestine, cancer of 601
type of: Rectum, cancer of 856
Intestine, obstruction of 602
causes of: Intestine, cancer of
601; Intussusception 604;
Rectum, cancer of 856:
Volvulus 1062
causing Abdominal swelling 55;
Vomiting 1065
Intestine, tumors of 602
see also index entry Intestine,

cancer of
Intoxication 602
Intra- 602
Intracavitary therapy 602
type of Radiation therapy 846
Intracerebral hemorrhage 602
Intractable 603
Intramuscular 603
Intraocular pressure 603
Intrauterine contraceptive device:
see index entry IUD
Intrauterine growth retardation
603
Intravenous 603
drug abuse: Drug dependence
378
see also index entry
Intravenous infusion
Intravenous infusion 603
uses of: Feeding, artificial 443;
Rehydration therapy 859
Intravenous pyelography:
type of Pyelography 840
intrinsic factor:
absence of: Anemia,
megaloblastic 103; *disorders of
the stomach 943*
production of: Stomach 943
Introitus 603
Intron A 1106
Intropin 1106
Introvert 603
and Jungian theory 613
Intubation 603
Intussusception 604
cause of: Peutz-Jeghers
syndrome 788
causing Intestine, obstruction
of 602
Invasive 604
In vitro 604
In vitro fertilization (IVF) 604
and Surrogacy 957
in treatment of Infertility 41,
586
In vivo 605
Involuntary movements 605
involuntary muscle:
type of Muscle 706
Iodine 605
deficiency of: Goiter 494
dietary: *minerals and main food
sources 690; recommended daily
dietary allowances (RDA) of
selected minerals 19*
radioactive: Radiation 844
sensitivity to: Pyelography 840
in treatment of Thyroid cancer
984
Iodo 1106
Iodochlorhydroxyquin 1106
Iodoquinol 1106
Ion 605
production of: Radiation 844
Ionamin 1106
Ionax 1106
Ionil 1106
ionizing radiation:
type of Radiation 844
*radiation units 845*
Iopanoic 1106
Ipecac 606
Ipodate 1106
Ipratropium 606

Ipsatol 1106
IQ 606
and Intelligence 594
measurement of: Intelligence
tests 595
Iridectomy 606
Iridencleisis 606
Iridocyclitis 606
Iris 606
disorders of: *disorders of the eye
431;* Eye injuries 432;
Rheumatoid arthritis,
juvenile 871; Uveitis 1033
part of Eye 429; Uvea 1033
and Pupil 838
tearing of: Eye injuries 432
Iritis 606
type of Uveitis 1033
Iromin-G 1106
Iron 606
deficiency of: Anemia, iron-
deficiency 102
dietary: *minerals and main food
sources 690; recommended daily
dietary allowances (RDA) of
selected minerals 19*
excess of: Blood transfusion
190; Hemochromatosis 528;
Hemosiderosis 531; Siderosis
905
and Melena 673
Iron-deficiency anemia:
Anemia, iron-deficiency 102
Irradiation:
Radiation hazards 845
uses of: Radiation therapy 846;
Sterilization 939
Irrigation, wound 606
*irrigation techniques 607*
Irritable bladder 606
causing Incontinence, urinary
580
a *disorder of the bladder 177*
treatment of: Hyoscyamine 552
Irritable bowel syndrome 607
causing Abdominal pain 50;
Constipation 300; Diarrhea
356
a *disorder of the intestine 600*
treatment of: Fiber, dietary 452;
Hyoscyamine 552; Methyl-
cellulose 684; Propantheline
824; Psyllium 834
Ischemia 607
and Transient ischemic attack
1005
ischium:
part of Pelvis 778
islets of Langerhans:
part of Pancreas 765
Ismelin 1106
Iso-Bid 1106
Isocarboxazid 607
Isoclor 1106
Isoetharine 1106
Isofluorophate 1106
Isoflurane 1106
Isolation 608
and Quarantine 842
Isoniazid 608
causing Hepatitis, chronic
active 532
in treatment of Tuberculosis
1014

Isopropamide 1106
Isoproterenol 608
Isoptin 1106
Isopto Carbachol 1106
Isopto Carpine 1106
Isopto Cetamide 1106
Isopto P-ES 1106
Isordil 1106
Isordil Sublingual 1106
Isordil Tembids 1106
Isosorbide dinitrate 608
Isotope scanning:
Radionuclide scanning 27, 848
Isotretinoin 608
Isoxsuprine 608
Isuprel 1106
Itching 608
medical term: Pruritus 828
treatment of: Calamine 223;
Trimeprazine 1011
-itis 609
IUCD:
see index entry IUD
IUD 609
and *failure rates of contraceptives
304*
use of: Contraception 302;
*methods of contraception 303*
IVF:
see index entry In vitro
fertilization
IVP 609
type of Pyelography 840

# J

Jakob-Creutzfeldt disease:
Creutzfeldt-Jakob syndrome
319
Janimine 1106
Jaundice 610
causes of: Cholangiocarcinoma
272; Cholangitis 272;
Cholecystitis 273; Cholestasis
274; Cirrhosis 282;
Leptospirosis 635;
Metabolism, inborn errors of
682; Spherocytosis,
hereditary 927; Yellow fever
1086
causing Urine, abnormal 1029
in infants: Hemolytic disease of
the newborn 539; Newborn
727; Prematurity 817
and Pigmentation 795
treatment of: Phototherapy 793
Jaw 610
deformities of: Prognathism
823; Receding chin 854
deformities, treatment of:
Orthognathic surgery 752
disorders of: Burkitt's
lymphoma 219; Jaw,
dislocated 610; Jaw, fractured
610; Temporomandibular
joint syndrome 969
and Malocclusion 661
upper jaw: Maxilla 668
see also index entry jaw
muscles
Jaw, dislocated 610
Jaw, fractured 610

Jaw, fractured (continued)
    treatment of: Wiring of the
        jaws 1078
jaw muscles:
    anatomy of: *location of the
        temporomandibular joint 969*
    involuntary contraction of:
        Trismus 1011
Jealousy, morbid 611
Jejunal biopsy 611
    in diagnosis of Malabsorption
        659
Jejunum 611
    part of Intestine 601
Jellyfish stings 611
Jenamicin 1106
Jenner, Edward:
    *landmarks in drug development 32*
    history of Medicine 670
Jet lag 611
Jigger flea:
    Chigoe 262
Jock itch:
    Tinea 988
Joggers' nipple 613
jogging:
    causing Joggers' Nipple 613;
        Running injuries 877
Joint 613
    disorders of: Dislocation, joint
        364; Effusion, joint 392;
        Ehlers-Danlos syndrome 392;
        Gout 495, *496*; Neuropathic
        joint 723; Osteoarthritis 753;
        Osteochondritis dessicans
        753; Rheumatic fever 869;
        Rheumatoid arthritis 870;
        Subluxation 951
    examination of: Arthroscopy
        133
    examples: Ankle joint 111;
        Elbow 393; Hip 538; Knee
        621; Shoulder 902; *structure of
        the shoulder 903*; Suture 957;
        Wrist 1082
    false: Pseudarthrosis 828
    in Finger 455; Jaw 610; Skull
        914; Spine 932; Toe 933
    fusion of: Arthrodesis 132
    *types of joints 612*
    and *movement 698*
Joint replacement:
    medical term: Arthroplasty 133
    types of: Finger joint
        replacement 456; Hip
        replacement 539; Knee joint
        replacement 622
Joule 613
Jugular vein 613
    part of *circulatory system 281*
    and Vena cava 1043
Jumpers' knee 613
Jungian theory 613
Junk food 613
Juvenile arthritis:
    Rheumatoid arthritis, juvenile
        871

# K

Kabikinase 1106
Kahlenberg solution 1106

Kala-azar 614
    type of Leishmaniasis 633
Kanamycin 1106
Kantrex 1106
Kaochlor 1106
Kaolin 614
    use of: Poultice 812
Kaon 1106
Kaopectate 1106
Kaposi's sarcoma 614
    feature of AIDS 76
Karaya gum 1106
karyotype analysis:
    following Amniocentesis and
        chorionic villus sampling
        42
Kasof 1106
Kato 1106
Kawasaki disease 614
Kay Ciel 1106
Keflex 1106
Keflin 1106
Kefzol 1106
Keloid 614
    type of Scar 882
    *a disorder of the skin 910*
Kemadrin 1106
Kenacort 1106
Kenalog 1106
Keralyt 1106
Keratin 614
    as constituent of Hair 503;
        Nail 714; Skin 909
    constituent of: Sulfur 954
Keratitis 614
    causing Eye, painful red 433
    *a disorder of the cornea 308*
Keratoacanthoma 614
    type of Skin tumor 913
Keratoconjunctivitis 614
Keratoconjunctivitis sicca 615
    *a disorder of the cornea 308*
Keratoconus 615
    *a disorder of the cornea 308*
Keratolytic drugs 615
Keratomalacia 615
    *a disorder of the cornea 308;
        disorder of the eye 431*
Keratopathy 615
    *disorders of the cornea 308*
Keratoplasty:
    Corneal graft 308
Keratosis 615
    leading to Skin tumors 913
    treatment of: Fluorouracil 460
Keratosis pilaris 615
Keratotomy, radial 615
Kerion 616
Kernicterus 616
Ketamine 1106
ketoacidosis:
    causing Vomiting 1065
    type of Acidosis 63
Ketoconazole 616
ketones:
    excess of: Ketosis 616
Ketoprofen 616
Ketosis 616
    treatment of: Insulin 594
Ketrax 1106
Kidney 616
    disorders of:
        Glomerulosclerosis 491;
        *disorders of the kidney 618;*

Nephrocalcinosis 718;
    Nephrosclerosis 718
    drainage of: Nephrostomy 719
    function of: Acid-base balance
        63; *the function of the kidney
        617*; Urine 1027; Water 1070
    investigation of: Kidney
        function tests 619; Kidney
        imaging 619; Renal biopsy
        860
    part of Urinary tract 1025; *the
        urinary system 1028*
    part of: Nephron 718
    removal of: Nephrectomy 718
    study of: Nephrology 718
kidney, artificial:
    Dialysis 352; *procedure for
        dialysis 353*
Kidney cancer 617
    type of: Wilms' tumor 1078
Kidney cyst 618
    diagnosis of: Ultrasound
        scanning 1020
Kidney failure:
    alternative term: Renal failure
        860
Kidney function tests 619
Kidney imaging 619
Kidney, polycystic 619
Kidney stone:
    Calculus, urinary tract 224
Kidney transplant 619
    *procedure for a kidney transplant
        620*
    in treatment of Renal failure
        861
    type of Transplant surgery 1005
Kidney tumors 619
    diagnosis of: Ultrasound
        scanning 1020
Kie Syrup 1106
killer cell:
    and Histocompatibility
        antigens 541; Interferon 598
    part of Immune system 571; *the
        adaptive immune system 573*
    type of Lymphocyte 657
Kilocalorie 621
    and Calorie 226; Joule 613
Kilojoule 621
    and Joule 613
Kinesed 1106
kissing:
    and Sexual intercourse 898
    in spread of AIDS 78;
        Mononucleosis, infectious
        693; Syphilis 961
kiss of life:
    alternative term: Artificial
        respiration 134
Klebcil 1106
Kleer compound 1106
Kleptomania 621
Klinefelter's syndrome 621
Klonopin 1106
K-Lor 1106
Klor-con 1106
Klorvess 1106
Klotrix 1106
Klumpke's paralysis 621
K-Lyte 1106
Knee 621
    disorders of: Chondromalacia
        patellae 275; *location of knee*

joint effusion 392; Jumpers'
        knee 613; Knock-knee 622;
        Lyme disease 654
    *simple knee-jerk reflex 857*
    part of Skeleton 909; *bones of the
        skeleton 908*
    parts of: Cruciate ligaments
        321; Meniscus 676; Patella
        774
    surgery on: Meniscectomy 676
    see also index entry Joint
kneecap:
    medical term: Patella 774
Knee joint replacement 622
Knock-knee 622
    example of Valgus 1037
    and Walking 1067
Knuckle 623
    and Metacarpal bone 682
Koch, Robert:
    and Diagnosing disease 24;
        Microbiology 685
Koilonychia 623
Kolantyl 1106
Kolyum 1106
Komed 1106
Konakion 1106
Kondremul Plain 1106
Konsyl 1106
Koplik's spots 623
Koromex 1106
Korsakoff's psychosis:
    Wernicke-Korsakoff syndrome
        1076
K-Phos 1106
Krabbe's disease:
    type of Leukodystrophy 637
Kraurosis vulvae:
    type of Vulvitis 1066
Kretschmer, Ernst:
    and Somatotype 923
Kronofed 1106
Kronohist 1106
K-Tab 1106
Kudrox 1106
Kuru 623
    type of Slow virus disease 918
KU Zyme 1106
Kwashiorkor 623
Kwell 1106
Kwildane 1106
KY Jelly 1106
Kyphoscoliosis 623
Kyphosis 623
    *a disorder of the spine 933*

# L

Labetolol 624
Labia 624
    enlargement of:
        Pseudohermaphroditism 829
LaBID 1106
Labile 624
Labor:
    see index entry Childbirth
labyrinth:
    inflammation of: Labyrinthitis
        624
    part of Ear 384
Labyrinthitis 624
    symptoms of: Vertigo 1048;

Vomiting 1065
Laceration 624
　type of Wound 1081
Lac-Hydrin 1106
Lacril 1106
Lacrimal apparatus 624
　*functions of the lacrimal apparatus*
　*625*
lacrimal glands:
　part of Lacrimal apparatus 624
Lacrisert 1106
Lactase deficiency 624
　causing Food intolerance 463;
　　Lactose intolerance 625
Lactation 625
　and Breast-feeding 207
　suppression of: Bromocriptine
　　213
lacteals:
　part of Lymphatic system 655
Lactic acid 625
　causing Cramp 318
Lactocal-F 1106
Lactose 625
Lactose intolerance 625
　cause of: Lactase deficiency 624
　causing Diarrhea 356
Lactulose 625
Lamaze method:
　use of: Prepared childbirth 819
Lambliasis 625
　alternative term: Giardiasis 486
Laminectomy 625
Lanacort 1106
Lance 626
Lancet 626
Landsteiner, Karl:
　*landmarks in surgery 33*
language:
　and Speech 925; Speech
　　disorders 926; Speech
　　therapy 926
Laniazid 1106
Lanolin 626
　in treatment of Chapped skin
　　258
Lanorinal 1106
Lanoxicaps 1106
Lanoxin 1106
Lanugo hair 626
Laparoscopy 626
　in diagnosis of Abdominal pain
　　55; Ovary, cancer of 760;
　　Salpingitis 880
　uses of: *investigating infertility*
　　*587; sterilization, female 940*
Laparotomy, exploratory 626
　in diagnosis of Abdominal pain
　　50; Peritonitis 785
large cell carcinoma:
　type of Lung cancer 651
large intestine:
　see index entries Colon;
　　Intestine
Larobec 1106
Larodopa 1106
Larotid 1106
Larva migrans 626
　causing Toxocariasis 1000
Larylgan 1106
Laryngeal nerve 626
　*location of laryngeal nerves 627*
Laryngectomy 627
Laryngitis 627

causing Hoarseness 543
laryngomalacia:
　causing Stridor 947
　a *disorder of the larynx 629*
laryngopharynx:
　part of Pharynx 789
Laryngoscopy 627
　in diagnosis of Hoarseness 543
　*procedure for laryngoscopy 628*
　in treatment of Choking 272
　use of: Intubation 603
Laryngotracheobronchitis 627
　feature of: Tracheitis 1001
Larynx 627
　edema of: Pharyngitis 789
　*disorders of the larynx 629*
　*location of larynx 628*
　narrowed: Stridor 947
　removal of: Laryngectomy 627
Larynx, cancer of 628
　causing Hoarseness 543
Lasan 1106
Laser 629
Laser surgery 35
Laser treatment 629
　uses of: Cervicitis 254; Cervix,
　　cancer of 256; Glaucoma 490;
　　Heart surgery 522; Laser
　　surgery 35; *use of a laser 630;*
　　Retinal detachment 868;
　　Tattooing 966
Lasix 1106
Lassa fever 629
　Other new diseases 45
Lassitude 630
　feature of Sleeping sickness 917
　Tiredness 989
Lateral 630
Laudanum 630
Laughing gas 630
Laurence-Moon-Biedl syndrome
　630
LAV 630
　modern term: HIV 541
Lavage, gastric 630
Laxative drugs 630
　examples: Lactulose 625;
　　Methylcellulose 684; Psyllium
　　834
Lazy eye 631
$LD_{50}$ 631
LDL:
　see index entry low-density
　　lipoprotein
Lead poisoning 631
　causing Neuropathy 724
Learning 631
Learning disabilities 632
Ledercillin VK 1106
Leech 632
Leeuwenhoek, Antonj van:
　development of Microscope 685
　history of Medicine 670
　*landmarks in diagnosis 25*
left-handedness:
　and Stuttering 950
　type of Handedness 506
leg:
　bones of: Femur 445; Fibula
　　453; *location of the fibula 454;*
　　Tibia 987
　disorders of: Bow leg 198;
　　Femur, fracture of 445; Leg,
　　shortening of 633; Paraplegia

770; Restless legs 866; Shin
　splints 901
joints of: Ankle joint 111; Hip
　538; Knee 621
muscles of: Calf muscles 226;
　Quadriceps muscle 842
see also index entry Foot
leg, artificial:
　type of Limb, artificial 640
Leg, broken:
　Femur, fracture of 445
　Fibula 454
　Tibia 987
Legionnaires' disease 45, 632
Leg, shortening of 633
Leg ulcer 633
　treatment of: Calamine 223
Leiomyoma 633
Leishmaniasis 633
　causes of: Protozoa 828; Sand-
　　fly bites 881
Lens 633
　disorders of: Cataract 240; Lens
　　dislocation 634
　*location of the lens 634*
　part of Eye 429
　removal of: Cataract surgery
　　240; *procedure for cataract*
　　*surgery 241*
　see also index entries Contact
　　lenses; Glasses
Lens dislocation 634
　causing Double vision 371
　feature of Marfan's syndrome
　　664
Lens implant 634
　in Cataract surgery 240
Lente 1106
Lentigo 634
　type of Nevus 726
Leprechaunism 634
Leprosy 634
　treatment of: Dapsone 333;
　　Rifampin 874
Leptospirosis 635
　and Rats, diseases from 853;
　　Waterborne infection 1071
Lesbianism 635
Lesion 635
Lethargy 635
　Tiredness 989
Leucovorin 1106
Leukemia 635, *636*
　and Radiation hazards 846;
　　Strontium 949
　treatment of: Anticancer drugs
　　115; Bone marrow transplant
　　195; *performing a bone marrow*
　　*transplant 196;*
　　Mercaptopurine 681;
　　Radiation therapy 846
Leukemia, acute 635
　*leukemia 636*
Leukemia, chronic lymphocytic
　637
　*leukemia 636*
Leukemia, chronic myeloid 637
　*leukemia 636*
Leukeran 1106
Leukocyte 637
　type of Blood cell 183
Leukodystrophies 637
Leukoplakia 638
　associated with Mouth cancer

697; Tongue cancer 995
Leukorrhea:
　Vaginal discharge 1035
Leuprolide 1106
Levamisole 1106
Levlen 1106
Levobunolol 1106
Levodopa 638
　in treatment of Parkinson's
　　disease 773
　type of Synthetic drug 37
Levo-Dromoran 1106
Levonorgestrel 638
Levophed 1107
Levorphanol 1107
Levothroid 1107
Levothyroxine 638
　a synthetic Thyroid hormone
　　987
Levsin 1107
Levsinex 1107
LH 638
　see also index entry Luteinizing
　　hormone
LH-RH 638
　abbreviation for Luteinizing
　　hormone-releasing hormone
　　653
Liability insurance, professional
　638
Libido 638
　loss of: Sexual desire, inhibited
　　898
Librax 1107
Libritabs 1107
Librium 1107
Lice 638
　eggs of: Nit 728
　type of: Pubic lice 835
Licensure 638
Lichenification 638
Lichen planus 639
Lichen simplex 639
Lidex 1107
Lid lag 639
Lidocaine 639
　in treatment of Cardiac arrest
　　234; Ventricular tachycardia
　　1046
　type of *local anesthetic 106*
Lidoflazine 1107
Life expectancy 46, 639
　and Diabetes mellitus 351
life span:
　and Aging 74; Biological limits
　　46
Life support 640
　method of: Ventilation 1044;
　　*technique of artificial ventilation*
　　*1045*
　using Ventilator 1045
Ligament 640
Ligation 640
Ligature 640
light:
　effects of: Sunburn 954;
　　Sunlight, adverse effects of
　　955; Suntan 955
　intolerance to: Photophobia 793
　protection from: Sunscreens
　　955
　sensitivity to: Photosensitivity
　　793
　type of: Ultraviolet light 1021

Lightening 640
Light treatment:
  medical term: Phototherapy 793
Limb, artificial 640
  *types of artificial limb 641*
Limb defects 640
  type of: Phocomelia 792
Limbic system 640
Limbitrol 1107
limb prosthesis:
  Limb, artificial 640; *types of*
  *artificial limb 641*
Limp 641
  and Walking 1067
Lincocin 1107
Lincomycin 641
Lindane 641
Linear accelerator 641
  use of: Radiation therapy 846
Lioresal 1107
Liothyronine 1107
Liotrix 1107
Lip 641
Lip cancer 642
  cause of: Tobacco smoking 992
Lipectomy, suction 642
  type of Body contour surgery
  191
Lipid disorders 642
Lipid-lowering drugs 642
  examples: Cholestyramine 275;
  Gemfibrozil 478; Lovastatin
  650; Probucol 822
Lipids 642
  and Cholesterol 275; Fats 442
Lipoatrophy 642
Lipo-Hepin 1107
Lipoma 642
lipoproteins:
  and Cholesterol 275; Fats and
  oils 442
  excess of: Hyperlipidemia 553
Liposarcoma 642
Lipotriad 1107
Lipreading 642
  and Cochlear implant 286;
  Deafness 334
Liquaemin 1107
Liqui-Doss 1107
Liquid petrolatum:
  Mineral oil 689
Liquid Pred 1107
Liquifilm 1107
Liquiprin 1107
Lisp 642
Listeriosis 642
Lister, Joseph:
  *landmarks in surgery 33*
Lithane 1107
Lithium 643
  in treatment of Mania 663;
  Manic-depressive illness 663
Lithobid 1107
Lithonate 1107
Lithotabs 1107
Lithotomy 643
  types of: Nephrolithotomy 718;
  Pyelolithotomy 840;
  Ureterolithotomy 1023
Lithotomy position 643
Lithotripsy 39, 643
Lithotriptor 644
  use of: Lithotripsy 39, 643
Livedo reticularis 644

Liver 644
  *disorders of the liver 646*
  investigation of: Liver biopsy
  645; Liver function tests 648;
  Liver imaging 648
  *liver structure and function 645*
  removal of: Hepatectomy,
  partial 532; Hepatectomy,
  total 532
Liver abscess 645
  diagnosis of: Ultrasound
  scanning 1020
  feature of Amebiasis 92
Liver biopsy 645
liver bypass:
  type of Shunt 904
Liver cancer 647
  associated with Polycythemia
  807
  *a disorder of the liver 646*
Liver, cirrhosis of:
  Cirrhosis 282
  *a disorder of the liver 646*
liver damage:
  *disorders of the liver 646*
liver disease:
  *disorders of the liver 646*
Liver disease, alcoholic 647
  *a disorder of the liver 646*
  *effects of alcohol on the liver 21*
Liver failure 647
  causes of: Cirrhosis 282;
  Mushroom poisoning 707
  *a disorder of the liver 646*
  treatment of: Lactulose 625
Liver fluke 648
Liver function tests 648
Liver imaging 648
Liver transplant 648
  in treatment of Liver failure 647
Living will:
  Will, living 1077
Lobe 649
Lobectomy 649
Lobectomy, lung 649
  in treatment of Lung cancer 651
Lobotomy, prefrontal 649
*local anesthetics 106*
Lochia 649
  foul-smelling: Puerperal sepsis
  836
Locked knee:
  Knee 621
Lockjaw 649
  medical term: Trismus 1011
  symptom of Tetanus 975
Locomotor 649
Loiasis 649
Loin 649
Lomotil 1107
Lomustine 1107
Long, Crawford:
  *landmarks in surgery 33*
Loniten 1107
Loose bodies 649
  feature of Osteochondritis
  dissecans 753
Lo/Ovral 1107
Loperamide 649
Lopid 1107
Lopressor 1107
Lopressor HCT 1107
Loprox 1107
Lopurin 1107

Lorazepam 649
Lorcainide 1107
Lorcet 1107
Lordosis 650
  *a disorder of the spine 933*
Lorelco 1107
Loroxide-HC 1107
Lotion 650
Lotrimin 1107
Lotrisone 1107
Lotusate 1107
Lou Gehrig's disease 650
  type of Motor neuron disease
  696
louse:
  see index entry Lice
Lovastatin 650
low blood pressure:
  see index entry Blood pressure
low blood sugar:
  see index entry blood glucose
  levels
low blood volume:
  see index entry blood volume
low body temperature:
  medical term: Hypothermia 562
low-density lipoprotein (LDL):
  and Cholesterol 275; Fats and
  oils 442
  constituent of Globulin 490
  excess of: Hyperlipidemia 553
Loxapine 1107
Loxitane 1107
Lozol 1107
LSD 650
  and Serotonin 895
Lubrin 1107
Ludiomil 1107
Ludwig's angina 650
Lufyllin 1107
Lugol's solution 1107
Lumbar 650
  part of Spine 932
Lumbar puncture 650
  in diagnosis of Sleeping
  sickness 917; Subarachnoid
  hemorrhage 950
Lumbosacral spasm 650
Lumen 650
Lumpectomy 650
  type of Mastectomy 666
lump in the throat:
  medical term: Globus
  hystericus 490
Lunacy 650
Lung 650
  disorders of: Breathing
  difficulty 210, 211; *disorders of*
  *the lung 652*
  function of: Breathing 209;
  Respiration *864, 865*
  investigation of: Lung imaging
  652; Pulmonary function
  tests 836
  *location and structure of the lungs*
  *651*
  part of Respiratory system 865
  removal of: Lobectomy, lung
  649; Pneumonectomy 803
Lung cancer 651
  cause of: Tobacco smoking 991
  and Pneumoconiosis 803
  type of: Small cell carcinoma
  918

Lung, collapse of:
  Atelectasis 140
  Pneumothorax 804
Lung disease, chronic obstructive
652
lung fibrosis:
  types of: Interstitial pulmonary
  fibrosis 599; Pulmonary
  fibrosis 836
lung function tests:
  Pulmonary function tests 836
Lung imaging 652
lung, removal of:
  in Heart-lung transplant 520,
  *521*
  medical terms: Lobectomy,
  lung 649; Pneumonectomy
  803
lung transplant:
  and Heart-lung transplant 520,
  *521*
  in treatment of Cystic fibrosis
  328
Lung tumors 652
  type of: Lung cancer 651
Lupron 1107
Lupus erythematosus 653
  causing Hyperlipidemia 553;
  Keratoconjunctivitis sicca
  615; Raynaud's phenomenon
  853
  feature of: Photosensitivity 793
  treatment of: Plasmapheresis
  801
  type of Autoimmune disorder
  145
Lupus pernio 653
Lupus vulgaris 653
Luride 1107
Luteinizing hormone (LH) 653
  effect on Ovulation 760
  and Oral contraceptives 747
  production of: Pituitary gland
  797
  type of Gonadotropin hormone
  494
Luteinizing hormone-releasing
  hormone (LH-RH) 653
Luxated tooth 653
Lyme disease 653
  Other new diseases 45
Lymph 654
  and Lymphatic system 655;
  *structure and function of the*
  *lymphatic system 656*
Lymphadenitis 654
  causing Glands, swollen 488
Lymphadenopathy 654
  common term: Glands, swollen
  488
Lymphangiography 654
Lymphangioma 654
Lymphangitis 654
Lymphatic system 655
  disorders of: Burkitt's
  lymphoma 219; Glands,
  swollen 488; Hodgkin's
  disease 543; Lymphangitis
  654; Lymphedema 655;
  Lymphoma 657; Lymphoma,
  non-Hodgkin's 657;
  Mononucleosis, infectious
  693
  investigation of:

Lymphangiography 654
*structure and function of the lymphatic system 656*
Lymphedema 655
Lymph gland 655
medical term: Lymph node 655
Lymph node 655
enlargement of: Glands, swollen 488; Mononucleosis, infectious 693
and Lymphatic system 655; *structure and function of the lymphatic system 656*
tuberculosis of: Scrofula 887
Lymphocyte 655
part of Immune system 571; *the adaptive immune system 573*
production of: Spleen 933
type of Blood cell 184
Lymphogranuloma venereum 657
type of Sexually transmitted disease 898
Lymphoma 657
types of: Burkitt's lymphoma 219; Hodgkin's disease 543; Lymphoma, non-Hodgkin's 657
treatment of: Methotrexate 683; Procarbazine 822
Lymphoma, non-Hodgkin's 657
Lymphosarcoma 657
alternative term: Lymphoma, non-Hodgkin's 657
Lypressin 657
Lysergic acid 1107
Lysis 657
lysozyme:
production of: Lacrimal apparatus 624
Lyteers 1107

# M

Maalox 1107
Macro- 658
Macrobiotics 658
Macrodantin 1107
Macroglossia 658
macrophage:
definition of: Macro- 658
function of: Lymph node 655
macula:
see index entry macula lutea
macula lutea:
disorders of: Macular degeneration 658; Retinal detachment 868; Retinal hemorrhage 868
function of: Color vision 292
Macular degeneration 658
a *disorder of the eye 431; disorder of the retina 867*; Vision, disorder of 1054
Macule 658
Mafenide 1107
Magan 1107
Magnesium 658
Magnesium citrate 1107
Magnesium gluconate 1107
Magnesium hydroxide 1107
Magnesium oxide 1107
Magnesium salicylate 1107

Magnesium sulfate 1107
Magnesium trisilicate 1107
Magnetic resonance imaging (MRI):
see index entry MRI
magnetic resonance spectroscopy:
use of: MRI 700
Magsal 1107
Malabsorption 658
causing Rickets 874; Weight loss 1073
feature of *disorders of the pancreas 766*; Whipple's disease 1077
Maladjustment 659
Malaise 659
Malalignment 659
bone: Fracture 466
teeth: Malocclusion 661
Malar flush 659
Malaria 659
cause of: Protozoa 828
prevention and treatment of: Chloroquine 270; *preventing malaria 23*; Primaquine 821; Pyrimethamine 841; Quinine 842
transmission of: *insect-borne diseases 592; the spread of malaria 660*
Malathion 1107
male gender:
and Chromosomal abnormalities 277; Genetic disorders 484; Inheritance 590; Sex determination 897; Sex hormones 897
male pattern baldness:
treatment of: Hair transplant 504; Minoxidil 689
type of Alopecia 88
male sterilization:
Vasectomy 1040
Malformation 660
congenital: Birth defects 172, 173
Malignant 660
Malignant melanoma:
Melanoma, malignant 673
Malingering 661
Mallet finger:
alternative term: Baseball finger 161
Mallet toe 661
malleus:
bone in Ear 384
example of Ossicle 752
Mallory-Weiss syndrome 661
causing Vomiting blood 1065
Malnutrition:
causes of: Infectious disease 582; Macrobiotics 658
causing Immunodeficiency disorders 575
effect on Growth, childhood 499
see also index entry Nutritional disorders
Malocclusion 661
treatment of: Orthodontic appliances 750
Malpighi, Marcello:
and Microscope 685
Malpractice:

and Liability insurance, professional 638
Malpresentation 661
Mammary gland:
see index entry Breast
Mammography 22, 662
in diagnosis of Breast cancer 206
and Regular check-ups 22
Mammoplasty 662
*procedure for mammoplasty 663*
Mandelamine 1107
Mandible:
common term: Jaw 610
Mandibular orthopedic repositioning appliance 662
Mandol 1107
Mania 663
treatment of: Antipsychotic drugs 119; Lithium 643
type of Psychosis 833
Manic-depressive illness 663
treatment of: Antipsychotic drugs 119; Lithium 643
type of Psychosis 833
Manipulation 663
Mannitol 663
Manometry 664
Mantadil 1107
Mantoux test 664
type of Tuberculin test 1013
manubrium:
part of Sternum 940
MAOIs:
see index entry monoamine oxidase inhibitors (MAOIs)
Maolate 1107
Maprotiline 664
Marasmus 664
and Kwashiorkor 623
Marax 1107
Marbaxin-750 1107
Marble bone disease:
alternative term: Osteopetrosis 755
Marburg disease:
Other new diseases 45
Marcaine 1107
March fracture 664
Marezine 1107
Marfan's syndrome 664
leading to Aneurysm 107; Lens dislocation 634
Marflex 1107
Marijuana 664
causing Withdrawal syndrome 1080
constituent of: THC 977
Marital counseling 665
and Sex therapy 897
Marplan 1107
Marrow, bone:
Bone marrow 195
Marsupialization 665
Masculinization:
alternative term: Virilization 1050
and Sex determination 897
Masochism 665
and Sadism 878; Sadomasochism 878
Massage 665
and Physical therapy 793; *techniques of physical therapy 794*

Mast cell 665
function of: Histamine 540; Hypersensitivity 555; Inflammation 588
Mastectomy 666
as part of Sex change 896
in treatment of Klinefelter's syndrome 621
Mastication 667
Mastitis 667
resulting from cracked Nipple 728
Mastocytosis 667
Mastoid bone 667
inflammation of: Mastoiditis 667
Mastoiditis 667
Masturbation 668
and Orgasm, lack of 750; Sex therapy 898
Materna 1107
Maternal mortality 668
and Childbirth 263
Maxibolin 1107
Maxidex 1107
Maxiflor 1107
Maxilla 668
part of Skull 913
Maxitrol 1107
Maxzide 1107
Mazanor 1107
Mazindol 1107
McArdle's disease 668
Measles 668
prevention of: Immunization 571; *typical childhood immunization schedule 574*; Vaccine 1034
symptom of: Koplik's spots 623
Measurin 1107
Meatus 669
Mebaral 1107
Mebendazole 669
Mecamylamine 1107
Mechlorethamine 1107
Meckel's diverticulum 669
Meclan 1107
Meclizine 669
Meclocycline 1107
Meclofenamate 669
Meclomen 1107
Meconium 669
indicating Fetal distress 448
passing by Newborn 726
Medial 670
median lethal dose:
abbreviation for: $LD_{50}$ 631
Median nerve 670
part of Brachial plexus 198
Mediastinoscopy 670
Mediastinum 670
Medicaid 670
medical ethics:
and Confidentiality 296; Ethics, medical 422; Hippocratic oath 539
Medical examiner 670
medical history:
in Diagnosis 351
Medicare 670
Medication 670
and Drug 376
Medicine 670
and Forensic medicine 465

Medicolegal 671
Medicone 1107
Medigesic 1107
Medihaler-Epi 1107
Medihaler-Ergotamine 1107
Medihaler-Iso 1107
Mediplast 1107
Mediquell 1107
Meditation 671
　and Relaxation techniques 859
Medrol 1107
Medrol Enpak 1107
Medrol Oral 1107
Medroxyprogesterone 671
Medrysone 1107
Medulla 671
Medulla oblongata 671
　part of Brain stem 203
Medulloblastoma 671
Mefenamic acid 671
Mefoxin 1107
Mega- 671
Megace 1107
Megacolon 671
megaloblastic anemia:
　Anemia, megaloblastic 103
Megalomania 672
-megaly 672
Megestrol 672
Meibomian cyst:
　alternative term: Chalazion 256
meibomian glands:
　part of Eye 430
Meibomianitis 673
Meigs' syndrome 673
Meiosis 673
　and Chromosomes 280
　mechanism of meiosis 672
Melancholia 673
Melanex 1107
Melanin 673
　and color of Hair 503;
　　Pigmentation 794; Skin 910
　deficiency of: Pallor 765;
　　Vitiligo 1060
　in prevention of Sunburn 955
melanocytes:
　producing Melanin 673
melanocyte-stimulating hormone:
　production of: Pituitary gland
　　797
Melanoma, juvenile 673
　type of Nevus 726
Melanoma, malignant 673
　as complication of Lentigo 634
　diagnosis of: Skin biopsy 912
　of eye: disorders of the eye 431;
　　Eye tumor 433
　type of Nevus 726; Skin cancer
　　912
Melanosis coli 673
Melarsoprol 1107
Melasma:
　alternative term: Chloasma 270
melatonin:
　and Biorhythms 172
　production of: Pineal gland 795
Melena 673
　causes of: Esophageal varices
　　419; Peptic ulcer 780
　and Rectal bleeding 855
Melfiat 1107
Melioidosis 673
Mellaril 1107

Melphalan 674
Membrane 674
　of Cell 245
membranes, rupture of:
　as complication of Version 1047
　premature: Childbirth,
　　complications of 265
　use of: Induction of labor 581
Memory 674
Memory, loss of:
　medical term: Amnesia 94
Menadiol 1108
Menadione 1108
Menarche 674
Mendelian inheritance:
　Inheritance 590
Menest 1108
Meniere's disease 674
　a disorder of the ear 385
　effect on Balance 156; Walking
　　1068
　treatment of: Meclizine 669;
　　Promethazine 823
Meninges 675
　of Brain 201; Spinal cord 929
　protrusion of: Meningocele 675
Meningioma 675
Meningitis 675
　causing Stiff neck 941
　as complication of Mastoiditis
　　667; Mumps 703; Pleurodynia
　　802
　prevention of: Rifampin 874
Meningocele 675
　type of Spina bifida 928, 929
Meningomyelocele:
　Myelocele 710
Meniscectomy 676
Meniscus 676
　part of Knee 621
Menogaril 1108
Menopause 676
　and Osteoporosis 756; Varicose
　　veins 1038
Menorrhagia 676
　at menopause: Polycystic ovary
　　807
　symptom of Endometriosis 405
Menotropins 677
　type of Gonadotropin hormone
　　494
Menstrual extraction 677
　use of: Abortion, elective 57
menstrual pain:
　medical term: Dysmenorrhea
　　383
menstrual periods:
　see index entry Menstruation
Menstruation 677
　cessation of: Amenorrhea 93;
　　Menopause 676; Virilism
　　1050
　and Sanitary protection 881
　start of: Menarche 674
　see also index entries
　　Menstruation, disorders of;
　　Menstruation, irregular
Menstruation, disorders of 678
　cause of: Polycystic ovary 807
　examples: Amenorrhea 93;
　　Dysmenorrhea 383;
　　Menorrhagia 676;
　　Menstruation, irregular 678
Menstruation, irregular 678

symptom chart 679
mental age:
　and Intelligence tests 595
mental disorder:
　and Commitment 294; Consent
　　298; Mental illness 678;
　　Mental retardation 678
mental handicap:
　and Mental retardation 678
Mental hospital 678
Mental illness 678
Mental retardation 678
　causes of: Cerebral palsy 248;
　　Chromosomal abnormalities
　　277; Down's syndrome 372;
　　Fragile X syndrome 468;
　　Klinefelter's syndrome 621;
　　Rubella 877; Spina bifida 928;
　　Sturge-Weber syndrome 949;
　　Toxoplasmosis 1001;
　　Tuberous sclerosis 1014;
　　Turner's syndrome 1016
Menthol 1108
Mepenzolate 1108
Mepergan 1108
Meperidine 680
Mephenytoin 1108
Mephobarbital 1108
Mephyton 1108
Mepivacaine 1108
Meprobamate 680
　causing Withdrawal syndrome
　　1080
Meptazinol 1108
Mequitazine 1108
Mercaptopurine 681
Mercury 681
Mercury poisoning 681
　causing Minamata disease 689
Merthiolate 1108
Merzbacher-Pelizaeus disease:
　type of Leukodystrophy 637
Mesantoin 1108
Mescaline 681
　causing Hallucination 504
　source of: Peyote 788
Mesenteric lymphadenitis 681
Mesentery 681
mesomorphic body type:
　a Somatotype 924
Mesoridazine 1108
Mesothelioma 681
Mesothelium 681
messenger RNA:
　see index entry RNA
Mestinon 1108
Mestranol 681
Metabolism 681
Metabolism, inborn errors of 682
Metabolite 682
Metacarpal bone 682
　part of the skeletal structure of the
　　hand and wrist 506; Skeleton
　　909
Metamucil 1108
Metandren 1108
Metaplasia 683
Metaprel 1108
Metaproterenol 683
Metaraminol 1108
Metastasis 683
　and Cancer 227;
　　Carcinomatosis 234;
　　Secondary 889; Tumor 1015

Metatarsal bone 683
　part of Foot 463; skeleton of the
　　foot 464; Skeleton 909
Metatarsalgia 683
Metatarsophalangeal joint 683
Metatensin 1108
Metaxalone 1108
Meted 2 1108
Methacycline 1108
Methadone 683
　in treatment of Withdrawal
　　syndrome 1080
Methamphetamine 1108
Methane 683
Methanol 683
Methantheline 1108
Metharbital 1108
Methazolamide 1108
Methdilazine 1108
Methenamine 1108
Methergine 1108
Methicillin 1108
Methimazole 683
Methocarbamol 683
Methohexital 1108
Methotrexate 683
Methoxsalen 683
Methoxyflurane 1108
Methscopolamine 1108
Methsuximide 1108
Methyclothiazide 684
Methylbenzethonium 1108
Methyl alcohol:
　alternative term: Methanol 683
Methyl-CCNU 1108
Methylcellulose 684
Methyldopa 684
Methylergonovine 1108
Methyl-glyoxalbis-
　guanylhydrazone 1108
Methylphenidate 1108
Methylprednisolone 684
Methyl salicylate 1108
Methyltestosterone 1108
Methyprylon 1108
Methysergide 684
Meticorten 1108
Metimyd 1108
Metoclopramide 684
Metocurine 1108
Metolazone 684
Metoprolol 684
Metreton 1108
Metronid 1108
Metronidazole 684
Metryl 1108
Metyrapone 1108
Metyrosine 1108
Mevacor 1108
Mexate 1108
Mexiletine 684
Mezlocillin 1108
Micantin 1108
Miconazole 684
Micrainin 1108
Micro- 684
Microangiopathy 684
Microbe 685
　alternative term:
　　Microorganism 685
Microbiology 685
Microcephaly 685
Micro-K 1108
Micronase 1108

Micronefrin 1108
Micronor 1108
Microorganism 685
  study of: Microbiology 685
Microscope 685
  *types of microscope 686*
Microsurgery 35, 687
  in treatment of Nerve injury
    719
  uses of: Plastic surgery 801;
    Skin and muscle flap 912
microwave ovens:
  and Food and Drug
    Administration 461;
    Radiation 845
Micturition:
  alternative term: passing Urine
    1027
Midamor 1108
Midazolam 1108
Midbrain 687
  part of Brain stem 203
Middle ear:
  part of Ear 384
Middle-ear effusion, persistent
    688
  and Otitis media 758
Middle-ear infection:
  alternative term: Otitis media
    757
Mid-life crisis 688
Midol 200 1108
Midrin 1108
Midwifery 688
Migraine 688
  and Oral contraceptives 748
  treatment of: Ergotamine 416;
    Methysergide 684;
    Propranolol 824
  type of Headache 507
Milia 689
  in Newborn 727
Miliaria 689
  alternative term: Prickly heat
    821
Milk 689
  abnormal production of:
    Galactorrhea 472
  and Bottle-feeding 197; Breast-
    feeding 207; Expressing milk
    427
  secretion of: Breast 205
  source of Vitamin D 1059
Milk-alkali syndrome 689
Milkinol 1108
Milk of magnesia 689
Milk teeth:
  alternative term: Primary teeth
    822
Milpath 1108
Milprem 1108
Milrinone 1108
Miltown 1108
Minamata disease 689
  cause of: Mercury poisoning
    681
mind:
  alternative term: Psyche 830
Mineralization, dental 689
Mineralocorticoid 689
Mineral oil 689
Minerals 689
  *minerals and main food sources
    690*

and Nutrition 736; Trace
  elements 1001
*recommended daily dietary
  allowances (RDA) of selected
  minerals 19*
Mineral supplements 689
Minilaparotomy:
  method of Sterilization, female
    940
Minimal brain dysfunction 689
minipill:
  type of Oral contraceptive 747
Minipress 1108
Minnesota Multiphasic
  Personality Inventory:
  type of Personality test 787
Minocin 1108
Minocycline 689
Minoxidil 689
Mintezol 1108
Miochol 1108
Miosis 690
Miscarriage 690
  increased risk of: *alcohol and
    pregnancy 83*
  *types of miscarriage 691*
Mites and disease 691
Mitomycin 1108
Mitosis 691
  and Chromosomes 280
Mitotane 1108
mitral incompetence:
  alternative term: Mitral
    insufficiency 692
Mitral insufficiency 692
  disorder of Heart valves 523
mitral regurgitation:
  alternative term: Mitral
    insufficiency 692
Mitral stenosis 692
  associated with Malar flush 659
  disorder of Heart valves 523
mitral valve:
  disorders of: Mitral
    insufficiency 692; Mitral
    stenosis 692; Mitral valve
    prolapse 692
  part of Heart 514
Mitral valve prolapse 692
mitral valvotomy:
  type of Heart surgery 522
Mitrolan 1108
Mittelschmerz 692
Mity-Quin 1108
Mixtard 1108
Moban 1108
Mobidin 1108
Mobigesic 1108
Mobilization 692
Modane 1108
Modern diagnostic techniques
    26-31
Modern surgical treatment 34-35
Modicon 1108
Modrastane 1108
Moduretic 1108
moisturizer:
  type of Emollient 399
Molar:
  *structure and arrangement of teeth
    967*
  third molar: Wisdom tooth 1078
Molar pregnancy 693
Mold 693

causing Alveolitis 90; Rhinitis,
  allergic 872
and Diet and disease 358
group of Fungi 470
Mole:
  cancerous: Melanoma,
    malignant 673
  type of Nevus 726
Molecule 693
Molindone 1108
Mol-Iron 1108
Molluscum contagiosum 693
Mongolian spot 693
  type of Nevus 726
Mongolism 693
  modern term: Down's
    syndrome 372
Moniliasis:
  alternative term: Candidiasis
    230
Monistat 1108
Monitor 693
  use of: Coronary care unit 309;
    Intensive care 38, 595
monoamine oxidase inhibitors
  (MAOIs):
  group of Antidepressant drugs
    116
Monoarthritis 693
Monobenzone 1108
Monocid 1108
Monoclonal antibody:
  Antibody, monoclonal 115
monocytes:
  types of Blood cell 182;
    Phagocyte 789
Mono-Gesic 1108
Mononucleosis, infectious 693
Monorchism 694
monosaccharide:
  type of Carbohydrate 232
Monosodium glutamate 694
Monosulfiram 1108
mons pubis:
  *location of labia 624*
Monteggia's fracture 694
Montezuma's revenge 694
  alternative term: Travelers'
    diarrhea 1007
  type of Gastroenteritis 476
mood:
  abnormalities of: Affective
    disorders 73; Cyclothymia
    326; Delirium 338;
    Depression 344; Mania 663;
    Manic-depressive illness 663;
    Postpartum depression 810;
    Premenstrual syndrome 818;
    SADS 879
  and Euphoria 423
  medical term: Affect 73
Moon face 694
  feature of Cushing's syndrome
    325
MORA:
  abbreviation for Mandibular
    orthopedic repositioning
    appliance 662
Morbid anatomy 694
Morbidity 694
Morbilli:
  alternative term: Measles 668
Morning-after pill:
  method of Contraception,

postcoital 306
morning sickness:
  Vomiting in pregnancy 1065
Moron 694
Moro's reflex:
  example of Reflex, primitive
    857
Morphea 694
Morphine 694
  derivative of: Heroin 535
Morquio's syndrome:
  type of Mucopolysaccharidosis
    700
Mortality 695
  see also index entries Death;
    death rates
morula:
  in *the process of fertilization 446*
Mosaicism 695
  causing Turner's syndrome
    1016
Mosquito bites 695
  causing Malaria 659
  Insects and disease 592
motilin:
  a Gastrointestinal hormone 477
Motion sickness 696
  treatment of: Hydroxyzine 551;
    Meclizine 669; Promethazine
    823
Motor 696
motor cortex:
  function of: Cerebrum 251
  and Movement 699
motor fibers:
  of Nerve 719; Spinal cord 929;
    Spinal nerves 931
Motor neuron disease 696
Motor system disease:
  alternative term: Motor neuron
    disease 696
Motrin 1109
Mountain sickness 696
Mouth 697
  and Oral hygiene 748
  part of: Palate 765
Mouth cancer 697
  and *alcohol-related disorders 85;*
    Tobacco smoking 992
Mouth, dry 697
Mouth-to-mouth resuscitation:
  Artificial respiration 134
Mouth ulcer 699
Mouthwash 699
Movement *698*, 699
  abnormal: Dyskinesia 382
  causing Motion sickness 696
Moxalactam 1109
Moxibustion 699
MRI 28, 699, 700
  *three-dimensional magnetic
    resonance imaging 16*
  *how MRI works 29*
  type of Imaging technique 568;
    Scanning technique 882
MS 700
  abbreviation for Multiple
    sclerosis 701
MS Contin 1109
Mucocele 700
Mucolytic drugs 700
  use of: Cough remedies 316
Mucomyst 1109
Mucopolysaccharidosis 700

Mucosa 700
  alternative term: Mucous
    membrane 700
Mucous membrane 700
Mucus 700
  in Mucocele 700
  secretion of: Mucous
    membrane 700; Stomach 942;
    Trachea 1001
Mucus method of contraception:
  Contraception 302
Multiple myeloma 701
Multiple personality 701
  and Split personality 934
Multiple pregnancy:
  Pregnancy, multiple 816
Multiple sclerosis 701
  causing Optic neuritis 746;
    Paralysis 769; Retrobulbar
    neuritis 868; Strabismus 944
  features of Demyelination 340;
    features of multiple sclerosis 702
Multivitamin 702
Mumps 702
  complications of: Mastitis 667;
    Orchitis 749; Pancreatitis 767
  effect on Parotid glands 773;
    Salivary glands 880
  prevention of: Immunization
    571; typical childhood
    immunization schedule 574
Münchausen's syndrome 703
Murine Plus 1109
Murmur 703
Murocel 1109
Murocoll-2 1109
Muromonab CD3 1109
Muro's Opcon-A 1109
Muro Tears 1109
Murray, Joseph:
  landmarks in surgery 33
Muscle 703
  and Aerobics 72
  the body's muscles 704
  disorders of: disorders of muscle
    705; Muscle spasm 706;
    Muscular dystrophy 706;
    Myalgia 708; Myasthenia
    gravis 708; Myopathy 713;
    Myositis 713; Myotonia 713;
    Rhabdomyolysis 869; Strain
    944
  removal of: Myectomy 709
  tone of: Tone, muscle 995
  type of Tissue 989
muscle enzymes:
  abnormal levels of: Muscular
    dystrophy 706; Myocardial
    infarction 712
  types of Enzyme 410
Muscle-relaxant drugs 706
Muscle spasm 706
  causing Torticollis 998
  feature of Tetany 975; Multiple
    sclerosis 701; Myoclonus 712
muscle tumor:
  disorders of muscle 705
  types of: Fibroid 453;
    Leiomyoma 633; Myoma 713;
    Rhabdomyosarcoma 869
muscle wasting:
  and Atrophy 143
  feature of Motor neuron
    disease 696; Neuropathy 724;

Peroneal muscular atrophy
  786
  of Quadriceps muscle 842
Muscular dystrophy 706
  causing Paralysis 769
  inheritance of: Genetic
    disorders 483; Sex-linked 897
  a disorder of muscle 705
  types of muscular dystrophy 707
Musculoskeletal 707
Mushroom poisoning 707
  type of Food poisoning 463
Mutagen 707
Mutamycin 1109
Mutation 708
  cause of: Mutagen 707
  of Gene 479; Oncogenes 743
Mutism 708
Myadec 1109
Myalgia 708
Myambutol 1109
Myasthenia gravis 708
  causing Paralysis 769
  a disorder of muscle 705
  treatment of: Neostigmine 718;
    Plasmapheresis 800;
    Pyridostigmine 841
Mycelex 1109
Mycetoma 709
Mycifradin 1109
Myciguent 1109
Mycitracin 1109
Mycolog 1109
Mycolog II Cream 1109
Mycology:
  study of Fungal infections 470;
    Fungi 471
Mycoplasma 709
  causing Pneumonia 803, 804
Mycosis 709
  alternative term: Fungal
    infections 470
  and Fungi 470
Mycosis fungoides 709
Mycostatin 1109
Myco-Triacet 1109
Mydfrin 1109
Mydriacyl 1109
Mydriasis 709
Myectomy 709
Myel- 709
Myelin 710
  breakdown of: Demyelination
    340; Multiple sclerosis 701
Myelitis 710
Myelocele 710
  type of Spina bifida 928, 929
myelofibrosis:
  alternative term: Myelosclerosis
    710
Myelography 710
Myeloma, multiple:
  Multiple myeloma 701
myelomatosis:
  alternative term: Multiple
    myeloma 701
Myelomeningocele:
  Myelocele 710
Myelopathy 710
Myelosclerosis 710
Myiasis 710
Myidil 1109
Myidone 1109
Mykinac 1109

Mylanta 1109
Myleran 1109
Mylicon 1109
Myo- 710
Myobid 1109
Myocardial infarction 710
  causing Shock 901
  and Coronary heart disease 309
  a disorder of the heart 517
  features of myocardial infarction
    711
Myocarditis 712
  a disorder of the heart 517
myocardium:
  muscle of Heart 514
Myochrysine 1109
Myoclonus 712
  type of Spasm 924
Myofacial pain disorder:
  alternative term:
    Temporomandibular joint
    syndrome 969
Myoflex 1109
Myoglobin 712
  constituent of: Iron 606
Myoma 713
  a disorder of muscle 705
Myomectomy 713
  in treatment of Fibroid 453
Myopathy 713
Myopia 713
  associated with Retinal
    detachment 867; Retinal tear
    868
  treatment of: Contact lenses
    301; why glasses are used 489
myosarcoma:
  a disorder of muscle 705
Myositis 713
  causing Shin splints 901
  types of: Dermatomyositis 346;
    Polymyositis 808
Myotomy 713
Myotonia 713
Myringitis 713
Myringoplasty 713
Myringotomy 713
Mysoline 1109
Mysteclin-F 1109
Mysteclin-F Syrup 1109
Mytrex 1109
Myxedema 713
  causing Dementia 339
  feature of Hypothyroidism 563
  and Ground substance 498
  a disorder of the thyroid gland 986
Myxoma 713
  a disorder of the heart 517

N

Nabilone 1109
Nadolol 714
Nafcillin 1109
Nail 714
  constituent of: Keratin 614
  disorders of: fungal diseases 471;
    Ingrown toenail 589;
    Koilonychia 623;
    Onychogryphosis 743;
    Onycholysis 743
Nail-biting 714

causing Hangnail 506
Nalbuphine 1109
Naldecon 1109
Nalfon 1109
Nalidixic acid 714
Naloxone 714
Naltrexone 714
Nandrolin 1109
Nandrolone 714
Naphazoline 714
Naphcon 1109
Naprosyn 1109
Naproxen 714
Naqua 1109
Naquival 1109
Narcan 1109
Narcissism 715
  type of Personality disorder 786
Narcolepsy 715
  a disorder of Sleep 915
  symptom of: Sleep paralysis
    917
  treatment of: Pemoline 778
Narcosis 715
Narcotic drugs 715
  abuse of: Drug dependence
    378; Withdrawal syndrome
    1078
  antagonist of: Naltrexone 714
  examples: Codeine 286; Heroin
    535; Meperidine 680;
    Methadone 683; Morphine
    694; Opium 745; Oxycodone
    761; Pentazocine 780;
    Propoxyphene 824
  group of Analgesic drugs 97
  overdose, effects of: Drug
    poisoning 379; Respiratory
    arrest 865; Respiratory
    distress syndrome 865
  overdose, treatment of:
    Naloxone 714; Ventilation
    1044
  use of: Pain relief 764
Nardil 1109
Nasahist 1109
Nasal congestion 715
  associated with Nasal discharge
    715
  feature of Cold, common 287;
    Rhinitis 872; Rhinitis, allergic
    872
Nasalcrom 1109
Nasal discharge 715
  associated with Nasal
    congestion 715
  causes of: Cold, common 287;
    Influenza 588; Nasopharynx,
    cancer of 716; Rhinitis 872;
    Rhinitis, allergic 872
Nasalide 1109
Nasal obstruction 715
Nasal septum 715
  deviated: Nasal obstruction
    715; Submucous resection
    951
  part of Nose 731
  perforated: a disorder of the nose
    732; Wegener's
    granulomatosis 1072
Nasogastric tube 715
  using a nasogastric tube 716
nasolacrimal ducts:
  part of Lacrimal apparatus 624

Nasopharynx 716
  part of Pharynx 789
Nasopharynx, cancer of 716
  a *disorder of the nose* 732
Natabec 1109
Natafort 1109
Natalins 1109
Natamycin 1109
National Institutes of Health:
  NIH 728
Naturacil 1109
Natural childbirth:
  alternative term: Prepared
  childbirth 818
Nature's Remedy 1109
Naturetin 1109
Naturopathy 716
Nausea 716
  and Vomiting 1062
Navane 1109
Navel 716
  medical term: Umbilicus 1021
ND-Stat 1109
Nearsightedness:
  medical term: Myopia 713
Nebcin 1109
Nebulizer 716
Neck 716
  *anatomy of the neck* 717
  stiffness of: Neck rigidity 717;
  Stiff neck 941; Subarachnoid
  hemorrhage 950
  support of: Collar, orthopedic
  289
Neck dissection, radical 717
Neck rigidity 717
Necrolysis, toxic epidermal 717
Necrophilia 717
Necropsy 717
  alternative term: Autopsy 147
Necrosis 717
necrotizing ulcerative gingivitis:
  alternative term: Vincent's
  disease 1049
  complication of Gingivitis 487
needle sharing:
  and spread of AIDS 76; HIV
  541
negative feedback:
  in *endocrine system* 403
  and Homeostasis 544
NegGram 1109
Nematodes 717
  common term: Roundworms
  876
Nembutal 1109
Neo-Calglucon 1109
Neo-Cortef 1109
NeoDecadron 1109
Neologism 717
Neomycin 717
Neonate 717
  see also index entry Newborn
Neonatologist 717
Neonatology 718
Neoplasia 718
  formation of Tumor 1015·
Neoplasm 718
  alternative term: Tumor 1015
Neo-Polycin 1109
Neoquess 1109
Neosar 1109
Neosporin 1109
Neostigmine 718

Neo-Synalar 1109
Neo-Synephrine 12 Hour 1109
Neo-Tears 1109
Neotep 1109
Neothylline 1109
Nephrectomy 718
  in treatment of Kidney cancer
  618
Nephritis 718
Nephroblastoma:
  type of Kidney cancer 617
Nephrocalcinosis 718
Nephrocaps 1109
Nephrolithotomy 718
Nephrologist 718
Nephrology 718
Nephron 718
  part of Kidney 617
Nephropathy 718
  *disorders of the kidney* 618
Nephrosclerosis 718
Nephrosis:
  Nephrotic syndrome 719
Nephrostomy 719
Nephrotic syndrome 719
  causing Hyperlipidemia 553
  a *disorder of the kidney* 618
  treatment of:
  Hydrochlorothiazide 550
Neptazane 1109
Nerve 719
  disorders of: Nerve injury 719;
  Neuralgia 720; Neuritis 722;
  Neuroma 723; Neuropathy
  723; Neurotoxin 725
  surgical destruction of:
  Sympathectomy 959
  types of: Cranial nerves 318;
  Spinal nerves 931
  see also index entries Nervous
  system; Neuron
Nerve block 719
  type of Local anesthetic 106
Nerve injury 719
Nerve, trapped 720
  example: Carpal tunnel
  syndrome 238
Nervous breakdown 720
nervous exhaustion:
  alternative term: Neurasthenia
  722
Nervous habit 720
Nervous system 720, *721*
  anatomy of: Autonomic
  nervous system *146, 147*;
  Brain 199; Central nervous
  system 247; Cranial nerves
  318; Peripheral nervous
  system 784; Plexus 802;
  Spinal cord 929; *location of the
  spinal cord 930*; Spinal nerves
  931
  functions of: Hearing 511, *512*;
  Memory 674; Movement 699;
  Pain 763, 764; Reflex 857;
  Sensation 892; Smell 918; *the
  sense of smell 919*; Speech 925;
  Taste 965; Thought 979;
  Touch 998; *the sense of touch
  999*; Vision 1052; *the sense of
  vision 1053*
  and interaction with hormones:
  Neuroendocrinology 722
  see also index entries Nerve;

Neuron
Nestabs FA 1109
Netilmicin 720
Netromycin 1109
Neuralgia 720
  treatment of: Carbamazepine
  231
neural tube:
  in Embryo 397
Neural tube defect 722
  types of: Anencephaly 104;
  Spina bifida 928
Neurapraxia 722
Neurasthenia 722
Neuritis 722
Neuroblastoma 722
Neurocutaneous disorders 722
Neurodermatitis 722
Neuroendocrinology 722
Neurofibromatosis 722
  type of Neurocutaneous
  disorder 722
*neurologic sensory testing 893*
Neurologist 723
Neurology 723
Neuroma 723
Neuron 723
  anatomy of: Myelin 710;
  *structure of a neuron 724*
  transmission of impulses:
  Calcium 224;
  Neurotransmitter 725;
  Potassium 812; Sodium 922;
  Synapse 960
  see also index entries Nerve;
  Nervous system
Neuropathic joint 723
Neuropathology 723
Neuropathy 723
  causing Footdrop 464; Paralysis
  769; Pins and needles
  sensation 796
neuropeptides:
  examples: Endorphins 405;
  Enkephalins 408
  type of Neurotransmitter 725
Neuropsychiatry 725
Neurosis 725
  assessment of: Personality tests
  787
  and Suicide 953
  type of Mental illness 678
Neurosurgeon 725
Neurosurgery 725
Neurosyphilis 725
  complication of Syphilis 961
neurotensin:
  type of Gastrointestinal
  hormone 477
Neurotoxin 725
Neurotransmitter 725
  examples: Acetylcholine 62;
  Endorphins 405; Enkephalins
  408; GABA 472;
  Norepinephrine 730;
  Serotonin 895
  and Neuron 723; *how
  neurotransmitters work 726*;
  Synapse 960
Neutrogena 1109
neutrons:
  type of Radiation 844
Nevus 726
  and Pigmentation 795

a *disorder of the skin* 910
Newborn 726
  assessment of: Apgar score 124;
  Reflex, primitive 857; *types of
  primitive reflex 858*
  blood test: Guthrie test 502
  disorders of: Birth defects 172;
  Birth injury 173; Hemolytic
  disease of the newborn 529;
  Jaundice 610
  feces of: Meconium 669
Niacin:
  deficiency of: Pellagra 776
  part of the Vitamin B complex
  1058
Niacinamide 1109
Nickel 727
Niclocide 1109
Niclosamide 727
  *drugs used to treat worm
  infestations 1080*
Nico-400 1109
Nicobid 1109
Nicotine 727
  and Tobacco smoking 992;
  Withdrawal syndrome 1080
Nicotinic acid 727
  part of Vitamin B complex 1058
Nico-vert 1109
Nifedipine 727
Niferex 1109
Nifurtimox 1109
Night blindness 727
  cause of: deficiency of Vitamin
  A 1057
  a *disorder of the eye 431*
  feature of Retinitis pigmentosa
  868
Nightmare 727
Night terror 727
  causing Sleepwalking 917
NIH 728
Nilstat 1109
Nimodipine 1109
Nipple 728
  and Breast-feeding 207
  discharge from: Colostrum 293;
  Galactorrhea 472
  disorders of: Joggers' nipple
  613; Paget's disease of the
  nipple 763
  part of Breast 205
Nit 728
  egg of Lice 638
Nitrate drugs 728
  group of Vasodilator drugs
  1041
Nitrites 728
Nitro-Bid 1109
Nitrodisc 1109
Nitro-Dur 1109
Nitrofurantoin 728
  causing Hepatitis, chronic
  active 533
Nitrofurazone 1109
Nitrogen 728
  in Scuba-diving medicine 888
Nitrogen mustard 1109
Nitroglycerin 729
Nitrol 1109
Nitrolingual spray 1109
Nitropress 1109
Nitrospan 1109
Nitrostat 1109

Nitrous oxide 729
common term: Laughing gas 630
Nizoral 1109
NMR 729
alternative term: MRI 699
Nocardiosis 729
nociceptors:
receptors for Pain 763
Noctec 1109
Nocturia 729
causes of: Cystitis 328; Heart failure 519; Prostate, enlarged 825
Nocturnal emission 729
Node 729
type of: Lymph node 655
Nodule 729
feature of Fibrositis 453
Noise 729
causing Deafness 333
and Presbycusis 820
Nolahist 1109
Nolamine 1109
Noludar 1109
Nolvadex 1109
Noma 730
Nonaccidental injury:
common term: Child abuse 263
non-A, non-B hepatitis:
type of Hepatitis, viral 533
non-Hodgkin's lymphoma:
Lymphoma, non-Hodgkin's 657
Noninvasive 730
Nonoxynol 1109
nonrapid eye movement (NREM) sleep:
see index entry NREM sleep
Nonspecific urethritis 730
treatment of: Oxytetracycline 761
type of Chlamydial infection 270; Sexually transmitted disease 898; Urethritis 1024
and Urinary tract infection 1026
Nonsteroidal anti-inflammatory drugs 730
examples: Diflunisal 359; Ibuprofen 566; Indomethacin 581; Ketoprofen 616; Meclofenamate 669; Mefenamic acid 671; Naproxen 714; Piroxicam 796; Tolmetin 994
in treatment of Inflammation 588; Rheumatoid arthritis 871
Norcet 1109
Nordette 1109
Norepinephrine 730
type of Neurotransmitter 725
see also index entry Epinephrine
Norethindrone 731
Norethynodrel 1109
Norflex 1109
Norgesic 1109
Norgestrel 731
Norinyl 1110
Norlestrin 1110
Norlutate 1110
Norlutin 1110
Normodyne 1110
Norpace 1110

Norpace CR 1110
Norpramin 1110
Nor-Q-D 1110
Nortriptyline 731
Noscapine 1110
Nose 731
damage to lining of: Cocaine 285
disorders of: Nasal congestion 715; Nasal discharge 715; Nasal obstruction 715; Nosebleed 731; Nose, broken 732; disorders of the nose 732; Rhinitis 872; Rhinophyma 873
function of: Smell 918; the sense of smell 919
and Nasopharynx 716
part of: Nasal septum 715
reshaping of: Rhinoplasty 873
Nosebleed 731
feature of Yellow fever 1086
Nose, broken 732
Nose reshaping:
medical term: Rhinoplasty 873
Nostrilla 1110
Notezine 1110
notochord:
part of Embryo 397
Novafed 1110
Novafed A 1110
Novahistine DMX 1110
Novocain 1110
Novolin L, N, R 1110
NPH Insulin 1110
NREM (nonrapid eye movement) sleep:
and sleep patterns 915; Sleepwalking 917
type of Sleep 914
NSAIDs:
see index entry Nonsteroidal anti-inflammatory drugs
NSU:
abbreviation for Nonspecific urethritis 730
Nubain 1110
Nuclear energy 732
and Radiation 844
Nuclear magnetic resonance:
alternative term: MRI 699
Nuclear medicine 733
Nucleic acids 733
breakdown of: Uric acid 1025
as constituents of Chromosomes 279; Genes 478, 480
function of: Protein synthesis 827
and Genetic code 481
manufacture of: Vitamin B complex 1059
in Nucleus 735; Viruses 1050, 1051
types of: DNA 369; RNA 875
Nucleus 735
atomic: Nuclear energy 732; Radiation 844
cellular: Cell 245
constituents of: Chromosomes 279; Nucleic acids 733
Nucofed 1110
Numbness 735
associated with Pins and

needles sensation 796
symptom chart 734
symptom of Carpal tunnel syndrome 238; Cervical osteoarthritis 252; Multiple sclerosis 701; Raynaud's disease 853; Stroke 947; Transient ischemic attack 1005
type of Sensation, abnormal 893
Numorphan 1110
Nupercainal 1110
Nuprin 1110
Nurse 735
Nursing:
Breast-feeding 207
Nursing care 735
Nursing home 735
Nutracort 1110
Nutraplus 1110
Nutrient 736
types of: Carbohydrates 232; Fats and oils 441; Fiber, dietary 452; Minerals 689; Proteins 827; Trace elements 1001; Vitamin 1056; Water 1070
see also index entries Nutrition; Nutritional disorders
Nutrition 736
and Calorie 226; Diet and exercise 18; Energy requirements 407; Food additives 461
the four food groups and recommended daily servings 737
of infants: Feeding, infant 443
recommended daily dietary allowances (RDAs) of selected vitamins and minerals 19
see also index entries Nutrient; Nutritional disorders
Nutritional disorders 737
and Anorexia nervosa 112; Diet and disease 357; Food additives 461; Food allergy 461; Food-borne infection 461; Food fad 462; Food intolerance 462; Food poisoning 463; Malabsorption 658
examples: Alcohol-related disorders 84; Amblyopia 92; Anemia 100; Beriberi 165; Caries, dental 236; Keratomalacia 615; Kwashiorkor 623; Marasmus 664; Night blindness 727; Obesity 738; Osteomalacia 755; Pellagra 776; Rickets 874; Scurvy 888; deficiency or excess of Vitamin A 1057; deficiency of Vitamin $B_{12}$ 1058; deficiency or excess of Vitamin B complex 1058; deficiency or excess of Vitamin C 1059; deficiency or excess of Vitamin D 1059; deficiency or excess of Vitamin E 1060; deficiency of Vitamin K 1060; Wernicke-Korsakoff syndrome 1076
see also index entries Nutrient;

Nutrition
Nydrazid 1110
Nylidrin 1110
Nymphomania 737
Nystagmus 737
a disorder of the eye 431
and Vertigo 1048
Nystatin 737
Nystex 1110

# O

oat cell carcinoma:
alternative term: Small-cell carcinoma 918
Obermine 1110
Obesity 738
associated with Diabetes mellitus 349; Hiatal hernia 538
and Diet and disease 358; Weight 1073; Weight reduction 1075
feature of Pickwickian syndrome 794
Obetrol 1110
Obsessive-compulsive behavior 738
and Phobia 792; Superego 955
Obstetrician 739
Obstetrics 739
Obstructive airways disease:
Lung disease, chronic obstructive 652
occipital bone:
part of Skull 914
structure of the skull 913
occipital lobe:
part of Cerebrum 250
Occiput 739
Occlusal 1110
Occlusion 739
Occult 739
Occult blood, fecal 739
Occupational disease and injury 739
Health hazards 511
safety at work 740
Occupational medicine 740
Occupational mortality 741
Occupational therapy 741
Octoxynol 1110
Ocular 741
Oculogyric crisis 741
Oculomotor nerve 741
functions of cranial nerves 318
Ocusert 1110
Oedipus complex 741
and Psychoanalytic theory 831
Ogen 1110
Oils:
Fats and oils 441
Ointment 741
Olecranon 741
part of Elbow 393; Ulna 1019
olfactory bulb:
part of Olfactory nerve 742
Olfactory nerve 741
location of olfactory nerve 742
function of: functions of cranial nerves 318; the sense of smell 919

Oligo- 742
Oligodendroglioma 742
Oligohydramnios 742
Oligospermia 742
Oliguria 742
    and Urine, abnormal 1027
Olive oil 742
-oma 742
Omentum 742
Omeprazole 1110
Omnipen 1110
Omnipen-N 1110
omphalitis:
    infection of Umbilical cord 1021
Omphalocele 742
    alternative term: Exomphalos
    426
Onchocerciasis 742
    the cycle of onchocerciasis 743
    and disorders of the retina 867
Oncogenes 742
    in Viruses 1052
Oncologist 743
Oncology 743
Oncovin 1110
Onlay, dental 743
    use of: Restoration, dental 866
Onychogryphosis 743
Onycholysis 743
Onychosis 743
Oophorectomy 743
-opathy 744
Open heart surgery 744
Operable 744
operant conditioning:
    and Learning 631; Reflex 857
    type of Conditioning 295
Operating room 744
Operation 745
Ophthaine 1110
Ophthalmia 745
Ophthalmologist 745
Ophthalmology 745
Ophthalmoplegia 745
Ophthalmoscope 745
    use of: Eye, examination of 430
Ophthetic 1110
Ophthochlor 1110
Ophthocort 1110
Opiate 745
opiate receptors:
    and Endorphins 405
Opium 745
    solution of: Laudanum 630
Opportunistic infection 745
    examples: Fungal infections
        470; Pneumocystis
        pneumonia 803
    feature of Immunodeficiency
        disorders 575
Optic atrophy 746
    and Nystagmus 737
Optic disk edema 746
    and Papilledema 768
Optician 746
Opti-clean 1110
Optic nerve 746
    disorders of: Blindness 181;
        Optic atrophy 746; Optic disk
        edema 746; Optic neuritis
        746; Retrobulbar neuritis 868;
        Vision, disorders of 1054
    functions of: functions of the
        cranial nerves 318; Eye 429; the

sense of vision 1053; the
    visual fields 1056
Optic neuritis 746
Opticrom 1110
Optigene 3 1110
Optilets-M-500 1110
Optimine 1110
Optimyd 1110
Optometrist 746
Optometry 746
Orabase HCA 1110
Orajel 1110
Oral 746
Oral contraceptives 747
    adverse effects of: Edema 391;
        Thrombosis 981
    Contraception, hormonal
        methods 305
    methods of contraception 303
    failure rates of contraceptives 304
    in treatment of Premenstrual
        syndrome 818
Oral hygiene 748
oral phase:
    and Fixation 457
    in Psychoanalytic theory 831
Oral surgeon 748
Oral surgery 748
Oramide 1110
Orap 1110
Orasone 1110
Orazinc 1110
Orbit 748
    location of orbit 749
    part of Skull 914
Orchiectomy 749
    in treatment of Prostate, cancer
        of 825; Testis, cancer of 972
Orchiopexy 749
    in treatment of Testis,
        undescended 974
Orchitis 749
    causing Infertility 586;
        Oligospermia 742
    as complication of Pleurodynia
        802
    feature of Mumps 703
Oretic 1110
Oreticyl 1110
Oreton Methyl 1110
Organ 749
    displacement of: Prolapse 823
    framework of: Stroma 949
    preservation of:
        Cryopreservation 323
    reversed: Situs inversus 908
Organ donation 749
    and Transplant surgery 1005
organelles:
    parts of Cell 245
Organic 750
Organic brain syndrome:
    Brain syndrome, organic 204
"organic" food:
    Health food 511
Organism 750
    cloning of: Clone 284
organ transplants:
    and Organ donation 749;
        Transplant surgery 1005
Orgasm 750
    facilitation of: Pelvic floor
        exercises 777; Vibrator 1049
    and Masturbation 668; Sexual

intercourse 898, 899
    see also index entry Orgasm,
        lack of
Orgasm, lack of 750
    and Psychosexual dysfunction
        832
    treatment of: Sensate focus
        technique 891; Sex therapy
        897
    see also index entry Orgasm
Orgatrax 1110
Orinase 1110
Ornade 1110
Ornex 1110
Ornithosis 750
Orphan drugs 750
Orphenadrine 750
Ortho- 750
Orthodontic appliances 750
    how orthodontic appliances work
        751
    in treatment of Malocclusion
        661
Orthodontics 751
Orthodontist 752
Orthognathic surgery 752
    in treatment of Prognathism
        823
    type of Oral surgery 748
Ortho-Novum 1/35 1110
Ortho-Novum 1/50 1110
Ortho-Novum 7/7/7 1110
Ortho-Novum 10/11 1110
Orthopedics 752
Orthopedist 752
Orthopnea 752
Orthoptics 752
Orudis 1110
Os 752
Os-cal 1110
Osgood-Schlatter disease 752
Osmoglyn 1110
Osmosis 752
osmotic pressure:
    of Blood 182
    and Plasma proteins 801
Ossicle 752
    bones of Ear 384
    surgery on: Stapedectomy 938;
        Tympanoplasty 1016
Ossification 752
Osteitis 752
osteitis deformans:
    alternative term: Paget's
        disease 762
osteitis pubis:
    disorder of Pelvis 778
Osteo- 753
Osteoarthritis 753
    feature of: Loose bodies 649
    following Femur, fracture of
        445; Lordosis 650;
        Meniscectomy 676
    treatment of: Ibuprofen 566;
        Indomethacin 581;
        Ketoprofen 616;
        Meclofenamate 669;
        Piroxicam 796
    type of Arthritis 132
osteoblasts:
    function of: Bone 193
    and Osteopetrosis 755
Osteochondritis dissecans 753
Osteochondritis juvenilis 754

and disorders of the spine 933
    type of: Perthes' disease 787
Osteochondroma 754
osteoclastoma:
    type of Bone tumor 195
osteoclasts:
    function of: Bone 193
    and Osteopetrosis 755
Osteodystrophy 754
Osteogenesis imperfecta 754
Osteogenic sarcoma:
    Osteosarcoma 756
Osteoid osteoma 754
Osteoma 754
Osteomalacia 755
    and deficiency of Vitamin D
        1059
Osteomyelitis 755
    a disorder of the bone 194
    and disorders of the spine 933
Osteopathic medicine 755
Osteopetrosis 755
Osteophyte 755
    feature of Baseball elbow 161;
        Osteoarthritis 753
Osteoporosis 756
    diagnosis of: Densitometry 340
    and Menopause 676;
        Parathyroid glands 771;
        disorders of the spine 933
    leading to Femur, fracture of
        445
    treatment of: Estrone 422;
        Hormone replacement
        therapy 546; Vitamin
        supplements 1060
Osteosarcoma 756
Osteosclerosis 757
    alternative term: Myelosclerosis
        710
Osteotomy 757
    in treatment of Knock knee 623;
        Perthes' disease 787
Ostomy 757
Ot- 757
Otalgia 757
    common term: Earache 384
OTC 757
Otic-HC 1110
Otitis externa 757
    a disorder of the ear 385; ear
        infection 758
Otitis media 757
    complication of: Labyrinthitis
        624
    a disorder of the ear 385; ear
        infection 758
Otobiotic 1110
Otocort 1110
Otolaryngologist, head and neck
    surgeon 758
Otoplasty 758
Otorhinolaryngology 759
Otorrhea 759
    common term: Ear, discharge
        from 386
Otosclerosis 759
Otoscope 759
Ototoxicity 759
Otrivin 1110
Ouabain 1110
Outpatient treatment 759
Ovarian cyst 759
Ovary 759

**Ovary** (continued)
part of *endocrine system 403;*
Reproductive system, female
862, 863
function of: *the sources and main*
*effects of selected hormones 546*
removal of: Hysterectomy 565;
Oophorectomy 743;
Sterilization, female 940
see also index entry Ovulation
Ovary, cancer of 760
Ovcon 1110
Overbite 760
Overcrowding, dental 760
causing Malocclusion 661
over-the-counter:
OTC 757
Overuse injury 760
and Running injuries 877
Overweight:
Obesity 738
Ovral 1110
Ovrette 1110
O-V Statin 1110
Ovulation 760
failure of: Infertility 586;
Polycystic ovary 807
and *the process of fertilization*
*446;* Menstruation 677
painful: Mittelschmerz 692
suppression of: Contraception
304; Dysmenorrhea 383
Ovulen 1110
Ovum 761
and Ovulation 760
Oxacillin 761
Oxalid 1110
Oxandrolone 761
Oxazepam 761
Oxprenolol 1110
Oxsoralen 1110
Oxtriphylline 761
Oxybenzone 1110
Oxybutynin 1110
Oxycodone 761
Oxygen 761
and Breathing 209; Hemoglobin
528; Lung 650
form of: Ozone 761
insufficient: Hypoxia 564;
Mountain sickness 696;
Suffocation 953
Oxygen therapy 761
in treatment of Respiratory
failure 865
oxyhemoglobin:
in Blood cells 183
form of Hemoglobin 528
Oxymetazoline 761
Oxymetholone 1110
Oxymorphone 1110
Oxyphenbutazone 1110
Oxyphencyclimine 1110
Oxyphenonium 1110
Oxytetracycline 761
Oxytocin 761
production of: Pituitary gland
797
use of: Induction of labor 581
Ozena 761
Ozone 761
absorption of Ultraviolet light
1021
depletion of: Pollution 807

## P

P-200 1110
PABA 762
constituent of Sunscreens 955
Pabalate 1110
Pacemaker 762
and Cremation 319
interference with:
Transcutaneous electrical
nerve stimulation 1003
in treatment of Heart block 516;
Stokes-Adams syndrome 942
pacinian corpuscle:
function of: Sensation 892
*types of receptor 854*
Paget's disease 762
and Osteosarcoma 756
Paget's disease of the nipple 763
disorder of the Nipple 728
Pain 763, 764
and Endorphins 405;
Enkephalins 408;
Neurotransmitter 725
type of Sensation 892
types of: Abdominal pain 50,
*51;* Back pain 150, *253;* Chest
pain 259, *260;* Earache 384;
Facial pain 434; Headache
507, *508;* Referred pain 857;
Toothache 996
see also index entry Pain relief
Painful arc syndrome 763
and Rotator cuff 876; Tendinitis
970
Painkillers:
medical term: Analgesic drugs
97
see also index entry Pain relief
Pain relief 764
in childbirth: *pain relief in labor*
*and delivery 265*
drug methods: Analgesic drugs
97; Anesthesia, local 106;
Nonsteroidal anti-
inflammatory drugs 730
natural: Endorphins 405;
Enkephalins 408
nondrug methods:
Acupuncture 66; Cordotomy
307; Sympathectomy 959;
Transcutaneous electrical
nerve stimulation 1003
and Sports, drugs and 935
Palate 765
Palliative treatment 765
Pallor 765
palpation:
use of: Examination, physical
424
Palpitation 765
causes of: Alchohol
dependence 83; Anxiety 122;
Arrhythmia, cardiac 129;
Cardiomyopathy 236
and Ectopic heart beat 389
Palsy 765
alternative term: Paralysis 769
Pamabrom 1110
Pamelor 1110
Pamine 1110
Panacea 765

**Pancreas** 765
disorders of: Pancreas, cancer
of 766; *disorders of the pancreas*
*766;* Pancreatitis 767
imaging of: Pancreatography
767
*location of the pancreas 766*
part of Digestive system 359;
Endocrine system 402, *403*
and production of Glucagon
492; Hormones 547; *the*
*sources and main effects of*
*selected hormones 546;* Insulin
594
removal of: Pancreatectomy 767
Pancreas, cancer of 766
*a disorder of the pancreas 766*
Pancrease 1110
Pancreatectomy 767
in treatment of Pancreas,
cancer of 766; Pancreatitis 767
Pancreatin 767
Pancreatitis 767
causing Renal failure 860
*a disorder of the pancreas 766*
Pancreatography 767
methods of: CT scanning 323;
ERCP 415; Ultrasound
scanning 1019; X rays 1083
Pancrelipase 767
Pancuronium 1110
Pandemic 767
and Epidemic 410
Panic attack 768
feature of Panic disorder 768;
Phobia 792
Panic disorder 768
feature of: Panic attack 768
Panmycin 1110
Panoxyl 1110
Panoxyl AQ 1110
Panthenol 1110
Pantopon 1110
pantothenic acid:
part of Vitamin B complex 1058
Panwarfin 1110
papain:
type of Enzyme 410
Papanicolaou method:
see index entry Cervical smear
test
Papaverine 768
Papilla 768
of Tongue 995
Papilledema 768
Papilloma 768
papilloma virus:
as Carcinogen 233
causing Wart 1069; Warts,
genital 1070
Pap smear:
see index entry Cervical smear
test
Papule 768
common term: Pimple 795
feature of Acne 64
Par-/para- 768
Para-aminobenzoic acid 768
constituent of Sunscreens 955
Paracentesis 768
Paraffinoma 768
Paraflex 1111
Parafon Forte 1111
Paraldehyde 768

**Paralysis** 768
alternative term: Palsy 765
types of: Hemiplegia 528;
Paraplegia 770; Quadriplegia
842
Paralysis, periodic 769
paralytic ileus:
Ileus, paralytic 568
Paramedic 769
Paramethadione 1111
Paramethasone 1111
Paranoia 769
cause of: Sleep deprivation 916
feature of: Personality disorder
786; Psychosis 833
symptom of: Delusion 339
Paraparesis 770
type of Paralysis 768
and Walking 1068
Paraphilia:
common term: Deviation,
sexual 348
Paraphimosis 770
as complication of Phimosis 791
a disorder of the Penis 780
treatment of: Circumcision 282
Paraplegia 770
cause of: Spinal injury 930
type of Paralysis 769
parapraxia:
common term: Freudian slip
468
Parapsychology 770
Paraquat 770
type of Pesticide 788
Parasite 770, 771
Parasitology 771
Parasuicide:
Suicide, attempted 953
Parasympathetic nervous system
771
component of: Vagus nerve
1037
*functions of the autonomic nervous*
*system 146*
part of Autonomic nervous
system 147
Parathion 771
Parathyroidectomy 771
Parathyroid glands 771
disorders of:
Hyperparathyroidism 554,
*555;* Hypoparathyroidism
561; Parathyroid tumor 771
part of Endocrine system 402,
403
and production of Hormones
547; *the sources and main effects*
*of selected hormones 546*
removal of: Parathyroidectomy
771
Parathyroid tumor 771
Paratyphoid fever 772
type of Typhoid fever 1017
Paré, Ambroise:
*landmarks in surgery 33*
Paregoric 1111
Parenchyma 772
and Stroma 949
Parenteral 1111
Parenteral nutrition:
type of Feeding, artificial 443
Paresis 772
type of Paralysis 768

Paresthesia 772
  common term: Pins and
    needles sensation 796
Parietal 772
parietal lobe:
  part of Cerebrum 250
Parkinsonism 772
  feature of Shy-Drager
    syndrome 904
  see also index entry
    Parkinson's disease
Parkinson's disease 772
  a *disorder of the brain 202*
  causes of: Designer drugs 346;
    Neurotransmitter 725
  features of: Paralysis 769;
    Rigidity 875; Tremor 1008
  treatment of: Amantadine 92;
    Anticholinergic drugs 115;
    Bromocriptine 213; Levodopa
    638; Trihexyphenidyl 1011
  type of Degenerative disorder
    337
Parlodel 1111
Parmine 1111
Parnate 1111
Paromomycin 1111
Paronychia 773
Parotid glands 773
  types of Salivary glands 880
Paroxysm 773
  alternative terms: Seizure 890;
    Spasm 924
Parsidol 1111
Parturition 773
  common term: Childbirth 263
passage, blocked:
  medical term: Occlusion 739
passage, narrowed:
  medical term: Stenosis 939
Passive-aggressive personality
  disorder 773
  type of Personality disorder 786
passive smoking:
  causing Lung cancer 651
  and Tobacco smoking 992
Pasteur, Louis:
  germ theory of disease: Bacteria
    154; Bacteriology 155;
    Diagnosing disease 24;
    *landmarks in diagnosis 25;*
    Medicine 671
  and *landmarks in drug
    development 32;* Pasteurization
    774
Pasteurization 774
Patau's syndrome:
  type of Trisomy 1012
patch tests:
  and *allergy and the body 87*
  in diagnosis of Dermatitis 345
  types of Skin tests 913
Patella 774
  disorders of: Chondromalacia
    patellae 275; Jumpers' knee
    613
  part of Knee 621
Patent 774
Patent ductus arteriosus 774
  complication of: Endocarditis
    402
  leading to Heart failure 519
  type of Heart disease,
    congenital 518

Paternity testing 774
  and Blood groups 188;
    Histocompatibility antigens
    541; Serology 895
  *paternity testing using DNA
    fingerprints 775*
Pathibamate 1111
Patho- 775
Pathocil 1111
Pathogen 775
  causing Infection 581;
    Infectious disease 582
  examples of: Bacteria 153;
    Fungi 470; Protozoa 827;
    Viruses 1050
  type of Microorganism 685
Pathogenesis 775
Pathognomonic 775
Pathological 775
pathological anatomy:
  alternative term: Morbid
    anatomy 694
Pathologist 775
Pathology 775
Pathology, cellular 775
  type of Cytology 330
Pathophysiology 775
  type of Physiology 794
-pathy 775
Pavabid 1111
Pavacen 1111
Paveral 1111
Pavulon 1111
Paxipam 1111
PBZ 1111
PCNU 1111
Peak flow meter 775
  in assessment of Asthma 137;
    Bronchospasm 217
  use of: Pulmonary function
    tests 836
Peau d'orange 775
  as symptom of Breast cancer
    206; Elephantiasis 396
Pectoral 776
*pectoral muscles 776*
Pediacof 1111
Pediaflor 1111
Pediamycin 1111
Pediatrician 776
  and Neonatologist 717
Pediatrics 776
  branch of Neonatology 718
Pediazole 1111
Pedicle 776
Pediculosis 776
  infestation with Lice 638; Pubic
    lice 835
Pedophilia 776
Peduncle 776
peer groups:
  in Adolescence 69
  and Behavior problems in
    children 162
Peer review 776
Peganone 1111
Pellagra 776
  cause of: deficiency of Vitamin
    B complex 1058
pelvic colon:
  alternative term: Sigmoid colon
    905
Pelvic examination 776
  in investigation of *disorders of*

the cervix 255; Pelvic
    inflammatory disease 777
  *procedure for pelvic examination
    777*
Pelvic floor exercises 777
  in prevention of Uterus,
    prolapse of 1032
  in treatment of Incontinence,
    urinary 580
Pelvic infection 777
  see also index entry Pelvic
    inflammatory disease
Pelvic inflammatory disease 777
  causes of: Chlamydial
    infections 270; Gonorrhea
    495; IUD 609
  causing Abdominal pain 54;
    Ectopic pregnancy 389;
    Infertility 586; Intercourse,
    painful 598
Pelvic pain:
  type of Abdominal pain 50
Pelvimetry 777
Pelvis 777
  assessment of: Pelvimetry 777
  and Childbirth, complications
    of 265
  components of: Coccyx 286;
    Sacrum 878
  part of Abdomen 50; Skeleton
    909; *bones of the skeleton 908*
Pemoline 778
Pemphigoid 778
  a *disorder of the skin 910*
Pemphigus 778
  a *disorder of the skin 910*
Penapar VK 1111
Penbutolol 1111
Penecort 1111
Penfluridol 1111
Penicillamine 779
Penicillin drugs 779
  discovery of: *landmarks in drug
    development 32;* Antibacterials
    and antibiotics 36
  effect on Bacteria 154
  group of Antibiotic drugs 114
  in treatment of Infectious
    disease 584, 585
Penicillin V 1111
Penile implant 779
  and Sex change 896
  in treatment of Impotence 578
Penile warts:
  type of Warts, genital 1070
Penis 778
  and Circumcision 282;
    Intercourse, painful 598;
    *painful intercourse in men 596*
  functions of: Ejaculation 392;
    Erection 415; Sexual
    intercourse 898, 899
  part of Reproductive system,
    male 862, *863*
  parts of: Foreskin 466; Urethra
    1023; *location of the urethra
    1024*
Penis, cancer of 780
  associated with Smegma 918
Penntuss 1111
Pentaerythritol 1111
Pentamidine 1111
Pentazocine 780
Pentids 1111

Pentobarbital 780
Pentostatin 1111
Pentothal 1111
Pentoxifylline 780
Pentrax 1111
Pen-Vee K 1111
Pepcid 1111
Peppermint oil 780
pepsin:
  in Stomach 943
Peptic ulcer 780
  causing Peritonitis 785; Pyloric
    stenosis 841
  *sites and causes of peptic ulcer 781*
  perforated: Abdomen, acute 50
  recurrent: Zollinger-Ellison
    syndrome 1088
  a *disorder of the stomach 943*
  treatment of: Antacid drugs
    113; Gastrectomy 475; Ulcer-
    healing drugs 1018;
    Vagotomy 1036
Peptide 782
  as constituent of Proteins 827
  constituent of: Amino acids 94
Pepto Bismol 1111
Perception 782
  false: Hallucination 504
Percocet 1111
Percodan 1111
Percogesic 1111
Percorten 1111
Percussion 782
  use of: Examination, physical
    424; *types of physical
    examination 425*
Percutaneous 782
*percutaneous renal biopsy 860*
Perdiem 1111
Perforation 782
Pergolide 1111
Pergonal 1111
Peri- 782
Periactin 1111
Periarteritis nodosa 782
  type of Arteritis 131
Pericarditis 782
  associated with Dialysis 354;
    Lupus erythematosus 653;
    Pleurodynia 802; Rheumatoid
    arthritis 871
Pericardium 783
  part of Heart 514
Peri-Colace 1111
Perimetry 783
Perinatal 783
Perinatologist 783
Perinatology 783
Perineum 783
  incision in: Episiotomy 414
Periodic fever 783
  alternative term: Familial
    Mediterranean fever 439
Periodontal disease 783
Periodontics 783
Periodontitis 783
  causing Toothache 997
  as complication of Gingivitis
    487
  treatment of: Curettage, dental
    325
periodontium:
  inflammation of: Periodontitis
    783

Period pain:
    medical term: Dysmenorrhea
        383
periods:
    medical term: Menstruation 677
    see also index entries
        Menstruation, disorders of;
        Menstruation, irregular
Periosteum 784
    inflammation of: Periostitis 784
    part of Bone 192
Periostitis 784
    causing Shin splints 901
Peripheral nervous system 784
    components of: Cranial nerves
        318; Spinal nerves 931
    disorders of: Neuropathy 723
        and Nerve 719
    part of *nervous system 721*
Peripheral vascular disease 784
    causing Leg ulcer 633
    and Tobacco smoking 992
    treatment of: Angioplasty,
        balloon 110; Isoxsuprine 608;
        Papaverine 768;
        Pentoxifylline 780;
        Vasodilator drugs 1041
Peristalsis 785
    in Digestive system 359;
        Esophagus 420; Intestine 601;
        Ureter 1023
    and Muscle 706
    stimulation of: Vagus nerve
        1037
Peritoneal dialysis:
    type of Dialysis 354
Peritoneum 785
    inflammation of: Peritonitis 785
    part of Abdomen 50
Peritonitis 785
    causing Ileus, paralytic 568;
        Shock 901
    as complication of Appendicitis
        127; Dialysis 354; Peptic ulcer
        780; Puerperal sepsis 836;
        Typhoid fever 1017
Peritonsillar abscess:
    alternative term: Quinsy
Peritrate 1111
Permanent teeth 786
    and Eruption of teeth 416;
        *structure and arrangement of
        teeth 967*
Permapen 1111
Permethrim 1111
Permitil 1111
Pernicious anemia 786
    cause of: deficiency of Vitamin
        B$_{12}$ 1058
    causing Dementia 339
    feature of: Achlorhydria 62
    a *disorder of the stomach 943*
    type of Anemia, megaloblastic
        103; Autoimmune disorder
        145
Pernio 786
Peroneal muscular atrophy 786
    type of Neuropathy 724
Perphenazine 786
Persa-Gel 1111
Persantine 1111
persecution:
    and Delusion 339; Paranoia 769
Personal health care 18

Personality 786
    assessment of: Personality tests
        787
    changes in: Dementia 339;
        Personality disorders 786
    and Intelligence 594
    theories of: Freudian theory
        468; Jungian theory 613;
        Psychoanalytic theory 831
Personality disorders 786
    and Suicide 953; Suicide,
        attempted 954
    treatment of: Psychoanalysis
        831; Psychotherapy 833
Personality tests 787
Perspiration 787
    production of: Sweat glands
        958
Perthes' disease 787
    type of Osteochondritis
        juvenilis 754
    and Walking 1067
Pertofrane 1111
Pertussin 1111
Pertussis 787
    prevention of: DPT vaccination
        373; Immunization 571;
        *typical childhood immunization
        schedule 574*
Peruvian balsam 1111
Perversion:
    alternative term: Deviation,
        sexual 348
Pes cavus:
    common term: Clawfoot 283
pes planus:
    common term: Flatfoot 458
Pessary 788
    in treatment of Uterus,
        prolapse of 1032
Pesticides 788
    causing Pollution 807
Petechiae 788
    feature of Purpura 839;
        Radiation sickness 846
Petit mal 788
    type of Epilepsy 413
Petrogalar 1111
Petrolatum 1111
Petroleum jelly 788
PET scanning 25, 29, 788
    type of Imaging technique 570
    use of: Brain imaging 203
Peutz-Jeghers syndrome 788
Peyote 788
    source of Mescaline 681
Peyronie's disease 788
Pfizerpen VK 1111
pH 788
    see also index entry Acid-base
        balance
Phagocyte 789
    and Immunoglobulins 576
    part of Immune system 571; *the
        innate immune system 572*
    in Spleen 933
    type of Blood cell 183
Phalanges 789
    part of Finger 455; Foot 463; *the
        skeleton of the foot 464; the
        skeletal structure of the hand
        and wrist 506; Skeleton 909; the
        bones of the skeleton 908; Toe
        993; anatomy of the toes 994*

Phallus 789
    see also index entry Penis
Phantom limb 789
    following Amputation 96
Pharmaceutical 789
    see also index entry Drug
Pharmacist 789
Pharmacokinetics 789
Pharmacologist 789
Pharmacology 789
Pharmacopeia 789
Pharmacy 789
pharyngeal pouch:
    type of Esophageal
        diverticulum 418
Pharyngitis 789
    a disorder of the Pharynx 789
    symptom of: Sore throat 924
Pharyngoesophageal
        diverticulum 789
    alternative term: Esophageal
        diverticulum 418
    causing Swallowing difficulty
        958
    a disorder of the Pharynx 790
Pharynx 789
    common term: Throat 980
    disorders of: Pharyngitis 789;
        Pharynx, cancer of 790
    part of: Nasopharynx 716
    *location of the pharynx 790*
Pharynx, cancer of 790
Phazyme 1111
Phenacemide 1111
Phenaphen 1111
Phenazine 1111
Phenazopyridine 790
phencyclidine:
    common term: Angel dust 108
Phenelzine 790
Phenergan 1111
Phenergan D 1111
Phenformin 1111
Phenindamine 1111
Pheniramine 1111
Phenobarbital 790
Phenol 1111
Phenolphthalein 1111
Phenothiazine drugs 790
    causing *disorders of the retina 867*
    examples: Perphenazine 786;
        Prochlorperazine 822;
        Promazine 823
Phenoxybenzamine 1111
Phenprocoumon 1111
Phensuximide 1111
Phentermine 790
Phentolamine 1111
Phenurone 1111
phenylalanine:
    causing Phenylketonuria 791
    detection of: Guthrie test 502
Phenylbutazone 790
Phenylephrine 791
Phenylketonuria 791
    causing Mental retardation 678;
        Short stature 902
    diagnosis of: Guthrie test 502
    and Pigmentation 794
    type of Metabolism, inborn
        errors of 682
Phenylpropanolamine 791
Phenyltoloxamine 1111
Phenytoin 791

Pheochromocytoma 791
Pheromone 791
Phimosis 791
    causing Urine retention 1029
    complication of: Paraphimosis
        770
    a disorder of the Penis 780
phisoHex 1111
Phlebitis 791
    alternative term:
        Thrombophlebitis 981
Phlebography 792
    alternative term: Venography
        1044
Phlebotomy 792
    alternative term: Venesection
        1044
Phlegm:
    historic usage: Humors 548
    medical term: Sputum 936
Phobia 792
    causing Panic attack 768
    treatment of: Behavior therapy
        163
Phocomelia 792
    type of Limb defect 640
Phosphates 792
    type of Ion 605
Phospholine Iodide 1111
phospholipids:
    types of Fats and oils 442;
        Lipids 642
Phosphorus poisoning 792
Photocoagulation 793
Photophobia 793
    feature of Conjunctivitis 297;
        Corneal abrasion 307;
        Keratitis 614
Photosensitivity 793
    following Skin peeling,
        chemical 913
    and Pigmentation 795
    a *disorder of the skin 910*
Phototherapy 793
    in treatment of Psoriasis 830;
        Vitiligo 1060
    type of: PUVA 839
Phrenic nerve 793
Phrenilin 1111
Phyllocontin 1111
Physical constraints 47
Physical examination:
    Examination, physical 424
Physical medicine and
        rehabilitation 793
Physical therapy 793
    *techniques of physical therapy 794*
Physician 793
Physiology 794
Physiotherapy:
    alternative term: Physical
        therapy 793
physique:
    medical term: Somatotype 923
Physostigmine 794
Phytonadione 794
Piaget, Jean:
    and developmental Psychology
        832
Pica 794
    feature of Pregnancy 813
Pickwickian syndrome 794
PID:
    abbreviation for Pelvic

inflammatory disease 777
Pigeon toes 794
Pigmentation 794
Piles 795
    medical term: Hemorrhoids 530
Pill, birth-control:
    see index entry Oral
    contraceptives
Pilocarpine 795
Pilocel 1111
Pilonidal sinus 795
Pilopine HS Gel 1111
Pimozide 795
Pimple 795
Pincus, Gregory:
    landmarks in drug development 32
Pindolol 795
Pineal gland 795
Pinguecula 795
Pinkeye 795
    medical term: Conjunctivitis
    297
Pink puffer 795
    and Emphysema 400
Pinna 795
    part of Ear 384
Pins and needles sensation 796
    type of Sensation, abnormal
    893
Pinta 796
Pinworm infestation 796
Piperacillin 1111
Piperazine 796
    in treatment of Ascariasis 136
Piperonyl butoxide 1111
Pipracil 1111
Pirenzepine 1111
Pirmenol 1111
Piroxicam 796
pitchblende:
    source of Radium 848; Uranium
    1022
Pitocin 1111
Pitressin 1111
Pituitary gland 796
    disorders of: disorders of the
    pituitary gland 797; Pituitary
    tumors 797
    function of: the sources and main
    effects of selected hormones 546;
    hormones secreted by the
    pituitary gland 797
    and Hypothalamus 562
    part of Brain 199; endocrine
    system 403
    removal of: Hypophysectomy
    561
Pituitary tumors 797
    causing Galactorrhea 472;
    Tunnel vision 1015
    diagnosis of: Skull X ray 914
    treatment of: Hypophysectomy
    561
    type of Brain tumor 204
    type of: Prolactinoma 823
Pityriasis alba 798
    and Pigmentation 794
Pityriasis rosea 798
pityriasis versicolor:
    alternative term: Tinea
    versicolor 989
PKU test:
    alternative term: Guthrie test
    502

Placebo 798
    and Drug 377; Trial, clinical
    1008
Placenta 798
    and stages of birth 264;
    Childbirth 265; Chorionic
    villus sampling 276;
    Intrauterine growth
    retardation 603
    development of: Embryo 397;
    the developing embryo 398; the
    process of fertilization 446;
    Implantation, egg 578;
    Pregnancy 813
    functions of: Fetal circulation
    447; the sources and main effects
    of selected hormones 546; effects
    of hormones during pregnancy
    815
    position of: Ultrasound
    scanning 1019
Placenta previa 799
Placidyl 1111
Plague 799
    transmission of: Rats, diseases
    from 853
Plantar wart 799
    type of Wart 1069
Plants, poisonous 800
Plaque 800
    and Atherosclerosis 140; arterial
    degeneration in atherosclerosis
    141; diet and atherosclerosis 20
Plaque, dental 800
    causing Calculus, dental 224;
    Caries, dental 236; Gingivitis
    487; Periodontitis 783
    detection of: Dental
    examination 342; Disclosing
    agents 362
    development of plaque 801
    removal of: Floss, dental 459;
    Oral hygiene 748;
    Toothbrushing 997
Plaquenil 1111
Plasma 800
    constituents of: Plasma
    proteins 801
    exchange of: Plasmapheresis
    800
    part of Blood 182; constituent of
    blood 183
    use of: Bleeding, treatment of
    179
Plasmapheresis 800
    in treatment of Purpura 839
Plasma proteins 801
Plasminogen activator:
    alternative term: Tissue
    plasminogen activator 989
Plaster of Paris 801
    use of: Cast 239; fractures: types
    and treatment 467
Plastic surgeon 801
Plastic surgery 801
-plasty 801
Platelet 801
    as constituent of blood 183
    deficiency of: Bleeding
    disorders 178; Purpura 839;
    Thrombocytopenia 980
    function of: Blood clotting 185;
    Hemostasis 531
    type of Blood cell 184

Platinol 1111
Platyhelminth 801
    causing Tapeworm infestation
    964; Worm infestation 1081
    common term: Flatworm 458
Play therapy 801
Plegine 1111
Plethora 801
Plethysmography 801
    in diagnosis of Peripheral
    vascular disease 785
Pleura 802
    and Lung 651
Pleural effusion 802
    as complication of Pneumonia
    803; Tuberculosis 1014
    feature of Lung cancer 651
Pleurisy 802
    associated with Pneumonia 803
Pleurodynia 802
    causing Pleurisy 802
    type of Myositis 713
Plexus 802
    examples: Brachial plexus 198;
    Solar plexus 923
Plicamycin 1111
Plication 802
Plummer-Vinson syndrome 802
Plutonium 802
    source of Radiation 844
PMS:
    Premenstrual syndrome 818
Pneumaturia 802
Pneumo- 802
Pneumoconiosis 802
    causing Occupational mortality
    741
    and safety at work 740
    type of Dust disease 381;
    Occupational disease and
    injury 739
Pneumocystis pneumonia 803
    feature of AIDS 76;
    Immunodeficiency disorders
    575
    type of Opportunistic infection
    746
Pneumonectomy 803
    in treatment of Lung cancer 651
Pneumonia 803, 804
    causing Pleurisy 802
    as complication of Pertussis 787
    a disorder of the lung 652
    types of: Legionnaires' disease
    632; Pneumocystis
    pneumonia 803
Pneumonitis 804
Pneumothorax 804
    as complication of Tuberculosis
    1014
    a disorder of the lung 652
    and Pleura 802
Pocket, gingival:
    cause of: Periodontitis 783
Podiatrist 805
Podiatry 805
Podophyllin 805
    in treatment of Warts, genital
    1070
Poison 805
Poisoning 805
    as method of Suicide 953
    treatment of: Antidote 117;
    Antivenin 120; Charcoal 258;

Lavage, gastric 630
Poison ivy:
    type of Plant, poisonous 800
poison oak:
    type of Plant, poisonous 800
poison sumac:
    type of Plant, poisonous 800
Polaramine 1111
Polio:
    abbreviation for Poliomyelitis
    806
Poliomyelitis 806
    causing Leg, shortening of 633;
    Paralysis 769
    effect on Walking 1067
    prevention of: Immunization
    571; typical childhood
    immunization schedule 574;
    Vaccine 1034
    type of Myelitis 710
pollen:
    and Allergy 86; allergy and the
    body 87; Rhinitis, allergic 872
Pollution 807
Poly- 807
Polyarteritis nodosa:
    alternative term: Periarteritis
    nodosa 782
Polycarbophil calcium 1111
Polycillin 1111
Polycystic disease of the kidney:
    Kidney, polycystic 619
Polycystic ovary 807
Polycythemia 807
    a disorder of the blood 186
    causing Plethora 801
    treatment of: Venesection 1044
Polydactyly 808
Polydipsia 808
    common term: Thirst, excessive
    979
Polyestradiol 1111
Polyethylene glycol 1112
Poly-Histine CS 1112
Poly-Histine D 1112
Poly-Histine DM 1112
Polyhydramnios:
    alternative term: Hydramnios
    549
polymorphonuclear leukocyte:
    type of Blood cell 183
Polymox 1112
Polymyalgia rheumatica 808
    associated with Temporal
    arteritis 968
Polymyositis 808
    causing Rhabdomyolysis 869
    type of Myositis 713
Polymyxins 808
polyneuritis:
    type of Neuropathy 724
polyneuropathy:
    type of Neuropathy 724
Polyp 808
Polypeptide 808
    constituent of: Amino acids 94
    type of Peptide 782
Polypharmacy 808
polyploidy:
    type of Chromosomal
    abnormality 277
polyposis coli:
    alternative term: Polyposis,
    familial 808

Polyposis, familial 808
  complication of: Intestine,
    cancer of 601
  treatment of: Colectomy 288
Poly-Pred 1112
polysaccharide:
  type of Carbohydrate 232
Polythiazide 1112
polyunsaturated fats:
  and Diet and disease 357
  in treatment of Xanthomatosis
    1083
  types of Fats and oils 442
Polyuria:
  common term: Urination,
    excessive 1026
Poly-Vi-Flor 1112
Polyvinyl alcohol 1112
Poly-Vi-Sol 1112
Pompholyx 808
Pondimin 1112
Pons 808
  part of Brain stem 203
Ponstel 1112
Pontocaine 1112
population growth:
  and Birth control 172
Pore 809
Porphyria 809
  features of: Photosensitivity
    793; Urine, abnormal 1029
portal circulation:
  and Liver 644
  part of Circulatory system 282
Portal hypertension 809
  cause of: Cirrhosis 282
  leading to Esophageal varices
    419
  a disorder of the liver 646
Port-wine stain 810
  type of Hemangioma 526;
    Nevus 726
Positron emission tomography
  (PET):
  see index entry PET scanning
Postcoital contraception:
  Contraception, postcoital 306
Posterior 810
  alternative term: Dorsal 371
postinfarction syndrome:
  alternative term: Dressler's
    syndrome 374
Postmaturity 810
Postmortem examination 810
  alternative term: Autopsy 147
Postmyocardial infarction
  syndrome 810
  alternative name: Dressler's
    syndrome 374
Postnasal drip 810
Postnatal care 810
Postnatal depression:
  alternative term: Postpartum
    depression 810
Postpartum depression 810
Postpartum hemorrhage 811
  causing Maternal mortality 668
Post-traumatic stress disorder 811
Postural drainage 811
  in treatment of Bronchiectasis
    214
Postural hypotension:
  type of Hypotension 561
Posture (body) 812

Posture (drug) 1112
Potassium 812
  deficiency of: disorders of muscle
    705; Paralysis, periodic 769;
    Tetany 975
  sources of: minerals and main
    food sources 690
  type of Ion 605; Mineral 689
Potassium chloride 1112
Potassium citrate 1112
Potassium clavulanate 1112
Potassium gluconate 1112
Potassium iodide 1112
Potassium permanganate 812
Potency 812
  of Drug 376
Pott's fracture 812
  affecting Ankle joint 111; Fibula
    454; Tibia 988
Poultice 812
Povan 1112
Povidone-iodine 1112
Pox 812
  alternative term: Syphilis 961
Pragmatar 1112
Pralidoxime 1112
Pramet 1112
Pramilet 1112
Pramosone 1112
Pramoxine 1112
Prax 1112
Praziquantel 812
Prazosin 812
Precancerous 812
  and Cervix, cancer of 254
Precef 1112
Pred Forte 1112
Predisposing factors 813
Pred Mild 1112
Prednisolone 813
Prednisone 813
Preeclampsia 813
  alternative term: Toxemia of
    pregnancy 998
  leading to Eclampsia 388
  type of Toxemia 998
Prefrin 1112
Pregnancy 813
  and Braxton Hicks' contractions
    205; Cervical incompetence
    252; Genetic counseling 40,
    481; Pregnancy, false 815;
    Pregnancy, multiple 815, 816;
    Prenatal technology 40-43;
    Prepared childbirth 818; Stria
    946, 947; Twins 1016;
    Vomiting in pregnancy 1065
  causing Abdominal swelling 55;
    Menstruation, irregular 678
  complications of: Antepartum
    hemorrhage 113; Diabetic
    pregnancy 251; Ectopic
    pregnancy 389; Hydramnios
    549; Miscarriage 690; types of
    miscarriage 691; Placenta
    previa 799; Postmaturity 810;
    Preeclampsia 813;
    Prematurity 817; Pulmonary
    embolism 836; Pyelonephritis
    840; Rh incompatibility 871;
    how Rh incompatibility occurs
    872; Varicose veins 1038
  confirmation of: Pregnancy
    tests 816

risks during: alcohol and
    pregnancy 83; Pregnancy
    drugs in 814; Tobacco
    smoking 992
  stages of: Embryo 397; the
    developing embryo 398;
    Fertilization 447; the process of
    fertilization 446; Fetus 448;
    development of the fetus 449;
    effects of hormones during
    pregnancy 816; stages and
    features of pregnancy 814
  tests during: Amniocentesis 42,
    95; Chorionic villus sampling
    42, 276; Fetal heart
    monitoring 448; Fetoscopy
    42, 448; Prenatal care 818;
    prenatal screening procedures
    819; Ultrasound scanning 41,
    1019; how ultrasound scanning
    works 1020
  termination of: Abortion,
    elective 57
  see also index entry Childbirth
Pregnancy, drugs in 814
  and alcohol and pregnancy 83;
    Tobacco smoking 992;
    Teratogen 971
Pregnancy, false 815
Pregnancy, multiple 815, 816
  diagnosis of: Ultrasound
    scanning 1019
  leading to Prematurity 817
  and Twins 1016
Pregnancy tests 816
Pregnyl 1112
Prelone 1112
Prelu-2 1112
Preludin 1112
Premarin 1112
Premature ejaculation:
  Ejaculation, disorders of 393
Prematurity 817
  feature of Pregnancy, multiple
    816
  and Respiratory distress
    syndrome 865
  treatment of: Incubator 39, 580;
    Ventilation 1045
Premedication 818
  and Sedation 890
Premenstrual syndrome 818
  treatment of: Metolazone 684;
    Progesterone drugs 823;
    Vitamin supplements 1060
Premolar 818
  and Eruption of teeth 416;
    Permanent teeth 786;
    structure and arrangement of
    teeth 967; tooth eruption 417
Prenalterol 1112
Prenatal care 818
  prenatal screening procedures 819
  see also index entry Pregnancy
Prenatal diagnosis 41
Prenatal technology 40
Prenatal treatment 43
Prenate 90 1112
Prepared childbirth 818
  and Relaxation techniques 859
Prepuce:
  common term: Foreskin 466
Presalin 1112
Presbycusis 819

associated with Tinnitus 989
  a disorder of the ear 385
  type of Deafness 333
Presbyopia 820
  a disorder of the eye 431
Prescription 820
Preservative 820
  type of Food additive 461
pressure measurement:
  scientific term: Manometry 664
Pressure points 820
Pressure sores 820
  alternative term: Bedsores 162
Prevalence 820
  and Incidence 579
  prevalence of various chronic
    conditions in the US 821
Preventive dentistry 820
  and Oral hygiene 748; Public
    health dentistry 835
Preventive medicine 22-23, 820
Priapism 821
  cause of: Testosterone 974
  feature of Leukemia, chronic
    myeloid 637
  a disorder of the Penis 780
Prickly heat 821
  causes of: disorders of the skin
    910; Sweat glands 958
Prilocaine 1112
Primaquine 821
Primary 821
  and Secondary 889
Primary teeth 822
  and Eruption of teeth 416;
    Teeth 966; Teething 966; tooth
    eruption 417
Primatene Mist 1112
Primaxin 1112
Primidone 822
primigravida:
  Gravida 498
Primodone 822
Principen 1112
Pro-Banthine 1112
Probenecid 822
Probucol 822
Procainamide 822
Procaine 822
Procan SR 1112
Procarbazine 822
Procardia 1112
Prochlor-Iso 1112
Prochlorperazine 822
Procidentia 822
  and Uterus, prolapse of 1032
Proctalgia fugax 822
Proctitis 822
  associated with Gay bowel
    syndrome 478
  causing Rectal bleeding 855
  treatment of: Suppository 956
Proctocort 1112
Proctofoam HC 1112
Proctoscopy 822
  in diagnosis of Hemorrhoids
    530; Proctitis 822
  and Sigmoidoscopy 906
Procyclidine 822
Prodrome 822
Progens 1112
Progeria 822
Progestasert 1112
Progesterone drugs 823

constituent of Oral
contraceptives 747
examples:
Hydroxyprogesterone 551;
Levonorgestrel 638;
Medroxyprogesterone 671;
Megestrol 672;
Norethindrone 731;
Norgestrol 731
use of: Hormone replacement
therapy 546
Progesterone hormone 823
function of: *the sources and main
effects of selected hormones 546;
effects of hormones during
pregnancy 815*
production of: Ovary 759;
Placenta 798
type of Sex hormone 897
Progestin 823
alternative terms: Progesterone
drugs 823; Progesterone
hormone 823
Proglycem 1112
Prognathism 823
*types of malocclusion 661*
Prognosis 823
Progressive muscular atrophy 823
type of Motor neuron disease
696
Progynon 1112
Pro-Iso 1112
prolactin:
excess of: Prolactinoma 823
production of: Pituitary gland
797
Prolactinoma 823
Prolamine 1112
Prolapse 823
types of: Disk prolapse 364;
Rectal prolapse 855; Uterus,
prolapse of 1032
Prolixin 1112
Proloprim 1112
Promazine 823
Promethazine 823
Promist 1112
Prompt 1112
Pronation 824
Pronestyl-SR 1112
Propacet 100 1112
Propafenone 1112
Propantheline 824
Prophene 65 1112
Prophylactic 824
Propine 1112
Propoxyphene 824
Propranolol 824
Proprietary 824
and Generic drug 481
Proprioception 824
and Balance 156; Sensation 892
Proptosis 824
alternative term: Exophthalmos
426
Propylene glycol 1112
Propylhexedrine 1112
Propylthiouracil 824
Prorex 1112
ProSobee 1112
Prostaglandin 824
and Selenium 890
excess production of: *disorders
of the uterus 1031*

Prostaglandin drugs 824
uses of: Abortifacient 57;
Induction of labor 581
Prostaphlin 1112
Prostate, cancer of 824
treatment of: Diethylstilbestrol
359; Hypophysectomy 561;
Orchiectomy 749;
Prostatectomy 825, *826*
Prostatectomy 825, *826*
in treatment of Prostate, cancer
of 824; Prostate, enlarged 825
Prostate, enlarged 825
causing Hydronephrosis 551;
Incontinence, urinary 580;
Irritable bladder 606;
Nocturia 729; Renal failure
860; Urinary tract infection
1026; Urine retention 1029
treatment of: Prostatectomy
825, 826
Prostate gland 825
inflammation of: Prostatitis 827
part of Reproductive system,
male 862
Prostatism 826
and Prostate, enlarged 825
Prostatitis 827
causing Hematuria 527
as complication of Nonspecific
urethritis 730
treatment of: Flavoxate 458;
Trimethoprim 1011
Prosthesis 827
Prosthodontics 827
Prostigmin 1112
Prostine/15M 1112
Prostin VR 1112
Proteins 827
abnormal: Genetic disorders
482
analysis of: Electrophoresis 396;
*protein analysis 30*
constituents of: Amino acids
94; Peptide 782
dietary: Nutrition 736;
Vegetarianism 1042
dietary deficiency of:
Kwashiorkor 623; Marasmus
664; Nutritional disorders 737
types of: Albumin 81; Antibody
115; Enzyme 410; Globulin
490; Immunoglobulins 575;
Plasma proteins 801
in urine: Albuminuria 81;
Proteinuria 827
see also index entry Protein
synthesis
Protein synthesis 827
and Genetic code 481; *what
genes are and what they do 480;
steps in protein synthesis 828*
Proteinuria 827
cause of: Nephrotic syndrome
719
in pregnancy: Preeclampsia 813
type of: Albuminuria 81
protons:
and Radiation 844
Protoplasm 827
Protostat 1112
Protozoa 827
causing Infectious disease 583;
*protozoal infections 585*

types of Microorganism 685
Protriptyline 828
Protropin 1112
Proventil 1112
Provera 1112
Proximal 828
Prurigo 828
Pruritus 828
common term: Itching 608
pruritus ani:
*a disorder of the anus 121*
type of Itching 608
pruritus vulvae:
common term: Vaginal itching
1035
type of Itching 609
Pseud-/pseudo 828
Pseudarthrosis 828
Pseudo Bid 1112
Pseudocyesis:
common term: Pregnancy, false
815
Pseudodementia 829
Pseudoephedrine 829
Pseudoepidemic 829
and Sick building syndrome
904
Pseudogout 829
Pseudohermaphroditism 829
and Hermaphroditism 534
type of: Testicular feminization
syndrome 971
Pseudohist 1112
Psilocybin 829
type of Hallucinogenic drug
505
Psittacosis 829
treatment of: Oxytetracycline
761
type of Ornithosis 750
Psoas muscle 829
Psoralen drugs 829
use of: Phototherapy 793;
PUVA 839
Psoriasis 830
effect on Pigmentation 794
*a disorder of the skin 910*
treatment of: Anthralin 113;
Methotrexate 683;
Methoxsalen 683;
Phototherapy 793;
Prednisolone 813; PUVA 839
Psorigel 1112
Psych- 830
Psyche 830
Psychedelic drugs 830
alternative term:
Hallucinogenic drugs 504
Psychiatric treatment 39
types of: Behavior therapy 163;
Psychoanalysis 830;
Psychotherapy 833
Psychiatrist 830
Psychiatry 830
Psychoanalysis 830
basis of: Freudian theory 468;
Psychoanalytic theory 831
and Dream analysis 373;
Resistance 863; Transference
1004
in treatment of Obsessive-
compulsive behavior 739;
Personality disorders 786
type of Psychotherapy 833

Psychoanalyst 831
and Psychoanalysis 830
Psychoanalytic theory 831
associated with Freudian
theory 468
basis of Psychoanalysis 830
and Oedipus complex 741
Psychodrama 832
Psychogenic 832
Psychologist 832
Psychology 832
Psychometry 832
types of: Intelligence tests 595;
Personality tests 787
Psychoneurosis 832
alternative term: Neurosis 725
Psychopathology 832
Psychopathy 832
modern term: Antisocial
personality disorder 119
Psychopharmacology 832
Psychosexual disorders 832
see also index entry Sexual
problems
Psychosexual dysfunction 832
see also index entry Sexual
problems
Psychosis 833
causes of: Designer drugs 346;
LSD 650; Postpartum
depression 810
common terms: Insanity 591;
Mental illness 678
treatment of: Antipsychotic
drugs 119; Psychoanalysis
831
Psychosomatic 833
Psychosurgery 833
Psychotherapist 833
Psychotherapy 833
in treatment of Depression 344;
Panic disorder 768;
Personality disorders 786;
Schizophrenia 884
Psychotropic drugs 834
Psyllium 834
Pterygium 834
Ptomaine poisoning 834
alternative term: Food
poisoning 463
Ptosis 834
Ptyalism 834
Puberty 834
and Adolescence 69; Growth,
childhood 499; Menstruation
677; *changes of puberty 835*;
Sexual characteristics,
secondary 898
Pubes 835
Pubic lice 835
pubis:
part of Pelvis 778
Public health 835
and Preventive medicine 820
Public health dentistry 835
Pudenda:
alternative term: Genitalia
485
Pudendal block 835
type of Nerve block 719
Puerperal sepsis 835
and Postnatal care 810
Puerperium 836
Pulmonary 836

pulmonary circulation:
part of Circulatory system 280, 281
pulmonary edema:
cause of: Heart failure 519
type of Edema 391
Pulmonary embolism 836
causing Pulmonary hypertension 837; Shock 901
complication of Thrombosis, deep vein 982
a *disorder of the lung 652*
type of Embolism 396
Pulmonary fibrosis 836
type of: Interstitial pulmonary fibrosis 599
Pulmonary function tests 836
type of: Spirometry 932
using Peak flow meter 775
Pulmonary hypertension 836, 837
causing Heart failure 519; Pulmonary insufficiency 837
complication of Bronchitis 215; Emphysema 400; Septal defect 894
Pulmonary insufficiency 837
Pulmonary stenosis 837
causing Heart failure 519
a *type of congenital heart disorder 518*
Pulp, dental 838
Pulpectomy 838
in Root-canal treatment 875
Pulpotomy 838
Pulse 838
abnormal: Arrhythmia, cardiac 130; Palpitation 765
as measure of Heart rate 520
weak: Shock 901
Pump, infusion 838
Pump, insulin 838
pump oxygenator:
alternative term: Heart-lung machine 520
punch biopsy:
a *biopsy of the cervix 254*
following Cervical smear test 253
Punchdrunk 838
following Concussion 295
punch grafting:
type of Hair transplant 504
Pupil 838
constriction of: Miosis 690
dilation of: Mydriasis 709
part of Eye 429; Iris 606
*location of the pupil 839*
Purinethol 1112
Purodigin 1112
Purpura 839
cause of: Thrombocytopenia 980
causing Petechiae 788
feature of Bleeding disorders 178
type of: Schonlein-Henoch purpura 885
Purulent 839
Pus 839
collection of: Abscess 58; Boil 191; Pustule 839
formation of: Sepsis 894; Suppuration 956
symptom of Infection 581

Pustule 839
alternative term: Pimple 795
PUVA 839
in treatment of Mycosis fungoides 709; Psoriasis 830; Vitiligo 1060
type of Phototherapy 793
P.V. Carpine 1112
P-V-Tussin 1112
Pyelitis:
alternative term: Pyelonephritis 840
Pyelography 839
in investigation of Calculus, urinary tract 225; *disorders of the kidney 618*; Urinary tract infection 1026
type of Imaging technique 568; Kidney imaging 619
types of: *intravenous pyelogram 569*; *retrograde pyelogram 840*
Pyelolithotomy 840
Pyelonephritis 840
a *disorder of the kidney 618*
pyknic body type:
associated with Cyclothymia 327
and Somatotype 924
pyloric sphincter:
disorder of: Pyloric stenosis 840
part of Stomach 943; *location of the stomach 942*
type of Sphincter 927
Pyloric stenosis 840
complication of Peptic ulcer 780
a *disorder of the stomach 943*
Pyloroplasty 841
and Vagotomy 1036
Pyo- 841
Pyocidin-Otic 1112
Pyoderma gangrenosum 841
Pyrantel 841
Pyrazinamide 841
Pyrethrins 1112
Pyrexia:
common term: Fever 449
Pyrexia of uncertain origin 841
Pyridiate 1112
Pyridium 1112
Pyridium Plus 1112
Pyridostigmine 841
Pyridoxine 841
part of Vitamin B complex 1058
Pyrilamine 841
Pyrimethamine 841
Pyrogen 841
causing Fever 449
Pyromania 841
Pyrroxate 1112
Pyrvinium 1112
Pyuria 841

# Q

Q fever 842
cause of: Rickettsia 874
type of Pneumonia 803
Quackery 842
quadrantectomy:
type of Mastectomy 666
Quadriceps muscle 842
and Patella 774

Quadrinal 1112
Quadriparesis 842
Quadriplegia 842
cause of: Spinal injury 930
type of Paralysis 769
Quarantine 842
Quazepam 1112
Quelidrine 1113
Questran 1113
Quibron 1113
Quibron-T/SR 1113
Quickening 842
Quinacrine 842
Quinaglute 1113
Quinamm 1113
Quindan 1113
Quinestrol 842
Quinethazone 1113
Quinidine 842
Quinine 842
in treatment of Cramp 318
Quinora 1113
Quinsy 842
Quiphile 1113

# R

R & C 1113
Rabies 843
transmission of: Cats, diseases from 243; Dogs, diseases from 370
Racet 1113
Rachitic 843
see also index entry Rickets
Rad 844
radiation Dose 371
a *radiation unit 845*
radial artery:
blood supply to Hand 505
Radial nerve 844
branch of Brachial plexus 198
and Humerus 548
Radiation 844
adverse effects of: Cancer 227; Carcinogen 233; Cataract 240; Leukemia, acute 635; Lung cancer 651; Occupational disease and injury 739; Radiation and disease 45; Radiation hazards 845; Radiation sickness 846; Sunlight, adverse effects of 955
and Environmental medicine 409; Half-life 504; Infrared 588; Nuclear energy 732; *radiation units 845*; Radiolucent 848; Radiopaque 848; Ultrasound 1019; Ultraviolet light 1021
uses of: CT scanning 26, 323; *performing a CT scan 324*; Dental X ray 342; Imaging techniques 568; *imaging the body 569*; Interstitial radiation therapy 599; Intracavitary therapy 602; Nuclear medicine 733; PET scanning 29, 788; Radiation therapy 38, 846, *847*; Radioimmunoassay 847; Radiology 848;

Radionuclide scanning 27, 848; Scanning techniques 882; X rays 1083; *X-ray examination 1084; using X-rays to look at the body 1085*
see also index entry Radioactivity
Radiation hazards 845
and Occupational disease and injury 739
see also index entries Radiation; Radioactivity
Radiation sickness 846
Radiation therapy 38, 846, *847*
causing Lymphedema 655
in treatment of Leukemia 637; Lung cancer 651; Retinoblastoma 868
*radiation units 845*
radical mastectomy:
complication of: Lymphedema 655
type of Mastectomy 666; Radical surgery 846
Radical surgery 846
Radiculopathy 847
radioactive implants:
uses of: Interstitial radiation therapy 599; Intracavitary therapy 602; Radiation therapy 846
Radioactivity 847
and Half-life 504
sources of: Plutonium 802; Radium 848; Radon 849; Strontium 949; Technetium 966; Uranium 1022
see also index entry Radiation
radioallergosorbent test (RAST):
see index entry RAST
Radioimmunoassay 847
type of Immunoassay 575
Radioisotope scanning:
Radionuclide scanning 848
Radiologic technician:
X-ray technician 1084
Radiologist 848
Radiology 848
Radiolucent 848
Radionuclide scanning 27, 848
type of Imaging technique 570; Scanning technique 882
uses of: *imaging the body 569*; Liver imaging 648; Thyroid scanning 987
using Technetium 966
Radiopaque 848
Radiotherapy:
see index entry Radiation therapy
Radium 848
see also index entry Radiation
Radius 849
broken: Radius, fracture of 849
and Humerus 547; Ulna 1019; Wrist 1082
part of Skeleton 909; *bones of the skeleton 908*
Radius, fracture of 849
Radon 849
see also index entry Radiation
Ranitidine 849
Rape 849
causing Sexual desire, inhibited

898; Vaginismus 1036
*age when victimized by rape 850*
*incidence of reported rape 850*
rapid breathing, abnormal:
　medical term: Hyperventilation
　558
rapid eye movement (REM) sleep:
　see index entry REM sleep
Rash 850
*symptom charts 851, 852*
RAST 853
　type of Immunoassay 575
Rats, diseases from 853
　examples: Lassa fever 629;
　　Leptospirosis 635; Plague
　　799
Raudixin 1113
Rauwiloid 1113
Rauwolfia serpentina 1113
Rauzide 1113
Raynaud's disease 853
　treatment of: Nifedipine 727
　type of Peripheral vascular
　　disease 784
Raynaud's phenomenon 853
　feature of Rheumatoid arthritis
　　870; Scleroderma 886
　treatment of: Prazosin 812
RBC (red blood corpuscle):
　see index entry Blood cells
reading difficulty:
　a Learning disability 632
　medical term: Dyslexia 382
Reagent 854
recall:
　stage of Memory 674
Receding chin 854
　treatment of: Cosmetic surgery
　　313
Receptor 854
　and Stimulus 942
recessiveness (genetics):
　and Gene 481; Inheritance 590
Recombinant DNA 854
　and Genetic engineering 484
Reconstructive surgery:
　Arterial reconstructive surgery
　　130
　Plastic surgery 801
Recovery position 854
*first aid: the recovery position 855*
Rectal bleeding 855
　and Feces, abnormal 443;
　　Occult blood, fecal 739
rectal cancer:
　see index entry Rectum, cancer
　of
Rectal examination 855
　in diagnosis of Hemorrhoids
　　530; Rectal bleeding 855;
　　Rectum, cancer of 856
　techniques of: Proctoscopy 822;
　　Sigmoidoscopy 906
Rectal prolapse 855
Rectocele 856
　and Uterus, prolapse of 1032
Rectum 856
　disorders of: Proctitis 822;
　　Rectal bleeding 855; Rectal
　　prolapse 855; Rectum, cancer
　　of 856; Ulcerative colitis 1018
　part of Intestine 601
　see also index entry Rectal
　　examination

Rectum, cancer of 856
　diagnosis of: Rectal
　　examination 855
　symptoms of: Occult blood,
　　fecal 739; Rectal bleeding 855
red blood corpuscles (RBCs):
　see index entry Blood cells
Red eye 857
　alternative term: Conjunctivitis
　　297
Redisol 1113
Reducing:
　Weight reduction 1075
Reduction 857
　in treatment of Fracture 466
Referred pain 857
　Pain 763, *764*
Reflex 857
　and *pain 764*
Reflex, primitive 857
*types of primitive reflex 858*
Reflux 857
　associated with
　　Glomerulosclerosis 492
　causing Esophagitis 419
　type of Nephropathy 718
　type of: Acid reflux 63
Refraction 858
　testing of: Eye, examination of
　　430; Vision tests 1054; *types of
　　vision tests 1055*
Regenerative cell therapy 858
Regitine 1113
Reglan 1113
Regonol 1113
Regression 858
　cause of: Frustration 470
　and Fixation 458
Regroton 1113
Regurgitation 858
　see also index entry Reflux
Rehabilitation 858
Rehydration therapy 858
Reimplantation, dental 859
Reiter's syndrome 859
　complication of Nonspecific
　　urethritis 730
Rela 1113
Relapse 859
Relapsing fever 859
Relaxation techniques 859
　examples: Meditation 671; Yoga
　　1086
releasing factors:
　example: Luteinizing hormone-
　　releasing hormone 653
　production of: Hypothalamus
　　562
Rem 859
　a *radiation unit 845*
Remegel 1113
Remission 859
Remsed 1113
REM (rapid eye movement) sleep:
　and Dreaming 373; Nightmare
　　727; *sleep patterns 915*
　type of Sleep 914
Renal 860
Renal biopsy 860
Renal cell carcinoma 860
　type of Kidney cancer 617
Renal colic 860
　cause of: Calculus, urinary tract
　　225

complication of Lithotripsy 644
Renal failure 860
　as complication of Rheumatoid
　　arthritis, juvenile 871
　symptoms of: Thirst, excessive
　　979; Urine, abnormal 1029
Renal transplant:
　Kidney transplant 619
Renal tubular acidosis 861
Renese 1113
Renin 861
　and Angiotensin 110
　production of: Kidney 617
Renography 861
replantation microsurgery:
*techniques of microsurgery 687*
Reportable diseases 861
*incidence of some reportable
　diseases in US 862*
*top 20 reportable diseases in US in
　1986 862*
repression:
　as Defense mechanism 336
　in Psychoanalytic theory 831
　and Resistance 863
Reproduction, sexual 862
Reproductive system, female 862
*female reproductive system 863*
Reproductive system, male 862
*male reproductive system 863*
Rescinnamine 1113
Resection 863
Reserpine 863
Resident 863
Resistance 863
Resorcinol 1113
Resorption, dental 863
Respbid 1113
Respinol-G 1113
Respiration 864, *865*
　and Breathing 209; Respiratory
　　system 865
Respirator:
　Ventilator 1045
Respiratory arrest 865
*first aid: artificial respiration 134*
Respiratory distress syndrome
　865
　complication of Prematurity 817
　a *disorder of the lung 652*
　treatment of: Ventilation 1045
Respiratory failure 865
　causes of: Asthma 138;
　　Emphysema 399; Flail chest
　　458; Tobacco smoking 992
　causing Hypoxia 565
　treatment of: Ventilator 1045
Respiratory function tests:
　Pulmonary function tests 836
Respiratory system 865
　function of: Breathing 209;
　　Respiration 864, *865*
　parts of: Alveolus, pulmonary
　　90; Bronchus 217; Diaphragm
　　muscle 354; Epiglottis 412;
　　Larynx 627; *location of larynx
　　628;* Lung 651; Mouth 697;
　　Nasopharynx 716; Nose 731;
　　Pharynx 789; *location of the
　　pharynx 790;* Rib 873; *anatomy
　　of the ribs 874;* Trachea 1001
Respiratory therapy 866
Respiratory tract infection 866
Restless legs 866

causing Insomnia 593
Restoration, dental 866
Restoril 1113
Restricted growth:
　Short stature 902
Resuscitation:
　Artificial respiration 134
　Cardiopulmonary resuscitation
　　236
Retainer 866
　type of Orthodontic appliance
　　751
Retardation:
　Mental retardation 678
Retet 1113
Reticular formation 866
　and Arousal 129;
　　Consciousness 298;
　　Unconsciousness 1022
　location of: Brain stem 204
reticulocyte:
　type of Blood cell 182
Reticulogen 1113
Reticulosarcoma 866
　modern term: Lymphoma,
　　non-Hodgkin's 657
Retin-A 1113
Retina 866
　disorders of: *disorders of the eye
　　431; disorders of the retina 867*
　function of: Vision 1052; *the
　　sense of vision 1053*
　part of Eye 428; *anatomy of the
　　eye 429*
Retinal artery occlusion 866
Retinal detachment 867
　causing Floaters 459
　following Retinal tear 868
Retinal hemorrhage 868
Retinal tear 868
Retinal vein occlusion 868
Retinitis 868
Retinitis pigmentosa 868
　causing Night blindness 727;
　　Tunnel vision 1015
Retinoblastoma 868
　type of Eye tumor 433
Retinoic acid 1113
Retinoids:
　Vitamin A 1057
Retinol 868
　form of Vitamin A 1057
Retinopathy 868
Retractor 868
Retrobulbar neuritis 868
retrograde ejaculation:
　causing Infertility 586
　an *ejaculatory disorder 393*
retrograde pyelography:
　type of Pyelography 840
Retrolental fibroplasia 868
Retroperitoneal fibrosis 869
Retrosternal pain 869
retroverted uterus:
　alternative term: Uterus, tipped
　　1032
Retrovir 1113
retroviruses:
　example: HIV 541
　types of Viruses 1052
　*viruses and disease 1051*
Rett's syndrome 869
Reye's syndrome 869
　and Influenza 588

Rhabdomyolysis 869
rhabdomyomas:
*disorders of muscle 705*
Rhabdomyosarcoma 869
*a disorder of muscle 705*
Rh blood group:
type of Blood group 187
and Hemolytic disease of the
newborn 43, 529; Rh
incompatibility 871, *872*;
Rh₀(D) immune globulin
873
Rhesus (Rh) factors:
see index entry Rh blood group
Rheumatic fever 869
affecting Heart valve 523
following Scarlet fever 883
and *disorders of the heart 517*
Rheumatism 870
types of: Osteoarthritis 753;
Polymyalgia rheumatica 808;
Rheumatoid arthritis 870
Rheumatoid arthritis 870
associated with Raynaud's
phenomenon 853; Restless
legs 866
treatment of: Azathioprine 149;
Gold 494; Ibuprofen 566;
Indomethacin 581;
Ketoprofen 616;
Meclofenamate 669;
Methotrexate 683;
Penicillamine 779; Piroxicam
796; Prednisolone 813;
Prednisone 813
Rheumatoid arthritis, juvenile 871
Rheumatoid spondylitis:
Ankylosing spondylitis 111
Rheumatologist 871
Rheumatology 871
Rhindecon 1113
Rh incompatibility 871
causing Hemolytic disease of
the newborn 43, 529
*how Rh incompatibility occurs 872*
Rhinitis 872
Rhinitis, allergic 872
Rhinolar 1113
Rhinophyma 873
feature of Rosacea 876
Rhinoplasty 873
Rhinorrhea 873
Rhinosyn 1113
Rh isoimmunization 873
Rh₀(D) immune globulin 873
and Rh incompatibility 872
Rhythm method:
Contraception, periodic
abstinence 305
Rib 873
anatomy of: *anatomy of the ribs
874*; Skeleton 909; *bones of the
skeleton 908*; Thorax 979;
*anatomy of the thorax 980*
disorders of: Flail chest 458;
Rib, fractured 873; Tietze's
syndrome 988
Rib, fractured 873
Riboflavin 874
part of Vitamin B complex 1058
ribonucleic acid (RNA):
see index entry RNA
Rickets 874

cause of: deficiency of Vitamin
D 1059
and Osteomalacia 755
Rickettsia 874
causing Q fever 842; Rocky
Mountain Spotted Fever
875;
Typhus 1017
and Infectious disease 582
Rid 1113
Ridaura 1113
Riedel's thyroiditis:
type of Thyroiditis 987
Rifadin 1113
Rifamate 1113
Rifampin 874
Rigidity 874
Rigor 875
symptom of Fever 449
Rigor mortis 875
Rimactane 1113
Rimactane INH 1113
Ringing in the ears:
medical term: Tinnitus 989
Ringworm 875
medical term: Tinea 988
Ritalin 1113
Ritodine 875
Ritodrine 1113
River blindness:
medical term: Onchocerciasis
742
RNA 875
function of: *what genes are and
what they do 480*; Protein
synthesis 827; *steps in protein
synthesis 828*
type of Nucleic acid 733
Robaxin 1113
Robaxisal 1113
Robicillin VK 1113
Robimycin 1113
Robinul 1113
Robitet 1113
Robitussin 1113
Rocaltrol 1113
Rocephin 1113
Rock, John:
*landmarks in drug development 32*
Rocky Mountain Spotted Fever
875
cause of: Rickettsia 874
rodent ulcer:
alternative term: Basal cell
carcinoma 160
Roentgenography:
Radiology 848
X rays 1083
Roentgen, Wilhelm Conrad:
*landmarks in diagnosis 25*
discoverer of X rays 1083
Roferon-A 1113
Rolaids 1113
role models:
in Adolescence 69
Role-playing 875
Ronase 1113
Rondec 1113
Rondomycin 1113
Root-canal treatment 875, *876*
rooting reflex:
example of Reflex, primitive
857
*types of primitive reflex 858*

Rorschach test 876
Rosacea 876
causing Rhinophyma 873
Roseola infantum 876
Rotator cuff 876
part of Shoulder 902
Roughage:
Fiber, dietary 452
Roundworms 876
*diseases caused by roundworms
(nematodes) 877*
transmission of: Cats, diseases
from 243
and Worm infestation 1081
Roxanol 1113
RP-Mycin 1113
Rubber dam 876
Rubella 876
and Abortion, elective 57
causing Birth defects 173;
*disorders of the ear 385*; Heart
disease, congenital 518;
Infection, congenital 582
Rubeola 877
alternative term: Measles 668
Rubramin 1113
Rufen 1113
Running injuries 877
Rupture:
Hernia 534
Ru-Tuss 1113
Ru-Vert-M 1113
Rynatan 1113
Rynatuss 1113

# S

Sac 878
Saccharin 878
type of Artificial sweetener 135
Sacralgia 878
Sacralization 878
Sacroiliac joint 878
inflammation of: Sacroiliitis 878
part of Pelvis 778
Sacroiliitis 878
Sacrum 878
and Coccyx 286
pain in: Sacralgia 878
part of Pelvis 778; Skeleton 909;
*bones of the skeleton 908*;
*structure of the spine 932*
Sadism 878
feature of Sadomasochism 878
Sadomasochism 878
SADS 879
Safeguard 1113
Safe period:
Contraception, periodic
abstinence 305
"Safe" sex 879
and prevention of AIDS 79
*safety at work 740*
SalAc 1113
Salicylic acid 879
Salicylsalicylic acid 1113
Saligel 1113
Saline 879
saline laxative:
type of Laxative drug 631
Saliva 879
excessive: Ptyalism 834;

Salivation, excessive 880
insufficient: Mouth, dry 697
production of: Salivary glands
880
Salivary glands 880
producing Saliva 879
types of: Parotid glands 773
Salivation, excessive 880
type of: Ptyalism 834
Salmonella 880
causing Food poisoning 463;
Paratyphoid fever 772;
Typhoid fever 1017
salmon patch:
alternative term: Stork bite 944
Salpingectomy 880
Salpingitis 880
associated with Peritonitis 785
as complication of Nonspecific
urethritis 730
Salpingography:
Hysterosalpingography 565
Salpingo-oophorectomy 880
Salsalate 1113
Salt 881
solution of: Saline 879
see also index entry salt
(sodium chloride)
salt (sodium chloride):
compound of Sodium 922
excess of: Diet and disease 358;
Hypertension 557
loss of: Dehydration 338;
Diarrhea 356; Heat cramps
525; Heat disorders 525; Heat
exhaustion 525; Urination,
excessive 1025
retention of: Edema 391
Saluron 1113
Salutensin 1113
Salve 881
Sand-fly bites 881
and Insects and disease 592
Sandimmune 1113
Sanitary protection 881
Sanorex 1113
Sansert 1113
Sarcoidosis 881
variant of: Lupus pernio 653
Sarcoma 881
type of Tumor 1015
Sarna Lotion 1113
SAS-500 1113
SAStid 1113
Satric 500 1113
Saturated fats:
and Diet and disease 357
types of Fats and oils 441
satyriasis:
and Nymphomania 737
Savacort 50 1113
Scab 881
Scabene 1113
Scabies 881
Scald 881
*first aid: treating burns 220*
*type of Burn 219*
scalded skin syndrome:
cause of: Staphylococcal
infections 938
type of Necrolysis, toxic
epidermal 717
Scaling, dental 881
in treatment of Gingivitis 487;

Periodontitis 784; Vincent's disease 1049
use of: Oral hygiene 748; Periodontics 783; Preventive dentistry 820
Scalp 881
dermatitis of: Cradle cap 317; Dandruff 332
ringworm of: Tinea 988
swelling of: Cephalhematoma 247; Sebaceous cyst 889; Vacuum extraction 1034
Scalpel 882
scanning electron microscope (SEM):
type of Microscope 685, 686
Scanning techniques 882
types of Imaging technique 568
types of: CT scanning 26, 323; *performing a CT scan 324; magnetic resonance imaging (MRI) 700;* MRI 28, 699; PET scanning 29, 788; Radionuclide scanning 27, 848; Ultrasound scanning 30, 41, 1019; *how ultrasound scanning works 1020*
uses of: Diagnosing disease 24-29; *imaging the body 569*
Scaphoid 882
part of Wrist 1082
Scapula 882
and Acromioclavicular joint 65
part of Shoulder 902; *structure of the shoulder 903;* Skeleton 909; *bones of the skeleton 908*
Scar 882
abnormal types of: Adhesion 68; Desmoid tumor 347; Fibrosis 453; Keloid 614
formation of: Healing 510
Scarlatina 882
alternative term: Scarlet fever 883
Scarlet fever 883
associated with Strep throat 945
cause of: Streptococcal infections 945
Schamberg's Lotion 1113
Schilling test:
in diagnosis of Anemia, megaloblastic 104
Schistosome 883
causing Schistosomiasis 883
type of Flatworm 458; Platyhelminth 801
Schistosomiasis 883
type of Waterborne infection 1071
Schizoid personality disorder 884
and Somatotype 924
Schizophrenia 884
type of Psychosis 833
Schönlein-Henoch purpura 885
type of Purpura 839
Sciatica 885
and *symptoms and treatment of disk prolapse 365; Spondylolisthesis 935*
Sciatic nerve 885
disorder of: Sciatica 885
Scintigraphy 885
alternative term: Radionuclide scanning 848

Scirrhous 886
Sclera 886
damage to: Eye injuries 432
disorders of: Osteogenesis imperfecta 754; Scleritis 886; Scleromalacia 886
part of Eye 429
Scleritis 886
Scleroderma 886
symptom of: Raynaud's phenomenon 853
Scleromalacia 886
sclerosing cholangitis:
type of Cholangitis 272
Sclerosis 886
Sclerotherapy 886
in treatment of Portal hypertension 810; Varicose veins 1038
Scoliosis 886
affecting Walking 1067
*a disorder of the spine 933*
Scopolamine 887
Scorpion stings 887
Scotoma 887
type of Vision, disorder of 1054
Scot-Tussin 1113
scratching:
cause of: Itching 609
causing Lichenification 638; Lichen simplex 639
Screening 887
types of: Cancer screening 230; Mammography 22, 662; *prenatal screening procedures 819*
uses of: Prenatal care 818; Preventive medicine 820; Screening high-risk groups 22
Scrofula 887
Scrotum 887
disorders of: Hydrocele 550; Pseudohermaphroditism 829; Varicocele 1038
part of Reproductive system, male 862
and Testis 972
Scuba-diving medicine 887
and Air embolism 80; Barotrauma 159; Decompression sickness 335
*recompression chamber for diving accidents 888*
Scurvy 888
and Bleeding disorders 178
cause of: deficiency of Vitamin C 1059
symptoms of: bleeding Gums 502; Pallor 765
Sealants, dental 889
use of: Bonding, dental 192
Seasickness 889
type of Motion sickness 696
Seasonal affective disorder syndrome:
SADS 879
Sebaceous cyst 889
Sebaceous glands 889
disorders of: Acne 63; Blackhead 175; Dermatitis 345; Seborrhea 889
part of Skin 910
producing Sebum 889

Seborrhea 889
Seborrheic dermatitis:
type of Dermatitis 345
Sebulex 1113
Sebulon 1113
Sebum 889
overproduction of: Seborrhea 889
production of: Sebaceous glands 889
Secobarbital 889
Seconal 1113
Secondary 889
tumor: Metastasis 683
secondary sexual characteristics:
Sexual characteristics, secondary 898
second teeth:
Permanent teeth 786
secretin:
effect on Gallbladder 473
type of Gastrointestinal hormone 477
Secretion 889
Sectral 1113
Security object 889
and Attachment 143
Sedapap-10 1113
Sedation 890
Sedative drugs 890
Seffin 1113
Seizure 890
causing Respiratory arrest 865
feature of: Epilepsy 412; Withdrawal syndrome 1080
types of: Grand mal 497; Petit mal 788; Seizure, febrile 890
Seizure, febrile 890
Seldane 1113
Seldene 1113
Selegiline 1113
Selenium 890
deficiency of: Kwashiorkor 623
type of Trace element 1001
Selenium sulfide 1113
self:
psychoanalytic term: Ego 392
self-esteem:
exaggerated: Egomania 392; Superiority complex 956
low: Inferiority complex 586
Self-help organizations 1090-1095
self-hypnosis:
method of Hypnosis 559
Self-image 891
self-love:
Narcissism 715
Self-mutilation 891
Selsun 1113
SEM (scanning electron microscope):
type of Microscope 685, 686
Semen 891
and Ejaculation 392
production of: Reproductive system, male 862, 863
Semen analysis 891
in diagnosis of Azoospermia 149; Oligospermia 742
use of: *investigating infertility 587*
Semen, blood in the 891
Semets 1113
Semicid 1113
semicircular canals:

function of: Balance 156
part of Ear 384
seminal fluid:
constituent of Semen 891
production of: Reproductive system, male 862
seminal vesicles:
part of Reproductive system, male 862, 863
seminiferous tubules:
part of Testis 972
Seminoma:
type of Testis, cancer of 972
Semustine 1113
Senile dementia:
Dementia 339
Senility 891
Senna 891
Senokot 1113
Sensate focus technique 891
type of Sex therapy 897
Sensation 892
interpretation of: Perception 782
see also index entries Hearing; Smell; Taste; Touch; Vision
Sensation, abnormal 893
sensation, distorted:
Illusion 568
sensation, loss of:
alternative term: Numbness 735
induction of: Anesthesia 104; Anesthesia, dental 104; Anesthesia, general 104; Anesthesia, local 106; Nerve block 719
type of Sensation, abnormal 893
Senses:
and Sensation 892
see also index entries Hearing; Smell; Taste; Touch; Vision
Sensitization 893
sensorineural deafness:
assessment of: Hearing tests 513
type of Deafness 333
type of: Presbycusis 819
Sensory cortex 893
and Sensation 892
Sensory deprivation 893
causing Hallucination 504
sensory fibers:
of Nerve 719; *nervous system 721;* Spinal cord 929; Spinal nerves 931
sensory receptors:
function of: Sensation 892
part of *nervous system 721; types of receptor 854*
Separation anxiety 893
causing Nightmare 727; Phobia 792
Sepsis 894
Septal defect 894
type of Heart disease, congenital 518
Septicemia 894
causing Septic shock 895
and Puerperal sepsis 835; Sepsis 894; Toxemia 998
Septic shock 895
causes of: Septicemia 894; Toxemia 998

Septisol 1113
Septra 1113
Septum 895
 of nose: Nasal septum 715
 part of Heart 514
Sequela 895
Sequestration 895
Ser-Ap-Es 1113
Serax 1113
Serentil 1113
Serology 895
Serophene 1114
Serotonin 895
 excess of: Carcinoid syndrome
  234
 type of Neurotransmitter 725
Serpasil 1113
Serpasil-Apresoline 1113
Serpate 1114
Sertürner, Friedrich:
 landmarks in drug development 32
Serum 895
Serum sickness 896
 cause of: Hypersensitivity 557
Sevin 1114
Sex 896
 see also index entries female
  gender; male gender; Sexual
  intercourse
Sex change 896
 in treatment of Transsexualism
  1006
Sex chromosomes 896
 abnormal number of:
  Chromosomal abnormalities
  277
 and Inheritance 589; Sex
  determination 897
 types of Chromosome 279
Sex determination 897
 see also index entry Sex
  chromosomes
Sex hormones 897
Sex-linked 897
 and Genetic disorders 482;
  unifactorial genetic disorders
  483; Inheritance 590; X-linked
  disorders 1083
Sex therapy 897
 in treatment of Psychosexual
  dysfunction 833
 type of: Sensate focus
  technique 897
Sexual abuse 898
 types of: Child abuse 263; Rape
  849
Sexual characteristics, secondary
 898
 development of: Puberty 834;
  changes of puberty 835; Sex
  determination 897
sexual desire, exaggerated:
 medical term: Nymphomania
  737
Sexual desire, inhibited 898
 treatment of: Sensate focus
  technique 892; Sex therapy
  897
 type of Psychosexual
  dysfunction 832
Sexual deviation:
 Deviation, sexual 348
Sexual dysfunction:
 Psychosexual dysfunction 832

Sexual intercourse 898, 899
 and Child abuse 252;
  Deviation, sexual 348; Incest
  579; Rape 849; Sexually
  transmitted diseases 898
 after Hysterectomy 565
 painful: Intercourse, painful
  596; painful intercourse in men
  596; painful intercourse in
  women 597
 during Pregnancy 813
 see also index entry Sexual
  problems
Sexuality 898
 in Psychoanalytic theory 831
 types of: Bisexuality 174;
  Heterosexuality 537;
  Homosexuality, male 544;
  Lesbianism 635
Sexually transmitted diseases 898
 and Contact tracing 302; Rape
  850
 examples: AIDS 44, 76; incidence
  of new cases of AIDS in the US
  900; Chancroid 258;
  Chlamydial infections 270;
  Gonorrhea 495; incidence of
  gonorrhea in the US 900;
  Herpes, genital 536;
  Lymphogranuloma
  venereum 657; Nonspecific
  urethritis 730; Pubic lice 835;
  Syphilis 961; incidence of
  primary and secondary syphilis
  in the US 900; Trichomoniasis
  1009; Warts, genital 1070
Sexual problems 900
 examples: Ejaculation,
  disorders of 393; Impotence
  578; Infertility 586;
  investigating infertility 587;
  Intercourse, painful 596;
  painful intercourse in men 596;
  painful intercourse in women
  597; Orgasm, lack of 750;
  Psychosexual dysfunction
  832; Sexual desire, inhibited
  898; Transsexualism 1006;
  Vaginismus 1036
 treatment of: Penile implant
  779; Sensate focus technique
  891; Sex therapy 897
Sézary syndrome 901
shaking:
 medical term: Tremor 1008
Shellfish poisoning:
 Food poisoning 463
Shigellosis 901
shin bone:
 medical term: Tibia 987
Shingles:
 Herpes zoster 901
Shin splints 901
 type of Running injury 877
Shivering 901
 and regulation of Temperature
  968
Shock 901
 first aid: shock 902
 types of: Anaphylactic shock
  98; Electrical injury 394;
  Septic shock 895; Shock,
  electric 902; Toxic shock
  syndrome 998

Shock, electric 902
 first aid: electrical injury 395
 type of Electrical injury 394
 use of: ECT 388
Shock therapy 902
 type of: ECT 388
shock-wave treatment:
 medical term: Lithotripsy 39,
  643
Short stature 902
 and Growth, childhood 499
 treatment of: Growth hormone
  501; Nandrolone 714
Shoulder 902
 disorders of: Frozen shoulder
  469; Painful arc syndrome
  763; Shoulder, dislocation of
  902; Shoulder-hand
  syndrome 903
 muscles of: Deltoid 339; Rotator
  cuff 876
 structure of the shoulder 903
 a type of joint 612
Shoulder blade 903
 medical term: Scapula 882
Shoulder, dislocation of 903
 and Klumpke's paralysis 621
Shoulder-hand syndrome 903
Shunt 903
 and procedure for dialysis 353
 in treatment of Hydrocephalus
  550; Portal hypertension 810;
  Spina bifida 928
Shy-Drager syndrome 904
SIADH 904
Siamese twins 904
 type of Twins 1016
Sibling rivalry 904
Sick building syndrome 904
Sickle cell anemia 904
 a disorder of the blood 186
 type of Anemia, hemolytic 102
Sick sinus syndrome 905
 type of Arrhythmia, cardiac 129
Side effect 905
 of Drugs 378
Siderosis 905
SIDS 905
 abbreviation for Sudden infant
  death syndrome 952
Sievert 905
 a radiation unit 845
Sight:
 see index entry Vision
Sigmoid colon 905
 examination of: Sigmoidoscopy
  906
 part of Colon 290; Intestine 601
Sigmoidoscopy 906
 in diagnosis of Colitis 289;
  Intestine, cancer 602;
  Ulcerative colitis 1018
Sign 906
 and Symptom 959; Syndrome
  960
 type of: Vital sign 1056
Silain gel 1114
Silicone 906
 implant: types of implant 576;
  Mammoplasty 662;
  Mastectomy 666
Silicosis 906
 a disorder of the lung 652
 type of Pneumoconiosis 802

Silvadene 1114
Silver nitrate 906
Silver sulfadiazine 906
Simeco 1114
Simethicone 906
Simpson, James:
 landmarks in surgery 33
Simron 1114
Sine-Aid 1114
Sinemet 1114
Sinequan 1114
Sinew 906
 medical term: Tendon 970
Singers' nodes 906
 a disorder of the larynx 629
single photon emission
 computerized tomography
 (SPECT):
 type of Radionuclide scanning
  848
Singlet 1114
Sinoatrial node 907
 abnormal functioning of: cardiac
  arrhythmia 129; Sick sinus
  syndrome 905; Sinus
  tachycardia 908;
  Supraventricular tachycardia
  956
 and Pacemaker 762
 part of Heart 515
Sinubid 1114
Sinufed 1114
Sinulin 1114
Sinus 907
 see also index entry Sinus,
  facial
Sinus bradycardia 907
 type of Arrhythmia, cardiac 129
Sinus, facial 907
 effect of pressure on: Aviation
  medicine 148; Barotrauma
  159
 inflammation of: Sinusitis 907
Sinusitis 907
 cause of: Cold, common 287
 treatment of: Decongestant
  drugs 336; Naphazoline 714;
  Oxymetazoline 761;
  Phenylpropanolamine 791
Sinus tachycardia 908
 type of Arrhythmia, cardiac 129
Sinutab 1114
Situs inversus 908
Sjögren's syndrome 909
 causing Keratoconjunctivitis
  sicca 615; Mouth, dry 699
Skelaxin 1114
skeletal muscle:
 type of Muscle 703; the body's
  muscles 704
Skeleton 909
 bones of the skeleton 908
Skin 909
 aging of: Age spots 74; Aging
  74; the practical effects of aging
  75; Wrinkles 1082
 color of: Melanin 673;
  Pigmentation 794
 disorders of the skin 910
 function of: Sensation 892;
  Touch 998; sense of touch 999
 structure of: Sebaceous glands
  889; Sweat glands 958
 study of: Dermatology 345

Skin allergy 911
Skin and muscle flap 911
  use of: Plastic surgery 801
Skin biopsy 912
  type of Biopsy 170
Skin cancer 912
  cause of: Sunlight, adverse
    effects of 955
  treatment of: Cryosurgery 323;
    Radiation therapy 846
Skin graft 912
  use of: Plastic surgery 801
Skin infections:
  disorders of the skin 910
Skin peeling, chemical 913
Skin tag 913
Skin tests 913
  in diagnosis of Allergy 87;
    Rhinitis, allergic 872
  type of: Tuberculin tests 1013
Skin tumors 913
  disorders of the skin 910
  type of: Skin cancer 912
  treatment of: Radiation therapy
    847
Skull 913
  operations on: Burr hole 221;
    Craniotomy 319; Trephine
    1008
  part of Skeleton 909; bones of the
    skeleton 908
  parts of: Fontanelle 461; Jaw
    610; types of joints 612; Maxilla
    668; Sinus, facial 907;
    Sphenoid bone 927; Suture
    957
Skull, fractured 914
  diagnosis of: Skull X ray 914
  type of Head injury 507
Skull X ray 914
slapped cheeks' disease:
  medical term: Fifth disease 454
SLE (systemic lupus
  erythematosus) 914
  see also index entry Lupus
    erythematosus
Sleep 914
  disorders of: Insomnia 593; Jet
    lag 611; Narcolepsy 715;
    Nightmare 727; Night terror
    727; Sleep apnea 916;
    Sleepwalking 917
  and Dreaming 373; Snoring 922
  ejaculation during: Nocturnal
    emission 729
  sleep patterns 915
Sleep apnea 916
  causing Insomnia 593
  feature of: Snoring 922
Sleep deprivation 916
Sleeping drugs 916
  types of: Barbiturates 157;
    Benzodiazepine drugs 164
sleeping sickness (form of
  encephalitis):
  medical term: Encephalitis
    lethargica 401
Sleeping sickness (tropical
  disease) 916
  cycle of sleeping sickness 917
  transmission of: Tsetse fly bites
    1013
  type of Trypanosomiasis 1013
Sleep paralysis 917

  feature of Narcolepsy 715
Sleep terror:
  Night terror 917
Sleepwalking 917
"slimming disease":
  medical term: Anorexia nervosa
    112
Sling 917
  first aid: arm sling 918
Slipped disk:
  Disk prolapse 364
Slipped femoral epiphysis:
  Femoral epiphysis, slipped 444
Slit lamp 917
  use of: Eye, examination of 430
Slo-Bid 1114
Slo-Phyllin 1114
Slo-Phyllin GG 1114
Slough 917
Slow FE 1114
Slow-K 1114
Slow virus diseases 917
  types of: Creutzfeldt-Jakob
    syndrome 319; Kuru 623
Small-cell carcinoma 918
  type of Lung cancer 651
small intestine:
  parts of: Duodenum 380; Ileum
    568; Jejunum 611
  surgical opening into:
    Ileostomy 566
  see also index entry Intestine
Smallpox 918
Smear 918
  types of: Blood smear 189;
    Cervical smear test 252;
    procedure for a cervical (Pap)
    smear 253
Smegma 918
Smell 918
  function of Cerebrum 251;
    Nose 731; Olfactory nerve
    742
  the sense of smell 919
  and Taste 965
Smelling salts 919
Smoking:
  of Marijuana 664
  see also index entry Tobacco
    smoking
smooth muscle 704
  type of Muscle 706; the body's
    muscles 704
Snails and disease 920
Snakebites 920
  first aid: snakebite 921
Sneezing 921
Snellen's chart 921
  use of: Eye, examination of 430
Snoring 922
  associated with Sleep apnea
    916
snow blindness:
  type of Keratopathy 615
Snuff 922
  causing Mouth cancer 697
Sociopathy 922
  modern term: Antisocial
    personality disorder 119
Sodium 922
  type of Ion 605
  see also index entry Salt
Sodium bicarbonate 922
sodium chloride:

  see index entry salt (sodium
    chloride)
Sodium citrate 1114
Sodium fluoride 1114
Sodium iodide 1114
Sodium nitrite 1114
Sodium salicylate 922
Sodium thiosulfate 1114
soft chancre:
  alternative term: Chancroid
    258
  type of Ulcer 1018
soft palate:
  part of Palate 765
  and Uvula 1033
Soft-tissue injury 922
Soiling 922
  type of: Encopresis 401
Solar plexus 923
Solatene 1114
Solfoton 1114
Solganal 1114
Solu-Cortef 1114
Solu-Medrol 1114
Solvent abuse 923
Soma 1114
Soma Compound 1114
Somatic 923
Somatization disorder 923
Somatoform disorders 923
Somatotype 923
Somatrem 924
Somnambulism:
  Sleepwalking 917
Somophyllin 1114
Somophyllin CRT 1114
Somophyllin-T 1114
sonography:
  alternative term: Ultrasound
    scanning 1019
Soothe 1114
Soprodol 1114
Sorbitrate 1114
Sore 924
Sore throat 924
  causes of: Pharyngitis 789;
    Tonsillitis 996
Sotalol 1114
Space medicine 924
Sparine 1114
Spasm 924
spastic colon:
  alternative term: Irritable bowel
    syndrome 607
Spasticity 924
  and Muscle 705
Spastic paralysis 924
  feature of Cerebral palsy 249
  type of Paralysis 769
Spatulate 924
Specialist 924
Specific gravity 924
  and Density 340
Specimen 924
  and Biopsy 170; Staining 938
SPECT 925
  type of Radionuclide scanning
    848
Spectacles:
  Glasses 488
Spectazole 1114
Spectinomycin 1114
Spectrobid 1114
Spectrocin 1114

Speculum 925
  use of: procedure for a cervical
    (Pap) smear 253; D and C 332;
    procedure for pelvic examination
    777
Speech 925
  delay in: Developmental delay
    347
Speech disorders 926
  types of: Aphasia 125;
    Dysarthria 382; Dysphasia
    383; Dysphonia 383;
    Stuttering 950
speech, esophageal:
  following Laryngectomy 627
Speech therapy 926
  following Stroke 949
  in treatment of Stuttering 950
Sperm 926
  abnormal production of:
    Azoospermia 149;
    Oligospermia 742; Infertility
    586; investigating infertility 587
  investigation of: Semen
    analysis 891
  production of: Reproductive
    system, male 862, 863; Testis
    972
  role of: Fertility 447; the process
    of fertilization 446
Spermatocele 927
Spermatozoa:
  Sperm 926
sperm duct:
  medical term: Vas deferens
    1040
Spermicides 927
  introduction of: Suppository
    956
  use of: Contraception, barrier
    methods 304; Sponge,
    contraceptive 935
Sphenoid bone 927
  part of Skull 914; structure of the
    skull 913
Spherocytosis, hereditary 927
  a unifactorial genetic disorder 483
Sphincter 927
  of Anus 122; Esophagus 420;
    Stomach 943; location of the
    stomach 942
  type of Muscle 705
Sphincter, artificial 927
Sphincterotomy 927
Sphygmomanometer 927
  in measurement of Blood
    pressure 189
Spider bites 928
Spider nevus 928
  type of Telangiectasia 968
Spina bifida 928
  types of spina bifida 929
Spinal accessory nerve 929
  functions of cranial nerves 318
Spinal anesthesia 929
spinal canal decompression:
  Decompression, spinal canal
    335
Spinal cord 929
  part of Nervous system 720,
    721
  location of the spinal cord 930
  and Spinal nerves 931
  X ray of: Myelography 710

1173

Spinal fusion 930
Spinal injury 930
    type of: Whiplash injury 1077
Spinal nerves 931
    part of *nervous system 721*
Spinal tap:
    Lumbar puncture 650
Spine 932
    anatomy of: Coccyx 285;
    *anatomy of coccyx 286;* Disk,
    intervertebral 364; Sacrum
    878; Vertebra 1047; *location
    and structure of the vertebrae
    1048*
    *disorders of the spine 933*
Spirochete 932
    type of Bacteria 154
Spirometry 932
    type of Pulmonary function test
    836
Spironolactone 932
Spirozide 1114
Spleen 933
    overactivity of: Hypersplenism
    557
    removal of: Splenectomy 933
Splenectomy 933
Splint 934
    uses of: Splinting 934;
    Splinting, dental 934
Splinting 934
Splinting, dental 934
Split personality 934
    medical terms: Multiple
    personality 701;
    Schizophrenia 884
Spondylitis 934
Spondylolisthesis 935
    *a disorder of the spine 933*
    treatment of: Spinal fusion
    930
Spondylolysis 935
    causing Spondylolisthesis 935
Sponge, contraceptive 935
    causing Toxic shock syndrome
    1000
    type of Contraception, barrier
    method 305
spontaneous abortion:
    medical term: Miscarriage 690
Sporotrichosis 935
    type of Fungal infection 470
Sports, drugs and 935
Sports injuries 935
Sports medicine 936
"spotting":
    alternative term: Breakthrough
    bleeding 205
Spouse abuse 936
Sprain 936
    *first aid: sprains 937*
Sprue 936
    types of: Celiac sprue 245;
    Sprue, tropical 936
Sprue, tropical 936
S-P-T 1114
Sputum 936
Squamous cell carcinoma 937
    type of Lung cancer 651; Skin
    cancer 912
squamous cells:
    of Endothelium 407; Epithelium
    415
*squeeze technique 897*

Squint:
    medical term: Strabismus 944
SSKI 1114
Stable 938
Stadol 1114
Stage 938
    in diagnosis of Hodgkin's
    disease 544; Lymphoma,
    non-Hodgkin's 657
Staining 938
    using Gram's stain 497
staining, tooth:
    Discolored teeth 363
Stammering:
    Stuttering 950
Stanford-Binet test 938
    type of Intelligence test 595
Stanozolol 938
Stapedectomy 938
    in treatment of Otosclerosis 759
Stapes 938
    part of Ear 384
    removal of: Stapedectomy 938
Staphcillin 1114
Staphylococcal infections 938
Starch:
    type of Carbohydrate 232
Starvation 939
    causing Ketosis 616
    Diet and disease 357
Stasis 939
Staticin 1114
Statistics, medical 939
Statistics, vital 939
Statobex 1114
Statrol 1114
Status asthmaticus 939
Status epilepticus 939
    type of Epilepsy 413
STDs:
    abbreviation for Sexually
    transmitted diseases 898
Steatorrhea 939
Stein-Leventhal syndrome:
    Polycystic ovary 807
Stelazine 1114
Stenosis 939
stepping reflex:
    type of Reflex, primitive 857
Sterane 1114
stereoscopic vision:
    and Vision 1054; *the sense of
    vision 1053*
Stereotaxic surgery 939
    use of: Psychosurgery 833
Sterility 939
    and Infertility 586
Sterilization 939
Sterilization, female 940
Sterilization, male:
    Vasectomy 1040
Sternum 940
    *location of the sternum 941*
Steroid drugs 940
Steroids, anabolic 940
    abuse of: Sports, drugs and 935
Stethoscope 941
    invention of: *landmarks in
    diagnosis 25*
    use of: Auscultation 144; *types
    of physical examination 425*
Stevens-Johnson syndrome 941
    type of Erythema multiforme
    417

Stibocaptate 1114
Stibogluconate 1114
Sticky eye 941
Stiff neck 941
    feature of Meningitis 675
    types of: Neck rigidity 717;
    Torticollis 998
Stiffness 941
    after death: Rigor mortis 875
    of joints: Arthritis 132;
    Rheumatoid arthritis 870
    of muscles: Rigidity 875;
    Spasticity 924
    see also index entry Stiff neck
Stillbirth 941
    as complication of Postmaturity
    810
Still's disease:
    Rheumatoid arthritis, juvenile
    871
Stilphostrol 1114
Stimulant drugs 942
    abuse of: Sports, drugs and 935
    examples: Caffeine 222;
    Pemoline 778
    types of: Amphetamine drugs
    95
Stimulus 942
Stings 942
    types of: Insect stings 592;
    Jellyfish stings 611; Scorpion
    stings 887; Venomous bites
    and stings 1044
Stitch 942
stitch (surgical):
    Suturing 958
    *methods of suturing 957*
Stokes-Adams syndrome 942
Stoma 942
    in Colostomy 293; Ileostomy
    567
Stomach 942
    *disorders of the stomach 942*
    function of: *the digestive process
    360*
    hormones of: Gastrointestinal
    hormones 477
    investigations of: Barium X-ray
    examinations 158;
    Gastroscopy 478
    part of Digestive system 359
    removal of: Gastrectomy 475
    surgical opening into:
    Gastrostomy 478
stomach ache:
    Abdominal pain 50, *51, 53;*
    Indigestion 580
Stomach cancer 943
    *a disorder of the stomach 943*
Stomach imaging:
    Barium X-ray examinations 158
Stomach pump:
    Lavage, gastric 630
Stomach ulcer 944
    type of Peptic ulcer 780; *sites
    and causes of peptic ulcer 781*
Stomatitis 944
Stones 944
    types of: Calculus, urinary tract
    224; Gallstones 474
Stool 944
    alternative term: Feces 442
Stork bite 944
    type of Hemangioma 526

Stoxil 1114
Strabismus 944
    cause of: Retinoblastoma 868
Strain 944
    *first aid: strain 945*
Strangulation 945
Strangury 945
    feature of Urination, painful
    1027
Strapping 945
Strawberry nevus 945
    type of Hemangioma 526
Streptase 1114
Strep throat 945
    cause of: Streptococcal
    infections 945
Streptococcal infections 945
Streptokinase 945
Streptomycin 945
    causing Deafness 333
Streptozocin 1114
Stress 946
    associated with *hypertension 556*
    treatment of: Meditation 671;
    Meprobamate 680; Relaxation
    techniques 859
Stress fracture 946
    type of Running injury 877
stress incontinence:
    Incontinence, urinary 579
Stress ulcer 946
Stretcher 946
    *using a stretcher 947*
Stretch mark 946
    medical term: Stria 946
Stria 946
Stricture 947
Stridor 947
    feature of Croup 321;
    Epiglottiditis 412
    investigation of: Laryngoscopy
    627
Stroke 947
    *types and causes of stroke 948*
Stroma 949
Strongyloidiasis 949
    cause of: Roundworms 876;
    *diseases caused by roundworms
    (nematodes) 877*
Strontium 949
    source of Radiation 844
Strychnine poisoning 949
Stuart Natal, Stuart Prenatal 1114
Stuffy nose:
    Nasal congestion 715
Stump 949
    and Amputation 96; Limb,
    artificial 640; *types of artificial
    limb 641*
Stupor 949
    type of: Narcosis 715
Sturge-Weber syndrome 949
    *appearance of Sturge-Weber
    syndrome 950*
Stuttering 950
St. Vitus' dance 950
    modern term: Sydenham's
    chorea 959
Stye 950
Subacute 950
Subarachnoid hemorrhage 950
Subclavian steal syndrome 950
Subclinical 951
Subconjunctival hemorrhage 951

Subconscious 951
  and Consciousness 298;
    Unconscious 1022
Subcutaneous 951
subdural hematoma:
  type of Hematoma 527
Subdural hemorrhage 951
Sublimation 951
  and Psychoanalytic theory 831
sublingual glands:
  Salivary glands 880
Subluxation 951
submandibular glands:
  Salivary glands 880
Submucous resection 951
Subphrenic abscess 951
  type of Abscess 58
substance abuse:
  types of: Drug abuse 378; Drug
    dependence 378; Solvent
    abuse 923
Substrate 951
Succinylcholine 1114
Sucking wound 951
Sucralfate 952
  and Vitamin supplements 1060
Sucrets Cold Decongestant
  Formula 1114
Suction 952
  use of: Ventilation 1045
suction lipectomy:
  use of: Body contour surgery
    191
Sudafed 1114
Sudden death 952
  Death 335
  Sudden infant death syndrome
    952
Sudden infant death syndrome
  (SIDS) 952
  cause of: Sleep apnea 916
Sudeck's atrophy 952
Sufentanil 1114
Suffocation 953
Sugar:
  type of Carbohydrate 232
Suicide 953
Suicide, attempted 953
Sulamyd 1114
sulci:
  of Brain 199; Cerebrum 250
Sulf-10 1114
Sulfabenzamide 1114
Sulfacetamide 954
Sulfacet-R 1114
Sulfacytine 1114
Sulfadiazine 1114
Sulfadoxine 1114
Sulfamethizole 1114
Sulfamethoxazole 954
Sulfasalazine 954
Sulfinpyrazone 954
Sulfisoxazole 954
Sulfonamide drugs 954
  examples: Sulfacetamide 954;
    Sulfamethoxazole 954;
    Sulfasoxazole 954
  group of Antibacterial drugs
    36, 114
Sulfoxyl 1114
Sulfur 954
Sulindac 954
Sulphrin 1114
Sulqui 1114

Sultrin 1114
Sumox 1114
Sumycin 1114
Sunburn 954
sunlight:
  abnormal reaction to:
    Photosensitivity 793
  component of: Ultraviolet light
    1021
  effects of: Sunburn 955;
    Sunlight, adverse effects of
    955; Suntan 955
  protection from: Sunscreens
    955
  treatment with: Phototherapy
    793
  and Vitamin D 1059
Sunlight, adverse effects of 955
Sunscreens 955
  ingredient of: Para-
    aminobenzoic acid 768
Sunstroke 955
  type of Heat stroke 525
Suntan 955
Supen 1114
Superego 955
  and Freudian theory 468;
    Psychoanalytic theory 831
Superficial 955
Superinfection 955
Superiority complex 956
Supernumerary 956
Supernumerary teeth 956
Supination 956
  and Pronation 824
Suppository 956
  uses of: Abortion, elective 58;
    Constipation 300
Supprettes 1114
Suppuration 956
Suprarenal glands 956
  see also index entry Adrenal
    glands
Supraspinatus syndrome:
  Painful arc syndrome 763
Supraventricular tachycardia 956
  type of Arrhythmia, cardiac 129
Suramin 1114
Surbex 1114
Surfactant 956
  abnormality of: Sudden infant
    death syndrome 952
  deficiency of: Respiratory
    distress syndrome 865
Surfers' nodules 956
Surgeon 956
Surgery 956
  landmarks in surgery 33
  and Modern surgical treatment
    34-35; Operating room 744;
    Operation 745
  pain relief during: Anesthesia,
    dental 104; Anesthesia,
    general 104; techniques for
    general anesthesia 105;
    Anesthesia, local 106
  types of: Cosmetic surgery 313;
    Cryosurgery 323;
    Microsurgery 687;
    Neurosurgery 725; Plastic
    surgery 801; Transplant
    surgery 1005
Surmontil 1114
Surrogacy 957

Susceptibility 957
  and Histocompatibility
    antigens 540
  increase of: Immunodeficiency
    disorders 575
Sus-Phrine 1114
Sustaire 1114
Sutilains 1114
Suture 957
  of Skull 914
  type of Joint 612
  see also index entry Suturing
Suturing 958
  methods of suturing 957
Swab 958
Swallowing 958
  and Digestive system 359; the
    digestive process 360
Swallowing difficulty 958
  causes of: Esophageal atresia
    418; Esophageal spasm 419;
    Esophageal stricture 419;
    Esophagus, cancer of 420;
    Guillain-Barré syndrome 501;
    Larynx, cancer of 628;
    Myasthenia gravis 709;
    Pharynx, cancer of 790;
    Plummer-Vinson syndrome
    802; Tonsillitis 996
  investigation of: Barium X-ray
    examinations 158;
    Laryngoscopy 627
  and Spinal accessory nerve 929;
    Vagus nerve 1037
Sweat glands 958
  disorders of: Hyperhidrosis
    553; Hypohidrosis 560
  part of Skin 910; structure of skin
    909
  see also index entry Sweating
Sweating 959
  and Body odor 191; Heat
    disorders 525; Oliguria 742;
    Shy-Drager syndrome 904;
    Water 1070
  see also index entry Sweat
    glands
Sweeteners, artificial:
  Artificial sweeteners 135
Swimmers' ear 959
  medical term: Otitis externa 757
Sycosis vulgaris 959
  type of Folliculitis 460
Sydenham's chorea 959
  cause of: Rheumatic fever 869
Sydenham, Thomas:
  landmarks in drug development 32
Syllact 1114
sylvian fissure:
  part of Cerebrum 250
Symmetrel 1114
Sympathectomy 959
  in treatment of Raynaud's
    disease 853
Sympathetic nervous system 959
  and Hypothalamus 562
  part of Autonomic nervous
    system 147; functions of the
    autonomic nervous system 146
Sympatholytic drugs 959
  types of Vasodilator drugs 1041
Symphysis 959
Symptom 959
  and Sign 906; Syndrome 960

Symptothermal method:
  Contraception, periodic
    abstinence 305
Synacort 1114
Synalar 1114
Synalgos-DC 1114
Synapse 960
  structure of a neuron 724
Syncope 960
  common term: Fainting 435
Syndactyly 960
Syndrome 960
  and Symptom 959
syndrome of inappropriate
  antidiuretic hormone secretion:
    SIADH 904
Synemol 1114
Synkayvite 1114
Synophylate 1114
Synovectomy 960
synovial sheaths:
  of Hand 505; Tendon 970
Synovitis 960
Synovium 961
  inflammation of: Synovitis 960
  part of Joint 611; types of joints
    612
  removal of: Synovectomy 960
Synthetic drugs 37
Synthroid 1114
Syntocinon 1114
Syphilis 961
  complication of: Neurosyphilis
    725
  a Sexually transmitted disease
    898
  incidence of primary and secondary
    syphilis in the US 900
Syringe 962
Syringing of ears 962
Syringomyelia 962
System 962
Systemic 962
Systemic lupus erythematosus
  (SLE):
    type of Lupus erythematosus
    653
systemic sclerosis:
  alternative term: Scleroderma
    886
Systole 962
  and Diastole 357; Heart 515
systolic blood pressure:
  abnormally high: Hypertension
    557
  and Blood pressure 188

T

Tabes dorsalis 963
  as complication of Neuro-
    syphilis 725; Syphilis 961
Tabloid 1114
Tabron 1114
Tacaryl 1114
TACE 1114
Tachycardia 963
  symptom of Coronary heart
    disease 311
  type of Arrhythmia, cardiac 129
Tachypnea 963
tagamet 1114

T'ai chi 963
Talacen 1114
Talbutal 1114
Talipes 963
    effect on Walking 1067
Talwin 1114
Talwin Nx 1114
Tambocor 1114
Tamoxifen 963
Tampon 963
    causing Toxic shock syndrome
        998; Vaginal discharge 1035;
        Vaginitis 1036
    and tearing of Hymen 551
    type of Sanitary protection 881
Tamponade 963
    cause of: Pericarditis 783
Tan:
    alternative term: Suntan 955
Tandearil 1114
Tannin 963
Tantrum 964
    type of Behavioral problem in
        children 162
Tapar 1114
Tapazole 1114
Tapeworm infestation 964
    treatment of: Niclosamide 727;
        Praziquantel 812
    type of Worm infestation 1081
tar:
    as Carcinogen 233
    causing Occupational disease
        and injury 739; Squamous
        cell carcinoma 937
    in Tobacco smoking 992
Taractan 1115
Tarsalgia 964
Tarsorrhaphy 964
    in treatment of Corneal ulcer
        309
Tartar:
    alternative term: Calculus,
        dental 224
tartrazine:
    type of Food additive 461
Taste 965
    associated with Smell 918
    and Facial nerve 434;
        Glossopharyngeal nerve 492;
        Tongue 995
taste buds:
    part of Tongue 995
    and the sense of taste 965
Taste, loss of 965
Tattooing 966
Tavist 1115
Tay-Sachs disease 966
    a disorder of the brain 202
Tazicef 1115
Tazidime 1115
TB:
    abbreviation for Tuberculosis
        1013
T cell 966
    type of Blood cell 184;
        Lymphocyte 655
Tear-Efrin 1115
Tearisol 1115
Tears 966
    deficiency of:
        Keratoconjunctivitis sicca 615
    excess of: Watering eye 1072
    production of: Eye 430;

Lacrimal apparatus 624;
    functions of the lacrimal
    apparatus 625
Tears, artificial 966
Tears Naturale 1115
Technetium 966
Tedral 1115
Teebacin 1115
Teebaconin 1115
Teeth 966
    disorders of: Abrasion, dental
        58; Calculus, dental 224;
        Caries, dental 236;
        Crowding, dental 321; Dental
        emergencies 340; Discolored
        teeth 363; Erosion, dental
        416; Fluorosis 460; Fracture,
        dental 468; Impaction, dental
        576; Luxated tooth 653;
        Malocclusion 661; Overbite
        760; Overcrowding, dental
        760; Plaque, dental 800;
        Toothache 997; causes of
        tooth decay 238
    eruption of: Eruption of teeth
        416; Teething 966; tooth
        eruption 417
    examination of: Dental
        examination 341; Dental X
        ray 342
    extraction of: Extraction, dental
        428
    false: Bridge, dental 213;
        Denture 343; Prosthodontics
        827; Titanium dental
        implants 977
    repairs to: Bonding, dental 192;
        Crown, dental 321; Filling,
        dental 455; Inlay, dental 591;
        Onlay, dental 743;
        Pulpectomy 838;
        Reimplantation, dental 859;
        Restoration, dental 866;
        Root-canal treatment 876;
        Splinting, dental 934
    straightening of: Orthodontic
        appliances 750; how
        orthodontic appliances work 751
    structure and arrangement of teeth
        967
    types of: Permanent teeth 786;
        Primary teeth 822
Teeth, care of:
    Oral hygiene 748
teeth, grinding of:
    medical term: Bruxism 217
Teething 966
    and Eruption of teeth 416; tooth
        eruption 417
Tegafur 1115
Tegison 1115
Tegopen 1115
Tegretol 1115
Tegrin 1115
Telangiectasia 968
    type of: Spider nevus 928
Teldrin 1115
Temaril 1115
Temazepam 968
Temperature 968
    and Heat disorders 525
    high: Fever 449, 450; Heat
        stroke 525; Hyperthermia
        557; Hyperthermia,

malignant 557; Seizure,
    febrile 890
low: Hypothermia 562
measurement of: Thermometer
    978
during Ovulation 760
regulation of: Hypothalamus
    562; Shivering 901
Temperature method:
    Contraception, periodic
    abstinence 305
Temporal arteritis 968
    associated with Polymyalgia
        rheumatica 808
temporal lobe:
    location of the temporal lobe 969
    part of Cerebrum 250
Temporal lobe epilepsy 969
    treatment of: Psychosurgery
        833
    type of Epilepsy 412
temporomandibular joint:
    and Jaw 610; Skull 914
    location of the temporomandibular
        joint 969
Temporomandibular joint
    syndrome 969
Tempra 1115
Tenderness 970
Tendinitis 970
Tendolysis 970
    in treatment of Tenosynovitis
        971
Tendon 970
    disorders of: Running injuries
        877; Shin splints 901; Sports
        injuries 936; Tendinitis 970;
        Tenosynovitis 971;
        Tenovaginitis 971;
    surgery on: Tendolysis 970;
        Tendon repair 970; Tendon
        transfer 970
    type of: Achilles tendon 62
Tendon release:
    medical term: Tenolysis 970
Tendon repair 970
Tendon transfer 970
    in treatment of Talipes 963
Tenesmus 970
Teniposide 1115
Tennis elbow 970
    site of tennis elbow 971
Tenoretic 1115
Tenormin 1115
Tenosynovitis 971
Tenovaginitis 971
TENS:
    abbreviation for
        Transcutaneous electrical
        nerve stimulation 1003
Tension 971
    causing Fibrositis 453;
        Headache 507, 509
    feature of Anxiety 122;
        Premenstrual syndrome 818
    see also index entry Stress
Tenuate 1115
Tepanil 1115
Teramine 1115
Teratogen 971
    causing Birth defects 173
Teratoma 971
    and Testis, cancer of 972
Terazosin 1115

Terbutaline 971
Terfenadine 971
Terminal care:
    Dying, care of the 381
Termination of pregnancy:
    Abortion, elective 57
Terpin hydrate 1115
Terra-Cortril 1115
Terramycin 1115
Tessalon 1115
Testicle:
    see index entry Testis
Testicular feminization syndrome
    971
    and Sex determination 897
Testis 972
    disorders of: Epididymal cyst
        411; Epididymo-orchitis 411;
        Hydrocele 550; Monorchism
        694; Orchitis 749; Testis,
        cancer of 972; Testis, ectopic
        973; Testis, pain in the 973;
        Testis, swollen 973; Testis,
        torsion of 973; Testis,
        undescended 973; Varicocele
        1038
    part of endocrine system 403;
        Reproductive system, male
        862, 863
    producing Sperm 926;
        Testosterone 974
    removal of: Castration 239;
        Orchiectomy 749
Testis, cancer of 972
    treatment of: Orchiectomy 749
Testis, ectopic 973
    treatment of: Orchiopexy 749
Testis, pain in the 973
Testis, retractile 973
Testis, swollen 973
    causes of: Epididymal cyst 411;
        Hydrocele 550; Mumps 703;
        Orchitis 749; Spermatocele
        927; Varicocele 1038
Testis, torsion of 973
Testis, undescended 973
    causing Oligospermia 742
    treatment of: Orchiopexy 749
Test meal 974
    use of: Barium X-ray
        examinations 159
Testolactone 1115
Testosterone 974
    type of Androgen hormone 100
Testred 1115
Tests, medical 974
    and Cancer screening 230;
        Diagnosing disease 24-31;
        Diagnosis 351; Prenatal
        screening procedures 819;
        Preventive medicine 22-23;
        Screening 887
"test-tube baby":
    and In vitro fertilization 604;
        Treating infertility 41
Tetanus 975
    prevention of: DPT vaccination
        373
    symptom of: Trismus 1021
Tetany 975
    causes of: Hyperventilation
        558; Hypoparathyroidism
        561; Osteomalacia 755
    causing Spasm 924

Tetrabenazine 1115
Tetracaine 975
Tetrachloroethylene 1115
Tetracycline drugs 976
　adverse effects of: Discolored
　　teeth 364; Fanconi's
　　syndrome 440; Pancreatitis
　　767
Tetracyn 1115
Tetrahydroaminoacridine 976
tetrahydrocanabinol:
　abbreviation for THC 977
Tetrahydrozoline 976
Tetralogy of Fallot 976
　causing Heart failure 519
　a *type of congenital heart disease*
　*518*
Tetrex 1115
Texacort 1115
T/Gel 1115
Thalamus 976
　function of: Sensation 892
　part of Brain 199
Thalassemia 977
　a *disorder of the blood 186*
　type of Hemoglobinopathy 529
Thalidomide 977
　causing Phocomelia 792
　type of Teratogen 971
Thalitone 1115
Thallium 977
THC 977
　constituent of Marijuana 664
Theo-24 1115
Theobid 1115
Theoclear 1115
Theo-Dur 1115
Theolair 1115
Theo-Organidin 1115
Theophyl 1115
Theophylline 977
Theospan 1115
Theostat 1115
Theovent 1115
Theozine 1115
Theragran 1115
Therapeutic 977
Therapeutic community 978
Therapy 978
Thermography 978
Thermometer 978
　*medical thermometer 25*
Thiabendazole 978
　in treatment of Toxocariasis
　　1000: Trichinosis 1009
Thiamine:
　part of Vitamin B complex 1058
Thiamylal 1115
Thiethylperazine 1115
Thimerosal 1115
Thioguanine 1115
Thiopental 978
Thioridazine 978
Thiosulfil 1115
Thiosulfil-A 1115
Thiotepa 1115
Thiothixene 978
Thirst 978
Thirst, excessive 979
　medical term: Polydipsia 808
　symptom of Diabetes insipidus
　　349; Diabetes mellitus 349
Thiuretic 1115
Thoracic outlet syndrome 979

Thoracic surgeon 979
Thoracotomy 979
Thorax 979
　surgical opening of:
　　Thoracotomy 979
　*anatomy of the thorax 980*
Thorazine 1115
Thought 979
Thought disorders 979
　feature of Psychosis 833;
　　Schizophrenia 884
Threadworm infestation:
　alternative term: Pinworm
　　infestation 796
Thrill 980
Throat 980
　see also index entry Pharynx
Throat cancer:
　Pharynx, cancer of 790
Throat, lump in the:
　medical term: Globus
　　hystericus 490
Thrombectomy 980
Thromboangiitis obliterans 980
　alternative term: Buerger's
　　disease 218
thrombocyte:
　alternative term: Platelet 801
　*constituents of blood 183*
　type of Blood cell 184
Thrombocytopenia 980
　causing Purpura 839
　type of Bleeding disorder 178
Thromboembolism 981
Thrombolytic drugs 981
　examples: Streptokinase 945;
　　Tissue-plasminogen activator
　　989; Urokinase 1029
　in treatment of Myocardial
　　infarction 712; Thrombosis
　　981
Thrombophlebitis 981
　alternative term: Phlebitis 791
　and Thrombosis 981
　a Vein, disorder of 1043
Thrombosis 981
　an Artery, disorder of 130
　causes of: Oral contraceptives
　　748; Plaque 800; Raynaud's
　　phenomenon 853
　treatment of: Anticoagulant
　　drugs 116; Thrombolytic
　　drugs 981
　see also index entries
　　Thrombophlebitis;
　　Thrombosis, deep vein
Thrombosis, deep vein 981, 982
　as complication of Stroke 947
　complication of: Embolism 396;
　　Pulmonary embolism 836
　type of Peripheral vascular
　　disease 784
　a Vein, disorder of 1043
Thrombus 892
　surgical removal of:
　　Thrombectomy 980
Thrush 983
　medical term: Candidiasis 230
thumb:
　a Finger 455
　function of: Grip 498
　part of Hand 505; *the skeletal*
　　*structure of the hand and wrist*
　　*506*

weakness of: Carpal tunnel
　　syndrome 238
Thumb-sucking 983
　in adults: Regression 858
　causing Malocclusion 661
thymectomy:
　in treatment of Myasthenia
　　gravis 709
thymine:
　as constituent of Nucleic acids
　　733
　and *DNA and genetic disorders*
　　*40; what genes are and what*
　　*they do 480*
Thymoma 983
　associated with Myasthenia
　　gravis 709
Thymoxamine 1115
Thymus 983
　and Lymphocyte 657
　part of Immune system
　　tumor of: Thymoma 983
Thyrar 1115
Thyroglossal disorders 983
Thyroid cancer 983
　a *disorder of the thyroid gland 986*
　treatment of: Thyroidectomy
　　984
Thyroidectomy 984
　in treatment of Thyroid cancer
　　984
Thyroid function tests 984
Thyroid gland 985
　*disorders of the thyroid gland 986*
　and *the sources and main effects of*
　　*selected hormones 546*
　part of endocrine system 403
　producing Calcitonin 223;
　　Thyroid hormones 985
　removal of: Thyroidectomy
　　984
Thyroid hormones 985
　examples: Calcitonin 223;
　　Thyroxine 987
　and *the sources and main effects of*
　　*selected hormones 546;* Iodine
　　605; *disorders of the thyroid*
　　*gland 986*
Thyroiditis 987
　a *disorder of the thyroid gland 986*
　type of: Hashimoto's thyroiditis
　　507
Thyroid scanning 987
thyroid-stimulating hormone
　　(TSH):
　measurement of: Thyroid
　　function tests 984
　production of: Pituitary gland
　　797
Thyroid strong 1115
Thyrolar 1115
Thyrotoxicosis 987
　treatment of: Iodine 605
　type of *endocrine disorder 404*
Thyroxine 987
　type of Thyroid hormone 985
Tibia 987
　part of Skeleton 909; *bones of the*
　　*skeleton 908*
Tic 988
　symptom of Gilles de la
　　Tourette's syndrome 487
Ticarcillin 1115
Tic douloureux 988

alternative term: Trigeminal
　　neuralgia 1010
Ticks and disease 988
Ticlopidine 1115
Tietze's syndrome 988
Tigan 1115
Timentin 1115
Timolide 1115
Timolol 988
Timoptic 1115
Tinactin 1115
Tindal 1115
Tinea 988
　common term: Ringworm 875
　a *disorder of the skin 910*
　treatment of: Antifungal drugs
　　117
　type of Dermatophyte infection
　　346; Fungal infection 470
tinea pedis:
　common term: Athlete's foot
　　141
Tinea versicolor 989
Tingling 989
　alternative term: Pins and
　　needles sensation 796
　*symptom chart 734*
Tinidazole 1115
Tinnitus 989
　a *disorder of the ear 385*
　symptom of Labyrinthitis 624;
　　Meniere's disease 674; Otitis
　　media 758; Otosclerosis 759
Tinver 1115
Tioconazole 1115
T-Ionate P.A. 1115
Tiopronin 1115
Tipped uterus:
　Uterus, tipped 1032
Tiredness 989
　*symptom chart 990*
Tissue 989
　cultivation of: Culture 324
　hardening of: Sclerosis 886
　storage of: Cryopreservation
　　323
tissue death:
　and Ablation 57; Amputation
　　96
　types of: Gangrene 474;
　　Infarction 581; Necrosis 717
Tissue fluid 989
　constituent of: Water 1070
Tissue-plasminogen activator
　　989
Tissue-typing 990
　and Histocompatibility
　　antigens 540
　in Organ donation 749;
　　Transplant surgery 1006
Titanium dental implants 991
　*fitting dental implants 992*
Tixocortol 1115
T-lymphocytes:
　causing Graft-versus-heart
　　disease 497
　infected by HIV 541
　part of Immune system 571
　type of Blood cell 183;
　　Lymphocyte 655
TMJ syndrome:
　abbreviation for
　　Temporomandibular joint
　　syndrome 969

Toadstool poisoning:
  type of Mushroom poisoning 707
Tobacco chewing:
  Snuff 922
Tobacco smoking 991, *993*
  and Birth weight 174; Life
    expectancy 639; Pregnancy
    813; Smell 919
  causing Bronchitis 215;
    Coronary heart disease 311;
    Emphysema 399; Halitosis
    505; Leukoplakia 638; Lip
    cancer 642; Lung cancer 651;
    Mouth cancer 697;
    Myocardial infarction 712;
    Palpitation 765; Pancreas,
    cancer of 766; Penis, cancer
    of 780; Peripheral vascular
    disease 784; Pharynx, cancer
    of 790; Stroke 947; Tongue
    cancer 995; Vincent's disease
    1049
  constituent of: Nicotine 727
  Smoking and drinking 20-21
Tobramycin 993
Tobrex 1115
Tocainide 993
Tocography 993
Tocopherol:
  constituent of Vitamin E 1059
Tocopheryl acetate 1115
Toe 993
  anatomy of: Foot 463;
    Phalanges 789;
Toenail, ingrown:
  Ingrown toenail 589
Tofranil 1115
Toilet-training 994
  and Developmental delay 348;
    Encopresis 401; Enuresis 408;
    Soiling 922
Tolazamide 994
Tolazoline 1115
Tolbutamide 994
Tolectin 1115
Tolerance 994
Tolinase 1115
Tolmetin 994
Tolnaftate 994
Tomography 994
  type of X ray 1084
  *using X rays to look at the body*
  *1085*
-tomy 994
Tone, muscle 995
Tongue 995
  disorders of: Glossitis 492;
    Leukoplakia 638;
    Macroglossia 658; Tongue
    cancer 995
  functions of: Mastication 667;
    Speech 925; Swallowing 958;
    Taste 965
  part of Mouth 697
  removal of: Glossectomy 492
Tongue cancer 995
Tongue depressor 995
Tongue-tie 995
Tonic 995
tonic neck reflex:
  type of Reflex, primitive 857;
    *types of primitive reflex 858*
Tonocard 1115

Tonometry 996
  in diagnosis of Glaucoma 490
  in measurement of Intraocular
    pressure 603
  use of: Eye, examination of 430
Tonsil 996
  disorders of: Quinsy 842;
    Tonsillitis 996
  removal of: Tonsillectomy 996
Tonsillectomy 996
  in treatment of Tonsillitis 996
Tonsillitis 996
  complication of: Quinsy 842
tooth:
  see index entry Teeth
Tooth abscess:
  Abscess, dental 59
Toothache 996
  cause of: Caries, dental 236
Toothbrushing 997
  part of Oral hygiene 748
  and removal of Plaque, dental
    800
Tooth decay:
  medical term: Caries, dental
    236
Tooth extraction:
  Extraction, dental 428
Toothpaste:
  type of Dentifrice 342
Tophus 997
Topical 997
Topicort 1115
Topicycline 1115
Topsyn 1115
Torecan 1115
Tornalate 1115
Torsion 997
Torticollis 998
Totacillin 1115
Touch 998
  and Sensation 892
  *the sense of touch 999*
Tourette's syndrome:
  alternative term: Gilles de la
    Tourette's syndrome 487
Tourniquet 998
  type of: Esmarch's bandage 418
  use of: Venipuncture 1044
Toxemia 998
  leading to Septic shock 895
Toxemia of pregnancy 998
  alternative term: Preeclampsia
    813
Toxicity 998
Toxicology 998
Toxic shock syndrome 998
  cause of: Staphylococcal
    infection 938
Toxin 1000
  in blood: Toxemia 998
  causing Poisoning 805; Septic
    shock 895
  type of Poison 805
Toxocariasis 1000
  cause of: Roundworms 876;
    *diseases caused by roundworms*
    *877*
  type of Larva migrans 626
Toxoid 1000
  use of: Vaccine 1034
Toxoplasmosis 1000
  causing Birth defect 173;
    Blindness 181

and *disorders of the retina 867*
TPA:
  abbreviation for Tissue-
    plasminogen activator 989
Trabeculectomy 1001
Trace elements 1001
  types of Minerals 689
Tracer 1001
Trachea 1001
  disorders of: Tracheitis 1001;
    Tracheoesophageal fistula
    1001
  part of Respiratory system 865
  surgical opening into:
    Tracheostomy 1002
Tracheitis 1001
  a *disorder of the lung 652*
Tracheoesophageal fistula 1001
  associated with Esophageal
    atresia 418
Tracheostomy 1002
  in treatment of Choking 272;
    Ludwig's angina 650;
    Pharyngitis 789; Respiratory
    distress syndrome 865;
    Tetanus 975
  and Ventilation 1045
Tracheotomy 1002
Trachoma 1002
  a *disorder of the eye 431*
  treatment of: Oxytetracycline
    761
Tract 1002
Traction 1002
  *traction for femoral fracture 1003*
Traifed C 1115
Traimcin 1115
Training 1003
  and Fitness 457
Trait 1003
  and Gene 481
Trance 1003
Trancopal 1115
Trandate 1115
Tranquilizer drugs 1003
  types of: Antianxiety drugs 114;
    Antipsychotic drugs 119
  and Drug dependence 378;
    Withdrawal syndrome 1080
Transcutaneous electrical nerve
  stimulation 1003
  use of: Dying, care of the 381
Transderm-Nitro 1115
Transderm-Scop 1115
Transference 1004
  in Psychoanalysis 831
Transfusion:
  Blood transfusion 190
Transfusion, autologous 1004
  type of Blood transfusion 190
Transient ischemic attack 1005
  and Fainting 436; Stroke 947
  treatment of: Isoxsuprine 608;
    Papaverine 768
Transillumination 1005
Translocation 1005
  causing Trisomy 1012
  and Chromosomal
    abnormalities 277
  *effect of chromosomal translocation*
  *1004*
Transmissible 1005
Transplant surgery 34, 1005
  and Cyclosporine 326; Grafting

496; Immunosuppressant
  drugs 576; Organ donation
  749; Tissue-typing 990
  risks of: Graft-versus-host
    disease 497;
    Immunodeficiency disorders
    575
  *landmarks in surgery 33*
  types of: Bone marrow
    transplant 195; *performing a*
    *bone marrow transplant 196;*
    Corneal graft 308; Heart-lung
    transplant 520, 521; Heart
    transplant 522; Kidney
    transplant 619; Liver
    transplant 648
Transposition of the great vessels
  1006
  *types of congenital heart disease*
  *518*
Transsexualism 1006
  and Sex change 896
  type of Psychosexual disorder
    832
Transvestism 1006
Tranxene 1115
Tranylcypromine 1006
Trapezius muscle 1006
Trapped nerve:
  Nerve, trapped 720
Trasicor 1115
Trauma 1007
  leading to Post-traumatic stress
    disorder 811
Trauma surgery:
  alternative term: Traumatology
    1007
Traumatology 1007
Travase 1115
Travelers' diarrhea 1007
  type of Gastroenteritis 476
Travel immunization 1007
Trazodone 1008
Treatment 1008
  Treating disease 32-39
  Treating infertility 41
Trecator-SC 1115
Trematode 1008
Trembling:
  alternative term: Tremor 1008
Tremin 1115
Tremor 1008
  and Extrapyramidal system 428
Trench fever 1008
Trench foot:
  alternative term: Immersion
    foot 570
Trench mouth:
  alternative term: Vincent's
    disease 1049
Trental 1116
Trephine 1008
Tretinoin 1008
Trexan 1116
Triacetin 1116
Triad 1116
Triafed-C 1116
Trial, clinical 1008
  and Animal experimentation
    110
  type of: Controlled trial 306
  using Double-blind 371
Triamcinolone 1008
Triaminic 1116

Triamterene 1009
Triaprin 1116
Triavil 1116
Triazolam 1009
Triceps muscle 1009
Trichiasis 1009
Trichinosis 1009
    a disorder of muscle 705
Trichloracetic acid 1116
Trichlormethiazide 1116
trichobezoar:
    cause of: Trichotillomania 1010
    common term: Hairball 503
    type of Bezoar 166
Trichomoniasis 1009
    causing Nonspecific urethritis
        730; Vaginal discharge 1035;
        Vaginitis 1036
    treatment of: Metronidazole
        684; Suppository 956
    type of Sexually transmitted
        disease 898
Trichotillomania 1010
Triclocarban 1116
Triclosan 1116
Tricodene 1116
Tricuspid insufficiency 1010
    causing Heart failure 519
    disorder of a Heart valve 524
Tricuspid stenosis 1010
    disorder of a Heart valve 524
Tridesilon 1116
Tridihexethyl chloride 1116
Tridil 1116
Tridione 1116
Trientine 1116
Triethylenetetramine 1116
Trifluoperazine 1116
Triflupromazine 1116
Trifluridine 1010
Trigeminal nerve 1010
    functions of cranial nerves 318
    disorder of: Trigeminal
        neuralgia 1010
    location of the trigeminal nerve
        1011
Trigeminal neuralgia 1010
    type of Neuralgia 720
Trigesic 1116
Trigger finger 1010
    appearance of trigger finger 1011
    disorder of Tendon 970
triglycerides:
    formation of: Glycerol 493
    in Hyperlipidemias 553
    types of Fats and oils 442;
        Lipids 642
Trihexane 1116
Trihexyphenidyl 1011
Tri-Hydroserpine 1116
Trilafon 1116
Tri-Levlen 1116
Trilisate 1116
Trilostate 1116
Trimazosin 1116
Trimeprazine 1011
Trimethadione 1116
Trimethaphan 1116
Trimethobenzamide 1011
Trimethoprim 1011
    in treatment of AIDS 79
    used with Sulfamethoxazole
        954
Trimipramine 1011

Trimox 1116
Trimpex 1116
Trinalin 1116
Trind 1116
Tri-Norinyl 1116
Trinsicon 1116
Trioxsalen 1116
Tripelennamine 1116
Triphasil 1116
Triphed 1116
Tri-Phen-Chlor 1116
Triple antibiotic 1116
Triple Sulfas 1116
Triprolidine 1011
Trisoralen 1116
Trismus 1011
    feature of Tetanus 975
Trisomy 1011
    type of Chromosomal
        abnormality 277
    types of trisomy 1012
Trisomy 21 syndrome 1012
    alternative term: Down's
        syndrome 372
Trisoralen 1116
Tri-Vi-Flor 1116
Tri-Vi-Sol 1116
Trobicin 1116
Trochlear nerve 1012
    functions of cranial nerves 318
Trofan 1116
Trolamine 1116
Troleandomycin 1116
Tromethamine 1116
Tronolane 1116
Tronothane 1116
Trophoblastic tumor 1012
    type of: Hydatidiform mole 549
Tropicacyl 1116
Tropical diseases 1012
Tropical ulcer 1013
Tropicamide 1013
Trunk 1013
Truss 1013
    in treatment of Hernia 534
Trymex 1116
Trypanosomiasis 1013
    types of: Chagas' disease 256;
        Sleeping sickness 916
Trypsin 1116
Tryptophan 1116
Trysul 1116
Trypanosomiasis 1013
Tsetse fly bites 1013
    and transmission of Sleeping
        sickness 916
TSH:
    see index entry thyroid-
        stimulating hormone
T-Stat 1116
T-tube cholangiography 1013
Tubal ligation:
    method of Sterilization, female
        940
Tubal pregnancy:
    alternative term: Ectopic
        pregnancy 389
Tubercle 1013
Tuberculin tests 1013
Tuberculosis 1013
    as complication of
        Pneumoconiosis 803
    diagnosis of: Tuberculin tests
        1013

prevention of: BCG vaccination
    161
treatment of: Aminosalicylic
    acid 94; Ethambutol 422;
    Isoniazid 608; Pyrazinamide
    841; Rifampin 874
type of bacterial infection 584
type of: Lupus vulgaris 653
Tuberosity 1014
Tuberous sclerosis 1014
    type of Neurocutaneous
        disorder 722
Tubocurarine 1116
Tuboplasty 1014
    procedure for balloon tuboplasty
        1015
Tuinal 1116
Tularemia 1015
Tumbu fly bites 1015
    causing Myiasis 710
Tumor 1015
    alternative term: Neoplasm 718
    types of: Benign 164;
        Carcinoma 234; Malignant
        660; Metastasis 683; Sarcoma
        881
    see also index entry Cancer
Tumor-specific antigen 1015
Tums 1116
Tunnel vision 1015
Turner's syndrome 1016
    features of: Amenorrhea 93;
        Short stature 902
    and Sex chromosomes 896
    type of Chromosomal
        abnormality 277
Tussagesic 1116
Tussanil 1116
Tussar 1116
Tussend 1116
Tussionex 1116
Tussi-Organidin 1116
Tussi-Organidin DM 1116
Tussirex 1116
Tuss-Ornade 1116
Twin-K 1116
Twins 1016
    and Pregnancy, multiple 815,
        816
Twins, conjoined 1016
    alternative term: Siamese twins
        904
Twitch:
    feature of Dyskinesia 382
    types of: Fasciculation 441; Tic
        988
Tylenol 1116
Tylox 1116
Tympagesic Otic Solution 1116
Tympanometry 1016
Tympanoplasty 1016
    in treatment of Deafness 334
Tympanum 1017
    part of Ear 384
Typhoid fever 1017
    prevention of: Immunization
        574; guidelines for travel
        immunization 1007; Vaccine
        1034
    type of bacterial infection 584;
        Waterborne infection 1071
Typhus 1017
    cause of: Rickettsia 874
    transmission of: Rats, diseases

from 853
Typing:
    alternative term: Tissue-typing
        990
Tyzine 1116

# U

Ulcer 1018
    examples: Corneal ulcer 308;
        Genital ulceration 485; Leg
        ulcer 633; Mouth ulcer 699;
        Peptic ulcer 780
    feature of Basal cell carcinoma
        160; Noma 730; Pyoderma
        gangrenosum 841; Ulcerative
        colitis 1018
Ulceration 1018
Ulcerative colitis 1018
    features of: Proctitis 822;
        Pyoderma gangrenosum 841
    symptom of: Rectal bleeding
        855
    treatment of: Hydrocortisone
        550; Prednisolone 813;
        Prednisone 813; Sulfasalazine
        954
Ulcer-healing drugs 1018
    examples: Antacid drugs 113;
        Cimetidine 280; Famotidine
        440; Ranitidine 849;
        Sucralfate 952
Ulna 1019
    part of the Skeleton 909; bones
        of the skeleton 908
Ulna, fracture of 1019
    and Monteggia's fracture 694
Ulnar nerve 1019
    and Elbow 393; Funny bone 471
    part of Brachial plexus 198
Ultracef 1116
Ultrasound 1019
    type of Radiation 845
    use of: Lithotripsy 39, 643;
        Radiology 848
    see also index entries
        Ultrasound scanning;
        Ultrasound treatment
Ultrasound scanning 41, 1019
    type of Imaging technique 568;
        scanning technique 882
    how ultrasound scanning works
        1020
    use of: Diagnostic ultrasound
        30; imaging the body 569;
        Prenatal care 818; prenatal
        screening procedures 819;
        Radiology 848
Ultrasound treatment 1020
    use of: Physical therapy 793
Ultraviolet light 1021
    causing Sunburn 954
    and Sunlight, adverse effects of
        955
    type of Radiation 845
Umbilical cord 1021
    development of: Embryo 397
    and Newborn 727
umbilical hernia:
    disorder of Umbilicus 1021
    main types of abdominal hernia
        535

Umbilicus 1021
Unconscious 1022
  and Subconscious 951
Unconsciousness 1022
  brief: Concussion 295; Fainting
  435
  prolonged: Coma 294
Underbite 1022
undescended testis:
  Testis, undescended 973
Unibase 1116
Unilax 1116
Unipen 1116
Uniphyl 1116
Unipres 1116
Unisom 1116
United States Pharmacopeia
  (USP):
  Pharmacopeia 789
Unproco 1116
Unsaturated fats:
  types of Fats and oils 441
uracil:
  constituent of Nucleic acids 733
Uranium 1022
  source of Radiation 844
Urea 1022
  constituent of Blood 182; Urine
  1027
  constituent of: Nitrogen 729
  production of: Liver 645
Urecholine 1116
Uremia 1023
  feature of Renal failure 860
Ureter 1023
  obstruction of:
  Retroperitoneal fibrosis 869
  part of the urinary system 1028;
  Urinary tract 1025
Ureteral colic:
  Renal colic 860
Ureterolithotomy 1023
Urethra 1023
  disorders of: Hypospadias 561;
  Nonspecific urethritis 730;
  Urethral discharge 1024;
  Urethral stricture 1024;
  Urethritis 1024; Urinary tract
  infection 1025
  part of Penis 779
  location of the urethra 1024
Urethral dilatation 1023
  in treatment of Urethral
  stricture 1024
Urethral discharge 1024
  causes of: Gonorrhea 495;
  Nonspecific urethritis 730
Urethral stricture 1024
  causing Cystitis 329; Urinary
  tract infection 1026; Urine
  retention 1029
  complication of Nonspecific
  urethritis 730; Urethritis 1024
  treatment of: Urethral
  dilatation 1023
Urethral syndrome, acute 1024
Urethritis 1024
  causing Urethral stricture 1024
  type of Urinary tract infection
  1025
  type of: Nonspecific urethritis
  730
Urethrocele 1024
  and Uterus, prolapse of 1032

Urex 1116
urge incontinence:
  type of Incontinence, urinary
  579
-uria 1024
Uric acid 1025
  high blood level of:
  Hyperuricemia 558
uricosuric drugs:
  in treatment of Gout 496
Urinal 1025
Urinalysis 1025
  use of: Kidney function tests
  619
Urinary diversion 1025
  in treatment of Incontinence,
  urinary 580
  urinary diversion using ileal
  conduit 1026
urinary frequency:
  Urination, frequent 1027
urinary incontinence:
  see index entry Incontinence,
  urinary
Urinary tract 1025
  anatomy of: Bladder 175;
  anatomy of the bladder 176;
  Kidney 616; Ureter 1023;
  Urethra 1023; location of the
  urethra 1024; the urinary
  system 1028
  disorders of: disorders of the
  bladder 177; Calculus, urinary
  tract 224, 225; Hypospadias
  561; Incontinence, urinary
  579; disorders of the kidney 618;
  Nonspecific urethritis 738;
  Urethral discharge 1024;
  Urethral stricture 1024;
  Urethritis 1024; Urinary tract
  infection 1025; Urination,
  painful 1027
  function of: the function of the
  kidney 617; Urine 1027
  imaging of: Pyelography 839
  study of: Urology 1029
Urinary tract infection 1025
  causing Irritable bladder 606
  during Pregnancy 814
  treatment of: Nitrofurantoin
  728; Sulfamethoxazole 954;
  Sulfonamide drugs 954
Urination, excessive 1026
  at night: Nocturia 729
Urination, frequent 1027
Urination, painful 1027
  causes of: Cystitis 329;
  Gonorrhea 495; Herpes,
  genital 536; Urethritis 1024
Urine 1027
  constituents of: Urea 1022;
  Water 1070
  production and excretion of: the
  urinary system 1028
  testing of: Urinalysis 1025
  see also index entry Urine,
  abnormal
Urine, abnormal 1027
  examples: Anuria 121;
  Glycosuria 493; Hematuria
  527; Oliguria 742;
  Pneumaturia 802
  and Urination, excessive 1026
Urine retention 1029

Urine tests:
  Urinalysis 1025
Urised 1116
Urispas 1116
Uritabs 1116
Urobiotic-250 1116
Urodine 1116
Urogesic 1116
Urography 1029
  alternative term: Pyelography
  839
Urokinase 1029
Urologist 1029
Urology 1029
Uro-Phosphate 1116
Ursodeoxycholic acid 1029
Urticaria 1030
  of Newborn 727
  treatment of:
  Chlorpheniramine 271;
  Hydroxyzine 551;
  Promethazine 823;
  Pyrilamine 841
  type of Skin allergy 911
urticaria pigmentosa:
  alternative term: Mastocytosis
  667
USP (United States
  Pharmacopeia):
  Pharmacopeia 789
Uterus 1030
  disorders of: disorders of the
  cervix 255; disorders of the
  uterus 1031
  function of: Childbirth 263;
  stages of birth 264; Pregnancy
  813; stages and features of
  pregnancy 814
  part of Reproductive system,
  female 862, 863
  removal of: Hysterectomy 565
Uterus, cancer of 1031
  type of: Cervix, cancer of 254
Uterus, prolapse of 1032
  prevention of: Pelvic floor
  exercises 777
  treatment of: Hysterectomy
  565; Vaginal repair 1035
Uterus, retroverted:
  Uterus, tipped 1032
Uterus, tipped 1032
  tipped uterus 1033
Uticillin VK 1116
Uticort 1116
Utimox 1116
Uvea 1033
  inflammation of: Uveitis 1033
Uveitis 1033
  cause of: Herpes zoster 537
  causing Eye, painful red 433
  a disorder of the eye 431
UV light:
  abbreviation for Ultraviolet
  light 1021
Uvula 1033

—————————————

V

Vaccination 1034
  and Cowpox 317; Vaccine 36,
  1034

landmarks in drug development 32
  in prevention of Infectious
  disease 582
  see also index entry
  Immunization
Vaccine 36, 1034
  as method of Contraception 304
  see also index entries
  Immunization; Vaccination
Vacon 1116
Vacuum extraction 1034
Vagina 1034
  disorders of: Chlamydial
  infections 270; Rectocele 856;
  Urethrocele 1024;
  Vaginismus 1036; Vaginitis
  1036
  dryness of: Menopause 676;
  Sjögren's syndrome 909
  function of: Childbirth 263;
  stages of birth 264; the process of
  fertilization 446; Sexual
  intercourse 898, 899
  and painful intercourse in women
  597
  part of Reproductive system,
  female 862, 863
  structure of the vagina 1035
Vaginal bleeding 1034
  causes of: Antepartum
  hemorrhage 113; Postpartum
  hemorrhage 811;
  Menstruation 677
vaginal deodorants:
  causing Urination, painful
  1027; Vaginal itching 1035
Vaginal discharge 1035
  causes of: Candidiasis 230;
  Cervical erosion 251;
  Chlamydial infection 270;
  Gonorrhea 495; Nonspecific
  urethritis 730; Pelvic
  inflammatory disease 777;
  Trichomoniasis 1009; Uterus,
  cancer of 1032; Vaginitis
  1036
  and stages and features of
  pregnancy 814
Vaginal itching 1035
Vaginal repair 1035
  in treatment of Uterus,
  prolapse of 1032
Vaginex 1116
Vaginismus 1036
  causing Intercourse, painful
  598
  disorder of the Vagina 1034
  treatment of: Sex therapy 898
Vaginitis 1036
Vagitrol 1116
Vagotomy 1036
  in treatment of Peptic ulcer
  781
Vagus nerve 1037
  functions of cranial nerves 318
  effect on Heart 515
  overstimulation of: Vasovagal
  attack 1041
  surgical cutting of: Vagotomy
  1036
Valdrene 1116
Valergen 1116
Valertest 1117
Valgus 1037

Valisone 1117
Valium 1117
Valmid 1117
Valpin 1117
Valproic acid 1037
Valrelease 1117
Valsalva's maneuver 1037
in treatment of
Supraventricular tachycardia
956
Valve 1037
in Veins 1043
type of: Heart valve 523
see also index entries Heart;
heart valve abnormalities;
Heart valve surgery
Valve replacement 1037
see also index entry Heart
valve surgery
Valvotomy 1037
Valvular heart disease 1038
disorder of Heart valve 523
see also index entry heart valve
abnormalities
Valvuloplasty 1038
type of Heart valve surgery 524
Vancenase 1117
Vanceril 1117
Vancomycin 1038
Vanoxide-HC 1117
Vanseb 1117
Vaponefrin 1117
Vaporizer 1038
Varicella 1038
common term: Chickenpox 262
Varices 1038
type of: Esophageal varices 419
Varicocele 1038
causing Infertility 586;
Oligospermia 742
disorder of Testis 972
varicose ulcers:
type of Leg ulcer 633
Varicose veins 1038, 1039
causing Eczema 390
during Pregnancy 813
treatment of: Sclerotherapy 886
Variola 1039
alternative term: Smallpox 918
Varus 1039
vasa efferentia:
anatomy of: Epididymis 411;
Testis 972
Vasculitis 1039
Vas deferens 1040
anatomy of: Epididymis 411;
Reproductive system, male
862, 863; Testis 972
surgical cutting of: Vasectomy
1040
Vasectomy 1040
a method of contraception 303
Vaseline Petroleum Jelly 1117
Vasocidin 1117
VasoClear 1117
Vasocon 1117
Vasocon-A 1117
Vasoconstriction 1041
Vasodilan 1117
Vasodilatation 1041
Vasodilator drugs 1041
examples: Isosorbide dinitrate
608; Isoxsuprine 608;
Minoxidil 689; Nitroglycerin

729; Papaverine 768
in treatment of Ischemia 607
vasomotor rhinitis:
type of Rhinitis 872
Vasopressin 1041
alternative term: ADH 68
Vasosulf 1117
Vasotec 1117
Vasovagal attack 1041
causing Fainting 435
Vatronol 1117
vault cap:
type of Contraception, barrier
method 304
V-Cillin K 1117
VD 1041
alternative term: Sexually
transmitted disease 898
Vector 1041
and Zoonosis 1088; a selection of
zoonoses (diseases caught from
animals) 1087
Vecuronium 1117
Veetids 1117
vegan diet:
and Feeding, infant 444;
deficiency of Vitamin $B_{12}$
1058
type of Vegetarianism 1042
Vegetarianism 1042
causing Rickets 874
and Feeding, infant 444
Vegetative state 1042
Vein 1042
anatomy of: Valve 1037;
structure of a vein and artery
1043
part of Circulatory system 280,
281
X rays of: Venography 1044
see also index entry Veins,
disorders of
Veins, disorders of 1043
examples: Esophageal varices
419; Hemorrhoids 530;
Phlebitis 791; Retinal vein
occlusion 868;
Thrombophlebitis 981;
Thrombosis, deep vein 981,
982; Varicose veins 1038,
1039
Velban 1117
Velosef 1117
Velosulin 1117
Velvachol 1117
Vena cava 1043
part of Circulatory system 280,
281
Venereal diseases:
alternative term: Sexually
transmitted diseases 898
Venereology 1043
Venesection 1044
in treatment of Polycythemia
807
Venipuncture 1044
Venography 1044
in diagnosis of Thrombosis,
deep vein 982
Venomous bites and stings 1044
Ventilation 1044
technique of artificial ventilation
1045
and Tracheostomy 1002

see also index entry Ventilator
Ventilator 1045
in treatment of Respiratory
distress syndrome 865;
Respiratory failure 865
use of: Ventilation 1044
Ventolin 1117
Ventouse:
Vacuum extraction 1034
Ventral 1045
Ventricle 1046
of Cerebrum 250; Heart 514
Ventricular ectopic beat 1046
type of ventricular arrhythmia
1047
Ventricular fibrillation 1046
type of ventricular arrhythmia
1047
ventricular septal defect:
type of congenital heart disease
518; Septal defect 894
Ventricular tachycardia 1046
type of ventricular arrhythmia
1047
Ventriculography 1046
venule:
part of Circulatory system 280,
281
Vepesid 1117
Verapamil 1046
Vermox 1117
Vernix 1046
Verrex 1117
Verruca 1046
common term: Wart 1069
Verrusol 1117
Version 1046
Vertebra 1047
anatomy of: Coccyx 285;
anatomy of coccyx 286; Disk,
intervertebral 364; Sacrum
878; Skeleton 909; bones of the
skeleton 908; Spine 932;
location and structure of the
vertebrae 1048
disorders of: disorders of the
spine 933; Spinal injury 930;
Spondylolisthesis 935;
Spondylolysis 935
fusion of: Sacralization 878;
Spinal fusion 930
Vertebrobasilar insufficiency 1047
Vertigo 1047
causes of: disorders of the ear 385;
Labyrinthitis 624; Meniere's
disease 674
and Dizziness 367, 368
very low-density lipoprotein
(VLDL):
and Cholesterol 275; Fats and
oils 442; Hyperlipidemias 553
Vesalius, Andreas:
in history of Anatomy 99;
Medicine 670
Vesicle 1048
type of Blister 181
Vesprin 1117
vestibule:
part of Ear 384
Vestibulocochlear nerve 1048
and functions of cranial nerves
318; anatomy of the ear 384
location of the vestibulocochlear
nerve 1049

Viability 1049
Vibramycin 1117
Vibra-Tabs 1117
Vibrator 1049
Vicks 1117
Vicodin 1117
Vicon-C 1117
Vidarabine 1117
Vi-Daylin 1117
Villus 1049
part of Intestine 601
Viloxazine 1117
vimule cap:
type of Contraception, barrier
method 304
Vinblastine 1117
Vincent's disease 1049
Vincent's stomatitis:
alternative term: Vincent's
disease 1049
Vincristine 1117
Vindesine 1117
Vineberg, Arthur:
landmarks in surgery 33
Vioform 1117
Viokase 1117
Vira-A 1117
viral hepatitis:
Hepatitis, viral 533
type of Hepatitis 532
viral meningitis:
type of Meningitis 675
viral pneumonia:
type of Pneumonia 803, 804
Viranol 1117
Virazole 1117
Viremia 1049
Virginity 1049
Virilism 1049
cause of: Virilization 1050
Virility 1050
Virilization 1050
Virion 1050
Viruses 1050
Virology 1050
Viroptic 1117
Virulence 1050
Viruses 1050
causing disease: Infectious
disease 582; viral infections
583; viruses and disease 1051
study of: Virology 1050
Viscera 1052
visceral larva migrans:
alternative term: Toxocariasis
1000
type of Larva migrans 626
Viscosity 1052
Visine 1117
Vision 1052
aspects of: Accommodation 61;
Blind spot 181; Color vision
291; the sense of vision 1053;
Visual acuity 1055; Visual
field 1055; the visual fields
1056
and Child development 267,
268
function of Cornea 307; Eye
428; anatomy of the eye 429;
Optic nerve 746; Retina 866
study of: Ophthalmology 745
testing of: Eye, examination of
430; Vision tests 1054;

Vision (continued)
*types of vision tests 1055*
see also index entry Vision,
   disorders of
Vision, disorders of 1054
   causes of: *disorders of the cornea*
      *308; disorders of the eye 431;*
      *disorders of the retina 867*
   and Developmental delay 347;
      Vision, loss of 1054
   examples: Ambylopia 92;
      Anisometropia 111;
      Astigmatism 139; Color
      vision deficiency 292; Double
      vision 371; Floaters 458;
      Hyperopia 554; Myopia 713;
      Night blindness 727;
      Presbyopia 820; Strabismus
      944; Tunnel vision 1015
   treatment of: Contact lenses
      300; Glasses 488; *why glasses*
      *are used 489;* Keratotomy,
      radial 615
   see also index entries
      Blindness; Vision tests;
      Visual field
Vision, loss of 1054
   see also index entry Blindness
Vision tests 1054
   and Ophthalmology 745;
      Optometry 746
   types of: Evoked responses 424;
      Eye, examination of 430;
      Snellen's chart 921: *types of*
      *vision tests 1055*
Visken 1117
Vistaril 1117
Visual acuity 1055
   testing of: Eye, examination of
      430; Snellen's chart 921;
      Vision tests 1054; *types of*
      *vision tests 1055*
   and Visual field 1055, *1056*
   see also index entries Vision;
      Vision, disorders of
Visual field 1055, *1056*
   defects of: Hemianopia 527;
      Macular degeneration 658;
      Optic neuritis 746; Pituitary
      tumors 797; Retinal
      detachment 867; Retinitis
      pigmentosa 868
   testing of: Eye, examination of
      430; Vision tests 1054; *types of*
      *vision tests 1055*
Vital sign 1056
Vitamin 1056
   and Nutrition 736
   *recommended daily dietary*
      *allowances (RDAs) of selected*
      *vitamins 19*
   *vitamins and their sources in the*
      *diet 1057*
Vitamin A 1057
   and Carotene 238
   source of: Cod-liver oil 286
   see also index entry Vitamin
Vitamin B:
   Vitamin B$_{12}$ 1058
   Vitamin B complex 1058
   vitamin B$_1$:
      part of Vitamin B complex 1058
      see also index entry Vitamin
   vitamin B$_2$:

part of Vitamin B complex 1058
   see also index entry Vitamin
   vitamin B$_6$:
      part of Vitamin B complex 1058
      see also index entry Vitamin
Vitamin B$_{12}$ 1058
   synthetic form of:
      Hydroxocobalamin 551
   see also index entry Vitamin
Vitamin B complex 1058
   see also index entry Vitamin
Vitamin C 1059
   see also index entry Vitamin
Vitamin D 1059
   source of: Cod-liver oil 286
   see also index entry Vitamin
Vitamin E 1059
   see also index entry Vitamin
Vitamin K 1060
   as Hemostatic drug 531
   see also index entry Vitamin
Vitamin supplements 1060
   see also index entry Vitamin
Vitiligo 1060
   disorder of Pigmentation 794
Vitreous hemorrhage 1060
   cause of: Eye injuries 432
Vitreous humor 1061
   part of Eye 429
Vitron-C 1117
Vivactil 1117
Vivalin 1117
Vivisection 1061
   and Animal experimentation
      110
VLDL:
   see index entry very low-
      density lipoprotein
Vocal cords 1061
   disorders of: Hoarseness 542,
      543; Larynx, cancer of 628;
      *disorders of the larynx 629;*
      Singers' nodes 906; Stridor
      947; Voice, loss of 1061
   part of Larynx 628
Voice box:
   medical term: Larynx 627
Voice, loss of 1061
   alternative terms: Aphonia 125;
      Dysphonia 383
   *symptom chart 542*
Volkmann's contracture 1062
Volvulus 1062
   causing Abdominal pain 54;
      Intestine, obstruction of 602
Vomiting 1062, *1063*
   induction of: Ipecac 606
   projectile: Pyloric stenosis 841
   treatment of: Antiemetic drugs
      117; Perphenazine 786;
      Prochlorperazine 822;
      Promethazine 823
   Vomiting in pregnancy 1065
   see also index entry Vomiting
      blood
Vomiting blood 1065
   and Abdominal pain 54
   causes of: Cirrhosis 282;
      Esophageal varices 419;
      Mallory-Weiss syndrome 661;
      Peptic ulcer 780; Portal
      hypertension 810
Vomiting in pregnancy 1065
vomit, inhalation of:

causing Choking 272;
   *Pneumonia 804;* Pneumonitis
   804; Respiratory distress
   syndrome 865
Von Recklinghausen's disease
   1056
   alternative term:
      Neurofibromatosis 722
Vontrol 1117
Von Willebrand's disease 1066
   type of Bleeding disorder 178
Vosal 1117
VoSol HC 1117
Voxsuprine 1117
Voyeurism 1066
Vulva 1066
   and Bartholin's glands 160
   disorders of: Leukoplakia 638;
      Vaginal itching 1035; Vulva,
      cancer of 1066; Vulvitis 1066;
      Vulvovaginitis 1066
   part of Reproductive system,
      female 862
   parts of: Clitoris 284; Labia 624
Vulva, cancer of 1066
vulval dystrophy:
   causing Vaginal itching 1035;
      Vulvitis 1066
Vulvitis 1066
   causing Urethral syndrome,
      acute 1024
Vulvovaginitis 1066
Vytone 1117

# W

WAIS (Wechsler Adult
   Intelligence Scale):
   type of Intelligence test 595
Walking 1067
   in Child development 267
Walking aids *1068,* 1069
Walking, delayed 1069
   type of Developmental delay
      347
walking reflex:
   type of Reflex, primitive 857
Walleye 1069
   type of Strabismus 944
Wans 1117
Warfarin 1069
Wart 1069
   types of: Plantar wart 799;
      Warts, genital 1070
Wart-Off 1117
Warts, genital 1070
   treatment of: Podophyllin 805
   type of Sexually transmitted
      disease 898; Wart 1070
Wasp stings:
   type of Insect sting 592
Water 1070
   excessive loss of: Dehydration
      338; Diarrhea 356; Heat
      disorders 525; Heat
      exhaustion 525
   intake of: Nutrition 736; Thirst
      978; Thirst, excessive 979
   and Ion 606; Osmosis 753
   loss of: Sweat glands 958; Urine
      1027
   regulation of: ADH 68; Kidney

616; *the function of the kidney*
   617
   retention of: Edema 390; Water
      intoxication 1072
   therapeutic use of:
      Hydrotherapy 551
   see also index entry
      Waterborne infection
Waterborne infection 1071
   causing Diarrhea 356
   and Infectious disease 582;
      Preventive medicine 820;
      Staying healthy 17
Waterhouse-Friderichsen
   syndrome 1071
Watering eye 1072
   cause of: Ectropion 390
Water intoxication 1072
Water-on-the-brain:
   medical term: Hydrocephalus
      550
Water-on-the-knee 1072
   cause of: Bursitis 221
"waters, breaking of the":
   in Childbirth 265
Water tablets:
   medical term: Diuretic drugs
      366
Wax bath 1072
Wax, ear:
   Earwax 387
waxing:
   method of Hair removal 503
Weakness 1072
Weaning 1072
   and Feeding, infant 443
Webbing 1072
   of neck: Turner's syndrome
      1016
Wechsler tests:
   types of Intelligence tests 595
Wegener's granulomatosis 1072
Wehless 1117
Weight 1072
   and Obesity 738; Weight loss
      1073; Weight reduction 1075
   *weight tables 1073*
weightlessness:
   effects of: Environmental
      constraints 47; Space
      medicine 924
Weight loss 1073
   *symptom chart 1074*
Weight reduction 1075
Weil's disease:
   alternative term: Leptospirosis
      635
Welders' eye 1075
Wellcovorin 1117
Wells, Horace:
   and *landmarks in surgery 33*
Werdnig-Hoffmann disease 1075
   type of Motor neuron disease
      696
Werner's syndrome:
   type of Progeria 823
Wernicke-Korsakoff syndrome
   1076
   and deficiency of Vitamin B
      complex 1058
Wernicke's encephalopathy:
   *an alcohol-related disorder 85*
   stage of Wernicke-Korsakoff
      syndrome 1076

Westcort 1117
"wet dream":
  medical term: Nocturnal
    emission 729
wheals:
  feature of Urticaria 1030
Wheelchair 1076
Wheeze 1076
  associated with Breathing
    difficulty 210
  feature of Asthma 137;
    Bronchitis 214
Whiplash injury 1077
  cause of whiplash injury 1076
  injury to Neck 716
  type of Spinal injury 930
Whipple's disease 1077
  symptom of: Malabsorption 658
Whipple's operation 1077
  type of Pancreatectomy 767
Whipworm infestation 1077
Whitehead 1077
  medical term: Milia 689
white matter:
  of Brain 201; structure of brain
    200
  constituent of: Myelin 710
  and Gray matter 498
Whitfield's Ointment 1117
Whitlow 1077
Whooping cough:
  medical term: Pertussis 787
Wife beating:
  alternative term: Spouse abuse
    936
Wigraine 1117
Wigrettes 1117
Will, living 1077
Wilms' tumor 1078
  type of Kidney cancer 617
Wilpowr 1117
Wilson's disease 1078
  a disorder of the liver 646
Windpipe 1078
  medical term: Trachea 1001
Winstrol 1117
Wiring of the jaws 1078
  in treatment of Jaw, fractured
    611; Obesity 738
WISC (Wechsler Intelligence
  Scale for Children):
  type of Intelligence test 595
Wisdom tooth 1078
  and Eruption of teeth 416
  impacted: Impaction, dental
    577
  structure and arrangement of teeth
    967
Witches' milk 1078
Witch hazel 1117
Withdrawal 1078
Withdrawal bleeding 1078
Withdrawal method:
  alternative term: Coitus
    interruptus 287
Withdrawal syndrome 1078
  and Drug dependence 378
Womb:
  alternative term: Uterus 1030
wood alcohol:
  chemical term: Methanol 683
  type of Alcohol 81
Word blindness:
  alternative terms: Alexia 85;

Dyslexia 382
World Health Organization 1080
  and Preventive medicine 821
world population 172
Worm infestation 1081
  and Cats, diseases from 243;
    Dogs, diseases from 369
  treatment of: Antihelmintic
    drugs 118; drugs used to treat
    worm infestations 1080
Wound 1081
  first aid: wounds 1079
  and Healing 510
Wound infection 1081
  and Sepsis 894
Wrinkle 1082
  treatment of: Face-lift 434
Wrist 1082
  anatomy of: the skeletal structure
    of the hand and wrist 506
  movements of: types of joints
    612
  part of Skeleton 908
Wristdrop 1082
  cause of: damage to Radial
    nerve 844
  disorder of the Wrist 1082
Wry neck:
  medical term: Torticollis 998
Wyamycin S 1117
Wyanoids 1117
Wycillin 1117
Wydase 1117
Wygesic 1117
Wymox 1117
Wytensin 1117

# X

Xanax 1117
Xanthelasma 1083
Xanthoma 1083
  feature of Xanthomatosis 1083
Xanthomatosis 1083
X chromosome:
  and Chromosomal
    abnormalities 277;
    Inheritance 589; Sex
    determination 897; Sex-
    linked 897; Sperm 926
  type of Chromosome 279; Sex
    chromosome 896
  see also index entry X-linked
    disorders
Xerac 1117
Xerac BP 1117
Xeroderma pigmentosum 1083
Xerophthalmia 1083
  a disorder of the eye 431
Xerostomia 1083
  common term: Mouth, dry 697
Xiphisternum 1083
  part of Sternum 940
xiphoid process:
  alternative term: Xiphisternum
    1083
  part of Sternum 940
X-linked disorders 1083
  examples: Fragile X syndrome
    468; Klinefelter's syndrome
    621; Turner's syndrome 1016
  and Sex-linked 897

types of Genetic disorders 482;
  unifactorial genetic disorders
  483
X-Otag 1117
X-Prep 1117
X rays 26, 1083
  and Film badge 455; Radiation
    hazards 845; X-ray technician
    1084
  landmarks in diagnosis 25
  type of Radiation 844
  uses of: Angiography 109;
    Arthrography 133; Barium
    X-ray examinations 158; Bone
    imaging 194; three-dimensional
    bone imaging 27; Brain
    imaging 203; Chest X ray 259;
    Cholangiography 272;
    Cholecystography 274; CT
    scanning 26, 323; performing a
    CT scan 324; Dental X rays
    342; Digital subtraction
    angiography 26; ERCP 415;
    Heart imaging 519; Imaging
    techniques 568; imaging the
    body 569; Kidney imaging
    619; Liver imaging 648; Lung
    imaging 652; Mammography
    22, 662; Myelography 710;
    Pyelography 839; retrograde
    pyelogram 840; Radiation
    therapy 846; Radiology 848;
    Tomography 994;
    Venography 1044; X-ray
    examination 1084; using X rays
    to look at the body 1085
X rays, dental:
  Dental X rays 342
X-ray technician 1084
X seb 1117
Xylocaine 1117
Xylometazoline 1084

# Y

yang:
  see index entry Yin and yang
Yawning 1086
Yaws 1086
Y chromosome:
  and Chromosomal
    abnormalities 277;
    Inheritance 590; Sex
    determination 897; Sperm
    926
  type of Chromosome 279; Sex
    chromosome 896
Yeasts 1086
  causing Candidiasis 230;
    Fungal infections 470
  types of Fungi 470
Yellow fever 1086
  prevention of: Travel
    immunization 1007
  type of Tropical disease 1012
yellow skin:
  causes of: Carotene 238;
    Jaundice 610; Yellow fever
    1086
yin:
  see index entry Yin and yang
Yin and Yang 1086

in Chinese medicine 267;
  Macrobiotics 658
Y-Itch 1117
Yocon 1117
Yodoxin 1117
Yoga 1086
  and Relaxation techniques 859
Yohimbine 1117
Yohimex 1117
Yomesan 1117
Yutopar 1117

# Z

Zantac 1117
Zarontin 1117
Zaroxolyn 1117
Z-Bec 1117
Zeasorb-AF 1117
Zemo 1117
Zenate 1117
Zenker's diverticulum:
  disorder of the Pharynx 790
  type of Esophageal
    diverticulum 418
Zentinic 1117
Zentron 1117
Zephiran Chloride 1117
Zephrex 1117
Zetar 1117
Zide 1117
Zidovudine 1087
  in treatment of AIDS 79
Zinacef 1117
Zinc 1087
  deficiency of: Acrodermatitis
    enteropathica 65
  recommended daily dietary
    allowances (RDAs) of selected
    minerals 19
  sources of: minerals and main
    food sources 690
  type of Mineral 689; essential
    nutrients 736; Trace element
    1001
Zincfrin 1117
Zinc gluconate 1117
Zincon 1117
Zinc oxide 1087
  as constituent of Calamine 223
Zinc pyrithione 1117
Zinc sulfate 1117
Ziradryl 1117
Zollinger-Ellison syndrome 1088
  feature of: Peptic ulcer 780
Zone-A 1117
Zoonosis 1088
  a selection of zoonoses (diseases
    caught from animals) 1087
Zorprin 1117
Z-plasty 1088
  use of: Plastic surgery 801
Zygote 1088
  in the process of fertilization 446
Zyloprim 1117
Zymenol 1117

Allsport/Tony Duffy 47 /Michael King 47; American Society of Plastic and Reconstructive Surgeons, Inc., 179, 434, 758; AMI Portland Hospital (Ultrasound Dept.) 816; Argentum 467, 944, 951, 978, 1069, 1081

Mr. John Browett 539, 622, 1085; BUPA Fitness Centre 426; BUPA Medical Centre 205, 662

Cemax Inc. 27, 1085; Dr. M. Curling 253, 331

Dr. Richard Dawood 158, 193, 1084, 1085; Prof. P. Dieppe and Gower Medical Publishing 496; Dorling Kindersley/Paul Fletcher 1086; Dr. R. Doshi, Brook General Hospital 203, 490; Dr. Andrew Duncombe, St. Thomas' Hospital Medical School 186, 636

Edwards Laboratories, Orange County, California, 524; Mary Evans Picture Library 32

Dr. T. Fowler 91, 99, 200

Gibbs Dental Division 362, 801; Glaxo 390, 873; Mr. Brian Glenville 310

The Image Bank/Michael Salas 24; Institute of Orthopaedics, London, 75, 732, 753, 754, 756, 870, 1085

Mr. P. H. Jacobsen, Dental School, Cardiff 213; Dr. J. R. Jenner 365; Mr. R. P. Juniper 1078

KeyMed Ltd. 216, 330, 587, 781, 906

Sue Lloyd 487, 783; London School of Hygiene and Tropical Medicine 633, 660, 917

Mallinckrodt Institute of Radiology 16; Dr. Francis Mathey 103, 183, 927; Nancy Durrell McKenna 192, 197, 207, 257, 264, 572; Penny Miller/Down's Syndrome Association 372; Lorraine Miller, Hammersmith Hospital 193

National Medical Slide Bank 196, 254, 449, 471, 494, 514, 521, 559, 628, 630, 632, 633, 651, 656, 687, 693, 703, 715, 778, 817, 839, 875, 903, 928, 944, 948, 960, 977, 989, 995, 998, 1021, 1030, 1039, 1077, 1081

Vincent Oliver 162; Oxfam/Pat Diskett 36

Philips Medical Systems 24, 26, 30

Queen Elizabeth Military Hospital, Woolwich (Histopathology Dept., John Boyd Laboratories) 246, 382; Queen Square Imaging Centre/BUPA 700

Dr. I. R. Reynolds, Eastman Dental Hospital 217, 661, 751, 760; Ann Ronan Picture Library 25, 32

Science Photo Library 25, 26, 28, 43, 467, 565, 587; Science Photo Library/ Michael Abbey 21 /Dr. Tony Brain 503, 686 /Dr. Goran Bredberg 512 /Dr. Jeremy Burgess 33 /CDC 44 /CEA-Orsay/CNRI 29, 788 /CNRI 17, 20, 27, 34 41, 135, 801, 1044 /Dr. E. H. Cook 1050 /Dr. R. Damadian 28 /Division of Computer Research and Technology, National Institutes of Health 40 /Martin Dohrn 23, 38 /Don Fawcett 573 /Fawcett/Hirokawa/Heuser 1049 /Prof. C. Ferlaud/CNRI 1061 /Grave 999 /David Guyon, The BOC Group PLC 33 /Nancy Hamilton 80 /Jan Hinsch 278, 279 /Manfred Kage 31, 184 /King's College School of Medicine (Dept. of Surgery) 22 /David Leah 39, 580 /Francis Leroy 446 /Dr. Andrejs Liepins 31, 48 /R. Litchfield 87 /London School of Hygiene and Tropical Medicine 582 /Andrew McClenaghan 36 /Astrid and Hans-Frieder Michler 21, 724 /Mark Morgan 620 /NASA 46 /Ohio-Nuclear Corporation 26 /Omikron 965 /David Parker 37, 301 /Petit Format/CSI 1088 /Nestlé 42, 398 /John Radcliffe Hospital 34, 1018 /David Scharf 686 /Science Source 608 /Dr. Karol Sikora 229, 937 /Dr. Howard Smedley 847 /Sinclair Stammers 30 /St. Bartholomew's Hospital 392 /St. Mary's Hospital 247 /Dr. Rob Stepney 34 /James Stevenson 35, 496, 687, 963 /Alexander Tsiaras 31, 33, 35, 41, 133 /USDA 462 /US National Cancer Institute 77 /John Walsh 587, 686, 926 /Don Wong 430 /J. F. Wilson 1060; Prof. Crispian Scully, Dental School, University of Bristol 238, 342; Frank Spooner Pictures 45; Squibb Surgicare Ltd. 293, 567; St.

Bartholomew's Hospital 162, 168, 218, 244, 246, 273, 317, 396, 404, 578, 595, 614, 622, 673, 753, 804, 806, 840, 914, 961, 1011, 1020, 1062, 1069, 1070, 1085; St. John's Institute of Dermatology 63, 87, 174, 327, 345, 354, 950; St. Mary's Hospital Medical School (Audio Visual Services) 141, 236, 367, 521, 539, 547, 653, 654, 830, 889, 911, 914, 946, 968, 982, 987, 1002, 1085, 1086; Tony Stone/David Joel 16 /Chris Harvey 18; Dr. Paul Sweny 176, 225, 324, 353, 569, 643, 840, 1028

University of Washington School of Medicine/The Lancet 83; John Watney 80, 281; C. James Webb 545, 1009, 1025; Dr. David Wheeler 353; Dr. A. R. Williams, Charing Cross and Westminster Medical School 550; Dr. I. Williams 65, 132, 142, 219, 221, 289, 346, 380, 391, 427, 465, 467, 474, 537, 623, 743, 762, 768, 808, 834, 843, 912, 950, 1018, 1072; Jennie Woodcock 48; Women's Health Concern 663

Col. Robert M. Youngson 128, 241, 256, 321, 390, 634, 664, 834, 840

Zefa/Clive Sawyer 42

## ILLUSTRATIONS AND ADDITIONAL DESIGN

**Illustrators** Tony Graham, Karen Cochran, Paul Cooper, Sandra Doyle, Will Giles, Brian Hewson, Kevin Marks, Janos Marffy, Coral Muller, Frazer Newman, Nick Oxloby, Lynda Payne, Sandra Pond, Patricia Sempron, Mark Surridge, John Woodcock **Designers** Anne Cuthbert, Peter Blake, Thomas Keenes, Chris Scollen